CURRENT
Occupational &
Environmental
Medicine

fourth edition

Edited by

Joseph LaDou, MS, MD
Clinical Professor
Division of Occupational & Environmental Medicine
University of California, San Francisco

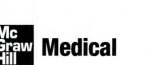
Medical

New York   Chicago   San Francisco   Lisbon   London   Madrid   Mexico City
Milan   New Delhi   San Juan   Seoul   Singapore   Sydney   Toronto

Current Occupational & Environmental Medicine, Fourth Edition

Copyright © 2007 by The McGraw-Hill Companies, Inc. All rights reserved. Printed in the United States of America. Except as permitted under the United States Copyright Act of 1976, no part of this publication may be reproduced or distributed in any form or by any means, or stored in a database or retrieval system, without the prior written permission of the publisher.

Previous editions copyright © 2004 by The McGraw-Hill Companies, Inc.; © 1997 by Appleton & Lange.

1 2 3 4 5 6 7 8 9 0 DOCDOC 0 9 8 7 6

ISBN-13: 978-0-07-144313-5
ISBN-10: 0-07-144313-4
ISSN: 1047-4498

Notice

Medicine is an ever-changing science. As new research and clinical experience broaden our knowledge, changes in treatment and drug therapy are required. The authors and the publisher of this work have checked with sources believed to be reliable in their efforts to provide information that is complete and generally in accord with the standards accepted at the time of publication. However, in view of the possibility of human error or changes in medical sciences, neither the authors nor the publisher nor any other party who has been involved in the preparation or publication of this work warrants that the information contained herein is in every respect accurate or complete, and they disclaim all responsibility for any errors or omissions or for the results obtained from use of the information contained in this work. Readers are encouraged to confirm the information contained herein with other sources. For example and in particular, readers are advised to check the product information sheet included in the package of each drug they plan to administer to be certain that the information contained in this work is accurate and that changes have not been made in the recommended dose or in the contraindications for administration. This recommendation is of particular importance in connection with new or infrequently used drugs.

This book was set in Adobe Garamond by Silverchair Science + Communications, Inc.
The editors were James F. Shanahan, Maya Barahona, and Peter J. Boyle.
The production supervisor was Catherine H. Saggese.
The text was designed by Eve Siegel.
The index was prepared by Coughlin Indexing Services.
R.R. Donnelley was printer and binder.

This book is printed on acid-free paper.

Authors' note: The conclusions and opinions expressed herein are those of the authors and do not necessarily represent the views and policies of the U.S. Food and Drug Administration or the California Department of Health Services.

INTERNATIONAL EDITION ISBN-13: 978-0-07-128658-9, ISBN-10: 0-07-128658-6
Copyright © 2007. Exclusive rights by The McGraw-Hill Companies, Inc. for manufacture and export. This book cannot be re-exported from the country to which it is consigned by McGraw-Hill. The International Edition is not available in North America.

Contents

Authors

John R. Balmes, MD
Professor of Medicine, University of California, San Francisco; Chief, Division of Occupational and Environmental Medicine, San Francisco General Hospital; Professor of Environmental Health Sciences, School of Public Health, University of California, Berkeley; Director, Northern California Center for Occupational and Environmental Health, UC Berkeley-UC Davis-UCSF
John.Balmes@ucsf.edu
Occupational Lung Diseases; Outdoor Air Pollution

Neal L. Benowitz, MD
Professor of Medicine, Psychiatry, and Biopharmaceutical Sciences; Chief, Division of Clinical Pharmacology and Experimental Therapeutics, University of California, San Francisco
Neal.Benowitz@ucsf.edu
Cardiovascular Toxicology; Smoking & Occupational Health

Paul D. Blanc, MD, MSPH
Professor of Medicine, Division of Occupational and Environmental Medicine, University of California, San Francisco
Paul.Blanc@ucsf.edu
Gases & Other Inhalants

Mahbub M.U. Chowdhury, MBChB, FRCP (U.K.)
Consultant in Occupational Dermatology, Department of Dermatology, University Hospital of Wales, Cardiff, United Kingdom
mmu.chowdhury@cardiffandvale.wales.nhs.uk
Occupational Skin Disorders

Jennifer H. Christian, MD, MPH
President/Chief Medical Officer, Webility Corporation, Wayland, Massachusetts
jennifer.christian@webility.md
Disability Prevention & Management

Richard Cohen, MD, MPH
Clinical Professor, Division of Occupational and Environmental Medicine, University of California, San Francisco
rcohenmd@pacbell.net
Injuries Caused by Physical Hazards

James E. Cone, MD, MPH
Assistant Clinical Professor, University of California, San Francisco; Director, Environmental and Occupational Disease Epidemiology, New York City Department of Health and Mental Hygiene, New York
jcone@health.nyc.gov
The Occupational Medical History

Rupali Das, MD, MPH
Assistant Clinical Professor of Medicine, University of California, San Francisco; Public Health Medical Officer, Occupational Health Branch, California Department of Health Services, Oakland, California
rdas@dhs.ca.gov
Routine Industrial Emissions, Accidental & Intentional Releases, & Hazardous Waste

Michael J. DiBartolomeis, PhD, DABT
Chief, Occupational Lead Poisoning Prevention Program and Research Scientist Supervisor II, California Department of Health Services Department of Health Services, Oakland, California
mdibarto@dhs.ca.gov
Health Risk Assessment

Michael L. Fischman, MD, MPH
Associate Clinical Professor and Assistant Chief, Division of Occupational and Environmental Medicine, Department of Medicine, University of California, San Francisco; Consultant in Occupational and Environmental Medicine and Toxicology, Fischman Occupational and Environmental Medical Group, Walnut Creek, California
michael.fischman@comcast.net
Building-Associated Illness

Allan J. Flach, PharmD, MD
Professor of Ophthalmology, University of California, San Francisco; Department of Veterans Affairs Medical Center, San Francisco, California
allan.flach@med.va.gov
Eye Injuries

Douglas P. Fowler, PhD, CIH
Visiting Lecturer in Industrial Hygiene, University of California, San Francisco; Distinguished Visiting Professor in Industrial Hygiene, Babes-Bolyai University, Cluj-Napoca, Romania; Principal Consultant, Fowler Associates, Redwood City, California
fowlrassoc@cs.com
Industrial Hygiene

Gary R. Fujimoto, MD
Adjunct Associate Clinical Professor of Emergency Medicine, Stanford University School of Medicine; Program Director, Occupational and Travel Medicine, Palo Alto Medical Foundation, Palo Alto, California
fujimotog@pamf.org
Occupational Infections

German T. Hernandez, MD, FASN
Assistant Clinical Professor of Medicine, University of California, San Francisco General Hospital Renal Center, San Francisco, California
ghernandez@medsfgh.ucsf.edu
Renal Toxicology

Robert J. Harrison, MD, MPH
Clinical Professor, Division of Occupational and Environmental Medicine, University of California, San Francisco
Robert.Harrison@ucsf.edu
Liver Toxicology; Chemicals; Multiple Chemical Sensitivity

Stephen Heidel, MD, MBA
Clinical Professor of Psychiatry, University of California School of Medicine, San Diego
stephen.heidel@sbcglobal.net
Occupational Stress

Franklin T. Hoaglund, MD
Professor Emeritus of Orthopedic Surgery, University of California, San Francisco
fhoaglund@aol.com
Musculoskeletal Injuries

Seichi Horie, MD, MPH, PhD
Professor, Department of Health Policy and Management, Institute of Industrial Ecological Sciences, University of Occupational and Environmental Health, Kitakyushu City, Japan
horie@med.uoeh-u.ac.jp
Injuries Caused by Physical Hazards

Fu Hua, MB, MPH, PhD
Deputy Dean and Professor, School of Public Health, Fudan University, Shanghai, China
hfu@shmu.edu.cn
Smoking and Occupational Health

Leslie M. Israel, DO, MPH
Associate Clinical Professor, Associate Occupational Medicine Residency Program Director, Center for Occupational and Environmental Health, Department of Medicine, Division of Occupational Medicine, University of California, Irvine
lisrael@uci.edu
Clinical Toxicology

Ira L. Janowitz, MPS, PT, CPE
Senior Ergonomics Consultant, University of California, San Francisco/Berkeley Ergonomics Program, Richmond, California
janowitz@comcast.net
Ergonomics & the Prevention of Occupational Injuries

Jacob Johnson, MD
Assistant Clinical Professor, Department of Otolaryngology—Head and Neck Surgery, University of California, San Francisco
jjohnson@ohns.ucsf.edu
Occupational Hearing Loss

Tushar Kant Joshi, MBBS, MS, MSc
Visiting Professor, Drexel University School of Public Health, Philadelphia; Head, Centre for Occupational and Environmental Health, Lok Nayak Hospital, New Delhi India
joshi_tk@rediffmail.com
Water Pollution

Elizabeth A. Katz, MPH, CIH
Associate Industrial Hygienist, HESIS, Occupational Health Branch, California Department of Health Services, Oakland, California
ekatz@dhs.ca.gov
Solvents

Jeffrey L. Kishiyama, MD
Associate Clinical Professor of Medicine, Department of Immunology, University of California, San Francisco
Jeffrey.Kishiyama@ucsf.edu
Clinical Immunology

Ware G. Kuschner, MD
Associate Professor of Medicine, Division of
  Pulmonary and Critical Care Medicine, Stanford
  University School of Medicine, Stanford,
  California; Staff Physician, Veterans Affairs Palo
  Alto Health Care System, Palo Alto, California
kuschner@stanford.edu
Gases & Other Inhalants

Joseph LaDou, MS, MD
Director, International Center for Occupational
  Medicine; Clinical Professor, Division of
  Occupational and Environmental Medicine,
  University of California, San Francisco
joeladou@aol.com
*The Practice of Occupational Medicine; The
Occupational Medical History; Workers'
Compensation; Environmental Exposures & Controls*

Robert C. Larsen, MD, MPH
Clinical Professor, Department of Psychiatry;
  Director, Center of Occupational Psychiatry,
  University of California School of Medicine,
  San Francisco
rlarsen@occupationalpsych.com
Occupational Stress

Gideon Letz, MD, MPH
Medical Director, State Compensation Insurance
  Fund, San Francisco, California; Occupational
  Medicine Physician, Kaiser Permanente Medical
  Center, San Francisco, California
galetz@scif.com
Disability Prevention & Management

Richard Lewis, MD, MPH
Director of Occupational Health, The Cleveland
  Clinic Foundation, Cleveland, Ohio
lewisr3@ccf.org
Metals

Howard I. Maibach, MD
Professor, Department of Dermatology, University
  of California, San Francisco
maibachh@derm.ucsf.edu
Occupational Skin Disorders

Melanie A. Marty, PhD
Chief, Air Toxicology and Epidemiology Section,
  Office of Environmental Health Hazard
  Assessment, California Environmental Protection
  Agency, Oakland, California
mmarty@oehha.ca.gov
*Routine Industrial Emissions, Accidental &
Intentional Releases, & Hazardous Waste*

Raymond K. Meister, MD, MPH
Assistant Clinical Professor of Medicine,
  Division of Occupational and Environmental
  Medicine, University of California, San
  Francisco; Public Health Medical Officer,
  California Department of Health Services,
  Occupational Health Branch, Occupational
  Lead Poisoning Prevention Program,
  Richmond, California
rmeister@dhs.ca.gov
Biological Monitoring

Andrew H. Murr, MD, FACS
Professor of Clinical Otolaryngology—Head and
  Neck Surgery, University of California, San
  Francisco School of Medicine; Chief of Service,
  Department of Otolaryngology—Head and
  Neck Surgery, San Francisco General Hospital
ahmurr@ohns.ucsf.edu
Facial Injuries

Willis H. Navarro, MD
Associate Clinical Professor of Medicine, Division
  of Hematology/Oncology, University of
  California, San Francisco
Willis.navarro@ucsf.edu
Occupational Hematology

Michael A. O'Malley, MD
Medical Director, Occupational and
  Environmental Medicine/Family Practice,
  Employee Health Services; Associate Clinical
  Professor, Division of Occupational and
  Environmental Medicine, University of
  California, Davis
maomalley@ucdavis.edu
Pesticides

Ana Maria Osorio, MD, MPH
Commander, U.S. Public Health Service; Regional
Medical Officer, U.S. Food and Drug
Administration-Pacific Region, Oakland, California
anamaria.osorio@fda.gov
*Female Reproductive Toxicology; Male Reproductive
Toxicology; Disease Surveillance Systems*

Franklyn G. Prieskop, MS, MA, CSP
Retired, Boston, Massachusetts
fgprieskop@hotmail.com
Occupational Safety

David M. Rempel, MD, MPH
Professor of Medicine, Division of Occupational
and Environmental Medicine; Director,
University of California San Francisco
Ergonomics Program, University of California,
San Francisco and Berkeley
drempel@itsa.ucsf.edu
Ergonomics & the Prevention of Occupational Injuries

Peggy Reynolds, PhD, MPH
Chief, Environmental Epidemiology Section,
Department of Health Services, Oakland,
California
preynold@dhs.ca.gov
Disease Surveillance Systems

Scott T. Robinson, MPH, CIH, CSP
ABM Industries, Inc., San Francisco, California
scorob@attbi.com
Hearing Loss

Julietta Rodríguez-Guzmán, MD, SOH, SS
Assistant Professor, Graduate Occupational Health
Program, Universidad El Bosque, Bogotá,
Colombia
juliettarodriguez@cable.net.co
Workers' Compensation

Rudolph A. Rodriguez, MD
Associate Professor of Clinical Medicine, University
of California, San Francisco; Clinical Director of
Nephrology, San Francisco General Hospital
rrodriguez@medsfgh.ucsf.edu
Renal Toxicology

Jon Rosenberg, MD
Assistant Clinical Professor of Medicine, University
of California, San Francisco; Public Health
Medical Officer, Division of Communicable
Disease Control, Infectious Diseases Branch,
California Department of Health Services,
Berkeley, California
jrosenbe@dhs.ca.gov
Clinical Toxicology; Solvents

Hope S. Rugo, MD
Clinical Professor of Medicine, University of
California, San Francisco; Director, Breast
Oncology Clinical Trials Program, UCSF
Comprehensive Cancer Center
hope.rugo@ucsfmedctr.org
Occupational Hematology; Occupational Cancer

Marc B. Schenker, MD, MPH
Professor and Chair, Department of Public Health
Sciences; Chief, Division of Environmental and
Occupational Medicine, University of California,
Davis
mbschenker@ucdavis.edu
Appendix: Biostatistics & Epidemiology

James P. Seward, MD, MPP
Clinical Professor of Medicine, University of
California, San Francisco; Medical Director,
Health Services Department, Lawrence
Livermore National Laboratory
seward1@llnl.gov
Occupational Stress

Dennis Shusterman, MD, MPH
Professor of Medicine, Occupational and
Environmental Medicine Program, University of
Washington, Seattle
dennis3@u.washington.edu
Upper Respiratory Tract Disorders

Yuen T. So, MD, PhD
Professor and Director, Neurology Clinic,
Department of Neurology and Neurosciences,
Stanford University Medical Center, Stanford,
California
ytso@stanford.edu
Peripheral Nerve Injuries; Neurotoxicology

Gina M. Solomon, MD, MPH
Assistant Clinical Professor of Medicine, University of California, San Francisco; Senior Scientist, Natural Resources Defense Council, San Francisco, California
gsolomon@nrdc.org
Environmental Exposures & Controls

Ken Takahashi, MD, PhD, MPH
Professor and Chair, Department of Environmental Epidemiology, Institute of Industrial Ecological Sciences, University of Occupational and Environmental Health, Kitakyushu City, Japan
ktaka@med.uoeh-u.ac.jp
Occupational Infections

Daniel T. Teitelbaum, MD
Adjunct Professor of Environmental Sciences, Colorado School of Mines; Associate Clinical Professor of Preventive Medicine, University of Colorado Health Sciences Center; Medical Toxicologist and Occupational Physician, Denver, Colorado
toxdoc@ix.netcom.com
Water Pollution

Dan J. Tennenhouse, MD, JD, FCLM
Lecturer in Legal Medicine, University of California, San Francisco School of Medicine
dantennenhouse@yahoo.com
Liability Issues in Occupational Medicine

Susan N. Tierman, MD
Assistant Clinical Professor, University of California, San Francisco; Medical Director, Occupational Health, ALZA Corporation and PSAGA West, Johnson & Johnson, Mountain View, California
susan.tierman@alza.com
Disability Prevention & Management

Marilyn C. Underwood, PhD
Senior Toxicologist and Chief, Site Assessment Section, Environmental Health Investigations Branch, California Department of Health Services, Oakland
munderwo@dhs.ca.gov
Routine Industrial Emissions, Accidental & Intentional Releases, & Hazardous Waste

Catharina Wesseling, MD, PhD
Instituto Regional de Estudios en Sustancias Tóxicas (IRET) Central American Institute for Studies on Toxic Substances (IRET), Universidad Nacional, Heredia, Costa Rica
cwesseli@una.ac.cr
Environmental Exposures & Controls

Gayle C. Windham, MSPH, PhD
Research Scientist, Division of Environmental and Occupational Disease Control, California Department of Health Services, Oakland
gwindham@dhs.ca.gov
Female Reproductive Toxicology; Male Reproductive Toxicology

Yuxin Zheng, MD, PhD
Deputy Director, Professor, National Institute for Occupational Health and Poison Control, Chinese Center for Disease Control and Prevention; Director, WHO Collaborating Centre of Occupational Health, Beijing, China
yxzheng@163bj.com
Biological Monitoring

Preface

The fourth edition of *Current Occupational & Environmental Medicine* (formerly *Occupational & Environmental Medicine*) continues to serve as a concise yet comprehensive resource for health care professionals in all specialties who are called on to diagnose and treat occupational injuries and occupational and environmental illnesses. The addition of a number of authors from Asia, Europe, and Latin America adds to the international dimension of the book. The basic practice of occupational health and safety professionals is remarkably similar in all regions of the world. The text provides recent references for every topic discussed, emphasizing review articles useful to clinicians. The reader is given a number of Web sites that provide information on a variety of topics.

COVERAGE & APPROACH TO THE SUBJECT

The book provides a complete guide to common occupational injuries and occupational and environmental illnesses, their diagnosis and treatment, and preventive and remedial measures in the workplace and community. Our aim is to help physicians understand and deal with the complexities of occupational and environmental medicine and at the same time to provide useful clinical information on common illnesses and injuries. The book expands the coverage of environmental medicine well beyond that of the earlier editions. To reflect the book's usefulness as a clinical resource, it is now published in the LANGE *Current* series. The series consists of practical, concise, and timely books in core specialties and key subspecialties that focus on essential diagnostic and treatment information.

SPECIAL AREAS OF EMPHASIS

- Detailed coverage of diagnosis and treatment of a broad spectrum of occupational injuries and occupational and environmental illnesses.
- Chapters on how to approach the patient, how to obtain information on toxicants, clinical toxicology, and immunology orient the clinician to the complexities of occupational and environmental medicine.
- New methods of disability management and the important role that physicians can play in preventing disability.
- Practical information on toxic properties and clinical manifestations of common industrial materials.
- Techniques to prevent workplace-related accidents and illness.

SPECIAL SUBJECTS IN SUPPORT

- The role of non-physician health and safety professionals and their interaction with physicians is examined; the importance of a team effort in developing health and safety programs in the workplace is emphasized.
- Chapters on the legal aspects of occupational and environmental medicine round out the book's comprehensive approach.

ORGANIZATION & HIGHLIGHTS OF EACH SECTION

Section I (Chapters 1 through 5) defines the practice of occupational medicine and orients the practitioner with an approach to the diagnosis of occupational illnesses. It offers guidance for identifying workplace exposures to toxic materials, putting this information to immediate clinical use, and applying it toward better health and safety practices in the workplace. This section presents a comprehensive discussion of disability prevention and management and considers some of the legal issues important in the practice of occupational medicine.

Section II (Chapters 6 through 12) concisely discusses common occupational injuries and their treatments. Noise-induced hearing loss and the impact of other physical hazards, such as heat, cold, and radiation, are examined. It also emphasizes the importance of ergonomics and discusses how ergonomic principles can be instituted in the workplace to prevent further work loss associated with injury and illness.

Section III (Chapters 13 through 26) is a comprehensive discussion of clinical toxicology arranged by organ system, with special emphasis on the environmental as well as workplace origins of toxic exposure. It thoroughly reviews commonly recognized environmental and occupational illnesses and highlights many clinical problems not often thought to be work related. Chapter 17, "Occupational Infections," includes a discussion of "Bioterrorism" and its implications in the workplace.

Section IV (Chapters 27 through 31) presents the most common toxic materials encountered in the workplace and community and the diagnostic and treatment recommendations appropriate to illnesses related to these materials. This section is designed to serve as an immediate reference source and clinical guide for the practicing health care professional. The discussion on pesticides, in particular, emphasizes the environmental as well as occupational exposures that may lead to illness.

Section V (Chapters 32 through 36) presents the roles and responsibilities of other, non-physician occupational health and safety professionals, including the industrial hygienist and the safety professional. The chapter on industrial hygiene includes a discussion of recommended exposure limits for common industrial materials. The chapter on biologic monitoring provides the information necessary for institution of medical surveillance programs and for interpretation of data obtained in such programs. Chapters on occupational stress and drug and alcohol abuse in the work setting consider programs for controlling and treating these problems.

Section VI (Chapters 37 through 45) provides a comprehensive discussion of environmental medicine and some of the complex societal issues that accompany industrialization and technologic advances throughout the world. Emphasis is placed on recognizing that some common "occupational" exposures are found also in homes and public locations and require the same high index of suspicion that is assumed when encountered in the workplace. Chapter 38, which includes discussion on accidental releases and hazardous waste, will be of particular interest to health care professionals. This chapter presents a discussion of "Chemical and Radiation Terrorism" and the role of health care professionals in prevention and management. Chapters 44 and 45 present the important areas of Disease Surveillance and Health Risk Assessment, vital to the practice of environmental medicine.

The Appendix concisely introduces biostatistics and epidemiology. These topics are important not only in research but also in clinical practice. Ultimately, all occupational and environmental physicians serve as clinical epidemiologists.

ACKNOWLEDGMENTS

This book brings together a faculty with a combined experience of 30 years of teaching the UCSF course entitled "Occupational and Environmental Medicine." Working with the many attendees of our courses made it possible to compile a text that emphasizes practical information for clinicians.

Joseph LaDou, MS, MD
San Francisco, California
October 2006

SECTION I.
Occupational Health

The Practice of Occupational Medicine

Joseph LaDou, MS, MD

The Occupational Safety and Health Act of 1970 (OSHAct) assures "every working man and woman in the United States safe and healthful working conditions." This act created the Occupational Safety and Health Administration (OSHA) and the National Institute for Occupational Safety and Health (NIOSH). At the time the OSHAct was passed, occupational medicine was one of the country's smallest medical specialties, with only a few residency-trained specialists in academic positions or consulting practices or employed by major corporations. Private practitioners provided care for occupational injuries, sometimes in industrial settings, but mostly as a part of other services provided in a private office or hospital setting.

Then, as a result of passage of the OSHAct and formation of OSHA and NIOSH, occupational medicine became the center of considerable attention by medical schools, hospitals, clinics, and physicians in many different specialties. Occupational medicine was even considered a career opportunity by medical students. Medical schools received financial support for training from NIOSH, and OSHA gave occupational physicians a voice in the increasingly regulated industrial setting.

OPPORTUNITIES IN OCCUPATIONAL MEDICINE

Occupational injuries and illnesses are among the five leading causes of morbidity and mortality in the United States and in most other countries. Injuries at work comprise a substantial part of the country's injury burden, accounting for nearly half of all injuries in some age groups. Occupational health professionals play an important role in prevention, recognition, and treatment of injuries and illnesses. Occupational physicians customarily practice as company doctors employed by corporations, as consultants to corporations, or as private practitioners. Occupational physicians generally practice within the framework of the workers' compensation system. Workers' compensation law places the occupational physician in a critically important role. The physician must determine that an injury or illness is caused by work, diagnose it, prescribe care, and assess the extent of impairment and the ability of the worker to resume work. Determinations that injuries or illnesses are the result of work are increasingly contentious.

When a compensation case results in litigation, occupational health professionals become important witnesses in resolving disputes. The physician asked to evaluate the worker in most states is designated an independent medical examiner (IME). The IME's evaluation is the highest level of evaluation the worker will encounter. Most requests for IME opinions come from insurers, but on occasion, plaintiff's attorneys, judges, and others may initiate an IME evaluation.

The Institute of Medicine (IOM) has stated that there is a critical shortage of specialty-trained occupational and environmental physicians in communities, in academic medical centers, and in public health and related agencies. Moreover, the IOM reports a severe shortage of front-line primary-care physicians who are willing and able to care for patients with occupational and environmental illnesses. The IOM concludes that data from the Bureau of Labor Statistics (BLS) were significant underestimates of occupational diseases, which emphasized the need for more and better diagnoses of occupational diseases by primary-care practitioners. The IOM recommends that "all primary-care physicians be able to identify possible occupationally or environmentally induced conditions and make appropriate referrals for follow-up."

Since passage of the OSHAct, U.S. employment has nearly doubled, from 56 million workers at 3.5 million work sites to 105 million workers at nearly 6.9 million work sites. Most of the labor force expansion during this period was in service-sector companies with fewer than 500 employees. Although these companies are not likely to employ occupational physicians, they do add to the demand for injury and illness care, as well as for health and safety consulting.

There are at least 55,000 occupational fatalities each year, ranking the workplace as the eighth leading cause of death. Since the early 1970s, more than 113,000 worker deaths were attributed to pneumoconioses. This number represents only a small portion of the total deaths attributable to occupational lung disease. The number of deaths from asbestos-related mesothelioma has been increasing steadily in the same time period, as are deaths with hypersensitivity pneumonitis as an underlying or contributing cause. Asthma is now the most common occupational respiratory disease. Population-based estimates suggest that approximately 20% of new-onset asthma in adults is work-related.

Occupational injuries are significantly underreported, yet 3.8 million recognized disabling injuries still occur per year. One-third of all injury cases result in loss of work. The human costs associated with occupational injuries and illnesses are staggering. Financial costs of occupational injuries and illnesses exceed $150 billion per year.

Occupational Medicine Practice

The vast majority of physicians who practice occupational medicine do so with knowledge gained by self-study, attendance at short courses, and practice experience. It is a disconcerting fact that workers' compensation fails to compensate most occupational injuries and illnesses, including fatalities. Only a small fraction of occupational diseases is covered by workers' compensation, and only a small fraction of people suffering from occupational illnesses ever receives workers' compensation benefits.

Either by law or by practice, compensation in many states is particularly limited for occupational diseases. The U.S. Department of Labor estimated in 1980 that "only 5% of those severely disabled from an occupational disease receive workers' compensation benefits." A number of studies since that time show that the rate of reporting of occupational diseases has not changed much.

More than half a million chemicals are found in work settings, and many millions of workers are exposed to these substances. Yet only 10,000 workers' compensation claims for illnesses caused by chemical exposure are filed each year. Workplace exposure to carcinogens accounts for about 5–10% of all cancer cases, yet less than 0.1% of cancer patients ever receive any settlement from employers. For example, NIOSH estimates that 16–17% of lung cancer cases in men and 2% of cases in women are work-related.

As many as 15,000 of the 100,000 commonly used industrial chemicals are carcinogenic to humans. Occupational exposures cause an estimated 20% of all cancers. Although occupational cancers are totally preventable, workers continue to be exposed to carcinogens possibly because few cases are reported, are awarded benefits, or are successful in litigation. With the exception of cancers caused by exposure to asbestos, fewer than 1% of occupational cancer cases ever receive workers' compensation benefits from employers.

There are those who contend that a lack of training in occupational medicine accounts for the failure to diagnose occupational diseases and eventually to compensate workers. Moreover, the long latency periods of many occupational diseases present a causation dilemma both for physicians and for insurers. The failure of workers' compensation law to properly recognize occupational diseases and the interests of the industries that insurers serve explain much of the failure to compensate workers who have occupational diseases. Another important contributing cause is the limited information available to physicians. Of the tens of thousands of chemicals in common commercial use in the United States each year (3000 of them in quantities of more than 1 million pounds per year), only 7% have been screened for toxicity, and fewer than half of those have been studied thoroughly. Although interest in occupational medicine is increasing across the country, the failure to diagnose occupational diseases and the lack of proper compensation of workers continue to be major social policy failures.

Residency and Other Training

NIOSH, in addition to its roles in supporting occupational health research and recommending occupational standards to OSHA, funds most training programs in occupational health and safety. NIOSH extramural funds support a training program that consists of a network of 16 regional education and research centers located at universities in 14 states and approximately 35 individual training project grants in 25 states. Every year approximately 500 students in occupational medicine, occupational health nursing, industrial hygiene, and safety sciences graduate from NIOSH-supported programs.

Most training programs in occupational medicine are associated with universities that have schools of public health, but some programs are found within specific departments (e.g., preventive medicine, community medicine, internal medicine, or family practice) within a medical school. There are 30 approved residency programs in the United States, down from 40 just 10 years ago.

The annual number of graduates from each residency program averages only slightly greater than two. This small number does not answer the requirement for academically trained occupational physicians, nor does it fill the vacancies in public health departments in many areas of the country.

Teaching Occupational Medicine

Among the half of medical schools that required the teaching of occupational medicine in 1985, the mean required curriculum time over 4 years was 4 hours. In the 9 years that followed, there was almost no change in the percentage of medical schools specifically teaching occupational health to medical students, although the number of schools requiring occupational health as part of the curriculum increased slightly. Moreover, the mean number of required hours of occupational health teaching to medical students increased by a disappointing 2 hours, from 4 to 6 hours. The mean number of faculty members per school who are teaching occupational health has remained unchanged since 1977. Short courses are designed for physicians who do not have residency training but who are making a major commitment to training in occupational medicine.

Distance learning of occupational medicine augments and soon may replace short-course programs. Computer-managed instruction offered at the Medical College of Wisconsin and the University of North Carolina provides distance-education master of public health (MPH) degree programs for physicians and nurses. Tulane University School of Public Health offers an Internet-based MPH degree program in occupational health that is designed for physicians, nurses, and other health professionals who work in occupational health programs or clinics.

Board Certification

The American Board of Preventive Medicine (ABPM) began board certification of specialists in occupational medicine in 1955. ABPM had certified a total of 3518 occupational physicians through 2005. Fewer than half of these board-certified occupational physicians are currently in practice. Although occupational medicine is the most popular of the ABPM certifications, it remains one of medicine's smallest specialties. The number of residency-trained occupational physicians certified by ABPM is not replacing the losses to retirement or retreats from the field. In 2005, 101 residency graduates qualified for board certi-

Table 1-1. Board certification in occupational medicine.[1]

	2000	2001	2002	2003	2004	2005
Residency trained	64	63	72	95	68	63
Alternate pathway	27	17	25	18	23	23
ABPM[2]	6	5	3	8	6	4
New certifications	97	85	100	121	97	90

[1]From American Board of Preventive Medicine, 2006.
[2]The American Board of Preventive Medicine (ABPM) allows physicians who hold other ABPM certifications to qualify for certification in occupational medicine with 2 years of full-time practice in occupational medicine.

fication, and 63 passed the certification examination (a pass rate of 62%) (Table 1–1).

In the same year, 38 physicians qualified through the alternate pathway, and 23 passed the certification examination (a pass rate of 61%). The alternate pathway is an equivalency of residency training approved by the ABPM but limited to physicians who graduated before 1984. The applicant must demonstrate competency in occupational medicine through practice and experience and must complete educational courses at the postgraduate level. As is readily apparent, the alternate pathway now excludes younger candidates and is dropping to inconsequential numbers. Applicants for board certification peaked at 331 in 1996. Less than half that number applied for board certification in 2005.

The total number of new board certifications in occupational medicine has fallen back below 100 per year. This small supply of new board-certified specialists is far below that which would be required merely to replace the loss by retirement of older board-certified physicians. For details on board certification, contact

American Board of Preventive Medicine, Inc.
330 South Wells Street, Suite 1018
Chicago, IL 60606-7106
Web site: www.abprevmed.org.

The Health and Safety Team

Health and safety programs ought to consist of a team made up of occupational health and safety professionals, and ideally, each company should use the team on a full- or part-time basis. However, employer acceptance of these team members varies widely. There is a long history of territoriality among the professionals, often to the detriment of the team concept. Safety professionals, with their more frequent contact with management, seek to protect their turf and authority. Occupational health nurses covet their autonomy and do not want to report to occupational physicians. Industrial hygienists often are seen as providing an engineering service to the employer that is required by law, whereas health professionals are more optional team members.

Occupational health nurses expanded their roles in many industries over the past 20 years, with increased involvement in health promotion, management and policy development, cost containment, research, and regulatory issues affecting the workplace. Their roles continue to expand with increased emphases on cost-effective policies and disability management. This partly explains why occupational health nurses are gradually taking over the industry positions formerly held by occupational physicians.

In contrast to the discouraging picture of occupational medicine training, occupational health nursing training is highly successful. Occupational health nursing is growing in numbers and influence in corporate health and safety. Approximately half the nurses working in industry belong to the American Association of Occupational Health Nurses (AAOHN). The majority of the AAOHN membership is certified in occupational health nursing through academic, practice, and continuing-education programs. For every occupational physician employed by a corporation in 1970, there were approximately five occupational health nurses. Today there appear to be more than 20 occupational health nurses for every occupational physician in the industry.

Training programs for many occupational health nurses now produce specialists with master's and doctoral degrees who compete for the consultative positions that are the highest level of practice for the occupational physician. More than 800 master-level and 40 doctoral-level occupational health nurses have been added to the workplace through NIOSH training programs. Other programs train occupational nurse practitioners who compete with occupational physicians in many clinical settings.

A few occupational physicians study ergonomics, occupational psychology, gerontology, and other disciplines envisioned as important career opportunities in the occupational health care of the future. For the most part, though, occupational physicians are not changing their behaviors in this increasingly competitive environment.

REFERENCES

Bureau of Labor Statistics Web site: www.bls.gov/home.htm.

LaDou J: Occupational medicine in the United States. Int J Occup Environ Health 2006;12:154 [PMID: 16722196].

Lax MB et al: Medical evaluation of work-related illness: A comparison of evaluations by a treating occupational medicine specialist and independent medical examiners. Int J Occup Environ Health 2004;10:1 [PMID: 15070020].

London L: Dual loyalties and the ethical and human rights obligations of occupational health professionals. Am J Ind Med 2005;47:322 [PMID: 15776476].

National Institute for Occupational Safety and Health Web site: www.cdc.gov/niosh/homepage.html.

Schulte PA: Characterizing the burden of occupational injury and disease. J Occup Environ Med 2005;47:607 [PMID: 15951721].

Smith GS et al: Injuries at work in the US adult population: Contributions to the total injury burden. Am J Public Health 2005;95:1213 [PMID: 15983273].

INTERNATIONAL OCCUPATIONAL HEALTH

Never in history has there been as much occupational injury and disease as exists in the world today. Occupational health should have high priority on the international agenda. Although many countries have improved working conditions to high standards, working conditions for the majority of the world's workers do not meet the minimum standards and guidelines set by the International Labor Organization (ILO) and the World Health Organization (WHO). Progress in bringing occupational health to the industrializing countries is painfully slow. In the poorest countries, there has been no progress at all.

OCCUPATIONAL INJURY AND DISEASE

The ILO estimates that the world's work force suffers more than 1 billion accidents every year. Occupational accidents cause permanent disabilities and economic losses amounting to more than 6% of national incomes. Well over two million people are killed by their work every year.

The WHO estimates that there are at least 250 million cases of occupational disease worldwide, with an unknown additional toll on national incomes. Occupational diseases are grossly underreported in all developing countries. In southern Africa, only about 2% of occupational disease is recognized and reported. The global epidemic of occupational diseases is occurring almost exclusively in the developing countries. There is general agreement that if these countries continue their current rate of industrial growth, the number of occupational injuries and disease cases will double by the year 2025.

The global epidemic of occupational injury and disease is aggravated by the rapid transfer of even more hazardous industries to industrializing countries. The opportunities for improvements in occupational health presented by globalization are outweighed by the shift in the health costs to workers with high-risk jobs, and this shift primarily affects migrant workers, women, children, and workers with temporary employment. Although international standards obligate employers to pay for occupational injuries and diseases, inadequate prevention, detection, and compensation make a mockery of these standards. The most important ILO Convention on Occupational Safety and Health in general (no. 155) has been ratified by only 42 of the 178 ILO member states. Only 23 countries have ratified the ILO Employment Injury Benefits Convention (no. 121), adopted in 1964, which lists occupational diseases for which compensation should be paid.

GLOBALIZATION

Globalization, the fast-paced growth of trade and cross-border investment, is a selective phenomenon. Many countries benefit from globalization, and many do not. A recent study showed that 24 countries that are home to three billion people, including China, Argentina, Brazil, India, and the Philippines, have substantially benefited from global trade in the past 20 years. National incomes in their economies grew by an average of 5% a year during the 1990s (compared with 2% in the developed countries), and their poverty rates declined. However, another two billion people live in countries that have become less rather than more integrated into the world community. In these countries—including Pakistan and much of Africa—trade has diminished in relation to national income, economic growth has been stagnant, and poverty has risen.

The 500 largest corporations account for 70% of world trade. They can and should be a powerful force in the provision of occupational and environmental health. The dominant role of multinational corporations in global manufacturing and trade carries with it a major responsibility for the economic development of countries. All too often, in the industrializing countries, the multinational corporations are interested only in taking advantage of free-trade privileges, wages as low as 11 cents an hour, a near-total absence of unions, and the disinterest or frank corruption of unstable or distracted governments. The experience of developed countries with the costs of occupational health is that a very substantial financial burden is being shifted to the industrializing countries through the process of globalization.

WORKING CONDITIONS

Workers in all countries are entitled to the basic benefits of federal labor and health and safety laws, including workers' compensation. At present, only a small minority of workers in Africa, Latin America, and Asia receives protection from such social security schemes.

The ILO reports that occupational health and safety laws cover only 10% of the population in developing countries and that such laws omit many major hazardous industries and occupations, including agriculture, fishing, forestry, and construction; small-scale enterprises; and the informal sector. Most small-scale enterprises in industrializing countries lack appropriate occupational health regulations and protective or control measures. Throughout the world, small-scale enterprises do not provide basic occupational health services and other primary medical care. Moreover, many small factories are located in the middle of or near residential areas. Small-scale industrial hazards threaten the health of workers' families and the adjacent community.

Much of the world's workforce is in the informal sector. The informal sector is an integral part of the economy of industrializing countries and includes unofficial self-employed workers whose activities range from hawking goods on the street to independent contracting and small family-run businesses. Although the work of these people is in many cases similar to that of formal-sector workers, what distinguishes the informal sector is the absence of rights and social protection, including access to health insurance, pension benefits, and protection under the federal labor and health and safety laws.

INTERNATIONAL AGENCIES

The WHO is responsible for the technical aspects of occupational health and safety, e.g., the promotion of medical services, medical examinations, and hygienic standards. The agency encourages national occupational health policies and strategies through World Health Assembly resolutions.

The ILO is an international coordinating body that plays an important role in promoting uniform policies for occupational health and safety in all countries. The ILO sets minimum standards in the field of occupational health and safety that have a strong ethical component. ILO conventions guide all countries in the promotion of workplace safety and in managing occupational health and safety programs, including Convention 81 (labor inspection), Convention 155 (occupational safety and health), Convention 161 (occupational health services), Convention 170 (chemical safety), and Convention 174 (prevention of major industrial accidents). ILO conventions and recommendations on occupational safety and health are international agreements that have legal force if they are ratified by the national government. More than half the 184 conventions adopted so far by the ILO have links to health and safety issues. The United States has ratified only 14 of them.

Helping the Industrializing Countries

Direct consultations with countries occur through WHO and ILO regional, country, and central offices. Some consultative services to developing countries also occur through the WHO network of 55 collaborating centers located throughout the world. The WHO and the ILO are required to provide direct consultation to developing countries when such countries request aid with their health and safety programs. In reality, the WHO and the ILO have limited budgets and personnel available to provide the required consultative services. Moreover, it is not clear that the WHO and the ILO could identify a model occupational health and safety program to recommend. Virtually all foreign models of health and safety programs require trained and experienced personnel to institute them and to provide continuing leadership. The overwhelming reality in the industrializing countries is that they lack trained personnel at every level.

Training of Occupational Health and Safety Personnel

Most industrializing countries have few trained occupational health and safety professionals, which presents a major obstacle to the implementation of regulations and policies and to the provision of occupational health services. Because of the shortage of formally trained occupational physicians, workers who have occupational diseases often remain unrecognized in industrializing countries. Thus, the rate of compensation for occupational diseases is one-tenth that of the developed countries, and a large majority of workers with occupational injuries do not receive rehabilitation or appropriate care to return to work. Industrial (occupational) hygienists are quite rare in industrializing countries, yet they are crucial to progress in occupational health. Regulatory standards cannot be implemented and enforced if there are no personnel trained in industrial hygiene. The few international training programs that exist today do not begin to provide the number and quality of occupational health and safety graduates required by the global industrial expansion. Over the next 20 years, the population of the developed countries will fall slightly, whereas the developing world will acquire two billion more people, many of them in countries that are currently political and economic failures. In such a world, occupational health is not likely to make much progress, and harmonization of work standards will remain an elusive goal.

REFERENCES

Catalogue of ILO Publications on Occupational Safety and Health: www.ilo.org/public/english/protection/safework/publicat/iloshcat/index.htm.

Delclos GL et al: A global survey of occupational health competencies and curriculum. Int J Occup Environ Health 2005; 11:185–198 [PMID: 15875895].

International Labor Organization (ILO) Web site: www.ilo.org.

International Occupational Safety and Health Information Center (CIS): www.ilo.org/cis.

LaDou J: International occupational health. Int J Hyg Environ Health 2003;206:303 [PMID: 12971685].

Rantanen J et al: The opportunities and obstacles to collaboration between the developing and developed countries in the field of occupational health. Toxicology 2004;198:63 [PMID: 15138031].

Rosenstock L et al: Advancing worker health and safety in the developing world. J Occup Environ Med 2005;47:132 [PMID: 15706172].

World Health Organization (WHO) Web site: www.who.org.

The Occupational Medical History

James E. Cone, MD, MPH, & Joseph LaDou, MS, MD

Most occupational physicians practice within the framework of the workers' compensation system. Workers' compensation law places the occupational physician in a critically important role. The physician must determine that an injury or illness is caused by work, diagnose it, prescribe care, and assess the extent of impairment and the ability of the worker to resume work. All physicians and other health care providers need to become familiar with workers' compensation laws in their states (see Chapter 3) and to learn more about the field of occupational medicine.

Accurately diagnosing occupational illnesses is important beyond the usual reasons for accuracy in medical diagnosis. This is a result of the public health, social, and economic implications of occupational disease for the community of workers in the same workplace or in other workplaces with similar exposures. In many states, the diagnosis of an occupational illness triggers additional responsibility on the part of the clinician. These responsibilities are primarily those of timely notification: informing the worker regarding the potential legal and other implications of the diagnosis, informing the workers' compensation insurer of the diagnosis and the basis for the clinician's opinion, and reporting to the appropriate public health or labor-related governmental agencies.

A differential diagnosis that appropriately includes occupational exposures as potential causes or exacerbating factors of the patient's presenting symptoms or suspected disease is a crucial first step in recognition. Only a very small percentage of occupational disease cases historically are reported to governmental public health surveillance systems in the United States. Table 2–1 outlines the barriers to accurate diagnosis.

THE OCCUPATIONAL HISTORY

The most important tool for the diagnosis of occupational illness is the occupational history. Figure 2–1 illustrates a quick survey of occupational health issues that are appropriate to raise in every initial evaluation. If answers to these questions are positive, more detailed follow-up questioning is necessary (Table 2–2).

Two lines of questioning are useful in occupational history taking: (1) Given a pattern of symptoms or organ system involved, what occupational exposures should be inquired about? (2) Given an exposure type

or occupation, what symptoms should be specifically reviewed?

The chief complaint and history of present illness may suggest potential diagnostic possibilities that lead to specific etiologic hypotheses. For example, a history of headache while at work suggests potential solvent or carbon monoxide exposure, and cough and wheezing while at work or predictably delayed after leaving work may suggest irritant or triggering allergen exposure. A history of fevers and back pain in a clinical laboratory worker or Mexican slaughterhouse worker suggests possible brucellosis. Additional sources of information may help to confirm or rule out hypothesized occupational etiology.

EMPLOYEE DOCUMENTS

Have the employee sign a release enabling you to obtain medical records from treating or consulting clinicians. These records may provide important clues about prior diagnoses, history of exposures, predisposing factors for illness, and the course and progress of the illness.

Other useful employee documents may include medical surveillance records from the employer, the National Institute for Occupational Safety and Health (NIOSH) Health Hazard Evaluation, and reports from the Occupational Safety and Health Administration (OSHA) and from employer or union industrial hygiene consultants. The company health and safety manager should cooperate in answering questions about similar illnesses in coworkers.

In many states, the clinician is required to report suspected or diagnosed occupational disease or injury on an approved form. Insurance companies also may require this prior to payment under the workers' compensation insurance rules, which vary from state to state. In some states, the statute-of-limitations clock starts running at the time a worker is notified by a clinician of a work-related cause for an illness.

THE OCCUPATIONAL HAZARD

When a patient's medical history suggests that occupational or environmental factors may be a primary or secondary cause or contributor to illness, the clinician

Table 2–1. Barriers to accurate diagnosis of occupational diseases.

Patient
- Inadequate training/knowledge of exposures in the workplace
- Lack of worker access to material safety data sheets (MSDSs)
- Resistance to reporting potential work-relatedness to clinician out of fear of loss of job, benefits
- Psychological denial that symptoms could be work related
- Influence of coworkers/spouse on reporting of symptoms to clinician
- Long induction period (the time between initial exposure to a cause of disease and the occurrence of disease)
- Long latency period (the time between occurrence of disease and its recognition, whether by medical testing or by symptoms)

Clinician
- Inadequate training/knowledge about exposures and diseases found in the workplace
- Inadequate time to conduct an occupational history
- Failure to consider occupational factors in differential diagnosis
- Lack of awareness of the legal requirements for reporting, notification
- Incentives in insurance systems to report diseases as work-related (reimbursement maximization) or not
- Perceived hassle of reporting to governmental or other surveillance systems

Societal
- Strong disincentives in insurance systems to recognition of occupational disease
- Lack of recognition of the scope and costs of occupational disease in the population in general
- Lack of funding of research into chronic diseases that may be occupationally related
- Historically, the relative isolation of occupational medicine from traditional medical care

Logistical barriers
- Loss of reports (e.g., in the copying, packaging, mail system, misfiling, and mis-sorting, errors in coding, data entry, and analysis) between the clinician and the surveillance system approaches 30% in some settings

---

should identify all potentially toxic materials or hazards in the workplace, home, or environment. Several helpful references are available to assist the clinician in identifying potential toxic exposures based on specific industry or occupational experience.

1. Grayson M: *Kirk-Othmer Encyclopedia of Chemical Technology,* 4th ed. (New York: Wiley InterScience, 2005); available through various vendors or available as *Kirk-Othmer* online at www3.interscience.wiley.com/cgi-bin/mrwho.

2. Lewis RJ: *Sax's Dangerous Properties of Industrial Materials,* 11th ed. (Hoboken, NJ: Wiley, 2005); also available on CD-ROM.

3. Stellman J (ed): *International Labour Organization Encyclopedia of Occupational Health,* 4th ed. (4 vols.). (ILO, 1999); free online at www.ilo.org/encyclopaedia/.

MATERIAL SAFETY DATA SHEET

The most readily available source of information on chemical ingredients in compounds available commercially is the *material safety data sheet* (MSDS). The law mandates that workers be provided access to MSDSs on all hazardous substances in a workplace (OSHA Hazard Communication Standard). The internet has multiple online databases of MSDSs that may be accessed by using any one of the search engines (e.g., www.google.com) and typing in the term *MSDS*. One Web site, www.ilpi.com/msds/index.html#Internet, maintains a list of databases that offer free MSDS access.

MSDSs, it must be remembered, are often outdated, incomplete, or inaccurate and thus may need augmentation by a call to the company toxicologist listed on the MSDS to obtain more complete, updated information.

Other sources of hazard information include

1. Poison control centers (1-800-222-1222) or www.aapcc.org/.

2. City, county, or state health departments (see their respective Web sites).

3. The National Institute for Occupational Safety and Health (NIOSH), 1-800-35NIOSH (see Web site at www.cdc.gov/niosh/homepage.html).

4. Agency for Toxic Substances and Disease Registry (see Web site at www.atsdr.cdc.gov/ for listing of toxicologic profiles and teaching case studies).

5. State health department resources include an excellent catalog of chemical fact sheets maintained by the New Jersey State Health Department (www.state.nj.us/health/eoh/rtkweb/rtkhsfs.htm) and an excellent series of chemical and ergonomic fact sheets for workers and clinicians from the California State Department of Health Services' Hazard Evaluation System and Information Service (HESIS) (www.dhs.ca.gov/ohb/HESIS/).

6. A unique resource with a focus on the toxicology of environmental chemicals subject to California's Proposition 65 is the California Office of Environmental Health Hazard Assessment (OEHHA) at www.oehha.ca.gov/.

7. Local academic centers of excellence in occupational and environmental health, which are often affiliated with schools of medicine, nursing, or public health [see Web site at www.niosh-erc.org/

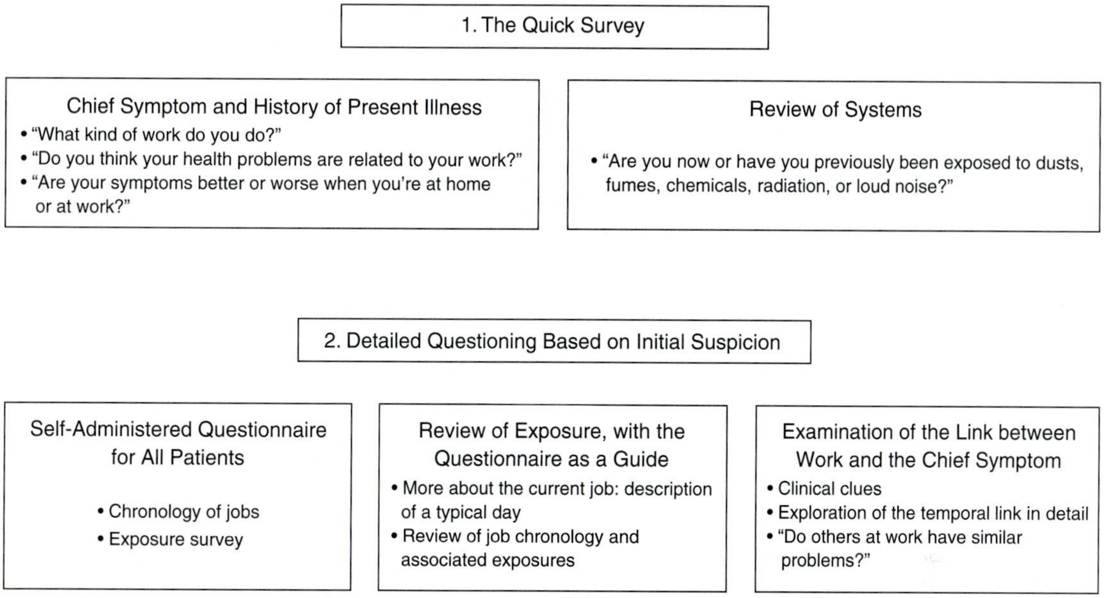

1. The Quick Survey

Chief Symptom and History of Present Illness
- "What kind of work do you do?"
- "Do you think your health problems are related to your work?"
- "Are your symptoms better or worse when you're at home or at work?"

Review of Systems

- "Are you now or have you previously been exposed to dusts, fumes, chemicals, radiation, or loud noise?"

2. Detailed Questioning Based on Initial Suspicion

Self-Administered Questionnaire for All Patients

- Chronology of jobs
- Exposure survey

Review of Exposure, with the Questionnaire as a Guide
- More about the current job: description of a typical day
- Review of job chronology and associated exposures

Examination of the Link between Work and the Chief Symptom
- Clinical clues
- Exploration of the temporal link in detail
- "Do others at work have similar problems?"

Figure 2–1. The initial clinical approach to the recognition of illness caused by occupational exposure.

for a list of NIOSH-sponsored educational resource centers and www-apps.niehs.nih.gov/centers/Public/List/list-ctr.htm for a list of current environmental health academic centers of excellence sponsored by the National Institute for Environmental Health Sciences (NIEHS)].

8. Workers' compensation insurance carriers (retained by the employer) may employ nurses, industrial hygienists, or physicians familiar with the problems at a particular work site.

9. Occupational medicine clinics or clinicians may be located by contacting the Association of Occupational and Environmental Clinics (AOEC) (www.aoec.org) or the American College of Occupational and Environmental Medicine (ACOEM) (www.acoem.org/).

10. Medical libraries in academic health centers, schools of public health, or hospital libraries can provide computer searches and lists of other resources regarding toxic hazards (e.g., www.lib.berkeley.edu/PUBL).

SOME USEFUL COMPUTER DATABASES

Multiple computerized databases are available without charge online through the National Library of Medicine (www.nlm.nih.gov/):

Medline, via PubMed (www.ncbi.nlm.nih.gov/entrez/query.fcgi), provides access to citations and abstracts for more than 12 million published articles going back to the mid-1960s, with links to full-text articles and other publications. This is a good place to start your search, either by exposure [agent by chemical name or Chemical Abstract Service (CAS) identifier], symptom, or suspected disease category or diagnosis. To efficiently obtain the most specific results for your query, you may use the supplementary tools provided by Medline, including the Medical Subject Headings (MeSH) database (www.nlm.nih.gov/mesh/MBrowser.html), which is an online vocabulary look-up aid available for use with MeSH. It is designed to help quickly locate descriptors of possible interest and to show the hierarchy in which descriptors of interest appear. Full-text links to many journals are also available from commercial vendors of Medline citations (e.g., Ovid Technologies, www.ovid.com). These may be accessed from hospital or university libraries. An increasing number of medical journals are available free via the Internet, often after a delay of 6 months to 2 years (see the Web site www.freemedicaljournals.com for an updated listing). A growing archive of freely accessible scientific publications on the Internet was available as of December 2005 from PubMedCentral (see Web site at www.pubmedcentral.nih.gov/).

TOXLINE (see Web site at http://toxnet.nlm.nih.gov/index.html) is the National Library of Medicine's extensive collection of online bibliographic information covering the biochemical, pharmacologic, physiologic, and toxicologic effects of drugs and other chemicals. It contains more than three

Table 2–2. Essential elements of the comprehensive occupational history and questionnaire.

Do the symptoms vary in relation to day of the week, or do they improve on vacations or weekends?

Current or most recent work and exposure history:
  Job title; type of industry; name of employer
  Duration of job; year/month started, year/month finished (if not currently employed); hours worked per day; hours worked per week; shift
  Description of job (what is a typical workday), especially the parts of the job the patient believes may be potentially hazardous
  Exposures to dust, fumes, radiation, chemicals, biologic hazards, or physical hazards

  Protective equipment used (clothes, safety glasses, hearing protection, respirator, or gloves). Are these appropriate for the exposure (e.g., latex gloves provide no protection from most solvents)? How often changed?
  For exposures that are potentially relevant to the chief complaint, what was the duration and intensity of exposure? For example, was dust so thick that it impaired visibility? Was paint applied with brush, roller, or sprayer? Is there a temporal relationship between exposure and onset of symptoms?

  Engineering controls (process enclosure, local exhaust ventilation, general ventilation, shielding, recent substitution of safer equipment or chemicals)

  History of military service:
    Were you in the military? If yes, where were you stationed? Which years did you serve? What was your job classification?

  Membership in a union; safety climate; supervisory relations; recent organizational changes; work stress; layoffs; speedup

  Epidemiologic evidence:
    Other employees at the workplace who have similar health problems

  Toxicologic evidence:
    Do chemically analogous exposures cause similar disease symptoms, even though the chemical in question may have little known toxicity?
    Participation in workplace medical monitoring (e.g., blood, urine, respirator program, chest radiograph)
    OSHA inspection results, other industrial hygiene inspections; ergonomic workstation evaluations

Prior work history
  Job chronology, working backward from the current or most recent job
  Relevant information as above for each significant job previously held

  Major types of exposures:
  Based on your knowledge of the exposures associated with specific occupations, inquire into potential exposures to:

  • Corrosive substances (acids, alkalis)
  • Dusts
  • Fibers (asbestos, fiberglass)
  • Gases
  • Heavy metals
  • Pesticides, insecticides, herbicides
  • Plastics (di-isocyanates, phthalates, acrylonitrile)
  • Petrochemicals
  • Physical agents (noise, heat, vibration, repetitive lifting or other motions)
  • Radiation (electromagnetic, x-ray, ultraviolet)
  • Solvents

million bibliographic citations, almost all with abstracts and/or indexing terms and CAS Registry Numbers. A search on the TOXLINE system will result in citations from Medline as well as specialized databases of abstracts from National Institutes of Health–funded grants and contracts and European journal indices.

HSDB (see Web site at http://toxnet.nlm.nih.gov/index.html), the Hazardous Substances Data Bank, is a toxicology data file containing more than 4500 records organized by individual chemical; it is also located on the National Library of Medicine's (NLM) Toxicology Data Network (TOXNET). It focuses on the toxicology of potentially hazardous chemicals. HSDB is organized by sections, including human exposure and health effects, industrial hygiene, emergency handling procedures, environmental fate, regulatory requirements, and related areas. Data are referenced and derived from a core set of books, government documents, technical reports, and selected primary journal literature. One strength of HSDB is that it is peer-reviewed by the Scientific Review Panel (SRP), a committee of experts in the major subject areas within the scope of the data bank. However, it is wise to check the most recent referenced data to see when the records were last updated.

IRIS is the Environmental Protection Agency's (EPA) Integrated Risk Information System (http://toxnet.nlm.nih.gov/index.html). IRIS is useful for looking up information such as reference doses, carcinogenicity, chronic noncancer health effects, and reproductive hazards of chemical substances. This database also tracks the current status of health hazard assessments by the EPA.

RTECS (Registry of Toxic Effects of Chemical Substances) was, until December 2001, a database of toxicologic information compiled, maintained, and updated by NIOSH. The maintenance of this resource was transferred to a private company in 2001 (see the following NIOSH Web site listing current vendors at www.cdc.gov/niosh/rtecs/RTECSaccess.html).

NIOSHTIC-2 is a bibliographic database of occupational safety and health publications, documents, grant reports, and other communication products funded by NIOSH (see Web site at www.2a.cdc.gov/nioshtic-2/nioshticabout.html).

Other databases are available by subscription on CD-ROM or DVD, via commercial vendors, or online via the Canadian Center for Occupational Safety and Health's CCINFOweb (www.ccohs.ca/).

Federal agencies such as the Occupational Safety and Health Administration (OSHA), EPA, NIOSH, NIEHS, and the Agency for Toxic Substances and Disease Registry (ATSDR) and state agencies such as California's OEHHA can be located at their respective Web sites best by typing in their name into one of the many Internet search engines or by checking one of the library-maintained occupational health resource links (e.g., www.lib.berkeley.edu/PUBL/tox.html). The top European occupational health and safety government agencies can be accessed at http://agency.osha.eu.int/OSHA.

ASSESSMENT OF THE WORKPLACE

The clinician often can best understand the potential contribution of workplace exposures to the patient's illness by visiting the workplace, although time constraints may limit the number of patients for whom this may be performed. This necessitates first obtaining the permission of the patient to contact the workplace, obtaining access to the workplace by contacting the employer's health and safety manager or, for smaller workplaces, the owner/manager. Your patient also may give you the name of a union shop steward or health and safety committee member who may be also of assistance in obtaining access to unionized work sites.

Information that may be obtained during a site visit includes a detailed description of the work processes, prior results of industrial hygiene sampling and medical surveillance, lists of toxic or hazardous materials used, and, most important, a guided tour of the work site with a focus on the specific work areas where the patient has been working. If the worker is employed by a large company with an organized health and safety program, discussion with an industrial hygienist on the company staff or, if unionized, at the international union may be useful for identifying other exposure information, control measures, and potential future monitoring to evaluate the effectiveness of control measures.

Alternatively, on referral from a clinician, a site visit may be conducted by an industrial hygienist connected with an academically based occupational health clinic, inspector from the Occupational Safety and Health Administration (OSHA), or inspector from another agency with appropriate jurisdiction.

OSHA referral may be particularly useful in situations where the clinician suspects that potential violations of OSHA standards may be occurring. Obtaining the assistance of a physical therapist, occupational therapist, or hand therapist experienced with workstation evaluation may be useful with ergonomic problems and repetitive-motion injuries in the workplace.

ENVIRONMENTAL FACTORS

Toxic exposures may occur as well in other environments of patients, including home, school, transportation, and recreational activities.

OTHER RESOURCES

1. Nongovernmental Organizations

Several useful Web sites track links to nongovernmental organizations' Internet resources in occupational and environmental health [e.g., Duke University's Occupational and Environmental Web Resource List at http://occ-env-med.mc.duke.edu/oem/index2.html and the New York Committee on Occupational Safety and Health's (NYCOSH) Occupational Safety and Health/ Industrial Hygiene Links page at www.nycosh.org/reference_library/osh-ih.html]. Also useful to consult are search-engine listings of occupational health resources (e.g., http://directory.google.com/Top/Health/Occupational_Health_and_Safety/Organizations/), where listings include organizations from the well known (e.g., American Public Health Association) to the lesser known (e.g., Baltic Sea Network on Occupational Safety and Health).

2. International Meetings

A list of international meetings is available at these Web sites:

www.ilo.org/public/english/protection/safework/cis/oshworld/events.htm

www.phs.ki.se/occupmed/news/upcomingevents.htm

www.cdc.gov/niosh/exhibits.html

International Internet resources for occupational health professionals include

World Health Organization (WHO) Occupational Health: www.who.int/occupational_health/en/

International Labor Office (ILO) Catalogue of CIS Publications: www.ilo.org/public/english/protection/safework/cis/products/index.html

English version of the *ILO Encyclopedia of Occupational Health and Safety:* www.ilo.org/encyclopaedia/

WHO/ILO Joint Effort on Occupational Health in Africa: www.sheafrica.info/

Association of Societies for Occupational Safety and Health (ASOSH): www.asosh.org/index.html

European Agency for Safety and Health at Work: http://agency.osha.eu.int/news/events/index_en.html

Occupational and Environmental Medicine Resource Index (links to OSH agencies): http://links.occhealthnews.net

NIOSH, EPA, ATSDR, Chemfinder, NLM, teaching materials: www.elsevier.com/homepage/sah/tox/greenberg.pdf

ENVIRONMENTAL HEALTH HISTORY

Pollution of air and water, contamination of food, releases from nearby industrial facilities or waste sites, and environmental hazards in the home environment are all common causes for concern among patients, community members, and public health officials. Physicians today are called on increasingly to address questions or problems related to environmental health. The environmental health history is becoming an important tool for evaluating patients, especially on initial clinician visits and for those with new-onset asthma or allergic rhinitis symptoms, dermatitis, symptoms suggesting potential lead or pesticide poisoning or exposure, as well as at least once during prenatal and well-baby visits. The CH^2OPD^2 mnemonic (*c*ommunity, *h*ome, *h*obbies, *o*ccupation, *p*ersonal habits, *d*iet, and *d*rugs) may be a useful starting point for a more focused environmental history. All physicians must understand the effects of common environmental exposures and the similarities and differences between environmental health and occupational health. Environmental health is discussed in Chapter 37.

REFERENCES

Dames S et al: Clinical problem solving: Don't know much about history. N Engl J Med 2005;352:2338 [PMID: 15930425].

De Rosa CT et al: Implications of chemical mixtures in public health practice. J Toxicol Environ Health 2004;7:339 [PMID: 15371239].

Haafkens J et al: Searching bibliographic databases for literature on chronic disease and work participation. Occup Med (Lond) 2006;56:39–45; e-pub Nov 11, 2005 [PMID: 16286433].

Kogevinas M: The importance of cultural factors in the recognition of occupational disease. Occup Environ Med 2005;62:286 [PMID: 15837846].

Meldrum M et al: The role of occupation in the development of chronic obstructive pulmonary disease (COPD). Occup Environ Med 2005;62:212 [PMID: 15778251].

NIOSH Compendium of Occupational and Environmental Questionnaires: www.cdc.gov/niosh/compend.html.

Payne-Sturges DC et al: Personal exposure meets risk assessment: A comparison of measured and modeled exposures and risks in an urban community. Environ Health Perspect 2004;112:589 [PMID: 15064166].

Poonai N et al: Barriers to diagnosis of occupational asthma in Ontario. Can J Public Health 2005;96:230 [PMID: 1591309].

Richardson RD, Engel CC Jr: Evaluation and management of medically unexplained physical symptoms. Neurologist 2004;10:18 [PMID: 14720312].

Santana VS: Beyond the duality of disease and illness in occupational medicine. Occup Environ Med 2005;62:284 [PMID: 15837844].

Schwela D, Hakkinen PJ: Human exposure assessment resources on the World Wide Web. Toxicology 2004;198:169 [PMID: 15138040].

Tarlo SM, Liss GM: Evidence-based guidelines for the prevention, identification, and management of occupational asthma. Occup Environ Med 2005;62:288 [PMID: 15837848].

Velez-McEvoy M: Occupational and environmental exposure history. AAOHN J 2004;52:146 [PMID: 15119811].

Workers' Compensation

Joseph LaDou, MS, MD, & Julietta Rodríguez-Guzmán, MD

Virtually every country provides some form of entitlements to workers or their survivors to assist them in the event of an occupational injury or illness. Workers' compensation is the form of social insurance broadly accepted in industrially developed countries. Most commonly, workers' compensation is embedded in a country's social security system. In the United States, however, the workers' compensation insurance system has almost no link with the Social Security System.

Workers' compensation laws share many characteristics on an international basis. There are, however, many important differences between the several federal and state systems in the United States. Workers' compensation systems are designed to ensure that the injured worker gets prompt but limited benefits and to assign to the employer sure and predictable liability. Physicians and other health care providers who render care for work-related injuries and illnesses must (1) understand the requirements of their state's workers' compensation system and (2) provide the necessary services both to treat the condition appropriately and efficiently and to ensure the flow of benefits to the worker.

Most occupational physicians practice within the framework of the workers' compensation system. Workers' compensation laws place occupational physicians in a critically important role. Physicians must determine that an injury or illness is caused by work, diagnose it, prescribe care, and assess the extent of impairment and the ability of the worker to resume work. Determinations that injuries or illnesses are the result of work are increasingly contentious. Workers' compensation fails to compensate many occupational injuries and illnesses, including fatalities. All physicians and other health care providers need to become familiar with workers' compensation laws in their states and to learn more about the field of occupational medicine.

The Department of Labor reports that occupational diseases affect 15–20% of all Americans. By either law or practice, compensation for occupational diseases in many states is particularly limited. The majority of individuals with known or suspected occupational disease do not file claims for workers' compensation wage replacement. Fewer than 10% of the workers reported by a health care professional as having a known or suspected occupational disease receive benefits. Workers who develop occupa-

tional diseases following long latency periods seldom receive the benefits to which they are entitled. More than 90% of asbestosis claimants are unjustifiably denied compensation. Similar problems exist in the reporting of occupational asthma, hypersensitivity pneumonitis, and related disorders. The most commonly reported reason for delay in diagnosis of occupational asthma is failure of the treating clinician to ask the relevant occupational history questions.

WORKERS' COMPENSATION LAW

The financial responsibility of the employer for the injury or death of an employee in the workplace was first established under Bismarck in Germany in 1884. Great Britain followed in 1897 with legislation requiring employers to compensate employees or their survivors for an injury or death regardless of who was at fault. Thus workers' compensation laws are the result of a historic compromise in which the employee gave up the right to sue the employer for negligence in exchange for the employer's agreement to pay the cost of medical care and to compensate the worker for time lost from work. By the beginning of the twentieth century, all European countries had workers' compensation laws. The workers' compensation movement did not begin in the United States until 1908, when a forerunner of the Federal Employees Compensation Act was passed. In 1911, the first states enacted their laws. These initial workers' compensation systems were far from the array of programs that deal with disability income loss, medical care, accident prevention, and vocational rehabilitation that characterize contemporary workers' compensation programs.

One of the major deficiencies in workers' compensation law is that its roots are in the past century at a time when occupational disease was not recognized. The system operates with relative success in the recognition and compensation of work-related injuries. However, far fewer than half of all occupational diseases are compensated under workers' compensation systems, and the reporting of occupational diseases by government agencies is also woefully inadequate. Consequently, preventive measures aimed at occupational diseases receive less attention than those directed at the causes of occupational injury.

13

Worker Benefits

The objectives of workers' compensation systems are to provide injured employees with an income following an injury and during recovery, to ensure injured workers a competitive position in the employment market, and to avoid lengthy and costly legal action. In the event of death, survivors are compensated for the loss of their income provider. An injured employee is automatically entitled to medical treatment and compensation, whether the incident is the fault of the employee or the employer. The cost of workers' compensation benefits is considered a cost of doing business and is passed on to purchasers of the product or service. In the case of governmental workers' compensation systems, the costs are included in the taxes collected by federal, state, and local governments.

To be compensable, an injury usually must "arise out of and in the course of employment (AOE/COE)." A work injury that activates or aggravates a preexisting condition also is compensable. Recurrence of an earlier compensable injury is also compensable. Depending on the jurisdiction, judicial action may be necessary to resolve questions of liability for self-inflicted injuries and suicidal acts. Similar determinations may be necessary for injuries occurring under the influence of alcohol or drugs, during entirely personal activity (not AOE/COE), and for violence at work.

Occupational diseases are the direct result of work or exposure to toxic substances or other environmental hazards in the workplace. Occupational disease claims have proliferated in recent decades. In some states, this resulted from judicial interpretations. In other jurisdictions, the increase is the result of "presumptions" that lead to the automatic acceptance of workers' compensation liability for certain diseases in designated worker groups. An example is the presumption in California law that heart disease in police and fire personnel, as well as some other uniformed services, is related to work and is covered by workers' compensation. In all areas of the United States, occupational disease claims are increasing as physicians become more familiar with the discipline of occupational medicine and more confident of their diagnoses of occupational diseases and begin to understand the causes of multifactorial diseases.

Many states recognize cumulative-injury claims as occupational illnesses when the worker has sustained repeated physical or mental injuries that eventually result in a disability. These broadened interpretations of illness and disability open workers' compensation systems to numerous claims of occupational stress. They also bring many new cases of repetitive-motion disorders, cardiovascular diseases, hearing loss, and emotional disturbance into the system. Occupational physicians play key roles in many states where their medical opinions are necessary to resolve issues surrounding compensability of such contentious cases as myocardial infarction and cerebrovascular accident, occupational exposure to toxic materials, and the occurrence of birth defects and other reproductive and developmental problems. Many physicians devote their practices to such forensic activities.

Payment benefits to workers or their families are of six types: (1) permanent total disability, (2) temporary total disability, (3) permanent partial disability, (4) temporary partial disability, (5) survivors' benefits, and (6) vocational rehabilitation benefits.

A. PERMANENT TOTAL DISABILITY

Permanent total disability covers workers who are so disabled that they will never be able to work again in an open labor market and for whom further treatment offers no hope of recovery. Most states compensate such individuals with two-thirds of their average wages subject to minimum and maximum limits. Because benefits are not taxed, this can amount to approximately 85–90% of take-home wages. States also may provide additional funds for dependents. Although some states limit the duration of payments, others provide compensation for the remainder of the injured worker's life.

B. TEMPORARY TOTAL DISABILITY

The majority of injured workers fall under the temporary total disability classification; that is, the worker is expected to recover with treatment but is unable to work for some period of time. Benefits are paid during the recovery period on the basis of the worker's average earnings. Minimum and maximum limits apply, and benefits of as much as two-thirds of gross or 80% of take-home wages are paid until the individual is able to return to work or reaches maximum recovery. There is a waiting period for this type of compensation, but it is paid retroactively if the worker cannot work for a certain number of days or if hospitalization is necessary. The waiting period serves as an incentive to return to work after less serious injuries. Thus, it is like a deductible provision in other forms of health insurance.

C. PERMANENT PARTIAL DISABILITY

Permanent partial disability occurs when an injured worker is disabled to the point that the worker has lost some ability to compete in the open labor market. In some jurisdictions, benefits compensate the injured worker for losses in future earnings and are divided into two categories: (1) scheduled injuries (e.g., loss of a limb, an eye, or hearing) and (2) nonscheduled injuries (e.g., back injury or tenosynovitis). The first is paid according to a schedule fixed by statute. Under this category, benefits are paid whether or not the individual is working. Payment usually is provided for a specified number of weeks, the length of which depends on which part of the body is damaged. Benefits are based on a percentage of earnings at the time of injury and again are subject to a minimum and a maximum amount. Nonscheduled injuries receive weekly benefit payments based on a wage-loss-replacement percentage. The percentage is derived from the difference between wages earned before and after injury. In some states, however, nonscheduled permanent partial disabilities are compensated as a percentage of the total disability benefits.

D. TEMPORARY PARTIAL DISABILITY

Temporary partial disability occurs when a worker is injured to the degree that the worker cannot perform his or her usual work but is still capable of working at some job during convalescence. Many insurers and employers view modified duty as a critical element of the treatment plan and rehabilitation of these injured workers. Under this category, the injured worker is compensated for the difference between wages earned before the injury and wages earned during the period of temporary partial disability, usually at two-thirds of the difference. Modified duty may save the worker from wage differentials by stopping the temporary partial disability payment.

E. SURVIVORS' BENEFITS

Dependent survivors of employees killed on the job are paid death benefits under workers' compensation. The method and size of payments vary widely among the various states, but all systems provide for a death benefit and some reimbursement for burial expenses.

F. VOCATIONAL REHABILITATION BENEFITS

Some level of rehabilitation is provided in all states even if unspecified by statute. Vocational and psychological counseling or retraining and job placement assistance are typical benefits. The goal is to return the injured worker to suitable, gainful employment.

Benefits from Other Sources

A number of benefits are available to workers from other sources.

A. SOCIAL SECURITY DISABILITY INSURANCE (SSDI)

Social Security supplements workers' compensation with monthly benefits for disability. Such benefits are available only after a 5-month waiting period and are calculated as if the disabled individual had reached Social Security retirement age. To be considered disabled, the injured person must be unable to work in substantial gainful employment. Furthermore, the disability must be expected to last more than 1 year or to result in premature death. SSDI combined with workers' compensation cannot exceed 80% of the worker's average earnings or the total family benefit under Social Security before the injury. If the combined compensa-

tion does exceed this amount, Social Security benefits are reduced accordingly, although some states will reduce workers' compensation benefits by all or part of the Social Security payments.

B. SECOND-INJURY FUNDS

Second-injury funds compensate workers for injuries that are exacerbated by a subsequent injury. Some states' second-injury funds compensate workers for flare-ups that do not necessarily lead to total disability. These funds are established and maintained by most states in the hope that the outcome will encourage employers to hire the handicapped or previously injured workers. The employer's compensation carrier makes payments for the second injury, and the fund reimburses the carrier for any additional costs.

Employers' Responsibilities

Employers are responsible for providing medical treatment and compensation benefits for employees injured at work or made ill from exposure to the workplace environment. The system is based on a premise of liability without fault; that is, regardless of whether the worker, the employer, or neither is at fault, the employer is still responsible for providing medical treatment and compensation benefits to the injured employee.

Workers' compensation insurance coverage is compulsory for most private employment except in New Jersey, South Carolina, and Texas. In these states, employers may decline coverage, but, in turn, they lose the customary common-law defenses against suits filed by employees (the "exclusive remedy" is the quid pro quo under which the employer enjoys immunity from being sued in exchange for accepting absolute liability for all work-connected injuries). Employees most likely to be exempt from coverage include domestic workers, agricultural workers, and casual laborers. Coverage also may be limited for workers in small companies with only a few employees (this number varies by state), nonprofit institutions, and state and local governments. Workers' compensation laws cover approximately 87% of all wage and salary workers.

A. DEMONSTRATION OF ABILITY TO PAY BENEFITS

Unless exempted by the law, employers must demonstrate their ability to pay workers' compensation benefits. There are three ways of accomplishing this: (1) insurance with a state fund, (2) insurance through a private carrier, or (3) self-insurance.

1. *State insurance funds.* The states have adopted two methods of meeting the problem of workers' compensation coverage. Some states require that employers insure through a state fund that operates as the exclusive

provider of insurance. Other states operate their funds in competition with private carriers. A few states do not permit an employer to be self-insured.

2. **Private insurance carriers.** Private workers' compensation insurance contracts have two purposes: (a) to satisfy the employer's obligation to pay compensation and (b) to ensure that the injured employee receives all the benefits provided by law. Once the contract is signed, the insurer is responsible for compensating the injured worker. The carrier's liability is not relieved by either the insolvency or death of the employer or any disagreement the carrier may have with the employer. Most state funds are similarly restricted.

3. **Self-insurance.** Large employers may decide to serve as their own insurers. This approach includes the responsibility for adjusting claims and paying benefits, although it is possible to contract these tasks out to companies that provide such services (third-party administrators). To qualify as a self-insurer, a company must demonstrate that it has the financial ability to pay all claims that reasonably may be expected. The state agency may require that a bond or other security be posted. Because this form of insurance is both time-consuming and requires financial reserves, smaller companies seldom can self-insure.

Companies choose to self-fund to reduce costs and to maximize cash flows. Because costs of benefits, claim reserves, litigation, and attendant administrative costs have spiraled in recent years, many companies have concluded that they could do as well as independent carriers while saving the cost of commissions and premium taxes and take advantage of greater cash flow and increased investment income rates. Self-insured employers are more likely to contest injury and illness claims than are privately insured employers or state insurance funds. This tendency to litigate may erase some of the cost savings that are realized by self-insurance.

B. PENALTIES FOR NOT HAVING INSURANCE

Employers often fail to provide workers' compensation insurance coverage for their employees. The cost of even one serious injury can deplete a company's entire annual income or even bankrupt it. Consequently, all but three states have made workers' compensation insurance mandatory. Otherwise, a company could be out of business even before a seriously injured employee is fully recovered.

There are heavy penalties for uninsured employers. They can be subject to fines, loss of common-law defenses, increases in the amount of benefits awarded, and payment of attorneys' fees. The biggest financial deterrent is that the employee may bring a civil suit against the employer. A number of states will force closure of an uninsured busi-

ness. All states have established uninsured employer's funds to which injured employees can apply for benefits. Applying to such a fund does not preclude the individual from also bringing action against the employer for penalties and legal fees. The uninsured employer is also required to reimburse the fund for benefits paid to injured workers.

Insurance Costs & Claims Expenses

The cost of workers' compensation insurance is rate-adjusted for all but the smallest employers—a process known as *experience rating.* When fewer injuries and illnesses occur, the employer profits from lowered workers' compensation insurance costs. Experience modification provides an automatic financial incentive for employers to provide their employees with a work environment that is free from the hazards that may result in compensation claims. The results of economic studies on the value of experience rating are conflicting, and there are numerous problems in the interpretation of available data. Nonetheless, it is a hallowed provision of workers' compensation systems. Most large employers are experience-rated, whereas small employers are typically insured in groups of similar companies. As the definitions of compensable injury are broadened, the intent and benefits of experience rating are diluted.

Approximately three-fourths of all compensable claims for workers' compensation benefits and one-fourth of all cash-payment benefits involve temporary total disability. Permanent total disability occurs in fewer than 1% of all compensable workers' compensation claims. Benefits paid in cash compensation are nearly equaled by medical and hospitalization benefits.

State and federal funds and self-insured employers each pay about one-fifth of all regular benefits, whereas private insurance companies pay the remaining three-fifths. The total costs to employers include the expenses of policy writing, claims investigation and adjustment, allocation to reserves to match increases in accrued liabilities, payroll auditing, commissions, premium taxes, and other administrative expenses and profit.

Employers are required to provide medical treatment as well as compensation benefits. The injured or ill employee is required to report the injury or illness as soon as possible. There is typically a statute of limitation that limits the employer's liability when an injury or illness is not reported promptly. It is considered that the requirement has been met if the employer is informed by someone other than the injured individual. The employer then must provide all medical care reasonably required to alleviate the problem. In fact, the law allows for treatment even when recovery is not possible; that is, palliative care that does not cure but only relieves.

In most states, there are no statutory limitations on the length of time or the cost of treatment, although states and private insurers are implementing a number of cost-containment strategies. These include (1) utilization review of inpatient and outpatient care, (2) hospital bill auditing of inpatient services, (3) medical bill auditing of practitioner and other services, and (4) preferred-provider networks for inpatient care (where fees are discounted) and outpatient care (where the emphasis is on optimization of outcome measures). Some jurisdictions are considering the disallowance of payment for services provided by physicians who own facilities where patients are referred for testing or treatment.

Workers in many states are permitted by state workers' compensation regulations to choose their own physicians. The choice may be any licensed physician or may be made from a list maintained by the employer or the state workers' compensation agency. Regardless of how the physician is chosen, the worker must submit to periodic examinations by a physician of the employer's choice. If either the employer or the worker is dissatisfied with the progress under the chosen physician's treatment, either can request, and often is allowed, to change physicians. Typically, an employee is permitted one such change for subjective reasons alone. In contrast, the employer can be required to prove to the state agency that a change is needed. Reasons for discharging a physician include incompetence, lack of reasonable progress toward recovery, inadequate or insufficient reporting by the physician, and inconvenience of the physician's practice location. If the employer selects the physician, an employee who is not satisfied with the treatment and progress may be permitted consultation with another physician at the employer's expense.

Although the employer must provide medical treatment for the injured employee, if the employee refuses reasonable treatment or surgery without justifiable cause, the employer is relieved of responsibility for any benefits related to injuries caused by the delay in or refusal of any treatment. When the suggested treatment or surgery entails a significant risk, the worker's refusal usually is considered justified.

ROLE OF THE OCCUPATIONAL HEALTH PROFESSIONAL

The occupational physician provides medical care to the injured or ill worker, typically in a clinic or hospital setting to which the patient has been referred by the employer. Other health care professionals are involved in many of the required activities of workers' compensation systems because medical treatment involves the services of physicians and nurses and, frequently, physical therapists. The occupational physicians must determine the work-relatedness of the injury or illness. The physician who takes a careful occupational health history, documenting the details of the events leading up to and including the event of the injury or illness, often will be the most important influence on the finder of fact (workers' compensation judge or referee) as to work-relatedness. The physician who provides treatment and follows the worker medically usually will be the most important influence on the finder of fact as to the nature and extent of the injury or illness.

All parties—the worker, the employer, and the insurer—benefit from an emphasis by the occupational physician on early return to work. The proper determination of work restrictions acceptable to the employer and the worker draws on the occupational physician's experience, his or her familiarity with the workplace and job description, and his or her rapport with both the worker and the employer. Moreover, through continuing care of the worker, the occupational physician determines when the worker has reached maximal medical improvement or maximal functional recovery. Insurers in many states ask the physician to determine the degree of "impairment" (measured by anatomic or functional loss), which the insurers will give to disability raters, workers' compensation judges, commissioners, or hearing officers. These nonmedical people make the decision as to "disability." Disability, unlike impairment, depends on the job and one's ability to compete in the open job market. Impairment does not necessarily imply disability. For example, the loss of the distal phalanx of the second digit on the left hand results in the same impairment rating in a concert violinist and in a roofer, but the disability is much greater for the musician. It is important to discuss impairment and disability separately. An individual with carpal tunnel syndrome may be disabled when considered for a job with repetitive hand movements but not for a job that does not require extensive use of the hands.

Insurers also may ask the physician to determine work restrictions (e.g., no overhead lifting for someone with shoulder problems or no working around moving machinery or at unprotected heights for someone with a balance problem) in order to match the impairment to specific jobs. In some instances, the exact physical restrictions are best determined by a functional-capacity evaluation. There are growing numbers of specialized centers that can assist physicians with both detailed job analyses and functional-capacity evaluations.

When an impairment evaluation is requested, the examining physician in most states must use the most current American Medical Association (AMA) Guides to the Evaluation of Permanent Impairment or the guides used in the physician's jurisdiction. Some states will send medical examiners their recommended guidelines for general medical and psychiatric assessments.

The diagnosis of occupational illness requires a careful and thorough history, review of prior medical records, and examination to determine the multifactorial nature of the case. The occupational physician may be required to state an opinion as to the validity of the workers' compensation claim and maybe even the percentages of the illness that are of work and nonwork origin. Apportionment is a legal device for distributing financial responsibility. It is intended to ensure that employers are only responsible for the portion of injuries or illnesses that actually were caused in their workplace. Apportionment applies only to permanent disability.

Physicians who are experienced with submission of current status and progress reports to employers and insurance companies can expand their experience to include disability evaluations. All physicians who treat injured workers should develop the experience and confidence to undertake impairment and disability evaluations. The physician who has been asked to do a disability evaluation should understand exactly what the requesting party wants to know and obtain and completely review copies of all relevant medical records, reports, and test results. In some states, physicians must be accredited to do these evaluations.

Many workers' compensation cases are settled with "continuing medical treatment" provided either within limits or as a lifelong benefit. The opinion as to the value of continued medical treatment and for what purpose it is to be rendered should be stated, along with recommendations for current treatment should it be different from treatment already given the employee by other physicians.

Independent Medical Examiner

When a compensation case results in litigation, occupational health professionals become important witnesses in resolving disputes. The physician asked to evaluate the worker in most states is designated an independent medical examiner (IME). The IME is the highest level of evaluation a worker will encounter. Most requests for IME opinions come from insurers, but on occasion, plaintiffs' attorneys, judges, and others may initiate an IME evaluation. The opinion of the IME likely will be the final opinion for the worker and determine the success or failure of his or her claim. The IME does not establish a legal doctor-patient relationship because the examination of the worker is not based on the worker's consent. The IME report should be complete and definitive and include diagnosis, cause of injury or illness, prognosis, maximal medical improvement status, permanent impairment, work capacity, and opinion on further clinical management. The IME must be prepared to testify at a deposition and, on rare occasion, in front of a workers' compensation judge or referee. The IME seldom sees the worker again and does not assume any responsibility for medical care.

Claims Disputes

Differences of opinion often arise over workers' compensation claims. Such disputes often result from issues of insurance coverage, work-relatedness of the injury or illness, provision of medical treatment, the worker's earnings capacity, and the extent of the disability. The last is the most common cause of disputes and requires the physician to provide expert medical opinion. Although the system was designed to be "no fault," a large number of claims are subject to disputes between the employer, the insurance carrier, and the worker. Because adjudication is cumbersome, costly, and time-consuming, tribunals have been established to hear claims disputes in the minimum time possible and at the least cost.

In most states, the initiation of a claim is by the worker, and the initial review is by the insurer. When there is a disagreement on the result, either party can apply for a hearing before the workers' compensation agency or court. If there is still dissatisfaction with the hearing officer's decision, an appeal can be made.

The states vary widely in their methods of hearing disputes, but the most commonly used methods are (1) a court-administered system, (2) a wholly administrative system, and (3) a combination of the two. The last is rapidly becoming almost as unwieldy as the common-law approach that it was designed to replace.

A. THE COURT-ADMINISTERED SYSTEM

In the court-administered system, the employer may be covered either by a carrier or by self-insurance. All injuries or illnesses resulting in more than 6 days of disability must be reported within 14 days, usually accompanied by a physician's report. (Time periods, exact procedures, fee percentages, and so on are drawn from one state for the purposes of example.) The state department of labor, through its workers' compensation division, decides whether the worker should receive compensation other than medical treatment. A form letter then is sent to the worker informing the worker of his or her rights in case additional benefits are decided on. Unless there is a complaint, the compensation agency takes no further action to ensure prompt payment, but the carrier must file notice when the claim is first paid. The system also requires that a settlement agreement be filed, even if the worker refuses to sign it. An administrative trial court reviews that agreement to determine whether the worker is receiving his or her just benefits. If so, the agreement is approved, and payments are made accordingly.

The employer has 10 days thereafter to file with the division certified copies of all relevant documents from the worker's file. If the division decides that the agreement does not provide sufficient benefits to the worker, the insurance carrier is required to adjust the agreement and have the court order modified. If the carrier refuses, the division advises the worker to take court action. Once the court has approved the settlement, it is binding on all parties if not contested within 30 days. However, the worker may go to trial court to contest the settlement at any time within 1 year of the injury. Compensation cases receive priority and usually are completed within 10 weeks. The case is heard by a trial judge and may be appealed to a civil court and from there even to the state supreme court if the judge's finding is unacceptable to the worker. The attorney may receive a set percentage of the award for his or her services.

B. THE WHOLLY ADMINISTRATIVE SYSTEM

Under a wholly administrative system, the workers' compensation board reviews claims made against covered employers. Injuries must be reported as soon as possible, and a claims adjudicator of a board located closest to the worker's home (again, using one state's system as an example) determines benefits or the denial of benefits. If the claim is denied, the worker is informed of the reason for denial and how to appeal. Either the government, without charge, or the worker's union assists in the appeal. Judgments can be appealed, in turn, to a board of review in all cases except those related to a rehabilitation decision.

The review boards are part of the department of labor but are totally disassociated from the workers' compensation division. In this example state, the review boards are composed of a chairperson and two members, one chosen by an employers' group and the other by an organization of workers.

The claimant must make an appeal within 90 days after the claims adjudicator's report has been received. The appeal may be in the form of a letter stating the claimant's objections, or it may be submitted on a two-page form used for that purpose. The review board studies the workers' compensation board file and any new information the board obtains in the course of its decision making. There is no hearing on the matter unless the claimant requests it, and such a request will be denied if the board decides that an appeal is not justified. If the board agrees to a hearing, it is held at a location that is convenient for the worker. The worker may have an attorney, but the appeals process does not include payment of the attorney's fees, that being the responsibility of the worker.

Although the decision of the review board is usually binding, it can be appealed further to the commissioners of the workers' compensation board within 60 days by a labor union on behalf of the injured worker or by an organization of employers on behalf of the injured worker or employer. If the chairperson of the review board believes that an important principle underlies the appeal, he or she may allow the worker to make an appeal within 30 days. Furthermore, if the decision of the review board is not unanimous, the worker is permitted to appeal to the commissioners on his or her own behalf within 60 days. The decision of the commissioners is binding and may not be appealed to the courts.

A medical review panel exists for medical issues only. This panel is composed of a chairperson appointed by the government and two physicians, one selected by the worker and one by the employer. Decisions by this panel are final. Many states sponsor less formal panels of physicians who interview and examine the claimant and then render opinions on disability, work restrictions, treatment, and prognosis.

C. THE COMBINATION SYSTEM

The workers' compensation agency under the combination system is composed of a seven-member appeals board that is responsible only for reviewing appeals and an administrative director who is responsible for the administrative functions of the agency. In California, for example, eight individuals are appointed by the governor and confirmed by the state senate.

Both the employer and the attending physician (again, using one state's system as an example) must file first reports of worker injury or illness with the state division of labor statistics and research. They are usually submitted through the employer's compensation carrier or adjusting agent and constitute the initiation of a claim. Furthermore, within 5 days of the injury, the employer must inform the injured worker, in simple terms, not only about the benefits to which he or she is entitled but also about the services available from the state division of workers' compensation. The employer is further required to inform the compensation system administrator, as well as the worker, about commencement and termination dates of benefits, nonpayment of benefits, and rejection of claims. The worker also must be informed that he or she can obtain an attorney, if desired. The worker further must be advised that any action must be taken promptly to avoid loss of compensation.

Thus the worker is informed of his or her rights, and because there are penalties for the unwarranted rejection of compensation, many claims are paid automatically. The division of workers' compensation becomes involved only if either the employer or the employee seeks adjudication from the workers' compensation appeals board. Such adjudication is initiated by the filing of a simple one-page form. The application must be filed within 1 year of the injury or by the date of the termination of benefits, whichever is longer. If the adjudication claim is related to further trauma resulting from the original injury, the application requirement is 5 years from the date of the original injury.

Although the system anticipates that a hearing will be held within 30 days of the application, this is seldom possible because of backlog. The hearings are conducted at several locations throughout the state and are assigned to a workers' compensation judge who makes the decision. Each judge usually reviews approximately 90 cases per month.

The hearings are designed to be informal, but often they cannot be distinguished from a nonjury court trial. The judges are knowledgeable in the workers' compensation process and are required to develop additional information if the evidence provided by the parties is inadequate. Medical information usually is presented in written reports. Once all the evidence is presented, the judge must present a written decision within 30 days.

If the employer or the employee is unhappy with the decision, he or she may file an appeal. This appeal is called a *petition for reconsideration* and must be filed within 20 days of the posting of the original decision. It is heard by a panel of three members of the appeals board. The panel is authorized to approve or deny reconsideration, issue a different decision based on the original evidence, or seek additional information, including consultation with an independent medical specialist.

The decision of this panel is final unless the dissatisfied party seeks a review within 45 days by submitting a petition for a writ of review to the appeals court. The court is empowered to deny the review without explanation. If a review is permitted, the appeals court studies the evidence, hears oral arguments, and presents a written decision. If the party bringing the appeal is still dissatisfied, that party may petition the state supreme court for a further hearing. However, state supreme courts rarely accept more than a few workers' compensation cases each year and only accept cases that contain precedent-setting issues.

In the most contested cases, both parties are represented either by attorneys or by expert lay representatives. On average, those representing the worker receive 9–15% of the award.

Reopening of Claims

Workers' compensation proceedings differ from civil lawsuits in one important aspect—the body that originally decided the award may alter its decision if the worker's condition changes or if there is other reason-

able cause. This process may be limited under certain conditions by state compensation laws, and most states establish a time limit beyond which a modification cannot be made. If the requirements of the law cannot be met, final decisions in compensating cases are as binding as those in any judicial proceeding.

There is a wide divergence among states as to benefit amounts, conditions that are compensable, processing of claims, settlement of disputes, and general economics of each system. Consequently, physicians who expect to be treating patients with occupational injuries and illnesses are well advised to learn how the workers' compensation system operates in the state in which they are practicing.

REFERENCES

Bernacki EJ: Factors influencing the costs of workers' compensation. Clin Occup Environ Med 2004;4:249 [PMID: 15182747].

Haines J et al: Workers' compensation for psychological injury: Demographic and work-related correlates. Work 2006;26:57 [PMID: 16373980].

LaDou J: Occupational medicine: The case for reform. Am J Prevent Med 2005;28:396 [PMID: 15831348].

LaDou J: World Trade Organization, ILO conventions, and workers' compensation. Int J Occup Environ Health 2005;11:210 [PMID: 15875900].

Leigh JP, Robbins JA: Occupational disease and workers' compensation: coverage, costs, and consequences. Milbank Q 2004; 82:689 [PMID: 15595947].

Physicians' Guide to the California Workers' Compensation System: www.dir.ca.gov/IMC/toc.pdf.

World Health Organization (WHO) International Classification of Functioning, Disability, and Health: www.who.int/icidh/index.htm.

Disability Prevention & Management   4

Gideon Letz, MD, MPH, Jennifer H. Christian, MD, MPH, & Susan M. Tierman, MD

Disability commonly is defined as absence from work or loss of work attributed to a medical condition. A diagnosis of a medical condition need not result in disability unless there also is a loss of functional capacity and ability to work. This chapter outlines the important role that physicians can play in preventing disability.

Disability episodes entail the use of sick leave, short- or long-term disability, family medical leave [Family and Medical Leave Act (FMLA)], workers' compensation benefits, and even disability retirement benefits and may result in job loss. Employers spend 6–8% of their total payroll for benefit programs that cover employees during medically related absence.

According to a recent survey of occupational physicians, fewer than 10% of work-related injuries should require workers to take more than a couple days off work. This contrasts markedly with the 24% of injured workers who receive temporary disability benefits. This suggests that up to 80% of paid temporary disability is medically unnecessary.

Delay in return to work is attributable to a variety of factors:

- The employer has a policy against light duty.
- The employer cannot temporarily modify a job.
- The treating physician is unwilling to force a patient back to work.
- The treating physician feels caught between the employer's and employee's versions of the situation.
- Too little information about the physical demands of the job has been provided to the treating physician.
- Either the injured worker, the employer, or both lack motivation to accomplish the return to work.

Most medically unnecessary disability days are the result of slow or inadequate communication between the physician and the employer, lack of temporary modified work or permanent work accommodations, legal disputes, and administrative delays.

Physicians are asked routinely by their patients to sign forms or write notes to authorize absence from work. However, very few of these requests require absence from work. Most of the time, absence from work is medically unnecessary but may be justifiable, depending on the circumstances (Table 4–1).

DELAYED RECOVERY: RISK FACTORS

The vast majority of workers who have work-related injury/illness and file a workers' compensation claim will be treated and return to work without unexpected delays. A small but important percentage of injured workers will experience delayed return to work with disability duration well beyond what would be predicted by the initial diagnosis.

Patients can begin developing a disabled mind-set after as little as 2–4 weeks off work. The observant clinician can see the patient's face change, his or her speech patterns alter, and his or her body language change as he or she starts wondering whether he or she will ever be able to work again, and the patient starts getting the idea that maybe he or she is now disabled. These reactions are uncommon in patients who are disabled by self-limiting problems such as recovery from elective surgery but are a serious risk in patients who are disabled owing to soft-tissue injuries and other kinds of self-reported conditions lacking objectively determinable indicators of biologic severity.

Long disability predicts a bleak outcome. The longer workers stay away from work, the more likely they are to be permanently disabled. By the time a worker has been off work for 3 months, the worker has only a 50% chance of ever returning to work. By 12 months, it is only approximately 2% (Figure 4–1).

Many studies document that a few injured workers account for a disproportionate percentage of workers' compensation costs. One study of workers' compensation claims in the United States found that 25% of all claims accounted for 97% of the total costs. When one considers only back pain claims, the statistics are even more striking. For example, one study found that 10% of low-back pain claims were responsible for 86% of the total costs for all types of workers' compensation claims.

These findings are consistent across both benefit programs and geographic jurisdictions. They are explained in part by the fact that severe injuries (e.g., head trauma and spinal cord injuries) require expensive treatments with prolonged rehabilitation and significant residual disability. However, the high-cost claims are not all biologically severe injuries and illnesses. In fact, many high-cost cases start out as minor musculoskeletal conditions such as lumbar sprain or upper extremity overuse but end up

Table 4–1. Medically justifiable/medically necessary absence from work.

Situation	Medically Justifiable?	Medically Necessary?
A fully recovered patient asks the doctor to delay his return to work for a week.	No	No
A pregnant patient with high blood pressure is confined to bed in order to prevent toxemia.	Yes	Yes
A patient with a mild back strain stays out of work because his doctor sent a note saying he can't lift 3-pound cartons.	Yes	No
A convalescing patient cannot go back to work because of a company policy against light duty.	Yes	No

in prolonged absence from work, often without objective pathology.

The term *delayed recovery* is applied to patients with unusually prolonged recovery that is disproportionate to objective clinical findings. These patients suffer physical, emotional, and financial hardship as a result of their prolonged absence from work. They are a source of frustration for the physicians who care for them because their symptoms cannot be explained easily and do not respond to standard therapeutic interventions. The costs associated with this group of patients

for medical treatment, wage replacement, and lost productivity have a significant negative impact. Given the high costs to society of lost productivity and the high human costs of disability to an injured worker, long-duration work disability is a serious public health problem.

Studies consistently show a poor correlation between physical impairment and duration of disability or return to work, as well as between traditional demographic variables (i.e., age, sex, education, etc.) and disability duration. This suggests that other variables explain the prolonged disability and delay in return to work. Many factors that appear to have predictive value are nonbiologic. For example, it is increasingly clear that the interaction between the worker and the work environment, such as job satisfaction and perceived stress, is key.

Current evidence suggests that understanding delayed recovery, chronic pain, and disability requires a biopsychosocial model that reflects a complex interaction between physical, emotional, social, and economic variables. Information in the medical and social science literature consistently identifies a number of specific factors that can be broadly categorized by their association with the injured worker/patient, the employer, or the treating physician.

REFERENCE

Harris I et al: Association between compensation status and outcome after surgery. JAMA 2005;293:1644 [PMID: 15811984].

1. The Injured Worker/Patient

There are a number of psychological factors, including personality traits, perceptions of the social environ-

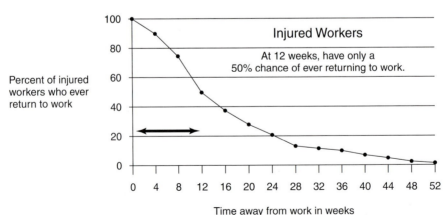

Figure 4–1. Time is of the essence.

ment, and attitudes or beliefs about illness, as well as history of psychiatric diagnoses and history of sexual and other abuse, that have been correlated with delayed recovery. For example, psychological distress and perception of severe disability are associated with poor outcomes, whereas a positive attitude about return to work does predict timely return to work.

Underlying depression is often an important etiologic factor in delayed recovery. Surveys of workers with chronic disability indicate that delayed recovery may be related directly to inadequate coping skills in response to life stressors and that disability can provide a socially acceptable way to express feelings such as depression. Unfortunately, treating physicians often fail to screen for psychiatric comorbidities, and even when such comorbidities are uncovered, many patients have either no coverage or inadequate access to mental health services, so depression often goes undiagnosed and untreated.

Delayed recovery usually involves chronic pain, although other subjective symptoms such as fatigue and paresthesias also may occur. The management of chronic pain is difficult for a number of reasons: Preexisting psychological distress (commonly anxiety/depression), individual differences in personality, and cultural background all can modulate the experience and reporting of pain symptoms. Beliefs about the etiology of the pain and social reinforcement of pain behaviors also can contribute to the delay in recovery and perpetuation of suffering and disability.

Secondary Gain

In reviewing the literature on delayed recovery, the powerful influence of social and psychological rather than medical factors is striking. Social and psychological forces can counteract the desire to get better and reinforce the disabled role. An individual is more likely to amplify and cling to particular symptoms (a behavior known as *somatization,* described in more detail below) when it results in secondary gain, that is, environmental reinforcement of illness behavior. Three types of secondary gain have been described:

- Sympathy, attention, and support (including financial)
- Being excused from responsibilities, obligations, duties, or challenges
- Ability to influence important people by virtue of their acceptance of the individual as sick/disabled

Immediately after an injury or illness, the outpouring of support from family, friends, and coworkers often reinforces the individual's feelings of dependency and entitlement. With the special status of disability, there are lessened expectations with regard to work, and family roles are changed. Often the disabled worker is excused from responsibilities in daily life. When the perception exists that work is causally related to the injury or illness, there is also a feeling of entitlement, that is, a sense that the individual has suffered an injustice and that society owes him or her something. This is amplified by any system that awards benefits contingent on proving disability.

Somatization

Somatization is a common reflection of emotional distress and presents with a preoccupation with and unconscious exaggeration of physical symptoms. It is the explanation for real symptoms in the absence of an identifiable physical disorder. Somatization explains much of what clinicians label as "nonspecific pain" in the low back, neck, hand, and chest, and it undoubtedly explains why many people with mild degenerative conditions file workers' compensation claims. It is estimated that 50–70% of patients with a diagnosable psychiatric disorder present initially with somatic (physical) symptoms that obscure the psychiatric distress (most commonly depression) from the physician's view.

When workers are faced with life changes (which may involve work, family, or personal issues) and have inadequate coping skills, somatization may result in disability and delayed recovery. An illness or accident can transform excessive stress, tension, and dependency needs into acceptable forms of disability that temporarily increase self-esteem, providing a more acceptable justification for existing symptoms (psychological secondary gain).

The willful faking of symptoms, known as *malingering,* is occasionally the cause of delayed recovery. True malingering (i.e., intentionally defrauding the insurance system) is rare but does occur. Differentiating a true malingerer from a patient with symptom magnification and chronic-illness behavior can be difficult. A common feature in both these groups is inconsistency between history, physical examination, and performance of standardized tasks. Erratic and variable grip-strength measurements and inconsistent results on range-of-motion testing should raise the index of suspicion. Waddell signs or similar validity checks on physical examination provide additional clues. Referral to an experienced forensically trained independent medical examiner may be necessary to distinguish between malingering and symptom magnification when there are persistent complaints in the absence of objective findings.

Wage Replacement

There are specific provisions of the workers' compensation system that may at times provide a perverse incentive relative to return to work.

1. Most jurisdictions provide wage replacement at something less than full pay. However, for low-wage workers, the fact that temporary disability benefits are not considered taxable income results in take-home pay that approximates their usual income.

2. The provision of financial compensation for permanent disability is a double-edged sword. For severely injured workers with significant residual impairment, monetary compensation is justified on the basis of decreased earning potential. However, the fact that increased severity of impairment is widely presumed to require longer duration of work absence and more extensive medical treatment provides an incentive to stay off work for susceptible employees. This perverse incentive is reinforced by legal representation because the attorney is paid on a contingency basis related to the dollar amount of the permanent disability award or settlement.

Medical-Legal Issues

Disputes often arise in the life history of a workers' compensation claim. Formal litigation may result in relation to a number of issues, including liability, causation, degree of impairment, apportionment of residual disability, or need for medical care. Once a claim is litigated, the resolution typically is delayed for a year or more, and during this time, the injured worker is not motivated to return to work because of the concern that it would affect his or her claim adversely. Typically, multiple physicians who order a wide variety of diagnostic tests evaluate the injured worker. This tends to reinforce the individual's belief that something is seriously wrong. There is also a tendency for these patients to amplify and exaggerate their subjective complaints when they view the physician as having the legal and administrative power to determine their benefits. The observation that patients often recover quickly after their case is settled provides further evidence that current compensation laws foster disability behavior.

2. Employer/Occupational Factors

A number of variables related to the work environment correlate with the risk of delayed recovery. In particular, recent studies have found that the workers' perceptions of the work environment are predictive—perceived stress in the work environment, quality of relationships, and job satisfaction, for example.

Firm size is another variable that seems to be a consistent predictor of disability duration, with larger employers associated with shorter duration of disability. A number of reasons have been suggested to explain this observation:

1. Smaller firms have higher turnover and less access to information about disability prevention.
2. The workers' compensation premium is experience-rated for larger firms, providing incentives for disability management.

3. Larger firms have greater flexibility in creating modified/transitional work.

3. The Treating Physician

Because most physicians (even occupational medicine specialists) never receive formal training in disability prevention and management, their lack of expertise in this area can create barriers to a return to work. When patients have persistent complaints, the physician's first response may be to order more diagnostic tests, often invasive in nature, rather than considering the nonmedical factors that may be fostering illness behavior and inhibiting return to work. Operating in the medical model and ignoring the psychosocial determinants of illness, the untrained provider prescribes more time off from work. This common therapeutic pattern actually may prolong recovery and further reinforce the sick role. If treatment goals are focused on alleviation of symptoms rather than on improvement of functional capacity, there is an increased risk that the patient will begin a downward spiral from anger and helplessness to depression, withdrawal, loss of identity, and finally into the sick role and chronic disability. Failure to include transitional work as an integral part of the treatment plan results in medically unnecessary time off work with resulting physical deconditioning and increased emotional distress. Lack of information about the physical demands of the job may frustrate physicians and make them less likely to release their patients to transitional work assignments.

Many physicians who treat patients with work-related injury/illness are not comfortable with the evaluation of patients' psychological status and the potential for psychosocial factors to create significant barriers to recovery. Referral for specialist evaluation should be considered whenever there are persistent complaints or when symptoms are unresponsive to standard medical treatment. Evaluation by a psychologist or other mental health professional can help the primary care physician to

1. Determine specific psychological and behavioral issues related to the patient's pain behavior and disability.
2. Provide insight on aspects of the patient's history and current situation that bear on the delayed recovery.
3. Recommend appropriate treatment goals and intervention strategies.

CLINICAL MANAGEMENT

People share three main pillars of identity: physical being, work or calling, and relationships. When any of the three are disrupted, it is destabilizing. If more than one is disrupted, it can cause a major alteration in one's sense of self.

> ***Bodily integrity.*** Loss of bodily integrity threatens identity and causes denial, anger, grief, depression, and uncertainty. People who lose a part of their body or even just a bodily function grieve for it and go through stages of adjustment as though a part of them has died. Acceptance is the final and necessary stage.

> ***Work.*** Work may be a calling, a trade, or simply a paycheck, but it is one of the most basic statements about one's self. For most people, the threatened or actual loss of work threatens identity and causes anxiety, depression, and loss of self-worth. Because work is so central to their lives, people may insist on returning to work before it is safe to do so because their identity is so wrapped up in their work.

> ***Relationships.*** People who are unable to work because of illness or injury have had two of their three identity pillars destabilized. They are apt to react to the combined disruption of their bodily integrity and their loss of work with a variety of psychological disturbances, and that puts strain on their third pillar—relationships. Family life is disrupted when the breadwinner is home sick. The sudden disappearance of all the daily social interchange with coworkers can create a significant vacuum in people's lives. Thus, loneliness is added to the list of problems caused by time off work. A significant fraction of disabled persons develop marital, family, and substance-abuse problems.

Ways to Improve Functional Outcomes

Whenever a patient develops a disabling illness or injury, the patient becomes anxious about the prognosis, particularly about the impact on life's activities. How the condition will interfere with everything from mobility and activities of daily living to work and recreation is a primary concern of anyone who is faced with a new medical condition. Physicians can foster patient trust and improve compliance if they are willing to devote time and attention to these concerns at every visit.

Accurate diagnosis and effective treatment are not the purpose of health care but rather a means to the end of restored/preserved comfort and function. A fundamental purpose of health care is to help people to get their lives back to normal. Anything that speeds this transition is a part of the healing process. In this context, answering questions and filling out forms that get patients safely back to their normal activities and work becomes an important part of the treatment process.

Assessing the Situation

These four "bedside" tests are useful in identification of overlooked or neglected issues that need attention.

A. The Return-to-Work Screening Test

By asking the patient the following three questions, this test identifies cases that require extra attention or referral:

1. It looks like you are going to have some problem with your [right hand, left foot, back, breathing, balance, vision, stamina, etc.] for a while. What impact will this have on your ability to do your regular work the usual way?
2. Have you figured out a way to work around this issue while you recover?
3. Will you have any problems with your boss or co-workers about modifying your job temporarily?

This test puts the burden on the employee (who is most familiar with the situation) to make the match between his or her current physical condition and what he or she knows of the job demands and work environment but also requires the employee to reveal potential conflicts or problems. Sometimes the answers will make it clear that this case requires extra attention.

B. The Grocery Store Test

This test is a quick way to sort out whether absence from work is medically required. The physician ponders this question: If this patient owned a "mom 'n pop" corner grocery store and had no one to cover for him or her while out of work, would this patient be able to find a way to get to work and be safe there? If yes because the patient could find a way to work comfortably and safely, then absence from work is probably not required medically, and the doctor should clear the patient for work with limits and restrictions as needed. If no because there is no known accommodation that would enable the patient to work, the doctor should specify in writing what the impediment to return to work is and let others decide whether they can remove it. If no because the patient must be home in bed all day, is too weak to leave the house, or needs to be in the hospital or other treatment facility, then there are clear medical reasons why the patient should not be released for work. These situations tend to improve rapidly, so it is wise to predict when the patient's functional status is likely to have improved enough to permit some functional work and to set up an appointment to reevaluate the return-to-work issue at that time.

C. The Obstacle Question

This test identifies environmental or logistical issues that are causing disability. The physician asks the patient this question: "What specifically is the obstacle preventing you from working today?" If the answer is not concrete enough, the physician asks again, "And what specific effect does this have on your ability to be at work today?"

This line of questioning shifts the focus away from justifying or rationalizing disability and puts the focus on finding a way around it. This question will uncover environmental and logistical barriers to a return to work. The identified obstacle needs to be addressed by the physician or referred to someone else in order to get this patient back to work.

Many problems uncovered by the obstacle question are simple to fix by the appropriate party once they are uncovered. In a couple of minutes, the physician, the medical office staff, the insurance adjuster, a nurse case manager, a physical therapist, a vocational rehabilitation counselor, or the employer's in-house medical, benefits, or safety staff may be able to solve it.

D. THE MOLEHILL SIGN

The molehill sign indicates when motivational issues are causing disability. This sign is named after the saying "making a mountain out of a molehill." If a seemingly minor health problem is having a major impact on the patient's daily life and work, the molehill sign is present. (A good measure of a person's commitment to something is the amount of inconvenience or discomfort he or she is willing to endure for it.)

A positive molehill sign points toward problems with motivation, meaning problems with incentives, intentions, feelings, beliefs, or the ability to cope. A search should begin for the underlying source of the apparently weak motivation. Every employee with apparently low motivation is a potentially productive one, especially if the situation is viewed as an opportunity for improvement. The person with the motivation problem is not always the person with the injury or illness. It also can be someone who has control over the resources and opportunities for recovery but refuses to use them. For example, a sizable fraction of patients with delayed recovery were in difficult supervisor-employee relationships.

REFERENCE

Boersma K, Linton SJ: Screening to identify patients at risk: Profiles of psychological risk factors for early intervention. Clin J Pain 2005;21:38 [PMID: 15599130].

Therapeutic Use of Rest & Activity

Regardless of the diagnosis, rest and activity prescriptions should be included as a formal element in every treatment plan. It may be useful to think of activity and rest (or lack of activity) as therapeutic drugs, with specific indications and contraindications.

A. REST

Rest has been known since antiquity to be beneficial in the healing process, and it is currently prescribed for everything from myocardial infarction to backache. It has dramatic analgesic effects for most musculoskeletal conditions and often is the only treatment necessary. In recent years, however, there has been an increasing awareness that too much rest can be harmful. Muscle fibers atrophy during immobilization with decreased cross-sectional area and potential for oxidative enzyme activity. Prolonged bed rest leads to loss of muscle mass (1.0–1.5% per day), cardiopulmonary deconditioning (15% loss of aerobic capacity in 10 days), bone mineral loss with hypercalcemia and hypercalciuria, and increased risk of thromboembolism.

B. EXERCISE

It is generally accepted that regular physical activity reduces risk and decreases morbidity and mortality from a wide variety of conditions. There is also abundant evidence that maintaining activity has significant psychological and social effects that are critical to the prevention of delayed recovery after work-related injury or illness.

1. Mobility & Activities of Daily Living—*Mobility* can refer to range of motion for an injured extremity or to postural states or degrees of ambulation. The term *activities of daily living* includes activities associated with personal care, eating, sexual activity, normal household activities, driving a car, and use of public transportation.

Early in the rehabilitation process, the activity prescription may be focused on mobility. After an ankle sprain, for example, there is an appropriate period for gradual increase in dependent positioning and weight bearing. With impingement of the shoulder, there are simple range-of-motion exercises that are recommended and certain movements (overhead reaching) to be avoided. For patients with acute low-back pain, the focus initially may be on gradually increasing periods of sitting, standing, and walking.

There is a consistent trend toward earlier mobilization, ambulation, and return to normal activity during recovery from a wide range of conditions from myocardial infarction and abdominal surgery to skeletal fractures and minor musculoskeletal conditions such as strain/sprain and tendonitis.

2. Structured Exercise—Clinical evaluation to identify specific dysfunction must precede development of a treatment plan. This includes a complete history and physical examination to document clinical signs and symptoms and physiologic testing when indicated, including both static and dynamic measurements of musculoskeletal function. Information related to the physical demands of job tasks is also essential in the development of a rehabilitation plan aimed at recovery of pertinent functions with appropriate endpoints.

The specifics of the initial exercise prescription should be based on objective findings and specific goals, and adjustments should be made based on response to treatment. Ideally, the physician and therapist are working closely enough so that the physician defines the general parameters and goals of therapy, but the physical therapist formulates the actual daily routine. Although general guidelines can be written for progression of therapy following a specific injury, exercise/activity prescriptions must be individualized.

3. Physical Therapy Endpoints—The initial goal of therapy is to decrease pain so that functional movement can be performed. During this phase of rehabilitation (ideally lasting less than 2 weeks), passive modalities may be beneficial (e.g., ice, heat, ultrasound, and electrical stimulation). These modalities may help to decrease inflammation and pain, thereby allowing patient reassurance and development of self-confidence. At this point, education regarding anatomy, pathophysiology, and body mechanics is emphasized. Once acute tissue injury has resolved and acute pain is under control, reconditioning should begin, and the injured worker must take a more active role in the rehabilitation process. The patient needs to understand that recovery and return to normal function are within the patient's control. Decreased use of passive modalities for pain relief is encouraged, and active exercises for neuromuscular mobilization, improved flexibility, muscular strength, and aerobic conditioning are emphasized.

1. Range of motion. The initial goal for most common musculoskeletal injuries is to regain range of motion (ROM). This is followed by a focus on muscular strength and then on power and endurance. Throughout the rehabilitation process, strength of uninjured parts and cardiovascular endurance should not be neglected. Improvement in ROM can be achieved with a combination of exercises that are performed passively, actively, or actively with assistance.

2. Strength. As the injured worker progresses with ROM, strengthening exercises can be initiated. During the early stages of active exercise, training can occur every day. As the workload increases to about 25% of the non-injured muscle group, the frequency should be reduced to every other day. This permits cellular adjustments in the muscle tissue that facilitate maximal strength gains.

Strength can be increased through a combination of isometric, isotonic, and isokinetic exercises. Isometrics can be used early when there is still a need to limit ROM and even can be used when the patient is immobilized to help control atrophy. With either isotonic or isokinetic exercise, strength should be developed initially by slow speed, low weights, and multiple repetitions. Once muscle strength is near 80% of the unaffected limb, the patient can begin working on power and endurance, which are improved by lifting weights more quickly at faster contractile velocities. In many cases, a strengthening program can be designed to reproduce the motions that are actually necessary to perform the specific job tasks at work (work hardening).

3. Cardiovascular fitness. Many injured workers are deconditioned, have a low physical work capacity, and are frequently overweight. Aerobic exercise can improve work capacity, provide endorphin release for pain control, facilitate weight loss, and improve overall cardiovascular fitness. Before initiating a cardiovascular fitness program, patients with significant chronic disease should be screened to rule out contraindications to aerobic exercise and should be monitored medically at least initially to ensure an appropriate protocol.

For maximal gain in cardiovascular fitness, the activity should use large muscle mass and be performed for a prolonged period in a continuous rhythmic fashion. Walking, swimming, jogging/running, cycling, and cross-country skiing are good examples. Other activities, such as figure skating and dancing, also can improve aerobic capacity and are less tedious than cycling or treadmill walking, but these activities do not provide as much control of intensity, and they should be employed cautiously until a base level of fitness is established. Jogging/running should be avoided in spine-injured patients because these activities transfer impact loading to the spine. Lower-impact cardiovascular activities, such as bicycling, swimming, walking, and stair climbing, are better choices. Exercise frequency of 3 days per week initially may be adequate for promoting strength and cardiovascular conditioning.

REFERENCES

Finnish Medical Society Duodecim: Physical activity in the prevention, treatment and rehabilitation of diseases: www.guideline.gov.

Hagen KB et al: The updated Cochrane Review of bed rest for low-back pain and sciatica. Spine 2005;30:542 [PMID: 15738787].

Moffett J, McLean S: The role of physiotherapy in the management of non-specific back pain and neck pain. Rheumatology (Oxf). 2006;45:371 [PMID: 16332949].

RETURN TO WORK

It is important to create an environment in which the worker will feel successful and be protected from reinjury. A failed effort to return to work creates a very high risk for prolonged disability. Returning people to their normal work with instructions to use common sense sets an expectation of self-care and recovery and produces better outcomes than do overly protective restrictions and limitations. Patients who have fears or anxieties about their return to work (RTW) may need a schedule that ensures success by starting slowly and increasing work demands steadily at regular intervals.

Returning someone to work every other day for the first week is one possibility. Whenever possible, the patient should be told that restrictions and limitations will be reduced progressively at each follow-up visit in order to set an expectation of progressive recovery of function. Most temporary restrictions and limitations should last no more than 90 days. Otherwise, the patient may need to be considered for permanent accommodations or some other long-term employment solution.

Patients who need reassurance or who are concerned about possible abuse by their employers should be offered extra support:

- Encourage patients to find an advocate at the company, who most likely will be in the medical, personnel, or safety department.
- Ask patients to call the physician or visit the office after the first day back at work to report progress and any problems.
- Ask patients to call the physician if they are having trouble during their on-the-job recovery.

The following approach to uncomplicated disability cases allows the physician to act as fact finder and medical advisor and to meet the employer or insurer's need for timely information without compromising the needs of the patient. It shifts the burden for determining the RTW date and arranging appropriate work to the employer, where it belongs.

1. Decide if any and all work is specifically contraindicated medically. Unless confinement to bed or home is medically indicated and required by the treatment plan, the employee should be cleared medically for on-the-job recovery.

2. Identify any obvious mismatch between the demands of the patient's regular job (or any proposed light-duty job) and the patient's condition.

   a. If the situation is unclear, request more information (e.g., job description including usual and proposed modified-duty tasks, data on physical demands of the proposed tasks/job, functional-capacity evaluation of patient by physical therapist, work-site inspection).

   b. Document sources of information; avoid relying solely on the patient or the employer.

   c. In the face of uncertainty, a referral is preferable to delay. Refer to someone with expertise in determining ability to work and supporting patients in modified duty. Alternatively, suggest an independent medical evaluation.

3. Three intervals are useful to those who need to make decisions:
   a. The time it will take until the medical condition is fully resolved.

   b. The time it will take for a "next step" improvement in functional capacity.
   c. The date of the patient's next appointment.

4. If a return to the usual job is not appropriate medically at present, describe the worker's current abilities and the circumstances under which the worker can safely/successfully participate in an on-the-job recovery program. The employer's (or insurer's) willingness and ability to eliminate obstacles and arrange an appropriate on-the-job recovery will determine the date when the employee actually gets back to work.

   a. Employers are more likely to find work when they are told what the employee can do. It is helpful if the physician mentions the parts of the usual job that the employee can now perform or provides examples of tasks that are medically appropriate.

   b. Describe any *medical restrictions*—what the patient should not be allowed to do or what the employer should do to accommodate the patient's restrictions. These are specific medical concerns or protective circumstances that allow patients to function safely at work during recovery. Determining restrictions is a medical issue. Medical restrictions should not be modified without physician agreement because the physician is concerned about a risk that the worker or employer may not see (Table 4–2).

   c. Describe the *functional limitations*—what the patient cannot or is unable to do. Limitations are the shortfall between the patient's current physical stamina, agility, strength, cognitive ability, etc., and the job. Functional limitations are not really a medical issue because all people have a limit to what they can do—their functional capacity. Physicians get involved because injured or ill patients' ability to do their normal jobs may have changed and because the physician's knowledge of the natural history of recovery is useful. It is usually safe for a worker and employer to mutually agree on a lessening of limitations (but not medical restrictions) as recovery progresses (see Table 4–2).

REFERENCES

American College of Occupational and Environmental Medicine (ACOEM): The attending physician's role in helping patients return to work after an illness or injury: www.acoem.org/guidelines/article.asp?ID=55.

Franche RL et al: Workplace-based return-to-work interventions. J Occup Rehabil 2005;15:607 [PMID: 16254759].

National Institute of Disability Management and Research (Canada): www.nidmar.ca/.

Webility Corporation: www.webility.md.

Young AE et al: A developmental conceptualization of return to work. J Occup Rehabil 2005;15:557 [PMID: 16254755].

Table 4-2. Examples of medical restrictions and functional limitations.

	Restrictions	Limitations
Person with a recent history of seizures	Should not work at heights because of risk of falling or under water	None: Fully capable of performing all tasks
Person with diabetes	Should avoid rotating shift work because of the adverse effects of circadian rhythm disruption on glycemic control	None: Fully capable of performing all tasks
Person recovering from inguinal hernia repair	May not lift more than (x) pounds for (y) weeks to avoid wound dehiscence and failure of surgical repair	Worker may or may not perceive him- or herself as fully capable of performing all tasks
Person with chronic shoulder pain and weakness caused by rotator cuff damage	None: Activity poses minimal medical risk of further damage	Incapable of lifting >10 lbs overhead; unable to tolerate frequent or repetitive overhead work

Functional Capacity

A key element in the RTW process is the physician's assessment of the injured worker's current functional status. Physicians generally include questions about the impact of the current medical problem on daily activities and function during the regular medical history and review of systems and then extrapolate that information to the work environment. Over time, most physicians develop a sense of the practical impact of particular medical conditions on functional ability. For example, the ability to drive a car, climb stairs, carry bags of groceries, or lift small children all can be related to work activities with similar functional demands. When the situation is unclear, a next step is to ask the patient to describe and demonstrate the activities that are currently a problem. The physician can assess the patient's level of effort and authenticity while observing the patient. Alternatively, the patient can be sent to the physical therapist for a functional-capacity evaluation (FCE). It is better to target the specific functions that are in question than request a comprehensive assessment of all possible functions.

Even the most sophisticated measurement tools and methods are only approximations of real-life functional capacity. However, understanding the distinction between capacity, current ability, tolerance, and risk will help to clarify the issues and provide a context for interpretation of functional-capacity testing data.

REFERENCES

Wind H et al: Assessment of functional capacity of the musculoskeletal system in the context of work, daily living, and sport: A systematic review. J Occup Rehabil 2005;15:253 [PMID: 15844681].

Wind H et al: The utility of functional capacity evaluation. Int Arch Occup Environ Health 2006;79:528 [PMID: 16416155].

Doctors' Oral & Written Reports

Employers and benefit administrators require doctors to communicate with them either orally or in writing. These reports may take the form of progress reports, medical releases, RTW slips, doctors' notes, or preprinted forms. Most commonly, doctors are asked to corroborate or verify the existence (or absence) of medical problems or to provide opinions on issues such as a patient's ability to return to work. These reports are based on the physician's medical knowledge but provide a basis for a practical or business decision by someone else. In other words, they serve nonmedical purposes that are highly significant to others.

Often the patient's comfort, safety, and income depend on the timeliness and accuracy of these reports. Moreover, the patient may see the doctor's answers to the employer and insurer's questions as an accurate description of the current and future situation.

Doctors' reports are often the required basis for decisions by others. Many governmental and private benefits programs require that information provided by treating physicians serve as the basis for eligibility and benefit decisions. These are sometimes called *medically driven programs.* The language of the doctor's answers is interpreted very precisely, and the decisions others make will be either "yes" or "no." Although medical issues are seldom black and white, employment and benefits decisions must be.

In the context of the workplace, a doctor's report may do the following:

1. Legitimize time off so that employers do not discipline patients for nonattendance.

2. Initiate wage-replacement benefits to employees who are/have been off work.

3. Corroborate the existence of a "qualifying disability" and thus the need for reasonable accommoda-

tion under the Americans with Disabilities Act (ADA).

4. Describe work capacity or limitations and restrictions.

5. Provide medical clearance, for example, for new jobs or hazardous assignments.

Delay in providing reports will delay the delivery of services and benefits. This can create financial hardship and slow a patient's recovery, thus leading to further disability and an increased risk of delayed recovery.

Medical Confidentiality

Information about what an employee can and cannot do at work and how that will change over time is not considered medically confidential, although it probably should be considered private and distributed on a need-to-know basis. Information about diagnosis, treatment, dates of service, etc., is medically confidential and should be handled in compliance with applicable state and federal laws.

Employers and insurers see the physician's duty to answer questions in a way that may differ from the way physicians see it. Employers see themselves as the customer along with the patient and think that their need for information is reasonable. They may be surprised and offended if a physician calls a request unethical and flatly refuses to give them any information. Physicians should treat employers courteously and provide them with appropriately limited information. In workers' compensation, both the employer and the benefits administrator have the right, by law, to at least some information about the alleged work-related injury or illness—enough for the employer to investigate the incident, manage its safety program, and make decisions on how to handle the claim. State laws vary on the extent or the lack of confidentiality. It is generally preferable to restrict the release of medical information to the employer's benefits or medical department, but other departments at some employers will insist on seeing medical details. Workers' compensation is specifically excluded from the Health Insurance Portability and Accountability Act of 1996 (HIPAA) regulations, although most physicians are not aware of this fact, and their office procedures will be set up to be HIPAA-compliant.

Disability benefits claim administrators need information about the condition causing a disability in order to manage the benefits claim. Many benefit policies are worded so that benefits are denied if the treating physician does not furnish information. The patient will need to authorize its release. Usually, an authorization to release medical information is part of the application form for benefits. Many medical offices prefer to get the patient to sign their own release, however. Under HIPAA, the physician is responsible for releasing the minimum necessary

information. HIPAA does not consider disability insurers to be a covered entity.

Physicians are asked a small number of predictable questions in disability claims. Traditionally, many employers and insurers have relied on doctors to decide when employees return to work. Today, enlightened employers and insurers make the RTW decision based on information about work capacity provided by physicians:

1. What are the medical findings, diagnosis, prognosis, treatment history, and plan? *Note:* Employers, as distinct from benefit administrators, do not need to know much of this except prognosis and functional capacity.

2. When will the employee be able to return to work? Full duty? Modified duty (also called *light, limited,* or *transitional work*)?

3. What are the patient's limits and restrictions?

4. Is the problem work-related?

5. Has the patient reached medical stability or maximum medical improvement?

6. Is there any permanent impairment?

Multiparty RTW Programs

Historically, employers and insurers have been very tolerant of employees who go off work on the various forms of disability leave, but this is changing. The idea that injured and sick employees should remain at home until they have recuperated fully and can do their regular job is becoming obsolete. RTW programs for workers' compensation cases continue to spread within the employer and insurance communities, although there is variation between companies in how actively, intelligently, and fairly the programs actually are operated.

In workers' compensation and the short- and long-term disability arena, the payers (employers and insurance carriers) are responsible for wage replacement in the form of temporary disability, permanent disability, and vocational rehabilitation benefits and therefore have a financial incentive to optimize the rehabilitation process and to facilitate a timely return to work. With the failure of "managed care" to control the escalating costs of workers' compensation medical services, workers' compensation insurance carriers are paying more attention to the 50% of the claims expense dollar that is spent on wage replacement. Given the magnitude of medically unnecessary temporary disability, interventions that address RTW barriers can be expected to provide significant return on investment.

Management of disability through RTW programs is by its nature a collaborative process. Because improving functional recovery and return to work is beneficial to all parties, implementation provides a sense of shared purpose among the key players (i.e., injured worker, employer, physician, and claims administrator) that fosters improved communication and improves outcomes.

Modified-work programs facilitate return to work for both temporarily and permanently disabled workers with a doubling of return to work among the workers who were offered modified work as compared with employees without access to any form of modified duty. The number of lost workdays per disabling injury also was cut in half when companies implemented modified-work programs. In most cases, modified work has been part of a broader program that simultaneously includes other interventions such as early reporting, use of treatment guidelines, and organizational and ergonomic modifications.

Program elements that appear to be important for a successful RTW program include

1. The establishment of better communications among the key players (i.e., medical providers, injured worker, supervisor, and claims administrator) in order to support the employee.

2. Management and front-line supervisor training and buy-in regarding the importance of the program to employee health and employer productivity.

3. Willingness of management to be flexible in modifying existing jobs or temporarily assigning employees to alternative jobs that are consistent with the injured employee's current physical limitations.

On occasion, work-site intervention programs have failed to produce the expected results. This can occur when employees or union representatives perceive that the only motivation for the RTW program is cost reduction without genuine interest in promotion of worker health and well-being. Workers and their supervisors will not want to participate if they see that the program pressures vulnerable people back to work prematurely, especially if it fails to protect them during recovery.

A major consulting opportunity for occupational physicians is to develop strategies for smaller employers who lack internal professional staff and often receive little assistance from workers' compensation insurers.

REFERENCE

Bernacki EJ et al: A preliminary investigation of the effects of a provider network on costs and lost time in workers' compensation. J Occup Environ Med 2005;47:3 [PMID: 15655406].

Bernacki EJ, Tsai SP: Ten years' experience using an integrated workers' compensation management system to control workers' compensation costs. J Occup Environ Med 2003;45:508 [PMID: 12762075].

Preplacement Examinations

The preplacement examination offers an important opportunity to prevent disability. In many clinical settings, these examinations account for the majority of patient encounters. The preplacement evaluation has evolved from being a preemployment, or exclusionary, examination to one that benefits both the employer and the employee.

Before passage of the ADA, many employers used the preemployment examination to deny work to applicants with handicaps. Whether an applicant was able to perform the job often was a secondary consideration. Applicants were disqualified if they had migraine headaches, diabetes, heart disease, etc., even if these illnesses did not interfere with the performance of the job. Since passage of the ADA in 1990, the medical examination follows rather than precedes the job offer. The medical examination is a targeted evaluation aimed at being job-related and consistent with business necessity. As such, the preplacement or postoffer examination is just one step in the process of hiring an applicant. The employer, the physician, and the applicant all have responsibilities in this process to make it successful.

The ADA defines a *physical disability* as an impairment that substantially limits a major life activity. A disability, however, is defined after mitigating measures are taken. For example, if someone is legally blind without glasses but can see normally with glasses or contacts, then the person is not considered disabled under the ADA. If a person's disability is corrected by medication, prosthetics, etc., then the resulting disability is defined after those steps are taken. However, some states allow that a person may be considered disabled even with a disability that can be corrected by medications, such as asthma, psychiatric illnesses, and seizure disorders. It is important to know the state laws that apply to one's practice. For instance, the ADA and most states exclude illegal drug or alcohol use and temporary disabilities such as pregnancy from protected status.

The Equal Employment Opportunity Commission (EEOC) has determined that one is considered disabled only if unable to perform a broad class of occupations rather than just one job. For example, if a person has back pain and is restricted to lifting no more than 50 pounds, he or she may be disabled for a warehouse position, but many jobs are available that may be performed with limited lifting. This person would not be considered disabled under the ADA.

A physician performing preplacement examinations needs to be familiar with certain definitions with regard to the ADA. The first is essential job functions. *Essential job functions* are the fundamental duties of a job, not ones that are performed as needed or occasionally. A physician should not determine which job functions are essential. It is the employer's responsibility to make that determination.

Essential job functions may be determined in several different ways. Job descriptions listing physical tasks and possible chemical and physical exposures as determined by a job-analysis specialist is one way. The judgments of employees and employer is another way. The amount of time spent on a specific job function is another. If leaving out a certain function changes the job in a significant way, then that is an essential function of the job.

With the job description in hand, the physician is able to perform the medical examination. There are some significant similarities and differences between a targeted preplacement examination and a general physical examination. With both, the history is paramount. Without a careful history, the physician will be unable to determine potential medical impairments. In a preplacement examination, the examining physician often has only one chance to elicit the necessary history, and that history should be job-related. Medical problems are only important if they directly affect the essential functions of the job. The preplacement examination is targeted on the functions necessary to perform the job rather than a general survey of the applicant's total health. All applicants of a given class must be given the same evaluation. This does not prevent more in-depth evaluation if an underlying disability or medical problem is found during the course of the examination.

Once the necessary physical examination and laboratory testing are complete, the physician needs to make a risk assessment. Is there no or low direct threat to health and safety if this applicant takes the job, or is there a moderate or highly likely direct threat to the applicant's or fellow employees' health and safety? This risk assessment will guide the physician when determining any work limitations and will enable the employer to provide reasonable accommodations.

Reasonable accommodation occurs if a candidate is unable to perform the essential functions of the job without some assistance. A reasonable job accommodation is an adjustment to the work environment that enables the disabled individual to perform the essential functions of the job. An applicant is not disqualified automatically if he or she is unable to perform the essential functions of the job. The employer must consider modifying the job or providing aids such as an amplified telephone to enable the applicant to perform the essential functions of the job. Ideally, this should be an interactive process between the applicant, employer, and physician. The physician should identify the work restrictions, and the employer and applicant should work together in good faith to determine effective and reasonable accommodation options.

It is the employer's responsibility to determine whether reasonable accommodation will result in undue hardship. For example, the employer has a right to expect reasonable job attendance. If a disability requires too much time off work during regular business hours, an employer may claim undue hardship. For example, it is not the responsibility of other employees to take over job tasks so that they work harder and longer than the disabled employee. Undue hardship must be based in fact and not based on speculation.

The employer first must interview the candidate to determine whether the candidate is the one most qualified for the position. All phases of the hiring evaluation of an applicant must be made before a preplacement examination is scheduled. If results of a physical agility test or background check are not yet available, and the results may affect the offer of employment, then the employer must wait. The preemployment examination is now legally a postoffer evaluation.

An employer may ask whether an employee can do the essential functions of the job and even ask about illegal drug use. Drug testing is not considered a medical examination under the ADA. The employer has the right to know about current illegal drug activity. An employer cannot ask about medications, medical conditions, or prior workers' compensation cases. Once the employer is satisfied that the job applicant is the best candidate, scheduling the preplacement examination may proceed.

The examining physician must understand what the applicant's position consists of prior to doing a preplacement examination. Ideally, the physician should have a copy of the job description outlining physical requirements and essential functions of the job before doing the examination. If the physician has neither a job description nor knowledge of the physical demands, he or she cannot determine whether an employee is qualified to perform the essential functions of the job with or without restrictions. The examining physician should not make a preplacement determination without adequate information about the physical and psychological demands of the job.

It is very helpful if the employer has accepted medical standards for a given position. Unfortunately, written medical standards are rarely available for most jobs. Medical standards are available for commercial drivers, airplane pilots, and public safety officers such as fire and police. Medical standards aid the physician in making reasoned decisions on whether an applicant can or cannot perform the job safely.

The physician may ask any medically pertinent questions if they are related to the job. Although an employer is unable to ask about back injuries, a physician can if the employee needs to lift on the job. Although musculoskeletal capacity can be extremely difficult to ascertain, the physician may gather whatever history or testing that is pertinent. For jobs with high aerobic demands, if a candidate describes anginal-type chest pain, has a family history of heart disease, and smokes, an evaluating physician may require the applicant to see a specialist for cardiac clearance. If the applicant has been evaluated for possible heart disease, the examining physician may obtain the pertinent medical records. The examining physician may ask for medical records from the treating physician only if it is needed to determine whether the applicant can perform the job safely. Rules of medical confidentiality apply to job applicants, and the employer is not allowed to know the nature of the inquiry, only the resulting limitations (see Chapter 5).

When performing a postoffer evaluation, a physician also should take into consideration federal OSHA and state OSHA medical surveillance requirements for the job. For example, if an employee falls under a hearing conservation program, the physician should obtain a baseline audiogram in anticipation that the employee will be enrolled in such a program. If a potential employee is required to wear a respirator on the job, a medical clearance for respirator use should be performed to ensure that the employee is able to wear a respirator safely. The examining physician has the right to gather all information necessary to make a reasoned decision.

Once the examination is completed and the pertinent medical information is obtained, a physician can determine three outcomes. The first is that the applicant is medically qualified. The applicant has no job restrictions that would preclude him or her from performing the essential functions of the job. The second outcome is that the applicant is qualified to perform the job with some accommodation. The physician needs to write down these restrictions; for example, the applicant is unable to lift greater than 50 pounds without assistance. The last outcome is that the employee is medically disqualified. A physician rarely determines that an employee is medically disqualified. This outcome usually occurs when an employee does not meet state or federal medical requirements for occupations that require driving a commercial vehicle, flying an airplane, or wearing a respirator. A public safety officer may fail to pass the accepted medical standards that are consistent with business necessity adopted by a municipality. These disqualifications are usually final, but most states allow the right of appeal and a second opinion if the candidate is rejected because of a medical condition. An employer can disqualify candidates that pose a direct threat to the health and safety of themselves or others. A recent U.S. Supreme Court decision upheld the right of an employer to disqualify candidates based on direct threat issues. The 2002 case involved a Chevron refinery preplacement applicant.

Mr. Echazabal was denied employment at an oil refinery because the company stated that the working environment presented a direct threat to his health. Mr. Echazabal sued under the ADA, which does not explicitly address the concern over the health and safety of the individual applicant. Chevron stated that its decision was based on an EEOC regulation that stated that a company need not hire someone in a position that was a direct threat to the job applicant's health and safety. The Supreme Court ruled that being qualified for a job means that you must be able to perform the essential functions of the job without undo risk to one's personal health and safety.

The U.S. Supreme Court stated that the ADA did not mean that an employee should be hired if he or she constitutes a direct threat to himself or herself or others. An employer can refuse to hire if the decision prevented lost time, health risks, and possible death of the employee. The refusal to hire was within the bounds of business necessity.

The ability to place work restrictions on or actually disqualify someone for a job will continue to be further defined as more cases are heard.

Fitness-for-Duty Evaluations

A fitness-for-duty examination is essentially the same evaluation and follows the same rules as a preplacement examination. The only difference is that a fitness-for-duty examination determines whether a previously hired employee who was able to perform the essential functions of the job is still able to perform these essential functions safely. Ideally, a fitness-for-duty evaluation will determine whether an employee is able to perform his or her job duties in a safe and efficient manner. It is also designed to help the employee to obtain appropriate treatment or reasonable accommodations so that the employee may continue his or her current occupation successfully. The employer may request a fitness-for-duty evaluation once the employee's own physician returns the employee to work to ensure that the employee can do his or her job functions safely without endangering himself or herself or others.

A fitness-for-duty evaluation usually is requested by a supervisor who has information that causes the supervisor to believe that an employee has a physical or psychological health problem that affects the employee's job performance or that the employee presents an imminent risk to himself or herself or others when doing the essential job functions. A fitness-for-duty evaluation is also requested when an employee makes threats against other employees, acts in a way that affects their job duties, or appears to have a physical impairment or disease that interferes with the employee's job duties. The courts have upheld the legal right of an employer to conduct fitness-for-duty evaluations. If an individual has health problems that seriously affect job performance, a fitness-for-duty examination is permitted to disclose the full extent of a disability.

To adequately determine an employee's fitness for duty, the evaluating physician must know both the psychological and physical requirements of the employee's job. The employer can provide a functional job description, or the physician can visit the workplace to see the job performed first hand. A manager or supervisor should clearly state to the physician the reason for the fitness-for-duty evaluation and the specific job functions that the employee is unable to perform. The employer must give the physician concrete examples of why this worker's performance may be linked to a physical problem.

The examining physician should have access to the employee's pertinent medical and personnel records in order to conduct an effective evaluation. If the employee refuses to sign a release of medical information, a fitness-for-duty examination can proceed in the absence of the records. The employer can require the fitness-for-duty evaluation as a condition of continued employment.

An employer needs to be explicit and communicate to the physician exactly what the employer is interested in. Is the company interested in whether the employee is a threat either to himself or herself or others or whether the employee is capable of violence? Is the major concern of the company over reasonable accommodations or what parts of the job the employee cannot perform safely? Is the illness work-related? If an employee is not fit for duty, what is the prognosis, the estimated time before an employee will be able to return to work? Are there specific treatment recommendations, and is the employee aware of these recommendations? If the physician does not know the questions, the physician may not provide the report the employer needs.

Once the employer has the physician's report, the employer has several options. Based on the impairments and functional limitations, the employer may

1. Return the employee to work.
2. Return the employee to temporary modified duty with an anticipated return to full work once treatment begins.
3. Place the employee in a permanent modified position.
4. Provide reasonable accommodations.
5. Perform disciplinary action if no medical cause for the behavior is found.
6. Medically terminate the employee.

If an employee is disabled and considered unfit for duty, the physician should clearly write out the physical limitations so that the employer can determine whether reasonable accommodation exists. An employer is required to make a good-faith effort to provide reasonable accommodation if the employee has physical or psychological limitations. If an employee does not have a serious health condition to explain why he or she is unable to perform the essential functions of the job, the problem is not a medical issue and should be addressed by the employer with progressive discipline. Poor job performance often is not caused by a medical condition. Many of these employees have character disorders and are not amenable to treatment. All the examining physician can do in these cases is make a reasoned assessment and refer the employee to a psychiatrist if needed to confirm whether a psychiatric diagnosis is causing the behavior and that a treatment is available to provide a reasonable prognosis. The physician performing a fitness-for-duty examination should be an evaluator and not assume treatment of the patient.

REFERENCE

Disability Studies Quarterly: www.dsq-sds.org_issue_pdf/dsp_2003 winter.pdf:52.

HEALTH & PRODUCTIVITY

Employee health and its effect on productivity are emerging as a critical focus for businesses and occupational health. Employers are realizing that the direct costs of insurance premiums are not what affects the bottom line. The indirect costs of absenteeism and "presenteeism" (lessened job performance owing to chronic health problems) are also a significant drain on company resources. Companies are recognizing that employees are their most important asset and often are not replaced easily. A healthy workforce is now seen as essential to long-term productivity. Companies traditionally believed that high performance was linked primarily to cognitive abilities. However, recent research demonstrates that in order to sustain business growth, employers must be aware of the effect of human health on performance. Employees must have optimal health to maintain optimal productivity.

Health care is not only a cost, but it is also an investment in the economic health of the company. Health care costs need to be targeted toward interventions that lessen health risks, decrease the incidence of new diseases, and mitigate the impact of chronic diseases on workers. Most companies are experienced at managing workers' compensation costs. The economic burden of workers' compensation is usually a small part of total health care costs. Businesses have not tried to manage private health costs in the same way that they have managed work-related health costs. With private health care premiums outstripping inflation, companies are now looking at strategies to reduce all health-related costs.

Measuring the effect of health on productivity is an emerging field. There are several surveys including the Stanford Presenteeism Scale, Work Performance Scales, and the Health and Performance Questionnaire that are used to quantify the amount of "presenteeism" owing to chronic conditions. When used thoughtfully, these questionnaires can give a company insight into the loss of employee productivity owing to chronic diseases and, more important, may point out what programs could improve the overall health of their specific workforce.

Occupational physicians and nurses understand the workplace and have substantial expertise in disability management. They understand the barriers that may occur before returning an employee back to work and the issues that may delay recovery or affect performance. Occupational physicians and nurses already play a pivotal role in workers' compensation disability management, decreasing workers' compensation costs and promoting an early safe return to work. An occupational health specialist is the key player in an integrated health management system. This system should encompass medical programs including return to work, reliance on evidence-based medicine protocols, treating minor non-work-related illnesses, and using employee assistance programs. There needs to be an internal process to change the work culture to one of total wellness and prevention, including supervisor training, the development of information systems to track and report trends, and data analysis to identify areas for opportunity.

By using a health and productivity questionnaire, the occupational health professional is able to analyze the health needs of a company. The medical depart-ment will know which chronic diseases affect their workplace and to what extent. The physician or nurse will be able to prioritize programs and determine what consulting and case-management systems will benefit the company most. Working with benefits and human resources, the physician or nurse can help the company to determine which health benefits need strengthening and what services should change based on the chronic health conditions and the medical risk factors of their specific workforce.

Companies realize that health insurance is a benefit that their employees count on. Rising health premiums are an increasingly serious concern of businesses. By monitoring the costs of health care and devising health strategies specific to the business, health care professionals create an opportunity for cost containment and an investment in human capital.

REFERENCES

Aldana SG et al: The effects of a worksite chronic disease prevention program. J Occup Environ Med 2005;47:558 [PMID: 15951715].

Collins JJ et al: The assessment of chronic health conditions on work performance, absence, and total economic impact for employers. J Occup Environ Med 2005;47:547 [PMID: 15951714].

Goetzel RZ et al: Health, absence, disability, and presenteeism cost estimates of certain physical and mental health conditions affecting U.S. employers. J Occup Environ Med 2004;46:398 [PMID: 15076658].

Liability Issues in Occupational Medicine

5

Dan J. Tennenhouse, MD, JD

While principles of medicine are similar everywhere, laws affecting occupational health liability are substantially different in every country and even in every state in the United States. This chapter will address primarily U.S. law because liability risk to occupational physicians is greater in the United States than anywhere else. Occupational health providers (licensed health care professionals) must make an effort to become familiar with their local and state laws that regulate the practice of medicine in general and occupational medicine in particular. For example, each state has its own occupational safety and health regulations, and knowledge of these regulations can help the provider to better protect both employers and employees. Each state also has specific reporting statutes that might create very strict legal duties for the provider (e.g., reporting of disorders characterized by lapses in consciousness or periods of confusion, pesticide poisoning, work-related injuries, etc.).

This chapter will specifically address occupational medicine law. Environmental law is a separate field that affects companies but carries little liability risk to occupational physicians that is not already encompassed within occupational medicine law.

NEGLIGENCE

A professional negligence (malpractice) action against a health care provider cannot succeed unless the following four elements are proved in a court of law:

1. The existence of legal duty on the part of the provider to protect the victim (the plaintiff) from harm.
2. A breach of that duty, which breach meets the legal definition of negligence.
3. Legal damages (harm) to the plaintiff compensable under the law.
4. A causal relationship between the negligence and the harm (i.e., that the negligent act substantially contributed to the harm suffered by the plaintiff).

A legal duty to the plaintiff exists when the provider makes a contract with the plaintiff to provide medical care and the plaintiff relies on that contract or when the plaintiff is a foreseeable victim of the provider's negligence toward a patient. In some circumstances, there may be no legal duty to the patient (worker) when the provider is required by a contract with the employer to perform a job-related evaluation of the worker without providing any treatment. In contrast, there may be a legal duty in some cases to persons other than the worker if the provider failed to protect them from injury caused by the worker. For example, prescribing a psychoactive medication for a worker without warning the worker not to drive or operate heavy equipment could expose the provider to liability from a coworker or from any member of the public who is injured by the medication-impaired worker.

Professional negligence, or malpractice, occurs when the provider fails to use the necessary care and have the skill ordinarily possessed and used in similar circumstances by other reputable providers with similar training and experience. The degree of care and skill ordinarily used in similar circumstances is a theoretical concept, sometimes called the *standard of care*. In a lawsuit, the standard of care is determined by the trier of fact (i.e., jury, panel of arbitrators, or judge in a nonjury trial), usually based on the testimony of expert witnesses. Any failure to meet this standard of care is professional negligence.

Damages are based on legally compensable harm to the plaintiff that may include monetary compensation for medical care, occupational rehabilitation, loss of full enjoyment of life, pain, emotional suffering, psychiatric injury, loss of occupational income, loss of future earning capacity, and the like. The purpose of a malpractice (civil) lawsuit is not to "do justice" or to "right a wrong," as in a criminal case, but instead is to compensate the plaintiff for injuries suffered. Inadequate as it may be, the law makes provision only for monetary compensation.

A causal relationship between the negligence and the harm exists when the negligence was a substantial (even if small) contributing factor to the plaintiff's injury. If the injury would have occurred to the same degree without the negligence, then there is no causal relationship, and the lawsuit must fail. For example, assume that a physician negligently fails to investigate a worker's chronic cough, exposing the worker to a risk of delayed diagnosis of lung cancer. Lung cancer nevertheless is discovered within 1 month but is in an advanced stage, and the worker soon succumbs to the cancer. There is little likelihood that the negligent delay in diagnosis would be found by a jury to be a legal cause of the worker's death. A 1-month delay in a diagnosis of terminal lung cancer probably would not affect the outcome in this case; however, there might be a very different legal outcome if the delay in diagnosis were 6 months.

If the worker contributed to his or her own injury by negligent noncompliance, the worker's own negligence would diminish the provider's negligence. Most states follow a scheme of proportionate fault, or comparative negligence, whereby a jury allocates fault on a percentage basis between provider and worker. The verdict, based on the extent of the worker's injury, is reduced by the percentage the worker was at fault.

Duty to Warn

Occupational providers have a legal duty to warn workers of increased risks when certain medical disorders or treatments affect their abilities to carry out workplace activities safely. For example, a worker who sometimes operates a crane is being treated for depression with trazodone. Known side effects of trazodone include blurred vision, incoordination, sedation, and syncope, any of which could cause an accident leading to injury to the worker and to others at the job site.

Failure to give adequate warning to the worker is negligence that exposes a provider to malpractice liability for injury to the worker unless the provider is a fellow employee protected by the workers' compensation exclusive-remedy rule. If the worker is involved in an accident arising from this failure to warn, and that accident injures a second person, the provider is also liable for that injury. Furthermore, if the second person is not a fellow employee, the workers' compensation exclusive-remedy rule would never apply.

If there may be a serious medical risk, providers should obtain a job description, either from a thorough verbal history taken from the worker or from the company's written job description. Such a job description will help the provider to recognize risks to the worker.

Occupational providers who initiate treatment also may have liability for choosing a treatment that causes increased risk owing to the nature of the worker's job if there were other appropriate treatment options that carry less risk. In this regard, the worker's job may, in effect, constitute a contraindication to the treatment chosen. For example, a worker who operates dangerous equipment complains of severe pain and is treated with a narcotic analgesic. The worker becomes drowsy on the job and accidentally injures a fellow worker. A malpractice lawsuit against the treating provider could be based on failing first to try to control the pain with a non-steroidal anti-inflammatory drug (NSAID) such as ibuprofen before exposing the worker to the side effects of the narcotic. Ignorance of the nature of the worker's job would be a weak defense.

Occupational physicians must describe the risks clearly to the worker and briefly document the warning. This responsibility should not be delegated to office staff. Workers may not take warnings from non-physicians seriously. The worker should be aware that the physician is documenting the warning in the medical record. If a worker is likely to be noncompliant, refuses to accept the warning, or may pose a serious hazard to other people, the physician also should contact and warn the worker's supervisor. This warning should clearly describe the job circumstances that may lead to increased risk of injury for that worker. However, the warning should not disclose any diagnosis or other private information about the worker that is unnecessary to warn the supervisor adequately. The physician should document the date, name of the supervisor, and nature of the warning given.

Occupational providers should be especially concerned about conditions that may affect

1. Body position (e.g., transient ischemic attack, vertigo, syncope, seizure, muscle weakness, etc.) for workers who work on a scaffold or other high place or close to bodies of water or to dangerous equipment, etc.

2. Judgment (e.g., mental disorder, organic brain injury, psychopharmaceutical, etc.) for workers who drive a vehicle, operate dangerous equipment, handle toxic substances, etc.

3. Level of consciousness (e.g., electrolyte imbalance, abuse substance, neurodepressive drug, sleep deprivation, etc.) for workers who operate a vehicle or dangerous equipment, work on a scaffold or other high place, handle toxic substances, etc.

4. Perception (e.g., loss of hearing, vision, touch, or temperature sensation, etc.) for workers who work around vehicles or dangerous equipment, rely on safety alarm systems, handle hot items, etc.

5. Reflexes (e.g., abuse substance, neurodepressive drug, neuropathy, etc.) for workers who operate a vehicle or dangerous equipment, etc.

6. Survival (e.g., myocardial infarction, cerebrovascular accident, pulmonary embolus, etc.) for workers who work alone, on a job site far from emergency medical services, on a scaffold or other high place, close to bodies of water or to dangerous equipment, etc.

A frequent concern for occupational physicians is liability from failure to warn a worker about potentially serious findings after conducting an examination on behalf of an employer or prospective employer. Physician liability depends on the legal technicality of whether or not the examining physician owed any legal duty to protect the worker from harm. If a duty is owed, the physician must warn the worker both of the possible seriousness of the finding and of the urgency of medical follow-up care. If no legal duty is owed, the physician has no liability irrespective of the outcome. Legal duty in this situation varies by state. Some states hold that the physician contracted only with the employer and never had a physician-patient relationship creating a legal duty. Every occupational physician who performs such examinations should be familiar with the applicable law of the state where the examination is performed. A better practice for physicians is to always warn every worker of the seriousness and urgency of any potentially dangerous medical findings in order to minimize avoidable injury without regard to legal issues.

The nature of the provider-employer relationship is paramount in determining the provider's own liability for negligence. The essential question is whether the provider is an employee or an independent contractor. If the provider is clearly an employee, negligence toward a fellow employee usually is encompassed by workers' compensation.

The workers' compensation system is the exclusive remedy available to workers who suffer job-related injuries and who cannot ordinarily sue their employers or coworkers for injuries sustained on the job. Because workers' compensation is the exclusive remedy, the worker also cannot sue for medical malpractice but must accept the workers' compensation award as the only compensation. The money damages awarded in a medical malpractice lawsuit could be many times greater than a workers' compensation award.

If the provider is an independent contractor, however, the provider can be sued directly by the worker for medical malpractice. The courts have not been eager to incorporate medical malpractice into the traditional areas encompassed by the workers' compensation exclusive-remedy scheme. Only if the provider is clearly and unequivocally a fellow employee are the courts likely to apply the exclusive-remedy provision of the workers' compensation system. For example, if the provider is giving medical services to the worker outside the scope of the employment arrangement, then an independent contractor status may be found by the court, thereby opening up the potential for a malpractice lawsuit.

Two tests are sometimes used by the courts to resolve the question of whether an occupational provider is an employee or an independent contractor. The control test determines how much independent decision making and control of actions are exercised by the provider. For example, the provider who is conducting a routine predeter-mined physical examination or who is providing care predetermined and formulated with management is deemed to be acting under the control of the employer and therefore is an employee. The provider who is making independent judgments, as any provider in private practice does, and who is not following preapproved functions or procedures is deemed an independent contractor. The indicia test determines whether the provider is treated as and functions as any other employee and so is actually under company control. Indicia of employee status are present if providers are required to keep regular working hours, are receiving the same benefits received by other employees, are required to report regularly to superiors, and must request and obtain authorization before acting outside existing protocols.

Because of the complexity of these rules and differences among the states (e.g., the "dual capacity" doctrine that applies in some states), the provider is well advised to consult with local legal counsel familiar with this area of law before making decisions that may affect the provider's status as an employee.

HARASSMENT/WRONGFUL TERMINATION ACTIONS

Lawsuits against companies for harassment of or discrimination against workers or prospective workers are epidemic, with many very large monetary awards. Lawsuits against companies for wrongful termination of workers are also epidemic. These legal actions usually involve employer actions based on poor judgment at supervisory or executive levels within a company that deprive a worker of job benefits by demotion, undesirable job assignment, termination, or constructive termination (creating allegedly impossible conditions under which to work and that force the worker to quit). Sometimes the employer actions involve retaliation against a worker for taking time off from work or for filing a workers' compensation claim.

A convenient reason for depriving a worker of job benefits is medical findings. If a provider states that a worker is unable to carry out essential job functions for medical reasons, the company has an excuse for taking action against the worker. This is not a legal problem for the provider unless evidence of some conspiracy can be shown. Unfortunately, evidence supporting the allegation of a conspiracy often exists.

1. A company official or supervisor suggests to a provider what medical findings would be desirable or should be reported (e.g., finding a reason to demote or terminate the worker or finding nothing wrong and returning the worker prematurely to work). This suggestion can take the form of a telephone call, memo, fax, or other communication

with the provider and often is recorded as a memo in the official's own files.

2. The provider then gives an opinion or makes a recommendation against the worker's interests without clear and well-documented medical reasons supporting that opinion or recommendation.

Providers implicated in such conspiracies may be liable not only for economic harm to the worker but also for punitive damages (i.e., extra damages awarded as punishment) for intentional misconduct. Examples of situations in which conspiracies might be shown include

1. A company official asks the provider to write up a report that overemphasizes medical limitations, describing the worker as not medically fit to continue the job or to assume responsibilities of a new job.

2. A company official asks the provider to return the worker to work prematurely or to lift specific work restrictions even though the provider believes that medical risks warrant further delay.

3. A company official insists that a worker who takes time off work for illness get an unnecessary psychiatric or other type of consultation (as harassment for the purpose of discouraging claimed illness).

Providers should be cautious of situations in which company officials make such recommendations or suggestions. They should refuse to discuss the possibility of providing opinions or recommendations for the convenience of the company. They always should have a reasonable medical basis and also clear documentation in support of all their opinions and recommendations. To show no concealment motive, every discussion or telephone conversation with a company official about a worker's medical status should be documented briefly in the worker's medical record in a neutral, objective manner.

MISREPRESENTATIONS

A. Misrepresentations to Insurers

A provider wrote a letter to an insurer stating that the patient needed surgery on a scar, that the surgery was "reconstructive" rather than "cosmetic," and that it would improve the patient's function. The patient's medical record and the patient's understanding of the purpose for the scar revision did not correlate with the provider's letter with regard to any improved function. In another example, a psychiatrist represented to an insurer that a patient with a chronic alcohol abuse disorder required hospitalization for acute psychotic manifestations related to alcohol abuse. In fact, the hospitalization was for alcohol dependence in an alcoholism recovery facility. In both these situations, the provider was aware that the proposed care was not covered by

the patient's insurance and that the misrepresentation could result in payment by the insurer.

Criminal fraud actions must have a statutory basis. For example, under California Penal Code Section 550, offering any written or oral statement in support of or in opposition to a claim for payment or any other insurance policy benefit knowing that the statement contains false or misleading information constitutes a felony. This code section also expressly applies to medical statements affecting workers' compensation claims. Similar statutes exist in other states.

Letters to insurers that are inconsistent with the medical records, with reports from other providers, or with the patient's understanding of the medical needs may create suspicion of fraud. Also, multiple inconsistent letters from the same provider may trigger suspicion of fraud.

B. Misrepresentations to Parties in Litigation

There is also a legal risk when a provider gives supporting evidence for parties who plan to call that provider as a witness or expert witness. For example, a physician was influenced by attorneys representing various parties in a lawsuit between the patient and her insurer over coverage. The physician reversed himself in his testimony. The patient lost her case, blamed the physician for making false statements that caused her to lose her case against her insurer, and sued the physician for the benefits she had sought from her insurer. The court said a physician has a duty to the patient of honest testimony on the patient's behalf. Providers can avoid this type of liability by always giving honest opinions in the first place and rejecting any prejudicial influences from self-serving attorneys, insurers, employers, or patients.

The litigation privilege protecting expert witnesses from lawsuit for statements made during testimony does not protect the witness from a lawsuit brought by the party that called the witness, only from a lawsuit by an adverse party [*Mattco Forge* v. *Arthur Young*, 6 Cal Rptr 2d 781 (1992)]. A party could sue its own witness for professional malpractice, fraud, breach of contract, and the like if dissatisfied with the expert witness' performance in support of the litigation. This usually means that the witness' testimony changed without good reason in the course of the litigation, surprising the attorney who called the witness.

Providers who write letters for insurance, workers' compensation, or litigation purposes should be certain that their statements are supported by and consistent with their medical record documentation. Once a provider takes a position, it is unwise to change that position without new documented information that clearly supports such a change. Patients should be informed of the content of a provider's letter so that they are not confused about the basis for any approval or denial of insurance benefits or about the medical issues in their workers' compensation claim or other litigation. If multiple providers are involved in a patient's care, review of another provider's report or even a telephone call to another provider prior to writing a letter can prevent dangerous inconsistencies.

Examples of situations creating an increased risk of fraud actions against providers include

1. The provider is asked to write a report that overemphasizes medical limitations, describing the employee as not medically fit to continue the job or to assume responsibilities of a new job.

2. The provider is asked to write a report that underemphasizes medical limitations, describing the employee's on-the-job injury as inconsequential so as to devalue a workers' compensation claim.

3. The treating provider always directs referrals to selected defense-oriented specialists in order to reduce workers' compensation risk.

4. The treating provider is told by someone who is not medically trained or who has not seen the patient to deny diagnostic or treatment services to an injured worker in order to reduce costs, even though the treating provider believes that the services are medically indicated.

5. The provider is asked to mislead an employee about a job-related injury or illness so as to prevent a workers' compensation claim.

EMPLOYEE RECORDS

Employee health information obtained through the efforts of the occupational health provider at the request of the company is the property of the company. Employers who pay for health care often believe that they are entitled to all information obtained and demand it from the provider. However, the occupational provider has certain professional responsibilities with regard to confidentiality. Employee medical information generally is not to be disclosed by either the employer or the provider to third parties without the consent of the employee. Releasing information from an employee's medical records without the employee's permission or other legal justification can result in an action by the employee for invasion of privacy and possibly an action by the provider's licensing board for unauthorized disclosure of a professional confidence. Furthermore, violation of medical confidentiality requirements imposed by federal law as part of the Health Insurance Portability and Accountability Act of 1996 (HIPAA) can carry additional penalties. Sometimes the distinction between employer and health care provider is blurred because the employer maintains a medical department with confidential files on its employees. If these medical files are not ordinarily accessible to non-medical personnel for non-medical purposes, such a medical department may be considered part of the health care team and, by implication, entitled to medical information without the express written authorization of the employee to release medical information to an employer. The provider who shares medical information with an employer's medical department knowing that, in fact, the information is being misused by the employer, however, may be violating the employee's right of confidentiality.

Employers often provide employees with medical examinations for the employer's own purposes. In such cases, information divulged to the employer should be limited to workplace-related findings. This includes the employee's ability to perform job functions but does not usually include medical diagnoses or other specific medical findings.

An employee who acquiesces to examination by company health providers may or may not be agreeing to disclosure of confidential medical information. To be certain that confidentiality requirements are met, it is prudent for the provider to have a written authorization from the employee before releasing any information to the employer. If such an authorization is always obtained prior to evaluation, disputes over an employer's right to confidential information without the employee's authorization can be avoided.

An employer who permits false or confidential employee information to be disseminated to company personnel can be liable to the employee for defamation or invasion of the employee's right to privacy. The provider may share liability with the employer if confidential medical information was disclosed without authorization.

In many states, the employees' right of access to their own health records is required by statute. Providers should be familiar with the laws in their state allowing patients to examine or receive copies of their records. In states where no such right of access exists by state law, access instead may be provided under HIPAA regulations. Occupational Safety and Health Administration (OSHA) regulations require employers dealing with toxic materials to make their records available to employees within 15 days after an employee's request to examine them. Documents that must be accessible include not only the employee's medical records but also environmental data about the workplace. An employee may even have access to the toxic exposure record of a fellow employee if such information is relevant to his or her own likelihood of toxic exposure.

LEGAL IMPLICATIONS OF THE AMERICANS WITH DISABILITIES ACT

The Americans with Disabilities Act (ADA) is intended to prevent discrimination against employees or applicants on the basis of a disability. The primary risks of a claim are to the employer rather than to the occupational provider; however, the provider can do much to help protect the employer. The ADA requires that employers not discriminate against a qualified individual with a disability because of the disability with regard to job application procedures, hiring, advancement, discharge, compensation, job training, and other privileges of employment. The ADA also requires the employer to make reasonable accommodations for a known impairment unless it would cause undue hardship (involve significant difficulty or expense).

The following definitions apply to the above ADA requirements:

Discriminate includes limiting an applicant or employee so as to affect job status or opportunities adversely.

Qualified individual with a disability is an individual with a disability who, with or without reasonable accommodation, can perform the essential functions of the employment. To determine what are *essential work functions,* the employer's judgment is considered along with any job description prepared before interviewing job applicants.

Disability is a physical or mental impairment that substantially limits one or more of the major life activities of an individual. It does not include individuals currently engaged in illegal use of drugs but does include those erroneously regarded as engaging in such use. *Disability* as used in the ADA includes emotional or psychiatric instability, a history of having filed workers' compensation claims, and even having disabled family members who require assistance necessitating rearrangement of work schedules. The definition of disability given in the ADA is so general and so vague that any chronic medical or psychiatric disorder should be considered a disability. New injuries and acute illnesses are probably not disabilities, but any residual impairment would be.

Reasonable accommodation includes making existing facilities accessible to and usable by disabled employees, job restructuring, modifying work schedules, reassignment, acquiring or modifying equipment, etc.

The ADA also requires that employers not inquire of or medically examine a job applicant about the nature or severity of a disability. Employers may require a medical examination, however, after an offer of employment to determine the applicant's ability to perform job-related functions. The employer may condition the job offer on the results if all persons offered the same job are required to be examined, and medical information is kept separate and confidential (except for notification of supervisors as to job restrictions, accommodations, and emergency care). Employers shall not, as a requirement, inquire of or medically examine an employee about the nature or severity of a disability unless the examination is shown to be job-related and consistent with business necessity.

If jobs or benefits are denied to individuals with disabilities because of a disability, the employer must show that the "qualification standards" are job-related, consistent with business necessity, and not correctable by reasonable accommodation. Qualification standards may require that the individual pose no direct threat to others in the workplace. *Direct threat* means a significant risk to the health or safety of others that cannot be eliminated by reasonable accommodation, for example, a crane operator with a poorly controlled seizure disorder.

An employer may prohibit use of illegal drugs and use of alcohol in the workplace, as well as being under their influence. Testing for illegal drugs is not a medical examination under the ADA. *Use of illegal drugs* is use, possession, or distribution of controlled substances except under supervision by a licensed health care professional.

If no reasonable accommodation is involved, the occupational provider can help to protect the employer by disclosing only the employee's ability to perform essential functions of employment and by not disclosing any diagnosis of a chronic medical or psychiatric disorder. If the employer does not possess knowledge of the disability, it cannot discriminate against the employee because of the disability. When the employee is unable to perform essential job functions, the occupational provider also can help the employer by assisting in determining if a reasonable accommodation can be offered. Employers may have little idea about what measures might be effective in enabling a disabled employee to perform the essential functions of employment.

CONTRACTUAL ISSUES BETWEEN PROVIDER AND EMPLOYER

Careful consideration of provisions in the contract between an occupational provider and an employer can offer an excellent opportunity to prevent legal problems. Legal counsel familiar with occupational medicine issues can assist in the preparation of these contracts. Consider asking legal counsel specifically to address the following issues in the contract.

1. Legal Responsibility

Two issues that should be addressed are the following:

1. Because there is no exclusive-remedy protection under workers' compensation law for independent contractors, the provider's relationship to the employer should be made clear in the contract.

2. Who is to bear the liability cost? Employers who bear no cost may believe that they have nothing to lose and have strong economic incentives to increase the providers' liability risk by pressuring them to write misleading letters, return employees to work prematurely, select medically inappropri-

ate care to reduce time off work, and the like. The contract should address such issues.

2. Illegal Employer Activity

The provider's unwillingness to participate in actions that may constitute harassment, discrimination, wrongful termination, or fraud can prevent involvement in major litigation against the employer. Some supervisors may attempt to misuse providers to harass or discriminate against employees, to assist them in wrongfully terminating employees, or to fraudulently deceive employees. The contract should clearly prohibit such conduct. Furthermore, occupational providers who are asked to make medical decisions about an employee's ability to work should have access to an accurate and adequate job description for the employee in order to render competent clinical judgments.

3. Confidential Patient Information

A frequent problem that is seldom addressed in contracts is the employer's right of access to confidential medical information about its employees. By specifying the employer's degree of access to information and how it may use such information, the contract negotiation becomes an opportunity to clarify the provider's right to protect patient confidentiality. HIPAA provisions may be cited as a basis for some of the confidentiality language of the contract.

4. Compliance with the Americans with Disabilities Act

Because of the risks of ADA claims against the employer, the contract should address such issues as the following:

1. If or how a diagnosis that could constitute a disability should be disclosed to the employer. Employers should be reminded that the ADA prohibits them from inquiring about an employee's or applicant's disabilities; therefore, they should not request a diagnosis of a chronic medical disorder.
2. How information about the employee's job functions will be made available to the provider.
3. How the provider should participate in decisions about reasonable accommodations to disabled employees.

5. Notification of Government Agencies or of Employees at Risk When a Dangerous Practice by the Employer Is Detected

Because providers may detect occupational conditions that adversely affect health, and because reporting of such conditions can cause economic harm to the employer, the contract should address the following issues:

1. Circumstances requiring the provider to notify appropriate agencies as specified in reporting statutes or when the public safety is otherwise endangered owing to conditions caused by the employer.
2. Circumstances requiring the provider to notify an employee who is personally endangered by occupational conditions.

IMPACT OF ETHICAL CODES ON OCCUPATIONAL HEALTH PRACTICE

Ethical issues frequently arise in occupational health practice, and consequently, ethical codes are likely to be cited as authority for some decisions by occupational health providers. Ethical codes, however, are not the law and have none of the force and effect of law. The provider's first duty is to know and follow the law. Only when the law permits a choice to be made can ethical principles guide medical decision making. Do not allow loosely written ethical codes to cause inappropriate decision making.

Occupational health providers often confront conflicts of interest between the health and safety needs of the employee or the public and the economic needs of the employer. Ethics codes tend to assume the employer always will act in its own interest and generally require the provider to protect the employee or the public. The law tends to be more flexible, accepting economic necessity for the employer as a factor that warrants consideration.

Ethical codes tend to be more loosely written than are laws, leaving much room for interpretation, and are not refined continuously in litigation as are laws. Such loose writing often takes the form of unclear or impractical language. For example, an ethical code that requires the "highest degree of care" by the provider sets an impossible standard, which, if set forth in a law, would render every provider negligent most of the time and drastically increase the cost of health care owing to high liability insurance premiums. As another example, an ethical code requiring that patient confidentiality be maintained at all times implies that no release of patient information can ever take place without express patient consent. Such an absolute ethical rule would be dangerous and impractical. The law, on the other hand, provides numerous necessary exceptions, such as for emergencies when the patient is unable to consent.

Occupational health providers should know the applicable law well enough to recognize when an ethical code overlaps the law and then follow only the law. Providers also should recognize that ethical codes usually require reasonable interpretation and should take care to apply them in a practical manner.

OCCUPATIONAL HEALTH NURSING

Nurses practicing in occupational settings usually are company employees. They commonly have more autonomy, however, than hospital-based nurses and frequently act without direct physician supervision. Because of this autonomy, the preceding discussions of the legal obligations and liabilities of occupational providers generally apply to occupational health nurses. To ensure that occupational health nurses are not operating outside the scope of licensed nursing practice or outside the umbrella of workers' compensation, the following guidelines should be followed:

1. The course and scope of the occupational health nurse's professional duties and activities should be defined by protocols outlining standardized nursing procedures. Each protocol should be in writing and should be jointly approved, dated, and signed both by a physician and by a company executive.

2. Each protocol for a function or duty of the occupational health nurse should clearly describe the specific procedure or action and the circumstances under which the procedure or action may be performed. Special consideration should be directed toward activities associated with an increased risk of employee injury such as evaluation of acute chest pain, chronic shortness of breath, chronic joint pain, unresolving infection, and the like.

3. Protocols for occupational health nurses should not include functions that are restricted by law to other health care professionals, such as prescribing or dispensing medications where limited by state law or performing surgical procedures.

4. Any special training or experience required of the occupational health nurse in order to perform a particular function or procedure should be described.

5. Procedures that require direct physician orders or direct supervision should be identified.

6. Circumstances requiring immediate notification of or referral to a physician or hospital emergency department should be specified.

7. Circumstances requiring physician review of the nurse's actions and when such review must take place should be specified.

8. Protocols should be reviewed on a scheduled periodic basis.

REFERENCES

Americans with Disabilities Act: www.usdoj.gov/crt/ada/adahom1.htm.

Geaney JH: The relationship of workers' compensation to the Americans with Disabilities Act and Family and Medical Leave Act. Clin Occup Environ Med 2004;4:273 [PMID: 15182749].

Health Insurance Portability and Accountability Act of 1996 (HIPAA): www.hhs.gov/ocr/hipaa.

London L: Dual loyalties and the ethical and human rights obligations of occupational health professionals. Am J Ind Med 2005;47:322 [PMID: 15776476].

Scheid TL: Stigma as a barrier to employment: Mental disability and the Americans with Disabilities Act. Int J Law Psychiatry 2005;28:670 [PMID: 16112732].

SECTION II.
Occupational Injuries

Musculoskeletal Injuries

6

Franklin T. Hoaglund, MD

Definitions of Common Orthopedic Conditions

The following definitions are suggested for the common occupational injuries.

A. STRAIN

A *strained* muscle, ligament, or tendon has been pushed or pulled to its extreme by forcing the joint beyond its normal range of motion. It commonly results from lifting a heavy weight or bearing an unexpected external force, usually traction force. By definition, the symptoms of strain should resolve within a few days to a week.

B. SPRAIN

A *sprain* is an injury in which a ligament has been stretched beyond its limit, causing tears or disruption in some fibers within the substance of the ligament. Reactive inflammation with associated edema and local venous congestion develops over hours to days. A complete tear of a ligament is sometimes called a *third-degree sprain.*

C. TENDINITIS

Tendinitis is inflammation of a tendon. It may be the result of a primary inflammatory disease, such as rheumatoid arthritis, or it may be secondary to a mechanical injury.

D. TENOSYNOVITIS

Tenosynovitis is inflammation of a tendon sheath.

E. BURSITIS

Inflammation of a bursa is known as *bursitis.* An example is olecranon bursitis caused by inflammation in the thin tissue planes between the skin and olecranon.

F. MYOSITIS

Myositis is inflammation of muscle. The inflammation may be primary, as in polymyositis, or secondary to mechanical injury, such as when a muscle has been overstretched.

G. ARTHRITIS

Arthritis indicates an abnormal joint caused by injury, disease, or congenital abnormality. Examples include posttraumatic arthritis, osteoarthritis, and congenital hip dysplasia.

H. REPETITIVE STRAIN INJURES

Repetitive strain injuries are related to cumulative trauma (primarily end-range repetitive movements that involve a forceful or a vibratory component). These cumulative traumas may lead to acute or chronic inflammation of the tendon, the muscle, the capsule, or the nerve with associated pain. This swelling leads to stenosis, which can entrap tendons, nerves, and vascular tissues. Cumulative trauma may involve the extremity (commonly the hand, wrist, elbow, or shoulder) or the trunk (low-back strain).

INJURIES OF THE NECK

Neck pain among workers usually has its origin in the cervical spine. For most young workers with single episodes of neck pain and stiffness, rapid recovery is expected based on the natural history of soft-tissue injuries or postural strains. Careful clinical evaluation with specific treatment is appropriate. Radiographic studies are seldom helpful but should be done to rule out significant pathology in patients with lingering symptoms.

Cervical Degenerative Disk Disease

Cervical degenerative disk disease is common in both men and women after 40 years of age. The cause is unknown. The most common site of degenerative change is at C5–C6, but more than one disk may be involved. In patients younger than 40 years of age, pain usually occurs before radiographic changes are evident. Soft-disk protrusion not seen by plain-film radiography can account for true radiculopathy with resulting pain in the arms. Long-standing and more severe changes eventually can produce encroachment on the spinal canal and cervical myelopathy. Most people older than 40 years of age have degenerative changes in their cervical spine but no symptoms.

Clinical Findings

A. Signs & Symptoms

Neck pain may be noted first after a whiplash injury or after an incident in which the neck has been put in an extreme position or held flexed or extended for long periods. Onset of pain can be acute or gradual. The work history may include awkward and prolonged positions such as driving or working at a computer terminal. History of prior injury with specific statement of dates and job relationship should be documented. Psychological factors such as job dissatisfaction and monotony may affect recovery from recurrent or chronic neck problems.

A common symptom is posterior neck pain or high interscapular pain after prolonged sitting with the head fixed in one position. Symptoms may be severe at night during recumbency. There is often little in the way of physical findings other than restricted head and neck motion. Upper extremity reflexes, circulation, and sensation are usually normal. Patients demonstrate some restrictions of motion and pain with the head in extreme extension, in full flexion, in chin rotation, or in lateral flexion. Upper extremity symptoms and reflex changes are infrequent but may be present.

Certain key clinical history and physical findings may raise suspicion of a possibly serious underlying condition of the spine. Unexplained weight loss, neck pain not improved with rest, fever, immunosuppression, or intravenous drug use may suggest disk space infection. Spine fracture should be suspected with a history of significant trauma such as a fall from height or a motor vehicle accident. Inflammatory arthritis of the spine can cause neck symptoms. Erythrocyte sedimentation rate is a useful laboratory test to help rule out nonmechanical sources of neck pain. A bone scan is also a useful survey test.

The remaining patients can be separated into two diagnostic categories based on location and characteristics of their symptoms.

1. The symptoms are regional and are located in the neck, shoulder, and upper arm. Often there can be a nonspecific headache. The neurologic examination is typically normal.

2. Radicular cervical spine problems are those with significant radiation of pain or numbness below the elbow or into one or several fingers but not the whole hand. The pattern should be along known nerve root innervation.

B. Imaging

Anteroposterior/lateral radiography of the cervical spine is indicated when a serious underlying condition is suspected. It may reveal narrowing of the disk space and production of osteophytes. The most frequently affected levels are C5 and C6, but any level may be affected. Patients in their thirties may have symptoms before radiographic signs are present; this is especially true for patients who have sustained rear-end automobile collisions. Specialized imaging studies, such as computed tomography (CT) and magnetic resonance imaging (MRI), are not usually indicated in the early course of treatment unless there is a suspicion of serious spinal pathology.

Differential Diagnosis

In patients with pain limited to the interscapular area, the possibility of dorsal spine disease, tumor, or infection should be considered. The more common cause is referral from cervical strain. Bone tenderness over the dorsal spine processes should alert the examiner to the need for a dorsal spine radiograph, although this also may be referral from the cervical spine. Tumors or infection of the cervical spine can produce constant pain symptoms but are much less common. Pancoast tumor or brachial neuritis may produce upper extremity radiculopathy that mimics cervical spine pathology.

Electrophysiologic tests are used to identify dysfunction of a spinal nerve root or to identify a primary muscle abnormality. These tests also may differentiate entrapment problems of the brachial plexus and median and ulnar nerves, as well as the presence of neuropathy, on the basis of metabolic abnormalities such as diabetes.

Treatment

Treatment methods are the same for radicular and regional neck problems for the first month. Patients should be instructed to avoid prolonged sitting with the neck in a fixed position, extreme positions of the head or neck, and activities that bring on symptoms, such as driving, which sometimes requires sudden and extreme head movement. They should be taught to perform gentle range-of-motion exercises while at work and, as symptoms abate, to do resistance exercises.

A soft cervical collar provides rest for the neck muscles by supporting the head, especially late in the day, and also will limit extremes of motion. Soft collars may be of benefit in the first week of treatment but are of no benefit longer term.

In more severe cases, cervical traction in slight flexion is helpful. A nonsteroidal anti-inflammatory drug (NSAID) or acetaminophen in conjunction with heat and massage is useful generally. Muscle relaxants and sedatives usually are not warranted. Occasionally, the patient needs acetaminophen with 30 mg codeine or Vicodin at bedtime. Sleeping in an easy chair, sitting up or with the torso at a 45-degree angle, minimizes discomfort associated with turning over from the recumbent position. Pain usually subsides with time and proper rest, and restricted neck motion gradually resolves.

Physical therapy in the form of heat, ultrasound, massage, and the like may reduce pain and muscle spasm and may help to restore normal range of motion. Job modifications including administrative and ergonomic adjustments (e.g., job rotation and workstation modification) to limit work activities that might aggravate neck problems should be instituted in the workplace to promote a return to work. Traction (either manual or home pulley systems) may be of benefit in the first week of treatment for acute neck problems but are of limited benefit longer term.

When patients have upper extremity radiculopathy and do not respond to conservative treatment, disk excision and anterior interbody fusion should be considered. Cervical spine fusions for cervical degenerative disk disease in the absence of radiculopathy have unpredictable results. Patients with definite findings of cervical myelopathy may require decompression by corpectomy or laminoplasty at more than one level.

REFERENCES

Carette S, Fehlings MG: Clinical practice: Cervical radiculopathy. N Engl J Med 2005;28;353 [PMID: 16049211].

Douglass AB, Bope ET: Evaluation and treatment of posterior neck pain in family practice. J Am Board Fam Pract 2004;17:S13 [PMID: 15575026].

INJURIES OF THE SHOULDER

Pain complaints in the neck or upper thoracic spine frequently are referred to the shoulder. The comprehensive evaluation of shoulder pain includes careful examination of the cervical and thoracic spine (Figure 6–1).

1. Impingement Syndrome of the Shoulder

The term *impingement syndrome* has replaced more diffuse diagnostic terms such as *bursitis* and *tendonitis* in the definition of shoulder pain following either repeated overuse or sudden overload. This pathology accounts for the vast majority of shoulder pain coming on spontaneously or associated with occupational stresses.

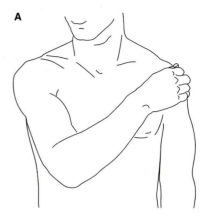

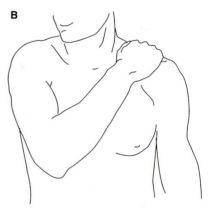

Figure 6–1. *A.* Patient putting opposite hand on side of pain to indicate shoulder pain. *B.* Patient identifying pain location in upper trapezius and upper interscapular area. Although patients sometimes refer to this area as their shoulder, the pain usually arises from the cervical spine.

In the normal shoulder, the coracoacromial ligament crosses the supraspinatus tendon of the rotator cuff. In some individuals, when a hand is brought from the side to an overhead position in forward flexion or abduction, there may be contact pressure or impingement of the acromion and coracoacromial ligament on the rotator cuff or the intervening bursa. The pathology starts with a subacromial bursitis and may progress to an irritation of the supraspinatus tendon or tendonitis. Further progression leads to the beginning of ulceration (partial-thickness tear) of the tendon, which can lead to a full-thickness discontinuity or rupture of the rotator cuff. The long head of the biceps projecting across the joint beneath the cuff to its origin on the supraglenoid tubercle may rupture. Paralleling these soft-tissue changes, the anteroinferior aspect of the acromion develops osteophytic lipping with further encroachment on the subacromial space.

Clinical Findings

A. Signs & Symptoms

The onset of anterior shoulder pain may be gradual or acute. Occasionally, the onset coincides with the start of new repetitive-motion work activities, especially overhead use of the shoulder. Patients may be unaware of the inciting activity. The pain may be expressed generally over some aspect of the anterior shoulder. In some cases, pain is limited to the lateral arm about the deltoid insertion on the humerus. Occasionally, pain is referred to the distal arm, elbow, and rarely, to the hand.

All levels of pain occur, including severe pain at rest caused by a tense subacromial bursa. Night pain is a frequent complaint that brings the patient to medical treatment.

On physical examination, patients begin to experience anterior shoulder pain when the arm is abducted at 30–40 degrees of elevation or brought above 90 degrees in a position of forward flexion. With the elbow flexed at 90 degrees, active external rotation usually does not cause discomfort. However, internal rotation (when the patient attempts to place his or her thumb on the opposite inferior angle of the scapula) is painful. With significant disruption of the rotator cuff, a patient may have no active elevation past 90 degrees of flexion. However, patients can have full-thickness tears of the rotator cuff without lost motion. Point tenderness anterior to the acromion over the subacromial bursa is common.

Posttraumatic impingement syndrome may occur after a minor injury to the arm or shoulder. The self-imposed immobilization of the shoulder predisposes the patient to the impingement syndrome because of imbalanced rotator cuff muscle function secondary to painful inhibition of normal motion.

B. Imaging

Plain x-rays include an anteroposterior (AP) view of the shoulder taken in internal and external rotation and an axillary and an outlet view. These may show some sclerotic change at the greater tuberosity or evidence of acromioclavicular (AC) joint degenerative arthritis. With massive disruptions of the cuff, the humeral head may be elevated in relationship to the glenoid cavity.

An MRI can determine the state of the cuff, as well as the presence of bicipital tendon pathology, labral tears, muscle atrophy indicating nerve injury, subluxation, dislocation, and virtually all soft-tissue change. However, it is not necessary to make a specific diagnosis of cuff tear if

the patient gets over the pain. With progressive age there is an increasing incidence of asymptomatic partial- or full-thickness cuff tears so that after 70 years of age most people have cuff tears.

Differential Diagnosis

Angina caused by myocardial ischemia may be confused with primary shoulder disease. Acute shoulder sepsis may mimic acute bursitis because of the comparable severity of pain. Sepsis usually is associated with systemic signs, such as an elevated erythrocyte sedimentation rate and white blood cell count, but is, in fact, quite rare. Osteoarthritis of the glenohumeral joint is not common and may be indistinguishable from some aspect of the impingement syndrome until plain radiographs are obtained. Pain from symptomatic degenerative arthritis of the acromioclavicular joint may be diagnosed or resolved by steroid injection into the joint.

Treatment

The goals of treatment are to resolve the patient's pain and restore normal muscle balance around the shoulder. This usually can be accomplished with nonoperative treatment. Patients with less severe symptoms can be started on anti-inflammatory medications, pendulum exercises, and shoulder rotator cuff exercises. Pendulum exercises are performed with the individual flexing at the waist, relaxing all shoulder girdle musculature, and dangling the involved arm in a pendulum-like fashion. This reduces the pressure on the impinged area and may increase the circulation to the tendon. Selective contraction of the internal and external rotator cuff muscles depresses the humeral head and reduces the pressure in the subacromial space. Patients are taught to do this using resistance exercises such as with an elastic band (Thera-Band), with the arm at the side, elbow flexed 90 degrees, applying force in internal and external rotation.

The fastest way to resolve impingement symptoms is to inject the subacromial space with corticosteroid and local anesthetic (e.g., triamcinolone 40 mg and 1% lidocaine 4 cc) (Figure 6–2). This mixture is injected with a no. 25 needle directed at the point of the shoulder toward the greater tuberosity 2.5 cm inferior to the anterolateral quarter of the acromion. The diagnosis is made when the patient's symptoms are relieved immediately. The patient then is started on progressive resistance exercises.

Patients who respond only temporarily to the injection or who develop recurrence after two or three injections and who have participated in proper exercises may be candidates for surgery or arthroscopic surgery to decompress the subacromial space. This includes removal of bone from the undersurface of the acromion and AC joint, bursectomy, and cuff debridement and repair as necessary.

Clinical Findings

A. SIGNS & SYMPTOMS

Acute anterior shoulder dislocation results from a specific injury and is associated with severe anterior shoulder pain. The patients may be aware of a configurational change in the shoulder. Patients guard against shoulder motion by holding the elbow flexed with the ipsilateral forearm in the opposite hand. Any attempt at motion is associated with severe pain. Posterior dislocations are less obvious.

B. IMAGING

AP and axillary radiographs are obtained in all suspected dislocations. Anterior dislocations will show the humeral head displaced inferiorly to the glenoid, confirming the diagnosis. In posterior dislocations, the humeral head is at the same level as the glenoid on the AP radiograph. The diagnosis can be confirmed with an axillary view, which shows the head posterior to the glenoid. Posterior dislocations may be missed in initial screening radiographs in the absence of an axillary view.

Treatment

Anterior and posterior dislocations are reduced by closed techniques immediately. Anterior dislocations can be reduced by various methods, including the Hippocratic maneuver. This technique involves gradual axial distraction to the arm in a position of forward flexion. Countertraction is applied to the axilla with the patient under intravenous analgesia [such as 40–100 mg meperidine HCl (Demerol)]. Gentle rotation of the arm into internal rotation frequently assists reduction. Confirmatory radiographs are obtained after reduction.

Following reduction, patients are immobilized with the elbow at the side and the arm in a position of 10 degrees of external rotation for 3 weeks (Figure 6–3). This position as compared with a sling and the arm in internal rotation is a new concept based on better anatomic contact between the torn labrum and the glenoid. Patients are allowed to return to their usual activities at 6–8 weeks. Long-term rates of success with this position of immobilization are unknown. If patients become recurrent dislocators, repair of the torn capsular attachment from the labrum of the glenoid anteriorly can be done arthroscopically, but the highest rate of success is with open surgery. Acute posterior dislocations usually require temporary immobilization in a position of slight abduction, shoulder extension, and external rotation to keep the humeral head reduced.

REFERENCES

Itoy E et al: A new method of immobilization after traumatic anterior dislocation of the shoulder: A preliminary study. J Shoulder Elbow Surg 2003;12:413 [PMID: 14564258].

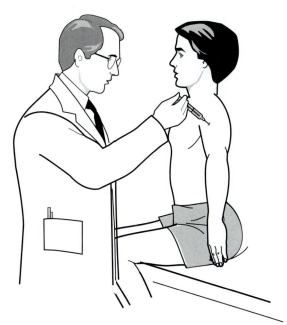

Figure 6–2. Lateral approach for subacromial injections. Needle should be positioned at an angle of 45 degrees downward and directed 45 degrees medially.

REFERENCES

Koester MC, George MS, Kuhn JE: Shoulder impingement syndrome. Am J Med 2005;118:452 [PMID: 15866244].

Trojian T et al: What can we expect from nonoperative treatment options for shoulder pain? J Fam Pract 2005;54(3):216 [PMID: 15755374].

2. Shoulder Dislocations

The anatomy of the shoulder contributes to the ease with which shoulder dislocations can occur. Stability of the large humeral head in the shallow 5- by 2.5-cm glenoid depends on shoulder capsule and specific ligament attachments to the margins of the glenoid. Excessive force applied in any direction may cause a dislocation. With forces applied to the arm held in a position of abduction and external rotation, the humeral head is driven forward, tearing the anterior and middle glenohumeral ligaments and capsule from the margin of the glenoid. The humeral head is driven out anteriorly and rests in a position anterior and inferior to the glenoid. Rarely, the humeral head can dislocate posteriorly with automobile accidents, grand mal seizures, or electroshock therapy. In young people with lax ligaments and psychiatric disabilities, it may be dislocated intentionally.

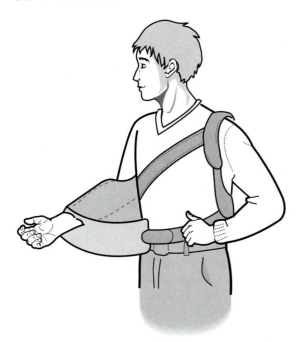

Figure 6–3. Patient immobilized with the elbow at the side and the arm in a position of 10 degrees of external rotation.

Mazzocca AD et al: Arthroscopic anterior shoulder stabilization of collision and contact athletes. Am J Sports Med 2005;33:52 [PMID: 15610999].

3. Anterior Shoulder Subluxation

With a similar mechanism of force application to the abducted external rotated shoulder, a partial capsular tear or a partial tear of the capsule glenoid attachment occurs in which the humeral head subluxes anteriorly and reduces spontaneously. The injury is usually associated with sporting activities. Some patients continue to have anterior shoulder pain with light activities or use of the arm overhead. If the patient is not responding to strengthening exercises of the shoulder internal rotators (pectoralis major and subscapularis muscles), shoulder reconstruction, such as repair of the capsule-glenoid attachment as in the Bankhart procedure, may be required.

4. Multidirectional Instability

People with ligamentous laxity may have shoulder joints that sublux easily in the anterior, posterior, or inferior direction. In the absence of injury, patients are asymptomatic. Following a minor injury in which the shoulder joint is subluxed forcibly, patients may continue to have shoulder pain with daily activities and symptoms of instability with different positions of the shoulder and arm.

Physical examination may demonstrate evidence of ligamentous laxity in the wrists, elbows, and knees. Shoulder examination will reveal laxity and excessive translation of the humeral head anterior and posterior. Patients may demonstrate the instability voluntarily.

Treatment is directed at educating the patient to adjust to the problem, altering his or her lifestyle, strengthening the shoulder, and delaying symptomatic activities. In some patients, surgical repair is directed at correcting the dominant directional instabilities.

REFERENCES

Gartsman GM, Hasan SS: What's new in shoulder and elbow surgery. J Bone Joint Surg Am 2005;87:226 [PMID: 15634837].

Lee MP: Open operative treatment for anterior shoulder instability: When and why? J Hand Ther 2005;18:384 [PMID: 16059865].

5. Thoracic Outlet Syndrome

Thoracic outlet syndrome is a group of symptoms and signs caused by compression of the neurovascular structures passing out of the chest and neck and beneath the clavicle to the axilla. Compression of the elements of the brachial plexus and/or subclavian vessels occurs in the interscalene triangle, behind or below the clavicle or subcoracoid space. Cervical ribs or congenital fibrous bands and rarely a nonunion or malunion of the clavicle can lead to thoracic outlet compression. The condition is uncommon, and the diagnosis is missed frequently. Women are affected more frequently than men, usually between the ages of 20 and 50 and before 30 years of age.

Clinical Findings

A. SIGNS & SYMPTOMS

Patients have pain and/or paresthesia radiating from the neck or shoulder and down to the forearm and fingers. They usually have difficulty with overhead activities. The hand may feel swollen or heavy. The lower trunk of the brachial plexus is involved more commonly, producing signs of numbness, tingling, and weakness in the ulnar-innervated intrinsic muscles. Patients also may have venous compression or arterial insufficiency from the outlet.

B. IMAGING

Plain radiographs of the cervical spine should be studied for congenital differences such as cervical ribs and long transverse processes or even hypoplastic first ribs. Apical lordotic chest views are indicated to rule out Pancoast-type tumors. Sophisticated MR angiographic or high-resolution CT scans may be helpful.

Differential Diagnosis

The diagnosis can be confused with cervical disk disease at the C7–T1 level (which is rare), which may produce a C8 radiculopathy. Compression of the ulnar nerve in the cubital tunnel or Guyon's canal usually can be distinguished by appropriate electromyography (EMG). Provocative maneuvers such as overhead exercise or standing in the military brace position will obliterate the ipsilateral radial pulse and produce symptoms. More important, one should look for the reproduction of symptoms with specific controlled movements, e.g., controlling the stretch on the brachial plexus through scapular depression, shoulder abduction (to 90 degrees), and external rotation or wrist/finger extension, followed by elbow extension with supination.

Treatment

The initial treatment is conservative and depends on appropriate postural strength training to reduce the mechanism of thoracic outlet compression. The reduction of obesity and general physical fitness are encouraged. Overhead activities or carrying heavy loads should be minimized.

The initial approach is to teach patients that posture is a primary cause of impingement and begin postural training and general upper extremity and shoulder exercise. Progress is measured in weeks or months.

Rarely, patients may require surgery that may include surgical release of the anterior scalene muscles and resection of the first rib or fibrous band. When symptoms caused by a clavicular malunion do not respond to conservative treatment, clavicular osteotomy is indicated.

REFERENCES

Brantigan CO et al: Use of multidetector CT and three-dimensional reconstructions in thoracic outlet syndrome. Hand Clin 2004;20:123 [PMID: 1500539].

Casbas L et al: Post-traumatic thoracic outlet syndromes. Ann Vasc Surg 2005;19:25 [PMID: 15714363].

Huang JH, Zager EL: Thoracic outlet syndrome. Neurosurgery 2004;55:897 [PMID: 15458598].

6. Clavicle Fractures

Clavicle fractures usually occur from a direct blow to the shoulder and rarely from falling on an outstretched hand. Middle-third fractures are most common. Distal-third fractures are infrequent.

Clinical Findings

A. SIGNS & SYMPTOMS

The proximal fragment of the clavicle is elevated by the action of the sternocleidomastoid; the weight of the shoulder displaces the distal fragment downward. Local swelling occurs from bleeding from the fracture site. The patient supports the involved extremity with the opposite hand. Rarely, a proximal fragment can perforate the skin, producing an open fracture. Plain radiographs of the clavicle are sufficient for diagnosis.

Treatment

Immobilization of the fracture is provided by the application of a figure-of-eight bandage or a sling and swath. It is doubtful that a figure-of-eight sling or even a plaster bolero will influence the fracture position.

Some mild cosmetic deformity usually is present. Open reduction with internal fixation is seldom indicated but may be necessary for an open fracture or a distal-third fracture occurring alone or in combination with a fracture of the neck of the scapula (floating shoulder). Conservatively treated distal-third fractures have a high rate of nonunion.

REFERENCES

Robinson CM, Cairns DA: Primary nonoperative treatment of displaced lateral fractures of the clavicle. J Bone Joint Surg Am 2004;86:778 [PMID: 15069143].

Zlowodzki M et al: Treatment of acute midshaft clavicle fractures. J Orthop Trauma 2005;19:504 [PMID: 16056089].

7. Fractures of the Proximal Humerus

Isolated fractures of the proximal humerus can occur after a direct fall onto the arm or elbow.

Clinical Findings

A. SIGNS & SYMPTOMS

Clinical symptoms include pain experienced over the proximal shoulder region or radiating the length of the arm. Local swelling is noted on examination from bleeding at the fracture site. Dissection of the hematoma may be noted onto the anterior chest after a few days. Evaluation is with plain radiographs of the scapula and shoulder. These include AP radiographs of the scapula and proximal humerus and a lateral scapular view. An axillary view is necessary to rule out a dislocation of the head fragment. If present, this requires reduction, usually by operative methods. Most proximal humeral fractures are displaced minimally.

Treatment

The four-part classification of proximal humeral fractures of Neer is helpful in deciding treatment. Nondisplaced or minimally displaced fractures of the surgical or anatomic neck of the greater or lesser tuberosities can be treated by temporary immobilization. Displaced fractures of one or both tuberosities are indicative of a rotator cuff tear. Displaced fractures may require surgical treatment by open reduction and internal fixation. Four-part fractures result in lost blood supply to the humeral head and may require prosthetic replacement. Instruction in early shoulder motion is required both for unfixed and for operated fractures. The goal of physical therapy is to restore normal range of motion and strength around the shoulder. Patients should be progressed from active range-of-motion to resistive exercises beginning with isometrics and progressing to isotonic exercises.

REFERENCE

Neer CS: Displaced proximal humeral fractures. Clin Orthop 2006;442:77 [PMID: 16394743].

8. Frozen-Shoulder Syndrome (Adhesive Capsulitis)

In patients with frozen-shoulder syndrome, there is marked restriction of glenohumeral joint motion, presumably in response to diffuse capsular inflammation. Etiology is unknown.

Clinical Findings

A. SIGNS & SYMPTOMS

These patients may be comfortable at rest, and symptoms are produced when they attempt to move the glenohumeral joint beyond that allowed by the inflammation and adhesions. All ranges of motion are limited. Loss of axial humeral rotation (internal and external rotation) with the elbow at the side is diagnostic. Adhesive capsulitis frequently is confused with loss of motion from rotator cuff pathology. In the latter situation, there is no loss of axial rotation.

Treatment

Resolution of pain from a frozen shoulder requires a short period of sling immobilization for pain relief. Shoulder motion will recover gradually over 6–18 months. Recovery of motion can be facilitated initially by distension of the glenohumeral joint with 30 cc fluid, saline with lidocaine, and triamcinolone diacetate 0.5 cc. This is followed by gentle manipulation of the arm into external rotation.

REFERENCES

Diercks RL, Stevens M: Gentle thawing of the frozen shoulder: A prospective study of supervised neglect versus intensive physical therapy in patients with frozen shoulder syndrome. J Shoulder Elbow Surg 2004;13:499 [PMID: 15383804].

Shrader MW et al: Understanding proximal humerus fractures: Image analysis, classification, and treatment. J Shoulder Elbow Surg 2005;14:497 [PMID: 16194741].

9. Acromioclavicular Joint Separation

Acromioclavicular joint injuries may result from falls or from direct trauma to the arm or shoulder. They are common in contact sports such as ice hockey and football.

Stability across the acromioclavicular joint is provided primarily by the conoid and trapezoid ligaments. These ligaments, which are connected to the undersurface of the clavicle, suspend the scapula in the upright position by their attachment at the base of the coracoid process. The less robust acromioclavicular ligaments and the attachments of the deltoid musculature between the clavicle and the arm provide additional stability. In minor injuries, the ligaments of the acromioclavicular joint are stretched, and with increased force, the coracoacromial ligaments are injured as well. In severe injuries, the deltoid can be partially avulsed from its origin at the clavicle or acromion.

Clinical Findings

Signs and symptoms include pain and tenderness over the acromioclavicular joint and deformity of the joint. Radiographs of the injured shoulder will rule out fracture of the clavicle or proximal humerus. Displacement of the acromioclavicular joint usually can be demonstrated on an AP view of the joint. Shoulder radiographs taken with the patient holding a weight or with traction applied to the humerus are rarely necessary.

Treatment

Treatment for most injuries consists of relieving symptoms by using a sling to immobilize the shoulder and support the weight of the arm. Patients may resume activity as comfort returns. Once the shoulder is stable in terms of decreased pain (4–6 weeks), physical therapy may be helpful for increasing strength. The usual residual of AC injuries is a mild cosmetic deformity caused by prominence of the distal end of the clavicle.

If there is severe disruption of the AC joint with detachment of the deltoid, surgery may be indicated. The deformity can be corrected by surgically detaching the coracoacromial ligament from the acromion and inserting it into the distal end of the clavicle, which is shortened by 1–2 cm. There is no urgency in deciding on surgical reconstruction because repair need not be done immediately. In general, the conservative and surgical approaches to treatment yield equivalent results, at least for the less severe disruptions.

REFERENCES

Dumonski M et al: Evaluation and management of acromioclavicular joint injuries. Am J Orthop 2004;33:526 [PMID: 1554085].

Montellese P, Dancy T: The acromioclavicular joint. Primary Care 2004;31:857 [PMID: 15544824].

INJURIES OF THE ELBOW, WRIST, AND HAND

1. Lateral Humeral Epicondylitis (Tendonitis of Common Extensor Origin or Tennis Elbow)

Lateral humeral epicondylitis received the designation "tennis elbow" because it was a common complaint among tennis players. The lesion can occur with any type of repetitive wrist dorsiflexion activity, such as may be suffered by any worker whose work calls for repeated forceful wrist extension, as in a power grasp. The pathologic process is thought to represent collagen necrosis at the attachment of the extensor carpi radialis brevis to the lateral humeral epicondyle and the extensor carpi radialis longus origin along the supracondylar line.

Clinical Findings

Patients may have ill-defined elbow symptoms or pain radiating into the dorsal aspect of the forearm. Symptoms may occur at night and at rest, but usually they are related to activity, especially grasping or wrist dorsiflexion. There is local tenderness over the lateral humeral epicondyle or distal to it in the common extensor origin. Sometimes there is pain at the distal third of the humerus at the origin of the extensor carpi radialis brevis.

On clinical examination, symptoms can be reproduced by asking the patient to dorsiflex the wrist against resistance (as in grasping the back of a chair and lifting) or to apply resistance against wrist dorsiflexion (Figure 6–4). Radiographic findings are normal. Tenderness at the lateral epicondyle is expected.

Differential Diagnosis

The symptoms of radial head osteoarthritis, which is rare, can resemble those of tennis elbow. Plain-film radiography usually will distinguish the two disorders.

A fractured radial head or neck caused by falling on an outstretched hand may cause similar symptoms. The history of the injury and plain-film AP and lateral radiographic views will establish the diagnosis of fracture.

Prevention

General strengthening of elbow and forearm musculature and proper instruction in the use of hand tools

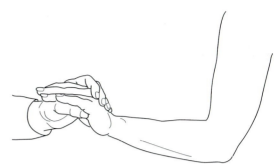

Figure 6–4. Physician testing dorsiflexion of a patient's wrist against resistance. Resulting lateral humeral epicondylar pain suggests tennis elbow.

and/or modification of the hand tool may prevent lateral humeral epicondylitis in workers at risk.

Treatment

A. GENERAL MEASURES

The lesion usually heals if the harmful activity is eliminated. Patients should be instructed to avoid dorsiflexion activities and carrying heavy objects with the elbow extended (some women carry their purses in this manner). Nonsteroidal anti-inflammatory drugs are helpful, especially for patients with night pain.

B. SPECIFIC MEASURES

Triamcinolone acetonide 40 mg injected into the most tender area of the epicondyle or common extensor origin usually is effective in relieving symptoms. Occasionally, a second injection is necessary. Complications of this treatment include fat necrosis and local skin atrophy. Loss of pigmentation (usually temporary) in darker-skinned patients may result from the injection.

Rarely is surgical release of the common extensor origin or extensor carpi radialis brevis necessary. As patients recover from an acute episode, forearm muscle strengthening is helpful. A Velcro sleeve around the proximal forearm to minimize contraction power of the extensor tendon of the extensor muscle mass, as used by some tennis players, also appears to be beneficial.

REFERENCES

Aoki M et al: Magnetic resonance imaging findings of refractory tennis elbows and their relationship to surgical treatment. J Shoulder Elbow Surg 2005;14:172 [PMID: 1578901].

Nirschl RP, Ashman ES: Tennis elbow tendinosis (epicondylitis). Instr Course Lect 2004;53:587 [PMID: 15116648].

2. Olecranon Bursitis

Olecranon bursitis is irritation and swelling in the normally occurring bursa between the olecranon prominence and the overlying skin. It is much more common in men, and trauma is usually a factor. Occasionally, the cause of the swelling is a low-grade infection, which must be considered prior to treatment. Swelling that develops over the olecranon process after hospitalization for any surgery may be gouty in origin.

Patients usually present with a history of gradual swelling and pain, although these symptoms may be acute after a direct blow to the olecranon process. Signs of increased warmth suggest a septic process. Sepsis can be present when symptoms are quite mild. Localized fluctuant swelling will be present with or without sepsis.

The use of a protective pad to avoid reinjury is sufficient treatment in most cases, and simple immobilization is adequate in mild cases. Aspiration and culture are indicated when sepsis is suspected. Aspiration is best performed by introducing the needle at least 2.5 cm away from the bursa and then tunneling beneath the skin before actual penetration. This technique may prevent secondary infection of a sterile bursa, which is a risk when direct penetration through overlying skin is used.

REFERENCE

Floemer F et al: MRI characteristics of olecranon bursitis. AJR 2004;183:29 [PMID: 15208103].

3. De Quervain Tenosynovitis (First Dorsal Wrist Extensor Compartment Tenosynovitis)

De Quervain tenosynovitis involves the first dorsal compartment of the wrist. Onset usually associated with overuse of the thumb, as in repetitive grasping. Rarely, an aberrant or extra tendon may be present in the sheath, which normally contains the abductor pollicis longus and the extensor pollicis brevis. The tenosynovial lining will show low-grade inflammation.

Clinical Findings

Patients in new job activities or those who engage in repetitive grasping complain of pain in an ill-defined area along the radial side of the base of the thumb, occasionally extending as far distally as the interphalangeal joint. Local swelling usually is present over the lateral aspect of the distal radius and may be present in the absence of pain. When the patient grasps the fully flexed thumb into the palm and then ulnar deviates the hand at the wrist, exquisite pain develops and repro-

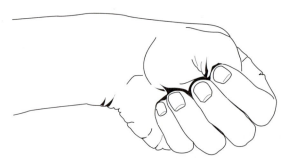

Figure 6–5. Finkelstein test. With the thumb clasped in the palm as shown, the wrist is deviated toward the ulna, producing pain over the first dorsal extensor compartment.

duces the patient's complaint (a positive Finkelstein test; see Figure 6–5). Crepitus frequently is present over the involved tendon sheath. There are no specific laboratory or radiographic findings.

Differential Diagnosis

Old nonunion of the navicular bone occasionally produces similar symptoms. Pain associated with osteoarthritis of the first carpometacarpal joint, which occurs in approximately 25% of white women older than 55 years of age, may mimic De Quervain tenosynovitis, which occurs in younger patients. Plain-film AP radiographs of the wrist will rule out carpometacarpal osteoarthritis (see below) and nonunion of the navicular bone.

Treatment

Most patients learn to limit their grasping activities, and the symptoms then resolve. Patients are instructed to decrease gripping activities and avoid unnecessary extension and abduction of the thumb.

The standard treatment is lidocaine 1 cc delivered locally with a 25-gauge needle to the common first dorsal extensor sheath; this is followed by triamcinolone acetonide 20 mg. With the needle in the proper position, no resistance to injection is encountered. Immobilization of the thumb in a splint can be helpful, as are NSAIDs.

In the rare patient who does not respond to local injection, surgical decompression of the common extensor sheath by incision may be necessary. This procedure may inadvertently injure the sensory branch of the radial nerve, even when it is performed with the aid of magnification. Pain associated with a sensory branch radial nerve neuroma is at least as bad as and usually worse than the original tenosynovitis. Symptoms in the majority of patients with tenosynovitis resolve after one cortisone injection.

REFERENCES

Richie CA 3d, Briner WW Jr: Corticosteroid injection for treatment of de Quervain's tenosynovitis. J Am Board Fam Pract 2003;16:102 [PMID: 12665175].

Tallia AF, Cardone DA: Diagnostic and therapeutic injection of the wrist and hand region. Am Fam Physician 2003;67:745 [PMID: 12613728].

4. Medial Epicondylitis or Flexor Pronator Syndrome

Medial epicondylitis or flexor pronator syndrome is caused by overuse of the finger flexors and the wrist flexors/pronators and occurs in sportsmen such as golfers and baseball pitchers, as well as in manual workers who do forceful repetitive work with the elbow flexed. Patients have exercise pain on the medial aspect of the elbow radiating to the forearm.

Physical findings include local tenderness over the medial epicondyle or common proximal flexor origin. The symptoms can be reproduced by resisted active wrist flexion.

Treatment is based on rest of the involved tissues and modified activity. The proximal forearm band to limit muscle contraction may be helpful. Steroid injection is useful. Extracorporeal shock therapy has provided conflicting results. The need for surgical relief is rare.

REFERENCES

Ciccotti MC, Schwartz MA, Ciccotti MG: Diagnosis and treatment of medial epicondylitis of the elbow. Clin Sports Med 2004;23:693 [PMID: 15474230].

Descatha A et al: Medial epicondylitis in occupational settings: Prevalence, incidence and associated risk factors. J Occup Environ Med 2003;45:993 [PMID: 14506342].

5. Cubital Tunnel Syndrome

The ulnar nerve may be trapped, irritated, or subluxed in its anatomic course through the cubital tunnel and its entrance to the forearm through the arch of origin of the flexor carpi ulnaris. Compression of the nerve in the canal may be related to old elbow injuries with enlarging osteophytes, cubitus valgus, or a nerve that subluxes out of the groove.

Clinical Findings

Patients present with aching pain in the medial aspect of the elbow and pain and recurrent paresthesias in the distribution of the ulnar nerve into the ulnar fingers. Symptoms frequently are aggravated by the position of elbow flexion or resting the elbow on a worktable.

Physical examination may reveal minimal findings. There may be a Tinel sign over the ulnar nerve in the cubital tunnel and weakness of the interossei and thumb adductor. Atrophy of these muscles is uncommon.

The differential diagnosis must exclude compression of the nerve in Guyon's canal. This diagnosis is excluded by the presence of numbness or history of numbness on the ulnar half of the dorsum of the hand.

Treatment

Treatment is conservative initially, and patients are taught to avoid pressure on the flexed elbow, flexion at night, or while working.

For patients with muscle atrophy of the interossei and those not responding to conservative management, surgical decompression of the nerve in the canal, medial epicondylectomy, or anterior transposition of the nerve submuscularly is indicated.

REFERENCES

Huang JH, Samadani U, Zager EL: Ulnar nerve entrapment neuropathy at the elbow: Simple decompression. Neurosurgery 2004;55:1150 [PMID: 15509321].

Sellards R, Kuebrich C: The elbow: Diagnosis and treatment of common injuries. Primary Care 2005;32:1 [PMID: 15831310].

6. Anterior Interossei Syndrome

The anterior interosseus branch of the median nerve innervates the radial half of the flexor digitorum profundus, the flexor pollicis longus, and the pronator quadratus. The syndrome occurs when there is injury or compression of this nerve.

Clinical Findings

The physical findings demonstrate the inability to pinch between the thumb and index finger. When there is involvement of the pronator teres, patients will have weakness of pronation against resistance. The diagnosis can be confirmed by EMG. Patients may present with an ill-defined pain in the anterior forearm, frequently with a history of a single strong contraction of the anterior forearm muscles resulting in subsequent motor loss.

Treatment

Tension must be released in the involved muscles to help decrease the impingement. Forearm pronation and thumb adduction movements should be minimized. If conservative treatment is unsuccessful, surgical decompression may be needed.

7. Trigger Finger or Thumb

Stenosing tenosynovitis of the flexor tendon to a finger or of the flexor pollicis longus to the thumb may produce pain when the digit or thumb is forcibly flexed or extended (Figure 6–6). Motion of the proximal interphalangeal (PIP) joint of the finger or the interphalangeal (IP) joint of the thumb produces the symptoms, which is a painful snap. This causes the joint to collapse suddenly much like a trigger.

The cause of the tenosynovitis may be repetitive finger flexion or direct trauma over the site of the stenosis on the metacarpal head in the distal palm. It is also associated with de Quervain disease, carpal tunnel syndrome, and rheumatoid arthritis. The patient's work history may reveal the source of the irritation.

Treatment

Kenalog (20 mg) with 1 cc 1% lidocaine is injected directly into the synovial sheath at the point of greatest tenderness and usually is curative. Patients not responding or developing recurrent symptoms may require surgical release of the tendon sheath.

REFERENCE

Ryzewicz M, Wolf JM: Trigger digits: Principles, management, and complications. J Hand Surg [Am] 2006;31:135 [PMID: 16443118].

8. Scaphoid Fractures

Scaphoid fractures occur in younger people from a fall on the outstretched hand. The scaphoid fractures against the unyielding anterior radiocarpal ligament. In

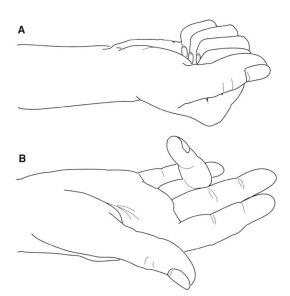

Figure 6–6. Trigger finger. *A.* The profundus tendons are completely flexed. *B.* An attempt at extension after flexion produces triggering or locking in flexion.

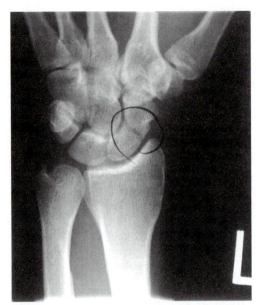

Figure 6–7. Fractured scaphoid in a 34-year-old man.

elderly patients with osteoporosis, the same mechanism of injury will produce a Colles fracture.

Clinical Findings

A. SIGNS & SYMPTOMS

The patient complains of pain at the base of the thumb or of wrist pain that may not be localized. On physical examination, there is tenderness to direct pressure over the tuberosity of the scaphoid.

B. RADIOGRAPH DIAGNOSIS

For any suspected carpal bone fracture or so-called wrist sprain, three radiographic views are obtained: posteroanterior (PA), lateral, and scaphoid views (Figure 6–7). With any wrist injury, look for subluxation of the scaphoid, in addition to scaphoid fracture or other fractures/dislocations. If a scaphoid fracture is suspected and the radiographs are negative, an MRI or bone scan may be necessary. The sensitivity of these tests has the advantage of making a definitive diagnosis sooner.

Treatment

When the scaphoid fracture is nondisplaced, treatment includes a thumb spica cast with a sugar-tong extension around the elbow to limit pronation and supination. Immobilization is continued until the fracture union is definite based on radiograph, usually at least 12 weeks. The restrictions imposed by cast immobilization can be avoided by percutaneous screw fixation of the scaphoid. For displaced fractures, open reduction and internal fixation usually are indicated.

REFERENCES

Brooks S et al: The management of scaphold fractures. J Sci Med Sport 2005;8:181 [PMID: 16075778].

Dias JJ et al: Should acute scaphoid fractures be fixed? A randomized, controlled trial. J Bone Joint Surg Am 2005;87:2160 [PMID: 16203878].

Pillai A, Jain M: Management of clinical fractures of the scaphoid: Results of an audit and literature review. Eur J Emerg Med 2005;12:47 [PMID: 15756078].

9. Nonunion of a Scaphoid

Symptoms from a scaphoid nonunion may occur long after the original injury. Late-onset symptoms may occur after a minimal wrist strain or reinjury. Radiography or MRI is necessary in patients with complaints of repeated wrist injury because of this possibility. Surgical treatment with bone grafting is necessary to repair a scaphoid nonunion.

10. Carpal Tunnel Syndrome

Carpal tunnel syndrome is a traumatic or pressure neuropathy of the median nerve as it passes through the carpal tunnel volar to the nine flexor tendons. The canal boundaries are the rigid transverse carpal ligament on the volar side and the carpal bones on the dorsal side.

Carpal tunnel syndrome affects patients of any age but is more common in women. Pregnancy increases the risk. Symptoms may appear after an injury, such as a direct blow to the dorsiflexed wrist or an injury associated with a Colles fracture. Rheumatoid arthritis, which causes inflammation in the sheath surrounding the flexor tendons, is one example of a space-occupying lesion that produces the encroachment. Rare hypothyroid patients with myxomatous tissue in this area are at risk for bilateral symptoms. While the cause of the syndrome is unknown in most cases, repetitive wrist and finger movements involved in work and hobby activities are frequently implicated.

Clinical Findings

In the absence of injury, patients can develop paresthesias in the median nerve distribution gradually and spontaneously (the distribution in the volar surface of the thumb and the index and long fingers). With progression of the syndrome, patients may be awakened at night with pain, tingling, burning, or numbness in this area of the hand. Characteristically, patients tend to stand up and massage the area or shake the wrist and fingers. Untreated carpal tunnel syndrome with progressively worsening symptoms may result in permanent damage to the median nerve with consequent persistent skin sensory deficit and thenar motor atrophy and weakness.

When patients are seen early, there is no evidence of thenar atrophy, and sensation remains intact. If a blood pressure cuff on the arm is inflated midway between arterial and venous pressure, venous engorgement occurs and elicits the symptoms. Patients who hold their wrists maximally flexed also will develop symptoms (Phalen's sign). The diagnosis is confirmed by nerve electrodiagnostic studies (nerve conduction studies and EMG).

Differential Diagnosis

Pain in the median nerve distribution with compression of the carpal tunnel should be distinguished from full median nerve compression occurring proximally. Occasionally, C6 radiculopathy from cervical disk disease may resemble this condition, but neurologic examination should distinguish between the two.

Treatment

Underlying conditions, such as rheumatoid arthritis or hypothyroidism, causing carpal tunnel should be treated. In the absence of signs of neuropathy, patients are instructed in reducing provocative or repetitive activities. Wrist splints holding the wrist in neutral are effective in alleviating symptoms. For patients not responding to rest and splinting, injections of cortisone into the carpal tunnel (with care to avoid injection into the median nerve) are beneficial. Patients who fail to respond to the preceding measures or whose symptoms recur may require carpal tunnel release, which is a well-documented and standardized procedure that is done endoscopically or by open surgery. When patients present with signs of nerve injury, constant numbness, loss of sensibility, or thenar atrophy, surgery is required. The diagnosis should be confirmed by electrodiagnostic studies before surgery is undertaken.

REFERENCES

Bland JD: Carpal tunnel syndrome. Curr Opin Neurol 2005;18:581 [PMID: 16155444].

Sevim S et al: Long-term effectiveness of steroid injections and splinting in mild and moderate carpal tunnel syndrome. Neurol Sci 2004;25:48 [PMID: 1522162].

Wasiak R et al: Geographic variation in surgical treatment for work-related carpal tunnel syndrome: Does improved return to work matter? Work 2006;26:3 [PMID: 16373974].

Werner RA, Franzblau A, Gell N: Randomized, controlled trial of nocturnal splinting for active workers with symptoms of carpal tunnel syndrome. Arch Phys Med Rehabil 2005;86:1 [PMID: 15640980].

11. Osteoarthritis of the First Carpometacarpal Joint

Osteoarthritis of the first carpometacarpal (CMC) joint occurs in about 25% of women older than 55 years of age. The cause is unknown. Although the condition is frequently asymptomatic, some patients are aware of pain at the base of the thumb when grasping, such as when unscrewing large glass jars, and there may be a clinical deformity of "squaring" of the base of the thumb at the CMC joint. Plain-film radiographs will demonstrate the osteoarthritic changes in the joint.

The differential diagnosis includes de Quervain tenosynovitis (discussed earlier), in which tenderness and swelling are more proximal, and old nonunion of the scaphoid. Acute fracture of the scaphoid occurs in younger patients and can be ruled out by plain-film radiographs.

Most patients will respond to instructions to avoid repetitive painful activities such as extreme positions of thumb abduction. Wearing an orthosis to immobilize the thumb can minimize symptoms.

Anti-inflammatory drugs are helpful for patients who experience pain at night. Rarely, patients may require a resection interposition arthroplasty or trapeziometacarpal arthrodesis.

REFERENCES

Day CS et al: Basal joint osteoarthritis of the thumb: A prospective trial of steroid injection and splinting. J Hand Surg 2004; 29:247 [PMID: 15043897].

Martou G, Veltri K, Thomas A: Surgical treatment of osteoarthritis of the carpometacarpal joint of the thumb: A systematic review. Plast Reconstr Surg 2004;114:421 [PMID: 1527780].

CLOSED TENDON AND LIGAMENT INJURIES IN THE HAND

1. Mallet Finger

A mallet finger (also known as *baseball finger* or *hammer finger*) is a deformity that occurs when there has been a disruption of continuity of the extensor tendon at the distal interphalangeal (DIP) joint. It occurs when excessive flexion force is applied to the forcibly extended DIP joint. A fracture of the distal volar articular surface of the second phalanx may occur with it.

Treatment

There is agreement that conservative splinting with only the DIP joint splinted in extensions or hyperextension for 6–8 weeks is effective even when initiated as long as 4 weeks after injury. Closed K-wire fixation may be required for more severe injuries or with associated fracture.

REFERENCES

Kalainov DM et al: Nonsurgical treatment of closed mallet finger fractures. J Hand Surg 2005;30:580 [PMID: 15925171].

Richards SD et al: A model for the conservative management of mallet finger. J Hand Surg 2004;29:61 [PMID: 14734074].

2. Ulnar Collateral Ligament Injury of the Thumb (Skier's or Gamekeeper's Thumb)

Forcible radial deviation of the thumb can cause partial or complete disruption of the ulnar collateral ligament with or without fracture. It is most common in skiers when the thumb is injured forcibly against the ski pole. British gamekeepers developed an occupational chronic injury twisting fowl necks. Diagnosis requires standard radiographs and stability testing of the thumb with the metacarpophalangeal (MCP) joint in full flexion. Splinting can be used for stable injuries or nondisplaced avulsion fractures. Open surgical repair should not be delayed when there is a question of instability.

REFERENCE

Cooper JG et al: Local anaesthetic infiltration increases the accuracy of assessment of ulnar collateral ligament injuries. Emerg Med Australas 2005;17:132 [PMID: 15796727].

INJURIES OF THE SPINE

Low-back problems affect virtually everyone at some time during their life. Low-back problems rank high among the reasons for physician office visits and are costly in terms of medical treatment and lost productivity at home and in the workplace. In industry, low-back problems account for 50% of all lost time from work. Seventy-five percent of all lost time is a result of a small number of patients (<10%).

Definition & Origin

Low-back pain is characterized as pain occurring in the lumbar region, buttocks, or proximal posterior thighs. Pain in this distribution may be a result of extraspinal causes such as abdominal vascular disease or pain referred from any pathologic process affecting abdominal organs, for example, peritoneal tumors, ovarian carcinoma, and renal lithiasis, and must be considered in medical history-taking and physical examination. Lumbar pain also may be referred from conditions in the dorsal spine, for example, compression fracture of the dorsolateral spine, infection, or tumor.

Pathology

The overwhelming majority of low-back pain complaints arise from pathology in the lumbar disk and its natural history of response to mechanical stress and aging. Minor or major disruptions of the disk and its anatomic attachments generate an inflammatory response that causes the pain. Free nerve endings are present in the posterior third of the annulus. Mild damage or small rents in the annulus may occur, or the nucleus pulposus can bulge outward into or through the annulus. Disk ruptures may occur in any direction, including into the subchondral plate of the adjacent vertebra. Protrusion or sequestration of a disk into the neural foramina or spinal canal can cause neuropathy. Disk ruptures begin in the teens and continue to occur into old age.

The normal disk's viscoelastic properties are lost as we age; it becomes inspissated, stiff, and fibrous. Altered mechanics from this may cause the marginal osteophytes, which occur at annulus vertebral attachments. The facet joints develop early osteoarthritic changes that progress to encroach on the spinal canal space. There is secondary hypertrophy of the ligamentum flava. The end result is spinal stenosis. Instability may occur, causing displacement of one vertebra on another (degenerative spinal listhesis) and further narrowing of the canal. The greatest changes usually occur where the most motion is at L4–L5 and L5–S1 but may occur at any lumbar or thoracic lumbar level. All spines have some abnormality by 50 years of age. Disk degeneration is associated with facet osteoarthritis at that level. Disk narrowing throughout the cervical, thoracic, and lumbar spine accounts for the major loss of sitting height into old age.

1. Low-Back Pain Caused by Disk Disease or Injury

In the United States, a specific identifiable injury is associated with the onset of symptoms in only 15% of workers. Symptoms may begin at any age, with a peak incidence in the third or fourth decade.

Clinical Findings

A. SIGNS & SYMPTOMS

The onset of symptoms may be gradual or sudden. Patients sometimes wake with back pain after a day of strenuous activity, or symptoms may be directly related to a specific fall or lifting incident. Pain is usually but not always associated with motion and may be located in the lower lumbar region, the lumbosacral angle, the midline, the sacroiliac joint region, or the medial buttock. With associated radiculopathy, patients may experience leg pain independently of back pain. Pain from an S1 radiculopathy may be felt in the posterior calf and lateral border of the foot. L4 radiculopathy produces pain below the knee or in the medial part of the

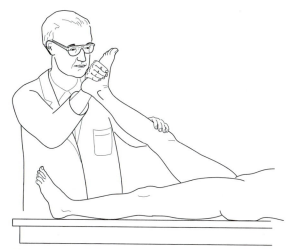

Figure 6–8. Straight-leg-raising test. The examiner's hand pushes the sole of the forefoot into dorsiflexion as the leg is raised passively.

leg, and L5 radiculopathy produces pain in the lateral calf and dorsum of the foot or in the great toe.

Restriction of back motion, common to all low-back-pain patients, is demonstrated on forward bending. Sciatic scoliosis, which is a list to the opposite side of a disk protrusion, may be present and is pathognomonic of an acute disk injury. Patients with severe disk problems avoid sitting and prefer standing or recumbency because intradiskal pressure is lower in the latter two positions.

With a disk that produces radiculopathy, straight-leg raising carried out passively by the examiner with the patient recumbent will cause back or leg pain, and the patient will guard against further elevation of the leg; this is considered a positive test (Figure 6–8). The degree of positivity is the angle of the elevated leg from the table, e.g., 45 degrees. S1 radiculopathy causes decreased or absent ankle jerk or decreased sensation along either the lateral border of the foot or the lateral three toes. L4 radiculopathy, which is less common, causes decreased or absent knee jerk and/or decreased sensation in the medial surface of the leg or pretibial region. L5 radiculopathy produces weakness of dorsiflexion of the great toe, hypoesthesia on the dorsum of the foot or great toe, or both (Figure 6–9).

B. IMAGING

Plain-film lateral and AP radiographic views of the entire lumbar spine are obtained with the patient standing. In addition, spot AP and lateral views of the two lowest disks are obtained with the patient recumbent and are used to rule out infection, tuberculosis, tumor, or fracture. Computerized axial tomographic (CAT)

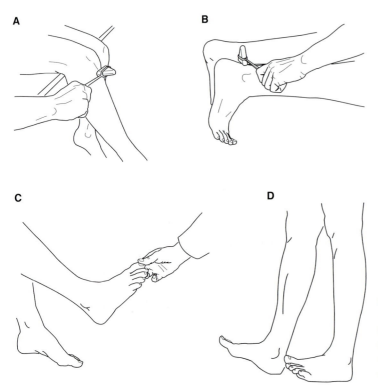

A

B

C

D

Figure 6–9. Reflex motor power physical examination checks L4, L5, and S1 radiculopathy. Knee jerk (*A*), ankle jerk (*B*), and big toe dorsiflexion (*C*) are shown. *D.* Patient walking on heels to demonstrate tibialis anterior motor power.

scan or MRI provides the most diagnostic information and should be performed if surgery is necessary.

Differential Diagnosis

Almost any pathologic process involving the spine, meninges, abdomen, pelvis, or retroperitoneal area can cause low-back pain. Physical examination should include evaluation for costovertebral angle tenderness, urinalysis to rule out renal disorders, abdominal examination for aneurysm, and evaluation of peripheral pulses to determine if there are vascular causes of back pain. If pyogenic infection of the disk space is suspected, gallium and technetium bone scans and an erythrocyte sedimentation rate are helpful in making this diagnosis; plain-film radiographs usually show no pathologic changes during the first 2 weeks of back pain caused by pyogenic sepsis. In tuberculosis of the spine, which has an insidious onset, plain films will show disk space collapse and endplate loss at the initial examination.

Ankylosing spondylitis (see below), which occurs primarily in males, may start in the latter part of the second decade. Chest expansion measured at the nipple line will be less than 2 cm. Plain radiographs will show sacroiliitis or early "squaring" of the lumbar vertebral bodies.

Deposits of tumor or multiple myeloma in the pedicles of vertebral bodies usually present with an early compression fracture. An MRI is superior for the diagnosis and staging of both focal and diffuse myeloma. Nonspinal causes of back and leg pain such as the piriformis syndrome also should be considered. Investigations for this would include MR neurography and interventional MRI.

A large or massive disk protrusion may produce cauda equina syndrome. Symptoms include urinary retention, sphincter paralysis, and perineal numbness. Cauda equina syndrome should be considered initially and ruled out in every patient with low-back pain. With any suspicion of cauda equina syndrome, an immediate MRI is done and immediate lumbar spine decompression carried out. There is no place for conservative treatment for cauda equina syndrome.

REFERENCES

Benzon HT et al: Piriformis syndrome: Anatomic considerations, a new injection technique, and a review of the literature. Anesthesiology 2003;98:1442 [PMID: 12766656].

Filler AG et al: Sciatica of nondisk origin and piriformis syndrome: Diagnosis by magnetic resonance neurography and interventional magnetic resonance imaging with outcome study of resulting treatment. J Neurosurg Spine 2005;2:99 [PMID: 15739520].

Prevention

Proper instruction about prevention of symptoms of degenerative disk disease should be mandatory for all new employees, regardless of their activity level. Education about body mechanics, lifting, bending, the hazards of prolonged sitting, and the deleterious effects of lack of exercise and obesity should be emphasized (see Chapter 4). Industrial workers with any degree of low-back pain should be given an opportunity for early medical evaluation to minimize progressive changes. Job activity should be designed to minimize prolonged sitting or standing and to avoid sitting while leaning forward and rotating. Employee selection using strength-performance criteria may be useful. There is no evidence that preplacement radiographs are helpful to either the employer or the employee for identifying individuals who may be at risk for developing low-back injuries. However, appropriate evaluation and counseling of individuals with previous back injury or surgery are valuable.

Treatment

A. Conservative Measures

Symptoms in 80–90% of patients with acute low-back pain or radiculopathy will resolve with conservative measures such as temporary bed rest, time, and avoidance of reinjury. Patients with severe pain should be instructed to remain in bed in the semi-Fowler position for a few days. Bed rest for 3–7 days has a positive effect on lost time from work. Early gentle activity, including walking, is encouraged as symptoms resolve. The safest effective pain medication is acetaminophen. For any patient with significant initial radiculopathy, return to full-time work should be based on resolution of symptoms. Progressive sitting as tolerated is appropriate as long as radiculopathy does not increase. For those who perform heavy labor, this prescription may be as long as 3–4 months.

Patients whose occupations involve light labor or who are self-employed and can adjust their work schedules may be allowed to work part time and then be encouraged to be recumbent during leisure time. Initial use of a lumbosacral corset is especially helpful for those whose occupations call for prolonged sitting or driving. As symptoms resolve, corset use is tapered gradually, and patients are taught progressive exercises.

At the appropriate time, a swimming program in which the individual uses either the backstroke or the sidestroke is encouraged.

B. Exercise

Exercise with early mobilization in the pain-free directions should be implemented as soon as possible. A stepwise program using exercise goals that are increased gradually over time is appropriate in uncomplicated cases of low-back problems. Progressive strengthening exercises for abdominal and back muscles may promote recovery and prevent prolonged disability caused by deconditioning. The focus of back exercises should be first to restore normal mobility and then to restore normal strength. Return-to-work interventions are helpful in reducing lost time and facilitating recovery of endurance.

C. Surgical Measures

Patients with radiculopathy who fail to respond to conservative treatment (as evidenced by persistent pain and persistently positive results in the straight-leg-raising test or by sciatic scoliosis with evidence of disk protrusion) are candidates for surgery. Surgery may consist of percutaneous nucleoplasty or diskectomy to relieve nerve root pressure. In rare cases, spinal fusion is added to the procedure if postlaminectomy instability is expected. Lumbar spinal disk replacement is being substituted for some patients in need of spinal fusion. Long-term results of disk replacement are unknown.

REFERENCES

Brodke DS, Ritter SM: Nonsurgical management of low-back pain and lumbar disk degeneration. Instr Course Lect 2005;54:279 [PMID: 15948456].

Hlobil H et al: Effectiveness of a return-to-work intervention for subacute low-back pain. Scand J Work Environ Health 2005; 31:249 [PMID: 16161707].

Lipson SJ: Spinal-fusion surgery: Advances and concerns. N Engl J Med 2004;350:643 [PMID: 14960739].

Nordin M et al: Nonspecific lower-back pain: Surgical versus nonsurgical treatment. Clin Orthop 2006;443:156 [PMID: 16462440].

2. Chronic Low-Back Pain

In a small percentage of patients without prominent sciatica or serious underlying conditions such as tumor or infection, persisting low-back pain is categorized as chronic when symptoms persist longer than 3–6 months. Preexisting depression or psychological problems, workplace dissatisfaction, contentious compensation claims, and even other types of chronic pain may be present.

Management of such patients is challenging and requires consideration of underlying psychiatric issues and encouragement that serious organic disease or neurologic injury is not present after appropriate imaging studies. Patients are guided with safe pharmacologic treatment, including antidepressive agents such as amitriptyline. The value of early exercise and return to work at a lower level temporarily and remaining active is emphasized. Any surgery in chronic back pain patients who do no have major spinal disease or radiculopathy is not indicated.

REFERENCES

Carragee EJ: Persistent low-back pain. N Engl J Med 2005; 352:1891 [PMID: 15872204].

Young S, Aprill C, Laslett M: Correlation of clinical examination characteristics with three sources of chronic low-back pain. Spine J 2003;3:460 [PMID: 14609690].

2. Spinal Stenosis

Spinal stenosis usually is caused by progressive degenerative disk and facet joint encroachment into the spinal canal and or neuroforamen. It may be the most common cause of leg pain in the elderly. Spinal stenosis in the younger patient may be caused by congenitally short pedicles with or without disk disease.

Disk degeneration at multiple levels causes narrowing of the thecal sac and nerve root impingement. Although involvement at more than one level is evident radiographically, patients usually present with single-root involvement. Standing and walking with the lumbar spine in extension further decrease the already compromised space in the spinal canal. With the spine flexed, as it is when seated, there is more space for the neural contents, and relief of symptoms occurs.

Clinical Findings

A. SIGNS & SYMPTOMS

Neurogenic claudication may be accompanied by ill-defined pain in the lower extremity or by pain that is distributed along a specific nerve root and felt while walking. Patients may experience difficulty in standing, such as when shopping or waiting in line. The symptoms typically are relieved with sitting, recumbency, or even standing with one hip and knee flexed and one foot raised on a stair or footstool.

There may be no physical findings, or there may be unilateral decreased reflex changes affecting the involved root or decreased power in the great toe extensor (L5). In some cases, there are symmetric signs with generalized areflexia. Patients should be asked to walk to reproduce symptoms and then be reexamined for reflex changes (the Gill walk test). Patients usually have negative results in the straight-leg-raising test.

B. IMAGING

Plain-film radiographs may show scoliosis or degenerative disk changes with associated osteophytic hypertrophy of the facet joints at one or more levels. In younger patients with congenital spinal stenosis, shortening of the pedicles may be seen on lateral radiographic views of the spine; however, this shortening may be best seen on CT scans.

CT scan or MRI of the spine will show encroachment on the theca or nerve roots caused by a combination of disk degeneration, osteophytic overgrowth of the facet joints, and ligamentous hypertrophy at one or more levels.

Differential Diagnosis

Patients with degenerative disease of the spine also may have degenerative arthritis of the hips or knees. The source of groin pain on hip motion is more likely to be the hip joint rather than lower lumbar spinal stenosis. Knee pain associated with degenerative arthritis is more localized. Vascular claudication can mimic neurogenic claudication but is associated with altered pulses and will require assessment by Doppler ultrasonography and treatment by vascular surgery. Tumors or infections of the spine may produce leg pain from radiculopathy.

Patients who have bladder or bowel dysfunction and who are suspected of having cauda equina syndrome will require immediate investigation. If the diagnosis is confirmed, surgical decompression is indicated on an emergent basis.

Treatment

Epidural corticosteroids frequently are effective for varying periods of time. Braces that keep the spine in flexion during walking or standing may be tried but tend to further weaken the paraspinal musculature. Patients who do not respond to epidural steroids after further time may require surgical decompression. Interlaminar decompression, laminectomy, foraminotomy, or facetectomy may be necessary at one or more levels. Preoperative spinal instability with spondylolisthesis or postdecompression instability must be assessed. If instability is significant, single or multiple-level spinal fusion may be necessary. Currently, internal fixation with pedicle screws offers the best fusion rate for pre- or postdecompression instability.

REFERENCE

Kornblum MB et al: Degenerative lumbar spondylolisthesis with spinal stenosis: A prospective long-term study comparing fusion and pseudarthrosis. Spine 2004;29:726 [PMID: 15087793].

3. Coccygodynia

The coccyx consists of three small segments of bone with articulations between them. The segments are connected to the sacrum by the sacrococcygeal joint. A direct fall onto the coccyx or a direct blow to the area can injure any of the articulations and cause coccygodynia. Pain at the lower tip of the spine may persist if the injury is aggravated by sitting. Symptoms can be reproduced by manual palpation of or direct pressure over the coccyx. Plain films will rule out fracture.

Patients should be instructed to sit with a small pillow under the midthighs so that the buttocks are raised from the chair. Anti-inflammatory drugs are helpful in relieving pain at night. A few patients require local anesthesia and cortisone delivered into the articulation.

REFERENCE

Hodges SD, Eck JC, Humphreys SC: A treatment and outcomes analysis of patients with coccydynia. Spine J 2004;4:138 [PMID: 15016390].

4. Spondylolysis & Spondylolisthesis

Spondylolysis, a defect in the pars interarticularis, may develop during childhood as a congenital anomaly or from an unhealed stress fracture. The defect may be familial, but some cases are associated with trauma (such as when a football lineman performs a blocking maneuver and puts the spine into forceful extension). The defect may allow spondylolisthesis or forward displacement of one vertebra on the next. In older age groups, spondylolisthesis may result from degenerative disk disease or facet arthritis. Displacement of L5 on S1 is the most common level seen in isthmic spondylolisthesis; displacement of L4 on L5 is most common in degenerative spondylolisthesis. Individuals with backache have no greater incidence of isthmic spondylolysis and spondylolisthesis than do individuals without backache. The presence of the lesion may not necessarily be the cause of the patient's back pain.

Clinical Findings

A. SIGNS & SYMPTOMS

Spondylolysis and spondylolisthesis may cause symptoms similar to those of degenerative disk disease. Patients with spondylolisthesis occasionally have bilateral posterior thigh pain and may experience radiculopathy caused by irritation of the nerve root as it passes the fibrocartilaginous buildup at the pars interarticularis (most commonly the fifth root in L5–S1 spondylolisthesis). In degenerative spondylolisthesis, there is no defect in the pars interarticularis, and the leg complaints emerge from secondary spinal stenosis and neuroforaminal narrowing.

Patients with a pars-defect spondylolisthesis may have tight hamstring muscles in both legs, as demonstrated on straight-leg raising. Local point tenderness over the spinous process of the involved vertebrae may produce exquisite tenderness or even radiation of pain in the distribution of the fifth nerve root (doorbell sign).

B. IMAGING

An angled AP radiograph (upshot view) of the two lowest vertebrae should demonstrate the defect in the pars

interarticularis. Oblique views also can demonstrate the pars defect, but they expose the patient to a large amount of radiation. Spondylolisthesis is obvious on lateral-view radiographs. CT scans will show the pars defect (double-facet sign) in spondylolysis and the elongated spinal canal in spondylolisthesis.

Treatment

Patients with spondylolisthesis or spondylolysis may or may not have other lumbar problems. They should be treated with conservative measures similar to those recommended for patients with disk disease (see above). For those who do not respond to conservative treatment, surgery may be indicated. This may consist of decompression of the root and transverse process fusion or anterior interbody fusion. For adolescents with spondylolisthesis of minimal degree, lateral fusion alone is sufficient. For patients with degenerative spondylolisthesis, the addition of internal fixation enhances the success rate.

REFERENCES

Hammerberg KW: New concepts on the pathogenesis and classification of spondylolisthesis. Spine 2005;30:4 [PMID: 15767885].

Kwon BK, Albert TJ: Adult low-grade acquired spondylolytic spondylolisthesis: Evaluation and management. Spine. 2005; 15:30 [PMID: 15767884].

5. Ankylosing Spondylitis

Ankylosing spondylitis affects approximately 1% of the white population and may be more prevalent in other groups, such as the southern Chinese. It is much more prevalent among males than females. Approximately 90% of affected patients have a genetic predisposition to the disease, as evidenced by the presence of HLA-B27, and symptoms develop in one of seven white patients who test positive for HLA-B27.

Clinical Findings

A. SIGNS & SYMPTOMS

Patients with ankylosing spondylitis experience spontaneous and gradual onset of low-back pain with associated restriction of spine motion, but this may be confused with disk symptoms occurring in the workplace. Symptoms frequently begin during the second decade and, apparently, are frequently missed during this period. Occasionally, patients will develop a markedly stiffened spine and not remember experiencing any pain. Rarely, the disease presents like sciatica, with back and leg pain.

Restricted back motion usually can be demonstrated on forward flexion, but muscle spasm from disk disease also may do this and is more common. Even in the early stages of the disease, maximal chest expansion measured at the nipple line is less than 5 cm. Stiffening of the spine becomes more obvious as the disease progresses, and normal dorsal kyphosis increases with flattening of the lumbar region and reduction of the normal lumbar lordosis. There may be involvement of the glenohumeral joints or hip joints, and rarely, a patient will have more peripheral joint involvement.

B. IMAGING

On plain-film radiographs of the back, the sacroiliac joints show erosions, sclerosis, and in more advanced cases, frank bony fusion. Lateral views of the lumbar spine in the early stages show "squaring" of the vertebrae (in which the normal slight anterior concavity has been filled with new bone as a result of inflammation beneath the anterior longitudinal ligament). In later stages, the classic bony bridging, or "bamboo spine," is evident.

Treatment

It is not possible to predict the extent of the spondylosis that will occur, but the goal of treatment must be to minimize symptoms, maintain a good spinal position with gravity, and avoid progression of thoracic kyphosis. The greatest risk of deformity is kyphosis, and the exercise programs are directed at spinal extension strengthening. Patients should be taught to lay prone, as well as over a longitudinal roll, to facilitate spinal extension. Treatment is aimed at relieving pain and preventing deformity. Traditionally, patients are treated with anti-inflammatory medication (NSAIDs). If this does not control symptoms effectively, anti–tumor necrosis factor (TNF) alpha drugs such as etanercept or infliximab are begun as first-line treatment. These drugs have a dramatic effect on symptoms and physical findings.

A worker with a stiff, ankylosed spine who complains of pain after a fall should be considered to have a fracture until it is proved otherwise. The fracture could increase the patient's spinal deformity, usually in flexion. Common fracture locations are the dorsolumbar junction and the cervicothoracic junction. It is necessary to obtain bone scans, repeat radiographs, or MRIs and to immobilize the patient to protect against flexion deformity. Immobilization may involve use of a halo-jacket device for fractures at the cervicothoracic junction or a brace at the dorsolumbar junction. Spinal stabilization with rods may be necessary. Total hip replacement can be done for the hip disease of ankylosing spondylitis.

REFERENCES

Braun J et al: Therapy of ankylosing spondylitis: II. Biological therapies in the spondyloarthritides. Scand J Rheumatol 2005; 34:178 [PMID: 16134723].

Sieper J, Rudwaleit M: How early should ankylosing spondylitis be treated with tumour necrosis factor blockers? Ann Rheum Dis 2005;64:61 [PMID: 16239391].

van der Heijde D et al: Assessment in Ankylosing Spondylitis (ASAS) International Working Group: A model for psoriatic arthritis and psoriasis? Ann Rheum Dis. 2005;64:108 [PMID: 15708922].

INJURIES OF THE HIP

1. Trochanteric Bursitis

Trochanteric bursitis is an uncommon disorder that may be caused by local contusion that results in bleeding into the trochanteric bursa. More commonly, however, the onset of symptoms is spontaneous. Symptoms consist of local tenderness and persistent pain with activity.

Trochanteric bursitis is often confused with hip arthritis because of referred joint pain from the latter and sometimes low-back pain. The diagnosis can be confirmed by administering an anesthetic into the trochanteric bursa.

Treatment

Local cortisone injection is usually successful in resolving the symptoms.

2. Osteonecrosis of the Femoral Head

Classic osteonecrosis was described in caisson workers who were subjected to severe atmospheric pressure changes, creating vascular blockage in the femoral head. However, standards for the rate of barometric pressure change (from data on navy divers) have been effective in eliminating pressure change as a cause. Today, osteonecrosis occurs in several groups: in patients with subcapital fractures that interrupt the blood supply; in a small number of patients taking high doses of cortisone (e.g., in less than 1% of those who undergo renal transplantation with concurrent cortisone therapy) and, less frequently, in patients taking low doses of cortisone; in patients with asthma; in patients with lupus erythematosus; and in drug abusers. It also occurs idiopathically. There is an association with high alcohol consumption.

One theory of pathogenesis is that a clotting abnormality or increased level of lipoprotein obstructs the small vessels of the femoral head producing an infarct. Increases in marrow pressure of the proximal femur have been documented in early osteonecrosis. As revascularization of the ischemic bone begins, there is overactivity of osteoclastic bone resorption compared with osteoblastic bone regeneration. This imbalance leads to weakening of subchondral bone at the interface of viable and dead bone, producing a fracture, and accounts for the mechanical symptoms secondary to deformity of joint contours.

Clinical Findings

A. SIGNS & SYMPTOMS

The onset of pain associated with activity is usually insidious. Occasionally, a specific event (e.g., putting the lower extremity in an extreme position) will precipitate pain. Infrequently, pain occurs at night. Patients limp with an antalgic gait on the affected side, and hip motion may be slightly restricted compared with a lesser involved or uninvolved opposite side. Symptoms can be elicited by movements at the extremes of hip motion—especially rotation.

Some patients with osteonecrosis have involvement of the opposite hip, knees, or shoulders. Involvement of both knees and shoulders may occur in the absence of hip disease.

B. IMAGING

An AP radiograph of the pelvis in the early stages of osteonecrosis will show mottling changes in the femoral head. Findings on plain-film radiographs are rarely normal. With progression of the disease, there is flattening of the femoral head (Figure 6–10). This flattening is a result of settling of a quadrant of the head—because of the fracture—between the vascular and avascular bone. The cartilage, which receives its nutrients via the surface from the synovial fluid, remains normal until late, and secondary osteoarthritic changes occur. MRI may show abnormalities before they are evident on CT scans or plain films.

Differential Diagnosis

Symptoms of osteonecrosis may be confused with those of early degenerative arthritis of the hip. The two disorders can be distinguished with plain films.

Treatment

Once the diagnosis is established, patients are started on alendronate 70 mg orally per week, which reduces osteoclastic activity and inhibits bone turnover. This regimen has been shown to prevent early collapse of the femoral head. Long-term results of this bisphosphonate treatment are being studied. Partial relief of symptoms may result from use of measures such as body-weight reduction, walking with a cane in the hand on the unaffected side, or walking with crutches. It is important to maintain normal range of motion and strength about the hip joint.

Attempts to decompress the proximal femur by early drilling of the femoral head and neck are used in the early stages.

Surgical treatment is indicated in symptomatic patients in whom the weight-bearing dome of the fem-

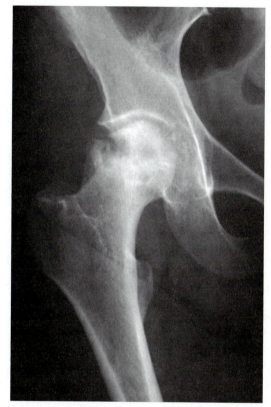

Figure 6–10. Advanced osteonecrosis of the femoral head.

oral head has collapsed. At the time of surgery, it is difficult to be certain of the damage to the acetabular cartilage, which, if present, would necessitate total hip replacement. Hemiarthroplasty, cemented or uncemented, or surface replacement of the femoral head and acetabulum usually is required.

The complications of hip replacement and hemiarthroplasty include loosening of the femoral or acetabular prosthesis, which is the most frequent adverse consequence, and infection on rare occasions. Sciatic or femoral nerve injury occurs rarely. Loose prostheses can be revised. An infected arthroplasty requires debridement of the prosthesis, appropriate antibiotics, and depending on whether the infection has been eradicated, reinsertion of a prosthesis.

REFERENCES

Beaule PE, Amstutz HC: Management of Ficat stage III and IV osteonecrosis of the hip. J Am Acad Orthop Surg 2004;12:96 [PMID: 15089083].

Lai KA et al: The use of alendronate to prevent early collapse of the femoral head in patients with nontraumatic osteonecrosis: A randomized clinical study. J Bone Joint Surg Am 2005;87: 2155 [PMID: 1620387].

3. Osteoarthritis of the Hip

The cause of primary osteoarthritis of the hip is an underlying genetic predisposition. Secondary osteoarthritis results from mechanical stress applied to an anatomically abnormal hip, such as in congenital hip disease where there is deficient acetabular coverage. Femoral head deformity in Legg-Perthes disease or slipping capital femoral epiphyses are infrequent causes of hip osteoarthritis.

The disease has a definite genetic basis but may be first noticed in the workplace. Repeated subliminal trauma to or overuse of the hip is debated as a causative factor.

Osteoarthritis of the hip occurs in 3–8% of whites, in whom most cases are primary. It is rare among Asians and blacks. Osteoarthritis secondary to congenital hip disease is quite common among native Japanese and is more likely to be symptomatic in the fourth, fifth, and sixth decades (younger patients than in primary osteoarthritis).

The earliest pathologic changes occur in the articular cartilage, with fibrillation, fissuring, and surface cartilage loss. This is followed by the body's attempt at repair through proliferation and replication of existing chondrocytes. Low-grade inflammatory changes occur in the synovium secondarily and in response to cartilage surface degeneration. As the disease progresses, osteophytic projections occur at the margins of the articular cartilage and the periosteum, and there is cartilage loss down to eburnated subchondral bone. This results in an incongruous relationship between the femoral head and acetabulum. Synovial and capsular thickening occurring along with the incongruous bony relationship contributes to restricted joint motion.

Clinical Findings

A. SIGNS & SYMPTOMS

Patients gradually become aware of pain with activity. The pain may be felt in the groin, proximal thigh, trochanteric region, or lateral buttock. Rarely, patients complain of pain only in the distal thigh or knee. Early in the course of the disease, patients may not be aware of a subtle hip limp (antalgic gait or abductor lurch during weight bearing on the affected side). As the disease progresses, they may be awakened at night with hip pain, which is usually what causes them to seek medical evaluation.

Restricted hip motion is seen on clinical examination. The earliest loss is internal rotation, followed by loss of abduction and flexion. With long-standing symptoms, patients may have obvious thigh atrophy.

B. IMAGING

Plain-film radiographs demonstrate the characteristic changes of osteoarthritis—joint space narrowing, subchondral sclerosis, and marginal osteophytes.

Treatment

In the early stages of the disease, an anti-inflammatory drug such as diclofenac sodium (Voltaren, 50 mg twice daily) or ibuprofen (800 mg three times daily) may provide symptomatic relief. Using a cane in the hand on the unaffected side or protecting the hip by using two crutches is beneficial. Patients who experience unrelieved pain at night or increasing symptoms will require total hip replacement.

REFERENCE

Zhang W et al: EULAR evidence-based recommendations for the management of hip osteoarthritis. Ann Rheum Dis 2005;64:669 [PMID: 15471891].

INJURIES OF THE KNEE, ANKLE, & FOOT

1. Prepatellar & Infrapatellar Bursitis

Local trauma, such as that resulting from a direct blow or from kneeling repeatedly (e.g., scrubbing floors), can produce prepatellar bursitis, characterized by pain, tenderness, and irritation of or bleeding into the pancake-shaped bursa overlying the patella. In no form of prepatellar bursitis is there evidence of knee joint effusion indicating intraarticular involvement.

Priests, carpenters who lay flooring, and other workers who kneel over the region of the tibial tubercle may experience similar trauma resulting in infrapatellar bursitis. Superficial infrapatellar bursitis causes diffuse swelling over the tibial tubercle and lower portion of the patellar ligament. Deep infrapatellar bursitis is dumbbell-shaped because the patellar ligament compresses its center.

The treatment of prepatellar or infrapatellar bursitis is usually symptomatic. Knee flexion and kneeling are avoided, and the knee may be splinted in extension when symptoms are severe. Occasionally, prepatellar bursitis may be septic and require diagnostic aspiration, antibiotic treatment, and surgical drainage.

2. Pes Anserinus Bursitis & Tibial Collateral Ligament Bursitis

Bursitis can occur beneath the tibial collateral ligament or beneath the pes anserinus insertion. The usual cause is kneeling or direct trauma.

Signs and symptoms include local pain and tenderness. Swelling may be minimal. The symptoms frequently are attributed to meniscal pathology because a torn meniscus produces similar symptoms. Plain radiographs are taken to rule out other bone lesions. The diagnosis can be confirmed by a local injection of 3 cc lidocaine with 40 mg Kenalog (triamcinolone acetonide), which also may be curative.

3. Chondromalacia Patellae

Chondromalacia patellae is characterized by fibrillation or roughening of the undersurface of the patellar articular cartilage, usually on the medial facet. It occurs much more frequently in growing females than in growing males, but it also may occur during the young-adult years. The articular cartilage changes generally are nonprogressive.

Symptoms of anterior knee pain may begin spontaneously or with a direct blow to the patella. They tend to be intermittent and usually are not associated with knee joint effusion. The pain occurs with activity, is usually more severe when descending than when ascending stairs, and is relieved by rest. It can be reproduced during clinical examination by depressing the patella at the patellofemoral groove against active quadriceps contraction. Other causes of knee disorders need to be ruled out by physical examination of the knee and plain-film radiographs.

In most cases of chondromalacia, treatment consists of instructing patients to do active isometric quadriceps exercises with the knee in extension and to protect the knee by avoiding kneeling, squatting, and activities that cause discomfort. An elastic patella support may be helpful. Tracking of the patella should be noted. Controlled contractions of the quadriceps with emphasis on the vastus medialis can be helpful. Symptoms generally are self-limited, lasting for just a few weeks. However, if the patella is frankly subluxing and causing articular damage at the patellofemoral joint, patellar realignment surgery may be necessary.

REFERENCE

Elias DA, White LM: Imaging of patellofemoral disorders. Clin Radiol 2004;59:543 [PMID: 15208060].

4. Popliteal Cyst (Baker Cyst)

A cystic swelling medial to the head of the gastrocnemius muscle in the popliteal fossa is almost always related to intraarticular pathology. Osteoarthritis and meniscal disease are common causes. The cysts are the result of the overflow of synovial fluid from the knee joint.

Clinical Findings

Symptoms include pain and a feeling of fullness in the popliteal fossa. Patients may not be aware of any ante-

rior joint symptoms, for example, the torn meniscus, osteoarthritis, and rheumatoid arthritis. Swelling from the cyst may wax and wane along with the amount of joint fluid in the anterior knee joint.

Treatment

Treatment is directed at the primary intraarticular problem.

5. Tears & Internal Derangements of the Meniscus

Traumatic injury to the meniscus may occur at any age, although it occurs most commonly in young male athletes. Some meniscal injuries result from an apparent minor twisting of the lower extremity or even from sudden twisting of the knee while squatting. Injuries are much more common in the medial than in the lateral, more mobile meniscus and can range in severity from those that cause little damage and manifest relatively minor pain to those that displace the large bucket handle of the meniscus and cause frank catching and locking of the joint. The meniscus becomes stiffer with age, and symptoms may result from degenerative tears that occur in the fourth or fifth decade.

Approximately 20% of patients with excised menisci develop radiographic changes of joint-space narrowing, and some progress to degenerative arthritis in the vacant compartment. Postmortem studies demonstrate that torn menisci left in place are unrelated to degenerative arthritis of the knee joint and, conversely, that degenerative arthritis of the knee joint can occur in the absence of meniscal injury. Therefore, there is no late risk of osteoarthritis from leaving a torn but asymptomatic meniscus in place.

Clinical Findings

Symptoms and signs of a torn meniscus include pain at the extremes of motion and local tenderness at the joint line over the involved meniscus. McMurray sign (rotation of the tibia on the femur when moving the knee from flexion to extension) is rarely positive. Diagnosis can be confirmed by MRI and, more definitively, by arthroscopic examination.

Treatment

After the initial pain decreases from the acute injury, active range-of-motion exercises should be progressed to resistance exercises. Patients who continue to manifest symptoms after a prolonged period of conservative therapy require surgery. When the tear is located peripherally, where there is vascularity and thus healing is possible, repair is accomplished through arthroscopy. Arthroscopic debridement is performed for marginal lesions. Because long-term osteoarthritis is associated with total meniscal excision, this procedure should be avoided.

6. Knee Ligament Injuries

Knee ligament injuries can result from indirect force such as a fall or misstep or from a direct blow. They are seen most commonly in young athletes who engage in contact sports, but they also occur in the workplace. The injuries range from simple strain to frank disruption in which the ligament is torn in its substance or avulsed from its bony attachment.

First-degree injury is a tear involving a few fibers of the ligament. The knee is tender on palpation but shows no instability and demonstrates no excessive motion when force is applied. Second-degree injury, which is a partial tear of the ligament, also causes no instability. Third-degree injury is a complete tear or disruption of the ligament that does result in joint instability. The different ligaments of the knee can be injured individually or in combination.

Diagnosis

Accurate diagnosis of knee ligament injuries requires considerable experience and depends on a careful history, a detailed physical examination of the joint, and special imaging techniques. Severe pain may interfere with proper physical examination, in which case MRI is indicated.

The most common knee ligament injuries are to the medial collateral and anterior cruciate ligaments or some combination of the two. Lateral collateral ligament and posterior cruciate ligament injuries are less common. Plain-film radiographs are obtained and usually are negative for bone injury. MRI can specify the nature and location of ligament disruption as well as provide evidence of injury to the meniscus, articular cartilage, and bone.

In addition to the usual evaluation of knee motion and detection of the presence of ecchymosis and local swelling, the various ligaments in the knee are tested by stressing the joint in different directions. Such stress can manifest instability and indicate which ligaments are involved. Valgus and varus stresses with the knee flexed at 15 degrees test the medial and lateral collateral ligaments, respectively. Anterior cruciate stability is tested by the anterior drawer, Lachman, and pivot-shift tests. The posterior drawer test is specific for the posterior cruciate ligament. Stress tests that can demonstrate opening of the joint also may be necessary.

Common Types of Knee Ligament Injuries

A. INJURIES OF THE MEDIAL COLLATERAL LIGAMENT

The most frequent mechanism of injury is indirect force that applies valgus stress to the knee. On examination, there may be evidence of local hemorrhage or

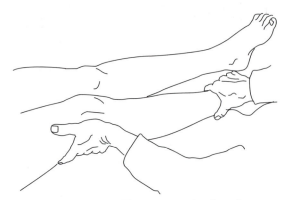

Figure 6–11. Collateral ligament testing for valgus stress to the knee.

effusion into the joint (Figure 6–11). Tenderness usually can be demonstrated at the site of ligamentous injury, at the site of attachment of the ligament in the region of the medial epicondyle, or along the ligament one handbreadth below the joint line at its distal attachment on the tibia. The degree of instability can be determined by applying valgus stress to the joint in full extension and at 20 degrees of flexion. Any instability detected by opening of the medial joint space is indicative of medial collateral ligament injury. Instability noted in full extension indicates medial collateral ligament injury plus additional injury involving the anterior cruciate ligament, the posterior capsule, or both.

B. INJURIES OF THE ANTERIOR CRUCIATE LIGAMENT

The mechanism of injury of the anterior cruciate ligament (ACL) is that of a force applied to a decelerating and twisting knee or sudden hyperextension. At the time of injury, patients experience a perceptible pop, followed by an effusion (blood that arises slowly and is maximal at 24 hours). The ACL is stretched or torn against the outlet of the bony intercondylar notch. The ligament usually is torn in its substance (interstitial) and rarely avulsed from either bony insertion. Anterior cruciate ligament injuries commonly accompany medial collateral ligament injuries when significant force is applied to the knee in abduction, flexion, and internal rotation. Medial menisci may be injured along with the medial collateral and anterior cruciate ligaments.

1. Signs & Symptoms—Physical examination reveals evidence of an intraarticular (bloody) effusion and pain with limited knee motion. The Lachman test will be positive. This involves flexing the knee 20 degrees and manually translating the leg forward (Figure 6–12). The amount of displacement will depend on whether there is a partial or complete tear and whether there is disruption of other joint capsule restraints.

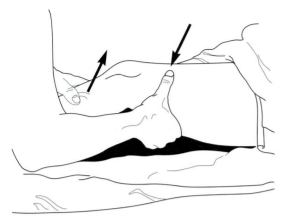

Figure 6–12. The Lachman test for anterior cruciate ligament insufficiency. The thigh is stabilized with a posteriorly directed force, and the tibia is subluxed anteriorly.

2. Imaging—An MRI can confirm specific ACL or other joint pathology.

Treatment

First- and second-degree medial collateral injuries can be treated symptomatically with crutches and a knee immobilizer. Third-degree injuries have been treated effectively with cast immobilization or cast bracing and rarely are treated by open surgical repair. The goal of treatment for medial collateral ligament tear is to restore normal range of motion and increase the strength of the muscles around the knee, particularly the vastus medialis.

In an athlete or a young person with a tear of the anterior cruciate ligament, arthroscopic intraarticular or open extraarticular ACL reconstruction usually is done. In any patient who is symptomatic with episodes of giving way, surgical reconstruction will restore stability. Guided physical therapy is important after ACL repair.

REFERENCES

Cummings JR, Pedowitz RA: Knee instability: The orthopedic approach. Semin Musculoskelet Radiol 2005;9:5 [PMID: 15812708].

Haddad FS, Oussedik SI: Cruciate ligament reconstruction. Hosp Med 2004;65:412 [PMID: 15287345].

Quarles JD, Hosey RG: Medial and lateral collateral injuries: Prognosis and treatment. Primary Care 2004;31:957 [PMID: 15544829].

C. OSTEOARTHRITIS OF THE KNEE

Osteoarthritis of the knee is a group of clinical entities including localized chondral defects and diffuse cartilage disease caused by biologic predisposition, injury, or biomechanical failure of hyaline cartilage. Genetic factors appear to be involved in the absence of specific insult, in which case the disease is termed *primary. Secondary* osteoarthritis may occur after injuries such as an intraarticular fracture, ligamentous instability, or meniscal injury.

Radiographic findings of knee osteoarthritis are common in the working population; they are found in at least 25% of the population older than 50 years of age.

1. Clinical Findings and Treatment—Minor strains of the mildly osteoarthritic knee may produce symptoms of pain, swelling, and restricted motion. Plain radiographs are diagnostic. The symptoms usually resolve within a couple of weeks with rest or modified activity. Acetaminophen or NSAIDs are helpful in reducing pain. Arthroscopy has no role in treatment of the osteoarthritic knee. For patients with persistent symptoms, oral glucosamine and chondroitin sulfate, local corticosteroid injection, or viscosupplementation (Figure 6–13) may be helpful. For advanced knee osteoarthritis, when patients cannot tolerate the limitations of walking or night pain, surgical treatment is offered. In younger patients, a realignment osteotomy can be done for varus or valgus deformity. Total knee replacement is the gold standard for older patients.

REFERENCES

Dervin GF et al: Effect of arthroscopic debridement for osteoarthritis of the knee on health-related quality of life. J Bone Joint Surg Am 2003;85:10 [PMID: 12533566].

Lingard EA et al: Predicting the outcome of total knee arthroplasty. J Bone Joint Surg Am 2004;86:2179 [PMID: 15466726].

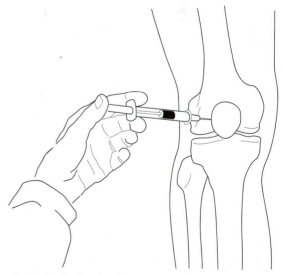

Figure 6–13. Needle placement into the intraarticular space of the knee. The needle is inserted from the lateral side beneath the patella with the knee in extension.

7. Ankle Sprains (Sprains of the Lateral Collateral Ligament Complex)

The lateral collateral ligament complex of the ankle consists of seven ligaments that attach the fibula to the tibia, talus, and calcaneus. An inversion injury with or without the foot in plantar flexion may strain or sprain the anterior talofibular ligament, which is the ligament most commonly injured. When this happens, tenderness will be present, as will local swelling at either the anterolateral neck of the talus or the tip of the fibula. A stronger external force may disrupt the posterior talofibular ligament, the calcaneofibular ligament, or the tibiofibular ligaments that account for the ligamentous stability of the ankle mortise.

Clinical Findings

Depending on the seriousness of the injury, pain can range in severity from minimal on weight bearing to severe enough to make walking impossible. Local swelling and tenderness will be present at the site of ligament damage. Fibular fractures or tibiofibular ligament disruptions can be ruled out with plain-film radiographs. Stress films of the ankle to determine the degree of tilt of the talus can be obtained but are not usually indicated.

Treatment

Treatment of ankle sprains usually consists of relieving the symptoms by supporting the ankle with an elastic bandage or adhesive strapping. Decreased weight bearing with crutches while maintaining a normal pattern of gait is usually successful. In more severe cases, the patient is immobilized for 2–3 weeks in a below-knee ankle-foot orthosis (AFO) that allows weight bearing, which is followed by appropriate exercise instruction. Prolonged immobilization is to be avoided. Surgery is not indicated unless there is ligamentous injury causing disruption of the ankle mortise. For patients treated conservatively with delayed recovery, the usual cause is muscle atrophy requiring judicious physical therapy.

In rare cases, a patient will have persistent instability that is impossible to predict at the initial evaluation. When this instability occurs, secondary end-to-end repair of the anterior talofibular ligament (Broström procedure) may be indicated.

REFERENCE

Anandacoomarasamy A, Barnsley L: Long-term outcomes of inversion ankle injuries. Br J Sports Med 2005;39:14 [PMID: 15728682].

8. Avulsion Fractures of the Fifth Metatarsal

Avulsion fractures of the tip of the fifth metatarsal are produced by inversion injuries to the foot and ankle, usually when the ankle is flexed. They occur commonly in athletes and dancers but also may occur in anyone who, for example, steps into a hole or trips.

In contrast with ankle sprain, an avulsion fracture does not cause tenderness about the fibular malleolus. Instead, it causes local tenderness and swelling over the base of the fifth metatarsal. Location of the fracture site can be confirmed by radiograph.

Treatment consists of relieving symptoms. Wearing a stiff-soled shoe, including a doughnut pad to relieve the pressure on the fracture site, is sufficient for patients whose symptoms are minimal. More severe injuries and symptoms may call for immobilization in a short-leg walking cast for 4–6 weeks. Nonunion of this fracture is rare. A true Jones fracture—a transverse fracture across the full base of the metatarsal—can result in delayed union and even nonunion.

REFERENCE

Rammelt S et al: Metatarsal fractures. Injury 2004;35:77 [PMID: 15315882].

9. Plantar Fasciitis (Medial Calcaneal Tubercle Bursitis)

Pain affecting the plantar aspect of the medial heel may develop spontaneously or may occur after direct trauma to the area or after impact on the heel. Patients are comfortable at rest, but pain returns with weight bearing and is especially severe when the patient gets out of bed in the morning.

Clinical examination reveals exquisite local tenderness over the medial calcaneal tubercle, which is the site of plantar fascial attachment. Lateral radiographs usually show a spur that projects from the calcaneus and has been present for many years. This suggests that the more recent local symptoms are due to bursitis in the area or to traction on the plantar fascia.

Wearing heel cushions can minimize impact on the heel and relieve symptoms. Use of a soft heel cup or local cortisone injection is helpful, as is the use of a shoe insert with a medial wedge that maintains the heel at a slightly varus angle and reduces traction on the plantar fascia. The use of a dorsiflexion brace worn at night should be tried. Conservative treatment is effective in more than 90% of patients.

REFERENCE

Cohen RS, Balcom TA: Current treatment options for ankle injuries: Lateral ankle sprain, Achilles tendonitis, and Achilles rupture. Curr Sports Med Rep 2003;2:251 [PMID: 12959705].

10. Interdigital Neuritis (Morton Neuroma)

Interdigital neuritis of the plantar digital nerve branches to the second or third interspaces is caused by inflammation and is not a true neuroma. The etiology is not proven but is likely related to mechanical factors. It occurs more frequently in middle-age women. Patients complain of pain and burning and tingling of the involved toes. Pain is produced by direct pressure on the neuroma, which is located between the second and third web spaces and is aggravated by dorsiflexing the toe, such as during the push-off phase of gait or when wearing high-heeled shoes. Patients frequently describe the pain as radiating into the toes.

On clinical examination, a small "click" usually can be felt as pressure is applied to the second and third web spaces while the examiner passively dorsiflexes the toes. The click may disappear temporarily after the initial manipulation. Diagnosis usually can be confirmed by local nerve block.

Treatment with metatarsal pads or low-heeled, well-fitting shoes should be tried. Surgical excision of the neuroma or release of the transverse ligament may be necessary.

REFERENCE

Thomson CE, Gibson JN, Martin D: Interventions for the treatment of Morton's neuroma. Cochrane Database Syst Rev. 2004;(3):CD003118 [PMID: 15266472].

11. Osteochondral Lesions of the Talar Dome

Osteochondral lesions of the medial or lateral aspect of the dome of the talus are usually the result of trauma, but ischemic necrosis and endocrine disorders may be responsible. Symptoms include pain, swelling, and catching about the ankle. Typical findings may include signs and symptoms similar to a lateral or medial ankle sprain.

Imaging

Standard plain radiographs of the ankle usually will identify the osteochondral defect; however, an MRI may be necessary.

Treatment

When osteochondral acute fractures are recognized initially, they are treated by immobilization. Displaced lesions with a free fragment may require replacement and fixation, which can be done arthroscopically. Chronic lesions are treated expectantly with temporary mobilization and observation. Patients not responding may require surgical treatment, such as fragment excision, replacement, drilling, or bone grafting.

REFERENCE

Schachter AK et al: Osteochondral lesions of the talus. J Am Acad Orthop Surg 2005;13:152 [PMID: 15938604].

Peripheral Nerve Injuries

7

Yuen T. So, MD, PhD

The term *peripheral neuropathy* encompasses a wide spectrum of disorders that involve sensory, motor, or autonomic nerve fibers. Clinically important diseases include nerve trauma, nerve entrapment, genetic disorders, nerve ischemia, and inflammatory neuropathies, as well as neuropathies associated with systemic diseases such as diabetes, alcoholism, collagen-vascular diseases, cancer, uremia, and hypothyroidism.

Occupational exposures affect peripheral nerves in two possible ways. First, excessive exposure to many industrial or environmental chemicals causes a generalized nerve disorder. This is characterized typically by simultaneous involvement of numerous peripheral nerves and manifests as a diffuse and symmetric clinical syndrome. Second, some occupations may predispose workers to physical injuries to peripheral nerves. Single nerves or spinal roots are affected in these instances, leading to a focal or localized pattern of neurologic symptoms and signs. The term *polyneuropathy* is used often to refer to the former, in contrast to *mononeuropathy* or *focal neuropathy,* which often is a result of physical injuries. Neurotoxins, diabetes, and alcoholism are examples of disorders that result in polyneuropathy. Neuropathies related to toxins are discussed in Chapter 24. This chapter is devoted to focal neuropathies.

GENERAL PRINCIPLES

Symptoms of focal neuropathies fall into two categories: motor and sensory disturbances. When severe enough, focal nerve injury leads to weakness and atrophy of muscles innervated by the affected nerve. The pattern of weakness is frequently the most useful clue for anatomic localization of nerve injuries. Sensory symptoms include hypesthesias (diminished sensation), paresthesias (altered sensation), and pain. The distribution of sensory dysfunction usually approximates the cutaneous innervation of the involved nerve and provides a useful clue for anatomic localization. A notable exception is pain. Pain may be caused by tendinitis, arthritis, or other rheumatologic or orthopedic disease. Even when it is caused by a nerve injury, its location may be distant from the site of nerve involvement (referred pain).

Even minor derangement of peripheral nerves causes paresthesias. It has been shown experimentally that abnormal firing of a single sensory nerve fiber may lead

to a perceptible tingling. Paresthesia is thus a sensitive indicator of neuropathy. Except in very severe nerve injuries such as trauma, marked loss of sensation is uncommon and is encountered rarely in the occupational setting. Patients may use the term *numbness* to refer to paresthesia rather than a true loss of sensation. Genuine loss of sensation (i.e., an elevated threshold of stimulus detection) is not easy to demonstrate by bedside examination without elaborate tools. As with sensory symptoms, the perception of weakness is very observer-dependent. Pain and sensory disturbances often mislead a patient to report weakness even when muscle strength is intact. Complaints of weakness always should be followed by careful clinical examination.

The temporal pattern of sensory symptoms provides useful diagnostic clues. Entrapment neuropathies such as carpal tunnel syndrome and ulnar neuropathy at the elbow typically cause tingling and numbness that fluctuate through the course of a day. The pressure within an anatomically confined space (carpal tunnel for median nerve and cubital tunnel for ulnar nerve) increases with flexion or extension of the joints. Increased pressure contributes to mechanical irritation and ischemia of the nerve leading to sensory symptoms. Careful inquiry frequently reveals a strong correlation between symptoms and physical activities or postures of the involved limb (Table 7–1). Such a history of exacerbation is useful in distinguishing entrapment neuropathies from the polyneuropathy of systemic diseases (e.g., diabetic and alcoholic neuropathies). The latter tends to give sensory symptoms that are relatively constant.

Some patients may be inherently more susceptible to physical injuries of peripheral nerves. Women, for example, usually have a smaller carpal tunnel size than men; the difference explains in part the increased incidence of carpal tunnel syndrome in women. Some polyneuropathies predispose peripheral nerves to mechanical injury. The most dramatic example is a hereditary disorder of peripheral nerve myelin called by the descriptive name of *hereditary neuropathy with increased liability to pressure palsy* (HNPP). A far more common example is encountered in patients with diabetes mellitus. Not only do many diabetic patients develop a polyneuropathy, but these patients also are more susceptible to entrapment neuropathies than the general population.

72

Table 7–1. Occupational entrapment neuropathies.

Syndrome	Entrapment Site	Occupational Predisposition
Carpal tunnel syndrome	Carpal tunnel (just distal to wrist crease)	Repetitive/forceful finger flexion or wrist movement Sustained abnormal wrist posture Others (see Table 7–2)
Ulnar neuropathy at elbow	Cubital tunnel or condylar groove	Elbow flexion Repetitive elbow movements Leaning on elbow
Ulnar neuropathy at wrist	At or near Guyon canal	Leaning on wrist Repetitive pounding with hands
Thoracic outlet syndrome	Anomalous cervical rib or fibrous band compressing lower trunk of brachial plexus	Carrying heavy objects (e.g. suitcases, bags) Sustained arm raising above shoulder

Approach to Patients

History taking should focus on the nature of sensory and motor symptoms. "Numbness," "tingling," "prickly," and "pins and needles" often are used interchangeably by patients. Pain, if present, should be documented by its character and location. The term *weakness* may mean different symptoms to different observers and never should be taken at face value. The distribution of symptoms is important. Asymmetric onset of symptoms or asymmetric pattern of involvement helps to confirm the focal nature of a neuropathy. The history taking also must include a detailed probe of all possible exacerbating factors. For upper extremity symptoms, these may include neck turning, coughing, driving, sleeping, carrying a heavy shoulder bag, or any prolonged or forceful use of the hands or arms. For lower extremity symptoms, these may include bending, twisting, Valsalva maneuver, prolonged walking, or standing.

Physical examination should include assessment of sensation, strength, and tendon reflexes in the affected limbs. Cutaneous sensation is tested by stimuli of light touch, pin prick, or cold temperature. Altered sensation in the distribution of an affected nerve can be very helpful. However, the sensory examination is subjective and depends on a patient's ability to observe and report. The clinician should resist the temptation to depend excessively on published maps of cutaneous innervation. They provide rough guidance at best. Muscle strength testing in the hands of skilled clinicians provides additional information. Each muscle should be tested individually. Focal weakness, if present, provides a reliable sign for localization of nerve lesion. Readers should refer to the many excellent texts on peripheral neuroanatomy.

Diagnostic Tools

Nerve conduction study and electromyography (EMG) are important laboratory tools in the evaluation of focal neuropathies. Nerve conduction studies are performed by electrical stimulation of a nerve at different sites along its course. Parameters such as nerve conduction velocity and response amplitude measure nerve function. In many focal neuropathies, the site of the lesion is identified by focal slowing in nerve conduction velocity or by reduction in amplitude of the nerve response. EMG is performed by inserting a needle electrode into skeletal muscles to record their electrical activities. Fibrillation potentials and positive sharp waves are seen in denervated muscle fibers. Denervation also may be indicated by a reduction in the number of recorded motor-unit action potentials. There are also electromyographic signs of reinnervation to help identify a chronic nerve lesion; in such cases, the amplitude and duration of the motor-unit action potentials are increased abnormally. Nerve conduction studies and EMG often are performed together. The term *electromyography* loosely refers to both tests, even though, strictly speaking, electromyography means only the needle electromyographic examination of muscles.

There are several drawbacks to nerve conduction and EMG studies. These tests are uncomfortable at best, with occasional patients tolerating them poorly. Another drawback is the need to use specialized and expensive equipment. Although simplified electronic devices have been advocated, especially in the setting of occupational health screening (e.g., screening for carpal tunnel syndrome), there is an unavoidable compromise in accuracy. Proper interpretation and performance of these tests require specialized training. Unfortunately, the expertise of providers varies greatly. Misleading conclusions may result from improper performance and interpretation of these tests.

Quantitative sensory testing employs specially designed equipment for delivery of calibrated vibratory, light touch, thermal, or electrical stimuli. The subject is asked to report perception of the stimuli according to a specific test paradigm. As with the bedside sensory examination, quantitative sensory testing depends on patient cooperation. Therefore, it does not provide truly objective information. There are two advantages to quantitative sensory testing. First, it reduces the interobserver variability and may be administered successfully by paramedical personnel. Second, it provides quantitative data that are suitable for comparison with the normal population and for longitudinal assessment of patients. Thermal sensation testing has an additional benefit of assessing small-diameter sensory nerve fibers that are not tested at all by conventional EMG and nerve conduction studies.

Ultrasonography is gaining acceptance in the imaging of peripheral nerves, especially for visualization of the nerve at sites of entrapment, such as the carpal tunnel and the ulnar groove. Ultrasonography typically reveals enlargement and change in the echogenicity of compressed nerve. Resolution of these abnormalities may follow successful decompression, providing a way to follow patients in the course of treatment.

Magnetic resonance imaging (MRI) and computed tomography (CT) are important adjunctive tools to evaluate focal neuropathies. They are employed most frequently to assess cervical and lumbar radiculopathies, conditions that mimic entrapment neuropathies. The advancement of technology has permitted unprecedented visualization of the spinal cord, nerve roots, and bony structures. The main limitation is their relative lack of specificity in diagnosing symptomatic disease. Asymptomatic but radiologically significant spondylitic disease is seen frequently in the normal population. Varying degree of MRI or CT abnormalities are encountered in more than 50% of asymptomatic subjects older than 50 years of age and in approximately 20% of those younger than 50 years of age. Thus imaging studies should never replace a careful clinical evaluation.

REFERENCES

Beekman R, Visser LH: High-resolution sonography of the peripheral nervous system: A review of the literature. Eur J Neurol 2004; 11:305 [PMID: 15142223].

Bonfiglioli R et al: Course of symptoms and median nerve conduction values in workers performing repetitive jobs at risk for carpal tunnel syndrome. Occup Med (Lond) 2006;56:115 [PMID: 16371398].

Ilkhani M et al: Accuracy of somatosensory evoked potentials in diagnosis of mild idiopathic carpal tunnel syndrome. Clin Neurol Neurosurg 2005;108:40 [PMID: 16311144].

OCCUPATIONAL FOCAL NEUROPATHIES

1. Carpal Tunnel Syndrome

Carpal tunnel syndrome is by far the most common entrapment neuropathy. The median nerve and the flexor

Table 7–2. Causes of carpal tunnel syndrome.

Reduced carpal tunnel size
Fractures
Gout
Rheumatoid
Tenosynovitis
Increased nerve susceptibility
Diabetes mellitus
Hereditary neuropathy with liability to pressure palsy
Uremia
Possibly other polyneuropathies
Extrinsic masses at or near carpal tunnel
Ganglia
Hematoma
Osteophytes
Other conditions
Acromegaly
Amyloidosis
Hypothyroidism
Pregnancy

digitorum tendons pass through the carpal tunnel. The transverse carpal ligament forms the roof of the tunnel. Symptomatic median nerve entrapment is associated with reduced carpal tunnel size, increased nerve susceptibility, extrinsic masses compressing the median nerve, and some systemic diseases (Table 7–2). The dominant hand is affected more often and more severely in most patients. Repetitive and forceful use of the hands and fingers exacerbate symptoms of carpal tunnel syndrome. As one might imagine, a number of occupations predispose workers to increased symptoms. A substantial proportion of cases also occur in patients who do not have an at-risk occupation or another identifiable risk factor.

If patient reporting is reliable, a confident diagnosis can be made just on the basis of the history. A diagnostically useful feature is intermittent paresthesia of the hand and fingers. Paresthesia may be worse at night, awakening the patient from sleep, or may be exacerbated after prolonged use of the hands. Paresthesia is often most prominent in the median-innervated fingers (the first three digits and the lateral half of the ring finger), although approximately half of all patients report symptoms in all five fingers. Pain usually is localized to the hand and wrist but also may be referred to the forearm and even the shoulder. Prominent pain may suggest another superimposed condition such as tenosynovitis or arthritis. Pain alone without paresthesia is seldom due to carpal tunnel syndrome.

Although it is common for patients to complain of hand weakness or an increased tendency to drop objects held in the hand, objective weakness is either absent or mild in the majority of patients. The finger flexor muscles responsible for hand grip are supplied by branches of the median nerve in the forearm and therefore are spared by a lesion at the carpal tunnel. Weakness is detectable in the median-innervated thenar muscles (abductor pollicis brevis and opponens pollicis) in severe cases. Likewise, thenar atrophy is seen only in advanced disease.

Increased tingling or numbness to percussion of the median nerve at the carpal tunnel (Tinel sign) or to 1-minute flexion of the wrist (Phalen sign) is present in approximately two-thirds of patients with carpal tunnel syndrome. However, they are not pathognomonic signs of carpal tunnel syndrome because false-positive results are common. Tendon reflexes, as well as the remainder of the neurologic examination, are normal unless a superimposed cervical radiculopathy or polyneuropathy is present.

Diagnostic Investigations

Nerve conduction and EMG studies can document the disorder when the history is uncertain, assess the severity of the nerve pathology, and provide confirmation as well as a baseline prior to treatment. Focal slowing of sensory nerve conduction velocity at the carpal tunnel is the earliest and most specific sign. Other median nerve conduction abnormalities are present in more severe cases. Ulnar nerve conduction studies should be performed as a control and should be normal unless a polyneuropathy or a concurrent ulnar neuropathy is present. Sometimes cervical radiculopathy may be present as a confounding factor. Needle EMG evaluation of the cervical myotomes should be carried out in such cases. Electrodiagnostic studies are abnormal in approximately 70–90% of patients with unequivocal carpal tunnel syndrome. The yield is probably lower in patients with only mild symptoms, although the sensitivity of the test is difficult to ascertain because of the absence of a suitable gold standard for comparison. Quantitative sensory testing (e.g., vibrometer, neurometer, etc.) and thermography have been used as alternatives to routine electrodiagnostic studies. Present data are inconclusive and do not support their routine use in patient management.

Treatment

The choice of treatment depends on the certainty of the diagnosis and the severity of symptoms and neurologic deficits. Most symptomatic patients benefit from prophylactic work restrictions in combination with partial immobilization using wrist splints. Additional benefits may be provided by injection of corticosteroids near the carpal tunnel. This should be performed by experienced personnel because injection injury to the median nerve is a rare but well-recognized complication. However, multiple injections are to be avoided because corticosteroids weaken the flexor tendons and predispose them

to later rupture. Short-term use of an oral steroid, such as 10–20 mg prednisone per day for 2 weeks, may give a modest temporary relief. Oral nonsteroidal anti-inflammatory agents, systemic diuretics, and pyridoxine (vitamin B_6) are of unproven benefit.

Persistent and disabling symptoms, neurologic deficits on physical examination, and moderate to severe nerve conduction abnormalities suggest moderate or advanced disease. Most of these patients eventually require surgical treatment. All that is needed in surgery is division of the transverse carpal ligament. Surgical dressings typically are removed in a few days, and most patients recover fully from the procedure within 6 weeks.

Incomplete relief of symptoms after surgery may be a result of incorrect preoperative diagnosis, incomplete section of the transverse ligament, or other causal etiologies that are untreated. Some patients develop recurrent symptoms after a period of initial success. Possible causes include postoperative fibrosis and progressive tenosynovitis. Degenerative arthritis, iatrogenic injury to the median nerve, and other complications such as complex regional pain syndrome are also possible after surgery. Patients on workers' compensation may have less-favorable treatment outcome.

REFERENCES

Bland JD: Carpal tunnel syndrome. Curr Opin Neurol 2005; 18:581 [PMID: 16155444].

Daniell WE et al: Work-related carpal tunnel syndrome in Washington State workers' compensation: Temporal trends, clinical practices, and disability. Am J Ind Med 2005;48:259 [PMID: 16142733].

El-Karabaty H et al: The effect of carpal tunnel release on median nerve flattening and nerve conduction. Electromyogr Clin Neurophysiol 2005;45:223 [PMID: 16083145].

Gooch CL, Mitten DJ: Treatment of carpal tunnel syndrome: Is there a role for local corticosteroid injection? Neurology 2005;64:2006 [PMID: 15985566].

2. Ulnar Neuropathy

Ulnar nerve dysfunction usually manifests as weakness and atrophy of the intrinsic hand muscles and tingling in the little and ring fingers. The presenting history is variable. Some patients present solely with paresthesia, whereas others present only with weakness and atrophy. Not infrequently, patients come to medical condition only after someone else, frequently a medical provider, notices atrophy of the intrinsic hand muscles. Sensory disturbances are often intermittent and vary from day to day. They may worsen with prolonged elbow flexion or with repetitive elbow flexion and extension. Most ulnar neuropathies are associated with little or no pain. Pain, if present, usually is referred to the elbow. Some patients may awaken at night with elbow pain and hand numbness. These nocturnal symptoms may be confused with those of carpal tunnel syndrome. Weakness of hand grasp and thumb pinch occasionally may be part of the presenting syndrome. Most patients, however, are only aware of a generalized loss of dexterity or strength and are unable to identify the specific weak muscles.

Advanced cases are readily diagnosed on physical examination. Muscle atrophy involves all the intrinsic hand muscles with the exception of those in the thenar eminence (innervated by the median nerve). Weakness is demonstrable with pinching using the thumb (adductor pollicis and first dorsal interosseous), abduction of the index finger (first dorsal interosseous), and abduction of the little finger (abductor digiti minimi). Most ulnar neuropathies are caused by a lesion at the elbow. In such cases, flexion of the ring and little fingers also may be weak (ulnar portion of flexor digitorum profundus). Diagnosis is difficult in milder cases. In many instances it is difficult to distinguish with certainty an ulnar neuropathy from a C8 radiculopathy. Other conditions, such as polyneuropathy and amyotrophic lateral sclerosis, also may be confused with ulnar neuropathy.

Diagnostic Investigations

Although most ulnar neuropathies are caused by an elbow lesion, the nerve also can be compressed at the palm or wrist (Table 7–3). Electrodiagnostic studies provide a reliable means for further anatomic localization. Nerve conduction study may reveal focal slowing of nerve conduction velocity at the site of lesion. The pattern of denervation on EMG studies complements the clinical examination and anatomic localization. MRI studies are also invaluable in identifying signal abnormality in the ulnar nerve or structural lesion of the nerve.

Table 7–3. Causes of ulnar neuropathy.

Ulnar neuropathy at the elbow
  Acute trauma (dislocation, fracture)
  Bony deformity near the elbow (old fractures, supracondylar spur, rheumatoid arthritis, osteoarthritis)
  Entrapment at cubital tunnel syndrome
  External compression (during anesthesias, repeated leaning on elbow)
  Soft-tissue constriction (scar tissue, tumors, masses)
  Leprosy
Ulnar neuropathy at or near wrist
  Acute trauma (dislocation or fracture)
  Bony deformity near the wrist (old fractures, rheumatoid arthritis, osteoarthritis)
  Entrapment at Guyon canal
  External compression (repeated pressure on the palm, e.g., bicycling, certain occupations)
  Soft-tissue constriction (ganglia, scar tissue, tumors, masses)

Treatment

For mild intermittent symptoms, a change of activity and avoidance of leaning on the elbow or the palm may be the only necessary treatment. An elbow pad or splint may help those with a lesion at the elbow. Conservative therapy should be accompanied by careful follow-up. Patients with more severe cases and those who fail conservative therapy are candidates for surgery. Surgery should be preceded by electrodiagnostic confirmation and localization. For those with a lesion at the elbow, the most commonly used procedures are medial epicondylectomy, simple decompression at the cubital tunnel, or anterior transposition of the ulnar nerve. Regardless of the procedure chosen, the most important determinant of outcome is the severity of ulnar neuropathy at the time of surgery. Success rate varies and is highest in those with minimal neurologic deficits.

REFERENCES

Beekman R et al: Ulnar neuropathy at the elbow: Follow-up and prognostic factors determining outcome. Neurology 2004; 63:1675 [PMID: 15534254].

Thibault MW et al: Use of the AAEM guidelines in electrodiagnosis of ulnar neuropathy at the elbow. Am J Phys Med Rehabil 2005;84:267 [PMID: 15785259].

Visser LH et al: Short-segment nerve conduction studies in ulnar neuropathy at the elbow. Muscle Nerve 2005;31:331 [PMID: 15635692].

3. Thoracic Outlet Syndrome

This is likely to be a heterogeneous syndrome. The classic neurologic syndrome is often called the *true neurogenic thoracic outlet syndrome.* This is a rare disorder with paresthesia in the ulnar aspect of the hand and forearm, selective wasting of the thenar eminence, and to a lesser extent, wasting of other intrinsic muscles of the hand. Prior to the advent of electrodiagnostic testing, most patients said to have this syndrome probably had either carpal tunnel syndrome or ulnar neuropathy. Another rare syndrome is caused by angulation and compression of the subclavian artery over an anomalous cervical rib. This is often called *vascular thoracic outlet syndrome.* Typical manifestations are intermittent arm claudication, coldness of the limb, and occasional embolic phenomena in the distal upper extremity.

The most common entity, however, does not fit the true neurogenic or vascular syndromes. These patients present with intermittent pain and paresthesia poorly localized in the arm. Symptoms may worsen with carrying heavy objects in the arm or holding the arm overhead for a prolonged period. There is little evidence to support the idea that vascular compression plays a significant role in this syndrome. Popular clinical tests such as supraclavicular bruit, Adson maneuver, hyperabduction maneuver, and costoclavicular maneuver are all tests for vascular compression and are of limited value. Moreover, positive tests occur in many normal individuals. The remainder of the clinical examination usually is normal. Electrodiagnostic testing is used primarily to exclude other entrapment neuropathies or cervical radiculopathy and is abnormal only in the true neurogenic thoracic outlet syndrome.

For most patients, treatment begins with avoidance of activities that worsen symptoms. Exercises designed to promote proper shoulder and neck posture may help. These consist of strengthening exercises of shoulder girdle muscles and full range of movements of the shoulder and neck.

REFERENCES

Huang JH, Zager EL: Thoracic outlet syndrome. Neurosurgery 2004;55:897 [PMID: 15458598].

Koknel Talul G: Thoracic outlet syndrome. Agri 2005;17:5 [PMID: 15977087].

McGillicuddy JE. Cervical radiculopathy, entrapment neuropathy, and thoracic outlet syndrome: How to differentiate? J Neurosurg Spine 2004;1:179 [PMID: 15347004].

Weir E, Lander L: Hand-arm vibration syndrome. Can Med Assoc J 2005;172:1001 [PMID: 15824402].

Eye Injuries

Allan J. Flach, PharmD, MD

The personal tragedy and economic loss associated with impaired vision or even blindness as a result of occupational eye injuries can be prevented by identifying workers at risk and instituting appropriate safety programs. Proper maintenance of tools and equipment by the employer and effective use of protective devices, such as safety glasses or face shields, by the employee will reduce the number of injuries, such as ocular contusions, trauma as a consequence of penetrating and nonpenetrating foreign bodies, conjunctival and corneal abrasions, lid lacerations, and optic nerve damage.

Recognition of the toxic effects of chemical agents and protection from those that may be splashed into the eyes are vital for prevention of visual damage. The ready availability of facilities for cleansing and irrigation of the face and eyes in the workplace is of the utmost importance because initial steps for treatment of chemical burns—especially those caused by strong alkalis and acids—must be carried out immediately by the employee, fellow workers, or anyone else near at hand. There is no time to wait for specialized medical care, so employee education programs for emergency care of chemical burns are essential.

The risks of ocular damage for x-ray technicians, glassblowers, welders, and other workers exposed to ionizing, infrared, and ultraviolet radiation have long been known, but damage caused by exposure to excessive amounts of visible light has been recognized only recently. Wearing protective lenses that filter the most offending wavelengths of visible light may become commonplace in the future.

ANATOMY & PHYSIOLOGY (Figure 8–1)

A brief review of ocular anatomy and function will help in understanding the mechanisms of several kinds of eye injuries and how they affect the visual system. The orbit, eyelid, and conjunctiva are protective mechanisms for the eye. The orbit and its bony rim offer excellent mechanical protection from injuries, with the exception of those coming from the direct anterior or temporal directions. The eyelid and conjunctiva are essential for normal maintenance of the smooth, moist, clear anterior surface of the cornea, which, in turn, is essential for clear vision. The normal blinking mechanism depends on the third cranial nerve to open the lids and the seventh cranial nerve to close them. Moistening of the conjunctiva by lacrimal fluid depends in part on activation of the reflex arc between the sensory fifth innervation of the anterior eye and the parasympathetic secretomotor fibers that accompany the seventh cranial nerve along the petrous temporal bone into the middle fossa and then through the orbit to the lacrimal gland. Moistening of the corneal epithelium is aided by mucus from the goblet cells of the conjunctiva, particularly those on the tarsus of the upper lid. Reflex tear production by the lacrimal gland helps to dilute and wash away irritating substances that find their way into the conjunctival sac. The rich blood supply of the conjunctiva and lid also helps in resisting and limiting infections of the anterior eye.

Internal structures of the eye can be conveniently divided into anterior and posterior segments. The anterior segment includes the cornea, anterior chamber, iris, lens, and ciliary body. These structures comprise the essential optical elements of the eye. The regular pattern of the collagen fibers and posterior endothelial layer of the cornea maintain its optical clarity. Because the cornea and lens are avascular, they require a specialized source of nutrition, which is provided by aqueous humor. The ciliary body produces aqueous humor at a nearly constant rate, bathing the lens and posterior surface of the cornea and then draining near the base of the cornea through the structures associated with the Schlemm canal. A normal rate of production and drainage of aqueous humor maintains the intraocular pressure at between 10 and 21 mmHg. Injuries causing sustained elevation of pressure can lead to significant glaucomatous visual field loss. The iris and its pupil adjust the amount of light entering the eye. Contraction of the ciliary muscle changes the shape of the lens, thereby allowing for accommodation (adjustment of focusing for seeing at different distances).

The posterior segment of the eye is the light-sensing portion of the visual system and contains the retina and its supporting vascular layer, the choroid. The retina has more than 1 million nerve fibers that arise from the ganglion cells and collect in the optic disc to form the optic nerve, which transmits visual information to the posterior visual system. These nerve fibers are second-

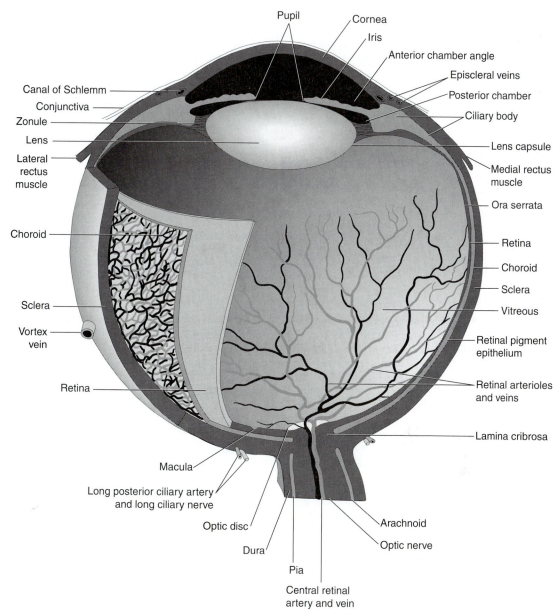

Figure 8–1. View of the inferior half of the right eye.

order neurons similar to the myelinated sensory tracts of the spinal cord and are not capable of healing with restoration of visual function following injuries such as penetrating wounds of the orbit or posterior orbital fractures involving the optic canal. Depending on the severity of the injury, the fibers may disappear partially or completely, resulting in either partial or complete atrophy of the optic disc (optic nerve). The optic chi-

asm, optic tracts, and visual radiations to the cortex usually are not involved directly in eye injuries except those involving the bones of the head and the intracranial structures.

Visual acuity depends on the optical clarity of the cornea, lens, and vitreous and proper functioning of the fovea, which is the avascular center of the retinal macula and is composed entirely of specialized cones that are color-sensitive and capable of resolving the finest images. If this small area (<0.5 mm in diameter) is damaged, no adjacent portion of the retina is capable of assuming the fine function that provides maximum visual acuity.

Eye injuries causing retinal detachment or vitreous hemorrhage can lead to loss of peripheral vision, and injuries of the extraocular muscles or their nerves can produce diplopia (double vision).

HISTORY & EYE EXAMINATION

Caution: For chemical burns (see "Chemical Burns of the Eye" below), emergency treatment should be started immediately, and the history and examination of the patient can proceed in due course. In cases of suspected ruptured or lacerated globe (see below), care must be taken to prevent further damage to the eye during transport to the hospital and initial evaluation.

History

The occupational medical history should include a variety of questions not always considered pertinent to general histories. In addition, the worker should be asked about vision before and after the injury and whether any visual loss was sudden or gradual. Sudden loss of vision without obvious injury may be caused by central retinal artery occlusion or ischemic damage to the optic nerve, occasionally caused by giant cell arteritis. These problems require emergency treatment. Progressive loss of vision following facial bone fractures or head injuries is sometimes a result of optic nerve damage, which may respond to surgery if recognized in time.

In cases of mechanical injury, the worker should be asked about previous tetanus inoculations and about the nature of the forces involved during the injury. Was the eye struck with a small, rapidly moving object that may have penetrated the globe, as sometimes occurs when a steel hammer strikes a steel tool? Or was the eye hit by a large, slowly moving object that may have caused a contusion injury or rupture of the globe? If the presence of a foreign body is suspected, the worker should be asked about the type of material that might be involved (a magnetic metal such as iron or steel, a nonmagnetic metal such as aluminum or copper, or an organic material such as wood) because this information is helpful for determining the method of treatment and for prognosis. Soluble metallic salts from iron- or copper-containing foreign bodies can cause irreversible toxic damage to the retina, best prevented by their prompt removal. Less soluble materials, such as aluminum, plastic, or glass, are associated with a better prognosis. Organic foreign bodies, such as pieces of wood or splinters of plant material, may introduce an intraocular infection that frequently is difficult to treat and has a very poor prognosis.

If a chemical burn is present or suspected, the type of chemical (alkali or acid) will influence how quickly and deeply it penetrates the eye. If eye injuries are thought to be caused by long-term exposure to chemicals, the various substances to which the worker is exposed should be identified and a Material Safety Data Sheet (MSDS) obtained for each, as described in Chapter 2. The worker also should be asked about exposure to aerosols, surfactants, detergents, dust, and smoke, which can damage the corneal epithelium.

Examination

Even if an injury is thought to have affected only one eye, both eyes should be examined carefully. If swelling prevents easy opening of the eyes for inspection, a sterile topical anesthetic can be instilled through nearly closed eyelids by applying the drops along the lid fissure. After a few minutes, smooth sterile retractors may be used carefully to lift the lids for eye examination.

A. EXTERNAL EYE EXAMINATION

1. Eyelids—Note symmetry of the lids of both eyes. Look for lacerations that cross the lid margins and for perforating wounds through the skin of the lid above or below the lid margin. Except in the case of a suspected ruptured or lacerated globe, the lid can be everted to search for foreign bodies on the upper tarsus. To evert the lid, the patient is asked to look down while the physician pulls gently on the lashes and applies mild pressure on the upper surface of the lid.

2. Orbits—Palpate the orbital rims, and note discontinuities and crepitus caused by subcutaneous air from fractures of the paranasal sinuses. In orbital fractures, injury to the inferior or superior orbital nerves as they pass through the floor or roof of the orbit can cause decreased sensibility of the lids and face.

3. Conjunctiva—To examine the conjunctiva, evert the lids by applying gentle pressure over the superior orbital rim of the upper lid or over the malar eminence of the lower lid, thereby avoiding direct pressure on the globe. Look for foreign bodies, hemorrhage, laceration, and inflammation.

Inflammation caused by trauma usually produces a watery discharge (tears), in contrast to the purulent mucoid discharge of bacterial conjunctivitis. Viral or chlamydial conjunctivitis is characterized by lymph follicles in the inferior fornix of the conjunctival sac along with a watery discharge. Preauricular lymph nodes are also frequently present.

4. Corneas—With a bright light, look at the light reflection on the normally smooth corneal surface. Irregularities indicate disruptions of the corneal epithelium. Because the cornea is normally clear and lustrous, the surface texture of the iris is seen easily and clearly. A corneal wound with incarceration of the iris also may be indicated by asymmetry of the pupil. A fluorescein paper strip moistened with sterile saline or a topical anesthetic can be used to stain the tears on the surface of the cornea. The stain diffuses into any area of disrupted epithelium and stains it bright green. The color is enhanced with a blue light. Details of the cornea and the anterior eye are much more easily examined with magnification such as a 2× to 4× loupe or (and preferably) with a slit lamp and microscope, if one is available.

5. Anterior chambers—The anterior chambers should appear deep and clear. Hyphema (hemorrhage into the anterior chamber) is almost always a sign of significant injury. Hypopyon (purulent material in the anterior chamber) is characterized by a white or gray layer of inflammatory cells at the chamber bottom. Hypopyon usually is caused by an infection following a penetrating injury or a bacterial or fungal corneal ulcer.

6. Pupils—The pupils should appear round, black, and equal in size. Pupillary reactions to light should be noted carefully. Normally, both pupils constrict and dilate equally and simultaneously when one pupil is stimulated by light. While the illuminated pupil is demonstrating the direct-light response, the unilluminated pupil is showing the consensual-light response. The direct-light responses of the two eyes can be compared by moving a flashlight back and forth between the eyes and pausing a few seconds at each eye to observe the pupil. Normally, each pupil constricts when illuminated; failure of one pupil to constrict but to dilate instead indicates the presence of an afferent pupillary defect (Marcus Gunn pupil), which may be the result of an optic nerve injury or extensive retinal damage on that side.

B. Test of Ocular Motility

If there are no severe eye injuries, the ocular movements may be tested safely by comparing the excursions in all directions to make sure that they are the same in both eyes. Limitation of upward or downward gaze occurs frequently in orbital floor fractures and may be the result of accompanying edema or mechanical restriction of the ocular muscles. It also can result from direct trauma to a muscle when a penetrating injury of the orbit occurs.

C. Ophthalmoscopic Examination

1. Red reflex—The presence of a good bright-red reflex demonstrates normal optical clarity of the eye. A direct ophthalmoscope with a good bright light is used to observe the red reflex (the red glow reflected from the fundus). Examination should take place in a darkened room with the instrument set at 0 or +1, and the eyes should be observed at arm's length, approximately 60 cm (2 ft), so that the reflex in both of them can be seen at the same time and compared. An opacity in the cornea, ante-rior chamber, lens, or vitreous or a gross change in the color of the retina will appear as a dark form against a red background or as a dull or absent red reflex.

2. Optic discs—The examiner should be as close to the patient as possible to maximize the relative size of the pupil. The optic discs should be examined for the presence of papilledema. Optic discs usually are well vascularized and have a good pink color. When nerve fibers in the optic nerve die as the result of various injuries, the blood supply to the disc decreases in proportion to the loss of fibers. The disc will show a faint pallor if only a few fibers are missing, or it may appear completely white as a result of optic atrophy following total destruction of the nerve.

3. Optic cups—The width of each optic cup is usually one-third or less the diameter of the whole optic disc. If it is as large as half the diameter, or if the optic cups are not similar in both eyes, there is an increased risk for glaucoma. Therefore, estimating the cup size is useful for screening patients for glaucoma.

4. Retinal vessels—The vessels should be examined along the upper and lower arcades proceeding from the optic disc, and the presence of hemorrhages, exudates, and other alterations in the appearance of the retina should be noted.

5. Maculae and foveae—Each macula should be checked for alterations in its usual relatively featureless appearance. Its center, the fovea, always can be located 2.5 disc diameters temporal to the optic disc. Its concave center usually shows a small, bright foveal light reflex.

D. Measurement of Intraocular Pressure

If a lacerated or ruptured globe is suspected, intraocular pressure should not be measured. In other injuries, pressure can be measured with a Schiotz tonometer or with an applanation tonometer, if one is available on a slit lamp. If a tonometer is not available, a general impression of extremely high or low intraocular pressure can be obtained by gently palpating each globe in turn with one finger of each hand through the closed upper eyelid. Comparison of the firmness of the two eyes is occasionally useful when the intraocular pressure is extremely high, as in angle-closure glaucoma.

Angle-closure glaucoma accounts for only approximately 5% of all glaucoma; it usually presents with acute aching pain in the involved eye with moderate redness of the globe and blurred vision, sometimes described as colored halos around bright lights. It occurs when the iris root touches the back of the cornea, blocking aqueous outflow and causing intraocular pressure to rise very rapidly, thus leading to the symptoms. Angle-closure glaucoma can occur only in eyes with anatomically shallow anterior chambers and narrow chamber angles. An attack of angle-closure glaucoma requires prompt treatment. The first approach is to lower the pressure medically with topical miotics such as pilocarpine 1–4% every 15 minutes for 1–2 hours. The production of aqueous humor is reduced with a topical ophthalmic β-adrenergic blocker and a carbonic anhydrase inhibitor. Intraocular pressure can be lowered quickly by increasing the osmolarity of the blood that moves water out of the vitreous humor, thus reducing the ocular volume and the intraocular pressure. Intravenous urea or mannitol infusions are effective, but oral ingestion of glycerin is as effective, safer, and more easily available. Subsequent attacks are prevented by making an opening in the peripheral iris (iridectomy), which passes aqueous humor directly from the posterior chamber to the anterior chamber, keeping the filtration angle open. The iridectomy usually is made with a laser.

Open-angle glaucoma accounts for most cases of glaucomatous visual loss (90%). Its onset is insidious, there is no pain, and visual symptoms are noticed only after severe irreversible loss of visual field has occurred. Therefore, it becomes the physician's responsibility to see changes in the optic cup. Asymmetric cups or cups as large as one-half the disc diameter are suspicious. Such changes are an indication to request visual fields. Early lowering of intraocular pressure is the only way to prevent loss of visual field. All adults should be encouraged to have their intraocular pressures measured every 1 or 2 years.

The remaining 5% of cases of glaucoma have a variety of causes. Contusion injuries to the eye can tear the iris root and the ciliary body's attachment to the sclera, damaging the filtration angle, reducing aqueous outflow, and raising pressure. This is called *angle-recession glaucoma.* Blood in the anterior chamber (hyphema) and inflammatory cells in cases of chronic inflammation, such as uveitis, can block aqueous outflow channels, causing secondary glaucoma.

Although many investigators discuss enhancing blood flow and neuroprotection as potential therapies, the only treatment of open-angle and secondary glaucoma proven effective is lowering of the intraocular pressure. This can be done by medically reducing the production of aqueous humor with a topical β-adrenergic blocker, a systemic carbonic anhydrase inhibitor, or a sympathomimetic drug. Parasympathomimetics, sympathomimetics, and prostaglandin analogues increase the outflow of aqueous humor. If these measures fail to lower the pressure adequately, a surgical procedure can be used to increase the drainage of aqueous humor into the subconjunctival space.

E. TEST OF VISUAL ACUITY

Visual acuity always should be tested and the results recorded before treatment is instituted. This is important both from the point of view of good care and for medicolegal reasons because patients do not always remember the amount of visual loss that occurred at the time of a severe injury. Visual acuity should be measured with a Snellen chart, if possible, or with a near-acuity card and recorded appropriately. Each eye should be tested separately, first without correction (glasses or contact lenses) and then with correction; each acuity measurement should be recorded for the right eye followed by the left. If a near-acuity card is used, it is important to record the distance at which the measurements were made and whether they were made with or without the patient's glasses. If visual acuity is poor and a refractive error is suspected, the chart or card can be read through a pinhole as a substitute for corrective lenses; an improvement in acuity will confirm the presence of a refractive error. If acuity is less than 20/200, the greatest distance at which fingers can be counted should be noted for each eye. If the patient cannot see the fingers well enough to count them, the greatest distance at which hand movements can be seen should be recorded. If vision is poorer than this, light perception can be tested with a bright flashlight held as close to the eye as possible, and the ability to perceive light in each of the four quadrants is recorded. If there is no light perception, it should be recorded as such. Visual acuity measured with a Snellen chart is based on a visual angle of 1 minute of arc; this is considered the best resolving power of the eye and is the standard used to design all types of test charts. The 20/20 letters are formed of black lines separated by white spaces, each 1 minute of arc wide; the whole letter is 5 minutes of arc high, measuring 8.7 mm (Figure 8–2). When letters of this size are read accurately at a distance of 20 ft (6 m), 20/20 vision is determined. Other letters on a chart increase in multiples of this standard dimension. The 20/200 letter is 10 times larger or 87 mm high and would appear the same size as a 20/20 letter when seen at a distance of 200 ft. Metric visual acuity charts use 6 m as the standard test distance; therefore, 6/6 = 20/20. The peak of the light-sensitivity curve of the eye is at a wavelength of about 555 nm. This means that our best vision is in yellow-green light.

There are two techniques for objectively estimating visual acuity—optokinetic nystagmus and visual evoked response—that may be useful in certain situations, particularly when the patient is unable or unwilling to respond to the usual subjective measures of visual acuity. Optokinetic nystagmus is a visually stimulated response to relatively large targets. These eye movements are observed in the intact visual system by passing an alternating series of dark and light stripes of equal width before the patient's eyes. Involuntary nystagmus is produced—slow following movement in the direction of movement of the stripes alternating with a

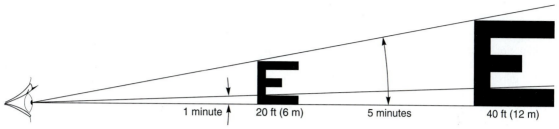

Figure 8–2. Measurement of visual acuity. Visual acuity measurements are based on a visual angle of 1 minute of arc subtending each part of a test letter. Each letter is made up of five equally sized black or white parts; therefore, the whole letter subtends a visual angle of 5 minutes of arc. The 20/20 letters are 8.7 mm high; the 20/40 letters are twice as large, or 17.4 mm high. This drawing is not to scale.

quick recovery movement. The stimulus is usually presented as a series of vertical stripes 1–2 cm in width on a handheld drum 10–15 cm in diameter. The drum is held 20–30 cm from the patient and turned slowly while observing the patient's eyes to see the induced nystagmus. The stripes also can be presented on a 50-cm-long cloth strip with the stripes running across the 10–12-cm width. Normally, the nystagmus can be induced in any direction, and its rate will vary with the speed of the stimulus.

The visually evoked response is an electroencephalographic recording over the visual cortex (occipital lobe) in response to visual stimuli. The stimulus can be a simple light flash giving an on-off response, or an estimate of visual acuity can be made by presenting an alternating pattern of dark and light squares in a checkerboard pattern on a television screen. The squares can be made progressively smaller until the response is no longer recorded, and the size of the smallest squares eliciting a cortical recording can be related to standard visual acuity measurements. The responses are involuntary and cannot be controlled by the subject; acuity measurements in the range of 20/400 to 20/20 have been recorded even in infants younger than 1 year of age. This technique usually is available through neuro-ophthalmologic or neurologic consultation. It can be particularly valuable when evaluating patients with compensation or forensic problems.

F. Test of Visual Fields

Visual fields should be tested, especially in patients with suspected head injury or a significant decrease in visual acuity. Each eye is tested separately by confrontation. The patient is asked to look at the examiner's eye while the examiner's hand moves toward the center of the visual field. The point at which the patient can accurately count fingers in each of the four quadrants is determined, and the results in the two eyes are compared carefully.

CHEMICAL BURNS OF THE EYE

Etiology & Pathogenesis

Strong alkalis and acids can cause the most severe and damaging chemical injuries to the eye and eyelids. Alkali burns are commonly caused by sodium and potassium hydroxide used as cleaning agents, by calcium hydroxide used in mason's mortar and plaster, and by anhydrous ammonia used in fertilizer. Battery acids and the strong acids used to clean metal in the electroplating industry are also common causes of severe eye injury.

Alkalis affect the lipid in cell membranes and thereby reduce the normal barriers to diffusion. This allows the chemical to penetrate rapidly the interior of the eye. Because alkalis are not neutralized quickly by tissue, their destructive action can continue for hours if they are not diluted and removed immediately by irrigation of the eye. In contrast, acids tend to be fixed by protein in tissues, and this neutralizes them in a relatively shorter period and keeps them from penetrating as deeply.

The corneal endothelium, which is essential for corneal clarity and good vision, is particularly vulnerable to chemical insult. There is often severe damage within the anterior chamber, including the aqueous outflow pathways, leading to glaucoma. Obliteration of the blood vessels of the conjunctiva and sclera can cause severe ischemia of the anterior eye, including the periphery of the cornea and the underlying ciliary body and iris. Ischemia, as well as the associated reduction in blood supply, is one of the major causes of the poor prognosis in patients with severe chemical burns.

Clinical Findings

The skin on the face and eyelids shows edema and erythema, sometimes associated with sloughing of the surface. Eye examination may require use of a topical anesthetic unless nerve damage is severe enough to cause anesthesia. The conjunctiva may be mildly hyperemic, show small hemorrhages, or be blanched and have the appearance of white marble. Testing the pH of the conjunctival surface with indicator paper will help to confirm the presence of acid (low pH) or alkali (high pH) injuries. The severity of injury (Table 8–1) usually is judged by the degree of corneal opacity using the normal clarity of the pupil as a guide. The cornea may appear gray or cloudy because of epithelial and stromal edema. If the cornea is not cloudy, the anterior chamber can be seen clearly. In some cases, the iris and pupil appear hazy and indistinct. Visual acuity is decreased in proportion to the severity of corneal damage. Injuries of the nasopharynx and upper respiratory passages frequently are found in association with aspiration of the chemical irritant.

Prevention

Chemical burns can be prevented by safety measures such as keeping chemicals in unbreakable containers and providing splash-protection shields and eyeglasses to employees who must handle chemicals. Workers at risk should be taught emergency treatment measures for themselves and their fellow workers.

Treatment

Emergency treatment (Table 8–2) should be started in the workplace by the patient or anyone immediately available. Any source of water (drinking fountain, hose, etc.) is adequate and should be used immediately to wash the eyes with copious amounts of water until the patient can be taken to an emergency facility. At least 1 L of saline or other isotonic solution then should be used to irrigate each eye carefully, with the lids held

Table 8–1. Classifications of chemical burns of the eye.

Classification	Clinical Findings
Mild	Erosion of the corneal epithelium Faint haziness of the cornea No ischemic necrosis of the conjunctiva or sclera
Moderate	Corneal opacity blurring details of the iris Minimal ischemic necrosis of the conjunctiva and sclera
Severe	Corneal opacity blurring the pupillary outline Severe ischemic necrosis and blanching of the conjunctiva and sclera

Table 8–2. Emergency treatment of chemical burns of the eye.

(1) **In the workplace:** Wash the eyes with copious amounts of water until the patient can be taken to an emergency facility.

(2) **In the emergency facility:**
   (a) Irrigate each eye with at least 1 L of saline or other isotonic solution, with the lids open to flush the conjunctival sac.
   (b) Use sterile topical anesthetic as necessary.
   (c) Remove particulate matter with cotton-tipped applicators.
   (d) Test the pH of the conjunctival surface, and continue irrigation until the pH approaches neutral.
   (e) Remove loose or damaged epithelium from the cornea and conjunctiva.
   (f) Dilate the pupil with cyclopentolate or scopolamine.
   (g) Give topical antibiotic drops, patch the eyes, and refer the patient to an ophthalmologist.

open to thoroughly cleanse the conjunctival sac. Use of a sterile topical anesthetic may be necessary.

Moist cotton-tipped applicators should be used to sweep the conjunctival surface free of particulate matter, such as the granules found in drainpipe cleaners and plaster. The pH of the conjunctival surface should be tested with pH test paper strips or urine pH test strips and irrigation repeated until the pH approaches the normal level of 7.0. As a general rule, there is no practical limit to the amount of irrigation that may be helpful. If there is any doubt about its efficacy, irrigation may be repeated for several hours while waiting for ophthalmologic consultation.

During irrigation, the gray color or cloudiness of the cornea may appear to clear, giving a false impression of improved clinical status. The change is usually a result of sloughing of the damaged corneal epithelium, which reveals the clearer corneal stroma underneath.

After irrigation is completed, cycloplegic drops (e.g., cyclopentolate or scopolamine) may be instilled to dilate the pupil and thus prevent posterior synechiae (adhesions between iris and lens). Antibiotic drops should be instilled before the eye is patched. The patch prevents blinking and should provide some comfort. The patient should be referred to an ophthalmologist.

Specific ophthalmologic treatment may include the use of topical corticosteroids and antibiotics to reduce the severe inflammatory response that occurs shortly after injury. These medications—particularly the corticosteroids—must be used with caution because they enhance the possibility of secondary infection and discourage the formation of new vessels in ischemic areas. Irrigation of the anterior chamber with saline solution may help to restore the pH to more normal levels. After the initial reaction subsides and the conjunctiva and cornea have epithelialized, the severity of the injury can be judged. A scarred cornea can be replaced by a corneal transplant, and a damaged lens (cataract) can be removed surgically and replaced with a clear synthetic lens. Glaucoma as a consequence of scarring of aqueous outflow pathways may be controlled medically—and if not, a surgical fistulization procedure may be done.

Prognosis

Emergency treatment of chemical burns usually is followed by a period of weeks or months of effort to rehabilitate the damaged ocular tissues. The degree of blanching or ischemia of the conjunctiva is an important factor influencing the final outcome. Ischemic damage, even in the presence of apparent healing, makes ultimate restoration of vision difficult. The survival of a corneal transplant depends on normal function of structures in the anterior eye. The survival of the cornea and the anterior segment of the eye are directly related to the degree of damage to the corneal endothelium, aqueous drainage pathways, and ciliary body. If the ciliary body fails to produce enough aqueous humor, the entire eye becomes soft and ultimately atrophies. In patients with severe burns, deep penetration and extensive destruction of ocular tissues can lead to perforation of the globe, infection, and loss of the eye. Milder burns in which chemical penetration is shallower may heal with little scarring.

THERMAL BURNS OF THE EYE & EYELID

Thermal burns of the eyelids and upper face may involve the eyes. However, in cases of flash burn caused by a sudden gas explosion, most individuals forcibly close their eyes, and this reflex lid closure usually protects the ocular surface. Direct contact with molten metal or glass can cause severe injury to the lids and even to the open eye. Thermal injury occurs rapidly at the time of contact. Tissue destruction is not progressive, as is the case with some chemical burns.

Eye examination may require topical anesthesia and careful use of lid retractors. Irrigation may be necessary to remove particulate matter, especially in injuries caused by explosions.

Depending on their severity, thermal burns of the eye structures are treated in the same manner as burns occurring elsewhere on the body (see Chapter 11). Extensive loss of lid skin can lead to exposure and drying of the cornea. This can be prevented by covering the eye with a transparent plastic sheet and sealing it to the surrounding skin with a sterile antibiotic ointment, thus producing a humidity chamber over the eye. Healing of lid skin frequently is followed by scarring, contraction, and distortion of the lids, which

result in some degree of exposure of the globe. Plastic surgery with skin grafting may be necessary to restore lid function.

REFERENCES

Arora R et al: Amniotic membrane transplantation in acute chemical burns. Eye 2005;19:273 [PMID: 15286672].

Daly M et al: Acute corneal calcification following chemical injury. Cornea 2005;24:761 [PMID: 16015102].

Fournier JH, McLachlan DL: Ocular surface reconstruction using amniotic membrane allograft for severe surface disorders in chemical burns. Int Surg 2005;90:45 [PMID: 15912900].

MECHANICAL INJURIES OF THE EYE & EYELID

Mechanical injuries range from superficial abrasions to complete disruption of the globe depending on the nature of the force striking the eye. Small, sharp, fast-moving objects can penetrate or lacerate the globe, whereas larger objects may exert enough compressive force to cause contusion injury or to rupture the eyeball.

Laceration of the Eyelid

Lid lacerations result from two common mechanisms: (1) contact with sharp, fast-moving objects such as glass or metal parts that cut the skin and subcutaneous tissues (partial-thickness lacerations) or involve the posterior layers, the tarsus, and the conjunctiva (full-thickness lacerations) and (2) avulsion injuries that are caused by blunt trauma (e.g., a blow to the malar eminence) and cause abrupt traction of the lid and tear it from its attachment to the medial canthal ligament. The type and extent of injury determine the method of treatment.

Partial-thickness lacerations can be closed by direct suturing with generally good results. Full-thickness lacerations require meticulous repair in two layers by an ophthalmic surgeon to accurately restore the continuity of the lid margin. If notching of the margin occurs with healing, the cornea may not be moistened adequately by tears and protected from abrasions and other trauma. Deep stab wounds above the upper lid may sever the levator muscle of the lid. The cut end of the levator is easier to retrieve and repair if surgery is performed immediately after injury. Inadequate repair can result in chronic ptosis. Severe damage to the upper lid and blinking mechanism also can place the patient at risk for superficial corneal injuries.

In avulsion injuries, lid structures that have pulled away from the globe should be examined carefully and placed as close to their anatomic positions as possible to protect the eye while the patient is awaiting treatment by an ophthalmic surgeon. Retention of avulsed lid structures is important. They frequently can be repaired and usually heal well because of their rich blood supply. It is difficult to substitute skin grafts or skin flaps for the normal lid structures, particularly the tarsal and conjunctival structures that are essential for normal functioning of the lid. Avulsion of the medial canthal ligament sometimes disrupts the lacrimal drainage system, and failure to repair it will result in epiphora (the overflow of tears).

Injuries to the Iris

Injuries to the iris can be caused indirectly by contusion and directly by perforating or penetrating injuries of the eye.

Contusion of the globe transmits force to the iris by the rapid displacement of aqueous humor. Because water is incompressible and the eye is essentially inelastic, these forces can be very large and destructive.

Iridoplegia is caused by damage to the pupillary sphincter. The pupil may react to light either directly or consensually and only slightly or not at all. The iris root, where it attaches to the ciliary body, may be torn, producing an iridodialysis. Sometimes the ciliary body with the iris root intact is torn away from its scleral attachment, producing an angle recession that can damage the aqueous outflow, causing a form of glaucoma.

Penetrating injuries, foreign bodies, stab wounds, corneal lacerations, and ruptured globes all may perforate, tear, or disrupt the iris. Iris tissue frequently herniates through corneal or scleral wounds.

Iris injuries usually do not require treatment other than incidental repair of the associated major injuries. Except for an increase in the amount of light entering an eye, it may have quite useful vision without an iris or with an iris with multiple holes. An eye with more than one pupil still sees only one image.

Injuries of the Retina

Retinal injuries are caused by both blunt trauma (contusion) and penetrating wounds. When the eye is struck in a contusion injury, the force is transmitted by the fluid contents throughout the interior of the globe. Posteriorly, the retina may become edematous in a discrete area, frequently including the macula—a condition called *commotio retinae* or *Berlin edema*. Vision is reduced but may improve to nearly normal when the edema clears. This process may require several weeks to a month to complete. Contusion injuries also cause forceful displacement of the vitreous, resulting in traction at its anterior attachment on the surface of the retina at the posterior edge of the ciliary body. This may disinsert the retina from the ciliary body or tear a hole in the peripheral retina. Hemorrhage may result, clouding the vitreous for a time.

Retinal tears or holes frequently cause retinal detachments, which require prompt surgical repair. Visual prognosis depends on macular involvement. If the macula is intact, vision is usually good; if the macula is detached for even a few days, the prognosis is apt to be poor. Penetrating injuries cause direct perforations and tears in the retina, causing hemorrhage and detachment. Treatment of retinal detachments requires localization and closure of the tears or holes. This is done by creating an adhesion and scar between the retina and the choroid surrounding the hole. A freezing probe placed on the scleral surface over the hole will cause an inflammatory reaction in the choroid that will adhere to the retina. Sometimes it is necessary to bring the scleral, choroidal, and retinal surfaces together. Usually this is done by placing an encircling band of silicone rubber around the entire globe; it also may be done by pushing them together from the inside by injecting a gas bubble into the vitreous space.

Ruptured or Lacerated Globe

If a ruptured or lacerated globe is present or suspected, placing a metal shield or other protective covering (e.g., the bottom half of a paper cup) over the injured eye will prevent external pressure from causing further damage during transport to the hospital. Patching the other eye will reduce ocular movements and thus help to prevent further trauma to the injured eye.

Visual acuity should be measured and recorded. Severe injuries almost always are associated with some degree of visual loss, lid swelling, orbital swelling, exophthalmos, and hemorrhage. If lid swelling is extreme, it may be necessary to use a sterile topical anesthetic and lid retractors to lift the lids away from the globe during initial examination.

If the cornea is clear and the pupil is round and reacts to light, the globe probably is intact. Global rupture usually is characterized by the presence of brownish or grayish tissue beneath the conjunctiva (subconjunctival hemorrhage), which is caused by exposure or herniation of uveal tissue, an irregular or disrupted corneal surface, or the presence of blood or gross alteration in the appearance of the iris and pupil. Pupillary light reflexes may be abnormal. The pupil pulled or peaked toward one side of the cornea usually indicates that the iris has herniated through a laceration in that direction.

Ophthalmoscopic examination may be difficult because of corneal irregularities and hemorrhage in the anterior chamber and vitreous. If the fundus can be examined and the disc and vessels appear relatively normal, gross disruption of the globe is unlikely. A bright red reflex usually indicates that the interior of the globe is intact. Intraocular pressure should not be measured if a ruptured or lacerated globe is suspected. A radiograph for detection of any radiopaque material in the region of the globe is an essential part of the initial examination.

Definitive examination and treatment should be performed by an ophthalmic surgeon. Until a surgeon is available, both eyes should be covered again, with a sterile eye pad used on the injured eye to minimize contamination. The patient should be supported with parenteral fluids and be considered a candidate for general anesthesia. The repair of a ruptured globe or corneal laceration usually is done under general anesthesia. A local anesthetic is not considered safe because the distortion from its injection might cause additional damage.

The eye is examined safely under anesthesia, usually with an operating microscope, and the repair is carried out by suturing the torn sclera or lacerated cornea. Exposed intraocular structures such as the iris or ciliary body may be replaced in the eye or excised depending on their condition. When the repair is complete, the eye is filled with saline or an electrolyte solution that simulates aqueous humor. Antibiotics are injected subconjunctivally after the globe is closed and are continued intravenously for 4–5 days to prevent infection that may have been introduced by the injury.

A ruptured globe has a grave prognosis for restoration of vision. Corneal lacerations have a better prognosis because their surgical repair usually is accomplished easily. If scarring occurs, corneal transplant can be performed.

Contusion Injuries

Blunt trauma to the eye causes various contusion injuries ranging in severity from ecchymosis of the eyelids (black eye) to major intraocular damage. Compression injuries of the anterior eye are characterized by corneal edema, anterior chamber hemorrhage, and increased intraocular pressure. These symptoms usually resolve without treatment. In some cases, however, return of normal intraocular pressure is followed several weeks or months later by another increase, which indicates the presence of angle-recession glaucoma. This is caused by a tear in the attachment of the iris and ciliary body from the internal surface of the sclera at the anterior chamber angle, damaging the aqueous outflow pathway. Patients with compression injuries always should receive follow-up care at the hands of an ophthalmologist so that angle-recession glaucoma can be detected and treated to prevent progressive damage to the optic nerve. Treatment usually begins with twice-daily drops of an ophthalmic β-blocker.

Hyphema (hemorrhage into the anterior chamber) frequently clears spontaneously, but secondary hemorrhage occurs after several hours or days in up to one-third of patients as a result of lysis of the thrombus in the injured vessels of the iris or ciliary body. Secondary hemorrhage frequently continues until the anterior chamber is completely filled with blood, during which time the intraocular

pressure may rise to 50–60 mmHg (normal 12–20 mmHg). Lysis and reabsorption of this blood clot may take many days and cause damage to the aqueous filtration pathways and subsequent glaucoma. Breakdown products of blood also can diffuse into the cornea, stain it, and cause long-term reduction of vision. If reabsorption of the blood clot is prolonged, it sometimes can be aspirated successfully. If not, the anterior chamber is opened, and the clot is removed directly. Secondary hemorrhages may require surgical treatment. The prognosis for good vision in patients with secondary hemorrhage is poor.

The prevention of secondary hemorrhages is difficult. Bed rest with binocular patching has been a standard treatment for many years. More recent experience comparing patients treated with bed rest and others allowed normal activity showed no significant difference in the incidence of secondary hemorrhages.

Aminocaproic acid has been used to retard fibrinolysis in the injured vessels to prevent secondary hemorrhages to the benefit of many patients. This treatment slows the lysis of the primary hyphema but, when given for 5–7 days, does reduce the occurrence of secondary hemorrhages. There are significant side effects, so use of aminocaproic acid must be considered carefully and monitored.

Retinal edema, particularly in the macula, causes acute reduction of vision. Vision usually improves with clearance of edema in a few days to several weeks. Clearance is not always complete, and there may be permanent damage to the macula. In ruptures of the choroid, blood spreads beneath the retina at the time of injury, and reabsorption of blood will reveal a crescent-shaped scar concentric with the optic disk. There is no treatment. Other contusion injuries include dislocation of the lens (partial or complete), traumatic cataracts, and tears in the region of the anterior attachment of the retina to the ciliary body, which lead to vitreous hemorrhages and detachment of the retina.

A damaged lens—either dislocated or cataractous—may reduce vision or may be displaced anteriorly, causing increased intraocular pressure by closing the aqueous filtration angle. In either case, the lens is removed by using one of the cataract surgery techniques. Vitreous hemorrhages are removed with a suction-cutting vitrectomy instrument. Following this procedure, the retinal detachment is repaired by creating an adhesive scar between the choroid and retina, usually by freezing through the scleral surface (cryotherapy) over the area of the retinal tear or hole. The sclera then may be buckled inward to push the adhesion against the retina. This is usually done by compressing the globe with an encircling band of silicone rubber. Sometimes, an intraocular gas bubble is used to push the retina, choroid, and sclera into contact.

Intraocular Foreign Bodies

An intraocular foreign body should be suspected on the basis of the occupational history, particularly if the worker complains of an irritating sensation in the eye and no superficial foreign body is found. For example, when steel tools are used to hammer other steel objects, the hammered steelwork hardens to a glassy surface from which small, sharp chips can fly and penetrate the globe with a minimum of discomfort at the moment of impact. Vision may be nearly normal if the entry wound is small. In cases such as this, in which a radiopaque foreign body is suspected, a radiograph should be taken. Ultrasonography usually will demonstrate nonradiopaque objects (e.g., glass and plastic). If a foreign body is found, referral to an ophthalmologist for further evaluation and early treatment is essential.

Failure to remove iron or copper foreign bodies can cause severe impairment or loss of vision owing to their toxic effects on ocular tissue. A retained iron or copper foreign body may dissolve away in several months to a year, but the damage done to the retina by the soluble metallic salts is irreversible, and marked visual loss—even blindness—results. The prognosis for these foreign bodies is good if they are removed before they have time to dissolve. Inert materials such as glass or plastic may cause mechanical damage to the eye, but in the absence of a local toxic reaction, the long-term prognosis is better. It is not necessary to remove every foreign body made of inert material; some of them may be left in place depending on their position in the globe and their effect on visual function. Iron-containing magnetic foreign bodies usually are removed with an ophthalmic magnet—sometimes through the entry wound or through a surgical incision made as close as possible to the foreign body. Nonmagnetic foreign bodies are removed with grasping instruments specially designed for ophthalmic microsurgery. Penetrating wounds caused by potentially contaminated objects such as agricultural implements or by wood fragments thrown from woodworking machinery can introduce severe intraocular infections that lead to complete disruption and loss of the globe; therefore, microbiologic studies and treatment with appropriate systemic and local antibiotics are required.

Injuries to the Orbit & Optic Nerve

Orbital floor ("blowout") fractures (see Chapter 9) frequently are associated with herniation of intraorbital contents into the fracture line. Usually there is severe edema within the orbit that restricts eye movements for 7–10 days. If restriction continues, surgical repair of the fracture may be indicated to free the entrapped extraocular muscles.

Facial bone and orbital fractures that extend to the posterior orbit may involve the optic canal, with damage to the optic nerve indicated by the presence of an afferent pupillary defect. Initial and later evaluations of the patient should include documentation of visual acuity. If there is progressive loss of vision, surgical decom-

pression of the optic nerve in the canal may preserve or, occasionally, even improve the remaining vision.

Orbital injuries may cause severe hemorrhage, marked exophthalmos of the globe, and a dramatic and abrupt increase in intraocular pressure owing to compression. Although this increased pressure usually is relieved by the normal dissipation of interstitial fluid in a short period of time, it occasionally results in occlusion of the central retinal artery or vein. Pressure sometimes can be reduced by the application of gentle external massage to the globe through the closed lids. Surgical lysis of the lateral canthus of the lids may be required.

Penetrating wounds can damage the optic nerve directly by advancing through the funnel-shaped orbit to reach its apex, where the nerve and its blood supply are trapped by the optic canal. Contusion of the nerve causes severe visual impairment and sometimes is treated with large doses of systemic corticosteroids in a manner similar to treatment of spinal cord injuries.

REFERENCES

Khaw PT et al: Injury to the eye. BMJ 2004;328:36 Review [PMID: 14703545].

Wirbelauer C: Management of the red eye for the primary care physician. Am J Med 2006;119:302 [PMID: 16564769].

Xiang H et al: Work-related eye injuries treated in hospital emergency departments in the US. Am J Ind Med 2005;48:57 [PMID: 15940717].

Injuries of the Corneal Epithelium (Abrasions & Superficial Foreign Bodies)

Abrasions of the corneal epithelium can be caused by superficial mechanical trauma (e.g., prolonged wearing of contact lenses), by the presence of a foreign body, or by exposure to ultraviolet radiation, chemicals, aerosols, dust, smoke, and other irritants. The occupational medical history should be taken, as described in Chapter 2.

Photokeratoconjunctivitis (welder's flash) is a specific ocular injury caused by unprotected exposure to ultraviolet radiation with wavelengths shorter than 300 nm (actinic rays). This radiation is generated by the welder's arc and damages the exposed corneal and conjunctival epithelium. Injuries are caused both by direct observation of the arc and in persons nearby who often are not wearing protective filters.

In the first few hours after exposure, there may be only mild discomfort and slight conjunctival redness. After a latent period of several hours—even as long as 6–8 hours—the injured epithelial cells slough, causing an acute onset of severe pain sometimes said to be "as though someone had thrown hot sand in my eyes." Marked tearing, photophobia, and blepharospasm (tightly closed lids) are usual.

Examination requires a sterile topical anesthetic, which may be introduced through nearly closed eyelids by placing several drops along the lid margins. When the eyes open, more anesthetic may be instilled, along with fluorescein from a sterile paper strip. The fluorescein will diffuse over the cornea where the epithelium has sloughed, staining it bright green—best observed with a blue light. Epithelial loss is confined to the area exposed in the lid opening.

Treatment consists of instillation of an antibiotic ointment and patching the eye or eyes to prevent lid movement or blinking. The epithelium will not heal rapidly and in some cases not at all if it is frequently wiped and disturbed by blinking. It will require 12–24 hours for healing to occur; in some cases, several days may be necessary. The eyes should be examined daily. Anesthetic drops and fluorescein help in following the progress of reepithelialization. Continue to patch with antibiotic ointment until healing has occurred. Corneal epithelium heals without scarring. Antibiotic solutions or ointments containing corticosteroids sometimes are recommended for the treatment of welder's flash burns. The steroids may speed clearing of the associated hyperemia and edema, but they increase the incidence of secondary bacterial, viral, and fungal infections. If steroids are used, frequent examination (every 12–24 hours) is essential to detect early signs of infection until healing occurs. In addition, prolonged use of topical steroids (10–14 days or more), even in low doses, can raise intraocular pressure and, in time, can cause significant glaucomatous field loss. This unpredictable response occurs in approximately 10% of the population. It is therefore probably best to avoid the routine or frequent use of topical corticosteroids in the treatment of corneal and conjunctival injuries and infections.

The patient should not be given anesthetic drops or ointment to use at home. Anesthetics slow and may even prevent epithelial healing, and when used in these circumstances, they have led to severe scarring of the cornea and even the loss of an eye.

These injuries are easily prevented by wearing adequate protective filters in the face masks for the welder and goggles or ultraviolet filter glasses by visitors and workers in nearby areas where the welding flash can be seen.

Symptoms and signs of corneal abrasions include severe ocular pain, tearing, and blurring of vision. Inspection of the anterior eye with a flashlight usually shows irregular light reflections on the corneal surface in the area of the abraded epithelium. Use of sterile topical anesthetic and fluorescein paper strips is helpful for further examination. The fluorescein dye diffuses into the area of disrupted epithelium, stains it bright green, and can be observed easily with a blue light. If further evaluation reveals normal pupillary reactions, a bright red reflex, and no disruption of the anterior segment, the injury usually is confined to the anterior external layer of the cornea.

Small foreign bodies on the surface of the cornea or conjunctiva may be seen directly or detected by evidence of damaged epithelium from the fluorescein stain. Foreign bodies usually can be removed with a cotton-tipped applicator, but a sharp instrument is helpful occasionally. The side bevel of a disposable hypodermic needle can be used to gently detach foreign bodies that are firmly attached to the corneal surface. Rust deposited in the anterior layers of the cornea frequently can be removed by the same gentle scraping maneuver. If all the foreign body or rust is not removed easily, it usually can be left to slough or absorb by itself without causing damage. After foreign bodies are removed, treatment is the same as for abrasions.

Abrasions are treated by applying a sterile ophthalmic antibiotic ointment effective against both gram-positive and gram-negative organisms (e.g., gentamicin, tobramycin, or a mixture containing bacitracin, polymyxin, and neomycin) and covering the affected eye with a patch dressing to keep the lids closed. Corneal epithelium usually heals promptly if the surface of the cornea is allowed to rest without blinking the lid. The initial process of healing is one in which the normal epithelial cells slide from the edge of the wound over the smooth surface of the cornea to fill the gap. The eyes should be inspected in 12–24 hours to determine if healing has occurred and to rule out corneal infection, which appears as a white or gray haze in the area of the wound. If the abrasion is not healed completely, a second application of the ointment and patch dressing for an additional 12–24 hours may be required. This process should be continued until the epithelial defect is healed. Scarring usually does not occur, and vision is restored to normal.

Caution: After the initial examination with topical anesthetic, sharp pain may return until the epithelium begins to heal. Under no circumstances should the patient be supplied with anesthetic drops or ointment to use during the healing process because topical anesthetics will delay healing and place the patient at risk for severe corneal infection and scarring. Antibiotic mixtures containing corticosteroids should not be used for treatment because they provide inadequate protection against bacterial infection and enhance the growth of viral and fungal pathogens.

Abrasions caused by fat-soluble petroleum products splashed into the eyes are treated initially by copious irrigation with water or saline solution to remove any remaining material. Staining with fluorescein will demonstrate the amount of epithelial loss, which may vary from a few punctate areas to complete denudation of the cornea. In either case, treatment is the same as outlined above. If the abraded area is large, the corneal stroma may appear slightly gray owing to some degree of edema. This clears rapidly with healing of the epithelium.

Exposure to aerosols (e.g., paint sprays), detergents, surfactants, dust, smoke, and vapors can produce both acute and chronic symptoms of abrasion. Acute symptoms almost invariably include marked tearing and blepharospasm, which act to protect the eyes and wash away the offending material. Treatment for acute symptoms is as for other abrasions (see above). Chronic exposure to low-level irritants causes fatigue of the lacrimal reflex and subsequent sensations of dryness and burning of the eyes. Some degree of redness is common. Irrigation with saline solution prevents most of these chronic symptoms. Adequate ventilation and avoidance of irritants in the workplace are obviously the best preventive measures.

Exposure to some chemical substances causes a delayed loss of corneal epithelium. For example, formaldehyde fumes cause diffuse damage to epithelial cells, leading to their accelerated sloughing with normal blinking. Fortunately, the abrasion will heal without scarring when the fumes are avoided subsequently. The long list of other substances that produce this effect includes butylamine, diethylamine, hydrogen sulfide, methyl silicate, mustard gas, osmium tetroxide, podophyllum resin, and sulfur.

INDIRECT INJURIES TO THE EYE

In massive crush injuries, compression of the abdominal and chest vessels can cause sudden vascular engorgement of the retina. This leads to marked edema and diffuse hemorrhages in the fundus and can result in permanent ocular damage. Purtscher retinopathy is one form of this condition. There is no treatment. The prognosis for vision depends on the amount of damage done to the macula or optic nerve. Slow improvement in vision occurs as hemorrhages absorb for periods of up to several months.

In fractures of the long bones, fat emboli can migrate to the retina and produce small embolic changes that have the appearance of cotton-wool spots and sometimes are associated with flame-shaped hemorrhages in the fundus. Fat emboli, thrombi from heart valve disease and endocarditis, and emboli from a variety of sources occasionally obstruct branches of the retinal artery and cause infarction of a segment of the retina. Cholesterol crystals shed from atheromatous plaques in the carotid arteries also may migrate to the retina and appear as glistening intraarterial bodies. In intravenous drug abuse, the injected drugs frequently contain inert substances such as talc, which may be seen in the retina as small white deposits. The prognosis for each of these conditions depends entirely on their location and whether or not the macula is involved. There is no ocular treatment. Clearing of the effects of these emboli—hemorrhages and edema—requires several weeks to a month. Cholesterol crystal emboli are an indication to investigate the patency of the carotid arteries.

Rarely, a septic embolus from a distant systemic infection causes endophthalmitis. Endophthalmitis generally has a poor prognosis. Specific diagnosis requires aspiration of vitreous fluid and sometimes aqueous humor for the isolation of organisms. Periocular injection of antibiotics adjacent to the scleral surface, occasionally intravitreal injection of appropriate doses of antibiotics, and intravenous antibiotics are the usual methods of treatment. The poor prognosis is a result of delay in diagnosis while the infection advances and of the unpredictable and sometimes poor ocular penetration of antibiotics.

SYMPATHETIC OPHTHALMIA

If the uveal tract (i.e., the iris, ciliary body, or choroid) of one eye is injured, the uninjured (sympathizing) eye may show inflammation. This rare disorder is thought to be an autoimmune inflammatory response and can be prevented by prompt, adequate treatment of the initial injury to minimize continuing trauma to the damaged uveal tissue. Sympathetic ophthalmia can cause complete loss of vision in both eyes if unrecognized and untreated early in its course. As soon as inflammation is seen in the sympathizing eye, treatment of both eyes with local corticosteroids (topical and periocular injections) and mydriatics should be started. Large doses of systemic corticosteroids are also used frequently.

OCCLUSION OF THE CENTRAL RETINAL ARTERY

Occlusion of the central retinal artery is characterized by sudden painless loss of vision and is considered an ocular emergency. Permanent loss of vision will result if the retina is deprived of blood for 30–60 minutes; consequently, arterial circulation must be restored as soon as possible.

Diagnosis is based on the history and eye examination. Occlusion usually is seen in older patients with arteriosclerosis or following embolism from the great vessels. It also can be caused by pressure from an unusually tight dressing over the eye, particularly when there is orbital edema or hemorrhage. If the visual loss is incomplete, the patient may be able to detect some light. Ophthalmic examination reveals a bloodless retina with thin and thready arteries. Early findings include a faint retinal edema that appears as a grayish or white discoloration and is particularly noticeable around the macula, allowing the normal red color of the choroid in the fovea to show through as a cherry-red spot. Later, red cells in the blood column of the arteries may separate into segments and appear as "boxcars." The veins also appear thinner than normal. The optic disc retains its normal pink color for several weeks, but the retinal edema becomes more apparent.

Although central retinal artery occlusions usually are not associated with increased intraocular pressures, the most effective treatment is immediate reduction of the normal intraocular pressure in an attempt to dislodge the embolus or thrombus thought to be obstructing the artery at a restricted area of the vessel as it passes through the scleral shell just posterior to the optic disc. The pressure can be reduced by using two fingers to alternately massage and press the globe through the closed lids. This maneuver should be repeated four or five times over 10–15 minutes to accelerate the expression of aqueous humor and applies intermittent pressure on the artery. The patient's use of a rebreathing bag will increase the amount of carbon dioxide in the cerebral and ocular blood vessels, sometimes effecting vascular dilation.

If these maneuvers fail, paracentesis of the anterior chamber may be indicated. After a topical anesthetic is given, the conjunctiva is grasped with fine-tooth forceps. An incision is made through the clear cornea at the periphery of the anterior chamber, with the sharp scalpel blade held in the plane of the iris so as not to touch either the iris or the lens. The blade then is turned slightly to allow some of the aqueous humor to escape abruptly. This lowers the intraocular pressure and sometimes restores circulation to the retina.

Anterior Ischemic Optic Neuropathy

This condition is characterized by an acute, painless loss of vision in individuals 50–70 years of age. The ischemia of the optic nerve is in or just behind the disc. The disc appears swollen or edematous at first, clearing with time and leaving various amounts of optic atrophy and usually a severe loss of vision. The same process in the 70- to 80-year-old age group may be a result of giant cell arteritis, frequently associated with temporal arteritis. Systemic steroids sometimes are helpful in the latter group to prevent involvement of the second eye.

OCCLUSION OF THE CENTRAL RETINAL VEIN

Occlusion of the central retinal vein produces painless visual loss and is seen most commonly in older patients with diabetes, hypertension, or other vascular occlusive diseases. Findings include a swollen optic disc, distended and tortuous retinal veins, and an edematous retina with flame-shaped hemorrhages.

There is no effective emergency treatment, although anticoagulants have been tried occasionally. An ophthalmologist should follow these patients. The prognosis for improvement of vision is slightly better for patients with an occluded retinal vein than it is for those patients with an occluded retinal artery.

REFERENCES

Garg SJ et al: Bone from an orbital floor fracture causing an intraocular foreign body. Am J Ophthalmol 2005;139:543 [PMID: 15767071].

Ghazi-Nouri SM et al Periorbital ecchymosis as a sign of perforating injury of the globe. Clin Exp Ophthalmol 2005;33:194 [PMID: 15807832].

Hagendon CL et al: Bilateral intraocular foreign bodies simulating crystalline lens. Am J Ophthalmol 2004;138:146 [PMID: 15234299].

EYE INJURIES CAUSED BY RADIATION EXPOSURE

See Chapter 12 for a description of the electromagnetic spectrum and a discussion of methods to prevent occupational exposure to radiation.

Injuries Caused by Ionizing Radiation

X-rays, beta rays, and other radiation sources in adequate doses can cause ocular injury. The eyelid is particularly vulnerable to x-ray damage because of the thinness of its skin. Loss of lashes and scarring can lead to inversion or eversion (entropion or ectropion) of the lid margins and prevent adequate lid closure. Scarring of the conjunctiva can impair the production of mucus and the function of the lacrimal gland ducts, thereby causing dryness of the eyes. X-ray radiation in a dose of 500–800 R directed toward the lens surface can cause cataracts, sometimes with a delay of several months to a year before the opacities appear. Treatment for these injuries is the appropriate oculoplastic repair of lid deformities and scarring. Deficiencies of tears and mucus can be improved by the topical use of artificial tears and protection from evaporation by wearing protective glasses with side shields that seal to the face. Radiation cataracts can be removed surgically by the appropriate standard technique.

Injuries Caused by Ultraviolet Radiation

Ultraviolet radiation of wavelengths shorter than 300 nm (actinic rays) can damage the corneal epithelium. This is most commonly the result of exposure to the sun at high altitudes and in areas where shorter wavelengths are readily reflected from bright surfaces such as snow, water, and sand. Exposure to radiation generated by a welding arc can cause welder's flash burn, a form of keratitis. After a latent period of several hours, the injured epithelial cells soften and slough, causing sudden onset of pain. Treatment of these injuries consists of applying antibiotic ointment and patches until the epithelial cells have had an opportunity to heal (see "Injuries of the Corneal Epithelium" above).

Wavelengths of 300–400 nm are transmitted through the cornea, and approximately 80% are absorbed by the lens, where they may cause cataractous changes. Accidental exposure to an inadequately shielded dental instrument used to accelerate the hardening of plastic fillings has caused significant lens opacities in dental personnel. Epidemiologic studies suggest that exposure to solar radiation in these wavelengths near the equator is correlated with an increased incidence of cataracts. They also indicate that workers exposed to bright sunlight in occupations such as farming, truck driving, and construction work appear to have a higher incidence of cataracts than do those who work primarily indoors. Experimental studies show that these wavelengths cause changes in the lens protein that lead to cataract formation in animals.

Cataract

Any opacity in the lens is called a *cataract*. Some degree of opacity is present in almost all lenses, and the significance of the changes depends solely on their effect on vision. Peripheral opacities, for example, that do not interfere with vision are of no clinical significance.

The lens is composed of lens protein arranged in an ordered pattern of cytoplasmic fibers produced by the lens epithelium. These cells continue to produce new fibers at a slow rate throughout life. The lens thus slowly increases in volume—mainly in thickness—pushing the iris forward.

Changes in the chemistry and hydration of the lens protein create various types of cataracts. These changes may be induced by a variety of agents, including near-ultraviolet radiation of 300–400 nm. These wavelengths are absorbed by the central lens fibers, causing the brownish discoloration of lenticular nuclear sclerosis. Ocular inflammation and corticosteroids, both topical and systemic, produce typical posterior subcapsular cataracts.

Types of Cataracts

A. Age-Related Cataracts

Age-related (senile) cataract is the most common type seen. Some degree of opacity is almost universal. The progress of change and the related reduction in vision is usually quite slow. Nuclear sclerosis—an increasing density in the central mass of protein—causes a myopic change that can be corrected by changing glasses for some years—in many instances restoring vision to near normal.

B. Congenital Cataracts

These can be unilateral or bilateral, and many are thought to be of genetic origin. Some are a result of maternal rubella during the first trimester of pregnancy. If the opacity prevents a clear view of the ocular fundus, surgical removal at an early age—even 2 months—is indicated to aid in the development of useful vision.

C. Traumatic Cataracts

Contusion injuries can cause opacities that may appear right away or may develop slowly over weeks or even months. Penetrating wounds can tear the lens capsule, allowing aqueous humor to soften lens protein, usually creating major opacities. These cataracts almost always need to be removed acutely—in many cases at the time of wound repair.

D. Secondary Cataracts

These changes result from inflammatory processes in the eye (uveitis) and usually begin by producing opacities just inside the posterior lens capsule. Similar changes occur in association with retinitis pigmentosa, glaucoma, and rarely, retinal detachments.

E. Cataracts Associated with Systemic Diseases

These are usually bilateral and may appear in patients with myotonia dystrophica, hypoparathyroidism, diabetes mellitus, and Down syndrome, as well as in many other less common conditions.

F. Toxic Cataracts

Lens opacities are reported following exposure to or ingestion of numerous chemicals. They are described at some length in *Grant's Toxicology of the Eye*. The most common cause at present is the use of corticosteroids, either topical or systemic.

Treatment

There is no effective medical treatment for cataract. Surgical removal usually results in significant improvement of vision in approximately 90% of patients. The results depend on whether other ocular changes are present, such as macular scars or optic nerve changes. Indications for surgery depend almost entirely on the needs of the individual patient to improve vision. Of course, a rapidly swelling acute traumatic cataract needs early surgery.

There are two commonly used methods of cataract extraction. The lens may be removed totally in its capsule—the intracapsular technique. Extracapsular extraction removes all the lens protein out of the lens capsular bag, leaving behind the entire capsule except for an anterior portion that was removed along with the lens epithelium.

The presence of the intact posterior capsule facilitates implantation of an intraocular lens behind the iris. This lens replaces the optical power of the patient's own lens. Complications of surgery are hemorrhage from the corneoscleral wound, infection, retinal detachment, and even damage to the macula from prolonged exposure to the light of the operating microscope.

Prognosis

The results of cataract surgery generally are excellent. Significant visual improvement is reported in nearly

90% of patients following extraction of age-related cataracts. The reduced expectations in eyes with injuries are a result of unpredictable intraocular complications such as retinal scarring and macular damage.

Injuries Caused by Visible Radiation (Light)

Visible light has a spectrum of 400–750 nm. If the wavelengths of this spectrum penetrate fully to the retina, they can cause thermal, mechanical, or photic injuries. Thermal injuries are produced by light intense enough to increase the temperature in the retina by 10–20°C (18–36°F). Lasers used in therapy can cause this type of injury. The light is absorbed by the retinal pigment epithelium, where its energy is converted to heat, and the heat causes photocoagulation of retinal tissue. Mechanical injuries can be produced by exposure to laser energy from a Q-switched or mode-locked laser, which produces sonic shock waves that disrupt retinal tissue.

Photic injuries are caused by prolonged exposure to intense light, which produces varying degrees of cellular damage in the retinal macula without a significant increase in the temperature of the tissue [usually no more than 1–2°C (1.8–3.6°F)]. Recent studies show that photic injuries are not burns in the literal sense but are damage from the light itself. Sun gazing is the most common cause of this type of injury, but prolonged unprotected exposure to a welding arc also can damage the retinal macula. When the initial retinal edema clears, there is usually some scarring that leads to a permanent decrease in visual acuity. The intensity of light, length of exposure, and age of the exposed individual are all important factors. The older the individual, the more sensitive the retina appears to be to photic injuries. Anyone who has had cataract surgery is much more vulnerable because filtration of light by the lens is impaired. In photic injuries caused by exposure to welding sources or other excessively bright light, treatment with systemic corticosteroids may be tried. A large initial dose of prednisone (60–100 mg) is tapered rapidly over a period of 10–14 days. This may reduce the acute edema or inflammatory response, but it is not always effective.

Wavelengths of 500–750 nm are most useful for vision and appear not to cause photic damage to the retina at exposures most commonly encountered. However, repeated exposure to bright sunlight by working outdoors for 3–4 hours each day can cause prolongation of the dark adaptation response, thereby reducing night vision.

Injuries Caused by Infrared Radiation

Wavelengths greater than 750 nm in the infrared spectrum can produce lens changes. Glassblower cataract is an example of a heat injury that damages the anterior lens capsule. Denser cataractous changes can occur in unprotected workers who observe glowing masses of glass or iron for many hours a day.

EFFECTS OF VIDEO-DISPLAY TERMINAL USE

In recent years, employees who spend 6–8 hours a day looking at video-display terminals have complained of eyestrain, headache, and general fatigue. The brightness of the light from such terminals is not great enough to produce any ocular injury. Posture, accommodative fatigue, and the early changes of presbyopia may contribute to feelings of eyestrain and physical stress. Measures to alleviate these problems associated with video-display terminal use are discussed in Chapter 12.

REFERENCES

Lombardi DA et al: Welding-related occupational eye injuries. Inj Prev 2005;11:174 [PMID: 15933411].

Rafnsson V et al: Cosmic radiation increases the risk of nuclear cataract in airline pilots: A population-based case-control study. Arch Ophthalmol 2005;123:1102 [PMID: 16087845].

Facial Injuries

Andrew H. Murr, MD

Despite the widespread use of personal protective devices and mechanical safeguards, injuries of the face occur with alarming frequency in the workplace. The severity of a facial injury usually is correlated directly with the type, direction, and energy of the injuring force. Superficial abrasions or lacerations commonly are associated with low-energy forces and usually are preventable with the use of appropriate protective devices. More severe injuries commonly are associated with equipment failure or improper use of high-speed or pressurized machinery. For example, the disruption of an air compressor or high-speed saw can result in dispersion of heavy particles at high energy, and the improper use of a sandblaster can result in penetration of the skin and eyes by small particles. Chain saws and other cutting tools can cause deep lacerations if protective gear is not used or if improper technique is employed. Not only do these occupational injuries of the face have the potential for severe physical deformity and disability, but major facial scars also have long-lasting psychological effects on the worker.

COMPREHENSIVE EARLY MANAGEMENT OF TRAUMATIC INJURIES

When encountering a patient with significant facial injury, the general principles used in the initial evaluation of patients with traumatic injuries should be applied. In localized injuries, this may involve a cursory review of systems, whereas in more severe injuries, a comprehensive assessment may require multiple radiographic studies and subspecialty consultations.

Steps for the initial management of traumatic injuries are as follows:

A. STABILIZE THE AIRWAY

The airway may be obstructed by blood, debris, loose dentures, teeth, or foreign bodies. An attempt should be made to remove these obstructions by suction or by direct instrumentation. The airway may be secured by positional changes if the patient is mobile. If a significant force has been delivered to the head and neck region by the trauma, cervical spine injury must be assumed until proven otherwise. In patients with such

trauma, cervical manipulation should be minimized. In most cases, gentle extension of the head with neck flexion will maximize the patient's upper airway. In the event positional changes are inadequate, a forward thrust of the tongue, either by direct traction on the tongue or by forward traction of the symphysis or angles of the mandible, may be adequate to open the airway. If the airway cannot be maintained satisfactorily, endotracheal intubation or tracheotomy should be accomplished.

B. CONTROL MASSIVE HEMORRHAGE

Massive hemorrhage ordinarily is best controlled by the application of packing or pressure. Careful clamping of bleeding vessels should be undertaken only if packing or pressure does not suffice. Clamping of bleeding vessels with small hemostats should be avoided in injuries along the distribution of the facial nerve, except in an ideal environment such as the operating room (Figure 9–1).

C. RULE OUT CARDIOPULMONARY INJURY

Early assessment of the patient's pulmonary and cardiac function is essential before attention to specific aspects of any maxillofacial trauma. The potential need for ventilatory support or fluid resuscitation should be evaluated soon after encountering the patient.

D. RULE OUT FRACTURE OF THE CERVICAL SPINE

In all traumas involving a significant force striking the head and neck, the stability of the cervical spine needs to be evaluated prior to manipulation of the head and neck. The head should be stabilized with sandbags or kept in a neutral position with a cervical collar until a cervical fracture is ruled out. In most cases, this would require radiographic imaging of the cervical spine or examination by a spine specialist.

E. RULE OUT OR TREAT ANY MAJOR NEUROLOGIC, THORACOABDOMINAL, AND ORTHOPEDIC INJURIES

In cases of dramatic injuries to the face, the focus of attention too easily falls to the most obvious site of injury. The patient's overall condition must not be jeopardized by undue attention to the maxillofacial region. A systematic review of the patient's injuries is needed, including careful examination for neurological

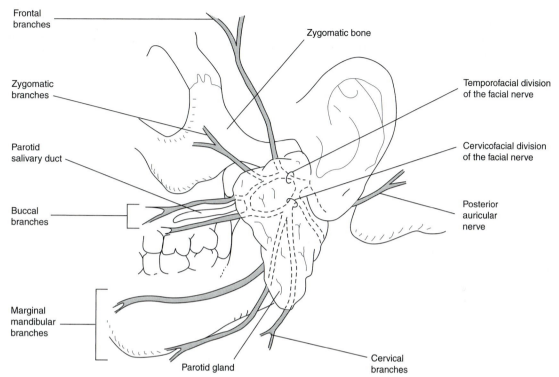

Figure 9–1. Course and distribution of the facial nerve branches after exiting the skull. Note the association of the buccal branch of the nerve with the parotid salivary duct.

injury and injury to the chest, abdomen, and/or extremities.

Only after completing these steps should a detailed and thorough evaluation of a facial injury be initiated.

MANAGEMENT OF SOFT-TISSUE INJURIES

Soft tissue may be damaged by blunt trauma or penetrating injury. The degree of damage usually is related to the amount of energy applied to the soft tissue and can vary dramatically with the etiologic agent. High-velocity penetrating materials, such as those from an explosion, frequently cause more massive soft-tissue injury than is immediately apparent because of late tissue necrosis. Continuing assessment is essential in such injuries because further debridement or repair may be needed as the true extent of destruction becomes apparent.

Diagnostic Considerations

In any soft-tissue injury of the face, an assessment for the involvement of certain vital deeper structures is essential.

A. FACIAL NERVE INJURY

The patient may complain of difficulty in moving parts of the face. All important facial motions must be evaluated. Ask the patient to wrinkle the forehead, close the eyes tightly, smile, and purse the lips. Failure to perform any of these movements in an otherwise cooperative patient suggests transection of the nerve. The nerve should be evaluated throughout its entire course to determine the site of injury. The presence of facial swelling or severe neurologic injury can mask a regional facial nerve palsy. The clinician should be suspicious of an injury if a laceration or penetrating trauma crosses the usual course of the facial nerve (see Figure 9–1). If complete hemifacial paralysis is noted, the injury to the nerve can be central, within the temporal bone or soon after the nerve exits the stylomastoid foramen.

It is useful to grade facial nerve function in all patients with head and neck trauma by using a standardized scale. Currently, the House-Brackmann scale is used widely and is relatively easy to remember. It is based on grading function on a 1–6 numerical scale and distinguishes function based on completeness of eye closure and the presence or absence of synkinesis.

After complete clinical evaluation and stabilization, a central or temporal bone injury is evaluated initially by computed tomographic (CT) scanning and/or magnetic resonance imaging (MRI). A CT scan is especially valuable in pinpointing the presence or absence of a temporal bone fracture. The patterns of temporal bone fracture can be divided into two major types: transverse fractures and longitudinal fractures. Facial nerve paralysis complicates up to 50% of transverse temporal bone fractures because the fracture line cuts across the internal auditory canal. Longitudinal fractures are more common, but because the fracture parallels the internal auditory canal, transection of the facial nerve is more unlikely. In certain cases, electrodiagnostic testing may be useful to evaluate the integrity of the facial nerve. Electroneurographic (ENOG) testing is the most objective of the electrical nerve tests for the facial nerve and measures the compound muscle action potential. The test compares the functioning side of the face with the nonfunctioning side, where a difference of greater than 90% is considered to be associated with a more guarded prognosis for recovery. Most peripheral nerve injuries in association with a laceration or penetrating trauma require direct exploration and repair of the nerve at the site of injury. For nerve injuries from direct laceration, early repair at the time of the initial laceration closure is desirable.

B. MEDIAL CANTHUS INJURY

A laceration that involves the medial canthal area may involve the lacrimal drainage system. With such injuries, the integrity of the ducts must be ensured by direct cannulation. Lacerations through this drainage system should be repaired and stented.

C. PAROTID DUCT INJURY

By massaging the parotid gland, saliva can be obtained through the caruncle of Stenson's duct located in the region of the second maxillary molar. Blood in the saliva flowing through this caruncle is a sign of injury to the parotid duct. Complete transaction of the duct would result in a lack of salivary flow on massage of the parotid gland. Significant injury to this duct requires exploration and repair with stenting in order to avoid subsequent salivary fistula formation. When injury to the duct is suspected in the presence of a laceration, a lacrimal probe can be used to cannulate the duct and to localize the injury in the laceration to allow a directed approach to exploration and repair. Injury to the parotid duct usually is accompanied by injury to its anatomic companion, the buccal branch of the facial nerve (see Figure 9–1). With such duct injuries, particular attention to facial nerve function is warranted.

Treatment

A. CARE OF LACERATIONS

The major goal of treatment of lacerations is to convert a contaminated wound into one that is as clean as a surgical incision. Sterile technique should be used in all cases.

1. Control of hemorrhage—Hemorrhage should be controlled by persistent pressure and/or packing. If this is inadequate, careful clamping of vessels with suture ligation or cautery can be used. Special attention to the regions involving the facial nerve, parotid duct, and lacrimal system is needed to avoid inadvertent injury to these important structures with hemostatic measures. If such an injury is of concern, formal exploration in the operating room should be considered.

2. Anesthesia—Sensory and motor function of the nerves of the face and neck must be assessed prior to induction of local or general anesthesia. An anesthetic should be administered before the wound is cleaned. Local anesthesia is best achieved by infiltration of a solution such as 1% lidocaine with 1:100,000 epinephrine. In certain cases, regional anesthesia using field blocks of specific nerves also can be used for facial wound repairs. If the repair is to be accomplished under general anesthesia and a nerve injury is suspected, a discussion with the anesthesia team requesting either no paralytic agents or short-acting paralytic agents should be accomplished well in advance so that electrical nerve stimulators or monitors can be used in the operating room if desired.

3. Wound cleaning and preparation for repair—After larger foreign bodies are mechanically removed from the wound, it is irrigated with copious amounts of normal saline solution to remove occult debris and bacteria. This can be done by using a blunt needle on a large syringe (e.g., a 19-gauge blunt needle on a 60-mL syringe) and forcefully irrigating the complete depth of the wound. In almost every case, primary closure of facial lacerations is recommended. Because the blood supply to the face is excellent, only obviously necrotic or nonviable tissue should be removed. The wound edge can be sharply débrided so that macerated edges are excised. This measure may require excision of some normal skin. Even a millimeter of debridement provides more viable uninjured tissue for closure. Débridement makes undermining of wound edges a requirement so that the tissue can be advanced to achieve closure. The edges are undermined in a plane between the dermis and subcutaneous tissue to a distance of 1–2 cm horizontally from the wound edge. No attempt should be made to straighten lacerations unless the laceration can be made to lie completely within or parallel to resting skin tension lines (Figure 9–2). These skin lines are similar to the lines of aging and are ordinarily directed in a perpendicular direction to the pull of facial muscles. A jagged laceration eventually is less apparent than one that is straight but crosses resting skin tension lines. Prior to wound closure, hemostasis must be meticulous.

4. Wound closure—Subcutaneous tissues are closed with absorbable suture of a suitable size, such as 3-0 or 4-0

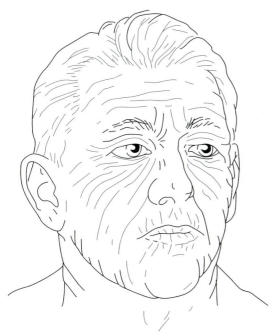

Figure 9–2. Lines of Langerhans, or the resting skin tension lines. Repair of lacerations should attempt to parallel these lines when possible.

chromic gut sutures. Synthetic monofilament suture also can be helpful when a longer period of tensile strength is desired. The skin is closed next with a subcuticular stitch of similar size. The needle enters the dermis and exits between the epidermis and dermis on one side, and it then enters between the epidermis and dermis on the opposite side and exits the dermis on that side. The knot is then tied. This technique results in the knot being placed below the surface and therefore not protruding between the skin edges. The wound already should be precisely approximated following closure of the subcuticular layer. The cuticular layer then is sutured with 5-0 or 6-0 monofilament nylon to achieve final closure. There should be no tension on the wound edges, and the cuticular stitch should not be used to close defects of more than 1 mm of skin. Larger defects require placement of more subcuticular sutures to remove all tension from the edges of the skin.

5. Wound dressings and follow-up care—The wound is dressed with an antibiotic ointment, and if appropriate, a tetanus toxoid booster should be given. Thereafter, the wound is cleaned three times daily with a sterile saline solution or hydrogen peroxide. Antibiotic ointment then is applied to help loosen eschar and facilitate epithelialization.

After the cuticular sutures have been in place for approximately 3–7 days, they are removed. Wound edges are treated with a substance that promotes adhesion, such

as tincture of benzoin, and adhesive strips are applied in a crisscross fashion to the wound edges. These strips should be maintained for at least 5 days, after which time tissue strength begins to develop as a result of the maturation of tissue collagen.

B. Special Considerations

1. Special structures—Nose, eyebrow, and mouth injuries require special attention in their repair because of their unique anatomy.

a. Nasal injuries. The anterior two-thirds of the nose is supported by several cartilaginous structures that can be lacerated along with the nasal skin in an injury. The complex relationship of these cartilages and the need to evaluate the soft tissues within the nasal passages often require evaluation by a specialist to obtain an optimal reconstruction of this structure. In simple lacerations with minimal cartilage damage, repair should include reapproximation of the cartilage by suture repair of the perichondrium or sometimes the cartilage itself with absorbable sutures. In some injuries, 4-0 clear nylon may be used as a permanent suture. The skin should be repaired as described earlier.

b. Eyebrow injuries. A laceration through the eyebrow requires special care to minimize injury to the hair follicles that may be exposed by the injury. Hair follicle injury from overzealous hemostatic measures or debridement may leave a large part of the eyebrow permanently devoid of hair. Minimal debridement or undermining of tissues should be performed in this region. Primary repair should focus on realigning the hairline as accurately as possible with the first cuticular sutures.

c. Mouth injuries. Lacerations or penetrating injuries through the skin that extend through the buccal mucosa or lips can be more difficult to repair. With full-thickness lacerations of the mouth, preparation of the wound is similar to other soft-tissue injuries. With most of these injuries, repair of the subcutaneous tissues, including the orbicularis oris, should be performed first with simple interrupted absorbable 3-0 or 4-0 sutures. Oral mucosa then is repaired with simple interrupted 4-0 chromic gut sutures up to the transition of oral mucosa to the vermilion. The skin laceration then should be repaired with subcuticular and then cuticular sutures, as described previously, focusing on reapproximating the vermilion border as accurately as possible. Even a small discrepancy of this border will be obvious to the casual observer when it is healed. After this is completed, the remainder of the vermilion is closed with 4-0 absorbable subcuticular interrupted sutures followed by epidermal closure using 5-0 nylon sutures in a simple interrupted fashion.

2. Delayed treatment—Unlike other locations, because of the face's exceptional blood supply, the delayed treatment of facial lacerations is similar to acute repairs in the absence of infection. If infection occurs, sutures are removed, the wound is opened, and wet-to-dry dressings are applied. When the wound has been cleansed of all purulent material and healthy granulation tissue is present, the preceding steps are used to reclose the wound.

3. Care of abrasions—Abrasive injuries can cause partial- to full-thickness loss of the epidermis. A full-thickness loss of skin results in an anesthetic area similar to that of a third-degree burn.

    a. Anesthesia. Anesthesia of a large abraded area can be achieved by local infiltration of an anesthetic solution such as lidocaine with epinephrine, by topical application of an anesthetic gel such as 4% lidocaine jelly or a eutectic mixture of local anesthetics (EMLA) cream, or by field block of specific nerves.

    b. Wound cleaning and repair. After adequate anesthesia has been achieved, the wound is cleaned by irrigation. Scrubbing with a soft scrub brush may be required to remove small embedded particles, but scrubbing should be undertaken carefully to avoid causing further injury. Small areas of full-thickness avulsion of less than 3 cm in diameter usually can be treated by mobilization of adjacent tissue or by rotation or advancement of local flaps. Larger areas of avulsion may require delayed skin grafting. Nevertheless, the goal usually is to obtain primary closure whenever possible. It is prudent to allow healing by secondary intention to occur and by allowing the wound to become mature and less contaminated prior to committing to flap-based closure in the acute period. To obtain the best color and texture match, the types of skin grafts and appropriate donor sites are chosen based on the location of the tissue loss. In addition, an attempt to preserve the facial aesthetic units with the use of flaps and skin grafting will help to maximize the benefit of the facial repair.

    c. Wound dressings and follow-up care. Partial-thickness abrasions are cleaned and covered with antibiotic ointment two to three times daily. For larger wounds, a semiocclusive dressing may be used to protect this region. These dressings should be changed as recommended by the manufacturer of the dressing. No treatment is needed for pigmentary changes that occasionally occur after injury because the pigment usually reverts to normal within 6–12 months. Sun exposure should be avoided because this may permanently pigment scars. The use of 30 SPF sunblock usually is recommended after about 14 days of healing if the patient is to be in the sun. Silicone sheeting sometimes is used as an occlusive dressing in patients with a tendency toward hypertrophic scarring in an attempt to minimize hypertrophic connective tissue formation.

C. CARE OF SKIN PENETRATED BY SMALL FOREIGN BODIES

Certain injuries may result in skin penetration of multiple small foreign bodies. Common examples include asphalt from an abrasive road "burn" or "rash," glass shards, and sand particles from a sandblast injury. These foreign bodies individually do not pose much of a problem, but they must be removed or they can result in a permanent tattoo. When foreign material is not removed completely from the wound, although the overlying skin may heal, the material often will cause chronic foreign-body reactions with eventual expulsion of the material through repetitive infections over long periods of time.

1. Wound cleaning and repair—Sparsely placed foreign bodies usually can be removed mechanically with a fine forceps. Magnification provided by a loupe or microscope frequently is necessary to achieve adequate removal. In certain cases, an orthopedic debrider may be used to mobilize these particles. Diffusely placed small foreign bodies, such as sand particles, may require removal by dermabrasion. Dermabrasion should be continued only to the depth necessary to remove the particles without causing a full-thickness injury. It is sometimes preferable to perform dermabrasion in a symmetric fashion so that the resulting pattern will be less noticeable.

2. Wound dressings and follow-up care—Care of these types of injuries following their cleaning and repair is the same as that described for partial-thickness abrasions.

D. CARE OF SCARRED FACIAL TISSUE

Scarring that results from facial injuries may require secondary revision. Assessment of the need for scar revision should be made only after the signs of acute inflammation have resolved, which usually requires 6–12 months. During this time period, dramatic improvement of scar appearance often occurs as the wound matures. It is usually best to delay reconstructive measures, such as Z-plasty, running W-plasty, and geometric broken-line closures, until the scar-revision stage of treatment. On occasion, a facial scar can be so dramatic that early revision is indicated because the eventual need for scar revision is apparent even after expected wound maturation. Proceeding with early reconstructive measures in these select patients will improve patient morale markedly. For hypertrophic scars, silicone sheeting can be used to decrease the hypertrophy. Occasionally, injected steroids can be used to help improve the long-term result.

MANAGEMENT OF FACIAL FRACTURES

In the evaluation of patients with facial injuries, the likelihood of a facial fracture can be determined by knowing the type and focus of force received in the facial injury and an understanding of the amount of force required to fracture the facial bones. The vulnerability of these facial bones varies considerably from the nasal bone, which requires minimal force to fracture, to the various skull-base fractures, or Le Fort fractures, which require a major blow to the midface.

Most facial fractures can be diagnosed on the basis of physical symptoms and signs alone. A hematoma points to a specific site of injury. Facial deformities secondary to depression of facial bone structures and impairment of sensory and motor functions of adjacent nerve structures are significant signs of a facial fracture.

General examination should include (1) assessment of facial symmetry and extraocular motility, (2) palpation of the orbital rims, frontozygomatic areas, zygomatic arches, and mandible, (3) evaluation of the dental occlusion, (4) determination of the stability and configuration of the nasal dorsum, and (5) evaluation of the three major cutaneous branches of the trigeminal nerve.

1. Nasal Fractures

Because of their prominent location and delicate construction, the nasal bones are the most commonly fractured structure in the facial skeleton. Fortunately, fracture of the nasal bones without displacement is often without consequence to the patient and sometimes does not require repair.

Clinical Findings

The most common finding in patients with nasal fractures is point tenderness over the nasal bones. Epistaxis frequently may be present following the injury. Periorbital ecchymosis may be noticeable, especially a day or two after injury. In more severe cases, the nasal dorsum is obviously deviated to one side or collapsed, and crepitation may be noted. Injury to the internal nasal structures also will be evident frequently. Inspection of the nasal vault may show an impaired airway on one side of the nasal septum with a corresponding concavity on the other side suggesting a traumatic septal deviation. With nasal trauma, hematomas can form between the septal cartilage and the perichondrium, devascularizing the septum. If not treated, they will result in septal cartilage destruction. Thus, it is critical to examine every patient with significant nasal trauma for a septal hematoma. A septal hematoma appears as a symmetric nasal septal convexity that is bluish in color and slightly soft to palpation. Early, if not immediate, incision and drainage may prevent the difficult sequela of septal necrosis with attendant collapse of nasal support. Lateral soft-tissue radiographs usually will confirm the diagnosis of nasal bone fracture.

Treatment & Prognosis

The presence of posttraumatic swelling can make assessment of the degree of nasal fracture displacement diffi-

cult. Often the decision to perform a reduction of the nasal fracture will be delayed until 3–5 days after the date of injury to allow soft-tissue swelling to regress. After 7–10 days, the nasal bones will have started to heal, and beyond that, closed reduction becomes increasingly difficult. As a general rule of thumb, after 3 weeks, surgical osteotomies often will be required to reduce a severe nasal fracture rather than a closed elevation of the nasal bones because of bone fixation through the healing process. Nondisplaced nasal fractures do not require treatment, but a small splint may be helpful for comfort. The nasal bone is not a weight-bearing structure; thus, closed reduction of a fracture without fixation is indicated for significantly displaced nasal fractures. Some surgeons prefer to wait until swelling has subsided substantially because they feel that more precise realignment of the nasal dorsum can be achieved at that time. However, performing closed reduction as soon as possible, preferably in the first 12 hours, rehabilitates the patient more rapidly. The use of closed reduction corrects the majority of gross abnormalities that result from the nasal injury. Definitive repair of any nasal deformity caused by nasal bone fractures may require an open reduction and repair, which is usually performed at least 3 months after the date of injury. Dislocation of the nasal septum should be addressed at the time of the repair of the nasal fracture. In more severe cases, immediate or delayed septoplasty may be required to reestablish an adequate nasal airway. Septal hematomas require immediate treatment to prevent infection and secondary necrosis of the septal cartilage. Treatment consists of draining the hematoma and using nasal packing to reapproximate the septal mucosa to the septal cartilage. Septal splints or through-and-through mattress sutures also may be used to treat this problem. A 7- to 10-day period of disability is expected after reduction of a nasal fracture. A nasal splint is worn for approximately 7 days. Glasses should not be worn in the immediate postoperative period because the nasal bones can be shifted by the pressure of the glasses resting on the nasal dorsum. Pressure or further injury to the nose must be avoided for at least 3 months following a nasal fracture.

2. Mandibular Fractures

Mandibular fractures usually occur from direct trauma to the jaw. Given the prominent location of the mandible, it is the second most common type of facial fracture. The majority of cases involve two fractures of this arch-shaped bone. The most frequent site of fracture is the region just below the condylar process.

Clinical Findings

Swelling and tenderness in the soft tissue overlying the fracture sites and pain with mastication are the most common signs of a mandibular fracture. Displacement of fracture fragments frequently results from the pull of the muscles of mastication causing malocclusion. Other symptoms and signs of a mandibular fracture may include a step-off deformity, instability of the dental arch, hypesthesia of the mental nerve, foul-smelling breath, trismus, or deviation of the jaw on opening. In certain cases of bilateral mandibular fractures, mobility of the anterior segment may allow collapse of the base of the tongue into the airway, resulting in airway obstruction. Anterior traction will correct this problem immediately, but these patients will require airway protection until the mandibular fractures are stabilized. In addition, particular attention should be paid to the patient's dentition. Fractured, chipped, or loosened teeth should be noted. Any avulsed teeth should be located because they may have been aspirated. Chest radiographs should be performed if the teeth cannot be found immediately. Plain mandibular radiographs or Panorex dental imaging will confirm the presence of the mandibular fractures and display the degree of displacement. CT scans can be quite useful to evaluate the presence and extent of condylar fractures and can be used to plan the treatment approach.

Treatment & Prognosis

The treatment algorithm for a mandibular fracture depends on the location, the number of fractures, and the availability of stable dentition. Single nondisplaced subcondylar fractures can be managed successfully with soft diet alone or a short period of intermaxillary fixation (IMF). Traditionally, definitive treatment of other mandibular fractures consists of closed reduction followed by IMF for 4–6 weeks. IMF relies on sufficient dentition to maintain good fixation after centric occlusion has been achieved. Open reduction and internal fixation using compression plating has allowed effective management of many types of fractures and is particularly useful for patients with little or no dentition. It also has offered an alternative technique that allows more rapid bone healing and earlier mobilization of the mandible than does IMF alone. Earlier function can minimize later temporomandibular joint (TMJ) dysfunction from prolonged inactivity because of the need for several weeks of IMF.

Chipped teeth require temporary coverage of pulp and dentin at the time of fracture therapy. Definitive repair of damaged teeth can be done later. Avulsed teeth should be placed in milk and replanted within the first 2 hours of avulsion. They can be stabilized to adjacent teeth during the period of IMF to allow them to heal.

The prognosis for return to function of the mandible following proper treatment is excellent. Subcondylar fractures that remain displaced may cause TMJ pain on

chewing and ultimately result in abnormal mobility of the joint. Rehabilitation devices to exercise the TMJ are available commercially and can minimize TMJ ankylosis. The period of disability after mandibular fractures is usually 4–6 weeks. If IMF is used, it may be maintained for 6 weeks. In these patients, return to active heavy labor may not be possible for 6–8 weeks. If rigid internal fixation techniques are used, return to active heavy labor can be somewhat earlier. Return to work requires individualization based on the type of injury, the type of repair, the job description, and other associated injuries.

3. Maxillary (Le Fort) Fractures

Maxillary fractures are classified as Le Fort I, II, and III fractures (Figure 9–3). These are uncommon fractures that require a very significant force striking the midface. The most common cause of these fractures is high-speed motor vehicle accidents. A Le Fort I fracture is a horizontal fracture of the palate and does not involve the orbits. A Le Fort II fracture traverses through the lateral buttress of the maxilla, the infraorbital rim, the orbital floor, the medial wall of the orbit, and the perpendicular plate of the ethmoid bone. A Le Fort III fracture has the characteristics of a Le Fort II fracture with the addition of frontozygomatic fractures and is known as a craniofacial dys-

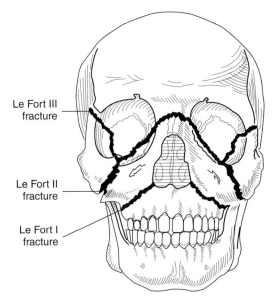

Le Fort III fracture

Le Fort II fracture

Le Fort I fracture

Figure 9–3. Maxillary fractures usually occur in patterns described by Le Fort. Le Fort fractures I to III are represented and extend into the skull base through the pterygoid plates. (Redrawn and reproduced with permission from Bailey BJ: *Head & Neck Surgery—Otolaryngology.* Philadelphia: Lippincott, 2006.)

junction fracture. All these fractures extend posteriorly through the pterygoid plates.

Clinical Findings

In patients with maxillary fractures, the midface usually is displaced posteriorly and inferiorly. This results in malocclusion, with the molar teeth meeting prematurely and the incisor teeth meeting with an open bite. In most patients, the entire midface appears to be flattened, and patients frequently present with epistaxis along with facial pain. The level of mobility in the midface depends on the type of fracture. To test for mobility, the forehead is stabilized by the palm of one hand, and the opposite thumb and forefinger are used to grasp the incisor teeth or palate. An attempt then is made to manipulate the palate. In Le Fort I fractures, only the palate is mobile. In Le Fort II and III fractures, findings may include mobility of the nasal dorsum and anterior malar face. These patients also may have hypesthesia of the infraorbital nerve, a nasal fracture, and cerebrospinal fluid rhinorrhea resulting from an associated fracture of the cribriform plate or anterior skull base. More severe cases may have concurrent mandibular fractures, nasoethmoidal complex fractures, or both. In patients with significant displacement of their maxillary fractures, the posterior displacement can impinge on the patients' airway, and they may require airway protection until definitive repair of the fractures takes place. In these patients with significant midface fractures, no tubes of any sort should be passed through the nose because the skull base can be penetrated with instrumentation, resulting in significant morbidity. Early ophthalmologic consultation to rule out globe injury or entrapment is indicated given the degree of force required to produce these fractures and their involvement of the bony orbital walls. Fine-cut CT scans in an axial and coronal plane are essential to define the exact extent of the injury and to assess the status of the orbital floor accurately.

Treatment & Prognosis

Management of maxillary fractures includes reduction of the midface and restoration of normal occlusion, followed by fixation. For best results, surgical intervention should occur during the 3–7 days after the traumatic injury. In extreme cases when the patient is unstable because of other associated injuries, repair can be delayed up to 14 or more days. The repair of maxillary fractures usually requires intranasal manipulations and the use of IMF; thus, a tracheotomy often is indicated to maintain the airway perioperatively. In most cases, closed reduction is performed initially using specialized forceps for grasping and mobilizing the midface to restore its normal position. Normal occlusion is ensured by the application of IMF. This step is followed by direct exposure of key points of the fracture, verification of reduction, and rigid fixation using titanium plates. Rigid fixation usually allows immediate removal of IMF for early function. Most cerebrospinal fluid leaks associated with midface fractures are self-limited and require no additional measures other than reduction of the fracture. Recovery from the surgery usually requires 2–3 weeks. A further period of rehabilitation of 1–2 months following these severe maxillofacial injuries often is necessary. Other associated injuries, such as brain or orthopedic injuries, commonly require more prolonged rehabilitation.

4. Zygomatic Fractures

The zygomatic complex is a prominent facial bone that forms the malar eminence, which gives projection to the cheek. This bone frequently is fractured by a direct blow to the cheekbone. This fracture previously was called the *tripod fracture,* but because more than three buttresses are fractured, it is more accurately named the *zygomatic complex fracture.* The entire bone usually is dislocated posteriorly, inferiorly, and medially (Figure 9–4). With such an injury, prominence of the malar eminence is lost, and this will result in an unsightly deformity if allowed to heal without reduction. In addition, the zygomatic complex helps to form the orbital floor; thus, untreated fractures with significant displacement may result in orbital complications such as enophthalmos.

Clinical Findings

Symptoms and signs include pain over the malar area, hypesthesia of the infraorbital nerve, step-off deformity of the infraorbital rim, flattening of the malar eminence, and lateral subconjunctival hemorrhage. A downward slant of

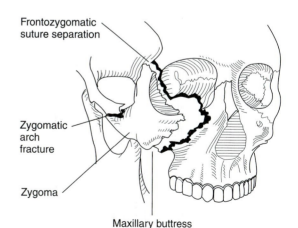

Frontozygomatic suture separation

Zygomatic arch fracture

Zygoma

Maxillary buttress

Figure 9–4. Fracture of the zygomatic complex usually results in medial, inferior, and posterior displacement. (Redrawn and reproduced with permission from Bailey BJ: *Head & Neck Surgery—Otolaryngology.* Philadelphia: Lippincott, 2006.)

the palpebral fissure may occur as a result of inferior displacement of the attachment of the lateral canthal tendon of the lower eyelid. Limited extraocular motility suggests involvement of the orbital contents. However, muscle contusion or neurapraxia of the third cranial nerve, as well as fracture of the orbital floor with entrapment of the inferior rectus muscle, can result in diplopia. In some cases, the eye is displaced backward or recessed in the orbit as a result of a relative increase in the volume of the bony orbit. This complication is called *enophthalmos;* if not corrected, it can result in significant long-term diplopia. The zygomatic arch may be displaced medially and impinge on the coronoid process, which can result in trismus or inadequate closure of the jaw. A standard facial axial and coronal CT scan should be obtained to screen for the presence of a zygomatic complex fracture. The CT scan is instrumental to determine the degree of displacement present and to assist in the reconstructive effort.

Treatment & Prognosis

Emergent treatment of zygomatic complex fractures usually is not required. In patients with significant periorbital trauma, ophthalmologic consultation to rule out significant orbital injury should be obtained in the early phases of patient management. If needed, repair of the fracture should be performed between 3–10 days after the injury. Although zygomatic fractures that are minimally displaced require no treatment, those that are symptomatic or have more than a few millimeters of displacement should be treated by open reduction and fixation. Incisions usually are made sublabially onto the anterior face of the maxilla and over the frontozygomatic suture. The zygoma is placed in its normal position, and rigid or absorbable plates are applied to maintain reduction. The orbital floor also must be evaluated carefully, and significantly displaced fractures should be repaired through an infraorbital or transconjunctival incision. If repairs are not made in patients in whom orbital volume is increased significantly because of the floor fracture, enophthalmos may occur after the swelling associated with the injury subsides. This late posttraumatic enophthalmos is difficult to repair. Reconstruction of the orbital floor may require the use of material such as bone or cartilage grafts or alloplastic materials to rebuild the floor and maintain the appropriate orbital volume. The prognosis for return to full function after a zygomatic complex fracture is excellent. Swelling usually will be resolved by 2 weeks after the injury. Light work can be resumed at that time. Heavy labor is best delayed until 4 weeks after repair. The malar area should be protected from possible recurrent injury for 3 months after repair.

5. Orbital Floor ("Blow-Out") Fractures

In certain cases, an orbital floor can be fractured without the other facial bones being injured. Classically, this frac-ture results from a focused blow to the globe without significant impact to the infraorbital rim or the zygomatic complex. The force is transmitted by the globe and fractures the weakest component of the orbit, the orbital floor.

Clinical Findings

In orbital floor fractures, periorbital swelling and eye pain may be the only presenting complaints. Entrapment of the inferior rectus muscle in the floor fracture can occur with subsequent diplopia and fixation of the globe when the patient attempts to look upward. As with zygomatic complex fractures, if there is significant displacement of the orbital floor into the maxillary sinus, enophthalmos may result.

The Waters radiographic view usually can demonstrate the orbital floor fracture. A teardrop deformity may appear beneath the orbital floor resulting from herniation of the orbital contents into the maxillary sinus below or hematoma formation in the mucosa of the sinus roof. An air-fluid level frequently is present in the maxillary sinus on the affected side. As with zygomatic complex fractures, an orbital CT scan is necessary to determine the exact extent of injury and the degree of displacement of the orbital floor.

Treatment & Prognosis

As with any periorbital trauma, ophthalmologic consultation to rule out vision-threatening orbital injury should be obtained as soon as possible. Surgical reconstruction of the orbital floor is required for entrapment of extraocular muscles, enophthalmos, or globe ptosis caused by the size of the orbital floor defect. In questionable cases, repair may be delayed 10–14 days in order to obtain a more accurate assessment of the degree of deformity or impairment of function as the traumatic swelling recedes. An infraorbital, subciliary, or transconjunctival incision is used to explore the orbital floor and repair it as needed. Alloplastic or autogenous implantable material often is needed to reestablish the orbital floor. The prognosis for return to full function after an orbital floor fracture is excellent. Periorbital swelling usually has resolved by 2 weeks after the injury or surgery. Light work can be resumed at that time. Heavy labor is best delayed until at least 4 weeks after surgical repair.

6. Nasoethmoidal Complex Fractures

With severe upper midface trauma, the entire nasal complex can be displaced posteriorly, causing collapse of the nasal bones into the ethmoidal sinuses. This type of injury also destabilizes the medial canthal ligaments, frequently resulting in posttraumatic telecanthus. In more severe cases, there may be an associated fracture of the anterior skull base and a potential for a cerebrospinal fluid leak.

Clinical Findings

Common symptoms and signs of nasoethmoidal complex fractures include facial pain, anosmia, watery rhinorrhea, flattening of the nasal dorsum, and downward, lateral, and anterior displacement of the medial canthus. A torn cribriform plate can cause cerebrospinal fluid rhinorrhea. Disruption of the medial canthal area with failure of apposition of the inferior lacrimal caruncle to the globe may result in epiphora, the uncontrolled flow of tears. An axial and coronal CT scan of the facial bones and paranasal sinuses is the study of choice to establish the diagnosis.

Treatment & Prognosis

Emergency reduction of nasoethmoidal complex fractures is only necessary in the rare event of uncontrolled bleeding or persistent cerebrospinal fluid rhinorrhea. Otherwise, treatment may be delayed until 5–7 days after injury; this allows adequate resolution of edema so that the medial canthal area can be restored to its normal position. Direct wiring or rigid fixation with microplates of the nasal and lacrimal bones is necessary. Nasal packing also may be required to maintain the normal position of the nasal bones.

The prognosis for return to normal function after nasoethmoidal fractures is excellent. A significant number of patients have persistent slight widening of the intercanthal distance, which usually is not functionally significant. The period of disability is usually 6–8 weeks and often is not as long as the disability from other associated injuries.

7. Frontal Sinus Fractures

The frontal sinus bones are extremely strong compared with the other facial bones; thus, fractures are relatively uncommon. Patients who have received sufficient force to fracture the frontal sinuses frequently have skull fractures and significant closed-head injury. The clinician should be aware that these sinuses vary greatly in their development, with 10% of the population having isolated unilateral development, 5% having rudimentary development, and 4% being without frontal sinuses on radiographic examination.

Clinical Findings

A contusion or laceration over the glabella may be the sign of an underlying fracture of the frontal sinus. Other symptoms and signs include pain, cerebrospinal fluid rhinorrhea or bloody rhinorrhea, flattening of the glabella, and in some cases, a step-off along the fracture line. A subperiosteal hematoma or soft-tissue swelling may obscure a depressed anterior table frontal sinus fracture during physical examination. These patients often display mental status changes as a result of concurrent intracranial injury. In one series, only 24% of patients with frontal sinus fractures were conscious at presentation. Axial and coronal CT scans are essential for the definitive diagnosis of fractures of both the anterior and posterior sinus walls.

Treatment & Prognosis

Emergency therapy ordinarily is not required. Surgical repair is indicated in patients with anterior or posterior wall fractures with significant displacement, frontonasal drainage tract compromise, or persistent cerebrospinal fluid leak. If the fracture is severely comminuted, the entire sinus may be removed and the frontonasal ducts plugged with autogenous material. In patients with extensive posterior table fractures, neurosurgical assistance will be needed intraoperatively. Anecdotal reports suggest that a mucocele can form many years following injury and may present as a brain abscess or as a mass with erosion of the frontal bones. Some authors advocate preventive treatment of these complications by obliteration of the frontal sinuses with fat or, if the posterior table is severely comminuted, with cranialization.

The period of recuperation after treatment of frontal sinus fractures is usually 4–6 weeks. The period of disability again usually is related more to associated injuries than to the frontal sinus injury.

REFERENCES

Bagheri SC et al: Comparison of the severity of bilateral Le Fort injuries in isolated midface trauma. J Oral Maxillofac Surg 2005;63:1123 [PMID: 16094579].

Biller JA et al: Complications and the time to repair of mandible fractures. Laryngoscope 2005;115:769 [PMID: 15867637]

Chang EL, Bernardino CR: Update on orbital trauma. Curr Opin Ophthalmol 2004;15:411 [PMID: 15625902].

Cruz AA, Eichenberger GC: Epidemiology and management of orbital fractures. Curr Opin Ophthalmol 2004;15:416 [PMID: 15625903].

Verschueren DS et al: Management of laryngotracheal injuries associated with craniomaxillofacial trauma. J Oral Maxillofac Surg 2006;64:203 [PMID: 16413891].

Hearing Loss

10

Jacob Johnson, MD, & Scott T. Robinson, MPH, CIH, CSP

Occupational hearing loss may be partial or total, unilateral or bilateral, and conductive, sensorineural, or mixed (conductive and sensorineural). Conductive hearing loss results from dysfunction of the external or middle ear, which impairs the passage of sound vibrations to the inner ear.

In the workplace, conductive and mixed hearing loss can be caused by blunt or penetrating head injuries, explosions, and thermal injuries such as slag burns sustained when a piece of welder's slag penetrates the eardrum. Sensory hearing loss results from deterioration of the cochlea usually because of loss of hair cells from the organ of Corti. Among the many common causes of sensory hearing loss are continuous exposure to noise in excess of 85 dB, blunt head injury, and exposure to ototoxic substances.

PHYSIOLOGY OF HEARING

Sound waves consist of alternating periods of compression and rarefaction within a medium such as air. The degree of this pressure variation has a correlation in the subjective awareness of loudness. Measurement of human hearing in terms of sound pressure level (SPL) in dynes per centimeter squared is cumbersome because of the differing sensitivity of the ear at the various frequencies. For this reason, a scale [decibels hearing level (dBHL)] allowing easy comparison among frequencies and individuals was developed. This scale is a logarithmic measurement of human hearing that, through standardization, has defined 0 dBHL as the faintest sound that the average normal-hearing person can detect. The human ear has a remarkable dynamic range of roughly 0–120 dB (10^6 SPL), which allows for detection of sound from the faintest noise to painful stimulation.

The frequency (or number of waves passing a point in a second) has a subjective correlate in pitch. The normal human cochlea is capable of detecting and encoding sound waves across the frequency range extending from approximately 20–20,000 Hz. The most important range for human speech reception is between 500 and 3000 Hz. Because isolated pure-tone waves seldom occur in nature, the cochlea is called on to analyze complex waveforms. The adult external auditory canal has a resonant frequency of about 3200 Hz and can amplify sound pressures of 10–20 dB in midrange frequencies.

There is considerable impedance to the passage of sound vibrations from air into the fluid-filled inner ear. To overcome this barrier, an impedance-matching mechanism known as the *conducting system* has evolved. This apparatus consists of the external auditory canal, tympanic membrane, and the three ossicles (malleus, incus, and stapes). The conducting system contributes approximately 45 dB to normal hearing.

The transduction of mechanical vibrations to nervous impulses by the inner hair cells takes place in the inner ear (cochlea) at the organ of Corti. At the organ of Corti, the hair cells rest on the frequency-encoding basilar membrane, and the stereocilia of the three rows of outer hair cells and the one row of inner hair cells oscillate against a tectorial membrane. The shearing action between the stereocilia and the tectorial membrane, caused by the traveling wave motion of the basilar membrane, results in an electrochemical process in the hair cells.

As the wave travels from base (high frequency) to apex (low frequency) along the basilar membrane, it reaches a peak amplitude that correlates directly with the frequency of the sound. Each point along the basilar membrane is frequency-specific (tonotopically organized). The electromotility of the outer hair cells enhances the frequency tuning and amplification of the traveling wave. The auditory nerve fibers innervating the hair cells also carry frequency selectivity.

EVALUATION OF HEARING

Test of Spoken Words

The simplest form of hearing evaluation may be performed in a quiet room without any sophisticated equipment. The patient is asked to repeat spoken words of increasing intensity while competing noises (the crumpling of paper or the sounds from a Bárány noise box) are presented to the opposite ear. Test results may be expressed as the ability to hear a soft whisper, loud whisper, soft-spoken voice, loud-spoken voice, or shout.

Tuning Fork Tests

Tuning fork tests should be performed with a 512 Hz tuning fork because frequencies below this level will elicit a tactile response.

A. RINNE TEST

In cases where the patient hears air conduction (tuning fork placed by the opening of the ear canal) better than via bone conduction (tuning fork placed on the mastoid bone), a sensorineural hearing loss or normal hearing is indicated. In cases where bone conduction is louder than air conduction, a conductive hearing loss is indicated.

B. WEBER TEST

When the tuning fork is placed on the forehead or front teeth, sound should lateralize toward the ear with a conductive loss and away from the ear with a sensorineural loss.

Pure-Tone Audiometry

Sensitivity to pure tones is measured at 250, 500, 1000, 2000, 3000, 4000, and 8000 Hz for both air conduction (head phones) and bone conduction (bone oscillator). Thresholds of hearing are expressed in decibels, with the normal range at each frequency from 0–20 dB. Because loud signals may stimulate the opposite ear, masking the contralateral ear with competing sound is necessary when asymmetry exists. When both air and bone conduction are decreased, a sensorineural hearing loss exists. Conductive losses are indicated by an "air-bone gap," in which the air-conduction threshold exceeds the bone-conduction threshold. Results may be presented numerically or shown graphically (Figures 10–1 to 10–5).

Bekesy Audiometry

Pure-tone thresholds also may be measured by Bekesy audiometry, in which the patient uses self-directed techniques that involve pressing and releasing a signal button. This procedure is used in some occupational screening programs, but it is generally not as reliable as procedures that are administered by an audiologist.

Speech Audiometry

Two routine tests are performed to assess speech reception and comprehension, which are the most important aspects of audition.

A. SPEECH RECEPTION THRESHOLD

The speech reception threshold (SRT) is the intensity (in decibels) at which the listener is able to repeat 50% of balanced two-syllable words known as *spondee words* (e.g., *baseball, playground,* and *airplane*). The threshold is usually in close agreement (usually within 6–10 dB), with an average of the pure-tone thresholds for frequencies between 500 and 3000 Hz. The normal range is between 0 and 20 dB, with losses of 20–40 dB termed

mild, 40–60 dB termed *moderate,* 60–80 dB termed *severe,* and greater than 80 dB termed *profound.*

B. SPEECH DISCRIMINATION SCORE

In the speech discrimination score (SDS), also referred to as *word recognition score,* monosyllabic words that are phonetically balanced are presented at intensities well above the threshold for speech reception (SRT plus 25–40 dB) in order to test speech comprehension. Results are expressed as a percentage of words repeated correctly. The normal range of SDS is 88–100%. Word lists are available for most languages. Significant depression of the SDS usually indicates socially significant disability.

Impedance (Immittance) Audiometry

The mechanical aspects of the middle ear sound transformer system can be assessed by tympanometry and acoustic reflex testing.

A. TYMPANOMETRY

Tympanometry employs an acoustic probe to measure the impedance of the eardrum and ossicular chain. Reduced middle ear compliance usually indicates a partial vacuum owing to auditory tube dysfunction, whereas noncompliance suggests either a tympanic membrane perforation or middle ear effusion. An increase in compliance suggests either laxity of the tympanic membrane or disruption of the ossicular chain.

B. ACOUSTIC REFLEX TESTING

Contraction of the middle ear muscles in response to a loud noise results in a measurable rise of middle ear impedance. Interpretation of acoustic reflex testing also may yield information regarding the integrity of the auditory portion of the central nervous system. It is also an indirect measurement of recruitment (the abnormal sensitivity to loud sounds) that frequently accompanies sensorineural hearing loss.

Evoked-Response Audiometry (Brain Stem Audiometry)

In patients who demonstrate unilateral or asymmetric sensorineural hearing loss, retrocochlear lesions (lesions of the eighth cranial nerve, brain stem, or cortex) must be ruled out. Evoked potentials, which typically are elicited in response to clicking noises and recorded via scalp electrodes, provide information about the location of sensorineural lesions. For individuals with normal hearing, as well as most patients with cochlear hearing losses, a series of five electro-encephalographic waves may be detected, representing the central auditory system from the eighth cranial nerve (wave 1) to the inferior colliculus (wave 5). The discovery of any significant delay or even a complete absence of response may indicate a cerebellopontine angle tumor (e.g., acoustic neu-

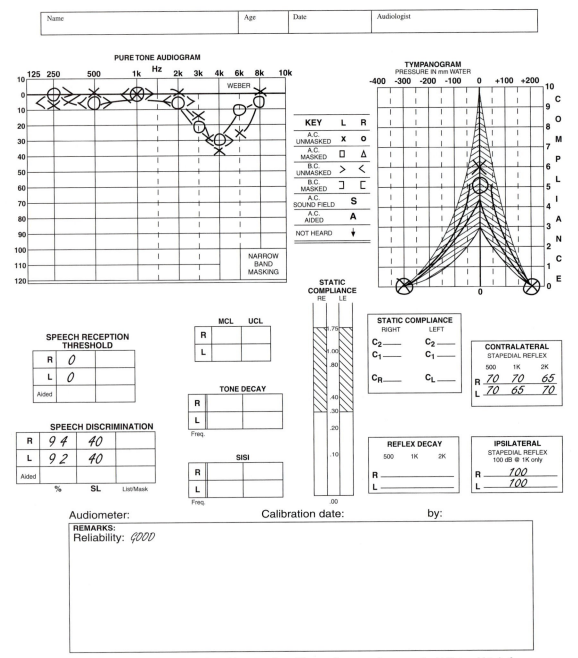

Name			Age	Date	Audiologist

PURE TONE AUDIOGRAM

TYMPANOGRAM
PRESSURE IN mm WATER

KEY	L	R
A.C. UNMASKED	X	O
A.C. MASKED	□	△
B.C. UNMASKED	>	<
B.C. MASKED	]	[
A.C. SOUND FIELD	S	
A.C. AIDED	A	
NOT HEARD	↓	

NARROW BAND MASKING

SPEECH RECEPTION THRESHOLD

R	0	
L	0	
Aided		

SPEECH DISCRIMINATION

R	9 4	40
L	9 2	40
Aided		
	%	SL	List/Mask

	MCL	UCL
R		
L		

TONE DECAY

R		
L		
Freq.		

SISI

R		
L		
Freq.		

STATIC COMPLIANCE
RE   LE

1.75
1.00
.80
.40
.30
.20
.10
.00

STATIC COMPLIANCE

	RIGHT	LEFT
C_2	—	C_2 —
C_1	—	C_1 —
C_R	—	C_L —

REFLEX DECAY

	500	1K	2K
R			
L			

CONTRALATERAL
STAPEDIAL REFLEX

	500	1K	2K
R	70	70	65
L	70	65	70

IPSILATERAL
STAPEDIAL REFLEX
100 dB @ 1K only

R	100
L	100

Audiometer: Calibration date: by:

REMARKS:
Reliability: *GOOD*

Figure 10–1. Normal to mild noise-induced hearing loss. The audiogram shows typical bilateral high-frequency sensorineural hearing loss, which is most severe at 4000 Hz. Note the normal speech discrimination score.

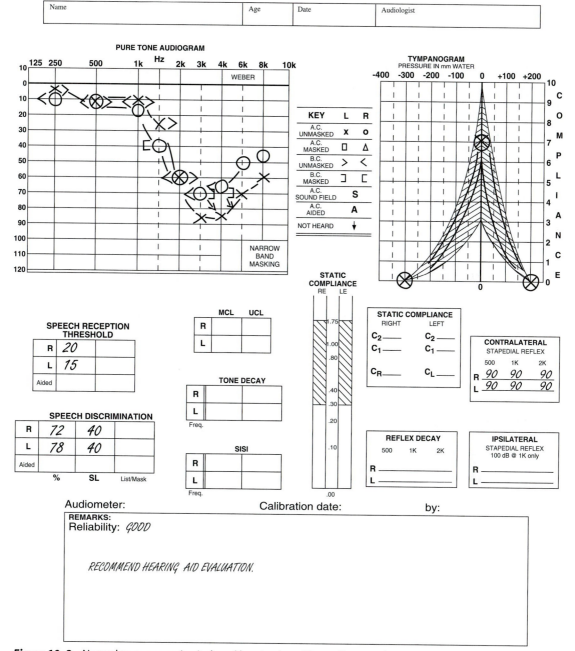

Figure 10–2. Normal to severe noise-induced hearing loss. The audiogram shows moderate to severe high-frequency sensorineural hearing loss but preservation of the lower tones. Note the moderate decrease in the speech discrimination score.

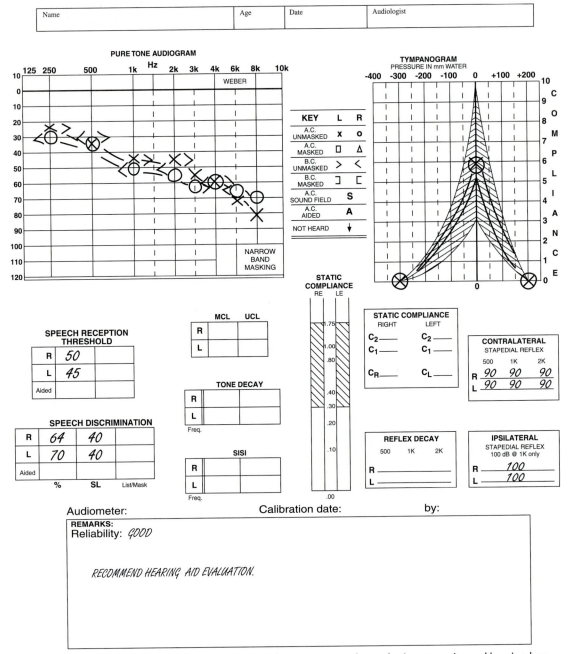

Figure 10–3. Presbycusis. The audiogram shows moderate to severe down-sloping sensorineural hearing loss. Note that the hearing threshold at 4000 Hz is better than at 8000 Hz, a pattern suggestive, but not diagnostic, of an aging change rather than exposure to noise.

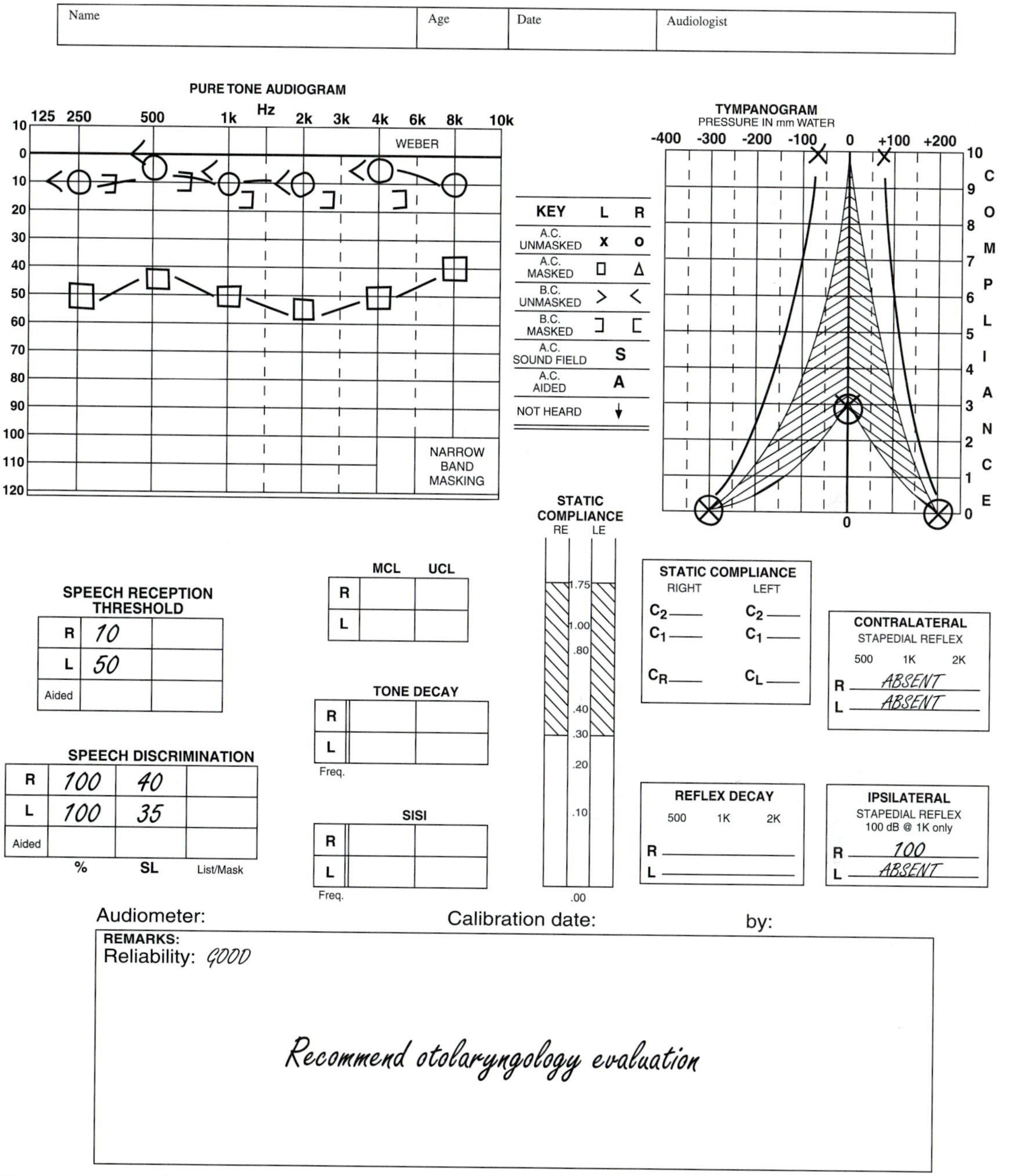

Name		Age	Date	Audiologist

PURE TONE AUDIOGRAM

Hz

WEBER

KEY	L	R
A.C. UNMASKED	X	o
A.C. MASKED	□	Δ
B.C. UNMASKED	>	<
B.C. MASKED	]	[
A.C. SOUND FIELD	S	
A.C. AIDED	A	
NOT HEARD	↓	

NARROW BAND MASKING

TYMPANOGRAM
PRESSURE IN mm WATER

C O M P L I A N C E

SPEECH RECEPTION THRESHOLD

R	10	
L	50	
Aided		

SPEECH DISCRIMINATION

R	100	40	
L	100	35	
Aided			
	%	SL	List/Mask

	MCL	UCL
R		
L		

TONE DECAY

R	
L	
Freq.	

SISI

R	
L	
Freq.	

STATIC COMPLIANCE
RE   LE

.75
.00
.80
.40
.30
.20
.10
.00

STATIC COMPLIANCE

RIGHT	LEFT
C_2 ___	C_2 ___
C_1 ___	C_1 ___
C_R ___	C_L ___

CONTRALATERAL
STAPEDIAL REFLEX

	500	1K	2K
R	ABSENT		
L	ABSENT		

REFLEX DECAY

	500	1K	2K
R			
L			

IPSILATERAL
STAPEDIAL REFLEX
100 dB @ 1K only

R	100
L	ABSENT

Audiometer: Calibration date: by:

REMARKS:
Reliability: GOOD

Recommend otolaryngology evaluation

Figure 10–4. Moderate conductive hearing loss. The audiogram shows a disparity between the thresholds of bone conduction and air conduction. This "air-bone gap" represents the degree of hearing impairment caused by dysfunction of the external or middle ear. Tympanogram shows an increase in left middle ear compliance. The audiogram is typical of a left ossicular chain disruption.

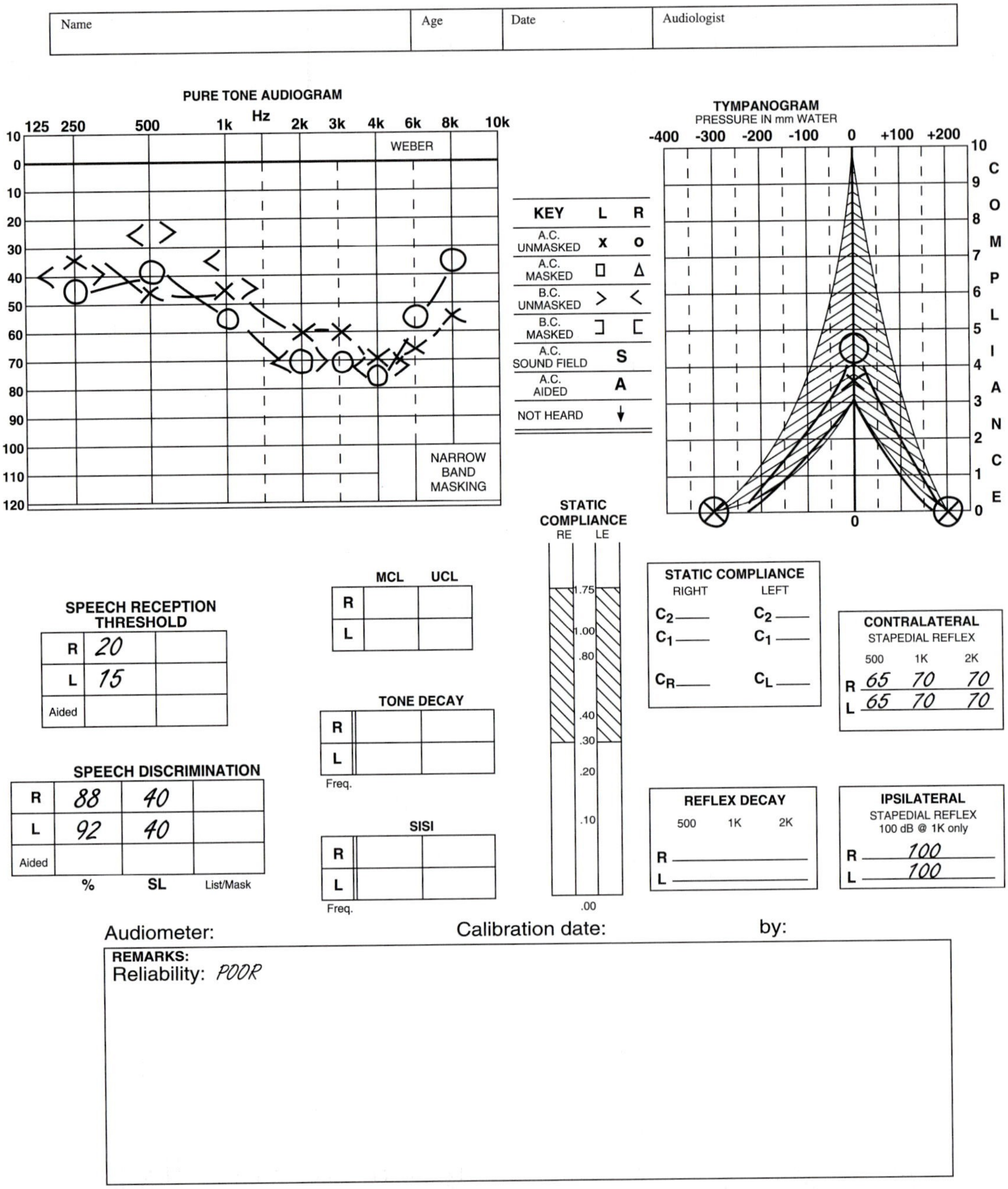

Name		Age	Date	Audiologist

PURE TONE AUDIOGRAM

Hz

125 250 500 1k 2k 3k 4k 6k 8k 10k

WEBER

TYMPANOGRAM
PRESSURE IN mm WATER

-400 -300 -200 -100 0 +100 +200

C
O
M
P
L
I
A
N
C
E

KEY	L	R
A.C. UNMASKED	X	o
A.C. MASKED	☐	Δ
B.C. UNMASKED	>	<
B.C. MASKED	⅃	⊏
A.C. SOUND FIELD	S	
A.C. AIDED	A	
NOT HEARD	↓	

NARROW BAND MASKING

STATIC COMPLIANCE
RE   LE

SPEECH RECEPTION THRESHOLD

R	20	
L	15	
Aided		

MCL   UCL

R		
L		

TONE DECAY

R		
L		

Freq.

SPEECH DISCRIMINATION

R	88	40	
L	92	40	
Aided			
	%	SL	List/Mask

SISI

R		
L		

Freq.

STATIC COMPLIANCE

	RIGHT	LEFT
C₂	C_2____	C_2____
C₁	C_1____	C_1____
CR	C_R____	C_L____

CONTRALATERAL
STAPEDIAL REFLEX

	500	1K	2K
R	65	70	70
L	65	70	70

REFLEX DECAY

	500	1K	2K
R			
L			

IPSILATERAL
STAPEDIAL REFLEX
100 dB @ 1K only

R	100
L	100

Audiometer: Calibration date: by:

REMARKS:
Reliability: *POOR*

Figure 10–5. Nonorganic hearing loss. The audiogram shows pure-tone thresholds that are significantly worse than the speech reception thresholds recorded on the same data.

roma) or a lesion of the brain stem. More definitive diagnosis of retrocochlear lesions requires computed tomographic (CT) scanning or magnetic resonance imaging (MRI).

Stenger Test

This test is useful for detecting feigned unilateral hearing loss. The Stenger principle states that when two tones of the same frequency but of different loudness are presented to both ears simultaneously, only the louder tone will be heard. When the louder tone is presented to the ear with a feigned hearing loss, the patient stops responding because the patient perceives that all the sound is coming from that side. Patients with true unilateral loss indicate that they continue to hear the sound in the opposite ear.

Otoacoustic Emissions

Otoacoustic emissions (OAEs) are a recent addition to objective hearing testing. OAEs are produced when the cochlea receives an external sound stimulus, and the mechanical properties of the outer hair cells act in a manner in which a measurable sound is produced and emanated laterally through the middle ear to be recorded in the external auditory meatus. There are two types of evoked OAEs used clinically today. They are transient-evoked otoacoustic emissions (TEOAEs) and distortion-product otoacoustic emissions (DPOAEs). Individuals with hearing better than 35 dB (TEOAEs) and 50 dB (DPOAEs) will produce OAEs in 99% of instances, unless there is middle ear pathology. Thus, if an individual generates OAEs but does not admit to hearing, a nonorganic origin must be assumed. OAEs are useful in occupational hearing loss because OAEs are rapid (30 seconds to 3 minutes), reproducible, frequency-specific (1000–10,000 Hz), and assess the injury to the outer hair cells caused by noise. However, since OAEs do not test inner hair cells, the auditory nerve, and higher auditory structures, their current role in occupational hearing loss will be in screening and supporting pure tone audiometry.

REFERENCES

Chan VS et al: Occupational hearing loss: Screening with distortion-product otoacoustic emissions. Int J Audiol 2004;43:323 [PMID: 15457814].

Seixas NS et al: Prospective noise-induced changes to hearing among construction industry apprentices. Occup Environ Med 2005;62:309 [PMID: 15837852].

Functional Hearing Test

The hearing in noise test (HINT) is a direct measure of functional speech perception in noise. This test has been validated for use in screening applicants for hearing-critical jobs. The HINT measures speech intelligibility in quiet and spectrally matched noise at suprathreshold levels using sentence materials. The sentences are presented in sets of 20 using an adaptive method to find the reception threshold for speech (RTS) level, where the sentences are repeated correctly half the time. The testing is done in quiet and three background-noise environments (noise front, noise right, and noise left). The noise level is fixed at 65 dBA, and the noise RTS, or signal-to-noise ratio, is the difference in decibels between the sentence level and the noise level. For the quiet test condition, an RTS of 28 dBA or lower is the passing criterion. In noise, the RTS is used to determine a percentile score based on norms for normal listeners. Some organizations use the 5% criterion guidelines (95% of normal listeners performed better than the subject on that task) as a passing score. Important issues must be considered when setting screening criteria. First, each employer must review the concept of hearing-critical tasks because these tasks often are performed in high-noise levels where normally hearing people cannot hear adequately and then determine their own criteria for passing based on the particular demands of the job. Second, noise-induced hearing loss is frequent in these noisy environments, and workers who acquire a hearing loss might not continue to meet the minimal auditory screening criteria. Third, adaptation strategies have to be considered when recruits or incumbents fail the screening test.

REFERENCE

Laroche C et al: An approach to the development of hearing standards for hearing-critical jobs. Noise Health 2003;6:17 [PMID: 14965451].

DIFFERENTIAL DIAGNOSIS OF SENSORINEURAL HEARING LOSS

Nonoccupational Hearing Loss

Before attempting to determine the extent of occupational hearing loss in a subject, the following nonoccupational hearing-loss disorders must be ruled out first.

A. PRESBYCUSIS

Presbycusis is a slow and progressive deterioration of hearing that is associated with aging and not attributable to other causes (see Figure 10–3). Presbycusis is associated with a variety of inner ear pathologies, including atrophy of the inner and outer hair cells and spiral ganglion in the basal turn of the cochlea. Other features that occur histologically include atrophy or degeneration of central auditory pathways and possibly mechanical changes in the cochlear duct affecting movement of the basement membrane. Usually the hearing loss is a gradual, symmetric, progressive, high-frequency sensorineural loss associated with gradually deteriorating speech discrimination.

B. HEREDITARY HEARING IMPAIRMENT

In developed countries, deafness has an important genetic origin, and at least 60% of the cases are inherited. Hereditary hearing impairment (HHI) can be conductive, mixed, or sensorineural impairment, and the pattern of inheritance can be dominant, recessive, X-linked, or mitochondrial. HHI is distinguished by a family history, consanguity, and physical findings consistent with a hereditary syndrome known to include hearing loss. Currently, more than 100 genes are involved in the different types of inherited deafness (syndromic and nonsyndromic). HHI is detected in early childhood, particularly if it is associated with syndromes (e.g., autosomal-recessive Usher syndrome, autosomal-dominant brachio-otorenal syndrome, or X-linked mixed hearing loss with stapes gusher). Autosomal-recessive nonsyndromic HHI also presents early and accounts for 80% of nonsyndromic hearing loss. A single gene locus, *DFNB1,* accounts for a high proportion of the recessive cases, with variability depending on the population. The gene involved in this type of deafness is *GJB2,* which encodes the gap-junction protein connexin 26. Connexins are transmembrane proteins that form channels that allow rapid transport of ions or small molecules between cells. Autosomal-dominant nonsyndromic HHI presents in early or middle adulthood and often is progressive. Genetic screening is available clinically for several of the nonsyndromic and syndromic mutations.

REFERENCE

Hereditary Hearing Loss Homepage (University of Antwerp and University of Iowa): webhost.ua.ac.be/hhh/.

C. METABOLIC DISORDERS

Progressive hearing loss may be related to diabetes mellitus, thyroid dysfunction, renal failure, autoimmune disease, hyperlipidemia, and hypercholesterolemia. These disorders may result in a sensorineural hearing loss that is bilateral, progressive, and high frequency.

In diabetes mellitus, the pathology is varied, involving primary neuropathy and/or small-vessels disease. Other metabolic disorders may involve pathology in the stria vascularis, which is important in maintaining the ion balance and the electrical potentials within the cochlea.

REFERENCE

Detaille SI et al: What employees with rheumatoid arthritis, diabetes mellitus and hearing loss need to cope at work. Scand J Work Environ Health 2003;29:134 [PMID: 12718499].

D. SUDDEN SENSORINEURAL HEARING LOSS

This is differentiated by its sudden onset, usually developing within 24 hours, in the absence of precipitating factors. The hearing loss is almost always unilateral. The hearing-loss pattern in sudden sensorineural hearing loss (SNHL) is variable. The degree of hearing loss is unpredictable, ranging from mild to severe. Vertigo is present is some cases of SNHL and suggests a more severe insult.

The etiology of SNHL is unknown; a viral cause, vascular insult, or inner ear membrane rupture (Reissner membrane, tectorial membrane) has been postulated. This disorder warrants a thorough evaluation in order to rule out any other known pathology.

The treatment of SNHL is debatable. The most common therapies are observation versus steroids (oral prednisone or intratympanic methylprednisolone). Vasodilators, anticoagulants, and diuretics also have been used in the treatment of some SNHL.

E. INFECTIOUS ORIGIN

This includes bacteria or viral infections, including meningitis and encephalitis, that may cause hearing loss. Spirochete infections such as congenital or acquired syphilis and Lyme disease can result in hearing loss and vestibular dysfunction. The congenital syphilis sufferer may develop symptoms in infancy or later in life that also may be associated with vestibular symptoms similar to Ménière syndrome; the hearing loss can be unilateral but usually is bilateral. Late syphilis may present a slowly progressive sensorineural hearing loss and also may exhibit associated vestibular problems.

Mumps may cause a rather severe, most typically unilateral sensorineural hearing loss. Other childhood viral exanthems also can cause sensorineural hearing loss. Congenital hearing loss also can be attributed to infectious origins such as rubella virus and cytomegalovirus.

F. CENTRAL NERVOUS SYSTEM DISEASE

Cerebellopontine angle tumors, especially acoustic neuroma, may present with progressive sensorineural hearing loss that is unilateral. This is in contrast to noise-induced hearing loss, where such hearing loss usually is bilateral. Patients with unilateral or asymmetric sensorineural hearing loss require further investigation to rule out these tumors. This investigation may require detailed audiometric studies and CT scan or MRI. Demyelinating diseases (e.g., multiple sclerosis) may present a sudden unilateral hearing loss that typically recovers to some degree.

G. MÉNIÈRE DISEASE (ENDOLYMPHATIC HYDROPS)

Ménière disease and its variants generally present a fluctuating low-frequency or flat unilateral sensorineural hearing loss, fullness or pressure in the affected ear, tinnitus, and episodic disabling vertigo. In the early stages, the hearing loss is usually low-frequency sensorineural, but over time it may progress to a flat severe hearing loss. Although the etiology is unknown, histopathology reveals a hydropic dilatation of the endolymphatic chambers of cochlea and membranous labyrinth.

H. NONORGANIC HEARING LOSS

Functional hearing loss for purposes of secondary gain is quite frequent. This may be seen in people with normal hearing and in those who embellish an existing organic hearing loss. With skillful audiometric techniques (as discussed previously), it is usually possible to distinguish organic from nonorganic hearing loss, but this may require referral to an audiologic center with considerable experience with this problem.

There are various indications of nonorganic hearing loss. Poor correlation between the speech reception thresholds and the average of the air conduction thresholds at 500, 1000, and 2000 Hz is the most common indication of functionality (see Figure 10–5). The speech reception thresholds are generally within 6 dB of the average of the "speech frequencies." Test-retest variability is also suggestive. In cases of suspected unilateral functional hearing loss, the Stenger test is useful. Evoked-response audiometry, otoacoustic emissions tests, or both also may be useful for objectively establishing hearing thresholds in patients unable or unwilling to cooperate with conventional testing.

NOISE-INDUCED HEARING LOSS

Etiology & Pathogenesis

Noise-induced hearing loss (NIHL) is a complex disease caused by an interaction between genetic and environmental factors. NIHL results mechanically from trauma to the sensory epithelium of the cochlea and metabolically from the generation of reactive oxygen species. The sensory epithelium of the cochlea consists of one inner row of stereociliated hair cells and three outer rows of stereociliated hair cells supported by supporting cells (Hansen and Deiter cells). The most obvious injury is to the stereocilia of the inner and outer hair cells (the electromechanical transducers of sound energy), which may become distorted or even disrupted under acoustically generated shearing forces of the tectorial membrane. All structures of the organ of Corti, however, can be affected. Vascular, chemical, and metabolic changes occurring in the sensory cells cause loss of stereocilia stiffness possibly as the result of contraction of the rootlet structures that anchor the stereocilia to the cuticular plate at the top of the hair cell.

Initially the vascular, chemical, and metabolic changes are potentially reversible, and given time, the hearing will recover. This is known as a *temporary threshold shift* (TTS). TTS can last for several hours. However, the condition in which continued noise exposure results in permanent loss of stereocilia with apparent fracture of the rootlet structures and destruction of the sensory cells, which are replaced by nonfunctioning scar tissue, is known as *permanent threshold shift* (PTS), and there is no recovery. The outer hair cells, which are important in tuning, generally are affected before the inner hair cells. A retrograde degeneration of cochlear nerve fibers occurs progressing centrally. Noise can involve other structures in the cochlea and

has been noted histologically, including vascular change in the area of the metabolically active stria vascularis. This results in a PTS. Because TTS may mimic PTS, individuals should be given audiometric tests after a recovery period of 12–24 hours following exposure to hazardous levels of noise. PTS may be caused by a brief exposure to extremely high-intensity sounds, but it is caused more commonly by prolonged repetitive exposure to lower levels of hazardous noise.

Susceptibility to NIHL is highly variable. While some individuals are able to tolerate high noise levels for prolonged periods of time, others who are subjected to the same environment can lose hearing rapidly. Risk of permanent hearing impairment is related to the duration and intensity of exposure (Table 10–1) as well as genetic susceptibility to noise trauma. Human twin studies and mammalian animal studies have shown that noise sensitivity does aggregate in families, and specific genes and proteins are being associated with vulnerability and resistance to NIHL. Contrary to expectations, recent studies have shown no major role for genetic variation of antioxidant enzymes in determining the susceptibility to NIHL and also indicate that the complexity of oxidative metabolism in the cochlea is greater than previously hypothesized.

Generally, prolonged exposure to sounds louder than 85 dBA (i.e., an 85-dB noise level determined by using the A scale) is potentially injurious. It has been estimated

Table 10–1. Relative intensity of common noises.

	Noise Level (dBA)
Recreational noise	
Normal conversation	50–60
Lawnmower	100
Motorcycle	110
Snowmobile	110
Firecrackers	150
Hunting weapons	160
Industry noise (average of many jobs)	
Printing and publishing	90
Truck transportation	90
Canning food products	100
Farm equipment	100
Textile mill	100
Lumber and wood products	100
Petroleum refining	110
Metal products	100
Mining, underground	110
Heavy equipment	110
Metal-tool operations	110
Military flight line	120

that more than 20 million production workers in the United States are exposed to hazardous noise that could result in hearing loss. Continuous exposure to hazardous levels of noise tends to have its maximum effect in the high-frequency regions of the cochlea. Noise-induced hearing loss is usually most severe around 4000 Hz, with downward extension toward the "speech frequencies" (500–3000 Hz) occurring only after prolonged or severe exposure. Interestingly, this tendency of noise-induced hearing loss to preferentially affect the high-frequency regions of the cochlea remains true regardless of the frequency of the injurious noise and may be related to the resonance of the ear canal.

The inner ear is partially protected from the effects of continuous noise by the acoustic reflex. This reflex, which is triggered when the ear is subjected to noise louder than 90 dB, causes the middle ear muscles (the stapedius and tensor tympani) to contract, thereby stiffening the conductive system and making it more resistant to sound entry. Because this protective reflex is neurally mediated, it is delayed in onset for a period ranging from 25–150 ms, depending on the intensity of the sound. Therefore, the biologic effect of sudden-impulse noise is not as dampened as the effect of continuous noise.

Acute Noise-Induced Hearing Loss

While most noise-induced hearing loss is a result of long-term exposure, acute noise-induced hearing loss (ANIHL) may result from a brief exposure to extremely loud noise. In some cases, this may follow intense impulse noises; in other cases, it may follow a single explosion. Blast injuries from explosions can result in pressures that injure middle ear structures such as the tympanic membrane. Blast injuries not only generate impulse noise but also may injure the ear though generation of overpressures and even hot combustion products that can disrupt the tympanic membrane. Although it is less common, an acute decrease in hearing also may occur following single periods of exposure to continuous noise. For example, several hours of unprotected exposure to a jet turbine producing sounds in the 120–140 dB range may result in permanent cochlear damage. Acute NIHL can result in temporary or permanent damage. Noise levels above 140 dB can result in permanent cochlear damage.

Clinical Findings

Patients with NIHL frequently complain of gradual deterioration in hearing. The most common complaint is difficulty in comprehending speech, especially in the presence of competing background noise. Because patients with noise-induced hearing loss have a high-frequency bias to their hearing loss, they hear vowel sounds better than consonant sounds. This leads to a distortion of speech sounds when they are listening to people with higher-pitched voices (e.g., women and children). Background noise, which is usually low frequency in bias, masks the better-preserved portion of the hearing spectrum and further exacerbates the problems with speech comprehension.

Noise-induced hearing loss frequently is accompanied by tinnitus. Most often patients describe a high-frequency tonal sound (ringing), but the sound is sometimes lower in tone (buzzing, blowing, or hissing) or even nontonal (popping or clicking). This sensation may be intermittent or continuous and usually is exacerbated by further exposure to noise. Tinnitus is usually most bothersome to patients when there is little ambient noise present. Therefore, some patients may complain of inability to fall asleep or to concentrate when in a quiet room.

On tuning fork examination, the patient hears air conduction better than bone conduction, which indicates a sensorineural hearing loss. When serial tuning forks from 512–4096 Hz are used, there is often a marked decrease in hearing in the higher frequencies. Audiometric examination usually reveals a bilateral, predominantly high-frequency sensorineural hearing loss, with a maximum drop of the pure-tone thresholds occurring at or around 4000 Hz on the pure-tone audiogram (see Figures 10–1 and 10–2).

The 4000 Hz notch, which frequently develops relatively early in the worker's exposure to hazardous noise, generally will move laterally as further exposure continues; thus lower and higher frequencies become affected somewhat later if the exposure continues. Because the most important thresholds for comprehension of human speech are between 500 and 3000 Hz, a significant decrease in speech discrimination threshold does not begin until frequencies of 3000 Hz and below are affected. The speech discrimination score is normal in the early stages of noise-induced hearing loss but may deteriorate as the loss becomes more severe. Because of great variability, noise-induced hearing loss cannot always be eliminated or established by the shape of the audiogram.

Most frequently, the hearing loss in NIHL is bilateral, although asymmetry can exist, particularly when the source of the noise is lateralized (e.g., rifle or shotgun firing). Tinnitus (ringing or buzzing) may or may not be present. Tinnitus is a subjective complaint, and measurements of tinnitus are based on the patient's ability to match the ringing in loudness and frequency. Often the tinnitus frequency matches the frequency of the hearing loss seen on the audiogram and is about 5 dB above that threshold in loudness. Tinnitus frequently is blocked out by ambient noise. Tinnitus in absence of hearing loss is probably not related to noise exposure.

Individuals who have acute noise-induced hearing loss can present with a variety of audiometric patterns, including temporary or permanent high-frequency neurosensory hearing loss, cupped neurosensory hearing loss (midfrequency), and flat neurosensory hearing loss. These patients frequently experience tinnitus, and a few will have symptoms of hyperacusis and, occasionally, vertigo.

Prevention

The Occupational Safety and Health Administration (OSHA) regulates exposure to noise at or above an 8-hour time-weighted average (TWA) of 85 dBA. Historically, 85 dBA has been characterized as the approximate biologic threshold above which permanent shifts in hearing are possible. The decision to make 85 dBA the regulated level of noise in the workplace was essentially a political one, representing a compromise between the need for protection of susceptible workers and the efficiency and expense of the industrial process. OSHA has mandated that the presence of occupational noise at or above an 8-hour TWA exposure of 85 dBA is the threshold that triggers the need to implement a hearing-conservation program.

REFERENCES

Carlsson PI et al: The influence of genetic variation in oxidative stress genes on human noise susceptibility. Hear Res 2005; 202:87 [PMID: 15811702].

Hong O: Hearing loss among operating engineers in American construction industry. Int Arch Occup Environ Health 2005;78:565 [PMID: 16021464].

A hearing-conservation program (HCP) is the recognized method of preventing noise-induced hearing loss in the occupational environment. While there is a tendency to think of "hearing conservation" as the provision of audiometric tests and hearing protection, much more is required. An effective HCP integrates the following program elements:

1. Noise monitoring
2. Engineering controls
3. Administrative controls
4. Worker education
5. Selection and use of hearing-protection devices (HPDs)
6. Periodic audiometric evaluations

Record keeping is also important, and OSHA requires that NIHL be recorded on the OSHA 300 Log of Injuries and Illnesses. If an employee's audiogram reveals a work-related standard threshold shift (10-dB shifts in hearing acuity) in one or both ears, and the employee's total hearing level is 25 dB or more above audiometric zero (averaged at 2000, 3000, and 4000 Hz) in the same ear(s) as the STS, then the employer must record the case in Section M(5) of the OSHA 300 Log. For the purposes of injury and illness recording, this sometimes may be referred to as a *recordable threshold shift* (RTS). It should be noted that prior to recording a hearing loss, employers may seek the advice of a physician or licensed health care professional to determine if the loss is work-related, make adjustments for presbycusis, and perform additional hearing tests to verify the persistence of the hearing loss. HCP elements are outlined briefly below.

A. NOISE MONITORING

If there is reason to believe that worker noise exposure will equal or exceed a TWA of 85 dBA, then noise monitoring is required. A sampling strategy must be designed to identify all workers who need to be included in the HCP. The noise present must be characterized in terms of frequency (predominantly high, predominantly low, or mixed), intensity (how loud it is), and type (continuous, intermittent, or impulse) using appropriate noise-monitoring instrumentation. Anytime there is any change in production, process, equipment, or controls, all noise monitoring tests must be repeated.

B. ENGINEERING CONTROLS

The information collected during noise monitoring (particularly octave-band analysis, which indicates the sound level at selected frequencies) may be used to design engineering noise controls. Designers conceptualize possible engineering solutions in terms of the source (what is generating the noise), the path [the route(s) the generated noise may travel], and the receivers (the workers exposed to the noise). The noise controls may involve the use of enclosures (to isolate sources or receivers), barriers (to reduce acoustic energy along the path), or distance (to increase the path and ultimately reduce the acoustic energy at the receiver) to reduce worker noise exposure. In general, engineering controls are preferred but are not always feasible because of their costs and limits in technology.

C. ADMINISTRATIVE CONTROLS

Administrative controls include (1) reducing the amount of time a given worker might be exposed to a noise source in order to prevent the TWA noise exposure from reaching 85 dBA and (2) establishing purchasing guidelines to prevent introduction of equipment that would increase worker noise dose. While simple in principle, the implementation of administrative controls requires management's commitment and constant supervision, particularly in the absence of engineering or personal-protection controls. In general, administrative controls are used as an adjunct to existing HCP noise-control strategies rather than as the exclusive approach for controlling noise exposure.

D. WORKER EDUCATION

Workers and management must understand the potentially harmful effects of noise in order to satisfy OSHA

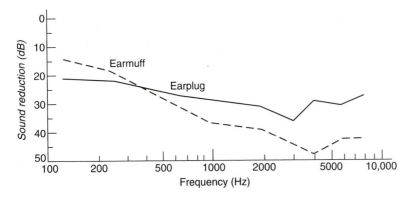

Figure 10–6. Comparison of the attenuation properties of a molded-type earplug and an earmuff protector. Note that the earplug offers greater attenuation of the lower frequencies, whereas the earmuff is better at the higher frequencies.

and, most important, to ensure that the HCP is successful in preventing noise-induced hearing loss. A good worker education program describes (1) program objectives, (2) existing noise hazards, (3) how hearing loss occurs, (4) purpose of audiometric testing, and (5) what workers can do to protect themselves. In addition, roles and responsibilities of the employer and the workers should be stated clearly. Training is required to be provided annually to all workers included in the HCP. Opportunities for maintaining awareness occur during periodic safety meetings, as well as during audiometric testing appointments when testing results are explained.

E. Hearing Protection Devices

Hearing protection devices (HPDs) are available in a variety of types from a number of manufacturers. There are three basic types of HPDs: (1) ear plugs, or *aurals* (premolded, formable, and custom-molded), (2) canal caps, or *semiaurals* (with a band that compresses each end against the entrance of the ear canal), and (3) ear muffs, or *circumaurals* (which surround the ear). Each of these types of devices has advantages and disadvantages that vary according to worker activity, equipment and facility noise characteristics, and the work environment (Figure 10–6). Selection of appropriate HPDs should include input from the industrial hygienist, the audiologist, the occupational medicine physician, and of course, the workers who will use these devices. Although the HCP is triggered by the presence of noise levels equal to or greater than an 8-hour TWA of 85 dBA, HPDs must attenuate worker exposure to an 8-hour TWA at or below 90 dBA, the OSHA 8-hour permissible exposure level (PEL) for noise.

It is important to note that—where hazardous noise levels are present—HPDs must attenuate exposure to an 8-hour TWA of 85 dBA or below for employees who have experienced a standard threshold shift. This requirement also applies to employees who have not yet had baseline audiograms. In general, the use of HPDs by employee exposed to TWA noise levels of 85 dBA or greater is recommended.

F. Audiometric Evaluations

Audiometric testing provides the only quantitative means of assessing the overall effectiveness of a hearing-conservation program. A properly managed audiometric testing program supervised by a certified audiologist or physician who is trained and experienced in occupational hearing conservation will detect changes in response to environmental noise that otherwise might be overlooked. Results of audiometric testing must be shared with employees to ensure effectiveness. The overall results or trends noted in an audiometric testing program can be used to fine-tune the HCP, that is, to determine which types of HPDs to offer to employees or to identify where additional employee training is needed.

Noise Reduction Ratings & Selection of Hearing-Protection Devices

All HPDs sold in the United States are assigned a standardized value known as the *noise reduction rating* (NRR). Manufacturers of HPDs are required by the Environmental Protection Agency to have various products tested in order to obtain an NRR prior to placing them on the market. While useful in making preliminary purchasing decisions, assigned NRRs must be viewed and applied cautiously. NRRs (listed in decibels) are based on laboratory attenuation data achieved under ideal conditions. Actual noise reduction achieved under field conditions using any HPD will be much lower than the assigned NRR. Adjustment of the assigned NRR may need to be made before a device is prescribed for field use. This is explained below.

A. Weighting-Scale Adjustment

Depending on the monitoring method used to determine noise exposure, an initial adjustment to the NRR of a selected device may be necessary. For example, if workplace noise levels are determined by using the C scale (dBC) on the monitoring instrumentation, the assigned

NRR may be subtracted directly from the actual measured TWA noise levels to determine the legal "adequacy" of the device selected relative to the regulatory 90-dBA TWA exposure criterion [or for employees who either (1) have standard threshold shifts or (2) have not yet had baseline audiograms, the 85-dBA TWA exposure criterion].

If workplace noise levels are determined by using the A scale (dBA) on the monitoring instrumentation, the assigned NRR must be reduced by 7 dB before being subtracted from the actual measured TWA noise levels to determine the legal "adequacy" of the device selected relative to the 90-dBA TWA exposure criterion [or for employees who either (1) have standard threshold shifts or (2) have not yet had baseline audiograms, the 85-dBA TWA exposure criterion].

The A-scale adjustment is necessary because this scale approximates the response of the human ear to speech frequencies and discounts much of the acoustic energy from the low and high frequencies that are present in the work environment. Because the C scale is essentially flat (unweighted) across the frequency spectrum, all the acoustic energy present is integrated into the measurement, and no adjustment is necessary.

B. DERATING

The effectiveness of HPDs depends on whether they are used properly. NRRs are obtained in the laboratory under ideal conditions and reflect the "best case" attenuation. To predict the NRR of HPDs during actual use more accurately (and conservatively), the product's NRR should be derated. In calculating the noise exposure to the wearer of a hearing protector at work, OSHA derates the assigned NRR (after weighting-scale adjustment) by one-half (50%) for *all* types of HPDs to determine the "relative performance." As a typical example, if a device has an NRR of 21 and workplace noise measurements were made using the A scale, then the predicted field attenuation or "relative performance" of the device would be $(21 - 7)/2 = 7$ dBA. Such a device would be expected to provide protection (per the legal OSHA 90-dBA PEL) where 8-hour TWA noise levels of up to 97 (90 + 7) dBA are present. As a worse-case example, failure to make an adjustment for A-scale noise measurements, along with a failure to apply a 50% derating, could lead an uninformed evaluator to falsely believe that this same HPD would provide protection in environments with 8-hour TWA noise levels of up to and including 111 (90 + 21) dBA. Workers in this situation would be at increased risk of sustaining a noise-induced hearing loss.

The National Institute for Occupational Safety and Health (NIOSH) recommends a variable scheme for derating NRRs. For example, earmuffs are derated 25%, formable earplugs are derated 50% (as shown above), and all other earplugs are derated 70%. This scheme may more accurately reflect the attenuation that can be expected for various types of HPDs under "real world" conditions.

Remember that the derating of an HPD is not required, but it does provide a conservative estimate of the likely field attenuation that will be provided.

C. COMBINING HPDs

HPDs may be combined (i.e., wearing earplugs and earmuffs) to provide more protection in high-noise environments. However, the NRRs of the combined devices are not added together to determine the total noise reduction. Under such circumstances, OSHA advises its inspectors that 5 dB is to be added after the weighting-scale adjustment is applied to the device with the *higher* NRR (again, OSHA does not require the 50% derating described earlier). This is a conservative approach to determining combined attenuation, and actual field attenuation (and protection) probably is higher. As a practical matter, double protection is inadequate when TWA noise exposures exceed 105 dBA.

D. HPD PROVISION VERSUS HPD ENFORCEMENT

When 8-hour TWA noise levels are equal to or greater than 85 dBA (a 50% noise dose) but below 90 dBA (a 100% noise dose), HPDs *must* be made available to the exposed workers. For 8-hour TWA noise dose levels at or above 90 dBA, however, HPDs must be provided to workers, *and* their proper use must be enforced by the employer [exceptions: (1) employees with standard threshold shifts must be provided with HPDs when the 8-hour TWA noise levels are equal to or greater than 85 dBA, and (2) employees who have not yet had baseline audiometric tests must be provided with HPDs]. A suitable variety of HPDs must be provided. The weighting-scale adjustment of the NRR must be applied, and it is advisable to apply a derating scheme that will adjust the NRR to ensure adequate protection of the worker.

REFERENCES

Daniell WE et al: Noise exposure and hearing loss prevention programs after 20 years of regulations in the United States. Occup Environ Med 2006;63:343 [PMID: 16551755].

Federal OSHA Noise Occupational Noise Exposure Standard (29 CFR 1910.95): www.osha.gov/pls/oshaweb/owadisp.show_document?p_table=STANDARDS&p_id=9735.

Middendorf PJ: Surveillance of occupational noise exposures using OSHA's Integrated Management Information System. Am J Ind Med 2004;46:492 [PMID: 15490475].

NIOSH: Noise and hearing loss prevention: www.cdc.gov/niosh/topics/noise/html.

US Department of Labor, Occupational Safety and Health Administration: www.osha.gov/SLTC/noisehearingconservation/index.html.

Treatment

There is no medical or surgical treatment available to reverse the effects of NIHL. After the diagnosis has been established by otologic examination and performance of an audiometric test battery, the physician should counsel the patient on the likely consequences of continued exposure to excessive noise and should recommend techniques for avoidance of further noise-induced damage. Hearing amplification is reserved for patients with socially impaired hearing.

Hearing aids must be fitted carefully to optimally meet the needs of the individual with regard to frequency bias and gain. In bilateral hearing losses, bilateral amplification usually provides more satisfactory rehabilitation. Whether or not to try hearing amplification is the patient's decision. A reasonable criterion for referral to a professional for hearing aid evaluation is a speech reception threshold greater than 25 dB or a speech discrimination score of less than 80% when words are presented at a normal conversation level of 50 dBHL. There are also some instances in which hearing aids may be recommended that will assist the patient to hear in certain circumstances such as lectures or group situations. In patients with high-frequency hearing loss and relatively normal low-frequency hearing, hearing aids generally are most helpful in those who have a significant hearing loss at 2000 Hz on the pure-tone audiogram. A borderline candidate may be an individual with normal hearing through 1500 Hz, a mild loss at 2000 Hz, and a moderate or greater loss at 3000 Hz and above.

Hearing aids are differentiated by their circuitry. The earlier basic type of hearing aid was the analog hearing aid. The analog hearing aid amplifies sound and generally is the least-expensive hearing aid. Unfortunately, the analog hearing aid amplifies all sounds, and although some filters can be inserted, they are not adjustable for varying situations.

Programmable hearing aids can retain various programs to allow the user to adjust to various noise environments. The user must be able to change to various formats depending on the auditory requirements in the environment.

The most advanced hearing aids, and the most expensive, are the digital hearing aids. These hearing aids modify incoming sound such that they can enhance speech and reduce ambient background noise automatically by analyzing spectral and temporal characteristics. They can allow greater gain before producing audible feedback (suppression). Digital hearing aids can allow for multiple and directional microphones.

Hearing aids are also differentiated by style. The largest and most powerful and adjustable is the behind-the-ear (BTE) aid. There is also an in-the-ear (ITE) aid, an in-the-canal (ITC) aid, and a completely in-the-canal (CIC) aid. The CIC is the smallest but is harder to adjust and is the least powerful.

Before purchasing a hearing aid, the patient should have a hearing aid evaluation and a trial period with the patient wearing the hearing aids in various circumstances.

A patient's willingness to wear a hearing aid will depend on many factors, including cosmetic considerations and concerns about the ability to insert the hearing aid and to manipulate its controls. Numerous other clever instruments, known as *assistive listening devices,* are available to enhance comprehension in small or large groups (e.g., at business meetings or conventions), with telephone use, and with various audio or visual media, such as television. Most of these devices work by wireless transmission of FM signals or infrared light beams. Aural rehabilitation classes designed to enhance the patient's ability to comprehend speech also may be helpful and usually are available in urban areas.

There is no cure for tinnitus resulting from noise-induced hearing loss, although numerous amelioration measures are available. In the absence of further inner ear injury, tinnitus will diminish gradually, usually over a course of weeks to months. A subtle degree of tinnitus often persists and is especially obvious when the patient is in a quiet room. For the few patients who find this to be extremely troublesome, masking the tinnitus with music or some other form of pleasant sound is often helpful. In patients with significant hearing loss, the most successful treatment may be appropriate hearing amplification. Modified hearing aids (tinnitus maskers) designed to produce masking noises generally have been of limited success. Use of biofeedback has helped some patients suppress their tinnitus. Psychiatric referral to manage associated depression sometimes is necessary.

Prognosis

Hearing in patients with NIHL generally will stabilize if the patient is removed from the noxious stimulus. If not, hearing will continue to deteriorate, ultimately resulting in severe hearing impairment or, in extreme cases, total deafness. Although adequate noise protection is essential and always should be recommended, other factors also may play a role in the patient's prognosis. Presbycusis can add to the noise-induced loss as the patient grows older, and preexisting noise-induced hearing loss also will cause the patient to be more susceptible to the adverse effects of ototoxic substances such as aminoglycoside antibiotics, loop diuretics, and antineoplastic agents used in the treatment of other disorders (see "Ototoxic Hearing Loss" below).

Future Therapies

In the mammalian auditory system, hair cell loss resulting from aging, ototoxic drugs, infections, noise, and other causes is irreversible and leads to permanent sensorineural hearing loss. To restore hearing, it is necessary to generate new functional hair cells. The advent of new approaches such as gene therapy, neural stem cell and embryonic stem cell transplantation, and genomics has lead to methods for inducing hair cell regeneration and repair in the mammalian cochlear and vestibular systems. Recently, a key transcription factor of hair cell development has been used via gene therapy to regenerate hair cells and improve hearing thresholds in deafened mice. This is the first demonstration of cellular and functional repair in the cochlea of a mature deaf mammal.

REFERENCES

Izumikawa M et al: Auditory hair cell replacement and hearing improvement by *Atoh1* gene therapy in deaf mammals. Nat Med 2005;11:271[PMID: 15711559].

Li H et al: Pluripotent stem cells from the adult mouse inner ear. Nat Med 2003;9:1293 [PMID: 12949502].

HEARING LOSS CAUSED BY PHYSICAL TRAUMA

Etiology & Pathogenesis

A broad spectrum of injuries may cause trauma to the ears. Blunt head injury is by far the most common cause of traumatic hearing loss. A blow to the head creates a pressure wave in the skull that is transmitted through bone in a manner similar to the way a pressure wave in air is carried by the conducting mechanism of the ear. The cochlear injury observed following blunt head trauma closely resembles both histologically and audiologically that which is induced by high-intensity acoustic trauma. Motor vehicle accidents are the major cause of blunt head trauma and account for about 50% of temporal bone injuries. Penetrating injuries of the temporal bone are relatively rare, accounting for fewer than 10% of cases. Other occupational causes of ear injury include falls, explosions, and burns from caustic chemicals, open flames, or welder's slag that enters the ear canal.

Examination & Treatment

In the conscious patient, hearing should be assessed immediately with a 512 Hz tuning fork. Even in an ear severely traumatized and filled with blood, sound will lateralize toward a conductive hearing loss and away from a sensorineural one. Complete audiometric examinations (see "Evaluation of Hearing" above) can be performed after the patient has been stabilized. Patients also should be checked for signs of vestibular injury (nystagmus) and facial nerve trauma (paralysis).

A. INJURIES CAUSING CONDUCTIVE HEARING LOSS

1. Blunt head trauma with or without temporal bone fracture may cause hematotympanum—a collection of blood in the middle ear. If this is the sole injury, hearing usually recovers over several weeks. Blunt head trauma on rare occasion may result in separation of the bones of the middle ear (ossicular chain disruption).

2. Burns sustained when a piece of welder's slag penetrates the eardrum often heal poorly, and chronic infection often results.

3. Barotrauma can result in a conductive hearing loss with fluid or blood behind the tympanic membrane. This is generally transitory and resolves in a few days to a few weeks.

4. Traumatic membrane perforations usually heal spontaneously if secondary infection does not develop (patients should be instructed not to get the ear wet during the healing period), although hearing loss may persist.

Conductive hearing loss that persists more than 3 months after injury is usually the result of a tympanic membrane perforation or disruption of the ossicular chain (see Figure 10–4). These lesions are suitable for surgical repair, usually on a delayed basis. Repair is by grafting the tympanic membrane or by reconstructing the ossicular chain with homograft or prosthetic materials or both.

B. INJURIES CAUSING SENSORINEURAL HEARING LOSS

Trauma to the inner ear results most commonly from blunt head injury. Labyrinthine concussion frequently occurs with transient vertigo, potentially permanent hearing loss, and tinnitus. Treatment is expectant, with vestibular suppressants such as meclizine offering symptomatic relief of vertigo.

Trauma also may cause rupture of the round or oval window membranes, which can lead to leakage of inner ear fluids into the middle ear (perilymph fistula). Most perilymphatic fistulas heal spontaneously. Persistent perilymphatic leakage is difficult to diagnose and requires surgical treatment, with autogenous material used to repair the defect. Most patients with surgically confirmed fistulas suffer recurrent episodes of vertigo and hearing loss, often temporally related to vigorous physical exercise.

C. INJURIES CAUSING MIXED CONDUCTIVE & SENSORINEURAL HEARING LOSS

Temporal bone injuries sometimes involve both the middle and inner ear, resulting in mixed, conductive, and sensorineural hearing loss. Fractures of the temporal bone tend to occur along lines that connect points of weakness in the skull base. Clinically, these fractures may be divided into two patterns: longitudinal and transverse. Longitudinal fractures are much more common (80% of cases) and usually result from a blow to the lateral aspect of the head. They frequently involve the structures of the middle ear but characteristically spare the inner ear, resulting in a conductive or mixed hearing loss. Transverse fractures are less common (20% of cases) and usually result from a severe occipital blow. Serious intracranial injury frequently accompanies transverse fractures. Typically, they traverse the inner ear and cause total sensorineural hearing loss and labyrinthine death. Fractures through the inner ear often are accompanied by severe vertigo that lasts for weeks or even months.

Temporal bone fractures are recognized clinically by the presence of blood, cerebrospinal fluid, or both in the ear canal or by the presence of blood in the middle ear behind an intact tympanic membrane. The ear canal should be cleaned carefully, using sterile suction to assess the integrity of the tympanic membrane. Under no circumstances should a recently traumatized ear be irrigated. Battle sign (ecchymosis over the mastoid region) is seen occasionally. Definitive diagnosis requires high-resolution CT scanning to demonstrate the fracture lines.

OTOTOXIC HEARING LOSS

Etiology & Pathogenesis

Ototoxic hearing loss is frequently the result of exposure to substances that injure the cochlea. Most ototoxins injure hair cells either directly or through disruption of other cochlear homeostatic mechanisms. In the vast majority of cases, ototoxic hearing loss stems from the use of medications such as aminoglycoside antibiotics (e.g., gentamicin), loop diuretics (e.g., furosemide), antineoplastic agents (e.g., cisplatin), and salicylates (e.g., aspirin).

In industries with noisy work environments, workers who are being treated with potentially ototoxic medications are at increased risk for hearing loss because the combination of some ototoxic drug treatments and noise trauma can lead to a greater degree of hearing loss than either would produce by itself. Aspirin, however, is probably not associated with an increased likelihood of NIHL. Patients with any type of preexisting sensorineural hearing loss, including NIHL, are considerably more susceptible to the ototoxic effects of medications.

Hearing loss also may result from exposure to ototoxic substances in the workplace. Heavy metals, including arsenic, cobalt, lead, lithium, mercury, and thorium, have documented ototoxic potential. Other chemicals that may be ototoxic include cyanide, benzene, aniline dyes, iodine, chlorophenothane, dimethyl sulfoxide, dinitrophenol, propylene glycol, methylmercury, potassium bromate, carbon disulfide, carbon monoxide, carbon tetrachloride, and industrial solvents such as styrene and toluene.

REFERENCE

Fechter LD: Promotion of noise-induced hearing loss by chemical contaminants. J Toxicol Environ Health A 2004;67:727 [PMID: 15192865].

Prevention

Workers who are exposed to or receiving ototoxic agents are at increased risk for NIHL. Medicinal ototoxins should be administered in the lowest dose compatible with therapeutic efficacy. Serum peak and trough levels should be monitored to reduce the risk of excessive dosages. Simultaneous administration of multiple ototoxic drugs should be avoided when possible to minimize synergistic effects. Persons with preexisting sensory hearing loss and compromised renal or hepatic function are at substantially increased risk. Identification of those at heightened risk of ototoxic hearing loss is important to avoid this complication. Audiometric evaluation and OAEs are appropriate to identify and monitor ototoxic exposure.

MEDICOLEGAL ISSUES

Calculation of Percentage of Hearing Loss

Several methods for calculating the percentage of hearing loss are in widespread use. The current method recommended by the American Academy of Otolaryngology and Head and Neck Surgery (AAO) is as follows: (1) The average hearing threshold level at 500, 1000, 2000, and 3000 Hz is calculated for each ear. (2) The percentage of the impairment for each ear (the monaural loss) is calculated by multiplying the amount by which the preceding average exceeds 25 dBA (low fence) by 1.5, up to a maximum of 100%, which is reached at 92 dBA (high fence). (3) The hearing handicap (binaural assessment) then should be calculated by multiplying the smaller percentage (better ear) by 5, adding this figure to the larger percentage (poorer ear), and dividing the total by 6.

The AMA Guides to the Evaluation of Permanent Impairment (5th edition) describe the same calculations for rating hearing impairment percentage as the AAO. In addition, the AMA guidelines have added a provision for tinnitus. "Tinnitus in the presence of unilateral or bilateral hearing impairment may impair speech discrimination. Therefore, add up to 5% for tinnitus in the presence of measurable hearing loss if the tinnitus impacts the ability to perform activities of daily living." The method recommended by the NIOSH is the same as the AAO except that 500 Hz is not included in the calculation. This frequently yields a higher estimate of the percentage of hearing loss. This method was used by the U.S. Department of Labor until February 1986, when the AAO method was adopted.

For the preceding calculations to be valid, the audiometer employed must be checked daily and calibrated periodically by an independent agency. The booth used for testing must meet the standards of background noise levels established by the American National Standards Institute (ANSI) in 1977.

A note of caution is needed regarding the calculation of percentage of hearing loss based on older audiograms. Different standards for the measurement of hearing were in use prior to establishment of the current standard by the ANSI in 1969. From 1964 to 1969, the standard of the International Standards Organization (ISO) was used; this is essentially the same as the current ANSI standard, and no conversion is needed. However, from 1951 to 1964, the standard of the American Standards Association (ASA) was used, and audiograms obtained in this period require conversion for use in the preceding formula. To convert an audiogram from the ASA to the ANSI standard, add 14 dB at 500 Hz, 10 dB at 1000 Hz, 8.5 dB at 2000 Hz, 8.5 dB at 3000 Hz, 6 dB at 4000 Hz, and 9.5 dB at 6000 Hz. If the 3000-Hz threshold was not measured in older audiograms, a three-tone average of 500, 1000, and 2000 Hz may be substituted.

Assessment of Impairment

As indicated previously, the normal range of speech reception threshold is between 0 and 20 dB, with losses of 20–40 dB termed *mild,* 40–60 dB termed *moderate,* 60–80 dB termed *severe,* and greater than 80 dB termed *profound.* Of course, the extent of disability suffered by the patient depends on many psychological, social, and work-related factors. Disability is a relative term. Assessment of the ability of an individual to do his or her job requires knowledge about the various duties performed by that individual. Some typical work-related issues for consideration include the amount of communication with coworkers and others that is required on the job, the type of communication (e.g., in person or via the telephone), and the need to hear alerting signals or emergency warning alarms.

To meet the Social Security Administration's guidelines for total disability as a result of hearing impairment, an individual must have either (1) an average hearing threshold of 90 dB or greater for the better hearing ear, based on both air and bone conduction at 500, 1000, and 2000 Hz or (2) a speech discrimination score of 40% or less in the better-hearing ear. In both cases, hearing must not be restorable by hearing amplification devices.

Compensation for Occupational Hearing Loss

An example of how occupational hearing loss is compensated is provided by the statistics of the U.S. Department of Labor. In the fiscal year 1999–2000, there were 6745 claims. The total cost to the federal government was $39,907,386, of which $8,982,139 was medical costs, and the average paid per claimant was $5917. The Department of Labor treats aggravated or accelerated hearing losses in the same manner as losses entirely precipitated or proximally caused by the patient's employment. In other words, the amount of preemployment hearing loss is not subtracted when the percentage of loss is calculated. In contrast, local and state government regulations frequently take into account the level of preexisting hearing loss and use formulas to correct for the anticipated progression of presbycusis when calculating compensation awards.

The relationship between NIHL and presbycusis is very debatable at this time. Many studies have tried to address the issue of the worker exposed to hazardous noise for a long period of time and his or her "presumed" hearing loss based on his or her age (presbycusis). The ISO published a report in 1990 that attempts to quantify that relationship. As with all large series, attempts to estimate hearing for individuals at a certain age are also based on determining the median or averages of large populations at that given age. There is much debate about whether epidemiologic hearing loss data can be applied to individuals.

Injuries Caused by Physical Hazards 11

Richard Cohen, MD, MPH, & Seichi Horie, MD

This chapter discusses health effects of occupational exposure to extreme temperatures (cold and heat), electricity, radiation, atmospheric pressure changes, vibration, and high-pressure injection. Hearing loss associated with exposure to noise is discussed in Chapter 10.

HYPOTHERMIA (COLD INJURY)

Cold injuries are classified as systemic or localized and as freezing (e.g., frostbite) or nonfreezing (e.g., immersion foot). Factors influencing the risk for these injuries include the atmospheric or water temperature, humidity, wind velocity, duration of exposure, type of protective equipment or clothing, type of work being performed and associated energy expenditure, and age and health status of the worker.

Workers at risk include both indoor and outdoor workers exposed to cold, such as meat packers and others who work with freezers, construction workers, cold-room personnel, fishermen, woodsmen, divers, mail carriers, firefighters, and road maintenance workers. The risk of hypothermia increases with age and also is increased if the employee is intoxicated with drugs or alcohol; is receiving medications such as barbiturates, antipsychotics, or reserpine; smokes; or has adrenal insufficiency, diabetes, myxedema, neurologic disease affecting hypothalamic or pituitary function or causing peripheral sensory impairment, peripheral vascular disease, or cardiovascular disease causing diminished cardiac output.

1. Systemic Hypothermia

Pathogenesis

Systemic hypothermia is reduction of the body's core temperature below 35°C (95°F). Hypothermia can occur at air temperatures up to 18.3°C (65°F) or in water up to 22.2°C (72°F).

When the body is exposed to cold environments, it has two types of normal physiologic reactions: (1) constriction of superficial blood vessels in the skin and subcutaneous tissue, resulting in heat conservation, and (2) increase in metabolic heat production through voluntary movement and by shivering. In cases of systemic hypothermia, cellular and physiologic functions are diminished. Oxygen consumption is decreased by approximately 7% per degree

Celsius, myocardial repolarization is slowed, and ventricular fibrillation is a major hazard.

Clinical Findings

The medical history should address the circumstances under which the patient was found, the probable duration of exposure, associated injuries or frostbite, preexisting medical conditions, alcohol or drug use, and recent changes in the level of consciousness. Because body heat is lost more quickly when a person is wet, immersed in water, or exhausted, these factors should be considered.

The onset of hypothermia often is insidious, without any specific characteristics. With profound hypothermia, there is often diminished memory, a decrease in or absence of shivering, and combativeness. Initial findings may include drowsiness, slurred speech, irritability, impaired coordination, general weakness and lethargy, recent diuresis, and puffy and cool skin and face.

Physical examination often reveals diminished neurologic reflexes, slow mental and muscular reactions, weak or nonpalpable pulse, arrhythmia, low blood pressure, and increased blood viscosity. Shivering and peripheral vasoconstriction begin with the core temperature at 35°C (95°F). Heart and respiratory rates and blood pressure decrease with reduced temperature. With mild hypothermia [33–35°C (91.4–95°F)], there is extensive shivering, which decreases as temperature drops to 33°C (91.4°F), wherein joint and muscle stiffness becomes more predominant.

Core temperature should be taken with a thermometer or thermocouple capable of measuring temperatures as low as 28°C (82.4°F), and esophageal or deep rectal measurement (15 cm) is best. The temperature may range from 25–35°C (77–95°F). Below 35°C (95°F), consciousness becomes dulled, causing disorientation, irrational thinking, forgetfulness, and hallucinations. Below 30°C (86°F), semiconsciousness and confusion may occur. Nerve conduction is slowed, although the central nervous system is protected from ischemic damage. The respiratory rate falls to 7–12 breaths per minute, and gastrointestinal motility slows or ceases. There may be hemoconcentration as a result of diuresis and loss of plasma volume. The latter occurs because of subcutaneous edema, which is accompanied by an elevation in corticosteroid levels. Loss of consciousness seldom occurs at temperatures above 28°C (82.4°F).

Table 11–1. Work warmup schedule for outdoor 4-hour period.[1-3]

°C (approx.)	°F (approx.)	No Noticeable Wind Max. Work Period (min)	No. of Breaks	5 mph Wind Max. Work Period (min)	No. of Breaks	10 mph Wind Max. Work Period (mm)	No. of Breaks	15 mph Wind Max. Work Period (mm)	No. of Breaks	20 mph Wind Max. Work Period (min)	No. of Breaks
−26 to −28	−15 to −19	(Norm. breaks)	1	(Norm. breaks)	1	75	2	55	3	40	4
−29 to −31	−20 to −24	(Norm. breaks)	1	75	2	55	3	40	4	30	5
−32 to −34	−25 to −29	75	2	55	3	40	4	30	5	Nonemergency work should cease	
−35 to −37	−30 to −34	55	3	40	4	30	5	Nonemergency work should cease			
−38 to −39	−35 to −39	40	4	30	5	Nonemergency work should cease					
−40 to −42	−40 to −44	30	5	Nonemergency work should cease							
−43 and below	−45 and below	Nonemergency work should cease									

[1]Adapted from the Saskatchewan Labour Department Health and Safety guidelines (www.labour.gov.sk.ca/safety/thermal/cold/Index.htm).
[2]Schedule applies to any 4-hour work period with moderate to heavy work activity, with warmup periods of 10 minutes in a warm location. It assumes that normal work practice provides for breaks in warm locations every 2 hours. It applies to workers in dry clothing. All temperatures are approximate. For limited physical activity, apply the schedule one step lower. For example, at −35°C (−30°F) with no noticeable wind (step 4), a worker at a job with little physical movement should have a maximum work period of 40 minutes with four breaks in a 4-hour period (step 5).
[3]Special warm-up breaks should be initiated at a wind chill cooling rate of about 1750 W/m²; all nonemergency work should have ceased at or before a wind chill of 2250 W/m².

Evaluation should include a complete blood count; measurement of blood glucose, renal and liver function tests, electrolytes, amylase, and alcohol and drug levels; urinalysis; urine volume; coagulation screen; sputum and blood cultures; thyroid function tests; arterial blood gas measurements with pH corrected for temperature [add 0.0147 pH unit for each degree less than 37°C (98.6°F)]; chest radiograph; and electrocardiograph (ECG). There may be evidence of metabolic acidosis, hypovolemia, elevation or depression of the blood glucose level, and renal failure. The ECG may show a pathognomonic J wave at the QRS-ST junction. The level of consciousness may worsen, and death may result from ventricular fibrillation or cardiac arrest.

Prevention

The risk of hypothermia is directly related to the wind-chill index, which includes both ambient temperature and wind velocity. Cold-stress guidelines are based on the wind velocity and temperature and are intended to prevent the core temperature from falling below 36°C (96.8°F) (Table 11–1).

The wind chill index (WCI) can be calculated from T and V, where T is the air temperature in Celsius (°C) and V is the wind speed at 10 meters height in kilometers per hour.

$$WCI = 13.12 + 0.6215T - 11.37V^{0.16} + 0.3965T \times V^{0.16}$$

The equivalent chill temperature t_{ch}, the temperature equivalent to that under calm wind (1.8 m/s), is given from

$$t_{ch} = (33 - WCI/22) \text{ °C}$$

When t_{ch} drops below −30°C, exposed flesh may freeze, and t_{ch} below −60°C may freeze skin within 1 to 2 minutes.

Ambient temperature is measured with a dry-bulb thermometer; wind velocity is measured with a standard wind gauge. Work and break schedules should take into account the expected wind velocity and temperature. Under high-risk weather conditions, workers should be under constant protective observation.

The required clothing insulation level (IREQ), duration limited exposure (DLE), and required recovery time (RT) can be calculated by the mathematical equation proposed in ISO/CD 11079 using physical activity, ambient temperature, radiant temperature, wind velocity, etc. Adequate insulating dry clothing to maintain core temperatures above 36°C (96.8°F) must be provided to workers if work is performed in ambient temperatures below 4°C (40°F).

Hypothermia can be prevented by wearing clothing specially designed to resist wind and rain but that also allows water vapor generated by perspiration to escape. Overheating when strenuous work is required in extreme cold can be prevented by wearing a number of thin layers of clothing that can be removed or donned as necessary. Wet garments should be replaced as soon as possible with dry ones, and constrictive garments should not be worn.

Jobs should be designed so that workers remain relatively active when exposed to cold environments and provided with dry, wind-protected, heated shelters for tasks involving stationary work positions. Outdoor workers should have heated rest facilities and hot food and hot drinks available. Workers should be trained to "keep warm, keep moving, and keep dry."

Workers exposed to the cold should be physically fit, without underlying vascular, metabolic, or neurologic diseases that place them at increased risk for hypothermia. They should be cautioned to avoid smoking and drug or alcohol use. New workers should be introduced into the work schedule slowly and instructed in the use of protective clothing, recognition of impending frostbite and early signs and symptoms of hypothermia, proper warming procedures, and first-aid treatment.

Treatment & Prognosis

In cases of mild hypothermia [rectal temperatures > 33°C (91.4°F)], patients who are young and otherwise healthy should be treated by rewarming in a warm bed or bath or with warm packs and blankets and with oral rehydration with warmed fluids (caffeine-free and nonalcoholic). Mildly hypothermic elderly or debilitated patients should be treated conservatively, using an electric blanket heated to 37°C (98.6°F). Treatment should increase in aggressiveness with decreasing core temperature, which in severe cases may call for both selected internal and external techniques (Figure 11–1).

Cardiac rhythm and rate should be monitored. Because the risk of death from ventricular fibrillation is high with severe hypothermia [<32°C (89.6°F)], treatment methods that may trigger fibrillation (e.g., central catheters, cannulas, or tubes) should be avoided unless their use is essential. However, patients who are comatose or in respiratory failure should be tracheally intubated. If cardiopulmonary resuscitation (CPR) is instituted, it should be continued until the patient has been rewarmed to at least 36°C (96.8°F). Evaluation for and treatment of localized areas of trauma and frostbite should be undertaken.

Measures should be instituted to correct acid-base deficiencies, normalize the serum potassium and blood glucose levels, increase the blood volume, maintain cardiac output and blood pressure, and provide adequate ventilation. Adequate cardiovascular support, acid-base balance, arterial oxygenation, and intravascular volume should be established as quickly as possible to minimize the risk of organ infarction during rewarming. Oxygen administration should begin prior to rewarming. Because most arrhythmias revert spontaneously to normal sinus rhythm as the patient rewarms, it is usually unnecessary to give antiarrhythmic agents unless there is a preexisting cardiac condition. Ventricular arrhythmias, however, should be treated as they are treated in a euthermic patient. Blood volume expansion with 5% dextrose–normal saline solution is recommended. Potassium-containing expanders should be avoided until the serum potassium levels are stable. If myxedema is an underlying factor, or if drug intoxication is present, appropriate treatment should be given. Localized areas of frostbite should be evaluated and managed as outlined under "Hypothermia of the Extremities" below.

Use of steroids or antibiotics is not recommended unless otherwise clinically indicated. Core temperature should be monitored frequently during and after initial rewarming because of the potential for delayed, repeat hypothermia.

Active internal rewarming for severe hypothermia is more effective than external rewarming.

A. ACTIVE EXTERNAL REWARMING METHODS

Although relatively simple and generally available, active external warming methods may cause marked peripheral dilatation that predisposes to ventricular fibrillation and hypovolemic shock. Either heated blankets or warm baths may be used for active external rewarming. Rewarming in a warm bath is most effective and performed in a tub of stirred water at 40–42°C (104–107.6°F), with a rate of rewarming of about 1–2°C (1.8–3.6°F) per hour. It is easier, however, to monitor the patient and to carry out diagnostic and therapeutic procedures when heated blankets are used for active rewarming. Forced-air rewarming [38–43°C (100.4–109.4°F)] is recommended when extracorporeal rewarming is not available; heated blankets are recommended for transport.

B. ACTIVE INTERNAL (CORE) REWARMING METHODS

Internal rewarming is essential for patients with severe hypothermia; extracorporeal blood rewarming [cardiopulmonary, arteriovenous (femorofemoral) or veno-

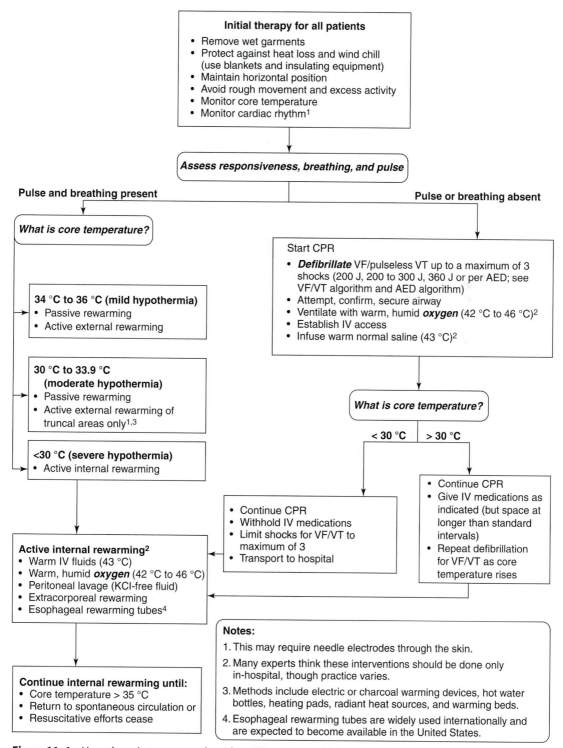

Initial therapy for all patients
- Remove wet garments
- Protect against heat loss and wind chill (use blankets and insulating equipment)
- Maintain horizontal position
- Avoid rough movement and excess activity
- Monitor core temperature
- Monitor cardiac rhythm[1]

Assess responsiveness, breathing, and pulse

Pulse and breathing present

What is core temperature?

34 °C to 36 °C (mild hypothermia)
- Passive rewarming
- Active external rewarming

30 °C to 33.9 °C (moderate hypothermia)
- Passive rewarming
- Active external rewarming of truncal areas only[1,3]

<30 °C (severe hypothermia)
- Active internal rewarming

Pulse or breathing absent

Start CPR
- *Defibrillate* VF/pulseless VT up to a maximum of 3 shocks (200 J, 200 to 300 J, 360 J or per AED; see VF/VT algorithm and AED algorithm)
- Attempt, confirm, secure airway
- Ventilate with warm, humid *oxygen* (42 °C to 46 °C)[2]
- Establish IV access
- Infuse warm normal saline (43 °C)[2]

What is core temperature?

< 30 °C   > 30 °C

- Continue CPR
- Withhold IV medications
- Limit shocks for VF/VT to maximum of 3
- Transport to hospital

- Continue CPR
- Give IV medications as indicated (but space at longer than standard intervals)
- Repeat defibrillation for VF/VT as core temperature rises

Active internal rewarming[2]
- Warm IV fluids (43 °C)
- Warm, humid *oxygen* (42 °C to 46 °C)
- Peritoneal lavage (KCl-free fluid)
- Extracorporeal rewarming
- Esophageal rewarming tubes[4]

Continue internal rewarming until:
- Core temperature > 35 °C
- Return to spontaneous circulation or
- Resuscitative efforts cease

Notes:
1. This may require needle electrodes through the skin.
2. Many experts think these interventions should be done only in-hospital, though practice varies.
3. Methods include electric or charcoal warming devices, hot water bottles, heating pads, radiant heat sources, and warming beds.
4. Esophageal rewarming tubes are widely used internationally and are expected to become available in the United States.

Figure 11–1. Hypothermia treatment algorithm. AED = automated external defibrillator; CPR = cardiopulmonary resuscitation; IV = intravenous; J = joules; VF = ventricular fibrillation; VT = ventricular tachycardia.

venous bypass] is the treatment of choice. If extracorporeal rewarming is not feasible, left-sided thoracotomy followed by pericardial cavity irrigation with warmed saline has been effective in patients with systemic hypothermia of less than 28°C. Repeated peritoneal dialysis may be employed with 2 L of warm [43°C (109.4°F)] potassium-free dialysate solution exchanged at intervals of 10–12 minutes until the core temperature is raised to about 35°C (95°F). Parenteral fluids (D$_5$ normal saline) should be warmed to 43°C (109°F) before administration. Heated, humidified air warmed to 42°C (107.6°F) should be administered through a facemask or endotracheal tube. Warm colonic and gastrointestinal irrigations are of less value.

Passive rewarming (insulation from cold) is of value only for mildly hypothermic patients or as first-aid management on the scene. Hypothermia victims without vital signs should not be pronounced dead until they have been rewarmed to a core temperature of 36°C (96.8°F) and are found to be unresponsive to continued CPR at that temperature.

Prognosis is directly related to the severity of metabolic acidosis; with low pH (6.6), elevated Pa$_{CO2}$ (8.0) and/or elevated potassium (4.0 mEq/L), the prognosis is poor. The prognosis is good for otherwise healthy patients but worsens with the presence of underlying predisposing problems or a delay in treatment.

2. Hypothermia of the Extremities

The cheeks, nose, earlobes, fingers, toes, hands, and feet are the areas most likely to develop ice crystals within the tissue, resulting in localized hypothermic injury. As skin temperature falls below 25°C (77°F), tissue metabolism slows, although oxygen demand increases if work continues. There may be tissue damage at 15°C (59°F) as a consequence of ischemia and thrombosis and at –3°C (26.6°F) as a consequence of actual freezing of the tissue.

Immersion foot (trench foot) is caused by a combination of cold temperature and exposure to water. This problem and chilblains (pernio) are nonfreezing injuries, whereas frostbite is a freezing injury. Predisposing factors for nonfreezing injuries include inadequate clothing and constricting garments. Those for frostbite include prior cold injuries, smoking, Raynaud phenomenon, and collagen-vascular disease.

Clinical Findings

A. CHILBLAINS (PERNIO)

Chilblains, also called *acute pernio,* consist of painful, erythematous, pruritic skin lesions caused by inflammation as a result of cold or dampness with cold. With prolonged exposure, this condition can progress to chronic pernio or "blue toes," characterized by erythematous, edematous, ulcerating lesions of the acral parts of the toes. Scarring, fibrosis, and atrophy can follow.

B. IMMERSION FOOT

There are three clinical stages: an ischemic stage, a hyperemic stage, and a posthyperemic recovery stage. Initially, feet are cold, numb, swollen, and waxy white or cyanotic. Between 2 and 3 days following removal from the cold, hyperemia occurs, along with intense pain, additional swelling, redness, heat, blistering, hemorrhage, lymphangitis, ecchymoses, and in some cases, sequelae such as cellulitis, gangrene, or thrombophlebitis. After 10–30 days, intense paresthesias sometimes occur and are accompanied by cold sensitivity and hyperhidrosis, which may persist for years. Tropical immersion foot occurring at higher temperatures is similar but usually has less intense symptoms with faster recovery.

C. FROSTBITE

In frostbite, freezing of superficial tissues (skin, subcutaneous) usually causes symptoms of numbness, prickling, and itching; skin is gray-white and hard. In severe cases, there may be paresthesias and stiffness, as well as injury to deeper tissues—bone, muscle, and nerve. Skin is often white and edematous. Deep frostbite may be followed by ulceration, necrosis, or gangrene.

Prevention

Keep skin dry and wear moisture-resistant hats, facemasks, earmuffs, scarves, gloves, mittens, socks, and boots. Wet or constrictive underwear should be replaced as soon as possible to prevent immersion foot. Pocket hand warmers may be used to warm extremities. Additional prevention guidelines are the same as for systemic hypothermia (see above).

Treatment

A. CHILBLAINS (PERNIO) AND IMMERSION FOOT

Treatment is intended to improve capillary circulation and includes elevating the extremities, gradually rewarming them by exposure to air at room temperature, and protecting pressure sites from trauma. Prazosin hydrochloride, 1 mg at bedtime, has been recommended for treatment and prophylaxis of pernio. Massage, ice, heat, and immersion should be avoided. Antibiotics are given if infection develops.

B. FROSTBITE

At the site of exposure, extremities can be rewarmed by removing wet gloves, socks, and shoes; drying the extremities and covering them again with dry clothing;

and either elevating them or placing them next to a warmer part of the body (e.g., placing the hands in the armpits). *Caution:* Rewarming should not be attempted if refreezing is likely prior to definitive therapy.

In cases of severe frostbite, hospitalization is recommended until the extent of tissue damage has been determined. The patient should be evaluated and treated, if necessary, for systemic hypothermia (see above).

Rapid rewarming of the frostbitten parts of the body can be accomplished by placing them in a moving water bath heated to 40–42°C (104–107.6°F) and leaving them there until thawing is complete but no longer (often 30 minutes). Dry heat is not recommended, and external heat should be discontinued once normal temperature has been reached. The patient should remain in bed with the affected parts elevated and uncovered at room temperature. Frostbitten parts should not be exercised, rubbed, or exposed to pressure. Dressings and bandages should not be applied. Whirlpool therapy at 37–40°C (98.6–104°F) twice daily for 15–30 minutes for three or more weeks helps to cleanse the skin and débrides superficial tissue. A combination of ibuprofen 200 mg four times daily and aloe vera can be used to prevent dermal ischemia.

Infection can be treated with povidone-iodine soaks, water soaks, whirlpool therapy, systemic antibiotics, or a combination of these methods. Tetanus antitoxin or a tetanus toxoid booster may be indicated.

Surgery generally should be avoided and amputation not considered until it is certain that the tissue is dead. Gangrenous and necrotic tissue should be treated by specialists.

Physical therapy can be instituted as healing progresses. The patient should be instructed to avoid exposure to the cold for several months and be advised of future hypersusceptibility to frostbite.

REFERENCES

Kampainen RR, Brunnette DD: The evaluation and management of accidental hypothermia. Respir Care 2004;49:192 [PMID:14744270].

Long WB 3rd et al: Cold injuries. J Long Term Eff Med Implants 2005;15:67 [PMID:15715518].

Ulrich AS, Rathlev NK: Hypothermia and localized cold injuries. Emerg Med Clin North Am 2004;22:281 [PMID:15163568].

DISORDERS CAUSED BY HEAT

Five medical disorders can result from excessive exposure to hot environments (in order of decreasing severity): heat stroke, heat exhaustion, heat cramps, heat syncope, and skin disorders. Among the many types of workers at risk are steel workers, oven and furnace operators, glassblowers, farmers, ranchers, fishermen, and construction workers.

A stable internal body temperature requires maintenance of a balance between heat production and loss, which the hypothalamus regulates by triggering changes in thirst, muscle tone, vascular tone, and sweat gland function. Production and evaporation of sweat are a major mechanism of heat removal (however, sweating causes loss of body water and sodium). The transfer of heat from the skin to surrounding gas or liquid (convection) or between two solids in direct contact (conduction) also may occur, but this decreases in efficiency as ambient temperature increases. The passive transfer of heat via infrared rays from a warmer to a cooler object (radiation) accounts for 65% of body heat loss under normal conditions. Radiant heat loss also decreases as temperature increases up to 37.2°C (99°F), at which point heat transfer reverses. At normal temperatures, evaporation accounts for approximately 20% of body heat loss, but at excessive temperatures, it becomes the most important means for heat dissipation. It, too, is limited as humidity increases and is ineffective at 100% relative humidity.

The scheduled and regulated exposure to heated environments of increasing intensity and duration (acclimatization) allows the body to adjust to heat by beginning to sweat at lower body temperatures, increasing the quantity of sweat produced, reducing the salt content of sweat, and increasing the plasma volume, cardiac output, and stroke volume while the heart rate decreases.

Health conditions that inhibit sweat production or evaporation and increase susceptibility to heat injury include obesity, skin disease, decreased cutaneous blood flow, dehydration, hypotension, cardiac disease resulting in reduced cardiac output, use of alcohol or medications that inhibit sweating, reduce cutaneous blood flow, or cause dehydration (e.g., atropine, antipsychotics, tricyclic antidepressants, diuretics, laxatives, anticholinergics, antihistamines, monoamine oxidase inhibitors, vasoconstrictors, and beta blockers), and use of drugs that increase muscle activity and thereby increase the generation of body heat [e.g., phencyclidine (PCP), lysergic acid diethylamide (LSD), amphetamines, cocaine, and lithium carbonate]. Infections, cancer, malnutrition, thyroid dysfunction, and other medical conditions characterized by debilitation and poor physical condition can reduce the effectiveness of the sweating mechanism and circulatory response to heat. Age and sex also affect susceptibility to heat injury. Older people do not acclimatize as easily because of their reduced sweating efficiency, and women generally generate more internal heat than men when performing the same task.

1. Heat Stroke

Heat stroke is a life-threatening medical emergency caused by thermal regulatory failure manifested by cerebral dysfunction with altered mental status, hyperpyrexia, abnormal vital signs, and usually, hot, dry skin. Heat stroke becomes imminent as the core (rectal) temperature approaches 41.1°C (106°F). It is most apt to occur following excessive exposure to heat; it occurs in one of two forms: *classic* or *exertional*. The classic form occurs under conditions of extreme heat among those with compromised heat-dissipation capability (elderly individuals, infants, and chronically ill or debilitated patients). Exertional heat stroke results from strenuous exertion in hot environments, often in unacclimatized individuals. Morbidity or mortality can result from cerebral, cardiovascular, hepatic, or renal damage.

Clinical Findings

Thermal regulatory failure is characterized by dizziness, weakness, nausea, vomiting, confusion, delirium, and visual disturbances; changes in mental status are its hallmark. Convulsions, collapse, or unconsciousness may occur. The skin is hot and initially covered with perspiration; later it dries. Blood pressure may be slightly elevated but becomes hypotensive. Core temperatures usually exceed 41°C (105.8°F). As with heat exhaustion, hyperventilation can occur and lead to respiratory alkalosis and compensatory metabolic acidosis. There also may be abnormal bleeding, renal failure, or arrhythmias.

Laboratory evaluation may reveal an increase in leukocytes because of dehydration; decreased serum potassium, calcium, and phosphorus levels; increased blood urea nitrogen levels; hemoconcentration; decreased blood coagulation; and concentrated urine with proteinuria, tubular casts, and myoglobinuria. Thrombocytopenia, increased bleeding and clotting times, fibrinolysis, and consumptive coagulopathy may be present. Myocardial, liver, or renal damage may be reflected in laboratory tests (Table 11–2).

Table 11–2. Accidental hyperthermia—clinical differential.

	Heat Cramps	**Heat Exhaustion**	**Heat Stroke**
Pathophysiology	Salt deficiency	Volume/electrolyte depletion	Thermoregulatory failure
Symptoms	Painful muscle cramps/ spasm Weakness Nausea Vomiting	Weakness Headache Syncope Nausea Vomiting Intense thirst (water depletion) Fatigue Muscle cramps (salt depletion) Malaise	Irritability Confusion Prodromal heat exhaustion Collapse Severe/sustained physical exertion (exertional heat stroke) Psychotic behavior
Objective findings	Euthermia	Core temperature ≤ 38°C (100.4°F) Profuse sweating Orthostatic vital signs Tachycardia Hyperventilation Tetany	Core temperature ≥ 40°C (104°F) Altered mental status—bizarre behavior Hot dry skin (classic heat stroke) Moist skin (exertional heat stroke) Coma Hypotension/shock Seizure Tachycardia Cyanosis Rales
Laboratory	Elevated creatine phosphokinase (CPK), creatinuria	Oliguria	Hyperuricemia CPK elevation Dissemination intravascular coagulation Respiratory alkalosis Hypokalemia Thrombocytopenia Myoglobinuria Hypoglycemia Transaminase elevation

Prevention

The American Conference of Governmental Industrial Hygienists (ACGIH) has developed an index of threshold limit values for exposure to heat in occupational settings. The values [wet-bulb globe temperature (WBGT)] are based on a formula (below) that includes the natural wet-bulb temperature T_{nwb}, the shielded dry-bulb temperature T_{db}, and black-globe temperature T_g, which are measurements that account for effects caused by solar radiant heat, air velocity, relative humidity, and ambient temperature. With direct exposure to sunlight:

$$WBGT = 0.7T_{nwb} + 0.2T_g + 0.1T_{db}$$

Without direct exposure to sunlight:

$$WBGT = 0.7T_{nwb} + 0.3T_g$$

Exposure limits take into account the type of work-rest regimen and the workload, including body position, movement, acclimatization, and limb use. These determine the heat load or metabolic rate, which is then related to the index to arrive at a recommended exposure standard for workers in a particular situation. In the absence of WBGT data, heat-index guidelines developed by the National Weather Service predict exposure risks according to ambient temperature and humidity (Figure 11–2). The standards are based on the assumption that workers are acclimatized and physically fit, are wearing appropriate clothing, and are supplied with adequate water and food. If these conditions are not met or the work environment cannot be controlled within the appropriate limits, calculation of the recommended sweat rate provided in International Standards Organization (ISO) 7933 or physiologic measurements of heart rate and core temperature provided in ISO 9886 should be performed by experienced personnel. Occupational heat exposure can be minimized with engineering controls such as air conditioning/cooling, fans, hot-air venting, reflective shielding, and spot cooling. Administrative controls such as limiting exposure duration may be necessary. Special cooled suits have been designed for hot environments. For additional information on the thermal comfort zone, see Chapter 12 and Figure 12–13.

In occupations in which workers are exposed to excessive heat, medical evaluation is recommended to identify individuals at increased risk for heat disorders caused by preexisting medical conditions or use of medications. Exposed workers should be trained to recognize early signs and symptoms of heat disorders and should be advised of the importance of proper attire, nutrition, and fluid intake. Employers should provide cool drinking water or electrolyte-carbohydrate solutions and should ensure that there are shaded rest areas close to the work site. For workers unacclimatized to heat, balanced electrolyte-carbohydrate solutions or 1% saline drinking water should be made available. Salt tablets are not recommended because their use may exacerbate or cause electrolyte imbalance. Organized athletic events should be managed with attention to thermoregulation; the WBGT index should be monitored, water consumption should be encouraged, and medical care should be immediately accessible.

Treatment

Treatment is aimed at rapid (within 1 hour) reduction of the core temperature and control of secondary effects. Evaporative cooling provides rapid and effective lowering of temperature and is accomplished easily in most emergency settings. Until medical care becomes available, the patient should be moved to a shady, cool place. Clothing should be removed, and the entire body should be sprayed with cool water [15°C (59°F)]; cooled or ambient air should be blown across the patient at high velocity (100 ft/min). The patient should be placed in the lateral recumbent position or supported in the hands-to-knees position to expose more skin surface to the air.

The cooling process should continue in the hospital with use of wet sheets accompanied by fanning. Immersion in an iced-water or cool water bath is effective for rapid cooling down to 39°C (102.2°F) (then stop immersion), but it has a greater potential for complications of hypotension and shivering and may impede other interventions. Other treatment alternatives include ice packs (groin, axilla, and neck) and iced gastric lavage, although these are much less effective than evaporative cooling. Treatment should continue until the core temperature drops to 39°C (102.2°F). Because of the risks of hypoxia and aspiration, intubation should be considered and 100% oxygen administered until the patient is cooled. The core temperature should continue to be monitored, although it usually remains stable after it has returned to normal. Chlorpromazine, 25–50 mg intravenously, or diazepam, 5–10 mg intravenously, can be used to control shivering and thus prevent an increase in heat. Antipyretics are contraindicated (Figure 11–3).

Patients should be monitored for hypovolemic and cardiogenic shock, either or both of which may occur. Attention should be paid to maintaining a patent airway, providing oxygen, correcting fluid and electrolyte imbalances, and supporting vital processes. Central venous or pulmonary artery wedge pressure should be assessed and intravenous fluids administered if indicated. If hypovolemic shock is suspected, 500–1000 mL of 5% dextrose in 1% or 0.5% normal saline solution may be given intravenously without overloading the circulation. Other medications appropriate for cardiovascular support should be considered.

Fluid output should be monitored with an indwelling urinary catheter, and fluid administration should maintain

The **Heat index** (HI) is the temperature the body feels when heat and humidity are combined. The chart below shows the HI that corresponds to the actual air temperature and relative humidity. (This chart is based upon shady, light wind conditions. **Exposure to direct sunlight can increase the HI by up to 15°F.**)

(Due to the nature of the heat index calculation, the values in the tables below have an error +/- 1.3°F.)

Temperature (F) versus Relative Humidity (%)

°F	90%	80%	70%	60%	50%	40%
80	85	84	82	81	80	79
85	101	96	92	90	86	84
90	121	113	105	99	94	90
95		133	122	113	105	98
100			142	129	118	109
105				148	133	121
110						135

HI	Possible Heat Disorder:
80°F – 90°F	Fatigue possible with prolonged exposure and physical activity.
90°F – 105°F	Sunstroke, heat cramps and heat exhaustion possible.
105°F – 130°F	Sunstroke, heat cramps, and heat exhaustion likely, and heat stroke possible.
130°F or greater	**Heat stroke highly likely with continued exposure.**

Figure 11–2. Heat index chart showing associated heat disorders.

a urine output of more than 50 mL/h. The patient should be monitored for complications, including renal failure (caused by dehydration and rhabdomyolysis), hepatic failure, or cardiac failure, respiratory distress, hypotension, electrolyte imbalance (hypokalemia), and coagulopathy. Elevated creatine phosphokinase (CPK), elevated liver enzymes, and metabolic acidosis are predictors of multiorgan dysfunction.

Because hypersensitivity to heat continues in some patients for prolonged periods following heat stroke, they should be advised to avoid reexposure to heat for at least 4 weeks.

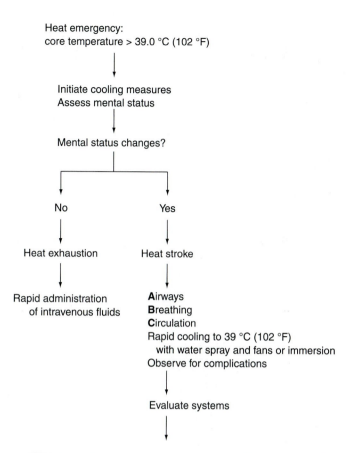

Heat emergency:
core temperature > 39.0 °C (102 °F)

↓

Initiate cooling measures
Assess mental status

↓

Mental status changes?

No ← | → Yes

No

↓

Heat exhaustion

↓

Rapid administration
of intravenous fluids

Yes

↓

Heat stroke

↓

Airways
Breathing
Circulation
Rapid cooling to 39 °C (102 °F)
   with water spray and fans or immersion
Observe for complications

↓

Evaluate systems

↓

Systems	Signs	Measures
Neurologic	Persistent coma Seizures Focal deficit	CT scan of the head Lumbar puncture Intubation Ventilatory support
Cardiovascular	Hypotension Congestive heart failure	Central line PA pressure line Fluids, medication as indicated
Hematologic	Petechiae Purpura Epistaxis Hematemesis	Monitor clotting studies Platelet and factor replacement DIC: administer heparin

Renal	Oliguria
	Anuria
		High creatine kinase level
		  and myoglobinuria: maintain
		  high urine output;
		  consider dialysis

Pulmonary	Decreasing P_{O_2} Increasing airway resistance	Consider ARDS PEEP support on ventilator

Figure 11–3. Algorithm for the management of heat emergencies. ARDS = acute respiratory distress syndrome; CT = computed tomography; DIC = disseminated intravascular coagulation; PA = pulmonary arterial; PEEP = positive end-expiratory pressure; P_{O_2} = partial pressure of oxygen.

2. Heat Exhaustion

In individuals performing strenuous work, prolonged exposure to heat and insufficient salt and water intake can cause heat exhaustion, dehydration, and sodium depletion or isotonic fluid loss with accompanying cardiovascular changes. Symptoms and signs may include intense thirst, weakness, nausea, fatigue, headache, confusion, a core (rectal) temperature exceeding 38°C (100.4°F), increased pulse rate, and moist skin. Symptoms associated with both heat syncope and heat cramps (see below) also may be present. Hyperventilation sometimes occurs secondary to heat exhaustion and can lead to respiratory alkalosis. Progression to heat stroke is indicated by a rise in temperature or a decrease in sweating.

Treatment consists of placing the patient in a cool and shaded environment and providing hydration (1–2 L over 2–4 hours) and salt replenishment—orally if the patient is able to swallow. Physiologic saline or isotonic glucose solution should be administered intravenously in more severe cases. At least 24 hours' rest is recommended.

3. Heat Cramps

Heat cramps result from dilutional hyponatremia caused by replacement of sweat losses with water alone. They are usually characterized by slow and painful muscle contractions and severe muscle spasms that last from 1–3 minutes and involve the muscles employed in strenuous work.

The skin is moist and cool, and involved muscle groups feel like hard, stony lumps similar to billiard balls. The temperature may be normal or slightly increased, and blood tests may show low sodium levels and hemoconcentration. Because the thirst mechanism is intact, blood volume is not diminished significantly.

The patient should be moved to a cool environment and given a balanced salt solution or an oral saline solution consisting of 4 tsp of salt per gallon of water. Salt tablets are not recommended. Rest for 1–3 days with continued salt supplementation in the diet may be necessary before returning to work.

4. Heat Syncope

In heat syncope, sudden unconsciousness results from volume depletion and cutaneous vasodilatation with consequent systemic and cerebral hypotension. Episodes occur commonly following strenuous work for at least 2 hours.

The skin is cool and moist and the pulse weak. Systolic blood pressure is usually under 100 mmHg. Treatment consists of recumbency, cooling, and rehydration. Preexisting medical conditions should be monitored and treated if necessary.

5. Skin Disorders Caused by Heat

Miliaria (heat rash) is caused by sweat retention resulting from obstruction of the sweat gland duct. There are three forms (listed here in increasing order of severity): miliaria crystallina, miliaria rubra, and miliaria profunda. As the site of duct obstruction becomes deeper in the skin, the severity increases and presentation varies (e.g., vesicles, erythema, desquamation, macules).

Erythema *ab igne* ("from fire") is characterized by the appearance of hyperkeratotic nodules following direct contact with heat that is insufficient to cause a burn. Intertrigo results from excessive sweating and often is seen in obese individuals. Skin in the body folds (e.g., the groin and axillas) is erythematous and macerated. Heat urticaria (cholinergic urticaria) can be localized or generalized and is characterized by the presence of wheals with surrounding erythema ("hives").

Treatment for these disorders consists of reduction or removal of heat exposure, reduction of sweating, and control of symptoms. Antihistamines may help to relieve pruritus in patients with urticaria. Corticosteroids are not beneficial.

REFERENCES

Glazer JL: Management of heatstroke and heat exhaustion. Am Fam Physician 2005;71:2133 [PMID:15952443].

Lugo-Amador NM et al: Heat-related illness. Emerg Med Clin North Am 2004;23:315 [PMID:15163570].

Sucholeiki R: Heatstroke. Semin Neurol 2005;25:307 [PMID: 16170743].

ELECTRICAL INJURIES

Electrical accidents comprise up to 4% of all fatal industrial accidents. Electricians, operators of high-power electric equipment and power generators, and maintenance personnel are at greatest risk for electric shock.

Physical contact with an energized electric circuit provides a pathway for electricity to traverse the body as it seeks a ground. Conductivity to the body is affected by skin moisture, as well as moisture on contacting surfaces (e.g., floors). Factors influencing the severity of electrical injury include the voltage (electrical force), amperage (current intensity), current type (alternating or direct current), duration of contact, area of contact, pathway of the current through the body, and amount of tissue resistance.

Electricity from alternating currents is more dangerous than that from direct currents. The alternating currents usually cause muscle tetanization and sweating, whereas the direct currents cause electrolytic changes in tissue. Most tissue damage is related to the heat produced by the electric current, and tissue resistance is largely influenced by the water content of the tissue. The vascular system and muscles are good conductors of electricity, whereas the bones, peripheral nerves, and dry skin have higher resistance.

A sudden exposure to intense electrical energy can cause not only tissue destruction and necrosis from heat and burning but also depolarization of electrically sensitive tissues such as nerve and heart. Alternating currents with voltages and frequencies as low as domestic circuits (100 V and 60 Hz) can produce ventricular fibrillation. High voltages (>1000 V) can cause respiratory paralysis. Most shocks involving currents exceeding 10,000 V are of such magnitude that the electrical force knocks the victim away from the power source, which reduces the electrical injury potential but often causes blunt trauma.

A tetanizing effect of voluntary muscles is greatest at frequencies between 15 and 150 Hz. Sustained grasp of the conductor does not usually occur at high voltages because the circuit probably arcs before contact with the victim, who is thrown back instead. Current above 20 mA can cause sustained contraction of chest respiratory muscles; alternating currents above 30–40 mA can induce ventricular fibrillation, whereas direct current is more likely to cause asystole. Lightning injuries differ from high-voltage electric shock injuries in that lightning usually involves higher voltage, briefer duration of contact, asystole rather than ventricular fibrillation, nervous system injury, a shock-wave characteristic, and multisystem pathologic involvement.

Clinical Findings

Exposure to electric current can cause shock, flash burns, flame burns, or direct tissue necrosis. Surface wounds covering heat-induced tissue necrosis are usually round or oval and well demarcated, and they may have a relatively innocuous yellow-brown appearance. A search must be made for both the entry and exit wounds to determine the electrical pathway through the body. Depending on the contact site and the pathway, there may be damage to nerves, muscles, or major organs such as the heart, brain, eye, kidney, and gastrointestinal tract.

In all cases, an ECG with a rhythm strip and a urine dipstick for blood and protein should be obtained, and the respiratory rhythm and rate should be checked. If organ, muscle, or nerve damage is suspected, appropriate diagnostic tests should be ordered such as urine myoglobin; CPK should be monitored for at least 24 hours if muscle symptoms occur or muscle injury is otherwise suspected. With muscle injury, the CPK level can be elevated significantly (>1000 U/L) but the MB fraction will be below 3% if there is no cardiac muscle injury. Occult fractures may occur following muscle tetany or blunt trauma. Patients should be observed for several days because some develop posttraumatic myositis with rhabdomyolysis.

Electrical injury causes increased vascular permeability, which may result in reduced intravascular volume and fluid extravasation in the area of internal injury. Hematocrit, plasma volume, and urine output should be monitored closely.

Acute- and delayed-onset central and peripheral nervous system complications are the most common sequelae of electrical injury. Cardiac complications usually consist of rhythm and conduction abnormalities, with rare infarction. Sepsis and psychiatric complications also occur.

Prevention

Electrical injuries can be prevented in industrial settings by making sure that electrical workers are properly qualified and trained to follow safety procedures involving the installation, grounding, and disconnection of power sources. Particular attention should be given to work requiring equipment manipulation during "live" operation. Nonconducting tools and clothing should be used whenever possible. Barricades and warning signs should be placed around high-voltage areas, and procedures to exclude other employees from these areas should be strictly enforced.

Workers should be instructed in the proper measures to free a victim from contact with electric current. If possible, the power should be turned off. If not, a nonconducting object such as a rope, a broom or other wooden instrument, or an article of clothing can be used to pull the victim away from the current and protect the rescuer from injury.

Treatment

Prior to CPR, first aid, or treatment, the patient must be separated from the "live" electric current. Power should be turned off and/or nonconductive devices should be used to separate the rescuer and patient from the current. The rescuer must be protected during this procedure. If necessary, CPR [including automated external defibrillator (AED) use] should be instituted until medical help arrives. Because the victim may have suffered spinal injury, extreme care must be taken during handling or transport. Smoldering clothes should be removed.

If major electrical injuries are suspected, the patient should be hospitalized and observed for secondary organ damage, impaired renal function, hemorrhage, acidosis, and myoglobinuria. Indications for hospitalization include significant arrhythmia or ECG changes, large burns, loss of consciousness, neurologic findings, pulmonary or cardiac symptoms, or evidence of significant deep-tissue/organ damage. A tetanus booster or antitoxin should be administered if indicated.

Superficial tissue damage and burns should be addressed. If major soft-tissue damage is suspected, surgical exploration, fasciotomy, or both must be considered. Gross myoglobinuria is a predictor for fasciotomy and/or amputation.

Lactated Ringer's solution should be administered intravenously at a rate sufficient to maintain urine output at between 50 and 100 mL/h. Continuous monitoring and prompt correction of acid-base or electrolyte imbalance are necessary if rhabdomyolysis occurs.

REFERENCES

Edlich RF et al: Modern concepts of treatment and prevention of lightning injuries. J Long-Term Effects Med Implants 2005;15:185 [PMID:15777170].

Moon SJ et al: Lightning-induced maculopathy. Retina 2005;25: 380 [PMID:15805923]

Selvaggi G et al: Rehabilitation of burn-injured patients following lightning and electrical trauma. Neurol Rehabil 2005;20:35 [PMID:15798354].

NONIONIZING RADIATION INJURIES

1. Injuries Caused by Radiofrequency & Microwave Radiation

Exposure

Injuries caused by the thermal effects of acute exposure to high levels of radiofrequency (RF) and microwave radiation have been documented. As with other thermal injuries, these injuries are characterized by protein denaturation and tissue necrosis at the site of thermal exposure, with an accompanying inflammatory reaction and subsequent scar formation. Nonthermal effects of low-level exposure have been demonstrated in some laboratory studies, but their significance in humans is not clear.

RF radiation and microwave radiation consist of energy in wave form traveling in free space at the speed of light. The radiation is defined in terms of frequency and intensity, with the frequency portion of the electromagnetic spectrum extending from 0–1000 GHz [1 Hz equals 1 wave or cycle per second (cps)]. Microwaves occupy only a portion of the frequency spectrum, that is, the portion between 300 MHz and 300 GHz (Figure 11–4).

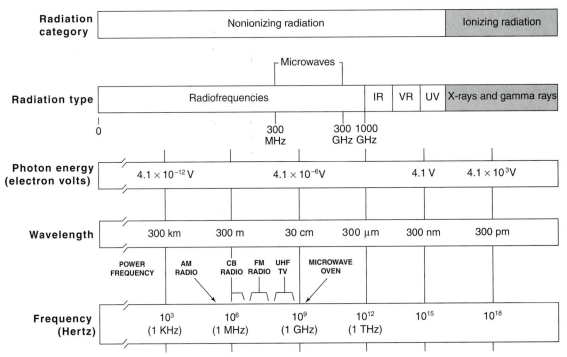

Figure 11–4. The electromagnetic radiation spectrum. GHz = gigahertz; IR = infrared radiation; kHz = kilohertz; MHz = megahertz; THz = terahertz; UV = ultraviolet light; VR = visible radiation (light).

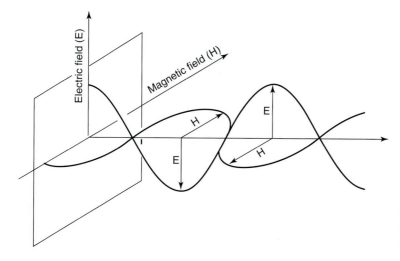

Figure 11–5. Electric field (E) and magnetic field (H) components of radiofrequency radiation.

RF radiation has insufficient energy to cause molecular ionization, but it does cause vibration and rotation of molecules, particularly molecules that have an asymmetric charge distribution or are polar in structure. It is composed of separate electric and magnetic field vectors, each perpendicular to the other and both perpendicular to the direction of the resulting electromagnetic wave (Figure 11–5). The electric field component is measured in volts per meter, the magnetic component in amperes per meter, and the resulting power density in watts per square meter.

Absorption of RF radiation depends on the orientation of the body in relation to the direction of the electromagnetic wave. Radiation at frequencies below 15 MHz and above 25 GHz are poorly absorbed and unlikely to cause significant thermally induced damage. Factors affecting conduction of RF radiation within the body include the thickness, distribution, and water content of the various tissues. As the water content increases, energy absorption and thermal effects increase. RF radiation can be modulated according to amplitude (AM) and frequency (FM) and can be generated in pulsed or continuous form. Pulsed waves are considered more dangerous.

The risk of thermal injury increases with higher intensities of radiation and closer proximity to the radiation source. Other factors that affect human susceptibility to RF radiation injury include environmental humidity and temperature, grounding, reflecting medium, tissue vascularity, increased temperature sensitivity of tissues (e.g., the testes), and lack of anatomic barriers to external radiation (e.g., the eye).

Occupational exposures are likely in any workplace where employees are near equipment that generates RF radiation, particularly equipment for dielectric heating (used in sealing of plastics and drying of wood), physiotherapy, radio communications, radiolocation, and mainte-

nance of aerial transmitters and high-power electrical equipment (Table 11–3). Injuries have been documented for acute exposure to energy levels exceeding 10 mW/cm². In most cases, the levels were greater than 100 mW/cm². Most studies of RF radiation effects in animals and other biologic test systems have not demonstrated thermally induced effects at energy levels below 10 mW/cm². In ani-

Table 11–3. Occupational radiofrequency and microwave exposures.

Sealing and heating equipment
    Automotive trades
    Furniture and woodworking
    Glass-fiber production
    Paper production
    Plastics manufacturing and fabrication
    Rubber product heating
    Textile manufacturing

Electrical equipment maintenance
    Radar
    Radio: AM, FM, CB
    Television: UHF and VHF
    Satellite
    Radio navigation
    Microwave generators and heat sources

RF applications
    Microwave tube testing and aging
    RF laser
    RF welding
    Medical diathermy and healing promotion

Power transmission line workers

mal studies, thermally induced effects include superficial and deep tissue destruction, cataract, and testicular damage.

Generally, acute high-level or long-term low-level exposures are not thought to cause cancer, but there is evidence for carcinogenesis in association with exposure to extremely low-frequency (ELF) radiation "magnetic fields" (<200 Hz). Current data indicate that ELF radiation causes childhood leukemia; accordingly, the International Agency for Research on Cancer has classified ELF radiation as a category 2B carcinogen ("possibly carcinogenic"). Although some studies have found an increased incidence of brain tumors, breast cancer (male), or leukemia in workers exposed to ELF radiation, most recent data regarding adult and occupational ELF radiation exposure do not indicate carcinogenic effects at any RF frequency. Similarly, teratogenicity has been questioned on the basis of findings of chromosomal changes in workers and an increase in the incidence of anomalies found in offspring of male physical therapists. However, because of conflicting study results, confounding exposures, and a lack of a verified biologic mechanism, the hypotheses of magnetic field–induced reproductive effects or teratogenicity have not been verified.

Although a number of health effects have been attributed to nonthermal and chronic RF exposures (including microwave and ELF radiation), current data do not support an association with cardiovascular, neurologic, or reproductive outcomes, with the possible exception of amyotrophic lateral sclerosis.

Literature is emerging regarding possible health effects associated with use of cell phones or mobile phones. Some studies of cell phone users have found nonspecific symptoms such as tension, depression, nausea, reduced concentration, headache, and vertigo. In vitro studies have reported altered expression of heat-shock protein (hsp 27) and genomic instability. Epidemiologic studies of cancer have had inconsistent results, with some finding increased rates of acoustic neuroma or brain cancer. Most of the recent authoritative reviews indicate that data are inadequate to draw any conclusions about health effects in relation to the use of cell phones.

Clinical Findings

Acute high-dose exposure usually is associated with a feeling of warmth on the exposed body part, followed by the feeling of hot or burning skin. The sensation of clicking or buzzing also may be present during the exposure. Other symptoms include irritability, headache or light-headedness, vertigo, pain at the site of exposure, watery eyes and a gritty eye sensation, dysphagia, anorexia, abdominal cramps, and nausea. Localized thermally induced masses may appear within days of exposure and consist of interstitial edema and coagulation necrosis.

The exposed skin has a sunburned appearance, with erythema and slight induration. There may be vesiculations or bullae. Blood pressure may be increased, and CPK levels may be elevated. Hematologic values, electroencephalographic and brain scan findings, sedimentation rate, and electrolyte values usually are within normal limits.

Beyond the immediately evident thermal injury, no further structural injury would be anticipated. In one case report, essential hypertension developed 1–3 months following exposure and then resolved with treatment. Symptoms of posttraumatic stress disorder have occurred, with emotional lability and insomnia persisting for as long as 1 year.

Differential Diagnosis

High-power equipment capable of generating RF and microwave radiation also might generate other forms of nonionizing radiation that should be considered. Chemical reactions caused by heat sources in the workplace should be investigated because thermal decomposition products of a heated hydrocarbon can cause the acute onset of similar symptoms, although blood pressure and CPK levels would not be expected to rise in such circumstances. Fear and anxiety resulting from the knowledge of a possibly damaging exposure also may cause many of the functional symptoms described earlier, although objective evidence of thermal injury and elevated CPK levels would not be expected.

Prevention

Exposure assessment should include the following factors: the distance between the power source and exposed workers, the peak power density at the time of exposure, the frequency and type of radiation wave (pulsed or continuous), and the duration of exposure (in minutes). Metal barriers around the energy source can be used to contain RF radiation. Intensity is proportional to $1/d^2$, where d is distance from the source. Accordingly, there is a rapid decrease in power density over distance, and specification of a "Personnel not allowed" area can provide an effective barrier. Procedures to deenergize equipment are recommended when employees are working close to exposed sources. Protective clothing generally is ineffective. Periodic environmental RF radiation measurements for equipment exposures are essential.

Treatment & Prognosis

Treatment is the same as for other thermal injuries. Thermal injuries usually heal without problems. If hypertension develops, it usually will resolve following a short course of antihypertensive therapy. Posttraumatic stress disorder and other psychological sequelae generally are responsive to short-term therapy.

2. Injuries Caused by Infrared Radiation

Infrared (IR) radiation covers the portion of the electromagnetic spectrum between visible and RF radiation (see

Figure 11–4). It has wavelengths between 750 and 3 million nm and is composed of three spectral bands—A, B, and C—that begin at 750, 1400, and 3000 nm, respectively. IR radiation is given off by any object having a temperature greater than absolute zero. Occupational exposures—in addition to sunlight—include processes in which thermal energy from IR radiation is used, such as heating and dehydrating processes, welding, glassmaking, and the drying and baking of coatings on consumer products.

Acute, high-intensity exposure to wavelengths shorter than 2000 nm can cause thermal damage to the cornea, iris, or lens. Thermal injury to the skin also can occur, but it is usually self-limited and results in an acute skin burn with increased pigmentation. Exposure to IR radiation has been associated with cataract formation, particularly among glassblowers and furnace workers.

Injuries can be prevented by shielding heat sources, using protective eye and skin wear, and monitoring exposure levels. Threshold limit values for exposure intensity are frequency-dependent in the biologically active wavelength spectrum of 750–2000 nm. Wavelengths in this range cause molecular excitation and vibration, resulting in heat that is absorbed by tissues and can cause thermal injury. In contrast, wavelengths exceeding 2000 nm are absorbed by water and are not biologically active because of the high water content of tissues.

3. Injuries Caused by Visible Radiation

Visible radiation (light) covers the portion of the electromagnetic spectrum between infrared and ultraviolet radiation (see Figure 11–4) and the wavelengths between 400 and 750 nm. The eye is the most sensitive target organ, with damage resulting from structural, thermal, or photochemical light-induced reactions. Workers at risk are those with prolonged or repeated exposure to intense light sources, including sunlight, high-intensity lamps, lasers, flashbulbs, spotlights, and welding arcs. Extremely intense light sources such as lasers also can cause pressure-induced (mechanical) retinal damage.

The retina is the usual site of injury and is most sensitive to the wavelengths of 440–500 nm (blue light), which cause a destructive photochemical reaction. Blue light is responsible for solar retinitis (eclipse blindness) and may contribute to retinal aging and to senile macular degeneration, which can result in visual field defects. Because the lens normally filters out wavelengths between 320 and 500 nm, it provides some protection of the retina from blue light. Individuals with aphakia (absence of the lens), who are more susceptible to retinal damage, should be cautioned against looking into the midday sun and other intense light sources and should be urged to wear spectacle filters when working in bright environments.

Short bursts of high-intensity light can cause heat-induced flash blindness, in which the temporary visual loss and afterimage are a result of bleaching of visual pigments.

As the light intensity and exposure duration increase, the afterimage persists longer. With mild to moderate exposures, symptoms of flash blindness resolve quickly.

Insufficient lighting or reflected light (glare) can cause asthenopia (eyestrain), visual fatigue, headache, and eye irritation. These problems are more likely to occur in people older than age 40. Symptoms are transient, and there is no indication that repeated episodes lead to ocular damage.

Contrast from surrounding light sources on areas of lesser intensity has led to complaints of asthenopia associated with video-display terminal use. This usually can be corrected by decreasing surrounding light intensities, using antiglare filters, and adjusting the contrast of the light on the screen.

Treatment of eye injuries is discussed in Chapter 8. Measures to prevent injury in workers at risk include preemployment evaluations for individuals with aphakia or a history of light sensitivity and medical surveillance to detect changes in visual acuity or early signs of ocular damage, use of goggles or face shields by welders, proper illumination of the workplace to reduce glare (see Chapter 12), and use of filters on intense light sources to eliminate blue-light wavelengths.

4. Injuries Caused by Ultraviolet Radiation

Ultraviolet (UV) radiation covers the portion of the electromagnetic spectrum between visible radiation and ionizing radiation (see Figure 11–4) and has wavelengths between 100 and 400 nm. The wavelengths are divided into three spectral bands—A, B, and C—with the A and B bands representing the longer wavelengths and producing most of the biologic effects (Table 11–4). Wavelengths shorter than 200 nm are biologically inactive; they can exist only in a vacuum or an inert gas atmosphere and are absorbed over extremely short distances in air. Wavelengths of 200–290 nm are absorbed primarily in the stratum corneum of the skin or the cornea of the eye, whereas the longer wavelengths can affect the dermis, lens, iris, or retina.

Because UV radiation has relatively poor penetration, the only organs it affects are the eye and skin. Eye injury is caused by thermal action from pulsed or brief high-power exposures, and skin damage is caused more commonly by photochemical reactions (including toxic and hypersensitivity reactions) from brief high- or extended low-power exposures. The thermal effects of protein coagulation and tissue necrosis are rapid in onset. The effects of chronic exposure include accelerated aging of the skin, characterized by loss of elasticity, hyperpigmentation, wrinkling, and telangiectasia.

UV injuries occur in occupations involving drying and curing processes, arc welding, or use of lasers or germicidal UV lights (Table 11–5), but by far the

Table 11–4. Ultraviolet light spectrum: ultraviolet A (UVA) and ultraviolet B (UVB) comparison.

	UVA	UVB
Wavelength	315–400 nm	280–315 nm
Penetration	Air, water, glass,	Air, quartz
Physical	quartz through eye	Anterior chamber
Biological	to retina	only
Health effects	Skin and eye injury require greater energy than UVB	Skin erythema at 280–315 nm Peak carcinogenicity at 280–320 nm Peak photokeratitis sensitivity at 270 nm Cataract
Proportion of natural background UV	97%	3%

Table 11–5. Workers potentially exposed to ultraviolet radiation.

Natural sunlight

Agricultural workers	Oil field workers
Brick masons	Open pit miners
Ranchers	Outdoor maintenance workers
Construction workers	Pipeline workers
Farmers	Police officers
Fishermen	Postal carriers
Gardeners	Railroad workers
Greenskeepers	Road workers
Horticultural workers	Sailors
Landscapers	Ski instructors
Lifeguards	Sports professionals
Lumberjacks	Surveyors
Military personnel	Other outdoor workers

Arc welding/torch cutting
Welders
Pipeline workers
Pipecutters
Maintenance workers

Germicidal ultraviolet
Physicians
Nurses
Laboratory technicians
Bacteriology laboratory personnel
Barbers
Cosmetologists
Kitchen workers
Dentists/Dental technicians

Laser
Laboratory workers

Drying and curing processes
Printers
Lithographers
Painters
Wood curers
Plastics workers

greatest proportion of injuries result from occupations that expose workers to natural sunlight during the peak time of UV energy dissemination, 10 AM to 3 PM. Factors affecting the severity of injury include exposure duration, radiation intensity, distance from the radiation source, and orientation of the exposed individual relative to the source and its wave-propagation plane. UV reflections from water and snow or their surrounding surfaces may increase exposure intensity.

Clinical Findings & Treatment

A. PHOTOKERATOCONJUNCTIVITIS (WELDER'S FLASH)

Ocular exposure to UV wavelengths shorter than 315 nm (especially wavelengths of 270 nm, to which the eye is most sensitive) can cause photokeratoconjunctivitis. Symptoms occur 6–12 hours after exposure and include severe pain, photophobia, a sensation of a foreign body or sand in the eyes, and tearing. After a latency period that varies inversely with the severity of the exposure, conjunctivitis appears, sometimes accompanied by erythema and swelling of the eyelids and facial skin. Slit-lamp examination may reveal diffuse punctate staining of both corneas.

Treatment consists of providing symptomatic relief, which may include ice packs, systemic analgesics, eye patches, and mild sedation. Local anesthetics should not be used because of the risk of further injury to the anesthetized eye. Symptoms usually resolve within 48 hours. Permanent sequelae are rare, and the eye does not develop tolerance to repeated exposure.

B. CATARACTS

Cataractogenesis (cortical) is attributed to both photochemical and thermal effects of intense exposure to UV wavelengths of 295–320 nm and usually appears within 24 hours. Cataract formation following repeated exposures to UV wavelengths longer than 324 nm has been reported but is not well documented. Treatment is by corrective surgery.

C. OTHER EYE INJURIES

The cornea and lens protect the retina from the effects of UV wavelengths shorter than 300 nm, but damage to the iris and retina is possible if individuals with aphakia are exposed to these wavelengths. In others, damage is possible with exposure to longer wavelengths or to high-power UV lasers. Treatment is supportive (Table 11–6). Two lesions of the bulbar conjunctiva have been associated with repeated exposures to UV radiation: pterygium (a benign hyperplasia) and epidermoid carcinoma.

D. ERYTHEMA

Absorbed UV radiation reacts with photoactive substances present in the skin and 2–24 hours later causes erythema (sunburn), the most common acute UV effect. Erythema is most severe following exposure to wavelengths of 290–320 nm and may be accompanied by edema, blistering, desquamation, chills, fever, nausea, and rarely, circulatory collapse.

Treatment of acute sunburn and any blistering that occurs is supportive and symptomatic and may include topical and mild systemic analgesics. Most symptoms subside within 48 hours. The resulting scaling, darkening of the skin (caused by increased melanin production), and thickening of the stratum corneum provide increased protection against subsequent exposures.

E. PHOTOSENSITIVITY REACTIONS

Two types of acute photosensitivity reactions of the skin can occur following exposure to UV radiation: phototoxic (nonallergic) and photoallergic reactions. Phototoxic reactions are much more common and frequently occur in association with use of medications such as griseofulvin, tetracycline, sulfonamides, thiazides, and preparations containing coal tar or psoralens. Phototoxicity may exaggerate or aggravate the effects of some systemic diseases, including

lupus erythematosus, dermatomyositis, congenital erythropoietic porphyria, porphyria cutanea tarda symptomatica, pellagra, actinic reticuloid, herpes simplex, and pemphigus foliaceus. Photosensitivity reactions may be characterized by blisters, bullae, and other skin manifestations.

Exposure to UV wavelengths above 320 nm after skin contact with furocoumarin-producing plants such as celery can cause phytophotodermatitis. A mild phototoxic reaction causes pigmentary changes along the pattern of points of contact, whereas bullae may result from a more severe inflammatory reaction. Photoallergic reactions to UV radiation occur in association with bacteriostatic agents and perfume ingredients, which cause skin irritation, erythema, and blistering. Treatment of photosensitivity reactions depends on the particular underlying or associative cause and ranges from symptomatic care in mild cases to hospitalization and use of systemic corticosteroids in cases of severe reactions.

F. PREMALIGNANT AND MALIGNANT SKIN LESIONS

Premalignant lesions associated with chronic exposure to UV radiation include actinic keratosis, keratoacanthoma, and Hutchinson melanosis. Malignant lesions associated with exposure are basal cell carcinoma (the most common), squamous cell carcinoma, and malignant melanoma. Hazardous UV wavelengths are thought to be between 256 and 320 nm. UV radiation also promotes carcinogenesis following exposure to some chemicals, including those found in tar and pitch. Increased risk for premalignant and malignant lesions occurs in fair-skinned individuals and in those who have repeated sunburns or tan poorly. Patients with a history of xeroderma pigmentosum are at greater risk for malignant melanoma.

Patients should be referred to a dermatologist for definitive diagnosis and treatment. Premalignant lesions may be treated by removal or use of topical medication. Treatment of malignant lesions may involve simple excision, radiation, or major surgery.

Prevention

Exposure guidelines are based on wavelength and irradiance. Exposed individuals should be counseled concerning photosensitizing agents. Welders should be urged to wear goggles or face shields to protect their eyes. Outdoor workers should be instructed to use sunscreen [broad spectrum with skin protective factor (SPF) 30] and protective clothing, and persons at increased risk because of preexisting medical conditions or excessive exposure should be examined periodically for the presence of premalignant or malignant lesions.

REFERENCES

Feychting M, Ahlbom A, Kheifets L: EMF and health. Ann Rev Public Health 2005;26:165 [PMID:15760285].

Table 11–6. Eye injuries caused by ultraviolet light.

Location	UV Effect
Conjunctiva	Conjunctivitis
Sclera	Hyperemia
Cornea	Keratitis
Cataracts	Lens
Aqueous	Toxic photochemicals
Vitreous	? Degradation in aphakics
Retina	Chromophore damage in aphakics

Hocking B, Westerman R: Neurological effects of radiofrequency radiation. Occup Med (Lond) 2003;53:123 [PMID:12637597].

Johansen C: Electromagnetic fields and health effects: Epidemiologic studies of cancer, diseases of the central nervous system and arrhythmia-related heart disease. Scand J Work Environ Health 2004;30(Suppl 1):1 [PMID:15255560].

Oliva MS, Taylor H: Ultraviolet radiation and the eye. Int Ophthalmol Clin 2005;45:1 [PMID:15632523].

Ramirez CC, Federman DG, Kirsner RS: Skin cancer as an occupational disease: The effect of ultraviolet and other forms of radiation. Int J Dermatol 2005;44:95 [PMID:15689204].

IONIZING RADIATION INJURIES

The two most significant health responses to ionizing radiation are the acute radiation syndrome that follows a brief but massive exposure and the chronic effects that are caused by a brief high-dose exposure or to high cumulative exposures. More than 200 significant radiation incidents have occurred since 1940 as a result of exposure to radioisotopes, x-ray generators and accelerators, radar generators, and similar sources of ionizing radiation. Because of the ubiquity of ionizing radiation in our environment, the effects of long-term low-dose exposures are more difficult to pinpoint, but clusters of illnesses have been found near nuclear test sites and in association with some occupations. Workers at risk, based on their history of exposures and resulting injury, include radiologists, uranium miners, radium dial painters, nuclear power plant operators, and military personnel. Table 11–7 lists other workers at risk based on the potential for exposure.

Ionizing radiation is emitted from radioactive atomic structures as energized particles (alpha, beta, proton, and neutron particles) that impart energy through collision with other structures or as high-energy electromagnetic x-rays or gamma rays. The different forms of ionizing radiation vary in natural source, energy, frequency, and penetrability, but they all share the ability to ionize incident materials and exist at the highest energies and frequencies of the electromagnetic spectrum (see Figure 11–4). Dislocation of an electron from an incident atom and the resulting biomolecular chemical reactions and instability can cause tissue damage. Table 11–8 summarizes the clinical effects of ionizing radiation.

External biologic exposure to x-rays, gamma rays, and proton and neutron radiation results in high absorption, whereas beta particles penetrate skin poorly and alpha particles do not penetrate at all. Internal exposure to alpha or beta particles by inhalation, implantation, or ingestion can result in serious acute or delayed injury. If radioactive contamination is suspected, decontamination procedures should be followed scrupulously during all phases of patient management.

As an emergency resource, the Oak Ridge Institute for Science and Education maintains 24-hour phone access to consultation regarding medical and health

Table 11–7. Potential occupational exposures to ionizing radiation.

Aircraft workers
Atomic energy plant workers
Biologists
Cathode ray tube makers
Chemists
Dental workers
Drug makers and sterilizers
Electron microscope makers and operators
Electrostatic eliminator operators
Embalmers
Fire alarm makers
Food preservers and sterilizers
Gas mantle makers
High-voltage electron, x-ray, vacuum, radar, klystron or television tube makers, users, repairmen
Industrial radiographers and fluoroscopists
Inspectors using—and workers in proximity to—sealed gamma ray sources (cesium 137, cobalt 60, iridium 192) and x-rays
Liquid-level gauge painters
Luminous dial painters
Military personnel
Oil well loggers
Ore assayers
Petroleum refinery workers
Physicians and nurses
Plasma torch operators
Plastics technicians
Prospectors
Radium refinery workers
Research workers, chemists, biologists, physicists
Thickness gauge operators
Thorium ore and alloy workers
Tile glazers
Uranium workers and miners
Veterinarians
X-ray aides and technicians
X-ray diffraction apparatus operators

physics problems associated with radiation accidents (865-576-1005).

1. Acute Radiation Syndrome

Acute radiation syndrome is a consequence of brief but heavy exposure of all or part of the body to ionizing radiation. The radiation disrupts chemical bonds, which causes molecular excitation and free-radical formation. Highly reactive free radicals react with other essential molecules such as nucleic acids and enzymes; in turn, this disrupts cellular function. The clinical presentation and severity of illness are determined by the dosage, body distribution, and duration of exposure. Tissues with the most rapid cel-

Table 11–8. Summary of clinical effects of ionizing radiation dosages.

	Subclinical Range	Therapeutic Range			Lethal Range	
	0–100 rem	100–200 rem (Clinical Surveillance)	200–600 rem (Therapy Effective)	600–1000 rem (Therapy Promising)	1000–5000 rem (Therapy Palliative)	>5000 rem (Therapy Palliative)
Incidence of vomiting	None	5% at 100 rem 50% at 200 rem	100% at 300 rem	100%	100%	100%
Delay time for vomiting	—	3 h	2 h	1 h	30 min	30 min
Leading organ affected	None	Hematopoietic tissue	Hematopoietic tissue	Hematopoietic tissue	Gastrointestinal tract	Central nervous system
Characteristic signs and symptoms	None	Mild nausea and moderate leukopenia	Severe leukopenia, diarrhea, nausea, purpura, hemorrhage, and infection; hair loss above 300 rem	Severe leukopenia, purpura, hemorrhage, infection, prostration, coma	Diarrhea, fever, and disturbance of electrolyte balance	Convulsions, tremor, ataxia, and lethargy
Critical period post-exposure	—	—	4–6 wks	4–6 wks	5–14 days	1–48 h
Therapy required	Reassurance	Reassurance and hematologic surveillance	Blood transfusion, antibiotics, and hematopoietic growth factors	Blood transfusion, antibiotics, hematopoietic growth factors, and consider bone marrow transplant	Maintenance of electrolyte balance	Sedatives
Prognosis	Excellent	Excellent	Good	Guarded	Hopeless	Hopeless
Convalescent	None	Several weeks	1–12 mos	Long		
Incidence of death	None	None	0–80%	80–100%	90–100%	90–100%
Time within which death occurs	—	—	2 mos	2 mos	2 wks	2 days
Cause of death	—	—	Hemorrhage and infection	Hemorrhage and infection	Circulatory collapse	Respiratory failure and brain edema

lular turnover are the most radiosensitive: reproductive, hematopoietic, and gastrointestinal tissues.

Clinical Findings

Although symptoms are unlikely with exposure to doses less than 100 cGy, abnormal laboratory findings may be seen at any dose over 25 cGy. For doses of 100–400 cGy, symptoms begin within 2–6 hours and may last up to 48 hours. For doses of 600–1000 cGy, symptoms begin within 2 hours and later merge into the illness phase. For those at Chernobyl who received more than 600 cGy, headache, fever, and vomiting developed within the first half hour. Within 6 days, severe lymphopenia developed, followed by severe gastroenteritis, granulocytopenia, and thrombocytopenia. For those in the lowest exposure group (80–210 cGy), slight lymphopenia occurred within a few days, followed by mild granulocytopenia and thrombocytopenia at 4 weeks.

Doses of 1000–3000 cGy can cause immediate gastrointestinal symptoms and massive fluid, blood, and electrolyte loss resulting from denudation of the gastrointestinal mucosa. Doses exceeding 3000 cGy are lethal. They cause progressive neurologic incapacitation associated with ataxia, lethargy, tremor, and convulsions. Death is almost immediate with the highest doses.

Some patients with acute radiation syndrome pass through four phases: prodrome, latent phase, illness, and recovery.

A. PRODROME

Symptoms and signs may include anorexia, nausea, vomiting, diarrhea, intestinal cramps, salivation, dehydration, fatigue, apathy, prostration, arrhythmia, fever, respiratory distress, hyperexcitability, ataxia, headache, and hypotension. Gastrointestinal and central nervous system findings predominate.

B. LATENT PHASE

The prodrome is sometimes followed by a period of relative well-being prior to the onset of illness. In cases of exposure to higher doses of radiation, the latent period is shortened or eliminated, and central nervous system or gastrointestinal effects predominate.

C. ILLNESS PHASE

Symptoms and signs in this phase may include fatigue, weakness, fever, diarrhea, anorexia, weight loss, hair loss, arrhythmia, ileus, ataxia, disorientation, convulsions, coma, and shock. Effects are primarily hematopoietic and a result of inhibition of hematopoietic stem cells. There may be a sequential decrease in lymphocytes, granulocytes, platelets, and erythrocytes. Leukopenia and thrombocytopenia may occur with secondary infection, hemorrhagic diathesis, or anemia. Cardiovascular collapse, pericarditis, and myocarditis have been reported. With doses exceeding 200 cGy, there may be reproductive system effects, including sterility, aspermatogenesis, and cessation of menses. Fetal and embryo toxicity or death also can occur.

D. RECOVERY PHASE

The prognosis for recovery from exposures of up to 600 cGy is good when appropriate therapy is given. For higher exposures, the prognosis worsens as the dose increases. Infection and sepsis are the major causes of morbidity and mortality in cases involving exposures below 1000 cGy, in which the major impact is hematopoietic.

Prevention

Occupational exposure to ionizing radiation should be monitored. The technology varies with the type of radiation and the target site. Personal exposure measurement devices include film badges (x-rays, gamma, and beta) or nuclear emulsion monitors (x-rays, gamma, beta, and neutrons), thermoluminescent dosimeters (beta, gamma, and neutron), and ionization dosimeters. A scintillation counter can be used to measure some radioisotopes in urine specimens or in tissue from target organs (e.g., urine tritium or ^{32}P, thyroid scintillation scan for ^{125}I). Environmental or area monitoring devices include the Geiger-Müller counter, ionization chamber, and scintillation detector. Where an exposure potential occurs, shielding with lead or other effective barrier can contain emissions.

To quantify risk from radiation exposure, a system of units has been created and revised many times. The International Commission on Radiological Units and Measurements (ICRU) has recommended that the older CGS (centimeter-gram-second) units be replaced by the equivalent SI (International System of Units) units, as shown in Table 11–9. Table 11–10 lists the recommended external exposure limits. The basis for the limits is what is referred to as the *acceptable risk*. This is thought to be 1 in 10,000 per year for workers with occupational exposures and 1 in 10,000–1,000,000 per year for the general public, based on estimated radiation-induced fatal cancers and serious hereditary disorders. Exposures can be prevented easily with the use of lead or other high-density material, which can enclose the source and/or shield the work area (e.g., lead blocks, cement, and leaded glass).

Treatment

The patient should be decontaminated, hospitalized, and placed under the care of hematologists and infectious disease specialists. Vital signs, fluid and electrolyte balance, and hematopoietic, gastrointestinal, and central nervous system functions should be monitored closely.

If the granulocyte counts fall below 1000/μL, prophylactic antibacterial agents, acyclovir, and antifungals have been recommended. If there is fever or suspected sepsis, antimicrobial agents by intravenous infusion should be started immediately. The choice of agents also should depend on the endemic pathogens at the particular hospital. Antimicrobial therapy should be continued until the granulocyte count exceeds 500/μL or until the patient has been afebrile for 5 consecutive days without evidence of infection. Reverse isolation should be maintained.

Granulocyte, platelet, and red cell transfusions may be necessary. Lymphocytes should be obtained immediately for HLA typing. Transfusions are recommended if the platelet count falls below 20,000/μL, the granulo-

Table 11–9. Radiation units.

Parameter	SI Units[1]	CGS Units[2]	Conversion
Activity = rate of decay (disintegration per second)	Becquerel (Bq)	Curie (Ci)	1 Ci = 3.7 × 1010 Bq 1 Bq = 2.703 × 10^{-11} Ci
Exposure (dose) = quantity of x-ray or gamma radiation at a given point	Coulomb (C)/kg of air	Roentgen (R)	1 C/kg of air = 3876 R 1 R = 258 MC/kg of air
Dose rate = dose per unit of time (counts per minute)	Coulomb (C)/kg of air/h	Roentgen (R)/h	Same as above
Absorbed dose = quantity of radiation absorbed per unit of mass	Gray (Gy) Joules (J)/kg	Rad Erg	1 Gy = 1 J/kg 1 Gy = 100 rads 1 rad = 0.01 Gy 1 rad = 100 ergs
Dose equivalent = absorbed dose in terms of estimated biologic effect relative to an exposure of 1 roentgen of x-ray or gamma radiation	Sievert (Sv)	Rem	1 Sv = 100 rem 1 rem = 0.01 Sv

[1]SI = International System of Units.
[2]CGS = centigram-gram-second system of units.

cyte count below 200/μL, or the hematocrit below 25%. Hematopoietic growth factors (filgrastim, sargramostim) have been effective in accelerating hematopoietic recovery. Bone marrow transplants have been used with questionable success in combating intractable hemorrhage and infection. They should be considered for patients exposed to 600–2000 cGy, and the decision about whether to use them should be made within a week of the radiation exposure.

Patients should receive supportive therapy as necessary for control of nausea, dehydration, and other symptoms. Ondansetron hydrochloride, 8 mg orally two or three times daily, has been recommended for nausea; chlorpromazine, 25–50 mg given deeply intramuscularly every 4–6 hours, is an alternative.

2. Acute Localized Radiation Injuries

Exposure of isolated skin and body parts to ionizing radiation will result in hair loss (doses above 300 cGy), erythema (above 600 cGy), dry desquamation (radionecrosis) (above 1000 cGy), and wet desquamation (above 2000 cGy). Pain and itching occur shortly after exposure and are followed by erythema and blister formation. In cases of severe localized burns, there may be tissue ischemia and necrosis.

Prevention is as for acute radiation syndrome (see above). Treatment is conservative and should not include surgery unless dictated by secondary complications. To conserve joint motion and prevent contractures, splinting and physical therapy may be required during convalescence. Injuries should be followed closely because the extent of tissue damage often is not readily apparent. Subsequent fibrosis, ulceration, infection, necrosis, or gangrene may occur and require surgery or more radical medical treatment.

3. Radionuclide Contamination

Skin contamination with radionuclides is rarely life-threatening. Immediate decontamination measures con-

Table 11–10. External radiation exposure limits.

Groups and Body Parts Exposed	Radiation Limit
Adults	5 rem (0.05 Sv) per year[1]
Whole body, head, trunk, arm above elbow, and leg above knee	or 2 rem (0.02 Sv) per year averaged over 5 years
Hand, elbow, arm below elbow, foot, knee, and leg below knee	50 rem (0.5 Sv) per year
Lens of eye	15 rem (0.15 Sv) per year
Skin (10 cm)	50 rem (0.5 Sv) per year
Pregnant women	0.05 rem (0.5 mSv) per month while pregnant

[1]Includes cumulative yearly (external) deep-dose equivalent and (internal) committed effective-dose equivalent.

sist of gently scrubbing the skin with soap and warm water and, if necessary, cutting the hair. Hair clippings, material removed by scrubbing, swabs of the nares and mouth, clothing, and personal effects should be saved for radioactivity analysis and dosage calculation.

For contaminated open wounds, gentle surgical debridement should be performed and wound irrigation considered. Depending on the type of radionuclide causing the injury, administration of a chelating agent may be indicated. For plutonium and alpha emitters, diethylenetriaminepentaacetic acid (DTPA) is effective and can be administered systemically, as well as in the wound irrigation solution. Blocking agents may also be considered, as in the case of radioiodines. Uranium and its associated radon daughter emissions are associated with lung cancer and probably reproductive effects, nonmalignant pulmonary disease, and nephritis.

4. Delayed Effects of High-Dose Radiation

Radiodermatitis often occurs in association with ionizing radiation therapy. The skin is dry, smooth, shiny, thin, pruritic, and sensitive, and there are signs of telangiectasia, atrophy, and diffuse pigmentation. The nails are brittle and striated.

Scarring in other tissues following high-dose exposure has led to endarteritis obliterans, dry-eye syndrome, myelopathy, pericarditis, hepatitis, nephritis, coronary artery disease, chromosomal injury, intestinal stenosis, pulmonary fibrosis, and cataracts.

Systemic exposure because of nuclear blast and/or fallout is associated with increases in thyroid neoplasms and leukemia. Cancers related to localized radioactivity include bone cancer from localized radioisotopes, thyroid cancer following childhood thymus irradiation, liver cancer associated with thorium dioxide, and lung cancer associated with radon decay products (radon daughters) in uranium miners. Leukemia has been reported in patients receiving radiotherapy for ankylosing spondylitis. Additional cancers associated with exposure to ionizing radiation include skin and breast.

Other effects of high-dose exposure include premature aging, shortening of the life span, and teratogenic (central nervous system deficit, mental retardation, and microcephaly) and reproductive abnormalities.

5. Effects of Low-Dose Radiation

Controversy continues over whether the risk for somatic and genetic disorders is increased significantly by cumulative low-dose exposures. The dose-response curve in the low-dose range cannot be determined at present, so most estimates of risk continue to be based on mathematical extrapolations from experiences with higher doses. Although developmental abnormalities are associated with doses as low as 10 cGy, and cancers are associated with levels below 100 cGy, the practical relevance of low-dose phenomena is extremely difficult to establish not only because of inconsistencies in the literature but also because the cumulative average exposure for people in the United States is approximately 8–10 cGy per lifetime (Table 11–11). Current data suggest that low cumulative exposure (50–100 mSv) is carcinogenic, but its risk depends on the total dose, cancer type, and age at exposure.

REFERENCES

International Commission on Radiation Protection: www.icrp.org.

National Council on Radiation Protection and Measurements: www.ncrp.com/comment.html.

Prasad KN et al: Health risks of low dose ionizing radiation in humans: a review. Exp Biol Med (Maywood) 2004;229:378 [PMID:15096649].

Radiation Emergency Assistance Center/Training Site (REACTS): www.orau.gov/reacts.

Sachs RK, Brenner DJ: Solid tumor risks after high doses of ionizing radiation. Proc Natl Acad Sci USA 2005;102:13040 [PMID:16150705]

US EPA Office of Radiation Protection: www.epa.gov/radiation.

LASER INJURIES

The energy of the laser source is transformed through atomic excitation into a coherent, collimated, monochromatic beam of radiation. Lasers operate at one wavelength, usually in the ultraviolet, visible, or infrared portion of the electromagnetic spectrum. They may emit radiation in continuous or pulsed waves.

Most industrial exposures to laser radiation occur in the construction industry, where lasers are used to provide alignment and grade levels on projects such as dam construction, tunneling, dredging, floor installation, and pipe laying. In the manufacture of electronics, laser use is increasing for welding, burning, and alignment. Intense laser sources are used to cut hard metals and diamonds, and less intense thermal applications include medical treatment.

Biologic effects occur at low intensities, although there is some variation with wavelength. Permanent injuries have not been associated with repeated low-intensity exposures. At high intensities, thermal or pressure-induced damage to the skin or eyes can occur. These injuries are more likely with lasers that have a high-intensity beam outside the visible light spectrum because the worker's proximity to the beam may not be apparent. Because of the thermal mechanism, any damage that occurs would be expected to be manifested immediately with the symptoms and signs of a corneal, retinal, or cutaneous burn. Exposure to ultraviolet (UV) lasers is more likely to cause corneal damage, whereas infrared and visible-light lasers are

Table 11–11. Average annual effective dose equivalent of ionizing radiations to a member of the US population.[1]

Source	Dose Equivalent[2]		Effective Dose Equivalent	
	mSv	mrem	mSv	%
Natural				
Radon[3]	24	2,400	2.0	55
Cosmic	0.27	27	0.27	8.0
Terrestrial	0.28	28	0.28	8.0
Internal	0.39	39	0.39	11
Total natural	—	—	3.0	82
Artificial				
Medical				
X-ray diagnosis	0.39	39	0.39	11
Nuclear medicine	0.14	14	0.14	4.0
Consumer products	0.10	10	0.10	3.0
Other				
Occupational	0.0009	0.9	< 0.01	< 0.3
Nuclear fuel cycle	< 0.01	< 1.0	< 0.01	< 0.03
Fallout	< 0.01	< 1.0	< 0.01	< 0.03
Miscellaneous[4]	< 0.01	< 1.0	< 0.01	< 0.03
Total artificial	—	—	0.63	18
Total natural and artificial	—	—	3.6	100

[1]Reproduced, with permission, from Beir V: Health Effects of Exposure to Low Levels of Ionizing Radiation. National Academy Press, 1990.
[2]To soft tissues.
[3]Dose equivalent to bronchi from radon daughter products. The assumed weighting factor for the effective dose equivalent relative to whole-body exposure is 0.08.
[4]Department of Energy facilities, smelters, transportation, etc.

more likely to injure the retina because of their ocular penetration. Eye symptoms of accidental high-intensity laser exposure include photophobias or a sudden visual flash followed by scotoma or shadow of unusual size and color. Visual acuity or fields may be reduced. Retinal changes, including edema, coagulation, hemorrhage, and opaque vitreous, can occur. Treatment for these laser injuries is the same as that for other ocular thermal injuries, with the addition of corticosteroids by some investigators.

To prevent injuries, exposure levels should be monitored. Threshold limit values for lasers have been established by the ACGIH and are based on intensity, wavelength, and exposure time. ANSI has developed a classification for lasers by degree of hazard, with class 1 representing no risk and class 4 representing a severe hazard, even from diffuse reflection. Evaluation of workers following laser exposures should include an assessment of exposure intensity, wavelength, duration, viewing angle, and ANSI laser hazard classification.

Individuals working in proximity to high-power lasers should be instructed in proper operating procedures and provided with protective eyewear designed for the specific wavelength of the laser. In some cases, the eyewear does not by itself offer sufficient protection owing to possible laser reflections. Other devices, including shields, barriers, and where possible, remote viewing equipment, should be used. Skin protection is also important when high-power lasers are used. If feasible, systems should be designed with the beam line totally enclosed and shielded.

Preplacement examinations are recommended for individuals who will work with class 3B and 4 lasers and should consist of, at a minimum, the medical history, tests for visual acuity (near and far) and refractive errors, visual fields, and inspection of the outer eye and skin. Because pathologic effects are not associated with long-term low-intensity exposures, periodic evaluation is not recommended for laser operators unless an acute high-intensity exposure occurs.

REFERENCES

Mainster MA et al: Assessment of alleged retinal laser injuries. Arch Ophthalmol 2004;122:1210 [PMID:15302664].

Tsuzuki A et al: A case of ocular injury from industrial laser burns. Jpn J Ophthalmol 2004; 48:172 [PMID:15060800].

ATMOSPHERIC PRESSURE DISORDERS (DYSBARISM)

Sudden shift to an environment of lower ambient pressure, as occurs with rapid ascension to the surface from deep-sea diving or with loss of cabin pressure while flying at high altitudes, causes decompression sickness. Compression sickness can occur following movement to an environment of higher ambient pressure, but the only common example of this is barotitis.

1. Decompression Sickness (Caisson Disease)

Decompression sickness results from mechanical and physiologic effects of expanding gases and bubbles in blood and tissue. When the body is exposed to an environment of higher than atmospheric gas pressure, as in tunneling or diving, it absorbs more of the inhaled gases than it does at sea level. Aided by its fat solubility, nitrogen concentrations increase in tissues, particularly those of the nervous system, bone marrow, and fat. Because the blood supply is poor in bone marrow and fat, nitrogen enters and leaves these tissues more slowly than oxygen or carbon dioxide does. As the surrounding pressure decreases (decompression), nitrogen expands and will form gas bubbles if there is insufficient time for its dissolution from tissues. Because oxygen and carbon dioxide have greater fluid solubility and move more easily between tissue compartments, their tendency for bubble formation is reduced. Remaining nitrogen gas bubbles are more symptomatic and destructive in less elastic structures or tissues (e.g., joints and central nervous system).

Most cases of decompression sickness have occurred after rapid ascension from sea depths in excess of 9 m (29.5 ft) or after sudden pressure loss at altitudes in excess of 7000 m (22,966 ft).

Clinical Findings

A complete evaluation of the systems affected—as determined by the history and physical examination—should be performed with appropriate x-rays and other diagnostic procedures. Anyone exhibiting signs or symptoms of decompression sickness within 48 hours of a high-pressure exposure should be given a compression test in which 100% oxygen at 3 atm is administered for 20 minutes in a hyperbaric chamber.

There are three types of decompression sickness, as described below. The type and severity of symptoms will depend on the age, weight/body fat, smoking status and physical condition of the patient, the degree of physical exertion, the depth or altitude before decompression, duration of compression, and rate and duration of decompression.

A. TYPE 1 DECOMPRESSION SICKNESS

This type, which has the best prognosis, affects the limbs and skin. Acute pain, usually around a frequently used joint, may be incapacitating and cause the patient to assume a stooped posture (the "bends"). Pain may begin immediately after decompression or up to 12 hours later and sometimes is accompanied by urticarial and bluish red mottling and itching of the skin ("diver's lice").

B. TYPE 2 DECOMPRESSION SICKNESS

Type 2 is more severe than type 1. Symptoms and signs of central and peripheral nerve damage may include vertigo, "pins and needles," paresthesias, hypoesthesia, ataxic gait, hyperreflexia, Babinski sign, paralysis or weakness of the limbs, headache; seizures; vomiting; visual loss or visual field defects, incontinence, impaired speech, tremor, and coma. Pulmonary manifestations (the "chokes") may include substernal pain, chest tightness, severe coughing, dyspnea, pulmonary edema, and shallow respirations. Cardiovascular findings include arrhythmia and hypertension.

Type 2 sickness, which is probably caused by gas bubbles in the central nervous system and spinal cord, may have significant sequelae, such as vascular obstruction and tissue infarction (which sometimes are accompanied by hemoconcentration, changes in osmotic pressure or lipid emboli, hemorrhagic infarcts of the lungs, ulcers of the colon, multifocal degeneration of white matter, and hypercoagulation of blood).

Pulmonary barotrauma and gas expansion in other tissues can cause arterial gas embolism, which is the second leading cause of death in divers (drowning is first). Types 1 and 2 decompression sickness also can occur with unpressurized descent from high altitude. Severity depends on the initial altitude and the rate of descent.

C. TYPE 3 DECOMPRESSION SICKNESS

The third type is characterized by aseptic necrosis of bone (osteonecrosis), which frequently involves the head or shaft of the humerus and less often involves the lower end of the femur and the tibial head. Osteonecrosis usually occurs 6–60 months following decompression and is asymptomatic unless there is joint involvement, which can cause permanent impairment. Radiographic examination may show bone sclerosis and mottling. Lesions are often symmetric.

Osteonecrosis may be the result of nitrogen bubbles obstructing the capillaries and has been reported in up to 50% of divers and underwater workers, although disability occurs in fewer than 3%. An increased incidence of memory deficits, retrograde amnesia, emotional instability, and other neurologic and psychiatric symptoms has been observed in divers with a history of multiple episodes of decompression sickness.

Prevention

Divers, underwater workers, and pilots should be screened to make that sure they are in good physical condition—not overweight and with no other conditions imposing an increased risk for dysbarism, such as vascular disorders, hypercoagulopathy, obstructive airways disease, pneumothorax, sinusitis, otitis media, dehydration, substance abuse, or recent bone fractures. Workers should receive training and education in proper compression and decompression procedures and in recognizing the symptoms and signs of decompression sickness.

Treatment

A. TYPES 1 AND 2 DECOMPRESSION SICKNESS

The patient should be placed in a supine position. For immediate first aid, 100% oxygen should be administered, and aspirin may be given for analgesia. The patient should be transported rapidly to an emergency facility that has a hyperbaric chamber for recompression and decompression. Information about the nearest facility and advice about recompression can be obtained 24 hours a day by calling the National Divers Alert Network (DAN) at 919-684-8111.

In the hyperbaric chamber, the patient is placed in an atmosphere of raised pressure. The pressure then is reduced at a slow rate, with decompression pressures and schedules determined on the basis of the duration and pressure exposure of the inciting incident. Compression protocols vary by provider; the U.S. Navy treatment schedules are commonly followed in the United States. Breathing 100% oxygen by mask, alternating with breathing normal, air should shorten the period of decompression. Some centers use oxygen-helium mixtures as an alternative to protocols requiring 100% oxygen in an effort to speed decompression without causing oxygen toxicity.

Corticosteroids, diuretics, or both can be used for cerebral or spinal edema. Volume depletion should be corrected with oral or parenteral fluids (normal saline or lactated Ringer's solution). In severe cases, anticoagulation with heparin or plasma volume expansion with low-molecular-weight dextran 40 is effective. Diazepam is used for treatment of confusional states and oxygen toxicity if oxygen is administered during treatment.

In cases of type 2 sickness, decompression may take several days. Careful monitoring should be maintained

to guard against oxygen toxicity of the lungs and central nervous system.

B. TYPE 3 DECOMPRESSION SICKNESS

Osteonecrosis and sequelae that are a result of chronic decompression sickness are treated in the same manner as those conditions arising from other causes.

2. Compression Sickness

When atmospheric pressure is increased, internal gases become compressed, usually with little effect. The only common form of compression sickness is barotitis. This can occur with descent of an aircraft from a high altitude, under water during diving descent, or during hyperbaric oxygen therapy, any of which causes a relative vacuum in the middle ear space if the auditory tube is already obstructed because of allergies or upper respiratory tract infection. Symptoms may include pain or a foggy feeling in the ears, dizziness, nausea, and vertigo. In more severe cases, the tympanic membrane may appear inflamed and retracted or ruptured.

Barotitis can be prevented in people at risk by avoiding high-pressure exposures or, for short exposures, by using decongestants. Barotitis is usually self-limiting but can be treated with decongestant nose drops, a nasal vasoconstrictor inhaler, or use of a Valsalva maneuver.

REFERENCES

Divers Alert Network: www.diversalertnetwork.org.

Petri NM, Andri D: Differential diagnostic problems of decompression sickness examples from specialist physicians' practices in diving medicine. Arch Med Res 2003;34:26 [PMID: 12604371].

Strauss MB, Borer RC Jr: Diving medicine: Contemporary topics and their controversies. Am J Emerg Med 2001;19:23 [PMID: 11326354].

DISORDERS CAUSED BY VIBRATION

Vibration occurs when mechanical energy from an oscillating source is transmitted to another structure. Every structure has its own natural vibration level, including the human body as a whole and each of its parts. When vibration of the same frequency is applied, resonance (amplification) of that vibration occurs, often with adverse effects. For example, at a frequency of 5 Hz, whole-body resonance occurs, and the body acts in concert with externally generated vibration and amplifies that effect.

1. Effects of Whole-Body Vibration

Truck and bus drivers, heavy-equipment operators, miners, and others exposed to long-term whole-body vibration have been reported to have a higher incidence of musculoskeletal, neurologic, circulatory, and digestive system disorders than does the general population. Low-back pain, intervertebral disk damage, and spinal degeneration are found frequently. European studies have found associated bony abnormalities (intervertebral osteochondrosis and calcification of intervertebral disks) and adverse reproductive effects (spontaneous abortion, congenital malformations, and menstrual changes). "Vibration sickness," characterized by gastrointestinal problems, decreased visual acuity, labyrinthine disorders, and intense musculoskeletal pain, also has been reported in these workers. Despite these reports, a relationship between exposure intensity or quantity and the disorders found in occupationally exposed groups has not been clearly defined. Although many questions remain unanswered regarding the effects of long-term whole-body vibration exposure, neurologic and spinal effects appear likely.

Although almost all clinical and experimental effects of whole-body vibration have occurred at frequencies less than 20 Hz, they also have been reported to occur at frequencies as high as 100 Hz, depending on other factors such as the amplitude, acceleration, duration, and direction (vertical or lateral) of the vibrating force. The International Standards Organization (ISO) has established guidelines for whole-body vertical vibration exposure times to various frequencies and accelerations, as shown in Figure 12–12 and discussed in Chapter 12. Not all investigators agree with existing exposure standards because of the many inconsistencies in the literature; however, prudence suggests that employers should try to minimize whole-body vibration exposures of their employees whenever possible by limiting the duration of exposure and choosing well-designed equipment that insulates workers from vibration.

2. Vibration-Induced White-Finger Disease (Hand-Arm Vibration Syndrome)

Vibration-induced white-finger disease [hand-arm vibration syndrome (HAVS)] is the most common example of an occupational injury caused by segmental vibration of the hands. In the United States, more than 1 million workers are estimated to have significant exposure to vibration from hand tools such as power saws, grinders, sanders, pneumatic drills, jackhammers, and other equipment used in construction, foundry work, machining, and mining. Although segmental vibration injury can occur with frequencies ranging from 5–1500 Hz, it usually occurs with frequencies of 125–300 Hz. Other factors affecting risk include the amplitude and acceleration of the equipment used and the duration of use. Cumulative trauma occurs most often with a work history of at least 2000 hours of exposure and usually over 8000 hours.

HAVS is characterized by spasms of the digital arteries (Raynaud phenomenon) caused by vibration-induced damage of the peripheral nerve and vascular tissue, subcutaneous tissue, bones, and joints of the hands and fingers. The pathologic process also may involve arterial muscle wall hypertrophy; demyelinating peripheral neuropathy; excess connective-tissue deposition in perivascular, perineural, and subcutaneous tissues; and microvascular occlusion. Attacks of vasospasm can last for minutes to hours and are more likely to occur with exposure to the cold and with strenuous physical exertion. The worker often is standing erect, with the hand held lower than the heart and maintained in a contracted position.

Clinical Findings

Attacks in severe cases can last from 15 minutes to 2 hours. They are usually easily reversible if the individual is removed from vibration exposure. Early symptoms consist of tingling followed by numbness of the fingers. The fingers later begin to turn white in a cold environment or when cold objects are touched. Intermittent blanching often starts with the tip of one finger but extends progressively to other fingertips and eventually to the tips and bases of all fingers on the exposed hands. With increasing severity of disease, blanching or cyanosis of the fingers may extend into the summer season. Return of blood circulation (reactive hyperemia, or "red flush") following each episode is accompanied by redness and swelling, acute pain, throbbing, and paresthesias.

In more advanced cases, there may be degeneration of bone and cartilage, with resulting joint stiffness, restriction of motion, and arthralgia. Manual dexterity may decrease and clumsiness increase. With greater intensities of vibration, the period between exposure to vibration and the appearance of "white finger" is shorter.

Diagnosis is based on exposure history and response to cold. Specific diagnostic tests can include finger systolic pressure response to cold stress, finger temperature response to cold, vibrotactile sensitivity and perception threshold measurements, ultrasonic measurements of blood flow, plethysmography, thermography, and other tests of localized vascular and neurologic function. Diagnostic staging is based on the Stockholm Workshop Scales, which consider both vascular and neurologic effects.

Differential Diagnosis

The diagnosis of HAVS is based on the occupational history of vibration exposures, the association of these exposures with episodes of Raynaud phenomenon (digital vasospasms), and exclusion of idiopathic Raynaud disease and other causes of Raynaud phenomenon, including trauma of the fingers and hands, frostbite, occlusive vascular disease, connective-tissue disorders, neurogenic disorders, drug intoxication, and exposure to vinyl chloride monomer.

Prevention

Segmental vibration can be prevented by using well-designed tools (see Chapter 12), wearing gloves to minimize vibration and keep the hands warm, and following a work-rest schedule that prevents long periods of exposure to vibration. Workers should be instructed about the early symptoms and signs of HAVS and advised of factors that may place them at higher risk, such as the use of vasoactive drugs and cigarette smoking. Exposure limits developed by the ACGIH rely on measurements of acceleration (of the tool) in each of three directional axes.

Treatment

In most cases, symptoms and signs disappear when the worker is removed from exposure to vibration. In other cases, attacks can be reduced in severity or stopped by massaging, shaking, or swinging the hands or by placing them in warm water or warm air.

For more intractable episodes, nifedipine, 30–40 mg/d, is effective; thymoxamine is an alternative. For more severe cases, stanozolol or prostaglandin E may be useful. Biofeedback training also has been suggested. Surgical sympathectomy may be considered for irreversible cases. For medical or surgical therapy, the patient should be referred to the appropriate vascular specialist or hand surgeon.

REFERENCES

Bovenzi M: Health effects of mechanical vibration. G Ital Med Lav Ergon 2005;27:58 [PMID:15915675]

Hagberg ML: Clinical assessment, prognosis and return to work with reference to work related neck and upper limb disorders. G Ital Med Lav Ergon 2005;27:51 [PMID:15915674]

International Standards Organization: www.iso.ch/iso/en/ISOOnline.frontpage.

HIGH-PRESSURE INJECTION INJURIES

Use of pressurized tools and systems in manufacturing and service industries occasionally results in severe injection injury. Common types of materials injected include hydraulic fluid, paint and paint thinner, grease, and fuel. The nondominant hand is the most common injury location, but other sites such as the orbit have been reported.

Pathogenesis

The type and amount of material injected, the anatomic location, and the velocity of injection determine the extent of injury. As an example of the effect of material type, paint and paint thinners often incite a large inflammatory response on a chemical basis, as well as having antibacterial properties. The amount of material injected determines the amount of localized tissue distension, which, in turn, determines the extent of vascular compromise. The site and velocity of injection affect the dispersion of the material injected along tissue layers as well as tissue penetration.

Pathologic response occurs in three stages. The first stage involves acute inflammation associated with vascular compromise from tissue distension. Gangrene and/or infection often complicates the first stage. The second stage involves chemically induced inflammation and foreign-body granuloma formation. The late stage involves tissue fibrosis and breakdown of skin overlying granulomas, resulting in ulceration and subcutaneous sinus formation.

Clinical Findings

With the initial event, the patient may feel a momentary stinging sensation; numbness and swelling are the initial symptoms. In fact, the initial appearance of the injury often does not reflect the severity of the injury. Also present will be a small puncture wound, from which some of the injected material may be oozing. Pressure exerted around the puncture may increase the amount of oozing.

Within a few hours, throbbing pain and pallor or cyanosis may develop. The pain sometimes is described as a burning sensation. Patients who do not seek immediate evaluation may present hours to several days later with leukocytosis and evidence of lymphangitis. Laboratory tests include radiography for evidence of radiopaque materials such as metals and xeroradiography for grease. CT scanning has been used to demonstrate localized edema, gas pockets, and globe distortion involved in orbital injection injuries.

Treatment

The goal of treatment is preservation of neurovascular structures. Aggressive decompression, debridement, and irrigation are recommended. Incision and debridement of devitalized tissues and removal of as much of the injected material should be done as soon as possible. Open debridement of all contaminated structures including tendon sheaths is recommended. Amputation may be required and is most frequent in injections involving paint or solvents. Pulsed-lavage irrigation, drainage, and open packing techniques have been used successfully. Delayed wound closure or closure by secondary intention is recommended.

Broad-spectrum antibiotic and tetanus prophylaxis, if indicated, should be provided. Early range-of-motion and intense physical therapy should be provided; twice-daily hand soaks in povidone-iodine and daily whirlpool treatments have been used successfully.

Initially, analgesics will be required, but local digital blocks should be avoided because of the risk of further vascular compromise. The value of steroid or dextran use has not been demonstrated for injection injuries, with the possible exception of steroids for high-pressure orbital injections, for which surgical debridement is more difficult or may not be appropriate.

REFERENCES

Luber KT et al: High-pressure injection injuries of the hand. Orthopedics 2005;28:129 [PMID: 15751366].

Ergonomics & the Prevention of Occupational Injuries

12

David M. Rempel, MD, MPH, & Ira L. Janowitz, PT, CPE

Ergonomics—also called *human factors engineering*—is the study of the physical and cognitive demands of work to ensure a safe and productive workplace. The function of specialists in ergonomics is to design or improve the workplace, workstations, tools, equipment, and procedures of workers so as to limit fatigue, discomfort, and injuries while also efficiently achieving personal and organizational goals. The goal is to keep the demands of the job within the physical and cognitive capabilities of employees.

Approach to Job Design

Ergonomists, industrial engineers, occupational physicians, and other health and safety professionals can work together to improve the design of jobs and workstations that have unsafe characteristics or have caused injury. Controlling errors, wasted movements, and tool and materials damage and improving quality are also important goals. The principles of job design and improvement discussed in this chapter are relevant to office and industrial settings, and examples are drawn from several areas. This chapter presents ergonomics approaches that can be applied in the workplace to prevent musculoskeletal disorders. These methods also play an important role in the management of musculoskeletal disorders (i.e., secondary prevention).

Approach to Prevention of Occupational Injuries

Health professionals should seek frequent opportunities to tour work areas and evaluate job procedures, equipment, and working conditions. The concepts presented here should be kept in mind during these tours, and problem areas and activities should be noted for later study and possible job redesign. Such tours should focus on work areas and tasks with high injury prevalence, high turnover, excessive absenteeism, high error rate, or other signs of a mismatch between workers and their jobs.

One way to redesign unsafe and unhealthy jobs is to restructure a job at a new skill level or new level of mechanization. This may involve job simplification (reduction of complexity of the job) or job enlargement (broader use of skills or a greater variety of tasks), and the aid of an ergonomist or an industrial engineer often will be necessary. These professionals should be concerned with employee health and safety as well as productivity because the two are often closely interrelated.

Structure of an Ergonomics Program

Most ergonomics programs contain the elements, in one form or another, set out in Figure 12–1. Health surveillance, the review of existing health data [e.g., workers' compensation data, Occupational Safety and Health Administration (OSHA) logs, and clinic or nursing station logs] or walkthroughs to identify jobs with excessive risk factors are used to identify and prioritize jobs or tasks associated with the highest risk of injury. Problem jobs also can be identified by discussing job tasks that are demanding with employees or by using risk-factor checklists. The next step is to perform a more detailed analysis of the high-risk job or task to identify and prioritize the risk factors. Then specific engineering or administrative strategies to reduce the most important risk factors are identified, discussed with the involved parties (workers, supervisors, engineering, facilities and maintenance, and management), and implemented on a pilot basis. The pilot intervention, which should last for 2 weeks to 2 months, is intended to ensure that the intervention is effective and does not cause unforeseen health problems or interfere with quality or productivity. Often a mock-up or prototype of the proposed workstation layout can be instrumental in uncovering potential problems as tasks are simulated.

In addition to the components in Figure 12–1, training in the components of an effective program and basic ergonomic methodologies should be provided to involved employees, supervisors, engineers, and health and safety staff. The training should include case studies based on current or recent tasks of concern. Training that simply presents abstract principles of good ergonomics is less effective than job-specific discussions.

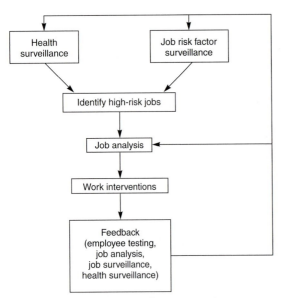

Figure 12–1. Components of an ergonomics program.

The health professional also should work with a committee within the organization to plan health and safety reviews and follow-up activities and to act as a resource for management. These committees should include ergonomists, industrial or process engineers, health and safety personnel, maintenance and facilities personnel, the affected employees, supervisors, and risk management personnel. Management support and appropriate assignment of responsibilities and follow-up are critical for success.

Various state and national governmental and non-governmental organizations have drafted ergonomics standards and guidelines for employers; Table 12–1 lists them. Many other countries and regions (e.g., Japan, Australia, and Canada) also have developed standards and guidelines related to ergonomics.

Cost-Effectiveness of Preventive Activities

Indirect costs of musculoskeletal disorders, such as replacement-employee wages, training costs for replacement workers, productivity reduction, and quality reduction typically add up to three to four times as much as the direct costs of medical, disability, and rehabilitation expenses. Improvements in workstation design and procedures often have a payback period of less than 1 year when the costs of the intervention are compared with the total costs of musculoskeletal disorders. Although job redesign usually focuses on reducing risk factors for common musculoskeletal disorders (e.g., wrist tendinitis or low-back pain), secondary benefits may include a reduction in acute injuries (e.g., fractures, lacerations, bruises, and strains). For example, an analysis of injuries in a petrochemical plant revealed that many of the contusions, burns, and strains/sprains occurred while operating valves that were in close proximity to structural steel and steam

Table 12–1. State and national ergonomics guidelines or standards.

Standard/Guideline	Organization	Issue
Hand Activity Limit ACGIH 2005	ACGIH	Upper extremity
Lifting Limit ACGIH 2005	ACGIH	Lifting
Vibration ACGIH 2005	ACGIH	Vibration
BSR/HFES 100	HFES	Computer workstations
NIOSH Lifting Equation	NIOSH	Lifting
CCR Title 8, Section 5110	California OSHA	All industry
Nursing Homes	Federal OSHA	Patient handling
Meat Packing 9400 [9241]	Federal OSHA	Meat packing
B11	ANSI	Design of machine tools
MIL-STD-1472F	US Department of Defense	Human engineering design criteria
ISO 9241, 9355, 14738	ISO	VDT, machine design
ISO 11228	ISO	Manual handling
EN 547, 614, 894, 1005	European Community	Safety of machinery

Abbreviations: ACGIH = American Conference of Government Industrial Hygiene; ANSI = American National Standards Institute; ASC = Accredited Standards Committee; HAL = hand activity limit; HFES = Human Factors and Ergonomics Society; ISO = International Standards Organization; MIL-STD = Military Standard; NSC = National Safety Council; TLV = threshold limit value.

lines. Subsequent measurements indicated that operating these valves required awkward postures and high forces. Most of these valves exceeded generally accepted civilian and military guidelines recommending an upper limit of 50 lb of tangential force applied to the hand wheel. Injuries often occurred when a worker's hands slipped off the hand wheel or valve wrench while attempting to operate the valve and came in contact with nearby hazards.

REFERENCES

Albers J et al: Identification of ergonomics interventions used to reduce musculoskeletal loading for building installation tasks. Appl Ergon 2005;36:427 [PMID: 15892937].

Goodman G et al: Effectiveness of computer ergonomics interventions for an engineering company: A program evaluation. Work 2005;24:53 [PMID: 15706072].

Hignett S et al: Finding ergonomic solutions: Participatory approaches. Occup Med (Lond) 2005;55:200 [PMID: 15857899].

van der Molen HF et al: Implementation of participatory ergonomics intervention in construction companies. Scand J Work Environ Health 2005;31:191 [PMID: 15999571].

PHYSICAL RISK FACTORS ASSOCIATED WITH MUSCULOSKELETAL DISORDERS

The National Institute for Occupational Safety and Health (NIOSH) and the National Academy of Sciences have reviewed the physical stressors or risk factors that are associated with upper extremity and neck disorders and low-back pain. These risk factors are

- The application of sustained or high forces
- Sustained awkward postures
- Rapid, repeated motions
- Contact stress
- Vibration
- Cold environment

Quantitative dose-response information for each of these risk factors and their relationship to specific disorders is limited. However, some data exist to help identify injury thresholds. For example, lifts associated with high compression, torsion, or shear forces on the spine have a greater potential to cause low-back pain. Repeated grip forces of greater than 10 N (1 kg) are associated with a greater risk of carpal tunnel syndrome. Table 12–1 includes some risk-assessment models. The American Conference of Governmental Industrial Hygienists (ACGIH) hand activity limit (HAL), the NIOSH lifting equation, and others are presented in more detail below.

The Strain Index, which estimates estimate the risk of injury to the distal upper extremity (elbows, wrists, and hands), uses the risk factors of intensity of exertion, duration of exertion, efforts per minute, hand/wrist posture,

speed or work, and duration per day. In a field test at a poultry plant, the Strain Index score was found to correlate well with the mean incidence rate of disorders of the distal upper extremities. The authors recommend that a score of 7 or above should trigger further investigation and possible intervention. Risk-assessment tools (e.g., Strain Index or ACGIH HAL) can be used before and after an intervention to assess the effect of the intervention on risk.

REFERENCES

David GC: Ergonomic methods for assessing exposure to risk factors for work-related musculoskeletal disorders. Occup Med (Lond) 2005;55:190 [PMID: 15857898].

Gell N et al: A longitudinal study of industrial and clerical workers: Incidence of carpal tunnel syndrome and assessment of risk factors. J Occup Rehabil 2005;15:47 [PMID: 15794496].

Violante FS et al: Relations between occupational, psychosocial and individual factors and three different categories of back disorder among supermarket workers. Int Arch Occup Environ Health 2005;78:613 [PMID: 16001210].

Werner RA et al: Risk factors for visiting a medical department because of upper extremity musculoskeletal disorders. Scand J Work Environ Health 2005;31:132 [PMID: 15864907].

WORKSTATION DESIGN PRINCIPLES

Reduce Sustained Awkward Postures

Tasks, tools, and workstations should be designed to prevent sustained awkward postures. There is nothing wrong with occasionally moving joints through their full range of motion at work. However, awkward postures that are sustained over several hours or repeated throughout the workday can pose a problem. Working with the hands above shoulder height for long periods can lead to shoulder, upper back, and neck disorders. Such sustained awkward shoulder postures may occur during construction work, automobile assembly and repair, and mail sorting. Sustained trunk flexion is seen often in agricultural or construction work. Work should be designed to prevent sustained

- Neck or trunk flexion, extension, or rotation
- Squatting
- Shoulder elevation, abduction, or flexion
- Elbow flexion
- Wrist extension or flexion
- Wrist ulnar or radial deviation
- Finger extension or wide finger spread

Awkward postures occur as a result of the interaction between the worker's anthropometry and the hand locations of the task or the visual target. Nearby machinery or material may get in the way of legs or arms, increasing reach distances. In general, the point of operation (the primary hand location for work) should be between waist and shoulder height and laterally between the shoulders. The point of operation should be in the lower area of this envelope if the materials or tools handled are heavy or if the hands have to be held in one area for a long period.

Reduce Contact Stress

Hard surfaces and edges may make convenient sites to rest the arm, but they can put pressure on tendons, nerves, bones, or bursa and lead to sore spots or soft-tissue disorders. If support surfaces are necessary (e.g., supporting arms during prolonged microscope use), the support should be rounded and padded to minimize the risk of contact stress and located so that it does not apply pressure on sensitive body regions (e.g., wrist or elbow).

Design Work Based on Anthropometric Data

One reason for physical stress on the job is the mismatch in size between the worker and the workplace, equipment, or tools. This mismatch may result in excessive forward bending and reaching for tools or materials, having to work bent over, having to work with one or both arms and shoulders held high for long periods, having to hold a heavy tool at some distance from the body for long periods, or having to sit in a position that is too low or too high.

Figures 12–2 and 12–3 show the critical body dimensions of adult men and women in the United States. Workplaces and machines should be designed so that larger workers (up to the 95th percentile) and smaller workers (down to the 5th percentile) can easily complete their tasks. That is, a well-designed work space accommodates the larger worker's body size, keeps supplies and control levers within comfortable reach and activation of the smaller worker, and accommodates the line of sight and hand and foot locations of a wide variety of employees.

The most important physical design rule for a sedentary job is that the operator be able to reach all frequently used items (e.g., parts, supplies, keyboards, tools, and controls) without leaning, bending, or twisting at the waist. Frequent reaching should be restricted to moderate movements of the arm, if possible. Figure 12–4 illustrates the forearm-only (preferable) and full-arm (satisfactory) reach limits for a North American population of men and women. Task designs that require movements outside the full-arm reach limits tend to increase the risks of shoulder, neck, and low-back problems.

A. Example

Women of average dimensions (50th percentile) can reach horizontally only about 74 cm (29 in), and short women (5th percentile) can reach horizontally only about 68 cm (27 in), as measured from the backrest of the chair when they are seated in an upright position. If a shelf of supplies or a panel of controls is 91 cm (36 in) in front of them (also measured from the backrest of the chair), they will have difficulty obtaining supplies or manipulating controls even when bending and twisting at the waist. Productivity will be reduced. The work area should be redesigned to reduce the reach distances to frequently used items or controls to within comfortable ranges.

The reach-envelope rules are particularly important if significant forces or weights are involved. The heavier the tool or work piece, the closer it should be to elbow height, unless the work piece or tool is otherwise supported. Continuously used tools, work pieces, or controls should be near elbow height and require little reach, within a "near reach zone" of 38 cm (15 in) from the shoulder.

Anthropometric data are used to place visual targets (e.g., computer screen, hard copy, or work piece), and the targets should be prioritized and located based on frequency of viewing. Frequently viewed targets should be directly in front of the operator and between eye level and 45 degrees below eye level.

Logically Locate Controls and Displays

Machine operation is most productive and least stressful when the machine does the work and the operator does the thinking. Controls (e.g., levers, switches, joysticks, and pedals) enable the operator to give a machine "orders" or feed it information. They also can provide feedback to the operator. Primary controls—those of greatest importance or used most often—should be located within the forearm-only reach limits (e.g., near reach zone), and other controls should be located within the full-arm (satisfactory) reach limits of the workstation, as shown in Figure 12–4.

The location of controls, displays, and other visual targets should be integrated with each other on a logical basis. Logical linkages suggest intuitive responses to the information displayed to the operator. In this manner, the control-display relationships can reduce the information-processing load on the operator and thus reduce stress and the rate of errors.

A. Example

If a steam turbine is to be monitored and operated, the primary displays should be in front of and below the eye level of the operator, and the turbine controls generally will be in front of and near the operator's hands. However, the control for rotational speed should be in proximity to and linked logically with its speed indicator display (e.g., the control and display should both be contained in a common area on the panel or linked by means of a color-coded line). Movement of the speed control upward or to the right also should move the speed indicator display upward or to the right. This will increase the stimu-

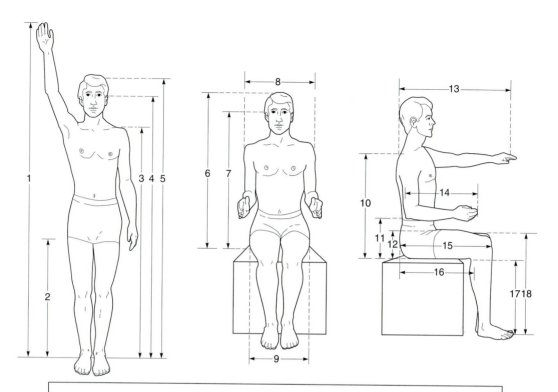

Male Body Dimensions (cm)

Dimension Number	Dimension Name	5th Percentile	50th Percentile	95th Percentile	Standard Deviation
1	Vertical reach	195.6	209.6	223.5	8.46
2	Crotch height	75.4	83.1	90.7	4.67
3	Shoulder height	133.6	143.6	154.1	6.22
4	Eye height	152.4	163.3	175.0	15.29
5	Stature	163.8	174.4	185.6	6.61
6	Height, sitting	84.5	90.8	96.7	3.66
7	Eye height, sitting	72.8	78.8	84.6	3.57
8	Shoulder breadth	41.5	45.2	49.8	2.54
9	Hip breadth, sitting	30.7	33.9	38.4	2.38
10	Shoulder height, sitting	57.1	62.4	67.6	3.18
11	Elbow height, sitting	18.8	23.7	28.0	2.78
12	Thigh clearance	13.0	14.9	17.5	1.36
13	Thumb tip reach	74.9	82.4	90.9	4.85
14	Elbow-fingertip length	44.3	47.9	51.9	2.31
15	Buttock-knee length	54.9	59.4	64.3	2.85
16	Buttock-popliteal length	45.8	49.8	54.0	2.50
17	Popliteal height	40.6	44.5	48.8	2.50
18	Knee height, sitting	49.7	54.0	58.7	2.73

Figure 12–2. Body dimensions for men. Corresponding weights are as follows: 5th percentile, 57.4 kg (126.3 lb); 50th percentile, 71 kg (156.2 lb); and 95th percentile, 91.6 kg (201.5 lb). Appropriate dimensions must be added for clothing and shoes.

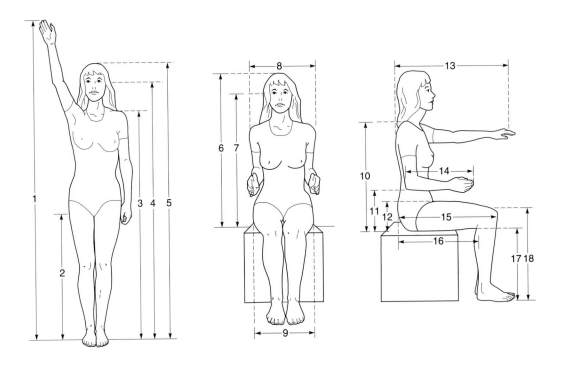

Female Body Dimensions (cm)

Dimension Number	Dimension Name	5th Percentile	50th Percentile	95th Percentile	Standard Deviation
1	Vertical reach	185.2	199.1	213.4	8.64
2	Crotch height	68.1	74.4	81.3	4.06
3	Shoulder height	123.9	133.3	143.7	6.00
4	Eye height	142.2	149.9	158.8	6.35
5	Stature	152.6	162.8	174.1	6.52
6	Height, sitting	79.0	85.2	90.8	3.59
7	Eye height, sitting	67.7	73.8	79.1	3.46
8	Shoulder breadth	38.4	42.0	45.7	2.24
9	Hip breadth, sitting	33.0	38.2	43.9	3.27
10	Shoulder height, sitting	53.7	57.9	62.5	2.66
11	Elbow height, sitting	16.1	20.8	25.0	2.74
12	Thigh clearance	13.2	15.4	17.5	1.31
13	Thumb tip reach	67.7	74.2	80.5	3.88
14	Elbow-fingertip length	40.0	43.4	47.5	2.28
15	Buttock-knee length	53.1	57.7	63.2	3.06
16	Buttock-popliteal length	43.5	47.5	52.6	2.76
17	Popliteal height	38.0	41.6	45.7	2.35
18	Knee height, sitting	46.9	50.9	55.5	2.60

Figure 12–3. Body dimensions for women. Corresponding weights are as follows: 5th percentile, 46.6 kg (103.5 lb); 50th percentile, 59.6 kg (131.1 lb); and 95th percentile, 74.5 kg (163.9 lb). Appropriate dimensions must be added for clothing and shoes.

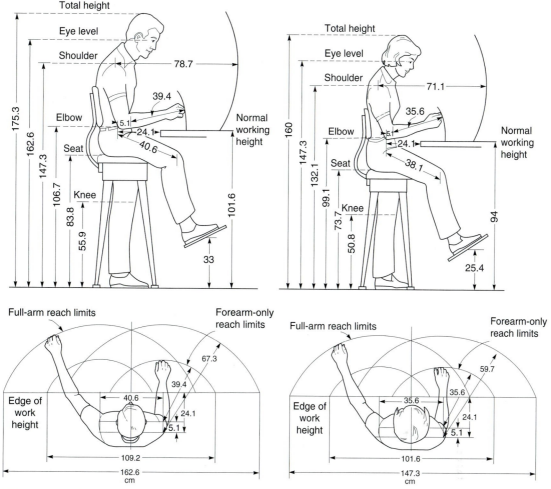

Figure 12–4. Forearm-only (preferable) and full-arm (satisfactory) reach limits for men and women in working areas shown in the horizontal and vertical planes. All dimensions are in centimeters.

lus-response compatibility of the two devices and improve the control capability of the operator.

Proper Design of Chairs

Common complaints that stem from improper seating include fatigue or ache in the back or lower parts of the body. The primary purpose of a chair is to provide comfortable but stable support for the weight of the body without localized pressure points. The chair must support the employee in the posture best suited for the task (e.g., slightly reclined for computer work or slightly forward-leaning for writing). Shifting body position over the course of the day is a natural way to distribute loads on the spine and maintain circulation in the buttocks and thighs; chair design should accommodate these postural variations.

If the seat pan is too deep [>41 cm (16 in)], the front edge can press against the back of the knees, particularly in short women. A shallow seat or a smoothly curved "waterfall design" front edge can eliminate this contact stress for shorter people. The seat pan should not be so concave that it restricts occasional changes of position. Many current chair designs have size adjustment features (e.g., sliding seat pans offering a range of depths or a choice of different size seat pans) for better fit. The seat should be soft enough to be comfortable but not so soft that changing posture or standing up is difficult.

Chair design also should provide sufficient lumbar support to maintain a comfortable degree of lumbar lordosis and assist in supporting the weight of the trunk. A chair should be easily adjustable while the operator is seated to offer a full range of seat heights, lumbar support height, and backrest slope. Without good support, general fatigue is more likely, and back pain may result.

The base of chairs should have five legs to reduce the likelihood of tipping over if the occupant leans backward. If the environment allows, the texture of material on the back and seat should be porous and slightly rough or nubby to allow some air circulation between the material and the body. If the chair has armrests, they should fit the employee or be adjustable in height and distance apart to provide good arm support while the occupant performs work tasks. Care should be taken in selecting furniture so that armrests do not strike parts of the work surface during normal chair movements, resulting in increased reach distances.

If it is necessary to adjust the chair seat height so that some employees' feet do not touch the ground, then a large, sturdy footrest must be provided to prevent the legs from dangling. Without stable foot support, a chair seat that is too high restricts circulation in the lower legs and makes it difficult to lean forward.

Types of Chairs

A. CHAIRS VERSUS STOOLS

A large proportion of the adult workforce can be accommodated by a chair that is adjustable from a seat height of 38–48.3 cm (15–19 in). Brief periods of sitting, for a highly mobile worker (e.g., laboratory or reception work), are best done on a tall stool with a seat height range of 53–72 cm (22–30 in). For people who move about frequently, it reduces leg and back fatigue to perch on a stool or padded "rest bar" whose height is nearly the length of the legs so that the upper body is not repeatedly raised and lowered whenever they sit and stand. Studies of office workers demonstrate reductions in lower extremity swelling and in cumulative load on the spine when employees alternate between sitting and standing for at least 2 hours during the workday.

B. CHAIRS WITH FORWARD-SLOPING SEATS

Chairs or stools with forward-sloping seats that do not use knee rests to support the legs hold promise for various classes of jobs and preferences of users. Forward-sloping seats are especially advantageous for users who must be extremely close to or leaning over their work, as is the case with some workers performing highly detailed office or repair work, dentists, surgeons, and the like. In addition to having adjustable heights and back support, these chairs should have an easily adjustable degree of slope and should provide for additional methods to prevent slipping out of the chair (e.g., high-

friction seat material and seat-pan contouring or "saddle" shaping). Such chairs are particularly appropriate for higher work surfaces, such as laboratory benches and reception counters [typically close to 100 cm (36–39 in) high], and seat height for forward-sloping and saddle chairs in these settings tends to be 57–76 cm (22.5–30 in).

C. CHAIRS THAT RECLINE

Chairs with a back support that reclines can transfer part of the upper body weight from the spine onto the backrest and can help to preserve lumbar lordosis. Reclining backward more than 20 degrees from vertical can lead to increased neck loading unless the visual target and controls of input devices are well positioned and a headrest is provided.

Proper Selection of Chairs

There are many well-designed chairs. The employer or ergonomics committee should obtain samples of two or three chairs appropriate for the task (with appropriate seat, backrest, and armrest adjustments and forearm support if needed) and meet the requirements of the workers (appropriate seat pan depth, backrest shape, casters versus glides, etc.) and ask the workers to try them out for at least a week. A briefer period for chair testing usually is insufficient because initial impressions often differ from long-term satisfaction. The opinion of the workers should be considered when a supply of new chairs is ordered.

Avoid Static Body Positions: Task Variation and Exercises

Workers who operate computers, control panels, and the like tend to hold their bodies in a fixed position for protracted periods in order to maintain a consistent physical relationship with the equipment. For example, data entry requires the maintenance of a fixed spatial relationship between the shoulders, hands, and the keyboard in order to strike the proper key each time without looking. In addition, computer users often maintain a rigid neck position for long periods looking at the copyholder or the computer monitor. Laboratory technicians and scientists working in biosafety cabinets are often in static postures for hours, performing highly precise tasks.

In jobs of this sort, measures should be taken to prevent pain and fatigue in the shoulders, neck, and back. Designing alternative tasks that can be performed after every 20–60 minutes of computer use can help to break up static postures. These can be short tasks (e.g., retrieving printouts or supplies, obtaining new hard copy or samples, or filing) that involve a few minutes of walking or standing. It may be necessary to use a timer or reminder software to remind the operator to get up out of the chair for a few minutes every 20–60 minutes.

A. EXAMPLE

The usual break schedule of data-entry operators in a government office (two 15-minute breaks plus lunch) was modified to add four additional 5-minute breaks during those hours that did not otherwise have a break. The employees were encouraged to use their break time to take a short walk or stretch. With more frequent breaks, employees reported less discomfort in the shoulders, upper arm, neck, and back. Even though 20 fewer minutes were worked per day, the productivity over an 8-hour shift remained the same.

Although there is no empirical evidence that exercises reduce the risk of musculoskeletal disorders, if specific exercises are recommended, they should be selected based on the following general guidelines:

1. Exercises should be designed to relieve static load of muscles following sustained awkward postures, highly repetitive tasks, or sustained fixed postures.
2. Exercises should target muscles in the upper and lower extremities, the shoulder girdle, the neck, and the lumbar and thoracic regions of the back.
3. Exercises should be designed to be performed at or near the workstation. They should not be so conspicuous that they call attention to the worker or cause embarrassment, nor should they significantly disrupt task performance.
4. Exercises should be performed throughout the day as the musculoskeletal fatigue builds up so that stress relief is timely and continuing.
5. Exercises should not present any obvious biomechanical or safety hazards. In employees with musculoskeletal disorders, there should be no contraindicated movements or positions involved.

COMPUTER WORKSTATIONS

Computer operators often complain of fatigue in the neck, upper back, shoulders, forearms, or wrists, especially when they use the computer for more than 4 hours per day. They also can experience visual fatigue or eyestrain from long-term viewing of the computer monitor. Appropriate setup and use of the computer workstation can help to reduce these aches and pains.

Adjust Chair First

The first step in adjusting a computer workstation is to adjust the seating. The seat height should be adjusted low enough that the operator's feet are firmly supported on the floor but not so low that the operator's weight is not evenly distributed over the seat pan. A large and stable footrest could be used, but only

when attempts to adjust the chair and workstation to a low enough height fail. Arm supports, which may be on the chair or the work surface, should comfortably support the forearms and remove loading from the wrist, elbows, and shoulders. Some computer users prefer to switch from sitting to standing during the day to promote posture changes; this requires workstations that adjust easily to a wide range of heights (Figure 12–5). Employees with neck, shoulder, or back problems may benefit from the ability to alternate between sitting and standing.

Proper Placement of Monitor & Documents

Primary visual targets (screens and/or hard copy) should be located in front of the operator, slightly (not more than 30 degrees) below eye level, and approximately 48–72 cm (20–30 in) away. If hard copy is used, a document holder should be placed either to one side of the screen or between the monitor and the keyboard. This will allow the operator to view the monitor with a minimum of neck flexion, extension, or rotation. Bifocal lens users are an exception to this recommendation; they usually need the primary display lower. Bifocal lens users may benefit from prescription monofocal lenses for computer use; these lenses permit a greater range of head postures. Eye care professionals should be informed of the type of work performed and the distance and location of the visual targets for consideration in their lens prescription.

Data-entry clerks look almost exclusively at the original data records (invoices, checks, etc.) they are recording. In this situation, it is the hard copy (preferably on a document holder) or an image of the hard copy that should be in front of the operator, and the monitor then should be positioned to one side or the other. If manual handling is required to turn pages, set aside checks or invoices, and the like, it may be necessary to compromise between optimal handling location and optimal viewing area.

A. EXAMPLE

In a data-processing office, checks were turned over one by one with the left hand while their amounts were entered on a computer keyboard with the right hand. The pile of checks was placed in front of the operator and near the screen. However, to turn the checks, the operators had to reach over the keyboard with their arm suspended, which caused shoulder pain. Moving the checks closer to the operator and to the left of the keyboard would have meant more twisting to the left. The checks were left in the same position, and padded armrests were provided to support the left forearm and take the load off the shoulder. The use of a numeric-only (smaller) keypad would allow for still better placement of the checks.

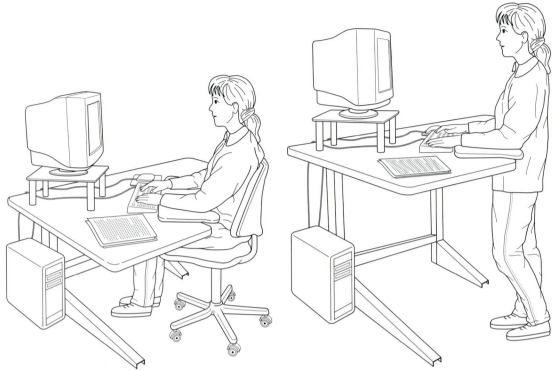

Figure 12–5. Computer-intensive work frequently involves the risk factor of static posture. To some extent, this can be mitigated with a rapidly adjustable sit-stand workstation. This workstation also can easily accommodate employees of different heights.

Eliminate Glare

The monitor should be positioned so that glare is minimized. There are several ways to reduce the glare:

1. Change the location of the monitor so that the light source is to the side of or above the computer user, not directly behind or in front. Move the monitor so that it is more than 2 m from a window.

2. Reduce the general illumination in the room to about 500 lux. This can be achieved by reducing the amount of overhead lighting (e.g., removing every other bulb or fluorescent tube), installing indirect lighting to direct light upward toward the ceiling, installing parabolic louvers for the fluorescent lights to direct the illumination straight downward, or controlling window illumination with shades, louvered blinds, and/or tinted window film.

3. Provide more illumination where needed with desk lamps ("task lighting") directed at the appropriate visual target. The goal is to have lighting as uniform as possible with a maximum ratio of 1:3 between the brightness of the computer screen and its immediate surroundings.

4. If steps 1 through 3 fail, use glare-reducing filters on computer screens. These filters are available in several designs, although the most effective are coated filters (e.g., polarized filters).

Another source of visual irritation is bright lights or unshaded windows. These can be partially or completely blocked.

In addition to taking measures to reduce glare, employers should encourage computer operators to look away from the screen from time to time (e.g., for 20 seconds every 20 minutes) to allow the eye muscles to relax and thus prevent visual fatigue and pain. Computer users who lean forward to see the screen may need their vision checked or the monitor moved closer.

Position of Input Devices

The keyboard and pointing device (e.g., mouse or trackball) should be positioned directly in front of and close to the computer user's shoulder to prevent sustained unsupported reach; however, it is also important to prevent sustained elbow flexion. The height of input devices should be adjusted so that the shoulders are not elevated and the wrists are relatively straight during use. The slope of the keyboard can be adjusted so that the wrists are not held in extension during keying. A thin keyboard will reduce wrist extension.

The use of a wrist rest has been associated with increased hand pain. If a wrist rest is used, it should be used during pauses in typing, not during keyboard use. It may be more appropriate to provide support to the forearms with the chair armrests, the desk surface, or forearm support boards.

People who use the computer for long hours and do not know how to touch type should take typing lessons. This will reduce the neck flexion associated with looking at the keyboard during typing. To reduce hand motions and mouse use, keystroke shortcuts can be used for frequently used commands (e.g., copy and paste) and repeated character sequences.

Alternative Keyboards & Pointing Devices

Alternative keyboards or pointing devices can reduce awkward wrist and forearm postures; however, there are limited empirical data to guide recommendations. Keyboard designs that split the keyboard in half, with some separation and tilt between the two halves, can reduce wrist ulnar deviation and forearm pronation. There is some evidence that a fixed-split keyboard can reduce hand pain and disorders among computer users in comparison with a conventional keyboard, but the beneficial effect may take weeks to be noticed. As with chairs, it is suggested that employees evaluate a different keyboard or mouse for at least a week while performing their usual tasks before making a decision about whether or not to use the device. A systematic evaluation by an ergonomics committee can be used to identify an appropriate set of input devices for use at the company.

For most computer work, pointing devices are now used more often than the keyboard. There are a number of different types and styles of pointing devices, including mice, trackballs, touch pads, pen/tablets, short sticks, and joysticks. For patients with right-hand pain, a switch to using the mouse with the left hand can be recommended; however, pain may develop in the left hand. A better solution is to provide several very different pointing devices and have the employee alternate between pointing devices on a daily or weekly basis.

HAND TOOL DESIGN AND SELECTION

Reduce Hand Force

The repeated application of high grip force to hold parts or to grip power tools is associated with tendon disorders of the forearm, muscle fatigue, and carpal tunnel syndrome. A classic example of a high-risk task is the sustained grip maintained by meat packers on a wet and slippery knife. Sustained or repeated pinch grip puts tendons at even greater risk than a power grip. Tasks and tools can be redesigned to reduce the force required to perform the tasks and to reduce the duration that force is applied during the task cycle.

Assembling parts with screws is usually performed with inline drivers. The high force required to hold and stabilize a powered driver when the screw tightens can be reduced by using a driver adjusted to the proper torque, antitorque clutches or bars, and screws appropriate for the task.

A. AVOID STATIC HOLDING POSITIONS

A production task might involve holding a work piece or tool continuously in one hand and working on it with the other. Reduction of fatigue may be accomplished by using a holding clamp or bench vise or, in the case of hand or power tools, by alternating hands or using self-locking tools. When sustained holding is still necessary, redesigning the tools or tool handles to achieve maximum comfort is helpful. For example, power tools can be suspended from cables or articulated with antitorque bars to decrease grip force and reduce the hand vibration. Heavy parts can be held with a jig or clamp so that the nondominant hand is not applying a constant grip force.

B. EXAMPLE

In a quality-control task, each part being checked was picked up and supported by the worker's left hand and forearm while testing clamps were attached and adjustments made. The job was redesigned so that each part was placed on a small, waist-high rolling rack that was pulled along by the worker, who then made attachments and adjustments with both hands.

Reduce Rapid, Repeated Motions

Tasks that require rapid hand and shoulder movements or movements that are repeated every few seconds throughout the day have been associated with tendon disorders. Exposures to these tasks can be controlled by limiting the number of hours per day that an employee performs these movements or by rotating employees between different tasks so that the same muscle-tendon-bone unit is not loaded all day.

Consideration also should be given to redesigning the task so that the distance moved is minimized, thereby reducing the speed necessary to complete the task. Experienced workers often know how to perform these tasks with smooth motions that reduce wasted energy and sudden impacts. Therefore, the experienced workers should be involved in teaching new hires the best work techniques.

Avoid Use of the Hand as a Tool

The palm of the hand should not be used as a hammer. Even frequent light tapping with the heel of the hand can cause injury to the nerves or arteries in the hand (e.g., hypothenar hammer syndrome). In sheet metal work, for example, the palm of the hand may be used for forcing parts together. A rubber mallet should be used instead.

Proper Design of Tool Handles

To avoid contact stress in the hands, tool handles should be designed so that the force-bearing area is as large as practicable and there are no sharp corners or edges. This means that handles should be either round or oval. Handles should have a high coefficient of friction in order to reduce hand-gripping forces needed for tool control. Pinch points should be eliminated or guarded.

Rigid, form-fitting handles with grooves for each finger usually do not improve the grip function unless they are sized to the individual's hand. Form-fitting, scalloped handles, which are often designed for the hand of a worker in the 50th percentile, will spread the

fingers of a small (5th percentile) hand too far apart for efficient gripping and will cause uncomfortable ridges under the fingers of a large (95th percentile) hand.

Many power tools (e.g., drills, sanders, and chain saws) are operated and controlled with two hands, and there is generally a primary handle with a trigger to provide for gripping by the dominant hand. If there is a secondary, stabilizing or antitorque handle, it should be adjustable to either side of the tool to permit use by either left-handed or right-handed people and permit the user to change the trigger hand from time to time to reduce fatigue.

Excessive use of a single finger for operating triggers on hand tools causes local fatigue and may result in a stenosing tenosynovitis, or "trigger finger." Triggers can be designed to be operated by two or more fingers at once or by a switch triggered by the foot. Locking buttons also can reduce sustained loading. Exposure to tool vibration will be addressed later in this chapter.

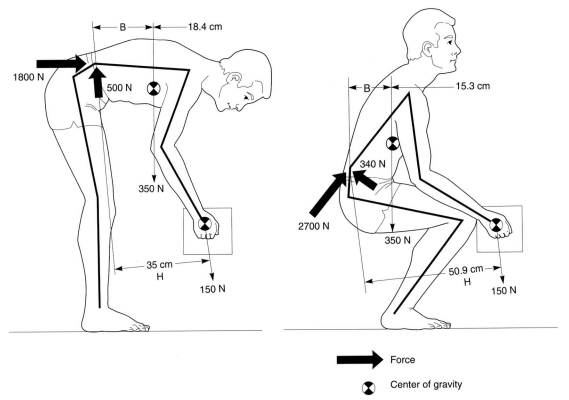

Figure 12–6. Forces on the base of the spine (L5–S1 forces) that result from two different methods of lifting a load weighing 150 N. When the lifting is done with the legs relatively straight, there is an L5–S1 shear force of 500 N and a spinal compression force of 1800 N. When the lifting is done with the knees bent, the L5–S1 shear force is only 340 N, but the spinal compression force is 2700 N. *B* = horizontal distance from the L5–S1 joint to the body's center of gravity; *H* = horizontal distance from the L5–S1 joint to the load's center of gravity.

REFERENCES

Gerr F et al: A randomized, controlled trial of postural interventions for prevention of musculoskeletal symptoms among computer users. Occup Environ Med 2005;62:478 [PMID: 15961625].

Heinrich J et al: A comparison of methods for the assessment of postural load and duration of computer use. Occup Environ Med 2004;61:1027 [PMID: 15550610].

Horgen G et al: A cross-country comparison of short- and long-term effects of an ergonomic intervention on musculoskeletal discomfort, eye strain and psychosocial stress in VDT operators. Int J Occup Saf Ergon 2005;11:77 [PMID: 15794875].

Nicholas RA et al: Workstyle and upper-extremity symptoms: A biobehavioral perspective. J Occup Environ Med 2005;47:352 [PMID: 15824626].

BIOMECHANICS OF LIFTING, PUSHING, & PULLING

Although a detailed biomechanical analysis of lifting, pushing, and pulling is beyond the scope of this chapter, some principles are included to illustrate basic mechanisms of injury and methods of injury prevention.

Principles of Lifting

Figure 12–6 illustrates the estimated forces on the base of the spine (L5–S1) that would result from two different methods of lifting a load of 150 N [approximately 15 kg (34 lb); 1 lb force = 4.44 N]. When the lifting is done with the legs relatively straight (lifting in a stooped position), there is an estimated anterior shear force at L5–S1 of approximately 500 N and a spinal compression force of 1800 N. When the lifting is done with the knees bent (lifting in a squatting position, or "lifting with the legs"), the L5–S1 shear force is only 340 N, but the spinal compression force rises to 2700 N. This assumes that the load is too bulky to fit between the knees, as is often the case in practice. A commonly repeated safety rule is to "lift with the legs" and keep the load close to the body, but a deep squat often makes it difficult, if not impossible, to do both. In the example illustrated in Figure 12–6, the horizontal

- Test the load; get help if needed.
- Plan the lift and the path you will take.
- Keep the load as close to the body as possible.
- Pivot and move your feet with a broad base of support to avoid twisting.
- Try to keep your movements smooth and coordinated.
- Keep the back in a straight line from "head to tail."

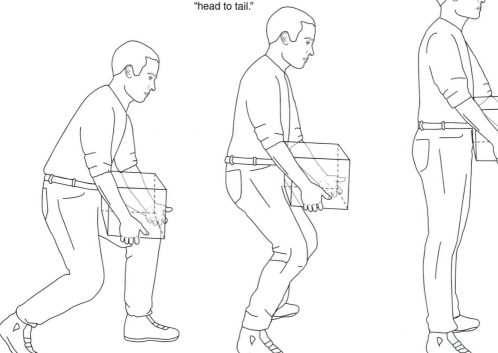

Figure 12–7. With good lifting technique, the spine is kept stable even when it must be tilted forward.

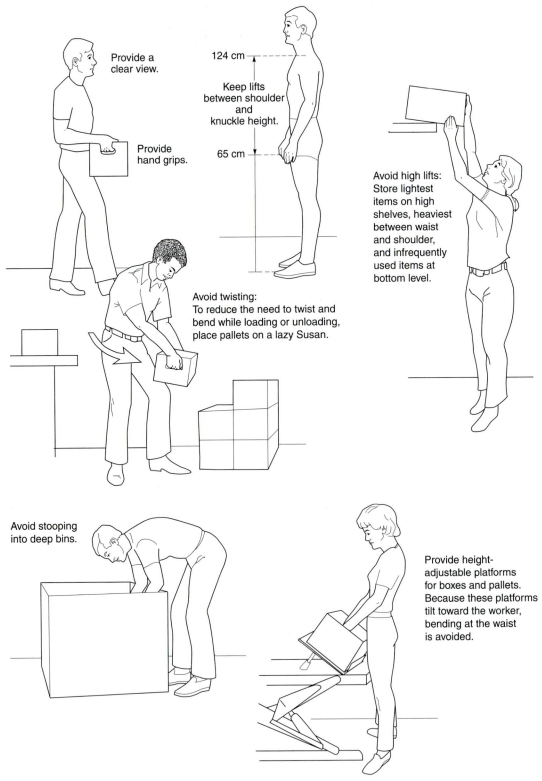

Provide a
clear view.

124 cm

Keep lifts
between shoulder
and
knuckle height.

Provide
hand grips.

65 cm

Avoid high lifts:
Store lightest
items on high
shelves, heaviest
between waist
and shoulder,
and infrequently
used items at
bottom level.

Avoid twisting:
To reduce the need to twist and
bend while loading or unloading,
place pallets on a lazy Susan.

Avoid stooping
into deep bins.

Provide height-
adjustable platforms
for boxes and pallets.
Because these platforms
tilt toward the worker,
bending at the waist
is avoided.

Figure 12–8. Suggestions for safe lifting.

distance H from the spine to the center of gravity of the load is longer in the squatting position than it is with a stooped lift. This causes the load to exert more torque on the spine, increasing the compressive force on the lower lumbar disks. Workers tend to avoid deep squats when lifting because squatting takes more time, requires more energy, is hard on the knees, and often results in poor balance. Optimal lifting styles (Figure 12–7) are those that

- Allow the load to be kept as close as possible to the spine.
- Offer a broad base of support for good balance.
- Allow the worker to see ahead and avoid obstacles.
- Allow the worker to retain a comfortable position ("neutral posture") of the spine, avoiding extremes of bending or twisting.

If possible, twisting should be avoided by turning the shoulders and hips together as a unit. Figure 12–8 offers several suggestions and guidelines for reducing the risk of injury with lifting tasks.

Principles of Pushing & Pulling

The estimated forces involved in pushing and pulling loads are illustrated in Figure 12–9. Pulling with a force of 350 N (80 lb) (the weight of the loaded cart times its coefficient of rolling friction) at a height of 66 cm (26.4 in) above the floor would result in a compressive force on the lumbar spine of about 8000 N, which is substantially above the NIOSH-recommended limit of

3400 N and even above the highest value (6400 N) that most workers can tolerate without injury.

The following are general guidelines to prevent injuries when pushing or pulling heavy loads: (1) Make certain that the area ahead of the load is level, offers adequate traction, and is clear of obstacles. If it is not level, some system of braking should be available. (2) Push the load, rather than pull it. This often will reduce spinal stress and in most cases will improve the visibility ahead. (3) Wear shoes that provide good foot traction. The coefficient of friction between the floor and the sole of the shoes should be at least 0.8 wherever heavy loads are moved. (4) When starting to push a load, brace the rear foot and shift the body weight forward. If the load does not start to move when a reasonable amount of force is applied, get help from a coworker or use a powered vehicle. (5) Pushing or pulling is easier when the handles of the loaded cart are at about hip height [81–114 cm (about 32–47 in) for a mixed-gender population] than when they are at shoulder height or above. Handles lower than the hips are awkward and difficult to use. Two vertical handles, or two sets of handles at different heights, allow workers of different stature to grasp the load at optimal points (Figure 12–10).

EVALUATING MANUAL MATERIALS HANDLING TASKS

Despite our entry into the "information age," manual materials handling is still a major cause of low-back pain and shoulder injuries. Efforts to address these with

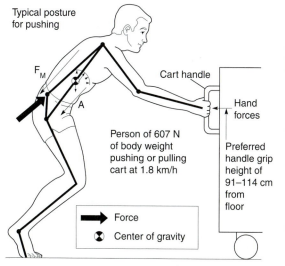

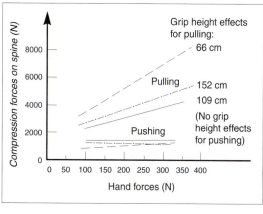

Figure 12–9. Forces involved in pushing and pulling loads. Pulling a force of 350 N (the weight of the cart times its coefficient of rolling friction) at a height of 66 cm above the floor causes a compression force on the lower spine of about 8000 N, which is substantially above the highest value (6400 N) that most workers can tolerate without injury.

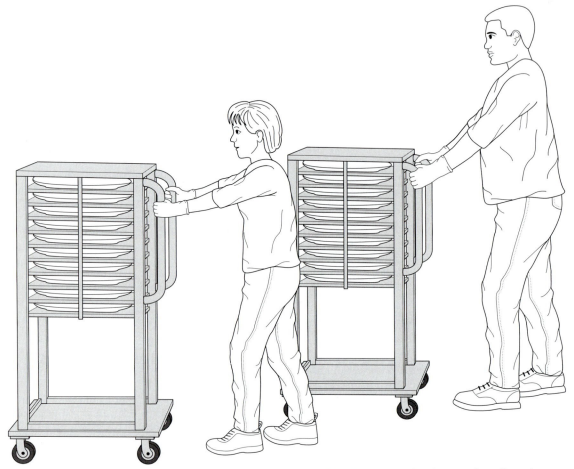

Figure 12–10. An example of a design of handles on a cart that will both accommodate large and small employees.

training programs directed at workers have largely failed. Although some of these injuries are associated with slips, trips, and falls while moving an object, most occur because the instantaneous or the cumulative load on the worker simply has exceeded his or her capabilities.

The attempt to set safe limits for manual material handling can be approached in four ways:

1. *Epidemiologic.* Identifying the risk factors by analyzing the distribution of injuries in a population.

2. *Biomechanical.* Estimating the forces applied to the body by manual materials handling tasks and comparing those with tissue tolerances derived from cadaver studies.

3. *Physiologic.* Estimating the energy requirements of manual materials handling tasks compared with the aerobic capacity of workers.

4. *Psychophysical.* Simulating a manual materials handling task in a controlled environment and recording the subjects' acceptance of fatigue or discomfort. These should be done with subjects who are representative of the population of interest in terms of age, physical condition, and gender. Maximum acceptable weights, forces, or distances for manual materials handling tasks can be estimated through this approach, although data on subsequent injuries usually are not collected because the study periods are so short (typically 1 day to 1 week).

NIOSH LIFTING EQUATION

Jobs in which lifting (as opposed to pushing, pulling, or carrying) is the predominant activity can be analyzed by using the NIOSH lifting equation (www.cdc.gov/niosh/pdfs/94-110.pdf). It considers that a person's ability to lift may be limited by either biomechanical or metabolic factors; that is, the limiting factor may be the resulting forces on the body (biomechanical) or the energy expenditure (endurance) demanded by repeated lifting. The equation attempts to synthesize the results of biomechanical, physiologic, psychophysical, and epidemiologic studies.

The NIOSH lifting equation aims to provide recommended weight limits (RWLs) that are protective of at least 75% of working women and 99% of working men. Even lifts falling within the RWL may exceed the capabilities of some workers, especially older women. The NIOSH lifting equation provides a ratio called the *lifting index,* which is calculated by dividing the actual weight lifted by the RWL. A lifting index of less than 1.0 is considered relatively safe for most workers.

The *load constant* [23 kg (51 lb)] is the highest RWL that would be possible, under ideal circumstances. The NIOSH lifting equation considers that the following factors, or "modifiers," reduce a worker's ability to lift and therefore would reduce the RWL. Each of these modifiers is a number between 0 and 1 that, when multiplied by the load constant, reduces the acceptable lifting weight. Figure 12–11 provides an example of dimensions used in the formula.

- The horizontal modifier considers the leverage exerted by the load being lifted from the fulcrum, the L5–S1 disk, to the center of gravity of the load. It should be determined at both the origin and destination of the lift. Greater horizontal distances reduce the weights that are safe to lift.

- The vertical modifier takes into account the amount of trunk bending necessary to perform the lift. Lifts that originate below or above knuckle height [76 cm (30 in) from the floor for the average person] are more difficult, so the recommended weight is reduced accordingly.

- The distance modifier is the vertical travel distance from the origin to the destination of a lift. Higher travel distances tend to increase both the biomechanical and metabolic loads of the lift.

- An asymmetry modifier takes into account the twisting of the torso while moving the object. The greater the amount of twisting, the higher is the probability of an injury. This modifier should be calculated at both the beginning and the end of the lift.

- The frequency modifier is calculated based on the average frequency of the lift, in lifts per minute, and is used to incorporate fatigue into the equation.

- A coupling modifier characterizes the grip as good, fair, or poor. A poor coupling, for example, would result in a modifier of 0.90, which would reduce the recommended weight limit by 10%.

ACGIH LIFTING GUIDELINES

The ACGIH has established a Threshold Limit Value (TLV) for lifting. This TLV recommends upper limits

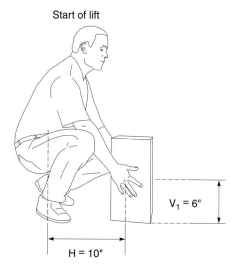

Start of lift

$V_1 = 6"$

$H = 10"$

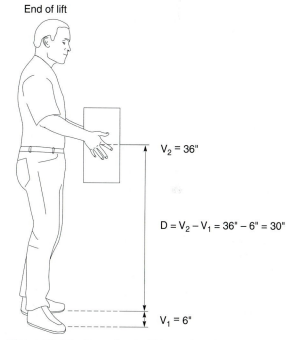

End of lift

$V_2 = 36"$

$D = V_2 - V_1 = 36" - 6" = 30"$

$V_1 = 6"$

Figure 12–11. Example of a lifting task and measurements used in the NIOSH lifting equation. The origin of *H* is taken from the point halfway between the ankles. *D* = distance modifier (in this case *D* = 30 in); *H* = horizontal modifier; *V* = vertical modifier.

Table 12–2. Moderate-frequency lifting >2 hours/day & <30 lifts/hour (in kilograms/pounds).

Horizontal Location/ Vertical Location	Close	Intermediate	Far
Shoulder & above	14/31	5/11	No known safe load
Knuckle to shoulder	27/59	14/31	7/15
Shin to knuckle	16/35	11/24	5/11
Floor to shin	9/20	No known safe load	No known safe load

Source: Based on American Conference of Governmental Industrial Hygienists (ACGIH): Physical Agents, 7th e. Publication no. 7DOC-734, 2005.

for repetitive lifting, with the goal of allowing the majority of workers to perform the task without developing back and shoulder disorders. It is intended to apply to two-handed lifts in which lifting without more than 30 degrees of rotation away from the sagittal plane. There are three tables used to calculate the TLV, chosen based on duration and lifting frequency per day. Each table is divided into four vertical zones of hand location ranging from floor level to 30 cm (12 in) above shoulder height. The three horizontal zones are defined in terms of distance of hand location in front of the midpoint between the observed worker's ankles.

Table 12–2 provides an example of the ACGIH TLV limits applied to moderate-frequency lifting. The TLV is a recommended weight limit, similar in concept to the NIOSH lifting equation–recommended weight limit, although the actual values do not always coincide. The NIOSH lifting equation (NLE) is based on a lower maximum permissible weight than the ACGIH lifting TLV (23 versus 34 kg) and allows for consideration of a smaller range of horizontal locations (i.e., distance from the load). However, the NLE considers trunk flexion and trunk twisting beyond 30 degrees and lifting frequencies greater than 360 per hour and includes consideration of grip quality (coupling) and vertical travel distance in its calculations. Neither approach is applicable to one-handed lifting, lifting in constrained postures, lifting in ambient high temperatures or humidity, poor traction underfoot, or lifting unstable objects with shifting loads, such as liquids. A comparison of the recommended weights for each approach by vertical location indicates that the ACGIH TLV tends to allow somewhat heavier lifts except near floor level.

PSYCHOPHYSICS AND LIFTING

Biomechanical, physiologic, and psychophysical approaches lend themselves to consideration of awkward and unusual postures more readily than do epidemiologic studies, in which working postures may vary widely. Some authors present recommended limits for a variety of lifting, pushing, and pulling tasks based on psychophysical testing. This involves having uninjured workers replicate a task for a few hours or days and report to the researchers what they feel they could comfortably perform over an 8-hour shift for a 5-day week (Table 12–3). These data can be used along with the other approaches or when a rough estimate of limits for lifting, pushing, and pulling tasks is needed. Unless otherwise noted, the applicability of psychophysical tables is limited to

- Task frequencies of no more than 4.3 lifts per minute
- Maximum acceptable forces for one-person manual handling

Table 12–3. Psychophysical limits for load lifting.

Height of Lift (cm)	Sagittal Plane Box Dimensions (cm)	Mean Lifting Limits[1] (N)	
		Men	Women
Floor-to-knuckle height when erect	30.5	296	194
	45.7	261	171
	61.0	236	152
Knuckle-to-shoulder height when erect	30.5	263	141
	45.7	233	129
	61.0	205	127
Shoulder-to-reach height when erect	30.5	221	120
	45.7	204	110
	61.0	195	112

[1]The values represent acceptable lifting limits (N) based on lifting frequency of once per minute sustained for 8 hours.

Table 12–4. Static strengths demonstrated by workers when lifting, pushing, and pulling with both hands on a handle placed at different locations relative to the midpoint between the ankles on the floor.

Test Description	Handle Location[1] (cm)		Mean Strength[2] (N)	
	Vertical	Horizontal	Men	Women
Lift—legs in partial squat	38	0	903	427
Lift—torso stooped over	38	38	480	271
Lift—arms flexed	114	38	383	214
Lift—shoulder high and arms out	152	51	227	129
Lift—shoulder high and arms flexed	152	38	529	240
Lift—shoulder high and arms close	152	25	538	285
Lift—floor level, close (squat)	15	25	890	547
Lift—floor level, out (stoop)	15	38	320	200
Push down—waist level	118	38	432	325
Pull down—above shoulders	178	33	605	449
Pull in—shoulder level, arms out	157	33	311	244
Pull in—shoulder level, arms in	140	0	253	209
Push out—waist level, stand erect	101	35	311	226
Push out—chest level, stand erect	124	25	303	214
Push out—shoulder level, lean forward	140	64	418	276

[1]Handle locations are measured in midsagittal plane, vertical from the floor and horizontal from the midpoint between the ankles.
[2]1 lb = 4.45 N.

- Using carts, bins, or boxes with good handles
- Distance of object handled from the front of the worker's body between 34 and 75 cm
- Vertical location of lift between 25 and 76 cm.

As in application of the NLE and ACGIH lifting TLV, there is no consideration of specific body mechanics or lifting technique because these can be expected to vary from worker to worker.

The University of Michigan has published three-dimensional biomechanical models that are designed to make lifting, pushing, and pulling analyses easy to calculate on a personal computer (3DStatic Strength Prediction Program, University of Michigan, www.engin.umich.edu/dept/ioe/3DSSPP/). The compression on the lower lumbar spine is estimated, as is the proportion of the industrial population capable of exerting a given force in a given direction. This model (like most in current use) is static and does not consider the additional force required to accelerate the object or the fatigue generated by repeating the activity over time. It is based on static strength testing of a large sample of working men and women (Table 12–4). Ergonomic and personal risk factors result in low-back pain, but psychosocial factors can influence low-back pain disability. Epidemio-

logic studies clearly indicate the role of mechanical loads on the etiology of occupational low-back pain.

Preplacement Tests

For jobs requiring strength for materials handling or other tasks, preplacement screening tests may be established to determine which applicants are likely to possess sufficient physical strength and work capacity to perform the essential tasks without injury to themselves or others. However, any such preplacement tests must evaluate body size, strength, and work-capacity traits relevant to and required by the tasks actually to be performed by the applicants. Otherwise, the test may be discriminatory against women or other physically small applicants. Typically, preplacement tests require subjects to perform the most physically demanding elements of the job. These tests should be designed carefully to establish job relevance.

Estimating Work Capacity

For workers who must expend high levels of energy (e.g., distribution center order selectors and agricultural workers), work capacity usually is defined in terms of their aerobic capacity. The proportion of a worker's maximum aero-

Table 12–5. Maximum heart rate and oxygen uptake for men and women in average physical condition.

Age (y)	Heart Rate (beats/min)		Oxygen Uptake (mL/kg/min)	
	Men	Women	Men	Women
20–29	190	190	34–42	31–37
30–39	182	182	31–33	25–33
40–49	179	179	27–35	24–30
50–59	171	171	25–33	21–27
60–69	164	164	23–30	18–23

bic capacity being used can be determined by measuring heart rate or oxygen uptake. Since heart rate and energy expenditure relate in a linear fashion except near the upper and lower levels of a person's capacity, heart rate monitoring of employees can be used to estimate the energy requirements of a job (Table 12–5). The heart rate at rest (HR_{rest}) is subtracted from the estimated maximum heart rate (220 – age) to yield heart rate reserve. The resting heart rate also is subtracted from the mean heart rate during working periods (HR_{work}) to form a ratio as in the following formula:

%HR range = % maximal aerobic capacity =
$[100\%(HR_{work} - HR_{rest})]/(HR_{max} - HR_{rest})$

If there is ever a question about whether an observed employee is exceeding his or her maximum work capacity on a given job, attention also should be paid to modifying the task, improving the work environment (especially ambient temperature), or both.

REFERENCES

Baker P et al: The effectiveness of a comprehensive work hardening program as measured by lifting capacity, pain scales, and depression scores. Work 2005;24:21 [PMID: 15706069].

Davis K, Marras W: Load spatial pathway and spine loading: How does lift origin and destination influence low back response? Ergonomics 2005;48:1031 [PMID: 16147419].

Jensen A, Dahl S: Stress fracture of the distal tibia and fibula through heavy lifting. Am J Indust Med 2005;47:181 [PMID: 15662637].

Jorgensen MJ et al: The effect of pallet distance on torso kinematics and low back disorder risk. Ergonomics 2005;48:949 [PMID: 16147414].

ENVIRONMENTAL FACTORS

The environment affects worker performance, health, and safety in a variety of ways. This discussion focuses primarily on physical aspects of the environment, although the social characteristics of the workplace (e.g., isolation versus overcrowding, being undervalued versus being appreciated, and organizational flexibility versus rigidity) often play a significant role in stress-related problems. For additional information regarding injuries caused by noise, temperature, and vibration, see Chapters 10 and 11.

Physical Hazards

Hazards come in many forms, including unguarded moving machinery or equipment, missing or poorly designed railings to protect workers from dangerous areas, and slippery or obstructed floors. The safety and health standards prepared by U.S. Occupational Safety and Health Administration (OSHA) outline the requirements for hazard elimination, as do many company safety regulations. Regular and consistent enforcement of these safety standards is essential.

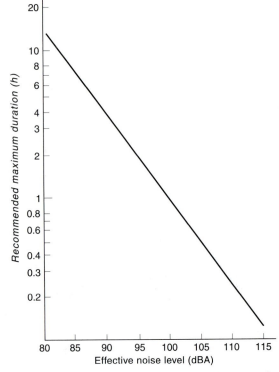

Figure 12–12. Recommended maximum duration of human exposure to various noise levels. Workers should not be exposed to sounds above 115 dBA. (ACGIH: *Threshold Limit Values for Chemical Substances and Physical Agents in the Work Environment.* American Conference of Governmental Industrial Hygienists, 2006.)

Noise

Workers frequently complain that there is too much noise and that this distracts them from their jobs. Loudness is directly related to the mechanical pressure transmitted to the eardrum, although the frequency and other characteristics of sound determine the degrading effect it has on performance. At a given intensity, lower frequencies are more likely to produce hearing impairments, whereas higher frequencies are more apt to interfere with concentration and thought processes. The less predictable and controllable the sound, the more annoying it is.

In quiet areas, some sound (e.g., soft music) may be preferable as a means of masking nearby conversations that otherwise might be distracting. *White noise* (sound spread uniformly over the full hearing spectrum) is sometimes used successfully in lieu of music but occasionally is found to be objectionable.

Sound levels above 50 dB may become increasingly intrusive, objectionable, and fatiguing depending on their frequency and predictability. Sound levels that exceed 85 dBA (as recorded on a sound level meter's A-weighted scale of frequency bands) and continue for as long as 8 hours may cause hearing loss. If noise levels routinely exceed 85 dBA, it is necessary to control the sound source or provide other means of hearing protection. Figure 12–12 shows the recommended maximum duration of human exposure to various noise levels. Workers should not be exposed to sounds above 115 dBA. Table 12–6 lists examples of the sound levels satisfying various communications needs.

Lighting

The amount of light required to perform a specific task without feeling visual fatigue is a function of the visual difficulty of the task at the desired work speed and quality and the visual acuity of the worker. Degree of visual difficulty typically is determined by (1) the contrast between the target and its background, (2) the spatial resolution, and (3) the size of the target. Visual acuity, even with corrected vision, varies with age. Table 12–7 shows the recommended ranges of illumination for various types of tasks.

As with computer work, it is critical to reduce objectionable glare in all workplaces. Glare may emanate directly from a bright light source or may be reflected off the shiny surfaces of machines, worktables, windows, displays, or tools. It can be reduced or eliminated by limiting light from the source or covering shiny surfaces with dull or nonreflective coatings.

A. EXAMPLE

In a garment plant, sewing machine operators complained of headaches and tired and itching eyes after lamps were installed on the far side of each machine.

Table 12–6. Preferred noise criterion (PNC) curves and sound pressure levels recommended for several categories of activity.

	PNC Curve[1]	Approximate Sound Pressure Level (dBA)[2]
Listening to faint musical sounds or using distant microphone pickup	10–20	21–30
Excellent listening conditions	≤20	≤30
Close microphone pickup only	≤25	≤34
Good listening conditions	≤35	≤42
Sleeping, resting, relaxing	25–40	34–47
Conversing or listening to radio or TV	30–40	38–47
Moderately good listening conditions	35–45	42–52
Fair listening conditions	40–50	47–56
Moderately fair listening conditions	45–55	52–61
Just acceptable speech and telephone communication	50–60	56–66
Speech not required but no risk of hearing damage	60–75	66–80

[1]PNC curves are used in many installations for establishing noise spectra.
[2]Voice sound frequencies are used to determine the approximate sound pressure levels. These levels are to be used only for estimates because the overall sound pressure level does not give an indication of the spectrum.

The purpose of the lamps was to improve visibility, but they had the opposite effect because their light reflected off the polished wood and metal sewing tables and the sewn material. Moving the lamps eliminated the glare and relieved the visual symptoms and headaches.

Temperature & Humidity

An elevated ambient temperature or humidity level increases the cardiovascular load of jobs requiring sustained heavy effort (repetitive materials handling), whereas a low temperature can reduce finger flexibility and accuracy substantially. The thermal comfort zone (Figure 12–13) is characterized by the ideal tempera-

Table 12–7. Recommended ranges of illumination for various types of tasks.

Type of Activity or Area	Range of Illumination[1]	
	Lux	Footcandles
Public areas with dark surroundings	20–50	2–5
Simple orientation for short temporary visits	>50–100	>5–9
Working spaces where visual tasks are only occasionally performed	>100–200	>9–19
Performance of visual tasks of high contrast or large size: reading printed material, typed originals, handwriting in ink, good xerography; rough bench and machine work; ordinary inspection; rough assembly	>200–500	>19–46
Performance of visual tasks of medium contrast or small size: reading pencil handwriting, poorly printed or reproduced material; medium bench and machine work; difficult inspection, medium assembly	>500–1000	>46–93
Performance of visual tasks of low contrast or very small size: reading handwriting in hard pencil on poor-quality paper, very poorly reproduced material; very difficult inspection	>1000–2000	>93–186
Performance of visual tasks of low contrast and very small size over a prolonged period: fine assembly, highly difficult inspection, fine bench and machine work	>2000–5000	>186–464
Performance of very prolonged and exacting visual tasks: the most difficult inspection, extra fine bench and machine work, extra fine assembly	>5000–10,000	>464–929
Performance of very special visual tasks of extremely low contrast and small size: some surgical procedures	>10,000–20,000	>929–1858

[1]The choice of a value within a range depends on task variables, the reflectance of the environment, and the individual's visual capabilities.

ture and humidity conditions for work. The comfort zone is affected by a number of factors in addition to temperature and humidity. Among these are air velocity (producing a wind-chill effect), workload, radiant heat sources, and amount and type of clothing. In general, the body's core temperature should not vary by more than 1°C (1.8°F) in either direction, and the preceding factors should be adjusted to accommodate this range.

Vibration

Vibration can be a hazard to the hands or spine. With the increasing interaction between workers and high-power tools, vibration at critical frequencies and accelerations has become an important source of injury and is associated with loss of equilibrium, nausea, hand-arm vibration syndrome (HAVS), and carpal tunnel syndrome. In addition, truck drivers and heavy equipment operators have an elevated risk of lumbar spinal disorders, hemorrhoids, hernias, and digestive and urinary tract problems, which may be a result of a combination of vibration, extended sitting, and truck loading and unloading.

Vibration of the hand and arm for extended periods, as occurs in the operation of hand power tools, such as chain saws, riveting hammers, sanders, pneumatic drills, power chisels, and grinders, may be a source of recurrent hand pain, numbness, and finger blanching or HAVS. HAVS involves the small blood vessels and nerves of the fingers and is exacerbated by exposure to vibration and cold. Workers also may have a decrease in touch sensitivity, fine finger dexterity, and grip strength. Continued exposure with severe disease can lead to gangrene of the fingertips. Other conditions linked to the use of vibratory hand tools include neuritis and decalcification and cysts of the radial and ulnar bones. Even after removal of vibration exposure, reversal of the disease will occur in only 50% of workers. Diagnosis, prevention, and treatment of HAVS are discussed in Chapter 11. The ACGIH has developed guidelines for vibration exposure.

The types of whole-body vibration that are of most concern to occupational health and safety analysts are those associated with operation of vehicles (e.g., buses, forklifts, and heavy construction equipment) and with operation of machinery (e.g., large punch presses, conveyors, and furnaces). The effect of vibration depends on its acceleration, duration, frequency, and direction (vertical or lateral) (Figure 12–14). Lower-intensity exposure (measured by surface-mounted accelerometers) can be

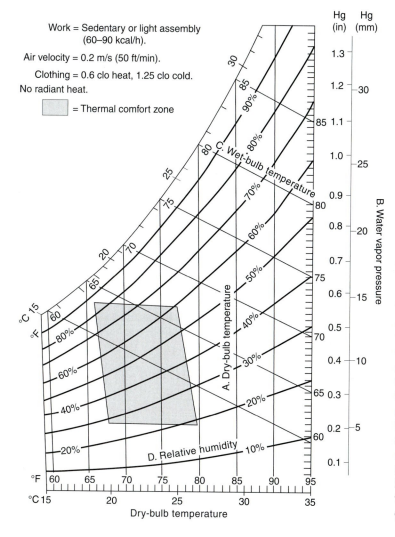

Work = Sedentary or light assembly (60–90 kcal/h).

Air velocity = 0.2 m/s (50 ft/min).

Clothing = 0.6 clo heat, 1.25 clo cold.
No radiant heat.

▨ = Thermal comfort zone

Figure 12–13. Thermal comfort zone. The dry-bulb temperature and humidity combinations that are comfortable for most people doing sedentary or light work are shown as the shaded area on the psychometric chart. The dry-bulb temperature range is 19–26°C (66–79°F), and the relative humidity range (shown as parallel curves) is 20–85%, with 35–65% being the most common values in the comfort zone. On this chart, ambient dry-bulb temperature (A) is plotted on the horizontal axis and indicated as parallel vertical lines; water vapor pressure (B) is on the vertical axis. Wet-bulb temperatures (C) are shown as parallel lines with a negative slope; they intersect the dry-bulb temperature lines and relative humidity curves (D) on the chart. In the definition of the thermal comfort zone, assumptions were made about the workload, air velocity, radiant heat, and clothing insulation levels. These assumptions are given in the top left corner of the chart. (ACGIH: *Threshold Limit Values for Chemical Substances and Physical Agents in the Work Environment.* American Conference of Governmental Industrial Hygienists, 2006.)

tolerated for longer periods without pain or injury than the high intensities; low-intensity vibrations of less than 1 Hz in fact may have a soothing effect.

Whole-body vertical vibration is a continuing problem for vehicle operators. The critical range of the torso's natural resonant frequency is 3–5 Hz, but discomfort can occur in the range of 2–11 Hz. Well-designed seats for bus and truck drivers will diminish the vibration in this critical frequency range by as much as 50%. However, older, stiffer seats can have an amplification effect of as much as 20%. In some buses or trucks, the lateral acceleration intensity may be twice the vertical intensity. Visual performance generally is impaired in the range of 10–25 Hz. Truck and bus seats usually do not transmit vertical vibrations in this frequency range, but other equip-

ment (e.g., overhead cranes, lumber mill saws, and conveying machinery) may.

REFERENCES

Blehm C et al: Computer vision syndrome: A review. Surv Ophthalmol 2005;50:253 [PMID: 15850814].

Maikala RV et al: Acute physiological responses in healthy men during whole-body vibration. Int Arch Occup Environ Health 2005;21:1 [PMID: 16175416].

Marrao C et al: Physical and cognitive performance during long-term cold weather operations. Aviat Space Environ Med 2005;76:744 [PMID: 1611069].

WEB SITES

American Conference of Governmental Industrial Hygienists (ACGIH): www.acgih.org.

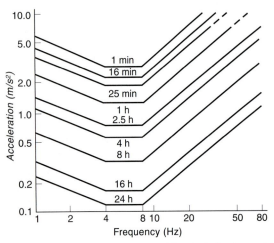

Figure 12–14. Maximum acceptable whole-body vertical vibration exposure times to various frequencies and accelerations. The shorter the vibration exposure, the higher the acceleration levels that can be tolerated. The least-acceptable range of frequencies at all accelerations and durations of exposure is from 4–8 Hz. (ACGIH: *Threshold Limit Values for Chemical Substances and Physical Agents in the Work Environment.* American Conference of Governmental Industrial Hygienists, 2006.)

Human Factors and Ergonomics Society (HFES): www.hfes.org.

National Institute for Occupational Safety and Health (NIOSH): www.cdc.gov/niosh.

ERGONOMICS GUIDES

A Strategy for Industrial Power Hand Tool Ergonomic Research: Design, Selection, Installation, and Use in Automotive Manufacturing (www.cdc.gov/niosh/pdfs/95-114.pdf)

Easy Ergonomics: A Guide to Selecting Non-Powered Hand Tools (www.cdc.gov/niosh/docs/2004-164/default.html)

US Federal OSHA Ergonomics (www.osha.gov/SLTC/ergonomics/index.html).

Ergonomics: Guidelines for Poultry Processing (www.osha.gov/ergonomics/guidelines/poultryprocessing/index.html)

Ergonomics: Guidelines for Retail Grocery Stores (www.osha.gov/ergonomics/guidelines/retailgrocery/index.html)

Ergonomics: Guidelines for Nursing Homes (www.osha.gov/ergonomics/guidelines/nursinghome/index.html)

Back Injury Prevention Guide in the Health Care Industry for Health Care Providers (www.dir.ca.gov/dosh/dosh_publications/backinj.pdf)

Ergonomics in Action a Guide to Best Practices for the Food-Processing Industry (www.dir.ca.gov/dosh/dosh_publications/Erg_Food_Processing.pdf)

Keys to Success and Safety for the Construction Foreman (www.dir.ca.gov/dosh/dosh_publications/foremanweb.pdf)

SECTION III.
Occupational Illnesses

Clinical Toxicology

Jon Rosenberg, MD, & Leslie M. Israel, DO, MPH

13

Toxicology is the study of physical and chemical agents and the injury they cause to living cells. All substances are potentially toxic. One objective of clinical and experimental studies in toxicology is to define the capacity of substances to produce harmful effects (i.e., toxicity), measure and analyze the doses at which toxicity occurs (i.e., the dose-response relationship), and assess the probability that injury or illness will occur under specified conditions of use (i.e., hazard and risk assessment).

A distinction is made between toxicity and hazard. An extremely toxic chemical that is in a sealed container on a shelf has inherent toxicity but presents little or no hazard. When the chemical is removed from the shelf and used by a worker in a closed space and without appropriate protection, the hazard becomes great. Thus the manner of use affects how hazardous the substance will be in the workplace.

TOXIC AGENTS & THEIR EFFECTS

Classification of Toxic Agents

Toxic agents can be classified or described in terms of the following.

A. Physical State of the Agent

The different physical states of toxic agents, with some examples of each, are shown in Table 13–1. A metal such as lead may be harmless in solid form, moderately toxic as a dust, and extremely toxic as a fume.

B. Chemical Structure of the Agent

Chemical structure can determine toxicity. Often one isomer, but not another, of a compound possesses tox-

icity. For example, aromatic amines are carcinogenic when substituted in other than the *para-* (*p-*) position. The stability of a substance and the presence of impurities, contaminants, or additives also can affect toxicity.

C. Size of the Agent (Nanotoxicology)

Nanosized materials, or nanoparticles, are materials less than 100 nm in size. *Nanotoxicology* is defined as the science and safety evaluation of engineered nanodevices and nanostructures. It is considered by some as a separate or specialized field of toxicology because materials not considered as toxic based on their basic properties may have unintended human health and environmental effects as a consequence of their small size. The possibility that particles like buckyballs, all-carbon molecules with chemical formula C_{60}, might have toxicologic effects unexpected based on their chemical composition, has created concerns that the field of nanotechnology might be growing too fast without adequate regulation. These concerns include a possible backlash against nanotechnology similar to that against genetically modified foods and organisms and the creation of a new type of chemical pollution from the release of nanoparticles from coatings or other products.

Their small size may facilitate absorption, particularly in the respiratory tract when airborne, and alter uptake and distribution to sites such as nervous system, bone marrow, lymph nodes, spleen, and heart. Because of their small size and corresponding large specific surface area, nanoparticles are thought to exhibit greater biologic activity when compared with larger particles. This increased biologic activity may cause positive (e.g., antioxidant activity, carrier capacity for therapeutics, penetration of cellular barriers for drug delivery), negative (e.g. toxicity, induction of oxidative

Table 13–1. Physical states of toxic substances.

Particulates
  Dusts
    Nuisance
      Calcium carbonate
      Cellulose (paper fiber)
      Portland cement
      Silicon
    Fibrogenic
      Silica
      Coal dust
    Fibers
      Asbestos
      Mineral wool
    Fumes
      Metal
      Polymer (polytetrafluoroethylene decomposition
        products)
Gases and vapors
  Butane, methyl bromide, ethylene oxide (gas)
  Hexane, trichloroethylene, benzene (vapor)
Liquids
  Elemental mercury
Solids
  Plastics

stress or of cellular dysfunction), or mixed effects. Toxicologic testing of nanoparticles is also affected by their size. Materials being tested need to be characterized by size, shape, and surface properties in addition to composition. The measurement of dose and of levels in biologic tissues may be difficult for some nanostructures. As a reflection of the increasing importance of this area, the journal *Nanotoxicology* was launched in 2005.

REFERENCE

Oberdorster G et al: Nanotoxicology: An emerging discipline evolving from studies of ultrafine particles. Environ Health Perspect 2005;113:823 [PMID: 16002369].

D. MEDIUM OF THE AGENT

The medium in which a toxic substance is found in part determines the population exposed and thus to some extent the hazard. Some toxic substances occur in a specific medium—for example, oxides of nitrogen in air (from vehicular exhaust), trihalomethanes in water (from chlorination), and nitrosamines in food (from nitrites). In the United States, several governmental agencies, including the Environmental Protection Agency (EPA), the Food and Drug Administration (FDA), and the Occupational Safety and Health Administration (OSHA), have developed regulations regarding exposure to toxic substances in various media.

E. SITE OF INJURY BY THE AGENT

Toxic agents can be described in terms of their effects on cellular (non-DNA-damaging agents) or genetic (DNA-damaging agents) material and on target organs (e.g., hepatotoxins and nephrotoxins).

F. MECHANISM OF ACTION OF THE AGENT

Toxic agents frequently are categorized on the basis of their mechanism of action. Asphyxiants, for example, deprive tissues of oxygen. Simple asphyxiants (inert gases) act by diluting or displacing oxygen without causing other toxic effects. In contrast, chemical asphyxiants such as cyanide and carbon monoxide actively interfere with the delivery or use of oxygen—cyanide by inhibiting cytochrome oxidase and other enzymes necessary for cellular utilization of oxygen and carbon monoxide by combining with hemoglobin to form carboxyhemoglobin, which decreases the oxygen-carrying capacity of the blood and inhibits release of oxygen to tissues.

G. CLINICAL EFFECTS OF THE AGENT

1. Onset of effects—Toxic effects can be immediate, as occurs with some irritants that cause direct damage to tissues at the point of initial contact, usually resulting in inflammation, or delayed, as with chemical carcinogens.

2. Reversibility of effects—Whether or not the toxic effects of a substance are reversible depends on the capacity of damaged cells to regenerate or recover. For instance, brain and other nervous system cells have little capacity to regenerate, whereas liver and muscle cells are more likely to regenerate or recover after injury.

Factors Affecting Clinical Response to a Toxic Agent

The following factors affect the dose-response relationship and the clinical response of humans to a toxic agent.

A. DURATION, FREQUENCY, AND ROUTE OF EXPOSURE

The severity of injury usually is related to the duration and frequency of exposure. The route of exposure often determines toxicity. For example, ethylene glycol is toxic when ingested but poses little threat in the workplace except when sprayed or heated.

B. ENVIRONMENTAL FACTORS

Toxicity is affected by atmospheric pressure, temperature, and humidity. For example, a concentration of carbon monoxide that has little effect at sea level can cause impairment of work capacity at an altitude of 5000 ft. Chemicals are absorbed more readily through skin that is injured or wet with perspiration and has increased blood flow in response to heat and humidity.

C. INDIVIDUAL FACTORS

Individual factors that determine "susceptibility" include racial and genetic background, age and maturity, sex, body weight, nutrition, lifestyle, immunologic and hormonal status, and presence of disease or stress. These factors are not independent of one another. For instance, genetic factors determine many of the other factors, and poor nutrition can affect immunologic status.

While much concern about the effect of age on individual susceptibility has focused on the fetus, the elderly also metabolize many chemicals less efficiently. As the work force ages, this may become an increasing concern.

The effect of nutritional deficiency on susceptibility to toxic agents has been of concern in developed countries primarily during war or famine, but it is relevant in developing countries as they industrialize. While toxicologic studies in animals readily demonstrate the effects of nutritional deficiency on susceptibility, the results of these studies are difficult to extrapolate to humans. The role of vitamins and minerals in chemical toxicity has been much debated.

There is controversy about the role of genetic factors and the development and use of genetic screening tests to identify individuals with increased susceptibility to toxic agents in the workplace. It is questioned whether such tests are accurate and whether job discrimination could result from their use as preemployment screening. Among the many genetic traits that might increase the risk of toxicity from exposure to chemicals or radiation, the most visible have been glucose-6-phosphate dehydrogenase (G6PD) deficiency, sickle cell anemia, and α_1-antitrypsin deficiency.

G6PD deficiency is an X-linked recessive disorder that primarily affects American black males and Mediterranean Jews. Affected individuals are susceptible to hemolysis from many drugs. Although some chemicals—notably naphthalene and arsine—can cause hemolysis following overexposure, there is no evidence that workers exposed to workplace-acceptable concentrations of these chemicals are at increased risk. Screening for G6PD deficiency thus is not supported by solid evidence.

Similarly, there is no evidence that any of the 7–13% of American blacks with sickle cell trait are at increased risk of hypoxia when working as airplane pilots or of hemolysis when working with hemolytic agents despite the fact that these "risks" have been cited to justify screening of individuals for these occupations.

Severe α_1-antitrypsin deficiency, when present in the rare homozygous condition, can lead to early emphysema in the absence of environmental agents. The more common heterozygous condition, which affects 4–9% of the U.S. population, may in combination with other factors place affected individuals at increased risk of developing emphysema from exposure to environmental agents.

TOXICOKINETICS, TOXICODYNAMICS, & TOXICOGENOMICS

Toxicokinetics is the study of the movement of toxic substances within the body (i.e., their absorption, distribution, metabolism, and excretion) and the relationship between the dose that enters the body and the level of toxic substance found in the blood or other biologic sample. *Toxicodynamics* is the study of the relationship between the dose that enters the body and the measured response. The magnitude of a toxic response usually is related to the concentration of the toxic substance at its site of action. *Toxicogenomics* is the study of the response of a genome to environmental stressors and toxicants. The recent sequencing of mammalian genomes has driven the development of toxicogenomic technologies, including microarray-based gene expression profiling, which allows the expression levels of thousands of genes to be measured simultaneously.

REFERENCE

Moggs JG: Molecular responses to xenoestrogens: Mechanistic insights from toxicogenomics. Toxicology 2005;213:177 [PMID: 15996808].

Bioavailability

The *bioavailability* of a toxic substance indicates the extent to which the agent reaches its site of action. If it is not in a "bioavailable form," as is the case with many orally ingested toxic substances that cause vomiting or diarrhea, it will be removed promptly. In other cases, some of the agent will be inactivated before it reaches the site of action. For example, when cyanide is taken orally, it is absorbed and passes to the liver, where the enzyme rhodanese may metabolize a portion of the ingested cyanide. On the other hand, if the cyanide in the form of gaseous hydrocyanic acid (HCN) is absorbed through the pulmonary circulation, it goes directly to the brain, where it may cause damage from hypoxia.

Cell Membrane Permeability & Cellular Barrier

Absorption, distribution, metabolism, and excretion all involve passage of toxic agents across cell membranes. Permeability depends on a toxic substance's molecular size and shape, solubility at the site of absorption, degree of ionization, and relative lipid solubility.

The distribution of some toxic agents is altered by unique cellular barriers, for example, the blood-brain barrier, the blood-testis barrier, and the placenta, which may exclude toxic substances. Many lipid-soluble toxic substances are stored in body fat. In an obese person with a fat content of 30–40%, this may form a stable reservoir for toxic substances, which then may be released slowly. Bone is an important deep reservoir for many heavy metals (especially lead) and for radioactive materials, and the effects of these materials can persist long after they have left the circulation.

Absorption

The rate of absorption depends on the concentration and solubility of the toxic agent. Agents in aqueous solution are absorbed more rapidly than those in oily suspension. Absorption is enhanced at sites that have increased blood flow or large absorptive surfaces (e.g., the adult lung and gastrointestinal tract, whose surfaces are the size of a tennis court and a football field, respectively).

A. Gastrointestinal Absorption

The amount of absorption through the gastrointestinal tract is usually proportionate to the gastrointestinal surface area and its blood flow and depends on the physical state of the agent. Most toxic substances are absorbed in the small intestine. Therefore, agents that accelerate gastric emptying will increase the absorption rate, whereas factors that delay gastric emptying will decrease it. Some toxic substances may be affected by gastric juice; for example, the acidity of the stomach may release cyanide products and form hydrogen cyanide gas, which is even more toxic than the cyanide salt.

B. Pulmonary Absorption

The most common route of occupational exposure is pulmonary absorption. Gaseous and volatile toxic substances may be inhaled and absorbed through the pulmonary epithelium and mucous membranes in the respiratory tract. Access to the circulation is rapid because the surface area of the lungs is large and the blood flow is great. The nasal hair, the cough reflex, and the mucociliary barrier help to prevent dust particles and fumes from reaching the lung.

The solubility of gases affects their absorption. Highly water-soluble gases such as ammonia and sulfuric acid are absorbed in the upper airways and cause marked irritation there. This serves as a warning and limits the injury to the lung. Noxious gases of low water solubility such as nitrogen dioxide and phosgene, which have few early warning properties, reach the lungs and cause delayed injury there.

C. Percutaneous Absorption

Many toxic substances pass through the skin, intact or broken. The amount of skin absorption generally is proportionate to the surface area of contact and to the lipid solubility of the toxic agent. The epidermis acts as a lipid barrier, and the stratum corneum provides a protective barrier against noxious agents. The dermis, however, is freely permeable to many toxic substances.

Factors that affect skin absorption include anatomic location, gender, age, condition (including hydration) of skin, personal hygiene, and environmental factors (e.g., temperature, humidity). Absorption is enhanced by toxic agents that increase the blood flow to the skin. It is also enhanced by the use of occlusive skin coverings (e.g., permeable clothes and industrial gloves) and topical application of fat-solubilizing vehicles. Hydrated skin is more permeable than dry skin. The thick skin on the palms of the hands and the soles of the feet is more resistant to absorption than is the thin skin on the face, neck, and scrotum. Burns, abrasions, dermatitis, and other injuries to the skin may alter its protective properties and allow absorption of larger quantities of the toxic substance.

REFERENCE

Semple S: Dermal exposure to chemicals in the workplace: Just how important is skin absorption? Occup Environ Med 2004;61:376 [PMID: 15031402].

D. Ocular Absorption

The eye is also a ready site of absorption. When chemicals enter the body through the conjunctiva, they bypass hepatic elimination and may cause severe systemic toxicity. This may occur when organophosphate pesticides are splashed into the eyes. Contact lenses, once thought to potentially enhance ocular absorption by serving as a reservoir for chemicals, in most cases serve as a barrier to the eye.

Distribution

Toxic substances are transported via the blood to various portions of the body. Some are removed by the lymph, and some insoluble compounds are transported through tissues such as the lung via cells such as macrophages. Most toxic substances enter the bloodstream and are distributed into interstitial and cellular fluids. The pattern of distribution depends on the physiologic and physicochemical properties of the material. The initial phase of distribution usually reflects the cardiac output and regional blood flow. Lipid-soluble agents that penetrate membranes poorly are restricted in their distribution, and their potential sites of action therefore are limited. Exceptions are the blood-brain and blood-testis barriers, which limit the distribution of water-soluble but not lipid-soluble chemicals to these organs. Distribution also may be limited by the binding of toxic substances to plasma proteins. Toxic agents can accumulate in higher concentration in some tissues as a result of pH gradients, binding to special cellular proteins, or partitioning into lipids. Some agents accumulate in tissue reservoirs, and this may serve to prolong the toxic action; for example, lead may be stored for years in bone and may be released later.

Metabolism

Toxic substances that are lipid-soluble may go through a series of metabolic conversions (biotransformation) to produce more polar (water-soluble) products and thereby enhance removal by urinary excretion. The most common site for biotransformation is the liver, but it also can occur in plasma, lung, or other tissue. Biotransformation may result in either a decrease (detoxification or inactivation) or an increase (activation) in the toxicity of a compound. Differences in the metabolism of toxic substances account for much of the observed differences between individuals and between animal species.

Biotransformation occurs in the liver by hydrolysis, oxidation, reduction, and conjugation. Microsomal enzymes play a key role in the process, and the activity of the microsomal enzyme system can be increased (induced) by many environmental and pharmacologic agents. Both normal individual differences in microsomal enzyme activity and susceptibility to induction are determined genetically and account for the marked variability in bioavailability of many toxic substances. Other factors that regulate key liver enzyme systems are hormones (which account for some sex-dependent differences) and disease states (e.g., the presence of hepatitis, cirrhosis, or heart failure). Because the activity of many hepatic metabolizing systems is low in neonates—particularly premature neonates—they may be much more susceptible to toxic substances that are inactivated by liver metabolism. Inefficient metabolizing systems, an altered blood-brain barrier, and inadequate mechanisms of excretion combine to make the fetus and neonate sensitive to the toxic effects of many agents.

Excretion

A. PATHWAYS AND MECHANISMS OF EXCRETION

Toxic substances are excreted either unchanged or as metabolites. Excretory organs other than the lungs eliminate polar (water-soluble) compounds more efficiently than they eliminate nonpolar (lipid-soluble) compounds. As discussed earlier, nonpolar compounds must be metabolized to more polar compounds before they can be eliminated renally. The kidney is the primary organ of elimination for most polar compounds and their metabolites. Excretion of toxic substances in the urine involves glomerular filtration, active secretion, and passive tubular reabsorption. Alkalization or acidification of the urine may change excretion of some agents dramatically. When tubular urine is more alkaline, weak acids are excreted more rapidly because they are ionized and passive tubular reabsorption is decreased. In contrast, when tubular urine is made more acidic, excretion of weak acid is reduced.

Many toxic substances metabolized by the liver are excreted first in the bile and later eliminated in the stool or reabsorbed into the blood and ultimately eliminated in the urine. Toxic substances also can be excreted in sweat, saliva, and breast milk, and there may be some minor removal in hair or skin.

B. CLEARANCE

Clearance is the rate at which a toxic agent is excreted, divided by the average concentration of the agent in the plasma. Most toxic substances are eliminated as a linear function of concentration; that is, a constant fraction of the toxic material is eliminated over time (per unit of time). If the point of saturation is reached, the body will no longer be able to eliminate a constant fraction of the material but instead will eliminate a constant amount per unit of time. Under these circumstances, the clearance becomes quite variable. Note that clearance is a measure not of how much is being removed but rather of the volume of fluid that is freed of the toxic agent per unit of time.

C. VOLUME OF DISTRIBUTION

The volume of distribution is calculated by dividing the dose of the toxic substance administered by the concentration in the blood. This volume is not necessarily a physiologic volume; it is merely an estimate of the degree of distribution of the toxic agent in tissues. The volume of distribution for most toxic agents depends largely on pH factors, protein binding, partition coefficients, and regional differences in blood flow and binding to special tissues.

D. HALF-TIME AND HALF-LIFE

The time it takes for the plasma concentration of a substance to be reduced by 50% is the *half-time*. For substances that are eliminated as a linear function (i.e., independent of concentration), the time it takes to eliminate 50% of the substance is the *half-life*. Calculation of half-life provides a means of estimating the dose that was absorbed. For a substance eliminated in linear fashion, approximately 90% of the amount in the body will be eliminated in 3.5 half-lives after the end of the period of exposure.

REFERENCES

Aubrecht J, Caba E. Gene expression: An emerging approach to investigate mechanisms of genotoxicity. Pharmacogenomics 2005;6:419 [PMID: 16004560].

The National Institute of Environmental Health Sciences (NIEHS) National Center for Toxicogenomics (NCT): www.niehs.nih.gov/nct/.

TESTS OF TOXIC EFFECTS

Much of our information about the toxic effects of different agents comes from studying various strains and species of animals. Toxic substances frequently cause effects in animals, some immediately after administration and others after a prolonged period. Acute effects are sometimes qualitatively quite different from chronic effects. For example, the acute effect of benzene is central nervous system depression, whereas its chronic effects are aplastic anemia and leukemia.

Although tests in animals are the most common methods of identifying agents that cause toxicity, the results are difficult to extrapolate to humans given the disparity among life spans (18–24 months for rodents versus 75 years for humans). In addition, different strains and species of animals may show both qualitative and quantitative differences in the pattern or intensity of response to a toxic agent. Even with the best statistical approaches and the best evidence of toxic responses in animals, there is no certain way of estimating the incidence of toxicity or determining the type of response to a toxic substance in a human population. Furthermore, there is no absolute certainty that safety factors for exposure to a toxic substance based on studies in animals would be valid for humans.

Another issue with animal or in vivo studies is the economic and practical feasibility of testing the approximately 80,000 chemicals in commerce and the large number of chemical mixtures. Therefore, in vitro test methods are being evaluated as an alternative to in vivo test methods.

Tests for Acute, Subacute, & Chronic Toxic Effects

Tests for acute effects usually are performed when there are no data available on the potential toxicity of a single exposure or a few exposures to a specific agent. An appropriate route of administration is chosen, and a specific endpoint (e.g., death of the laboratory animal) is selected. The signs and symptoms before death are observed, and the animal is later examined for gross and histologic damage to tissues. In some cases, topical application of an agent is used to test for skin or eye injury.

Tests for subacute or sublethal effects of a specific agent usually are performed during a period of 21–90 days in animals, with the route of administration chosen on the basis of anticipated human exposure. Two different species of rodents usually are involved in each test.

Tests for chronic effects are performed in animals when long-term human exposure to a specific agent is anticipated or a long latency period between exposure and toxicity is expected. Rats and mice usually are exposed from a few weeks of age until their premature death or their sacrifice at the end of the expected lifetime. Short-term tests for genotoxicity, including mutagenicity, are used to prioritize agents for long-term testing or to provide supportive data for the results of long-term testing.

Tests for Teratogenesis & Toxic Effects on Reproductive Organs

Teratologic tests involve exposing pregnant female animals to a specific agent at a critical time during pregnancy and then examining their offspring for malformations. Usually two or three species are used for comparison and controls. In reproductive studies, male and female animals are exposed to an agent and subsequently observed for reproductive failure or success. In cases of successful reproduction, the first- and second-generation offspring are also observed for their ability to reproduce. In cases of unsuccessful reproduction, male animals often are tested for sperm motility, count, and morphology.

IDENTIFICATION OF THE MECHANISMS OF TOXICITY

The best approach to understanding the mechanisms of a toxic effect involves three essential considerations: (1) the time course of the concentration of the active forms of a toxic agent at its active sites, (2) the kinetics of interaction between the active forms of the toxic compound and its active sites, and (3) the kinetics of the sequence of events resulting from the interaction that occurs before toxicity has been manifested. These observations then must be validated against experimental evidence in animals or epidemiologic studies in humans.

A special task force on toxicologic assessment has suggested six questions whose answers would lead to the development of protocols that would effectively identify the mechanisms of toxicity: What is the manifestation of the toxicity? What element causes the toxicity? What factors govern the concentration of the toxic element at its active sites? What is the physical or chemical nature of the reaction of the toxic substance at its active sites? What subsequent events lead to the manifestation of toxicity? How can toxicity be modulated?

The answers to these six questions are not simple. For example, toxicologists are not certain about the significance of tumors in animal species in which the incidence of spontaneous liver tumor is high. It is important to understand whether toxic agents act without further biotransformation or by direct interaction with an essential cellular constituent that maintains the integrity of the cell. Even if the parent toxic substance does not cause injury, an active metabolite (e.g., superoxide anion) may be detrimental to cell function.

The following types of research help to identify the mechanisms of action of specific toxic agents: (1) studying the effects of a particular type of pretreatment on the toxin-metabolizing enzyme systems in various organs and tissues, (2) analyzing the effects of inhibitors or inducers on activation or detoxification pathways at potential sites of metabolism, (3) elucidating the nature of the substrate cell, (4) studying the influence of genetic and environmental factors that affect potential toxic target sites, (5) reviewing the age and sex differences in the enzymes and target systems affected by a given toxic agent, and (6) determining the manner in which a toxic effect can be modulated, for example, by alteration in diet or manipulation of hormones.

REFERENCES

Bakand S et al: Toxicity assessment of industrial chemicals and airborne contaminants: Transition from in vivo to in vitro test methods: a review. Inhal Toxicol 2005;17:775 [PMID: 16195213].

Brent RL: Utilization of animal studies to determine the effects and human risks of environmental toxicants (drugs, chemicals, and physical agents). Pediatrics 2004;113:984 [PMID: 15060191].

Jonker D et al: Safety evaluation of chemical mixtures and combinations of chemical and non-chemical stressors. Rev Environ Health 2004;19:83 [PMID: 15329008].

Monosson E: Chemical mixtures: Considering the evolution of toxicology and chemical assessment. Environ Health Perspect 2005;113:383 [PMID: 15811826].

The National Toxicology Program Web site: http://ntp-server. niehs.nih.gov/.

TOXICOLOGIC RISK ASSESSMENT

Steps in Risk Assessment

Risk assessment is the characterization of the potential adverse health effects of human exposure to hazardous substances. It can be divided into the following steps:

Step 1. Hazard identification—(a) Description of the population exposed to a substance (population at risk). (b) Determination of the adverse health effects that would be caused by that substance (e.g., cancer and birth defects).

Step 2. Dose-response assessment—(a) Collection of epidemiologic and experimental dose-response data on the effects of the substance. (b) Identification of a "critical" dose-response relationship (discussed in detail below). (c) Quantitative expression of the dose-response relationship by mathematical extrapolation from high doses in animals to low doses in humans.

Step 3. Exposure assessment—Estimation of past, present, and future exposure levels of the population at risk and of actual doses received.

Step 4. Risk characterization—Estimation of the incidence of adverse health effects in the population predicted from the dose-response assessment (step 2) as applied to the exposure assessment (step 3).

Uncertainties Inherent in Risk Assessment

There are a number of uncertainties inherent in risk assessment for toxic substances: (1) Human data frequently are lacking or are limited because of an inability to detect low-incidence effects. Epidemiologic studies do not demonstrate causation or provide quantitative dose-response data, nor do they account for mixed and multiple exposures, a sufficient latency period for effects to be expressed, and differences between the populations studied. (2) Animal data are often of uncertain relevance to humans. A rational choice of the most appropriate species may not be possible. Toxicokinetic, toxicodynamic, and toxicogenomic data usually are lacking. The route, frequency, and duration of exposure may be different from those of the human population. The doses usually are much higher, and the animals studied are genetically homogeneous and free of exposure to other toxic substances. (3) The mechanisms of action for effects are poorly understood. (4) The exposure of the population at risk may not be quantified, and calculation of doses may not be possible.

Because of these uncertainties, the practice of quantitative risk assessment is sometimes criticized for being "unscientific." However, because human exposure to toxic substances may result in medical and public health risks, risk assessment often provides the only basis for decisions on how to manage potential risks. Methods for estimation of health risk assessment are discussed in Chapter 45.

DOSE-RESPONSE CURVES

A dose-response relationship exists when changes in dose are followed by consistent changes in response, as shown in dose-response curves. A number of toxicologic phenomena can be demonstrated by these curves. In Figure 13–1 the dose-response curves show the range of possible dose response relationships in an individual.

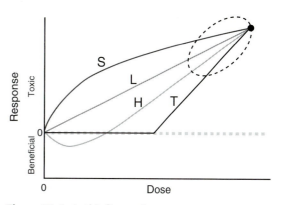

Figure 13–1. In this figure, dose-response curves are abbreviated as follows: H = hormetic (biphasic); L = linear (no threshold); S = supralinear; T = threshold. The dose-response curves show the range of possible dose-response relationships in an individual.

In Figure 13–2, the existence of a threshold is indicated by the arrow at the point where the curve intersects the dose coordinate. Doses below this point do not produce a response. Individuals who exhibit the response at doses well below the average or the mean are considered hypersusceptible (*H* in the figure), whereas those who respond only to doses well above the average or the mean are considered resistant (*R* in the figure).

In Figure 13–3, cumulative frequency curves are used to compare two doses of the same toxic substance to the dose that is lethal to 50% of the population (LD$_{50}$) and the dose that has an effect on 50% (ED$_{50}$). The ED$_{50}$ may, for example, represent an effect that is not harmful, such as odor. The ratio between comparable points on the curves (i.e., the ratio of LD$_{50}$ to ED$_{50}$) then will represent the margin of safety for odor as a warning against the lethal effect.

In Figure 13–4, cumulative frequency curves are used to compare the doses at which the same toxic effect is elicited by three different toxic substances (A, B, and C). Substance A is clearly the most toxic because at every dose level a greater percentage of the population exhibits the response to A than to substance B or substance C. The LD$_{50}$, the ED$_{10}$, and the threshold for

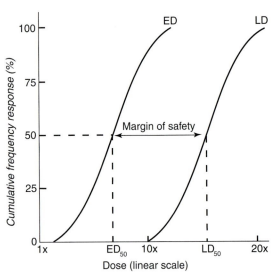

Figure 13–3. Dose-response curves comparing two doses of the same toxic substance. ED = effective dose; LD = lethal dose. The area between the ED and LD is the margin of safety.

A are all lower than the corresponding values for substances B and C. The comparison between substances B and C is less clear and demonstrates the need to consider the entire dose-response curves rather than individual points when comparing toxicities. Because the LD$_{50}$ of substance B is lower than that of substance C, at this dose substance B is more toxic than substance C. However, because the ED$_{10}$ of substance C is lower than that of substance B, at the lower dose substance C is more toxic than substance B. The shape of a dose-response curve is important for assessing the hazard of a toxic substance. A substance that has a low threshold and shallow dose-response curve (such as substance C) may be more hazardous at low doses, whereas a substance that has a steep dose-response curve (such as substance B) may be more hazardous as the dose increases. Adequate assessment of the hazard of a toxic substance requires evaluation of dose-response data over a wide range of doses.

REFERENCE

Oberemm A et al: How can toxicogenomics inform risk assessment? Toxicol Appl Pharmacol 2005;207:592 [PMID: 15990130].

DIAGNOSIS OF TOXIC EFFECTS

Different toxic substances often elicit similar clinical manifestations of toxicity. In some cases, the manifestations represent a response to more than one toxic agent,

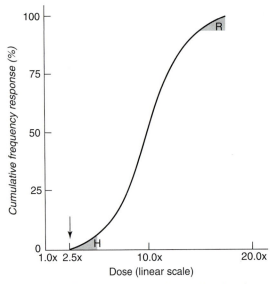

Figure 13–2. The existence of a threshold in this dose-response curve is indicated by the arrow. Doses below this point do not produce a response. Individuals who exhibit the response at doses well below the average or the mean are considered hypersusceptible (H), whereas those who respond only to doses well above the average or the mean are considered resistant (R).

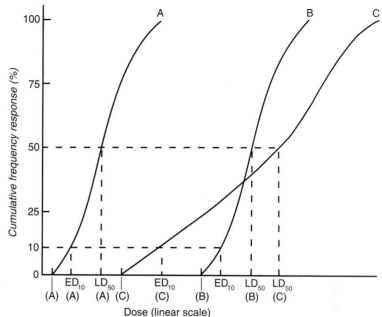

Figure 13–4. Dose-response curves comparing the doses at which the same toxic effect is elicited by three different toxic substances (A, B, and C).

a combination of toxic agents, or a chemical mixture and naturally occurring causes. In general, the manifestations of acute toxicity caused by high-dose exposures will be more specific than those of chronic toxicity or toxicity caused by low-dose exposures.

For example, patients with acute poisoning caused by a high-dose exposure to organophosphate pesticides may present with involvement of the autonomic nervous system (i.e., nausea, vomiting, diarrhea, increased lacrimation and sweating, bronchorrhea, bronchoconstriction, blurred vision, small pupils, and bradycardia), the neuromuscular system (i.e., fasciculations, cramps, weakness, and hyporeflexia), and the central nervous system (i.e., confusion, hallucinations, and depressed consciousness). The presence of small pupils with the rest of these findings is diagnostic of organophosphate poisoning. Cholinesterase activity in blood or plasma is likely to be extremely low, confirming the diagnosis. The poisoning is likely to be accompanied by a clear history of overexposure, such as that caused by exposure to a leak or spill from pesticide spraying equipment or by deliberate or accidental ingestion. In contrast, patients with chronic or low-level exposures to organophosphate pesticides usually have poorly defined clinical manifestations, such as mild diarrhea, sweating, myalgias, and malaise (findings that are virtually indistinguishable from those of influenza), and cholinesterase activity levels may be normal. ["Toxidromes" (i.e., symptom complexes of specific poisonings) for other substances are discussed under "Clinical Findings" in subsequent chapters.]

In some cases, the manifestations of toxicity as a consequence of high-dose exposure are totally different from those that are a consequence of low-dose exposure. For example, benzidine causes methemoglobinemia at high doses and bladder cancer at low doses. There are relatively few compounds that cause methemoglobinemia, and most cases can be attributed to a specific toxic substance in the workplace or the environment. However, bladder cancer has a number of known causes in addition to exposure to benzidine, and this makes it difficult to attribute bladder cancer to low-dose toxic exposure. With chronic exposure to low doses, toxic agents are more likely to cause an increase in the incidence of disorders already present in the population than they are to cause a novel disorder.

Because of this nonspecificity of clinical manifestations, a systematic approach to diagnosis is necessary and should include a greater emphasis on the history (general, occupational, and environmental), as discussed in Chapter 2. A list of possible toxic agents should be generated from the exposure history, and their toxicity should be reviewed. The results of physical examination and laboratory tests should be grouped according to findings related to each system or organ, and the findings then should be matched with findings caused by specific toxic substances. A search for causes other than exposure to toxic agents also should be made, and additional diagnostic tests should be ordered as necessary to rule out these other causes. Although biologic measurements of specific toxic substances may be helpful on occasion (see Chapter 36), they usually are not available soon enough for use in cases of acute poisoning, and it is often too late to measure them in cases of chronic exposure.

MANAGEMENT OF TOXIC EFFECTS

Management in most cases of toxicity consists of supportive care, symptomatic treatment, and removal from exposure to the toxic material. In cases of life-threatening toxicity, maintenance of cardiopulmonary function and fluid and electrolyte balance usually are indicated. Methods to enhance elimination, such as forced diuresis, hemodialysis, and hemoperfusion, have not been shown to be effective for treatment of poisoning owing to most toxic agents of industrial origin.

There are only a few specific methods of treatment or "antidotes." Chelating agents may reverse acute toxicity caused by some metals (e.g., lead, arsenic, and mercury), but they are less likely to affect subacute or chronic toxicity (see Chapter 27). Atropine and pralidoxime can be lifesaving in reversing the acute cholinesterase-inhibiting effects of organophosphate pesticides (see Chapter 31). In cases of acute cyanide or hydrogen sulfide poisoning, nitrites may be used to generate formation of cyanmethemoglobin or sulfmethemoglobin (see Chapter 30). Hydroxocobalamin (vitamin B_{12a}) is used in Europe and is currently being tested in the United States as an antidote for cyanide. Use of oxygen counters the effect and enhances the elimination of carbon monoxide (see Chapter 30).

REFERENCES

Altintop L et al: In acute organophosphate poisoning, the efficacy of hemoperfusion on clinical status and mortality. J Intensive Care Med 2005;20:346 [PMID: 16280408].

American Association of Poison Control Centers: The Toxic Exposure Surveillance System (TESS): www.aapcc.org/poison1.htm.

Blanusa M et al: Chelators as antidotes of metal toxicity: Therapeutic and experimental aspects. Curr Med Chem 2005;12:2771 [PMID: 16305472].

Ries NL, Dart RC: New developments in antidotes. Med Clin North Am 2005;89:1379 [PMID: 16227068].

Clinical Immunology

14

Jeffrey L. Kishiyama, MD

Immune hypersensitivity mechanisms play a part in many disorders of occupational medicine. A basic appreciation of the components and physiology of normal immunity is central to an understanding of the pathophysiology of hypersensitivity diseases of the immune system. This chapter reviews the primary immune response and the effector mechanisms, classifies the major mechanisms responsible for immune hypersensitivity disorders found in occupational medicine, lists some examples of these disorders, and concludes with a discussion of diagnosis and treatment of the hypersensitivity diseases often seen in the practice of occupational medicine.

OVERVIEW OF THE IMMUNE RESPONSE

The function of the immune system is to protect the host from invasion by foreign antigens by distinguishing "self" from "nonself" antigens. Such a system is necessary for survival in all animals. A normal immune response relies on the careful coordination of a complex network of specialized cells, organs, and biologic factors necessary for the recognition and subsequent elimination of foreign antigens. An abnormal, exaggerated immune response can cause hypersensitivity to foreign antigens with resulting tissue injury and the expression of a variety of clinical syndromes that are seen often in the practice of occupational medicine.

Innate & Adaptive Immunity

Living organisms have two levels of response to external invasion: (1) a nonspecific, innate system of natural immunity and (2) an adaptive system that is acquired and relies on immunologic memory (Figure 14–1). Innate immunity is present from birth and is nonspecific in its activity. The skin and mucosal barriers serve as the first line of defense of the innate immune system. Soluble factors, such as proteolytic enzymes, the complement system pathway, acute-phase proteins, cytokines, and leukocytes (including phagocytes and natural killer cells) provide additional layers of protection. Despite their lack of specificity, these components are essential because they are largely responsible for the natural immunity to a vast array of environmental microorganisms and foreign substances.

Higher organisms have evolved the adaptive immune system, which is triggered by encounters with foreign agents that have evaded or penetrated the innate immune defenses. The adaptive immune system has specificity for individual foreign antigens and immunologic memory, which allows for an intensified response on subsequent encounter with the same or closely related agent. Secondary immune responses are more rapid, larger, and more efficient than the primary response. Stimulation of the adaptive immune system triggers a complex sequence of events initiating the activation of lymphocytes, the production of antigen-specific antibodies and effector cells, and ultimately, elimination of the inciting substance. Although adaptive immunity is antigen-specific, the repertoire of responses is tremendously diverse, with an estimated 10^9 antigenic specificities.

Antigens & Immunogens

Foreign substances that can induce an immune response are called *antigens* or *immunogens*. Immunogenicity implies that the substance has the ability to react with antigen-binding sites on antibody molecules or T-cell receptors. Complex foreign agents possess distinct and multiple antigenic determinants, or "epitopes," that depend on the peptide sequence and conformational folding of immunogenic proteins. Most immunogens are proteins, although pure carbohydrates may be immunogenic as well. The immune response to a particular immunogen also may depend on the route of exposure to the foreign substance. Bloodborne substances are normally immunoglobulin-bound and removed via the reticuloendothelial system. Occupational allergen exposure through respiratory mucosal surfaces can lead to vigorous local production of immunoglobulin, along with recruitment, activation, and proliferation of leukocytes in involved tissues and regional lymphoid tissues.

Immunologic Effector Cells

A number of effector cells participate in immune defense and hypersensitivity reactions. These include mast cells, basophils, polymorphonuclear neutrophils, eosinophils, macrophages, monocytes, platelets, and lymphocytes. Depending on the type of immune response, many or all

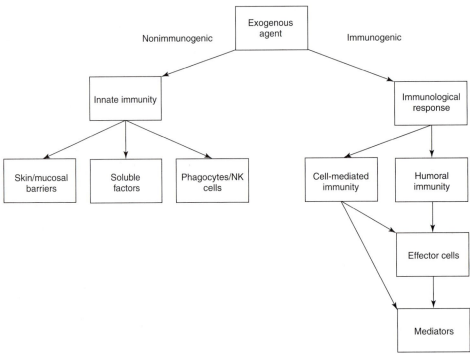

Figure 14–1. Host response to exogenous agents or exposures. NK = natural killer.

play a part. The effector cells have membrane receptors for various chemoattractants and mediators.

Lymphocytes are responsible for the initial specific recognition of antigen. They are functionally and phenotypically divided into B and T lymphocytes. Structurally, B and T lymphocytes cannot be distinguished visually from each other under the microscope; they can be enumerated by flow cytometric phenotyping or by immunohistochemical methods. Approximately 70–80% of circulating blood lymphocytes are T cells, and 10–15% are B cells; the remainder are referred to as *natural killer cells* (also known as *NK cells* or *null cells*).

The thymus-derived cells (T lymphocytes or T cells) are involved in cellular immune responses. B lymphocytes or B cells are involved in humoral or antibody responses. Both T and B lymphocytes are derived from precursor or stem cells in the marrow. Precursors of T cells migrate to the thymus, where they develop some of the functional and cell-surface characteristics of mature T cells. Through positive and negative selection, clones of autoreactive T cells are eliminated, and mature T cells migrate to the peripheral lymphoid tissues. There they enter the pool of long-lived lymphocytes that recirculate from the blood to the lymph.

T lymphocytes are heterogeneous with respect to their cell-surface markers and functional characteristics. Numerous subpopulations of T cells are now recognized. Helper-

inducer T cells (CD4) help to amplify B-cell production of immunoglobulin and amplify T-cell (CD8)-mediated cytotoxicity. Activated CD4 T cells regulate immune responses through cell-to-cell contact and by elaboration of soluble factors or cytokines.

Subsets of helper T cells can be identified on the basis of their pattern of cytokine production. T-helper type 1 (TH$_1$) cells produce gamma-interferon (IFN-γ) and tumor necrosis factor-beta (TNF-β), and T-helper type 2 (TH$_2$) cells produce interleukins 4, 5, 9, and 25, among others. Both subsets produce interleukin (IL)-2, IL-3, IL-10, IL-13, and granulocyte-macrophage colony-stimulating factor (GM-CSF). The TH$_1$ and TH$_2$ phenotypes represent diametrically opposed T-helper immune responses. The TH$_1$ subset of CD4 T cells promotes cellular immune responses to intracellular pathogens and underlies the pathogenesis of delayed-type hypersensitivity. TH$_2$ cells play a central role in immediate hypersensitivity and humoral immune responses because IL-4 and IL-13 promote immunoglobulin (Ig) E production and IL-5 is an eosinophil proliferation and differentiation factor. TH$_1$ and TH$_2$ responses mutually antagonize each other. Although other regulatory mechanisms clearly influence the balance between TH$_1$ and TH$_2$ responses, their polarity has led to the "hygiene hypothesis," a paradigm explaining the immunopathogenesis of atopic diseases.

Two subtypes of CD4+ T helper cells act as suppressor or regulatory T cells. T-helper type 3 (TH$_3$) and T regulatory 1 (Tr$_1$) cells synthesize immunomodulatory cytokines such as transforming growth factor-beta (TGF-β) and IL-10. The generation of these regulatory T cells is controlled by mucosal dendritic cells.

Cytotoxic or "killer" T cells are generated after mature T cells interact with certain foreign antigens. They are responsible for defense against intracellular pathogens (e.g., viruses), tumor immunity, and organ graft rejection. Most killer T cells express the CD8 phenotype, although in certain circumstances CD4 T cells can be cytotoxic. Cytotoxic T cells may kill their target through osmotic lysis, by secretion of TNF, or by induction of apoptosis, that is, programmed cell death.

B-cell maturation proceeds in antigen-independent and antigen-dependent stages. Antigen-independent development occurs in the marrow, where pre-B cells mature into immunoglobulin bearing naive B cells (cells that have not been exposed to antigen previously). In peripheral lymphoid tissues, antigen-dependent activation produces circulating long-lived memory B cells and plasma cells found predominantly in primary follicles and germinal centers of the lymph nodes and spleen. B cells are commonly identified by other surface markers in addition to surface immunoglobulins, including the receptor for the Fc portion of immunoglobulins, B-cell-specific antigens CD19 and CD20, and surface antigens coded for by the HLA-D genetic region in humans. All mature B cells bear surface immunoglobulin that is their antigen-specific receptor. The major role of B cells is differentiation to antibody-secreting plasma cells. However, B cells also may release cytokines and function as antigen-presenting cells.

Macrophages are involved in the ingestion, processing, and presentation of antigens for interaction with lymphocytes. In addition, they are effector cells for certain types of tumor immunity. Circulating monocytes are recruited to sites of inflammation, where they mature into macrophages. Both monocytes and macrophages contain receptors for C3b (activated bound complement) and the Fc portion of IgG and IgE, allowing for activation through antigen-specific and nonspecific immune pathways. Activation of these cells occurs after binding to immune complexes through exposure to various cytokines and after phagocytosis of antigen or particulates, such as silica and asbestos. They contain proteolytic enzymes and are able to synthesize proinflammatory mediators, including cytokines, arachidonic acid metabolites, and oxidative metabolites. Macrophages constitutively express toll-like receptor 4 (TLR$_4$), which can bind bacterial endotoxin, triggering cytokine release. It is hypothesized that macrophage-derived IL-12 and TNF modulate TH$_1$ and TH$_2$ differentiation, thereby affecting the expression of atopy and allergic disease.

NK cells are non-B, non-T lymphocytic cells, which can kill a wide spectrum of target cells. They are recognized by the presence of specific surface antigens (CD16 or CD56). NK cells are capable of binding IgG because of their membrane receptor for the IgG molecule (FcR). Antibody-dependent cell-mediated cytotoxicity (ADCC) occurs when an organism or a cell is coated by antibody and undergoes NK-cell-mediated destruction. Alternatively, NK cells can destroy virally infected cells or tumor cells without involvement of antibody.

Mast cells are basophilic staining cells found chiefly in connective and subcutaneous tissue. They have prominent granules that are the source of many mediators of immediate hypersensitivity and have 30,000–200,000 cell-surface membrane receptors for the Fc fragment of IgE. When an allergen molecule cross-links two adjacent mast cell surface–associated IgE antibodies, calcium-dependent cellular activation leads to the release of both preformed and newly generated mediators. Mast cells also have surface receptors for anaphylatoxins (activated complement fragments, C3a, C4a, and C5a), cytokines, and neuropeptides such as substance P. Activation by these non-IgE-mediated mechanisms may contribute to host immunity and provide ties between the immune and neuroendocrine systems. Mast-cell-deficient mice display a particular vulnerability to sepsis and rapid death after peritonitis possibly owing to insufficient TNF-α production during bacterial infection. Mast cells also appear in areas of wound healing and in fibrotic lung disease. Experimentally, mast-cell-derived mediators promote angiogenesis and fibrogenesis, suggesting that their presence in these sites is pathologically relevant. Neutrophils are granulocytes that phagocytose and destroy foreign antigens and microbial organisms. They are attracted to the site of antigen by chemotactic factors, including plasma-activated complement 5 (C5a), leukotriene B$_4$ (LTB$_4$), granulocyte colony-stimulating factor (G-CSF), GM-CSF, IL-8, and platelet-activating factor (PAF). They possess receptors for the Fc fragment of IgG and IgM antibodies (specific opsonins) and for C3b (nonspecific opsonin). Smaller antigens are phagocytosed and destroyed by lysosomal enzymes. Particles too large to be phagocytosed are destroyed by locally released lysosomal enzymes. Neutrophils contain or generate a number of antimicrobial factors, including oxidative metabolites, superoxide, and H$_2$O$_2$; myeloperoxidase, which catalyzes the production of hypochlorite; and proteolytic enzymes, including collagenase, elastase, and cathepsin B. Some or all of these factors may play a part in a number of hypersensitivity reactions, including the type I late asthmatic response, the type II cytotoxin reaction, and type III immune complex disease (see "Classification of Immune Hypersensitivity Disorders" below).

Eosinophils play both a proactive and a modulating role in inflammation. They are attracted to the site of the antigen-antibody reactions by PAF, C5a, chemokines, histamine, and LTB_4. They are important in the defense against parasites. When stimulated, they release numerous inflammatory factors, including major basic protein (MBP), eosinophil-derived neurotoxin, eosinophil cationic protein (ECP), eosinophil peroxidase, lysosomal hydrolases, and LTC_4. MBP destroys parasites, impairs ciliary beating, and causes exfoliation of respiratory epithelial cells; it may trigger histamine release from mast cells and basophils. Eosinophil-derived products may play a role in the development of airway hyperreactivity.

MEDIATORS OF IMMEDIATE HYPERSENSITIVITY

Mediators of immediate hypersensitivity are chemicals generated or released by effector cells following activation. They have various biologic activities and normally function in host defense, but they play a pathologic role in immune hypersensitivity. They may exist in a preformed state in the granules of mast cells and basophils or are newly synthesized at the time of activation of these and some other nucleated cells (Tables 14–1 and 14–2). A number of stimuli activate mast cells and basophils, including antigen-IgE interactions, binding of anaphylatoxins (C3a, C4a, C5a), lectins, neuropeptides, and certain drugs (morphine, codeine). Increased awareness of

Table 14–1. Mediators of immediate hypersensitivity.

Vasoactive and smooth-muscle constricting mediators
  Preformed
    Histamine
  Generated
    Arachidonic acid metabolites (PGD_2, LTC_4)
    PAF
    Adenosine
Chemotactic mediators
  Eosinophil-directed
    Eosinophilic chemotactic factor of anaphylaxis (ECFA)
    ECF oligopeptides
    PAF
  Neutrophil-directed
    High-molecular-weight neutrophilic chemotactic factor
    LTB_4
    PAF
Enzymatic mediators
  Neutral proteases
    Tryptase
    Chymase
  Lysosomal hydrolases
  Other enzymes
    Superoxide dismutase
    Peroxidase

the immunologic and physiologic effects of mediators has led to a better understanding of immunopathology and provides potential targets for future pharmacotherapies.

Preformed mediators include histamine, eosinophil, and neutrophil chemoattractants, proteoglycans (heparin, chondroitin sulfate), and various proteolytic enzymes. Histamine is a bioactive amine, packaged in dense intracellular granules, that when released binds to membrane-bound H_1, H_2, and H_3 receptors, resulting in significant physiologic effects. Binding to H_1 receptors causes smooth-muscle contraction, vasodilatation, increased vascular permeability, and stimulation of nasal mucous glands. Stimulation of H_2 receptors causes enhanced gastric acid secretion, mucus secretion, and leukocyte chemotaxis. Binding to H_3 receptors inhibits histamine release and synthesis. Histamine is important in the pathogenesis of allergic rhinitis, allergic asthma, and anaphylaxis.

Newly generated mediators include kinins, PAF, and arachidonic acid metabolites, including leukotrienes and prostaglandins. In many immune cells, arachidonic acid, liberated from membrane phospholipid bilayers, is metabolized either by the lipoxygenase pathway to form leukotrienes (LT) or by the cyclooxygenase pathway to form prostaglandins (PG) and thromboxanes A_2 and B_2 (TXA_2 and TXB_2). LTB_4 is a potent chemoattractant for neutrophils. LTC_4, LTD_4, and LTE_4 constitute slow-reacting substance of anaphylaxis, which has bronchial smooth muscle spasmogenic potency 100–1000 times that of histamine and which also causes vascular dilation and vascular permeability.

Almost all nucleated cells generate prostaglandins. The most important members are PGD_2, PGE_2, PGF_2, and PGI_2 (prostacyclin). Human mast cells produce large amounts of PGD_2, which causes vasodilatation, vascular permeability, and airway constriction. Activated polymorphonuclear neutrophils and macrophages generate PGF_{2a}, a bronchoconstrictor, and PGE_2, a bronchodilator. PGI_2 causes platelet disaggregation. TXA_2 causes platelet aggregation, bronchial constriction, and vasoconstriction.

Macrophages, neutrophils, eosinophils, and mast cells generate PAF, which causes platelet aggregation, vasodilatation, increased vascular permeability, and bronchial smooth-muscle contraction. PAF is the most potent eosinophil chemoattractant described and also plays a role in anaphylaxis. The kinins are vasoactive peptides formed in plasma when kallikrein, released by basophils and mast cells, digests plasma kininogen. They cause slow, sustained contraction of bronchial and vascular smooth muscle, vascular permeability, secretion of mucus, and stimulation of pain fibers. Kinins also may play a role in human angioedema and anaphylaxis.

Complement Cascades

The union of antigen with IgG or IgM antibody initiates activation of the classic complement pathway. Comple-

Table 14–2. Action of mediators in hypersensitivity reactions.

	Bronchial Constriction	Chemotaxis		Platelet Activation	Increased Vascular Permeability	Mucus Production	Increased Pruritus
		PMS	Eosinophil				
Histamine	X	X	X		X	X (nasal)	X
Leukotrienes							
C	X				X	X	
D	X				X	X	
E	X					X	
5-HETE		X					
PGD$_2$	X				X		
TXA$_2$	X			X			
Kallikrein					X		
PAF	X		X	X			
NCFA		X					
ECFA		X	X				

ECFA = eosinophilic chemotactic factor; 5-HETE = hydroxyeicosatetraenoic acid; NCFA = neutrophilic chemotactic factor; PAF = platelet-activating factor; PGD$_2$ = prostaglandin D$_2$; TXA$_2$ = thromboxane A$_2$.

ment-fixing sites on these immune complexes are exposed, allowing binding of the first component of the complement sequence, C1q. Other components of the complement sequence are subsequently bound, activated, and cleaved, eventually leading to cell lysis. Important by-products of the classic pathway include activated cleavage products, the anaphylatoxins C3a, C5a, and less potent C4a. C5a is a potent leukocyte chemotactic factor that also causes mediator release from mast cells and basophils. C4b and C3b mediate binding of immune complexes to phagocytic cells, facilitating opsonization.

Activation of the complement sequence by the alternative pathway is initiated by a number of agents, including lipopolysaccharides, trypsin-like molecules, aggregated IgA and IgG, and cobra venom. Activation of the alternative pathway does not require the presence of antigen-antibody complexes, nor does it use the early components of the complement sequence, C1, C4, and C2. Ultimately, owing to activation of the classic or alternative pathway, activation of the terminal complement sequence occurs, resulting in cell lysis and/or tissue inflammation.

Cytokines

Many immune functions are regulated or mediated by cytokines, which are soluble factors secreted by activated immune cells. Cytokines can be organized functionally into groups according to their major activities: (1) those that promote and mediate natural immunity, such as IL-1, IL-6, IL-8, TNF, and interferon (IFN)-γ, (2) those that support allergic inflammation, such as IL-4, IL-5, and IL-13, (3) those that control lymphocyte regulatory activity, such as IL-10, IL-12, and IFN-γ, and (4) those that act as hematopoietic growth factors, such as IL-3, IL-7, and GM-CSF (Table 14–3). This complicated network of interacting cytokines functions to modulate cellular function and immunologic responses. Many ongoing research investigations are focused on modulating cytokine responses as a way to control or treat disease processes.

Response to Antigen

The major immunologic responses to antigen include the elimination of antigen through antibody-mediated events (humoral response) and the direct killing of target cells by a subset of T lymphocytes called *cytotoxic T lymphocytes* (CTLs) (cellular response). The series of events that embody the immune response includes antigen processing and presentation, lymphocyte recognition and activation, cellular and/or humoral immune responses, and antigenic destruction or elimination (Figure 14–2).

A. ANTIGEN PROCESSING AND PRESENTATION

Most foreign immunogens are not recognized by the immune system in their native form and require capture and processing by specialized antigen-presenting cells.

Table 14–3. Major cytokines.

Cytokine	Major effects
IL-1	Endogenous pyrogen, lymphocyte activating factor
IL-2	Activation and expansion of antigen-specific lymphocytes
IL-3	Growth factor for hematopoietic stem
IL-4	Switch factor for IgE and IgG1, promotes TH_2 response
IL-5	Activates and enhances survival of eosinophils
IL-6	Promotes differentiation of B cells into plasma cells, stimulates production of acute phase reactants
IL-7	Promotes lymphocyte proliferation
IL-8	Chemotactic factor for neutrophils
IL-10	Inhibits antigen presentation, expression of MHC II and adhesion molecules
IL-12	Promotes TH_1 response, inhibits TH_2 response, activates NK cells
IL-13	Promotes IgE synthesis
IFN	Inhibits viral replication, stimulates MHC I expression
TNF	Cytotoxic for tumor cells, proinflammatory effects similar to IL-1
GM-CSF	Enhances proliferation, differentiation and survival for neutrophils, macrophages, megakaryocytes, eosinophils
TGF-β	Inhibits IL-2 responses, promotes wound healing and fibrosis

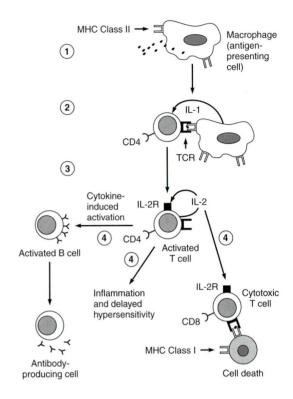

Figure 14–2. The normal immune response. (1) Antigen processing and presentation by antigen-presenting cells. (2) Recognition of antigen-MHC complex by CD4 T lymphocytes induces IL-1 secretion by antigen-presenting cells and subsequent cellular activation. (3) Activated T lymphocytes express IL-2 receptors and secrete IL-2, which upregulates IL-2 receptor expression in an autocrine fashion. (4) Activated CD4 T lymphocytes can stimulate CD8 cytotoxic T lymphocytes to mediate cellular cytotoxicity, B-lymphocyte activation, and differentiation into antibody-producing plasma cells, which mediate humoral immunity or delayed hypersensitivity and other inflammatory reactions.

Antigen-presenting cells include macrophages, dendritic cells in lymphoid tissue, Langerhans cells in the skin, Kupffer cells in the liver, microglial cells in the nervous system, and B lymphocytes. Following an encounter with immunogens, the antigen-presenting cells internalize the foreign substance by phagocytosis or pinocytosis, modify their parent structure, and display antigenic fragments of the native protein on their surface.

B. T-Lymphocyte Recognition and Activation

The recognition of processed antigen by specialized T lymphocytes known as "helper" T (CD4+) lymphocytes constitutes the critical event in the immune response. The helper T lymphocytes orchestrate the many cells and biologic signals that are necessary to carry out the immune response. Helper T lymphocytes recognize processed antigen displayed by antigen-presenting cells only in association with polymorphic cell-surface proteins encoded by the major histocompatibility (MHC) gene complex. Endogenously synthesized viral proteins are processed in association with MHC class I molecules, whereas exogenous foreign antigens that require an antibody-mediated response are expressed in association with MHC class II structures. All somatic cells express MHC class I, whereas only the specialized antigen-presenting cells can express MHC class II. Cytotoxic T lymphocytes (CD8+) recognize target cells bearing MHC class I complexed to antigen, whereas helper T lymphocytes expressing the CD4 antigen recognize antigen in the context of MHC class II.

Two signals are required for activation of these T lymphocytes: (1) binding of the antigen-specific T-cell receptor (CD3) to the antigen-MHC complex and (2) costimulation through CD28 (on T cells)–B7 (on antigen-presenting cells) interactions. These two signals induce the expression of IL-2 receptors on the surface of the CD4+ lymphocytes, as well as the production of various cell growth and differentiation factors (cytokines). Activated CD4+ T lymphocytes subsequently trigger the effector cells that mediate the cellular and humoral arms of the immune response.

C. ACTIVATION OF CYTOTOXIC T LYMPHOCYTES (CELLULAR IMMUNE RESPONSE)

CTLs eliminate target cells (virally infected cells, tumor cells, or foreign tissues), constituting the cellular immune response. These "killer" T lymphocytes release substances called *cytotoxins* that lead to cytolysis or destruction of infected target cells. CTLs arise from the antigen-driven activation and differentiation of resting mature small lymphocyte precursors. Activated CTLs manufacture a membrane pore-forming protein (perforin or cytolysin), IFN-γ, and TNF-β. Killing of target cells by CTLs requires direct cell-to-cell contact and proceeds sequentially by (1) adhesive interactions between CTLs and target cell, (2) activation of CTLs by antigen engagement of CTL receptors, (3) delivery of the lethal hit to target cells by poorly characterized mechanisms, and (4) programmed cell death of target cells.

D. ACTIVATION OF B LYMPHOCYTES (HUMORAL IMMUNE RESPONSE)

Activated helper T cells also may induce the growth and differentiation of B lymphocytes, which mediate the humoral or antibody-mediated response. Cytokines with growth and differentiation activity promote the proliferation and terminal differentiation of B cells into high-rate antibody-producing cells called *plasma cells*. B lymphocytes also may bind and internalize foreign antigen directly, process that antigen, and present it to CD4+ T lymphocytes. A pool of activated B lymphocytes may differentiate to form memory cells, which respond more rapidly and efficiently to subsequent encounters with identical or closely related antigenic structures. These secondary immune responses are more rapid and larger as a consequence of immunologic memory.

E. ANTIBODY STRUCTURE AND FUNCTION

The primary function of mature B lymphocytes is to synthesize antibodies. Antibodies are immunoglobulin molecules directed toward specific antigens. It has been estimated that the repertoire of immunoglobulin antigen specificities in the human body is 10^7. Immunoglobulins serve a variety of secondary biologic roles, including complement fixation, transplacental passive immunization of neonates, and facilitation of phagocytosis (opsonization),

all of which participate in host defense against disease. Circulating immunoglobulins have both a unique specificity for one particular antigenic structure and enough diversity to encounter a broad range of antigenic materials. This diversity arises from complex DNA rearrangements and RNA processing within B lymphocytes early in their ontogeny. All immunoglobulin molecules share a four-chain polypeptide structure consisting of two heavy and two light chains (Figure 14–3). Each chain includes an amino-terminal portion containing the variable (V) region and a carboxy-terminal portion containing four or five constant (C) regions. V regions are highly variable structures that form the antigen-binding site, whereas the C domains support effector functions of the molecules. There are five classes (isotypes) of immunoglobulins, which are defined on the basis of differences in the C region of the heavy chains.

IgG is the predominant immunoglobulin in serum. IgG antibodies are strong precipitins, and three subclasses—IgG_1, IgG_2, and IgG_3—can activate complement, qualities contributing to the pathogenesis of serum sickness and certain types of hypersensitivity pneumonitis (e.g., bird breeder's disease).

IgA is the predominant immunoglobulin on mucous membrane surfaces. It exists predominantly as a monomer in serum and as a dimer or trimer when secreted on mucous membrane surfaces. When the dimer or trimer passes through the epithelial cells to a mucous membrane surface, it acquires a smaller molecule called a *secretory piece* that stabilizes the molecule and prevents its degradation by proteolytic enzymes. IgA antibodies protect the host from foreign antigens on mucous membrane surfaces, but they do not fix complement by the classic pathway.

IgM is a pentamer that is found almost exclusively in the intravascular compartment. IgM antibodies are potent agglutinins and fix complement. They may mediate the trimellitic anhydride pulmonary anemia syndrome. IgD is a monomeric immunoglobulin. Its biologic function is unknown.

IgE is the heaviest immunoglobulin monomer, with a normal concentration in serum varying from 20–100 IU, but the concentration may be five times normal or even higher in an atopic individual. The Fc portion of IgE binds to receptors on the surfaces of mast cells and basophils. IgE antibodies play an important role in immediate hypersensitivity reactions such as nasal allergy and allergic asthma in veterinarians, laboratory animal handlers, and enzyme detergent industry workers.

F. HUMORAL MECHANISMS OF ANTIGEN ELIMINATION

Antibodies can induce the elimination of foreign antigen through a number of different mechanisms. Binding of antibody to bacterial toxins or foreign venoms promotes

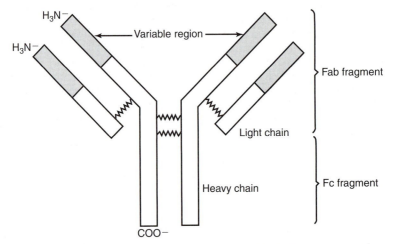

Figure 14–3. Structure of the immunoglobulin molecule. The immunoglobulin molecule is composed of two heavy and two light chains. The light chain and the amino-terminal (H₃N⁻) half of the heavy chain make up Fab, the antibody-binding fragment of the molecule. The carboxyl-terminal (COO⁻) halves of the heavy chains make up the Fc or crystalline half of the immunoglobulin molecule, which is responsible for the unique biologic activities of a given immunoglobulin class. Interchain disulfide bonds (⌇⌇⌇) bind the heavy and light chains.

elimination of antigen-antibody "immune complexes" through the reticuloendothelial system. Antibodies also can coat bacterial surfaces, allowing clearance by macrophages in a process known as *opsonization.* Some classes of antibodies can complex with antigen and activate the complement cascade, which culminates in lysis of the target cell. Finally, the major class of antibody, IgG, can bind to natural killer cells that subsequently complex with target cells and release cytotoxins through antibody-dependent cytotoxicity (ADCC).

CLASSIFICATION OF IMMUNE HYPERSENSITIVITY DISORDERS

Gell and Coombs devised a classification scheme to define the basic immunopathologic mechanisms of hypersensitivity by four distinct types of reactions (types I–IV) (Figure 14–4). Types I–III are all mediated by specific antibodies (humoral immune response), whereas type IV results from the actions of sensitized T lymphocytes (cell-mediated immune response). All defined mechanisms require an initial exposure to antigen, which induces a primary immune response (sensitization). Subsequent exposure to the same antigen (challenge) following a short lag period (usually at least 1 week) evokes the hypersensitivity response.

Elimination of foreign antigen by cellular or humoral processes is integrally linked to the inflammatory response, in which cellular messengers (cytokines) and antibodies trigger the recruitment of additional cells and the release of endogenous vasoactive and proinflammatory inflammatory mediators. Inflammation may have both positive and deleterious effects. Tight control of inflammatory mechanisms promotes efficient elimination of foreign substances and prevents uncontrolled lymphocyte activation and unregulated antibody production. Inappropriate activation or dysregulation of the system, however, can perpetuate inflammatory processes leading to tissue damage and organ dysfunction. Inflammation is responsible for hypersensitivity reactions and for many of the clinical effects of autoimmunity.

Type I: Anaphylactic or Immediate Hypersensitivity Reactions

These reactions are initiated by the interaction of antigen with specific IgE antibodies bound to mast cells and basophils with the subsequent release of inflammatory mediators. Examples of type I reactions in the practice of occupational medicine include allergic rhinitis and asthma seen in bakers and animal handlers and systemic anaphylaxis in beekeepers and health care workers (latex allergy).

Initial exposure to antigen in a genetically predisposed host leads to the synthesis of antigen-specific IgE by mature B cells, constituting the atopic state. Isotype switching to IgE production requires the cytokine IL-4, along with additional B lymphocyte activation and differentiation factors (IL-5, IL-6, IL-13). In contrast, IFN-γ, a TH_1 cytokine, inhibits IL-4-dependent IgE synthesis in humans. It has been hypothesized that the balance of IL-4 responses and those favoring IFN-γ may influence whether atopy develops in an individual.

Helper (CD4+) T lymphocytes play a central role in the induction of normal immune responses. Activated T lymphocytes that release TH_2-characteristic cytokines have been found at sites of inflammation in allergic airway disease and are believed to direct the immune response toward allergic inflammation.

Antigen-specific IgE binds to high-affinity Fc receptors on tissue mast cells and basophils as well as to low-affinity Fc receptors on lymphocytes, macrophages, eosinophils, and platelets, thus sensitizing these cells for future allergen encounters. On reexposure to allergen, the sensitized individual can mount an immediate hypersensitivity response. Mast cells, armed with antigen-specific IgE on their surfaces, can bind polyvalent allergen, cross-linking adjacent IgE molecules, thereby activating and degranulating the cell. Table 14–4 includes many occupational causes of immediate hypersensitivity reactions. Common environmental aeroallergens causing IgE-mediated reactions include pollen, house dust mites, mold, and animal dander. Activation of mast cells and basophils induces both the release of preformed mediators from cytoplasmic granules (i.e., histamine, chemotactic factors, and enzymes) and the synthesis and release of newly generated mediators (i.e., prostaglandins, leukotrienes, and PAF). Mast cells and basophils also have the ability to synthesize and release proinflammatory cytokines, growth factors, and regulatory factors that interact in complex networks.

The interaction of mediators with specific target organs and cells frequently induces a biphasic response: an early effect on blood vessels, smooth muscle, and secretory glands marked by vascular leakiness, smooth-muscle constriction, mucus hypersecretion, and a late response characterized by mucosal edema and the influx

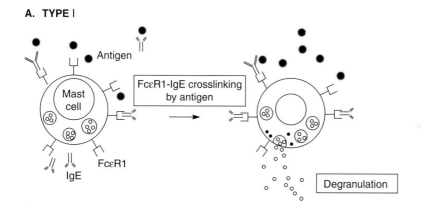

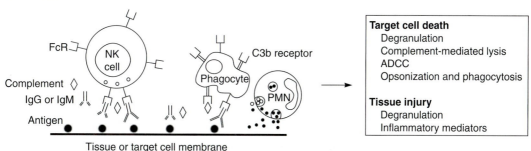

Figure 14–4. Hypersensitivity immune responses. **A:** Type I reaction. Mast cells and basophils bind IgE via high-affinity Fc receptors (FcεR1). Antigen binding and cross-linking of FcεR1-IgE complexes induce cellular degranulation and release of inflammatory mediators. **B:** Type II reaction. IgG or IgM antibodies against tissue or cellular antigens induces complement activation, which results in cell death and tissue injury. *(continued).*

C. TYPE III

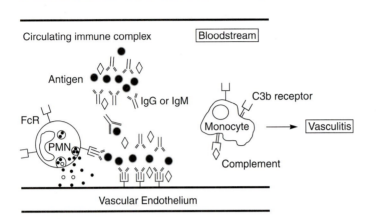

D. TYPE IV

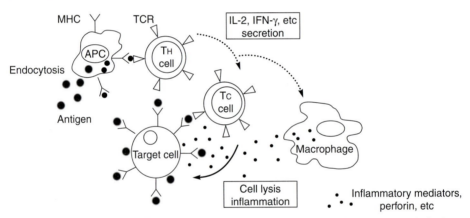

Figure 14–4. (continued) C: Type III reaction. Circulating immune complexes composed of soluble antigen and IgG or IgM deposit on vascular endothelium of various tissues, which activates the complement cascade. Polymorphonuclear leukocytes (PMNs) and other phagocytes are attracted to these sites of immune complex deposition via their Fc and C3b receptors and are induced to degranulate and phagocytose the complexes, resulting in local tissue injury and vasculitis. ***D:*** Type IV reaction. Via their T-cell receptors, helper T cells recognize target-cell antigenic peptides bound to antigen-presenting cells. This T-cell recognition results in the secretion of IL-2, IFN-γ, and other cytokines that are required for activation of tissue macrophages and cytotoxic T cells. Cytotoxic T cells recognize the same antigen bound to target cells and induce lysis by perforin and other molecules secreted by cytotoxic T cells. ADCC = antibody-dependent cell-mediated cytotoxicity; APC = antigen-presenting cell; Tc = cytotoxic T cell; TCR = T-cell receptor; TH = T-helper cell.

of inflammatory cells. The early-phase response occurs within minutes of an antigen exposure. In allergic rhinoconjunctivitis, the early-phase response is marked grossly by erythema, localized edema, rhinorrhea, and pruritus that result largely from the interaction of histamine with target tissues of the upper airway and con-

junctival mucosa. Histologically, the early response is characterized by vasodilatation, edema, and a mild cellular infiltrate of mostly granulocytes.

The late-phase response either may follow the early-phase response (dual response) or may occur as an isolated event (isolated late phase). Late-phase reactions

Table 14–4. Materials causally linked to rhinitis and asthma in the workplace.

	Allergen	Occupational Exposure
Plant material	Aromatic herbs, spices	Food industry workers
	Buckwheat	Food industry workers
	Carob bean flour	Food industry workers
	Coffee beans	Coffee Roasters
	Colophony	Solder workers
	Cotton	Cotton workers
	Fodder	Dairy farmers
	Grain dust	Bakers, millers
	Guar gum	Carpet manufacturers, pharmaceutical workers
	Henna	Hairdressers
	Hops	Brewers
	Latex	Health care workers, laboratory workers, housekeepers
	Obeche (African maple)	Sauna builders
	Sesame, fennel, anise seeds	Food industry workers
	Rose hips	Health food workers
	Tobacco	Tobacco workers
	Wood dusts	Construction workers, carpenters, sawmill workers, craftsmen
Animal and insect products	Animal danders	Veterinarians, farmers, zoo handlers
	Animal urinary proteins	Laboratory animal workers (rodents)
	Crustaceans	Food processors
	Food mites	Food handlers (especially handling cheese, poultry, chorizo, salty ham)
	Grasshoppers, midges	Laboratory workers
	Lactalbumin (cow's milk protein), egg proteins	Bakers, confectioners, food processors
	Live fish bait	Anglers
	Red spider mites	Nursery workers
	Storage mites	Grain workers, bakers
Fungi and mold		Farmers, gardeners, librarians, logging workers, vintners
Chemicals	Acid anhydrides	Plastic manufacturers
	Diacrylates	Auto body workers
	Diisocyanates	Polyurethane plastic and foam workers, spray painters
	Epoxy resins	Epoxy manufacturers
	Formaldehyde	Hospital workers, manufacturers, morticians
	Glutaraldehyde	Hospital workers, paper industry workers
	Persulfates (permanent wave solution)	Beauticians

(continued)

Table 14–4. Materials causally linked to rhinitis and asthma in the workplace. (Continued)

	Allergen	Occupational Exposure
Chemicals (cont.)	Reactive dyes	Dye manufacturers
	Sulfites	Food processors
Enzymes	β-Amylase	Bakers
	Bacterial enzymes	Detergent workers, pharmaceutical workers
	Lactase	Pharmaceutical workers
	Pectinase, glucanase	Fruit processors
Metals	Aluminum	Solder workers
	Chromium	Cement workers, tanners
	Cobalt	Hard metal workers
	Nickel	Metal workers
	Platinum salts	Catalyst manufacturers
	Stainless steel vapor	Welders
Pharmaceuticals	Antibiotics	Health care providers
	Corticotropin-releasing hormone	Pharmaceutical workers
	Psyllium	Health care providers

begin 2–4 hours after initial antigen exposure, reach maximal activity at 6–12 hours, and usually resolve within 12–24 hours. The late-phase response is characterized grossly by erythema, induration, heat, burning, and itching and microscopically by an influx of primarily eosinophils and mononuclear cells. There is strong circumstantial evidence suggesting that eosinophils are important proinflammatory cells in allergic airway disease, particularly asthma. Eosinophils are sampled frequently from the nasal mucosa of patients with allergic rhinitis and from the sputum of asthmatics. Products of activated eosinophils such as MBP and eosinophilic cationic protein are destructive to airway epithelial tissue and are associated with airways hyperreactivity. Epithelial disruption is a feature of patients with both atopic dermatitis and asthma. Immune cells infiltrating tissues in the late response may further elaborate cytokines and histamine-releasing factors that perpetuate the inflammatory response, leading to a sustained hyperresponsiveness and disruption of the target tissue (e.g., bronchi, skin, or nasal mucosa). As exposure to allergen persists, onset and resolution of the late-phase response becomes nebulous as chronic tissue inflammation develops. Late-phase reactivity has been found in atopic disease states, including allergic rhinitis and conjunctivitis, asthma, food-sensitive atopic dermatitis, and anaphylaxis. It is possible that dual asthmatic responses seen in individuals with detergent worker's asthma, tri-

mellitic anhydride asthma, and baker's asthma represent clinical examples of bronchial late-phase responses. Targeting the late-phase response with anti-inflammatory therapies, such as topical corticosteroids, remains a cornerstone of the medical management for allergic rhinitis and asthma. Immediate hypersensitivity can be demonstrated in vivo by a prick or intradermal skin test to specific antigen or in vitro by the radioallergosorbent test (RAST) or the enzyme-linked immunosorbent assay (ELISA).

Type II: Cytotoxic Reactions

In type II reactions, the antigen is a cell-surface protein or antigenic substance that binds covalently to a cell-surface protein (see Figure 14–4). In transfusion reactions, the antigen is a protein on the cell membrane of the incompatible erythrocyte. In some type II hypersensitivity disorders, a low-molecular-weight substance such as trimellitic anhydride (TMA), acting as a hapten, attaches to a host cell-surface protein that acts as a carrier. In the pulmonary disease–anemia syndrome, occurring in workers repeatedly exposed to high concentrations of volatile TMA, the chemical combines with an erythrocyte membrane protein or pulmonary basement cell membrane protein to form a complete antigen that, in turn, stimulates the formation of IgG or IgM antibody. On reexposure, cell-surface-bound antigen-antibody union takes place, facilitating phagocytosis or activating the terminal complement sequence leading to cell lysis. The Coombs test is helpful in demonstrating IgG antibody on the surface of red cells and leukocytes.

Type III: Immune Complex Reaction

Type III reactions depend on the union of soluble antigen with soluble IgG or IgM antibody and subsequent activation of the complement sequence with end-organ tissue damage (see Figure 14–4). In the Arthus reaction subtype, an immune complex is formed locally; in the second subtype, serum sickness, circulating complexes are deposited in various tissues.

Maurice Arthus, who injected bovine serum albumin intradermally into a previously immunologically sensitized rabbit, first described the Arthus reaction in 1903. Induration and erythema were noted at the injection site in 2 hours, peaked at 6 hours, and resolved in 12–24 hours. In some instances, necrosis developed at the site. The manifestations of the Arthus reaction are the result of binding of localized but not fixed antigen to circulating antibody, forming an immune complex in situ. This reaction may be operative in hypersensitivity pneumonitis. An example is pigeon breeder's disease. The antigen, serum dried in pigeon excreta, is inhaled, sensitizing the host and leading to IgG and IgM antibody formation. On subsequent exposure to inhaled antigen, localized alveolar immune complex formation occurs. The complex activates the complement cascade, with opsonin formation, enhancement of phagocytosis, and generation of C3a, C4a, and C5a anaphylatoxins, leading to vasodilatation and increased vascular permeability and facilitating the diffusion of other mediators and effector cells to the reaction site. The ingestion of immune complexes by polymorphonuclear cells causes activation of monocytes and macrophages and stimulates the release of lysosomal enzymes. PAF and thromboxane also can cause platelet aggregation and activation, leading to thrombus formation. In serum sickness, or *immune complex disease,* circulating antigen and IgG antibodies combine, forming immune complexes that in antigen excess form microprecipitates. These are filtered from the circulation at the postcapillary venule in tissues such as skin, kidney, joints, and lungs. Just as in the Arthus reaction, the complement cascade is activated, and tissue end-organ damage ensues. Clinical manifestations of serum sickness include generalized urticaria, polyserositis (i.e., arthritis, pleuritis, and pericarditis), fever, and nephritis.

Examples of circulating immune complex disease include classic serum sickness, which occurs 8–13 days after injection of the foreign serum or administration of drugs, and systemic lupus erythematosus, in which the antigen is host DNA. The presence of antibody in type III reactions may be demonstrated by the Ouchterlony gel diffusion technique.

Type IV: Cellular Immunity

Type IV delayed hypersensitivity reactions are not mediated by antibody; instead, they are mediated primarily by T lymphocytes (cell-mediated immunity). In contrast to type I reactions, which often occur within minutes of antigen challenge dose, type IV reactions require 24–72 hours to appear. Classic examples of type IV immunopathologic changes are the tuberculin skin test reactions and contact dermatitis.

CTLs that induce necrosis of antigen-bearing cells represent an important immune system function in the elimination of tumor cells, virus-infected cells, or transplanted cells bearing foreign proteins, but inappropriate activation or dysregulation of the system can result in immunologic tissue injury (type IV hypersensitivity). The histologic appearance of T-cell-mediated cytotoxicity is characterized by necrosis of affected cells and marked lymphocytic infiltration in affected tissues.

The activated T cells also promote the migration of mononuclear phagocytes into sites of antigen deposition and induce the activation and differentiation of macrophages (see Figure 14–4). Activated macrophages have increased capacity and efficiency for killing microorganisms. Type IV injury may result from the uncontrolled activation of tissue macrophages.

Contact dermatitis is a cutaneous type IV hypersensitivity reaction that usually occurs when low-molecular-weight (MW < 500) sensitizers haptenate with dermal proteins, forming a complete antigen. The complete antigen is recognized and bound by sensitized T cells that release cytokines, activating macrophages and promoting the subsequent inflammatory skin reaction. In addition, type IV hypersensitivity also may contribute to the pathogenesis of hypersensitivity pneumonitis. Antigens derived from mold spores or thermophilic actinomycetes bind with sensitized T lymphocytes to initiate the reaction. Patch testing with standard antigen-impregnated patches is used to demonstrate delayed-type contact sensitivity.

The Hygiene Hypothesis

Great attention has been drawn to changes in microbial exposure patterns by children and the possible link to the increased prevalence of allergic diseases in Western industrialized nations. Microbial interactions with innate and adaptive immune cells clearly shape defensive immune responses but also may modulate and regulate immune deviations responsible for hypersensitivity syndromes. Paradoxically, children raised on rural farms appear to have a decreased risk of hypersensitivity to environmental allergens, and children entered into day care at an early age appear to enjoy a lower risk of developing chronic asthma. It has been proposed that exposure to endotoxin or microbial by-products induces a shift in the TH_1-TH_2 balance, biased toward a TH_2 response to environmental allergens. TH$_2$ helper T cells play a central role in immediate hypersensitivity and humoral immune responses because IL-4 promotes IgE production and IL-5 is an eosinophil proliferation and differentiation factor.

REFERENCES

Chinen J, Shearer WT: Basic and clinical immunology. J Allergy Clin Immunol 2005;116:411 [PMID: 16083798].

Vandenbulcke L et al: The innate immune system and its role in allergic disorders. Int Arch Allergy Immunol 2006;139:159 [PMID: 16388196].

NONIMMUNE ACTIVATION OF INFLAMMATORY REACTIONS

Clinical symptoms and inflammatory reactions also can be initiated by nonimmunologic activation of cellular and humoral effector mechanisms. Substances such as plant-derived lectins (concanavalin A from the jack bean, phytohemagglutinins from the red kidney bean, and pokeweed mitogen), gram-negative polysaccharides, pneumococcal polysaccharides, fungal by-products, Epstein-Barr virus, trypsin, papain, silica, zinc oxide, and asbestos act as "pseudoantigens," nonimmunologically activating lymphocytes, macrophages, mast cells, basophils, and in some cases, the complement system. Nonspecific activators functioning in concert with specific antigens may play an important role in the induction of immune hypersensitivity reactions observed in many occupational immune disorders. Toxic constituents have been identified in many organic dusts, including endotoxin, mycotoxins, and volatile organic compounds, that have been implicated in occupational syndromes characterized by constitutional symptoms, fevers, and dyspnea. Some of these compounds have been studied in vitro and in vivo, demonstrating nonantigenic release of mediators and proinflammatory effects. Occupational exposure to organic acids, such as plicatic acid (red cedar) and abietic acid (colophony or resin), can cause airway epithelial cell desquamation, activation of complement, induction of bronchial hyperreactivity, and stimulation of afferent C fibers, inducing asthma and airways inflammation through toxic injury and neurogenic mechanisms.

Reactive airways dysfunction syndrome (RADS) is characterized by the acute emergence of bronchial hyperreactivity and symptoms of asthma after an acute exposure to high levels of respiratory irritants, usually toxic chemicals, smoke, or particulates. In contrast to the hypersensitivity syndromes, there is no latent period of sensitization.

IMMUNE HYPERSENSITIVITY OCCUPATIONAL DISORDERS

The most common occupational immune hypersensitivity disorders include allergic asthma or rhinocon-

junctivitis, hypersensitivity pneumonitis, and allergic contact dermatitis. The reactions depend on the host, the duration, the degree and type of sensitization, and the antigen.

Allergic asthma and allergic rhinitis occur when sensitized workers inhale specific antigen. Occupational asthma is probably one of the most prevalent of the immunologically mediated occupational disorders, although knowledge of its incidence is limited by the absence of a uniform definition of the disease, selection bias, underreporting, and differences in prevalence rates in different industries. In the United States and Japan, an estimated 2–15% of newly diagnosed adult asthma is a result of occupational exposure. Variable airflow limitation, bronchial hyperresponsiveness, or both as a result of conditions in a particular work environment mark occupational asthma. Histamine and arachidonic acid metabolites contribute to bronchoconstriction, but chronic airways obstruction also develops as a consequence of edema of bronchial mucosa, hyperplasia of bronchial smooth muscle, hypersecretion of mucus and sub–basement membrane thickening. Both occupational asthma and work-aggravated asthma are associated with wheezing, chest tightness, dyspnea, cough, or some combination of these symptoms. Bronchial hyperreactivity is characterized by a heightened sensitivity to both allergenic and nonallergenic stimuli. Nonspecific triggers for asthma include inhalation of cold, dry air, exercise, and exposure to respiratory irritants such as exhaust fumes, smoke, particulate matter, and strong odors.

Sensitization may result from a broad array of natural or synthesized chemicals that may appear in a diverse range of materials and processes. The list of documented causal agents has expanded rapidly over the past 5–10 years and now numbers more than 250 (see Table 14–4).

In general, atopic patients are predisposed to sensitization to large-molecular-weight inhalants (proteins) such as animal proteins, pollens, plant proteins, enzymes, mold spores, and house dust. There is no atopic predisposition to sensitization by low-molecular-weight chemicals such as toluene diisocyanate (TDI), TMA, or platinum salts.

Exposure to high-molecular-weight antigens generally induces classic type I IgE-mediated hypersensitivity reactions. Some low-molecular-weight compounds, such as anhydrides and platinum salts, act as haptens and induce specific IgE antibodies by combining with a cell-surface or carrier protein, whereas others, such as isocyanates, do not appear to induce specific IgE antibody or agent-protein complexes. Several clinical patterns have been observed after respiratory exposure to inhalants, including (1) acute bronchospasm with rapid resolution after removal of exposure, (2) late onset with the development of symptoms 4–6 hours after the exposure (often after a worker has returned home), or less commonly, (3) acute onset of continuous asthma symptoms without remission between early- and late-phase responses. In general, IgE-mediated reactions occur as isolated early-phase events or biphasic reactions, whereas IgE-independent reactions often occur as isolated late-phase or atypical asthmatic reactions.

Surveys among workers in high-risk occupations suggest that the etiologic agent or exposure is the most important risk factor for the development of occupational asthma. The incidence of allergic rhinitis or allergic asthma in workers with exposure to animal proteins is estimated to be between 20% and 30%. The prevalence of occupational asthma in workers exposed to anhydrides is estimated to be 20%, as compared with the National Health Interview Survey estimation of 5% in the general adult population in 1994.

A personal or family history of atopy and concurrent smoking are independent risk factors for IgE-mediated occupational asthma but do not appear to influence IgE-independent processes. Patients may develop occupational asthma early in the course of antigen exposure or may develop symptoms after 10 years of exposure.

Pathologic airway changes characterized by inflammatory cell infiltrates (primarily eosinophils), edema, hypertrophy of smooth muscle, subepithelial fibrosis, and obstruction of airway lumina by exudate or mucus are similar for patients with occupational asthma as for patients with other forms of asthma.

In principle, any agent that causes occupational asthma also could cause allergic rhinitis or allergic conjunctivitis. The sneezing, rhinorrhea, and nasal pruritus seen in allergic rhinitis are the result of tissue effects from early-phase mediators causing increased vascular permeability, tissue edema, stimulation of efferent C fibers, and mucus glandular secretions. Chronic nasal obstruction appears to be caused by the late-phase reaction with cellular recruitment and production of other inflammatory mediators. A phenomenon of priming has been observed, where frequent or chronic exposure to an allergen will lower the threshold for elicitation of symptoms. This appears to be caused also by the accumulation of inflammatory cells in the affected tissues. Recent studies estimate the cumulative prevalence of allergic rhinitis to be 20% in the general U.S. population. Occupational rhinitis can develop through both allergic and irritant mechanisms and may exist alone or be superimposed on allergic rhinitis caused by environmental pollens, dust mite, animal dander, or molds. Many patients with allergic rhinitis also will suffer from concomitant allergic conjunctivitis, manifest by conjunctival injection, eye pruritus, discharge, or discomfort. Although a non-life-threatening disorder, allergic rhinoconjunctivitis has a measurable impact on quality of life. In some quality-of-life surveys, its impact surpasses that of asthma because of its effect on physical, social, and emotional functioning and well-being at home, school, and work. Furthermore, uncontrolled rhinitis may lead to complications such as bacterial

sinusitis, cough, and asthma. Hypersensitivity pneumonitis is a parenchymal pulmonary disease resulting from sensitization and subsequent exposure to a variety of inhalant organic dusts and related occupational antigens. Sensitization to bacterial products, small amounts of serum present in the excreta of animals, thermophilic actinomycetes (e.g., *Micropolyspora faeni, Tectibacter vulgaris,* and *Thermoactinomyces sacchari*), fungi, and vegetable proteins has produced hypersensitivity pneumonitis. Examples include pigeon breeder's disease, farmer's lung, humidifier lung, malt worker's lung, mushroom worker's lung, and bagassosis. Occupational agents demonstrated to induce hypersensitivity pneumonitis include the diisocyanates found in most polyurethane paints, foams, and coatings and epoxies in most plastics. Hypersensitivity pneumonitis caused by plastics appears to have a more insidious course than does the classic farmer's lung. Prolonged treatment with systemic steroids may be required to clear inflammation and ventilatory impairment. The incidence varies with the type and frequency of antigen exposure and is not age-dependent. Sensitization is favored by the alveolar deposition of particulate antigen less than 5 μm in diameter.

With short-term high-level exposure to antigen, the acute disease is characterized by fever, cough, dyspnea, and myalgias that occur 4–12 hours after heavy exposure and remit within hours to days. The subacute or chronic form of the disease is associated with long-term low-level antigen exposure and induces an insidious onset of symptoms and eventually an irreversible restrictive ventilatory impairment.

Possible immune mechanisms operative in hypersensitivity pneumonitis include (1) a type III Arthus reaction in which specific antibody binds to antigen, forming immune complexes that, in turn, activate the complement system, (2) a type IV reaction in which sensitized T cells bind to antigen and then release cytokines, (3) nonspecific activation of immune hypersensitivity by lectins and lipopolysaccharide products of organic matter, and (4) any combination of the above.

There is evidence both to support and to reject the concept that hypersensitivity pneumonitis is a type III reaction. Up to 90% of patients have antigen-specific precipitins in their serum. However, 50% of similarly exposed asymptomatic subjects also have precipitins to the same antigens, which suggests that the precipitins merely may be markers of antigen exposure. Passive transfer of serum from a rabbit with hypersensitivity pneumonitis to a nonsensitized rabbit and subsequent aerosol challenge with antigen have failed to induce the reaction, suggesting that a type III response may not be operative in this species.

Recent evidence suggests that a type IV or cell-mediated immune reaction to inhaled antigen may play a more predominant role in the development of hypersensitivity pneumonitis. Histopathologic study of the lesions reveals infiltration with neutrophils, lymphocytes, and macrophages; noncaseating granulomas, giant cells, and fibrosis may be present. Granuloma formation favors the diagnosis of cell-mediated immune reaction; however, this also may be induced by nonphagocytosed antigen-antibody complexes. The lymphocytes of sensitized patients release cytokines when exposed to specific antigen. Experimentally, lesions resembling alveolitis can be induced by first sensitizing rabbits using methods favoring a cell-mediated immune response and then challenging with inhaled antigen. Furthermore, when rabbits are passively sensitized by lymphocytes from sensitized rabbits and then challenged, typical lesions consistent with alveolitis develop. These studies favor a type IV response.

It is possible that nonimmune activation of effector mechanisms of hypersensitivity may be operative. Lipopolysaccharides found in the cell walls of certain bacteria and fungi may activate the alternative complement pathway directly, leading to the release of anaphylatoxins that are also chemotactic for phagocytes. Lipopolysaccharides stimulate lymphocytes to release cytokines, including lymphocytotoxins and macrophage activators, resulting in local tissue inflammation and necrosis. Although this mechanism may play a part in hypersensitivity pneumonitis, it probably is not a primary role; studies demonstrate that sensitization must take place before a reaction occurs. It may be that hypersensitivity pneumonitis is a combination of a type III and a type IV immune response, possibly enhanced by nonimmune activation of effector mechanisms.

Although the diagnosis used to rely on finding IgG antibodies against offending agents, efforts now focus on finding an intense alveolar lymphocytosis on bronchoalveolar lavage (BAL). Lavage fluid in hypersensitivity pneumonitis is marked by increased numbers of CD8+ T cells, which often help to distinguish the syndrome from sarcoidosis, in which CD4+ T cells predominate, and idiopathic pulmonary fibrosis, which is characterized by a neutrophilic infiltration. Serum precipitins can be useful in bird fancier's disease and farmer's lung but can be an insensitive test for other etiologies owing to the lack of appropriate testing reagents for many antigens. Radiographic imaging and pulmonary function testing can establish interstitial involvement but BAL or histopathology sometimes may be necessary.

Allergic contact dermatitis (ACD) is a delayed hypersensitivity disorder caused by a variety of agents in the occupational setting, including latex, nickel, formaldehyde, potassium dichromate, thiurams, epoxy resins, mercaptos, parabens, quaternium-15, ethylenediamine, and cobalt. Rhus or poison oak allergic contact dermatitis is caused by cutaneous exposure to oils from the toxicodendron plants (see "Type IV: Cellular Immunity" above). Acutely, the dermatitis is characterized by erythema and induration with vesicle formation, exudation, and crusting in more advanced stages. Chronic ACD may be associated with fissuring, lichenification, or dyspigmentation. The face and hands are disproportionately affected because of their higher likelihood of exposure. Indeed, the appearance may resemble other forms of dermatitis, such as atopic dermatitis or irritant dermatitis. Overall, irritant dermatitis is four times more common than ACD. In contrast to agents causing ACD, irritant reactions are not characterized by a sensitization phase and do not result in an antigen-mediated inflammatory response.

ANTIGENS INDUCING OCCUPATIONAL IMMUNE HYPERSENSITIVITY DISORDERS

Antigens inducing occupational immune hypersensitivity disorders may be of animal, vegetable, or chemical origin. Table 14–4 lists and classifies reactions caused by a number of these agents. Immune hypersensitivity reactions occur when a sensitized worker encounters antigens in the work environment.

Animal Products

Occupational exposure to animal products may cause a type I immediate response manifested by symptoms of acute or chronic asthma and rhinitis. Animal danders and excreta, insects, shellfish, and animal enzymes induce IgE antibodies and type I reactions. Cat dander and saliva and dog dander antigens may induce occupational allergies in veterinarians and animal handlers. Mouse urine and rabbit and guinea pig epithelia may sensitize laboratory workers and cause respiratory allergy. Of 5641 workers who were exposed to animals at 137 laboratory animal facilities in Japan, approximately 25% had one or more allergic symptoms related to laboratory animals, most commonly rhinitis. Approximately 70% of workers developed symptoms during their first 3 years of exposure. The presence of atopy, the number of animal species handled, and the time spent in handling correlated significantly with the development of allergy. Bovine epithelial and urinary proteins have been demonstrated to cause asthma and rhinitis in farmers, as defined by immunologic tests and bronchial or nasal provocation. Insects, including the red spider mite and other arthropods, have induced occupational allergic disease in technicians and pest-control workers.

Alcalase, derived from *Bacillus subtilis*, is used in the manufacture of detergents in Great Britain and was at one time so used in the United States. As a result of daily exposure, atopic workers are particularly predisposed to sensitization and the development of IgE-mediated type I respiratory symptoms.

Vegetable Products

Castor bean, soy bean, and green coffee bean dust are potent antigens for some people, inducing a type I immediate response manifested as rhinitis and asthma. There are reports of patients living near castor bean processing plants who have developed severe asthma secondary to wind shifts resulting in inhalation of minute amounts of this dust. The inhalation of soybean dust released during the unloading of soybeans into a silo caused outbreaks of asthma in Spain. Installing filters on silos to prevent airborne dissemination of allergenic soybean dust eliminated these outbreaks. It is estimated that 10% of workers handling green coffee beans develop IgE-mediated symptoms, especially rhinoconjunctivitis. The antigenicity of the green coffee bean is destroyed by roasting. Workers who have an adverse immune response to green coffee bean dust are able to handle the roasted beans without difficulty.

An increasingly common problem and growing public health threat is hypersensitivity to natural rubber latex antigens derived from the commercial rubber tree *Hevea brasiliensis*. Between 1989 and 1993, the U.S. Food and Drug Administration received more than 1100 reports of injury and 15 deaths associated with latex allergy. Latex is a complex intracellular product, the essential functional unit of which is the rubber particle, a spherical droplet of polyisoprene coated with a layer of protein, lipid, and phospholipid. Numerous rubber proteins are potentially allergenic, although investigators have found several major antigens that seem to be particularly effective at generating an IgE response (Table 14–5). Latex antigens coat the surface of a number of common products, including gloves, catheters, and balloons. Latex or "dipped" rubber products (e.g., gloves and condoms) are produced through different processes than extruded or injection-molded hard-rubber products (e.g., tires) and are associated with a much higher risk for hypersensitivity reactions. Type I immediate hypersensitivity reactions to latex may range from mild to life-threatening and include systemic urticaria, rhinitis, conjunctivitis, bronchospasm, and anaphylaxis and may occur

Table 14–5. Major natural rubber latex allergens.

Hev b1	Rubber elongation factor
Hev b2	1,3-β-Glucanase
Hev b3	22–27-kD rubber particle protein
Hev b5	Acidic natural rubber latex protein
Hev b6.01	Prohevein
Hev b6.02	Hevein

following cutaneous, mucosal, or parenteral contact. Aerosol transmission of antigens is a commonly reported route of exposure. Workers at risk of latex allergy include health care workers and rubber industry workers. Since latex can be ubiquitous in certain settings, and since the incidence latex hypersensitivity may approach 1% in the general public, it can be difficult to establish the source and onset of sensitization. Furthermore, up to 3000-fold differences in allergen content have been noted when various brands of natural latex gloves were examined.

Risk factors for sensitization include increased exposure and atopy. Studies looking at nurses and surgeons have estimated the prevalence of latex hypersensitivity to range between 5% and 17%. The growing numbers of affected workers has been blamed on changes in latex processing and the increased number of exposed individuals because of body fluid exposure precautions in the last two decades. In 1998, Germany banned the use of powdered latex gloves, and the incidence of occupational latex allergy has decreased by 80%, demonstrating the impact of exposure-reduction measures. Allergic contact dermatitis also may be caused by latex exposure, although these type IV delayed hypersensitivity reactions are caused mostly by rubber additives such as thiurams, carbamates, benzothiazoles, thioureas, and amines. These rubber components are added to the plant-derived latex extracts during the manufacturing process as antioxidants, accelerating agents, or dyes. A curious condition, latex fruit syndrome, also has been seen in up to 52% of latex allergic patients. Immunologic cross-reactivity between latex allergens and those found in bananas, avocado, kiwifruit, and chestnuts and causes systemic hypersensitivity to these foods.

Five percent of workers in the western U.S. red cedar lumber industry develop asthma after a latent period of exposure that averages about 3–4 years. They exhibit bronchospasm to inhalation challenge with plicatic acid, a low-molecular-weight derivative of red cedar. Skin testing and RAST demonstrate IgE sensitivity in approximately 50% of affected workers, but positive results are also found in unaffected workers. Atopy does not predispose workers to sensitization. It is possible that some cases are caused by IgE-mediated processes. Other wood dusts also may cause occupational asthma, including oak, mahogany, zebrawood, and ash, but many sawmill workers also have significant exposure to molds as well. Colophony, a pine resin by-product (rosin) that is used as solder flux, causes both immediate and dual respiratory reactions in sensitized workers. The reaction is probably an IgE-mediated hypersensitivity to abietic acid.

In the United States, the most common agent causing occupational dermatitis is the oil from plants of the genus *Rhus* (poison oak, poison ivy, and poison sumac). Poison oak is found west of the Rocky Mountains; poison ivy and poison sumac are found to the east. The active principle is pentadecylcatechol, a low-molecular-weight substance that binds to one of the skin proteins, forming a complete antigen. Studies reveal that more than 90% of subjects are sensitized on exposure to these antigens. A subject will develop a type IV allergic contact dermatitis reaction 24–72 hours after challenge.

Respiratory symptoms secondary to exposure to flour dust occur in bakers. Potential allergens can be from cereal grain but also from mold spore contaminants, storage mites, egg proteins, or enzymes used in cooking and fermentation. The mean annual incidence of occupational respiratory diseases among bakery workers over a 10-year period in Finland was reported to be 374 per 100,000 workers, compared with a rate of 31 per 100,000 workers in general. Affected workers may exhibit (1) an immediate or (2) an immediate followed by a late-onset reaction; both are probably IgE-mediated. There is a direct relation between duration of exposure and the percentage of bakers who exhibit skin test reactivity.

Chemical Agents

Workers in industrial plants may be exposed to a wide variety of chemical agents. Two that have been studied extensively are the isocyanates and anhydrides. In contrast to biologic allergens, which are high-molecular-weight sensitizers, these agents are low-molecular-weight and must haptenate before becoming immunogenic. Isocyanates are used in the manufacture of pesticides, polyurethane foams, and synthetic varnishes. There are many case reports of obstructive airway problems related to toluene diisocyanate (TDI). These occur with equal frequency in atopic and nonatopic workers. The mechanism of obstructive airway disease has not been elucidated, but some hypotheses to explain the pathogenesis include the following:

1. *An irritant effect.* Evidence opposed to this hypothesis includes the latent period observed in many cases and the fact that all workers are not affected.
2. *Beta-adrenergic blockade.* In vitro studies demonstrate that TDI acts as a weak beta-adrenergic blocking agent.
3. *Immune hypersensitivity response.* This is suggested by the insidious onset of symptoms after a latency period of weeks to months, peripheral eosinophilia, and the induction of symptoms in sensitized workers on reexposure to minute quantities of the material. RAST and skin testing with a conjugate of a low-molecular-weight isocyanate with human serum albumin have demonstrated specific IgE antibodies and in some cases IgG antibodies; however, because the antibodies can be demonstrated in affected and nonaffected workers, they may better correlate with exposure and not with clinical disease. The ability to mount an immunologic response against isocyanates appears to be genetically determined because certain HLA genes have been linked to disease susceptibility.

Trimellitic anhydride (TMA) is used in the manufacture of plastics, epoxy resins, and paints. TMA dust or fumes have been associated with four clinical syndromes. In the TMA immediate-type reaction, the patient may have rhinitis, conjunctivitis, or asthma. The reaction requires a latent period of exposure before the onset of symptoms. IgE antibodies to trimellityl–human serum albumin (TMHSA) conjugates have been demonstrated. Although affected workers have no atopic predisposition, this is probably a type I reaction.

The late-reacting systemic syndrome (TMA flu) is characterized by cough, occasional wheezing, dyspnea, and systemic symptoms of malaise, chills, myalgia, and arthralgia. These reactions occur 4–6 hours after exposure to TMA. This may be a type III disorder in which immune complexes of IgG antibody and TMA protein conjugates are operative. Repeated exposure and a latent period of weeks to months are required before symptoms develop. IgG antibodies to TMHSA have been demonstrated.

The pulmonary disease–anemia syndrome develops after exposure to TMA fumes. It occurs after repeated high-dose exposure to the volatile fumes of TMA sprayed on heated metal surfaces to prevent corrosion. A Coombs-positive hemolytic anemia and respiratory failure are evident. This is an example of a type II cytotoxic reaction in which antibodies are directed toward TMA bound to erythrocytes and pulmonary basement membrane. High titers of IgG antibody to TMHSA and to a trimellityl-erythrocyte conjugate have been demonstrated.

The irritant respiratory syndrome occurs with the first high-dose exposure to TMA powder and fumes. Patients develop cough and dyspnea. Immune sensitization toward TMA conjugates has not been demonstrated.

Hexahydrophthalic anhydride (HHPA) is a component of some epoxy resin systems. A high fraction of HHPA-exposed workers displays nasal symptoms, and some of them have specific serum antibodies. Eleven subjects who were IgE sensitized against an HHPA–human serum albumin (HSA) conjugate and who reported work-related nasal symptoms had a significant increase of nasal symptoms and a decrease of nasal inspiratory peak flow after HHPA-HSA nasal provocation. The symptoms were associated with the presence of specific serum IgE and significant increases in eosinophil and neutrophil counts and in levels of tryptase and albumin in nasal lavage fluid, suggesting an IgE-mediated syndrome. Nine subjects who were not sensitized but complained of work-related symptoms and 11 subjects who were not sensitized and had no symptoms displayed no changes in any of these parameters following challenge. Another study reported that risk factors for the development of immunologically mediated respiratory disease caused by HHPA in 57 exposed workers included exposure level and the development of specific IgE or IgG antibodies.

Reactive metallic compounds are found in a wide range of industrial settings. Metallic salts are an important cause of immune hypersensitivity. After poison oak, nickel is the most common cause of contact dermatitis, a type IV reaction. There are also reports of asthma secondary to exposure to fumes of nickel and platinum salts. It is thought that these salts acting as haptens and binding with body proteins cause the induction of IgE immune sensitivity and, on subsequent exposure, bronchial asthma or dermatitis. Challenge studies with bronchial provocation by offending metallic substances have demonstrated bronchospasm and bronchial hyperreactivity after exposure to platinum salts, nickel sulfate, cobalt chloride, and vanadium. IgE-mediated hypersensitivity has been found with some but not all of these metallic compounds.

REFERENCES

Allmers H et al: Decreasing incidence of occupational contact urticaria caused by natural rubber latex allergy in German health care workers. J Allergy Clin Immunol 2004;114:347 [PMID: 15316514].

Taylor JS, Erkek E: Latex allergy: diagnosis and management. Dermatol Ther 2004;17:289 [PMID: 15327474].

Valks R et al: Allergic contact urticaria from natural rubber latex in healthcare and non healthcare workers. Contact Dermatitis 2004;50:222 [PMID: 15186377]

UNPROVEN & CONTROVERSIAL PRACTICES

Many patients complain of malaise and dysesthesia not associated with any measurable or demonstrable organ dysfunction. Practitioners of "clinical ecology" espouse the belief that many of these patients suffer from the controversial *syndrome of multiple chemical sensitivities*. This syndrome is defined by clinical ecologists as an "environmental illness" characterized by recurrent symptoms involving multiple organ systems as a response to exposure to a multitude of unrelated chemical compounds at doses below those generally regarded as safe in the general populace. Moreover, it is accepted by many of these practitioners that no single test of physiologic function correlates with symptoms. Many symptoms are nonspecific. A number of unsubstantiated "pseudoimmunologic" mechanisms have been proposed by clinical ecologists as the basis for this disorder, but none is consistent with a modern understanding of immunologic function. A well-publicized but similarly flawed theory of *Candida* hypersensitivity also may be cited by some patients as a cause for multiple nonspecific symptoms. There is no scientifically valid basis underlying this syndrome, and

it should not be confused with well-established local or systemic infections with *C. albicans*.

Disagreements between the traditional medical community and practitioners of clinical ecology center around the absence of any well-documented, controlled, reproducible studies that demonstrate that the dysesthesia is a result of chemical exposures rather than a misdiagnosed underlying disease (e.g., endocrinopathy, cancer, or collagen-vascular disease) or an undiagnosed psychiatric disorder. Such misdiagnosis can lead to significant cost in unnecessary diagnostic studies, litigation, morbidity, and even mortality. A full discussion of the issues surrounding this controversial aspect of occupational medicine is given in Chapter 43. Practitioners of clinical ecology rely on unproven or inappropriate diagnostic tests and therapies (Table 14–6). An unproven test is one that lacks proven validity and has not been subjected to properly designed, placebo-controlled, randomized clinical trials. Unproven procedures are tests or therapies incapable of diagnosing or treating any disease. Some of the tests and therapies are modifications of valid tests and therapies for well-specified existing allergic or immunologic disorders. Inappropriate procedures are those technically capable of diagnosing or treating an illness but not necessarily the symptoms experienced by the patient. Proponents of the inappropriate use of these tests and therapies claim that they are valid because they are used by "traditional" or "establishment" physicians. It is important for physicians specializing in occupational medicine to fully understand the basis and theories behind the unproven or inappropriate procedures and therapies used by many practitioners of clinical ecology so as to be able to inform patients about the validity and utility of the tests and treatments recommended. It is particularly important to recognize that a patient's perception of symptoms is that patient's reality, and every effort should be made to generate appropriate and effective diagnostic and treatment plans.

The California Medical Association Scientific Board Task Force on Clinical Ecology reviewed this subject in 1985, and its conclusion best summarizes the scientific knowledge to date: "No convincing evidence was found that patients treated by clinical ecologists have unique, recognizable syndromes, that the diagnostic tests employed are efficacious and reliable, or that the treatments used are effective."

REFERENCES

Niggemann B, Gruber C: Unproven diagnostic procedures in IgE-mediated allergic diseases. Allergy 2004;59:806 [PMID: 15230811].

Wuthrich B: Unproven techniques in allergy diagnosis. J Invest Allergol Clin Immunol 2005;15:86 [PMID: 16047707].

Table 14–6. Unproven and inappropriate tests and therapies.

Test or Therapy	Unproven	Inappropriate
I. Test		
Provocation neutralization	To determine nonspecific reactivity to an "offending" agent	
Applied kinesiology	To determine allergic reactivity to a food or chemical	
Cytotoxic leukocyte testing	To determine allergic reactivity to a food	
Electrodiagnosis	To determine allergic reactivity to a food	
Body/breath chemical analysis	To detect toxic chemicals in the body to account for symptoms	Diagnosis of "environmental" illness
Hair analysis	To detect toxic chemicals in the body to account for symptoms	Diagnosis of "environmental" illness
IgG antibodies or circulating immune complexes		Diagnosis of food allergy
Lymphocyte subsets, immunoglobulins, other immune system function tests		Alleged "multiple chemical sensitivity" without signs or symptoms of immunodeficiency
Pulse rate changes		Diagnosis of chemical, food, or alleged "food allergy"
Uncontrolled chamber challenges		Response to putative offending agents
II. Therapy		
Neutralization therapy	To "neutralize" symptoms caused by intake of offending agent	
Rotation diets	To prevent "sensitization" to a given food	
Acupuncture	To relieve allergic symptoms	
Orthomolecular therapy	To correct presumed deficiency of vitamins and/or minerals; to cure certain diseases	
Homeopathic remedies	To prevent or cure disease	
Removal of mercury amalgam	To treat mercury-induced symptoms or fatigue, malaise, etc.	
Multiple food elimination diets/chemical avoidance	To "boost" the immune response	"Boosting the immune system"
Anti-*Candida* therapy		"Treatment" of alleged release of immunotoxins from normal *Candida albicans* body flora
Clinical ecology		Symptoms allegedly arising from low-level exposure to organic and inorganic environmental chemicals (see Chapter 43)
Detoxification therapy		Symptoms allegedly arising from low-level exposure to organic and inorganic environmental chemicals (see Chapter 43)

DIAGNOSIS OF HYPERSENSITIVITY DISEASES IN OCCUPATIONAL MEDICINE

From the standpoint of both the patient and the employer, it is important to establish an early diagnosis. Many obstructive pulmonary problems that are reversible with proper early management become fixed disabilities with prolonged exposure to offending agents. Diagnosis of occupational hypersensitivity diseases should include both diagnosis of the hypersensitivity disease and establishment of a relationship between the disease and the workplace. The requirements for establishing the relationship to work generally are more stringent for medical situations than for field epidemiologic surveys. Although it is often possible to demonstrate a pattern of symptoms and signs suggesting occupational illness, confirmatory tests for occupational hypersensitivity diseases generally are not available. Occupational hypersensitivity diseases should be suspected in a person exposed at work to agents known to cause occupational disease, although the failure to identify a known agent does not rule out the disorder. An occupational history regarding possible past and current exposures should be obtained because early exposure to an agent may have induced chronic asthma.

History & Physical Examination

The initial workup should include a detailed history and physical examination and, when indicated, a chest film, pulmonary function tests, and a blood count (see Figure 20–4). The types of symptoms, aggravating and relieving factors, their temporal relationship with the work environment, and the effects of vacations and weekends should be noted. A history of improvement of symptoms during weekends and holidays and a worsening on return to work suggests but does not confirm occupational hypersensitivity disease. Late-onset respiratory reactions may not occur until a patient has returned home from work. The personal or family history of atopy (i.e., hay fever, allergic asthma, or atopic dermatitis) should be investigated. If there is bronchospasm, it is important to review medications the patient is currently receiving, including beta-blockers, aspirin, and nonsteroidal anti-inflammatory drugs, all of which may induce bronchial asthma; angiotensin-converting enzyme inhibitors may cause cough. The home environment should be reviewed, including any changes that have occurred, the presence of pets and molds, any recent moves, hobbies, and the use of tobacco by the patient or others in the household. Finally, a detailed occupational history should be elicited, including information regarding present and past employment. The assessment should include a detailed history of specific job duties and work processes for both the patient and coworkers. The frequency and intensity of exposures and peak concentrations of potential agents should be assessed. The investigator should review material safety data sheets for chemicals in the workplace, industrial hygiene data, and employee health records. At times it is helpful—with the employer's permission—to visit the work site.

Physical examination should focus on evaluation of the skin and the upper and lower respiratory tracts, but a full examination should be performed to identify signs of systemic or other medical illness. Evidence of atopy should be sought, including the presence of allergic facies, cobblestoning of the conjunctivae, pale and swollen mucous membranes, posterior pharyngeal lymphoid plaques, expiratory wheezing, and signs of atopic dermatitis. Evidence of clubbing, increased anteroposterior diameter of the chest, and the location and quality of skin rashes should be noted.

Laboratory Investigation

The diagnosis of occupational disease should be confirmed by objective data. A complete blood count demonstrating evidence of eosinophilia may aid in the diagnosis of atopy. The presence of eosinophilia on a stained smear of sputum or nasal secretions is consistent with asthma and allergic rhinitis, respectively. Total serum IgE level is often elevated in atopic patients, although this test is neither sensitive nor specific for establishing the diagnosis of atopy.

Baseline posteroanterior and lateral radiographs of the chest should be obtained in patients with pulmonary problems, noting increased anteroposterior chest diameter, flattening of the diaphragms, infiltrates, and evidence of bronchiectasis, hyperaeration, and diffuse micronodularity.

Pulmonary function studies before and after bronchodilator administration should be obtained in the case of pulmonary disorders; at a minimum, they should include forced expiratory volume in 1 second (FEV_1), forced vital capacity (FVC), forced expiratory flow between 25% and 75% of FVC (FEF_{25-75}), and peak expiratory flow rate (PEFR). Complete pulmonary function tests including lung volumes and diffusion capacity (DL_{CO}) determination may be helpful in ruling out a restrictive component of lung disease. Measurements of blood gases may prove helpful (see Chapter 20).

Measurement of bronchial hyperresponsiveness to pharmacologic agents including methacholine or histamine is an important step in the diagnostic workup. Bronchoprovocation challenge with pharmacologic agents is helpful in establishing increased nonspecific bronchial hyperreactivity, especially in patients who present without reversible obstructive patterns on their pulmonary function tests or in patients with cough as a sole manifestation of lung disease. In a methacholine challenge test, the subject performs serial spirometric maneuvers after inhaling increasing amounts of methacholine. If bronchial hyperreactivity is present, a detectable decrease in airflows or FEV_1 (a 20% decline is standard end point) will occur at low doses of methacholine. Asthmatics are up to 1000 times more sensitive than normal individuals to methacholine bronchoprovocation challenge. The absence of bronchial hyperresponsiveness after a person has worked for 2 weeks under normal working conditions virtually rules out the diagnosis of occupational asthma. The presence of bronchial hyperresponsiveness requires further testing to define the relationship of asthma to the workplace. Sensitization to antigen and pharmacologically induced bronchial hyperresponsiveness are associated with an 80% likelihood of immediate hypersensitivity to antigen in laboratory challenge.

Immunologic Tests

Based on the initial evaluation, specific immunologic tests may be ordered, including immediate allergy skin tests, patch tests, in vitro tests for IgE antibody, Ouchterlony gel diffusion tests, and provocative challenge with specific antigens.

A. Skin Tests

Epicutaneous (prick) and intradermal skin tests are helpful in establishing sensitivity to a number of inhalant protein antigens, including molds, house dust, animal dander, feathers, pollen, and extracts of suspected high-molecular-weight antigens in the work environment. Standardized occupational allergens are not available commercially at present. Skin tests are in vivo, rapid, cost-effective, and more sensitive and more specific than currently available in vitro RAST tests. Testing can be accomplished in 30–60 minutes at experienced centers. A positive skin test is marked by a pruritic wheal-and-flare reaction that peaks at 20 minutes, confirming the presence of antigen-specific IgE bound to skin mast cells. The initial wheal-and-flare reaction may be followed in 4–6 hours by an IgE-mediated late-phase reaction evidenced by erythema, induration, pruritus, and tenderness at the skin test site. Low-molecular-weight materials usually do not give a positive immediate skin test response unless they are linked to a protein carrier such as human serum albumin.

B. Patch Testing

Patch tests are useful in evaluating skin contact sensitivity (type IV delayed hypersensitivity). The test employs standard antigen-impregnated patches applied to the skin. The patches are removed after 48 hours, and the test sites are "read." A positive reaction consists of erythema, induration, and in some cases, vesiculation. A follow-up reading usually is done 24–48 hours after the first reading, allowing the technician to discriminate between delayed hypersensitivity and irritant reactions. In addition to antigens available in the standard antigen patch test kit obtained from the American Academy of Dermatology, suspected materials may be used from the work environment (see Chapter 18).

C. In Vitro Antibody Tests

RAST and ELISA are in vitro procedures that are used to detect antigen-specific IgE antibody. In these tests, inert particles coated with antigen are incubated with serum. If specific antibody is present, it binds to antigen on the surface of the particles. The complex is washed, incubated with radiolabeled or enzyme-labeled anti-IgE, and then washed again. The amount of anti-IgE measured by radioactivity or enzyme activity determines the amount of bound antigen-specific immunoglobulin. In vitro testing may be valuable in patients for whom appropriate skin testing reagents are unavailable or skin testing is not feasible. AlaSTAT (Diagnostic Products Corporation), Immuno-CAP (Pharmacia-UpJohn), and HY-TEC EIA (Hycor) are serologic tests approved by the FDA for use in the diagnosis of latex allergy in the United States.

D. Ouchterlony Gel Diffusion Test

This test is used to demonstrate IgG precipitating antibody to a specific antigen. Suspected antigens and the patient's serum are placed in separate wells cut into a gel-coated plate. The antigen and serum diffuse toward one another. If sufficient antibody is present, precipitin lines composed of antigen-antibody complexes form at some intermediate point. Detection of serum precipitins can confirm a type III hypersensitivity reaction. Precipitating antibodies specific for avian proteins and fungal antigens can be found in some cases of hypersensitivity pneumonitis.

E. Inhalation Challenge Tests

These tests are conducted by exposing the worker to the suspected antigen. *Caution:* Inhalation challenge studies are not without risk. Sensitized patients are susceptible to late-onset asthmatic reactions that may develop up to 12 hours after the initial challenge. These reactions often are refractory to bronchodilator treatment.

The challenge may be performed in the work environment or in a hospital laboratory situation. The patient probably should be hospitalized and observed for 12–24 hours after a laboratory challenge.

1. Work challenge—The patient is instructed to use a hand-held peak-flow meter to monitor and record peak expiratory flow rates four times a day for 2 weeks while at work and for an additional 2 weeks while away from work. There is good correlation with specific inhalation challenge; however, peak-flow diaries can be subject to patient bias and effort. Combining measurement of peak flow with serial measurements of bronchial hyperresponsiveness does not appear to improve sensitivity or specificity. The use of computerized peak-flow meters may improve accuracy but does not correct for patient effort. If initial peak-flow monitoring is suggestive of occupational asthma, a technician may be sent to the workplace to monitor hourly spirometry during the workday.

2. Laboratory inhalation challenge—This can be obtained in three ways: (a) After the worker's condition is stabilized off work, baseline tests are obtained; the worker is placed in a closed environment and asked to transfer suspected antigen dust, mixed in lactose powder, back and forth between two trays. (b) In another variation, the subject, in a hospital setting, is exposed to various volatile agents (e.g., solder, varnish) by actually working with the materials. In each of these challenges, pulmonary function tests are obtained immediately before and for several hours after exposure. (c) Aerosol inhalation challenge involves the administration of gradually increasing amounts of aerosolized suspected material while pulmonary function tests are monitored. A 20% or greater fall in FEV_1 is considered a positive response. False-negative inhalation challenge test results may occur if the incorrect agent or dose is used or if the patient has had an extended absence from work and has lost bronchial hyperresponsiveness.

Treatment

The diagnosis of occupational hypersensitivity disease has considerable economic implications for the worker and the worker's family, employers, and government agencies. Although pharmacotherapy can help to manage symptoms, it is environmental avoidance measures that are the cornerstone of any treatment plan. Safe or threshold levels of exposure are not well known or clearly defined for many agents. Complete removal of the worker from the workplace environment may be ideal but may place considerable economic hardships

on all involved. An attempt may be made to retrain workers for other roles within the same company or with another employer, to reduce exposure by improving ventilation or providing a respirator, or to make changes in the workplace to abide by existing laws. Public health agencies should be enlisted to begin surveillance programs when index cases have been identified. Patients who return to the same workplace require close medical monitoring and follow-up. Even after removal from the workplace, patients may continue to have chronic airways disease and require the use of medications. Experience with western red cedar (plicatic acid), TDI, and other low-molecular-weight substances reveals that at least half the patients will continue to have persistent, even worsening asthma despite removal from the source of exposure. Duration of symptoms greater than 6 months before removal is a strong risk factor for progressive disease even after removal from the workplace. Worker impairment and disability should be evaluated to determine if appropriate compensation is available.

REFERENCES

Becker AB: Primary prevention of allergy and asthma is possible. Clin Rev Allergy Immunol 2005;28:5 [PMID: 15834165].

Frew AJ: Advances in environmental and occupational diseases 2004. J Allergy Clin Immunol. 2005;115:1197 [PMID: 15940134].

Malo JL: Future advances in work-related asthma and the impact on occupational health. Occup Med (Lond) 2005;55:606 [PMID: 16314332].

Mapp CE et al: Occupational asthma. Am J Respir Crit Care Med 2005;172:280 [PMID: 15860754].

Occupational Hematology

15

Willis H. Navarro, MD, & Hope S. Rugo, MD

Occupationally related hematologic toxicity has occurred in cyclic fashion, historically associated with the development of the chemical industry and the advent of each world war. Common factors contributing to "epidemics" of toxicity have been the rapid introduction of many new chemicals and the exposure of large numbers of workers without adequate protection or education. As the toxicities of these agents gradually became known, regulation of their use was instituted, and exposure to some toxins such as radium has been eliminated. Hematologic toxins such as lead, benzene, arsenic, and arsine gas still exist; poisonings are still found in the workplace; and worker education is still inadequate. As new chemicals are introduced and new products become available, it is important to be aware of potential mechanisms of toxicity so that the epidemic poisonings of the past will not be repeated.

The study of hematotoxicity has improved our understanding of hematologic pathophysiology, taught important pharmacologic lessons, and introduced the concept of individual susceptibility to specific toxic agents. Observation of individual variations in susceptibility to toxic agents was made by recognizing that chemicals with oxidative potential could cause cyanosis and a life-threatening hemolytic anemia in some individuals at exposure levels that had little effect on the population at large. The normal population will manifest similar toxicities but only when exposed to much higher levels. Consequently, it is important to identify workers with increased sensitivity to certain chemicals and place them in jobs with less risk of contact with these specific toxic substances.

Exposure to hematotoxins may affect blood cell survival (denaturation of hemoglobin and hemolysis), metabolism (porphyria), formation (aplasia), morphology and function (preleukemias and leukemias), or coagulation (thrombocytopenia).

DISORDERS ASSOCIATED WITH SHORTENED RED BLOOD CELL SURVIVAL

METHEMOGLOBINEMIA & HEMOLYSIS PRODUCED BY OXIDANT CHEMICALS

Methemoglobin is formed by the oxidation of ferrous (Fe^{2+}) hemoglobin to ferric (Fe^{3+}) hemoglobin. It was first recognized in the 1800s, when coal tars were converted into individual chemicals that served as precursors for many products ranging from explosives to synthetic dyes and perfumes. Overexposure to these chemicals—which included anilines, nitrobenzenes, and quinones—was common, and little was known about their potential toxicity. Workers in these plants came to be known as "blue workers" because they suffered from "blue lip" as a result of the chronic cyanosis from toxic methemoglobinemia that developed in almost all of them. Gradually it was recognized that oxidation of hemoglobin was toxic to red blood cells and could be followed by an acute and life-threatening hemolysis known as *Heinz body anemia*. Heinz bodies are red blood cell inclusions that represent precipitated hemoglobin and are seen classically in individuals with a deficiency of glucose-6-phosphate dehydrogenase (G6PD) after exposure to an oxidant stress. Normal individuals exposed to large amounts of oxidant chemicals will develop methemoglobinemia and, occasionally, Heinz body hemolytic anemia. It is not understood why some chemicals may cause methemoglobinemia, hemolysis, or both, but the disorders are certainly related to individual susceptibility. Oxidative chemicals are common in industry, and it is important to know

208

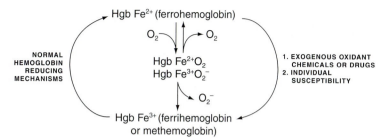

Figure 15–1. Oxidation of hemoglobin by the Embden-Meyerhof pathway.

what toxic agents have been implicated, to recognize the presenting signs and symptoms, and to be able to provide appropriate treatment when it is needed.

Despite the understanding of this phenomenon as new compounds were developed, for example, aniline and other coal tar derivatives, new cycles of toxicity were seen again. As new chemicals continue to be synthesized, awareness of their toxicity is necessary to avoid similar outbreaks of poisoning characterized by cyanosis and hemolysis. An understanding of the pathophysiology of this phenomenon is essential to handle this medical emergency correctly; it also will help in understanding the myriad therapeutic agents that may cause oxidative hemolysis in a susceptible individual.

Pathophysiology of Oxidant Hemolysis

Hemoglobin is unique in its ability to combine reversibly with oxygen without oxidizing its iron moiety. The small amount of oxidized hemoglobin or methemoglobin produced is readily reduced by an efficient enzyme system linked to energy provided by glucose metabolism via the Embden-Meyerhof pathway (Figure 15–1).

Methemoglobin is dangerous because of its inability to bind oxygen and because it increases the oxygen affinity of the remaining heme groups in hemoglobin tetramer, thereby decreasing oxygen delivery to the tissues. Oxidation results in denaturation of hemoglobin with the formation of precipitated hemoglobin (Heinz bodies) within the red cell. The presence of Heinz bodies alters the surface membrane of the red cell, causing increased rigidity and leakage. Macrophages in the reticuloendothelial system of the spleen and liver (the extravascular compartment) sense the altered red cell surface and remove Heinz bodies via partial phagocytosis (extravascular hemolysis). Because the red cell surface is unable to reseal and form a spherocyte (as in autoimmune hemolysis), the red cell remains intact as a cell with a piece missing, the so-called bite, or blister, cell. Heinz bodies also may be formed from a second form of denatured hemoglobin, sulfhemoglobin. Unlike methemoglobin, sulfhemoglobin is irreversibly associated with the heme moiety.

The development of methemoglobinemia or oxidative hemolysis in an individual exposed to an oxidant stress depends on the route of exposure, the specific chemicals involved, the dose and duration of exposure, and most important, individual susceptibility. Inborn structural abnormalities (unstable hemoglobins)—or, much more commonly, disorders of normal reducing capabilities such as the X-linked deficiency of the oxidation-reduction enzyme G6PD—cause some individuals to be much more susceptible to oxidant stress than others. There are many varieties of both these abnormalities. Recognition of these high-risk individuals in the workplace is important to reduce their chance of particularly toxic exposures.

The normal individual has less than 1% circulating methemoglobin. Ninety-five percent of methemoglobin formed daily by the autooxidation of hemoglobin is reduced by $NADH_2$ [nicotinamide adenine dinucleotide (reduced form)] generated by the dehydrogenation of phosphotriose by phosphotriose dehydrogenase. This reaction is catalyzed by NADH methemoglobin reductase (NADH cytochrome b5 reductase). A rare inborn deficiency of NADH methemoglobin reductase results in congenital cyanosis caused by methemoglobinemia (Figure 15–2).

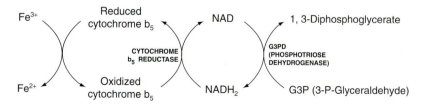

Figure 15–2. Reduction of hemoglobin by NADH-methemoglobin reductase (NADH cytochrome b_5 reductase).

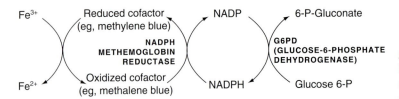

Figure 15–3. Reduction of hemoglobin by NADPH-methemoglobin reductase can be accelerated by a redox agent such as methylene blue.

An alternative methemoglobin reduction pathway exists that requires the presence of a redox cofactor such as methylene blue to achieve significant reducing capacity. In this reaction, nicotinamide adenine dinucleotide phosphate (NADPH) from the first two steps of the hexose monophosphate shunt converts methemoglobin to reduced hemoglobin. Because this pathway is normally responsible for so little reduction of methemoglobin, deficiency of the enzyme that catalyzes this reaction, NADPH methemoglobin reductase, does not result in methemoglobinemia or cyanosis. Because the formation of NADPH depends on G6PD, methylene blue, which is used to treat toxic and congenital methemoglobinemia, also can precipitate a hemolytic crisis in an individual with G6PD deficiency by competing for the NADPH necessary to maintain reduced glutathione, an essential protectant against erythrocyte oxidative stress. Additionally, methylene blue itself is an oxidant, but it is metabolized to the reducing agent leukomethylene blue. In normal individuals, the administration of a redox agent may increase the rate of reduction of hemoglobin dramatically so that it greatly exceeds that of the NADH-methemoglobin reductase reaction (Figure 15–3). This is the rationale for the effectiveness of methylene blue in toxic methemoglobinemia.

Two other pathways exist, but they reduce methemoglobin only to a small extent. Glutathione is responsible for conversion of less than 7–10% of ferrihemoglobin to ferrohemoglobin, and ascorbic acid in pharmacologic amounts also reduces oxidized hemoglobin. Because of the high redox potential of ascorbic acid, however, the rate of reduction is very slow, making it less effective in therapy. In physiologic concentrations, the contribution of ascorbic acid to methemoglobin reduction is insignificant.

1. Aniline

Historically, most work-related episodes of methemoglobinemia and hemolytic anemia were a result of exposure to aromatic nitro and amino compounds. These compounds are used most extensively as intermediates in the synthesis of aniline dyes; they are also used as accelerators and antioxidants in the rubber industry and in the production of pesticides, plastics, paints, and varnishes. Table 15–1 lists chemicals that are associated with methemoglobinemia and their industrial uses.

Many medicinal drugs are oxidants and can cause methemoglobinemia but will not be discussed here.

The clinical presentation of methemoglobinemia is exemplified by aniline toxicity. Aniline, used in the manufacture of dyes and in the rubber industry, is the most common and best-described aromatic amine. It is fat-soluble and readily penetrates the intact skin, even through clothing. The vapor form also may gain entry to the body through the lungs. Ingestion is rare in the industrial setting but causes serious toxicity when it does occur. Aniline is converted by hepatic microsomes to phenylhydroxylamine, which behaves as a catalyst in mediating hemoglobin oxidation. Hepatic clearance of phenylhydroxylamine is slow because its oxidized form, nitrosobenzene, is rapidly converted back to phenylhydroxylamine. Another clearance pathway gradually eliminates the amine from the body.

Clinical Presentation

Acute exposure usually is associated with spills or improper usage. Symptoms vary depending on the con-

Table 15–1. Chemicals associated with methemoglobinemia or oxidative hemolysis.

Chemical	Use
Aniline	Rubber, dyestuffs; production of MBI (methylene bisphenyl isocyanate)
Nitroaniline	Dyes
Toluidine	Dyes, organic chemicals
p-Chloroaniline	Dyes, pharmaceuticals, pesticides
o-Toluidine	Laboratory analytic reagent, production of trypan blue stain, chlorine test kits, test tapes, curing agent for urethane resins
Naphthalene	Fumigants used in clothing industry
Paradichlorobenzene	Fumigants used in clothing industry
Nitrates	Soil fertilizers
Trinitrotoluene	Explosives

Table 15–2. Symptoms of methemoglobinemia.

% Methemoglobinemia	Symptoms
10–30	Cyanosis, mild fatigue, tachycardia
30–50	Weakness, breathlessness, headache, exercise intolerance
50–70	Altered consciousness
>70–80	Coma, death

centration of methemoglobin (Table 15–2). Most cases are mild and transient and present as asymptomatic blueness of the lips and nail beds. In more severe cases, the patient will appear deeply cyanotic. Freshly drawn blood appears dark maroon-brown and does not become red after exposure to air. Pulse oximetry may indicate normoxia or mild hypoxia not reflective of the severity of methemoglobinemia. Arterial blood gases may show a normal oxygen tension (P_{O_2}) but co-oximetry will reveal methemoglobinemia reliably. Laboratory results may indicate hemolysis with an elevated reticulocyte count and variable degree of anemia. Examination of the peripheral blood smear shows evidence of reticulocytosis (polychromasia, possibly nucleated red cells) and may show bite or blistered red cells.

In chronic methemoglobinemia, polycythemia may be seen in response to chronic hypoxia. Hemolytic Heinz body anemia may or may not accompany methemoglobin formation or may follow resolution of cyanosis. Heinz bodies are detected easily by examining the peripheral blood smear stained with a supravital stain but will not be evident on a smear stained with Wright stain. Blood methemoglobin levels should be monitored closely.

Prevention

The most important safeguard in preventing oxidative hemolysis is to minimize atmospheric and cutaneous exposure to potentially oxidizing chemicals such as coal tar products. The identification of susceptible individuals such as those with G6PD deficiency may help to avoid significant toxicity in high-risk job situations. Screening for G6PD deficiency must be done either before a hemolytic episode or 1–2 months after the hemolysis has resolved. Young red blood cells, particularly reticulocytes, have normal G6PD levels in most G6PD-deficient individuals. During an acute hemolytic episode, older red blood cells are destroyed and replaced by young red blood cells. The result of a G6PD deficiency screen often will be normal in that acute setting. Biologic monitoring in the workplace may be done by measuring methemoglobin levels and reticulocyte counts (see Chapter 36).

Treatment

Treatment depends on rapid recognition of the problem. It is important to obtain as complete an exposure history as possible because it will guide treatment. The most important aspect of therapy is to ensure removal of the offending agent. Because of the fat-soluble nature of these compounds, it is essential that clothing be removed and the patient decontaminated thoroughly. For mild intoxication (<20% blood methemoglobin), observation should be sufficient to watch for progression of symptoms. For moderate to severe intoxication (>30% blood methemoglobin), 100% oxygen by mask is given to saturate the remaining hemoglobin, and the antidote, methylene blue, is administered. Care must be exercised in using methylene blue to avoid increasing methemoglobin from the oxidative potential of methylene blue itself.

For initial management, methylene blue should be given intravenously as a 1% solution at a dose of 1–2 mg/kg over 10 minutes. The maximal effect should be seen within 1 hour. If no response is evident by this time, administration of methylene blue may be repeated and exchange transfusion considered, although its role in methemoglobinemia has not been well defined. A patient who does not respond to methylene blue may have G6PD deficiency, and further administration could exacerbate hemolysis without altering hypoxia.

If the patient is improved after 1 hour, administration of methylene blue may be repeated at hourly intervals, either in intravenous form in the patient with altered consciousness or orally (50–100 mg) in an awake patient. Repeat doses should be given for symptoms, not solely on the basis of the methemoglobin level.

Ascorbic acid may be given in conjunction with the oral dose of methylene blue at a dose of 300–400 mg orally, although its role for this purpose remains controversial. Its onset of action is slow, and its potential for urine acidification may potentiate renal toxicity in patients who are actively hemolyzing.

2. Chlorate Salts

Chlorate salts, used primarily in pesticides and herbicides, cause an unusual form of methemoglobinemia and hemolysis that is unresponsive to methylene blue. Hemolytic anemia also has been seen in uremic patients undergoing hemodialysis when the water supply was found to contain chloramines, oxidant compounds made up of chlorine and ammonia now used in some public water supplies as a disinfectant. The denaturation of hemoglobin caused by chlorates is thought to be due to their direct oxidizing capacity and their ability to inhibit the hexose monophosphate shunt.

Treatment for poisoning with chlorates is supportive because there is no specific antidote. Exchange transfusion has been advocated for severe toxicity.

REFERENCES

Ash-Bernal R et al: Acquired methemoglobinemia: A retrospective series of 138 cases at 2 teaching hospitals. Medicine 2004; 83:265 [PMID: 15342970].

Bradberry SM: Occupational methaemoglobinaemia: Mechanisms of production, features, diagnosis and management including the use of methylene blue. Toxicol Rev 2003;22:13 [PMID: 14579544].

Watt BE et al: Poisoning due to urea herbicides. Toxicol Rev 2005;24:161 [PMID: 16390217].

HEMOLYSIS ASSOCIATED WITH EXPOSURE TO HEAVY METALS

After methemoglobinemia and oxidative hemolysis, transitional elements and heavy metals are the most important causes of work-related hemolytic anemia. These agents include arsenic, lead, mercury, copper, antimony, and others. The mechanism of hemolysis is unknown, but it is thought to be related to the affinity of these directly cytolytic metals to thiol groups such as are found on the surfaces of red blood cells and in the cysteine residues of hemoglobin. When the sulfhydryl-binding metals are exposed to red cells, the red cell membrane becomes permeable and takes on solute and water. This causes the red cell to swell and ultimately burst while in the vascular circuit (intravascular hemolysis).

1. Arsine

The most dramatic example of acute metal-induced hemolysis is that caused by arsine. Arsine is a volatile, colorless, nonirritating gas at room temperature [arsine's boiling point is −62°C (−79.6°F)]. It is usually produced accidentally by the action of acid on a metal contaminated with arsenic. However, arsine gas is now also used extensively in the growth and preparation of crystals and conducting devices in the semiconductor industry.

The toxicity of arsine may be best demonstrated by a case of two near fatalities. Two workers at a chemical manufacturing plant were cleaning a floor drain that had become clogged during a cleanup operation. Although the company had discontinued production of arsenical herbicides more than 5 years previously, a steel tank used to mix the chemicals had been left on a loading platform, where it collected rainwater. In attempting to open the drain, the two workers emptied water from the tank onto the floor with a drain cleaner containing sodium hydroxide, sodium nitrate, and aluminum chips. They then spent 2–3 hours working to unclog the drain, noting that the drain bubbled and gave off a sewer-like odor. By the next morning, both workers were hospitalized with acute hemolytic anemia.

Exposure was documented by the presence of arsenic in the drain as well as in the blood and urine of both patients. Each patient required multiple-unit exchange transfusions and fluid replacement; recovery took nearly a month for both.

Arsine gas was formed in this incident by the action of arsenic trioxide present in the storage tank and contaminated drain with hydrogen. Hydrogen was formed by the combination of sodium hydroxide and aluminum. Antimony also may be present with arsenic and under the same conditions can form stibine, a gas with toxicity similar to that of arsine. The toxicity of arsine here and in other reports is heightened by the fact that arsine is 2.5 times denser than air. This is particularly important in smelting and refinery work, where toxicity is likely to occur when workers are cleaning out large tanks containing acids and metal compounds.

The potential for arsine gas formation and exposure exists in a wide range of occupations and may be combined with exposure to stibine. Most occupational exposure occurs in the smelting, refining, and chemical industries. The respiratory tract is the most important portal of entry.

Chronic arsine poisoning has been described in workers at a zinc smelting plant and in workers engaged in the cyanide extraction of gold. These patients may be anemic, with chronic low-level hemolysis.

Clinical Presentation

A. SYMPTOMS AND SIGNS

Many manifestations of acute arsine poisoning are caused by acute and massive intravascular hemolysis. Appearance of symptoms may be delayed for 2–24 hours after exposure. Symptoms include nausea and vomiting, abdominal cramping, headache, malaise, and dyspnea. Patients often are alarmed by the presence of tea-colored urine that is not associated with pain on urination, causing them to seek medical attention. Physical examination may reveal the peculiar garlicky odor of arsine, fever, tachycardia, tachypnea, and hypotension. Later in the course of hemolysis, the patient may appear jaundiced, and there is often generalized nonspecific abdominal tenderness.

B. LABORATORY FINDINGS

The earliest laboratory finding may be hemoglobinuria. This occurs when the amount of free plasma hemoglobin exceeds normal haptoglobin binding and renal proximal tubular reabsorption. Accordingly, plasma haptoglobin levels fall, and free hemoglobin levels may be very high (>2000 mg/dL have been reported; normal: <1 mg/dL). The plasma may be brownish red from the presence of methemalbumin (oxidized hemoglobin bound to albumin). Although anemia may not be present on the first blood count, evaluation of the peripheral smear will reveal red cell fragmentation with marked poikilocytosis, basophilic stippling, and polychromasia. As the hematocrit falls, reticulocytosis develops. Total bilirubin is elevated, reflecting a rise primarily in the unconjugated or indirect form. When hemolysis is brisk, disseminated intravascular coagulation may occur, manifest as a low (or falling) fibrinogen level, a prolonged prothrombin time (caused by circulating fibrin split products), and the presence of schistocytes and thrombocytopenia. Renal function often is affected to various degrees, with an early rise in serum creatinine. This may be a result of both precipitated hemoglobin casts, causing renal tubular obstruction, and direct toxicity of arsine on the renal tubular and interstitial cells. Arsenic levels in blood and urine are useful as indicators of exposure rather than as guidelines for therapy.

Treatment

Initial therapy should include vigorous hydration to ensure adequate renal perfusion. For severe hemolysis with plasma hemoglobin levels greater than 400–500 mg/dL, exchange transfusion has been advocated. Repeated exchange is indicated for increasing levels of hemoglobin.

Renal function may be preserved with hydration. However, should renal failure develop, acute hemodialysis may be required. All patients must be monitored closely until all evidence of hemolysis has resolved, and renal function has stabilized. Some patients may be left with renal insufficiency or chronic failure requiring dialysis or transplantation. All survivors of acute arsine poisoning must be evaluated regularly for at least 1 year to watch for residual renal dysfunction. In chronic arsine poisoning, reduction of exposure or removal from exposure is the most important treatment.

2. Lead

Lead is more fully discussed with porphyria below. In addition to the suppression of erythropoiesis and heme synthesis described there, hemolytic anemia may be seen. Severe acute intravascular hemolysis is rare and usually is seen only with very high atmospheric exposure, as in power sanding and use of a blowtorch. The anemia of chronic lead toxicity is enhanced by shortened red cell survival as well as by inhibition of hemoglobin synthesis.

It has been suggested that the pathogenesis of lead-induced hemolysis is related to its marked inhibition of pyrimidine-5 nucleotidase. The hereditary homozygous deficiency of this enzyme is marked by basophilic stippling of erythrocytes, chronic hemolysis, and intraerythrocytic accumulations of pyrimidine-containing nucleotides. These nucleotides perhaps compete with adenine nucleotides in binding to the active site of kinases in the glycolytic pathway, thereby altering red cell membrane stability. Because lead causes an acquired deficiency of

this enzyme and the clinical findings are similar, severe toxicity has been likened to this hereditary disease.

3. Copper

Copper sulfate is used in India in the whitewashing and leather industry. Toxicity is primarily a result of accidental ingestion and suicide attempts and results in intravascular hemolysis, methemoglobinemia, renal failure, and often death. Hemolysis also has been caused by hemodialysis with water contaminated by copper piping. In vitro data suggest that multiple mechanisms are involved, including inhibition of glycolysis, oxidation of NADPH, and inhibition of G6PD. No specific treatment exists other than supportive therapy, with transfusions and hemodialysis as indicated.

REFERENCES

Chia SE et al: Association of renal function and delta-aminolevulinic acid dehydratase polymorphism among Vietnamese and Singapore workers exposed to inorganic lead. Occup Environ Med 2006;63:180 [PMID: 16497859].

Kim HS et al: The protective effect of delta-aminolevulinic acid dehydratase 1-2 and 2-2 isozymes against blood lead with higher hematologic parameters. Environ Health Perspect 2004;112:538 [PMID: 15064157].

THE PORPHYRIAS

The porphyrias are a group of disorders characterized by abnormalities in the heme biosynthetic pathway (Figure 15–4) that result in the abnormal accumulation of heme precursors. Although these are genetic disorders (inherited or sporadic) of enzymatic activity, acquired porphyria has been described following exposure to various toxins. Heme biosynthesis occurs chiefly in the liver and bone marrow and to a certain extent in nervous tissue. The rate-limiting step in heme biosynthesis is the synthesis of δ-aminolevulinic acid from glycine and succinyl-coenzyme A (CoA) via δ-aminolevulinic acid synthetase. This step is under negative feedback control by heme. Clinically, symptomatic porphyria can occur either as a result of inadequate enzymatic function along any step in heme biosynthesis or as a result of inappropriate overstimulation of δ-aminolevulinic acid synthetase, usually in the setting of decreased heme concentration.

The clinical syndromes of porphyria are characterized by neurotoxicity or cutaneous photosensitivity (both may occur). Neurotoxicity—typically abdominal colic, constipation, autonomic dysfunction, sensorimotor neuropathy, and psychiatric problems—is considered the result of direct toxic effects of the urine-soluble heme precursors δ-aminolevulinic acid and porphobilinogen on nervous

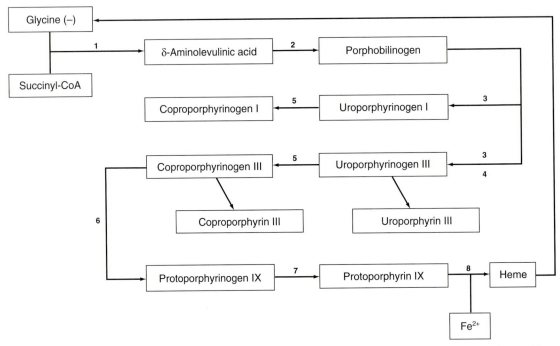

Figure 15–4. The heme biosynthetic pathway. Heme is a feedback inhibitor of enzyme (1) δ-aminolevulinic acid synthetase. Other enzymes are (2) δ-aminolevulinic acid dehydrase, (3) uroporphyrinogen I synthase, (4) uroporphyrinogen III cosynthase, (5) uroporphyrinogen decarboxylase, (6) coproporphyrinogen oxidase, (7) protoporphyrinogen oxidase, and (8) ferrochelatase.

tissue. Neurotoxicity also may be the result of heme deficiency interrupting nervous tissue homeostasis. Cutaneous photosensitivity is manifested as repetitive vesiculation, scarring, and deformity, with hypertrichosis of sun-exposed areas of the skin. This is the result of the relatively urine-insoluble heme precursors uroporphyrin III, coproporphyrin III, and protoporphyrin IX fluorescing in the skin following absorption of 400-nm wavelength electromagnetic radiation. These fluorescing porphyrias also can cause discoloration of teeth and occasionally hemolysis of erythrocytes in which porphyrins accumulate.

A number of industrial and environmental toxins have induced toxic porphyrias similar to porphyria cutanea tarda in people heavily exposed to the agents (Table 15–3). These toxins usually cause liver injury and deranged hepatic heme synthesis. Although the exact metabolic effects of these agents are not entirely understood, unregulated stimulation of δ-aminolevulinic acid synthetase usually is demonstrable.

1. Hexachlorobenzene

In an outbreak of acquired porphyria in Turkey between 1955 and 1958, more than 4000 people devel-

oped a cutaneous porphyria syndrome that resembled congenital erythropoietic porphyria approximately 6 months following ingestion of wheat containing the fungicide hexachlorobenzene. The wheat was intended for planting and contained 2 kg of 10% hexachlorobenzene per 1000 kg of wheat to control the fungus *Tilletia*

Table 15–3. Toxic substances associated with acquired porphyria in humans.

Toxin	Use
Hexachlorobenzene	Fungicide
2,4-Dichlorophenol	Herbicide
2,4,5-Trichlorophenol	Herbicide
2,3,7,8-Tetrachlorodibenzo-*p*-dioxin	Herbicide contaminant
o-Benzyl-*p*-chlorophenol	Cleanser and disinfectant
2-Benzyl-*p*-dichlorophenol	Commercial disinfectant
Vinyl chloride	Plastics
Lead	Paint compounds
Aluminum	Phosphorus binder

tritici. Affected people demonstrated cutaneous photosensitivity with skin hyperpigmentation, hypertrichosis, bullae, weakness, and hepatomegaly, a condition termed *kara yara,* or "black sore." Porphyrinuria was nearly universal, with the urine being pigmented red or brown. The mortality rate was 10%. Breast-fed infants younger than 2 years of age had a 95% mortality rate when ingesting mother's milk contaminated with the fungicide. These infants developed weakness, convulsions, and cutaneous annular erythema, a condition termed *pembe yara,* or "pink sore." Excess porphyrins could not be detected in the urine of these infants. A similar result occurs in animal models of hexachlorobenzene-induced porphyria. Infant rats and mice die of neurologic toxicity from hexachlorobenzene without porphyrinuria, whereas adult rats and rabbits develop cutaneous photosensitivity and porphyrinuria following prolonged exposure to the chemical.

A follow-up study between 1977 and 1983 examined 204 patients who had previously suffered from hexachlorobenzene porphyria. The mean age of these individuals was 32 years, and the mean time from hexachlorobenzene exposure was 7 years. The mean duration of cutaneous porphyria symptoms was 2.4 years. At the time of study, 71% of people had hyperpigmentation and 47% had hypertrichosis. Residual scarring on sun-exposed areas of the skin was evident in 87%. Other features included perioral scarring, small hands, arthritis, short stature, weakness, paresthesias, and myotonia. Seventeen patients still had red urine and demonstrated porphyrinuria (especially uroporphyrinuria). Hexachlorobenzene was measurable in 56 samples of human milk obtained from porphyric mothers at a mean value of 0.51 parts per million (ppm) (versus 0.07 ppm in controls).

The Turkish experience was the first associating exposure to an industrial chemical with acquired porphyria in humans. Not only were the symptomatic attack and mortality rates significant, but also the biochemical lesion persisted for decades in many survivors. The exact mechanism by which hexachlorobenzene induces porphyria remains to be elucidated. Most liver mitochondria of animals made porphyric by exposure to chlorinated benzenes, such as hexachlorobenzene, demonstrated increased activity of δ-aminolevulinic acid synthetase, the enzyme that controls the rate of porphyrin production. With the exception of mice made porphyric with diethyl-1,4-dihydro-2,4,6-trimethylpyridine-3,5-dicarboxylate, animal porphyric livers demonstrate an increased production of heme. Heme normally inhibits the activity of δ-aminolevulinic acid synthetase. This suggests that porphyrinogenic compounds are somehow interfering with the repressor signal of heme on δ-aminolevulinic acid synthetase. Other theories suggest that porphyrinogenic compounds induce δ-aminolevulinic acid synthetase by altering the intracellular oxidation state through action on the electron transport chain, thus stimulating succinyl-CoA production, depressing intracellular adenosine triphosphate levels, or both. In any event, the net result is overproduction of porphyrins mediated by unregulated δ-aminolevulinic acid synthetase activity.

The role of iron overload in the pathogenesis of hexachlorobenzene-induced porphyria has been examined. The suggestion that iron might be involved was based on the observation that 80% of patients with porphyria cutanea tarda—a disease associated with reduced hepatic uroporphyrinogen decarboxylase activity—have increased liver iron stores and increased levels of uroporphyrin I. Furthermore, decreasing hepatic iron stores by phlebotomy in patients with porphyria cutanea tarda often induces disease remission and a decrease in urinary uroporphyrin I excretion. In a porcine and human liver model, ferrous iron was found to markedly inhibit uroporphyrinogen III cosynthetase activity, enhance total porphyrin production, and greatly overproduce uroporphyrin I. In rats made porphyric with hexachlorobenzene, iron overload results in decreased production of liver heme, cytochrome P450, and cytochrome b5 and an absence of uroporphyrinogen decarboxylase activity. In addition, the nicotinic acid dehydrogenase (NAD):NADH ratio was more than twofold higher in sideritic rats made porphyric with hexachlorobenzene compared with nonsideritic rats. Furthermore, phlebotomized iron-deficient mice were protected from the porphyrinogenic effect of 2,3,7,8-tetrachlorodibenzo-*p*-dioxin.

Most authorities believe that iron plays a permissive rather than a causative role in porphyrias. This is based on the facts that not all patients with porphyria cutanea tarda are iron overloaded, that porphyria cutanea tarda is rare in patients with hemochromatosis, and that phlebotomy does not correct the biochemical lesion in patients with porphyria cutanea tarda. In addition, rats made porphyric by hexachlorobenzene did not require iron overload for porphyria to develop, although the porphyria was worsened by iron overload. Thus it remains unsettled whether iron overload is permissive or etiologic in patients exposed to porphyrinogenic toxins.

2. Herbicides

A number of herbicides clearly are associated with symptomatic porphyria. Twenty-nine patients exposed to 2,4-dichlorophenol and 2,4,5-trichlorophenol at a manufacturing plant exhibited chloracne; 13 had hyperpigmentation, 11 had hirsutism, and 5 had skin fragility. Eleven patients had increased excretion of urine porphyrins (uroporphyrin and coproporphyrin). Thus these patients had developed an acquired porphyria cutanea tarda-like syndrome after variable exposure to these herbicides. A follow-up study of 73 workers at this same herbicide plant 6 years later found no people with the porphyric syndrome and only one with persistent uroporphyrinuria. The authors of the follow-up study hypothesized that the decrease in the syndrome was a result of improved personal safety habits of the workers and decreased exposure to the chemicals. An alternative explanation is that the true porphyrinogenic agent is perhaps 2,3,7,8-tetrachlorodibenzo-*p*-dioxin, a by-product of 2,4,5-trichlorophenol, and that this contaminant had been effectively eliminated from the chemical stores at the factory. The contaminant was strongly implicated in an outbreak of acquired porphyria cutanea tarda, chloracne, and polyneuropathy in 80 industrial workers producing herbicides in Czechoslovakia.

3. Disinfectants

The commercial disinfectants *o*-benzyl-*p*-chlorophenol and 2-benzyl-4,6-dichlorophenol were implicated as a cause of acquired porphyria cutanea tarda in one woman exposed to these compounds.

4. Aluminum

A porphyria cutanea tarda-like syndrome has been described in patients with chronic renal failure being maintained on regular hemodialysis. Plasma and urine uroporphyrins are increased in these patients, whereas plasma and urine coproporphyrins are often low. Because aluminum is known to inhibit some heme synthetic enzymes, and because many chronic renal failure patients on hemodialysis are aluminum overloaded, aluminum has been implicated, but without proof, as the cause of porphyria in these patients.

5. Vinyl Chloride

Vinyl chloride is a known hepatotoxin used in the production of plastics. A study of 46 persons working in a polyvinyl chloride production plant revealed significantly elevated urinary coproporphyrin levels compared with normal controls. Exposure periods ranged from 2 to 21 years. The pathogenesis of coproporphyrinuria involves inhibition of coproporphyrinogen oxidase, inhibition of uroporphyrinogen decarboxylase, and perhaps induction of δ-aminolevulinic acid synthetase. Persons with excess urinary coproporphyrin production also manifested thrombocytopenia, splenomegaly, esophageal varices, scleroderma-like skin changes, Raynaud syndrome, and acroosteolysis.

6. Lead

Lead intoxication (blood lead level > 60 μg/dL in adults and > 25 μg/dL in children) causes symptoms and signs remarkably similar to those associated with acute intermittent porphyria. The classic acute intermittent porphyria triad is abdominal pain, constipation, and vomiting—all representing the neurotoxic effects of excess δ-aminolevulinic acid and porphobilinogen. This triad is seen with equal frequency in lead intoxication. Other shared characteristics include neuromuscular pains, paresis or paralysis, paresthesias, diarrhea, and seizures. The major differences between the two diseases are (1) an increase in neuropsychiatric signs in acute intermittent porphyria compared with lead intoxication and (2) anemia, which is present in lead intoxication but virtually absent in porphyria. The anemia of lead poisoning is a characteristic microcytic anemia with basophilic stippling of erythrocytes and sideroblasts in the bone marrow.

The biochemical features of lead poisoning demonstrate why these two diseases are so similar clinically. Patients with lead intoxication have markedly elevated urinary δ-aminolevulinic acid levels, as in acute intermittent porphyria. Mild lead poisoning (preanemia stage) is associated with normal porphobilinogen excretion, but once anemia occurs, excess urinary porphobilinogen becomes demonstrable. Although mild elevations of urine coproporphyrins and uroporphyrin I are present, fecal uroporphyrin and coproporphyrin are normal in patients with lead poisoning. These alterations in porphyrins are present only in patients with inorganic lead intoxication, not in patients with organic lead intoxication. Excess accumulation of protoporphyrin IX also has been found in erythrocytes of lead-intoxicated patients.

Lead poisoning is associated with greatly diminished activity of δ-aminolevulinic acid dehydrase in the brain, liver, kidney, and bone marrow. Because δ-aminolevulinic acid dehydrase is polymorphic, different individuals may have different levels of sensitivity to lead exposure depending on the particular form of the enzyme that is inherited. Lead also blocks the incorporation of iron into protoporphyrin IX by depressing the activity of ferrochelatase, an event most closely linked with the production of anemia and elevation of free erythrocyte protoporphyrin IX levels. Coproporphyrinogen oxidase activity is also depressed by lead. Thus the effect of lead on heme synthesis disruption occurs at multiple steps in the synthetic pathway, all of which occur in the mitochondrion.

TREATMENT OF TOXIC PORPHYRIAS

Because there is often no effective means of eliminating toxic environmental or industrial substances once they are incorporated into tissues, exposure to porphyrinogenic compounds must be avoided. Although no prospective data are available to support the use of phlebotomy for this purpose, this therapy may be of benefit in patients with toxic porphyria whose disease complex resembles porphyria cutanea tarda and in whom evidence of iron overload can be demonstrated. Patients with acute intermittent porphyria occasionally respond to high-dose carbohydrate infusions (400 g dextrose per day) or hematin infusions (3 mg/kg intravenously every 12 hours for 10–12 doses). However, the use of hematin infusions in toxic porphyria may not be of benefit because, as in the case of hexachlorobenzene, the toxic agent may be interrupting the negative-feedback signal by heme on δ-aminolevulinic acid synthetase.

For lead intoxication, prevention again is the best treatment. Unlike all other toxic porphyrias, specific therapy for lead intoxication is available with lead chelators (see Chapter 27).

REFERENCES

Anderson KE et al: Recommendations for the diagnosis and treatment of the acute porphyrias. Ann Intern Med 2005;142(6):439 [PMID: 15767622].

Kauppinen R: Porphyrias. Lancet 2005;365:241. [PMID: 15652607].

DISORDERS ASSOCIATED WITH DECREASED OXYGEN SATURATION

1. Carbon Monoxide Poisoning

Carbon monoxide is an odorless, colorless, nonirritating gas produced by the incomplete combustion of organic materials, particularly hydrocarbons. The workers at greatest risk are automobile mechanics (automobile exhaust systems), firefighters, and chemical workers exposed to methylene chloride (converted to carbon monoxide through in vivo metabolism).

Carbon monoxide binds to hemoglobin, forming carboxyhemoglobin, which decreases hemoglobin oxygen saturation and shifts the oxygen-hemoglobin dissociation curve to the left. Hemoglobin has an affinity for carbon monoxide that is 210 times greater than that for oxygen. Carbon monoxide also increases the stability of the hemoglobin-oxygen combination, thus inhibiting oxygen delivery to the tissues. In addition, carbon monoxide binds to the cytochrome oxidase chain, interfering with cellular respiration. These properties of carbon monoxide result in chemical asphyxiation.

Clinical Findings

Symptoms include general malaise, headache, nausea, dyspnea, vomiting, and alteration in mental status at high levels. Severe exposure may cause coma, seizures, arrhythmias, and death. Symptoms of anoxia may be prominent without cyanosis because of the cherry-red color of carboxyhemoglobin.

Laboratory findings at chronic low levels may show polycythemia; at higher levels, hypoxia is seen. Carboxyhemoglobin levels should be measured; a level less than 6% may cause impairment in vision and time discrimination; at 40–60% alterations in mental status and death may be seen. Blood carboxyhemoglobin levels can be elevated significantly both after intense exposures of short duration and after chronic low-level exposure.

Treatment & Prevention

Treatment depends on the degree of carboxyhemoglobin. At low levels without symptoms, removal from the source of exposure is sufficient. At higher levels or with symptoms, the treatment of choice is hyperbaric oxygen. Weaver et al. demonstrated a lower incidence of cognitive deficits in patients treated with three hyperbaric oxygen sessions during a 24-hour period starting within 24 hours of the end of carbon monoxide exposure. Oxygen markedly decreases the half-life of carboxyhemoglobin from 5–6 hours at room air to 90 minutes at 100% inspired oxygen by dilutional displacement of the carbon monoxide. Hyperbaric oxygen therapy decreases the half-life of carboxyhemoglobin further to 23 minutes at 3 atm. Prevention depends on adequate ventilation, with venting of combustion devices to the outside air.

REFERENCES

Domachevsky L et al: Hyperbaric oxygen in the treatment of carbon monoxide poisoning. Clin Toxicol. 2005;43:181 [PMID: 15902792].

Kao LW, Nanagas KA: Carbon monoxide poisoning. Med Clin North Am 2005;89:1161 [PMID: 16227059].

DISORDERS AFFECTING BLOOD CELL FORMATION & MORPHOLOGY

Premalignant and malignant hematologic diseases are linked to a variety of occupational exposures. Because the determination of cause and effect is very difficult to verify when the latency period is long and the exposure history is poorly documented, other methods for ascertaining this link have been explored. Cytogenetic study consists of examining the somatic chromosomes of hematologic cells in metaphase.

Cytogenetics

The chromosomal analysis of hematologic disorders is an important mechanism for classification and as a guide to prognosis and therapy. Cytogenetic analysis serves two purposes in occupational hematology: (1) to screen populations at risk for toxic exposure so that cryptic toxic agents can be identified and (2) in individual cases to identify diseases that might have been caused by exposure to mutagenic agents.

Abnormalities in chromosomes can be used as a marker for exposure to noxious environmental agents.

Through extensive epidemiologic study, certain abnormalities have been associated with specific diseases and prognostic categories. Toxic agents that are associated with chromosomal abnormalities in vivo are linked to the development of cancers and leukemias.

Cytogenetic analysis for hematologic disorders is best done by direct examination of cells obtained from bone marrow. Because these cells are continuously proliferating, it is relatively easy to examine those undergoing mitosis when the chromosomes are visible microscopically. High-resolution banding techniques are used to precisely identify deletions, translocations, inversions, and other structural chromosomal abnormalities.

Cells obtained from peripheral blood require artificial stimulation by a mitogen such as phytohemagglutinin and culture for 2–3 days to obtain enough cells in mitosis for analysis. Artifactual aberrations may be induced in cells that are manipulated after removal from the patient before fixing for analysis. The resulting risk of falsely abnormal evaluations increases the necessity and importance of well-matched and multiple controls.

Screening & Prevention

Cytogenetic analysis has been used as a screening tool to monitor industrial populations for early exposure to mutagenic chemicals and to identify possible mutagens. In this way, workers at risk might be removed from potentially dangerous conditions when the effects are still reversible. Peripheral blood lymphocytes rather than bone marrow must be used for obvious reasons of worker comfort, time, and cost.

The problem with using cytogenetics for monitoring is the relative insensitivity of the method to low levels of exposure. The only known dose-response relationship for exposure and somatic chromosome aberrations has been described with ionizing radiation. In a recent study of workers exposed to low levels (below exposure limits) of chemicals in a petrochemical plant in The Netherlands, cytogenetic monitoring by chromosomal banding techniques was carried out from 1976 to 1981. Results of these studies, published in 1988, found no increase in the frequencies of chromosome aberrations in the exposed populations compared with control populations. The authors concluded that the examination of peripheral blood lymphocytes for chromosomal aberrations is not sufficiently sensitive for routine monitoring of cytogenetics in workers exposed to low levels of the compounds.

Other techniques that have been evaluated in monitoring include sister chromatid exchange, the Comet assay, and the micronucleus assay, methods of evaluating chromosomal rearrangements of DNA. Although these techniques are faster and cheaper than cytogenetic analysis; the presence of detectable abnormalities by these assays, however, does not necessarily correlate with the incidence of chromosomal aberrations or the development of disease.

Further progress in methods to detect induced DNA damage is needed for cytogenetic analysis to be an adequate screening tool for large populations. With the advent of molecular biologic techniques, this should be possible in the future on a population-wide scale. At present, although individual health consequences cannot be estimated by population screening methods, abnormal chromosomal or cytogenetic findings clearly are an adverse sign when correlated with specific exposure risk data.

Relationship of Cytogenetic Abnormalities to Specific Diseases

Cytogenetic study provides a means of relating chromosomal aberrations in the bone marrow of a patient with preleukemia or leukemia to exposure to mutagenic agents. The population benefited includes workers exposed to industrial agents and radiation, as well as patients previously treated with chemotherapeutic agents or radiation. Many studies suggest that this population has a much higher incidence of chromosomal abnormalities than does a similar nonexposed group with the same diseases. In a summary of three retrospective studies of patients with de novo acute nonlymphocytic leukemia, individuals were grouped as nonexposed and exposed on the basis of occupation. Individuals who worked with insecticides, chemicals and solvents, metals or minerals, petroleum products, and ionizing radiation were considered exposed, whereas students, white-collar workers, and housewives were classified as nonexposed. Sixty-eight of 236 patients (29%) were found to be in the exposed group. Fifty-one of the 68 (75%) in the exposed group had abnormal karyotypes versus only 60 of 168 (36%) in the nonexposed group. In addition to this generalized increase in chromosomal aberrations, abnormalities in chromosomes 5 and 7 were observed in 37% of the exposed and in 12% of the nonexposed individuals.

These specific chromosomal abnormalities also have correlated positively with the development of leukemia after exposure to therapeutic mutagens (chemotherapy or radiation) used to treat other cancers. Specifically, a loss of the entire chromosome or of part of the long arm of either or both of these chromosomes has been seen. Although these chromosome abnormalities may occur in the absence of exposure to mutagens, patients with leukemias or preleukemic conditions with deletions involving chromosomes 5 or 7 should arouse a suspicion of prior exposure to chemical carcinogens or radiation, and this history should be sought vigorously. The prognosis for patients with abnormalities of chromosomes 5 or 7—or with multiple cytogenetic abnormalities when associated with prior exposure to mutagenic agents—is poor when compared with that of patients with a normal chromosome analysis.

Clearly, the greatest usefulness of cytogenetics is in the area of prevention and developing better techniques to assess future pathologic consequences of exposure at a time when effects still may be reversible. As more sensitive techniques are developed, they also may serve as a guideline for determining the threshold limit values for potential mutagens.

REFERENCES

Bonassi S et al: Chromosomal aberrations and risk of cancer in humans: An epidemiologic perspective. Cytogenet Genome Res 2004;104:376 [PMID: 15162068].

Maciejewski JP, Selleri C: Evolution of clonal cytogenetic abnormalities in aplastic anemia. Leuk Lymphoma 2004;45:433 [PMID: 15160903].

Palus J et al: Genotoxic effects of occupational exposure to lead and cadmium. Mutat Res 2003;540:19 [PMID: 12972055].

WORK-RELATED APLASTIC ANEMIA AND HEMATOLOGIC CANCERS

Hematologic cancers are discussed in detail in Chapter 16. In this section we discuss only aplastic anemia, myelodysplasia, and multiple myeloma, diseases not covered in Chapter 16.

1. Aplastic Anemia

Aplastic anemia, or medullary aplasia, is an acquired abnormality of the pluripotent hematopoietic stem cells resulting in pancytopenia (anemia, neutropenia, and thrombocytopenia). The average incidence of fatal aplastic anemia per year in the United States is approximately 2 per million and rises with age to an annual age-specific mortality rate of about 10 per million in people older than age 65. Approximately 50% of cases of aplastic anemia in North America and western Europe are idiopathic; most of the remainder are termed *secondary aplastic anemias* and may be caused by drugs, chemicals, radiation, infection, and immunologic mechanisms. A small percentage of cases are caused by hereditary diseases.

The largest category of secondary aplastic anemia is caused by therapeutic drugs; probably only a small fraction are a result of environmental and occupational causes. The drug most commonly implicated is chloramphenicol; other implicated drugs include acetazolamide, phenylbutazone, phenytoin, and sulfonamides—and there are many others. This section discusses only occupation-related cases of aplastic anemia.

Many cases of aplastic anemia develop after the occurrence of dysplastic morphologic changes in hematologic cells with associated chromosomal abnormalities. The incidence of acute nonlymphocytic leukemia in patients with aplastic anemia who survive 2 years

after diagnosis is approximately 5–10%; in patients with preceding dysplasia, the incidence may be higher. Chemicals that are capable of inducing bone marrow damage must be assumed to be potential leukemogens. It is difficult to link specific chemicals to the development of aplastic anemia because of the absence of a specific test for exposure and the frequency of multiple or unknown exposures. Only three agents are firmly established as a cause of aplastic anemia on a dose-dependent basis: benzene, ionizing radiation, and cytotoxic drugs such as antimetabolites and alkylating agents. Benzene and ionizing radiation are discussed at greater length in Chapter 16.

Benzene

Benzene was first described as a cause of fatal aplastic anemia in 1897. Early unregulated exposure to benzene—used widely as a solvent in the production of many products, including fabrics and pesticides—led to many cases of acute and chronic toxicity. Workers now at greatest risk of exposure are those involved in rubber manufacturing, shoemaking, petroleum and chemical production, printing, and steelworking.

Before 1950, benzene was the single most common cause of toxic aplastic anemia. With chronic doses of greater than 100 ppm, isolated cytopenias and aplastic anemia were common. The cytopenias usually resolved after termination of exposure; even with persistent exposure, spontaneous remissions have been described. At exposures of 100 ppm or higher, some workers will develop fatal aplastic anemia. Great variation in susceptibility to exposure has been seen, with evidence of poisoning sometimes appearing only after weeks or years. Cases of cytopenia also have been seen several years after exposure has been terminated; these cases are less likely to resolve with time and may be part of a preleukemic syndrome. In severe chronic poisoning, decreased red cell survival with hemolysis has been reported.

Toxicity is directly related to the amount and duration of exposure, although again there is individual variation in susceptibility. The current U.S. exposure limit is 1 ppm. The diagnosis is made by examination of the bone marrow after an abnormal complete blood count is reported. The bone marrow will reveal hypocellularity with fatty replacement, although islands of hypercellularity may be seen. Although cytogenetic abnormalities are associated with benzene exposure, specific chromosome changes are not. The initial prognosis in benzene-related aplastic anemia is better than that for idiopathic aplastic anemia; up to 40% of patients may recover completely after removal from the source of exposure. If hypocellularity persists for more than several months, recovery is not likely to occur. Exposure is also associated with the development of acute nonlymphocytic leukemia and chronic myelogenous leukemia—either de novo or in workers who have recovered from a bout of aplastic anemia—and in cases of irreversible aplastic anemia.

Treatment is supportive (i.e., with transfusions and such growth factors as erythropoietin, granulocyte colony-stimulating factor, and granulocyte-macrophage colony-stimulating factor). Drugs such as androgens to stimulate hematopoiesis have not been used extensively in benzene-induced aplastic anemia but should be tried when no other treatment option exists (such as bone marrow transplantation or colony-stimulating factors). Allogeneic bone marrow transplantation is the only known cure for irreversible aplastic anemia but is hampered by donor availability, higher mortality risk with increasing patient age, and the toxicity of the transplant regimen.

Ionizing Radiation

Ionizing radiation also has been associated with aplastic anemia in a dose-dependent manner. Internal exposure to absorbed alpha particles associated with aplastic anemia was demonstrated most strikingly in the radium watch dial workers who ingested radium by wetting their paintbrushes on their tongues. External exposure to radiation is much more common and may be in the form of whole-body exposure to a large dose, as in a nuclear accident or therapeutic radiation, or long-term exposure to small amounts, as may occur in the practice of radiology as a medical specialty.

Data from patients radiated for ankylosing spondylitis and from the survivors of the atomic bombings of Hiroshima and Nagasaki suggest that the risk of aplastic anemia is increased until 3–5 years after exposure, after which there is a marked decline in incidence. The most important late disturbance following irradiation of the bone marrow is leukemia. The ability to recover from a single dose of penetrating radiation depends on the fraction of surviving stem cells. Chromosomal aberrations are associated with exposure to ionizing radiation and rise in a linear manner as a function of the dose of radiation absorbed. The presence of these aberrations, including an increase in the number of sister chromatid exchanges, may signify excessive exposure but is not predictive of aplastic anemia or leukemia.

Strict regulation of exposure and monitoring with badges has virtually eliminated aplastic anemia caused by radiation except in cases of accidental overexposure. In this case, treatment again is primarily supportive. Recovery may be seen after a prolonged period of aplastic anemia lasting 3–6 weeks and may be predicted from the known total dose of radiation. If recovery does not occur, permanent injury to the stem cell population has resulted in chronic cellular hypoplasia or dysplasia or in leukemia. Treatment then may include bone marrow transplantation if a donor is available.

Other Chemicals

Aplastic anemia has been reported following exposure to a variety of other chemicals listed in Table 15–4. Toxicities often resolve completely with cessation of exposure. Again, individual susceptibility plays an important role, although it is poorly understood.

Two chemicals in particular deserve mention here. The aplastic anemia associated with trinitrotoluene may be accompanied by methemoglobinemia, oxidative hemolysis, liver damage, and dermatitis. The incidence of overexposure to arsenic has declined with its decreasing use over the past three decades. Fewer than 10 cases of poisoning are now reported annually in the United States. If arsenic-induced aplastic anemia or pancytopenia is suspected, laboratory confirmation of the exposure (see Chapter 27) should be obtained. Complete spontaneous recovery usually is seen if the patient is removed from the source of exposure within a few days to weeks.

REFERENCES

Brodsky RA, Jones RJ: Aplastic anaemia. Lancet 2005;365:1647 [PMID: 15885298].

Keohane EM: Acquired aplastic anemia. Clin Lab Sci 2004;17:165 [PMID: 15314891].

2. Myelodysplastic Syndromes

The myelodysplasic syndromes are a group of acquired genetic disorders of the blood-forming cells similar to cancer and characterized by ineffective hematopoiesis, clinically resulting in anemia, neutropenia, thrombocytopenia, or a combination of cytopenias. These syndromes are

Table 15–4. Chemicals reported to cause aplastic anemia in an occupational setting.

Chemical	Use
Benzene	Intermediate in the synthesis of fabrics, pesticides, rubber; solvent for glues, varnishes, inks, paints; octane booster for gasoline
Trinitrotoluene (TNT)	Production of explosives
Hexachloroclyclohexane (lindane) Pentachlorophenol Chlorophenothane (DDT)	Pesticide
Arsenic	Manufacture of glass, paint, enamels, weed killers, tanning agents, pesticides
Ethylene glycol monomethyl or monobutyl ether	Production of paints, lacquers, dyes, inks, cleaning agents

linked by the presence of bizarre hematopoietic morphology and the tendency to transform into acute leukemia. Most patients with myelodysplasia, however, do not develop leukemia, although specific syndromes associated with exposure to both occupational chemicals and cytotoxic drugs have a high incidence of progression to frank leukemia. Both benzene and ionizing radiation have been implicated in the development of myelodysplasia. Several case-control studies have suggested that other occupational risk factors, such as exposure to pesticides or solvents or employment in specific sectors such as farming, textile work, or the health professions, may be relevant. The median survival from these diseases is less than 12 months, and all patients eventually either develop leukemias or succumb to complications related to cytopenias. Exposure and treatment-related myelodysplasia is specifically associated with a high incidence of deletions involving chromosomes 5 and 7.

Myelodysplastic syndromes (MDS) are more common in men than in women, and 85% of patients are older than 40 years of age at the time of diagnosis. Laboratory features of MDS include cytopenias of various degrees and often an increase in the red blood cell mean corpuscular volume. The marrow usually reveals dysplasia in all three cell lines [granulocyte/erythroid/megakaryocyte (plateletforming)] and manifests abnormal marrow cellularity, usually hypercellular. There is an abnormal increase in the percentage of blast cells.

Several treatment options are available, although all have significant drawbacks. Allogeneic bone marrow transplantation (a transplant from a donor, usually a sibling or matched unrelated donor) is the only known cure but is limited primarily by patient age and carries a significant risk of treatment-related mortality. Transfusions and treatment of infections may be aided by the use of hematopoietic growth factors. The hypomethylating chemotherapy drug azacytidine is approved by the Food and Drug Administration for MDS, and two other agents, lenolidomide and decitabine, appear quite active, although none of these agents appears to be curative.

REFERENCES

Catenacci DV, Schiller GJ: Myelodysplasic syndromes: A comprehensive review. Blood Rev 2005;19:301 [PMID: 15885860].

Hofmann WK, Koeffler HP: Myelodysplastic syndrome. Annu Rev Med 2005;56:1 [PMID: 15660498].

Lawrence LW: Refractory anemia and the myelodysplastic syndromes. Clin Lab Sci 2004;17:178 [PMID: 15314893].

Stadler M, Ganser A: Treatment of myelodysplastic syndromes. N Engl J Med 2005;352:2134 [PMID: 15906434].

3. Multiple Myeloma

Multiple myeloma is a chronic leukemia of differentiated B cells (termed *plasma cells*) that accounts for 15% of all hematologic cancers. It is characterized by anemia, painful lytic and osteopenic bone disease, monoclonal immunoglobulin production (in serum or urine or both), hypogammaglobulinemia, and short survival. Patients also may have hypercalcemia, renal failure, or neuropathy. Treatment involves a variety of agents, including thalidomide, chemotherapy (with such agents as melphalan, vincristine, vinblastine, doxorubicin, cyclophosphamide, and carmustine), and corticosteroids with the goal of alleviating bone pain, correcting complications of the disease, and prolonging life. Autologous bone marrow transplantation soon after diagnosis appears to improve both disease-free and overall survival. This less toxic form of therapy is available to a wider range of patients up to age 70 years.

The peak incidence of multiple myeloma is between ages 55 and 65, and fewer than 2% of cases occur before the age of 40. Multiple myeloma is equally common in men and women but almost twice as common in blacks as in whites. The incidence of multiple myeloma has been increasing over the last three decades in North American and European men, but this rise has not been noted in the stable study populations in Minnesota and Sweden and simply may reflect an increase in our ability to diagnose the disease. The rise in incidence has aroused concern that myeloma might be associated with environmental or occupational factors.

Although there is no definitive link between occupational exposure and the risk of multiple myeloma, many epidemiologic studies suggest an association. Exposure to petroleum products, organic solvents, heavy metals, pesticides, and asbestos is implicated, but most studies are small and can be used only as a basis for hypotheses. Workers thought to be at risk include agricultural workers, chemicals workers, miners, smelters, stokers, and furniture workers.

Benzene is metabolized through a complex series of enzymatic steps that result in the production of oxygen radicals. These oxygen radicals have radiomimetic effects, which damage DNA and can induce hematopoietic cancer such as acute myelogenous leukemia.

An important association between high-dose radiation exposure and multiple myeloma has been observed in cohorts of controls and survivors of the atomic bombings of Hiroshima and Nagasaki for the period of 1950–1976. The relative risk for persons with an estimated air-dose exposure of 100 cGy or more was over four times higher than that of controls. This excess risk became apparent approximately 20 years after exposure. An association also has been proposed—but not confirmed—between the risk of multiple myeloma and exposure to low-dose radiation. At present, except in the case of high-dose radiation, there are insufficient data on which to base a firm conclusion about the relationship between exposure to ionizing radiation and the risk of developing multiple myeloma. Further large-scale incidence studies on this topic are needed.

REFERENCES

Baris D et al: Occupation, pesticide exposure and risk of multiple myeloma. Scand J Work Environ Health 2004;30:215 [PMID: 15250650].

Glass DC et al: Leukemia risk and relevant benzene exposure period. Am J Indust Med 2004;45:222 [PMID: 14748054].

Goldstein B: Benzene exposure and leukemia. Epidemiology 2004; 15:509 [PMID: 15232416].

TOXIC THROMBOCYTOPENIA

Unlike thrombocytopenia associated with toxicant-induced aplastic anemia, isolated toxic thrombocytopenia is a rare event. A number of toxic exposures have been reported that resulted in isolated thrombocytopenia (Table 15–5). In 1963, two cases of isolated thrombocytopenia were described in individuals exposed to the polymerizing agent toluene diisocyanate. In both, thrombocytopenia developed 14–22 days following a significant exposure that also induced bronchospasm. These patients developed thrombocytopenic bleeding with nadir platelet counts of 6000/μL and 30,000/μL. Bone marrow samples in both cases showed increased megakaryocytes. The pathophysiologic defect was enhanced peripheral platelet destruction, presumably on an immune basis (immune thrombocytopenic purpura). One patient responded transiently to corticosteroid therapy and then completely to splenectomy; the second patient had resolution of thrombocytopenia without any therapy.

Two more cases of toxin-induced immune thrombocytopenic purpura were described in 1969. Two children with significant turpentine exposure (one respiratory and cutaneous exposure, the second ingestion) developed petechiae and severe thrombocytopenia with increased bone marrow megakaryocytes. Both responded fully to corticosteroid therapy.

Insecticides can cause a selective megakaryocyte aplasia in people with significant inhalation or ingestion exposure. Isolated thrombocytopenia has been reported after exposure to 2,2-dichlorovinyl dimethyl phosphate, dieldrin, pyrethrin, hexachlorocyclohexane (lindane), and chlorophenothane (DDT). These patients demonstrated absent or decreased bone marrow megakaryocytes. Some megakaryocytes were vacuolated. Most patients received corticosteroids and responded with full platelet recovery.

A third form of toxic thrombocytopenia was described in 1984. Forty-six people exposed to vinyl chloride with evidence of toxic coproporphyrinuria also had thrombocytopenia. Although these patients were not described in detail, they appeared to have significant vinyl chloride liver toxicity, with esophageal varices and splenomegaly. The likely pathophysiologic mechanism of thrombocytopenia thus was enhanced peripheral platelet consumption caused by hypersplenism, although there were insufficient data presented to rule out an immune or megakaryocyte toxic mechanism.

Normal hemostasis depends both on the quantity of platelets present and on their ability to aggregate appropriately under physiologic stimulation. Qualitative disturbances in platelet function as a result of various occupational and environmental substances have been described. Some (but not all) pesticides, such as p,p-DDE [2,2-bis-(p-chlorophrenyl)-1,1-dichloroethylene] and Aroclor 1242 (a chlorinated biphenyl that is 42% chlorine), inhibit platelet aggregation in a dose-dependent manner by inhibiting platelet cyclooxygenase activity (an aspirin-like effect). Exposures to these substances could cause mucocutaneous bleeding in susceptible individuals. On the other hand, some environmental substances (e.g., methyl mercury, cadmium, and triethyl lead) induce platelet aggregation and could result in hypercoagulation. These qualitative platelet disturbances have not yet been reported in humans subject to occupational exposure and remain theoretical risks.

Table 15–5. Toxic agents associated with isolated thrombocytopenia.

Toxic Agent	Use	Mechanism
Toluene diisocyanate	Polymerizing agent	Immune
2,2-Dichlorovinyl dimethylphosphate Dieldrin Pyrethrin Hexachlorocyclohexane (lindane) Chlorophenothane (DDT)	Insecticide	Megakaryocyte hypoplasia
Turpentine	Organic solvent	Immune
Vinyl chloride	Plastics	Liver insufficiency with hypersplenism

OCCUPATIONAL EXPOSURE TO ANTICANCER DRUGS

Oncology nurses and pharmacists who prepare and administer chemotherapy to patients on a regular basis are at risk for exposure to potentially mutagenic agents. Data from a variety of sources are available on the mutagenic potential of many anticancer drugs. Epidemiologic studies link certain drugs (and radiation) to the development of secondary cancers; analytic in vitro methods of assessing mutagenicity offer corroborative evidence.

There are several obvious problems in assessing the risk to nurses. First is the low and intermittent exposure rate relative to the patients who receive these drugs therapeutically and who serve as in vivo models for the effects of heavy exposure. This limits the usefulness of epidemiologic data such as exposure rates and disease incidence when attempting to assess individual risks. Second, the methods for detecting exposure often are contradictory and may be cumbersome in time relative to work. For example, it may be difficult for nurses to obtain urine 6 hours after the end of a shift.

Methods for assessing risk include measuring blood and urine levels of drug, urine mutagenicity assays, cytogenetic monitoring and sister chromatid exchange studies, and environmental monitoring. Blood and urine levels may be difficult to interpret when drugs are metabolized rapidly. Studies evaluating oncology nurses versus control populations of other nurses or non-health care workers have been published with both positive and negative results using all the preceding methods. Clearly a combination of monitoring tools is required.

In addition to the preceding studies, which assess potential risk, the effect on human reproduction in terms of spontaneous abortion and teratogenic effects also has been examined. Again, the results are inconclusive but suggest an increase in both effects with frequent exposure. Information on safety practices is not available.

The agents implicated most commonly in mutagenic potential are those that are also implicated as causes of secondary cancers in patients receiving therapeutic drugs such as alkylating agents. Clearly, any cytotoxic drug should be handled with great care and with the goal of absolutely minimum exposure to personnel. This can be accomplished by worker education, gloves and protective clothing, laminar hoods for preparing drugs, and proper waste disposal. Periodic atmospheric checks and biologic monitoring can improve hygienic standards, but conclusions regarding the long-term health effects based on these results are not possible.

REFERENCES

Joseph LJ et al: Frequency of micronuclei in peripheral blood lymphocytes from subjects occupationally exposed to low levels of ionizing radiation. Mutat Res 2004;564:83 [PMID: 15474414].

Maffei F et al: Spectrum of chromosomal aberrations in peripheral lymphocytes of hospital workers occupationally exposed to low doses of ionizing radiation. Mutat Res 2004;547:91 [PMID: 15013703].

Miklacic S: Frequency of chromosomal lesions and damaged lymphocytes of workers occupationally exposed to x-rays. Health Phys 2005;88:334 [PMID: 15761294].

Occupational Cancer

16

Hope S. Rugo, MD

One of every two or three individuals in the industrialized world will develop some type of cancer during their lifetimes. The majority of cancers in adults are thought to be the result of a combination of factors, including environmental exposure, lifestyle, and genetic factors. Approximately 5–10% of all human cancers are thought to be caused by occupational exposure to carcinogens; however, the risks within an occupationally exposed population may be much higher.

The identification of occupational carcinogens is important at least in part because most occupational cancers are completely preventable with appropriate personnel practices and strict protective legislation. In this chapter the fundamental properties of occupational carcinogenesis are reviewed. Investigative methods used to identify possible carcinogens, general and specific strategies for prevention, and clinical presentations of well-described occupational cancers are covered in detail. A modified version of the International Agency of Research on Cancer's classification of occupational carcinogens is included in table form. Further classification of carcinogenic agents may be found on the Web site of the National Institute of Environmental Health Sciences (www.niehs.nih.gov/) and in the Report on Carcinogens (http://ehp.niehs.nih.gov/roc/toc10.html).

CARCINOGENESIS: FUNDAMENTAL PROPERTIES

Evidence suggests that cancers arise from a single abnormal cell. The initial stage in development of the abnormal cell appears to result from an alteration or mutation in the genetic material deoxyribonucleic acid (DNA). This alteration may occur spontaneously or may be caused by exogenous factors, such as exposure to carcinogenic chemicals or radiation. Whether a tumor develops from this altered cell may depend on a variety of factors, such as the ability of the cell to repair the damage, the presence of other endogenous or exogenous agents that foster or inhibit tumor development, and the integrity of the immune system.

Stages in Tumor Development

A variety of evidence indicates that cells undergo multiple heritable changes in the process of becoming a "cancer cell"; this process is termed *carcinogenesis*. Early

animal studies investigating the etiology of cancer cell growth hypothesized that tumor development involved at least two distinct stages: initiation and promotion. A classic example of this process is the mouse skin tumor model. In this model, a small dose of a carcinogen, known as the *initiator* [typically a polycyclic aromatic hydrocarbon (PAH)] is applied to the skin. Although large doses of PAH alone readily induced skin tumors, the smaller doses alone did not. However, application of a *promoter* such as croton oil following the initiator did result in tumor development. Interestingly, application of the promoter alone or prior to administration of the initiator did not result in skin tumors. A similar process has been implicated in the development of tumors in other organs, such as mouse liver and lung and rat trachea. For example, ingestion of a small quantity of various nitrosamines (initiators) followed by regular ingestion of polychlorinated biphenyls (promoters) results in production of liver tumors in mice. Clearly, there are limitations to the application of animal models of tumorigenesis to the etiology of common human tumors. However, these data have provided a framework to understand basic toxin-induced carcinogenesis (Figure 16–1).

From a functional point of view, it now appears helpful to view carcinogenesis as a stepwise process including initiation, promotion, and progression. Initiation is thought to result from an irreversible change in the genetic material (DNA) of the cell arising from interaction with a carcinogen that is a necessary, but not sufficient, condition for tumor development. It is this somatic mutation that sets the stage for tumor development and is the basis for the somatic-mutation theory of carcinogenesis.

Promotion consists of those processes subsequent to initiation that facilitate tumor development, presumably by stimulating proliferation of the altered cell. The mechanisms of promotion, sometimes referred to as *epigenetic mechanisms* (as opposed to the genotoxic or mutational effects of initiators), are incompletely understood. Promotion classically does not result from binding to and alteration of DNA but may result from production of or suppression of proteins that alter the way that DNA is transcribed. In the case of the mouse skin tumor model, croton oil appears to interact with membrane receptors to affect cellular growth and differentiation. Promotion typically yields a benign tumor or group of preneoplastic cells

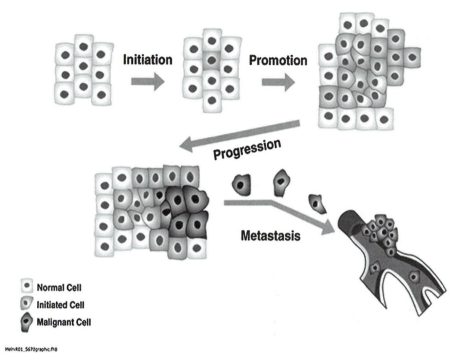

Normal Cell

Initiated Cell

Malignant Cell

MelnvR01_S67Ographic.fh8

Figure 16–1. Carcinogenesis progression.

that do not have the ability to invade stroma or metastasize; progression then creates those additional heritable changes necessary for the development of a malignant tumor.

This process is referred to as the *multistep* or *multistage model of carcinogenesis*. Most common adult cancers, such as colorectal cancer, are the results of multiple genetic and protein mutational changes. While it is clearly a simplistic categorization, carcinogens are often divided into initiating

agents, or genotoxic (DNA-reactive) "early stage" carcinogens, and promoting agents, or epigenetic "late stage" carcinogens. Table 16–1 lists the distinguishing features of initiating and promoting agents. Some agents (e.g., cigarette smoke) that seem to possess both initiating and promoting properties are termed *complete carcinogens*. However, it is clear that damage from cigarette smoke sets the stage for more efficient carcinogenesis with exposure to

Table 16–1. Distinctions between initiators and promoters of carcinogenesis.

Initiators	Promoters
Genotoxic	Not genotoxic; epigenetic mechanism
Carcinogenic alone	Not carcinogenic alone; active only after initiator exposure
Generally yield electrophilic compounds; highly reactive (often form free radicals)	Not electrophilic
Covalently bind to nucleophiles (e.g., DNA), leading to irreversible alteration in genetic material	Generally do not bind to nor alter DNA; often act by induction of cellular proliferation; effects may be reversible
Generally active in short-term tests (mutagenic)	Not active in short-term tests
Existence of threshold dose cannot be verified	Threshold probably exists
Single exposure may be sufficient to induce subsequent cancer	Repeated exposures required

toxins such as asbestos or nickel. Given the complexity of the multistage model and increasing experimental evidence that tends to blur the distinction between these categories, the value of categorizing specific agents probably is limited. In addition, owing to the time from exposure to an initiating agent to the subsequent development of visible cancer, identification of possible causative agents may be extremely difficult.

The mechanism by which carcinogen-induced alteration in DNA leads to initiation and ultimately to tumor development is related at least in part to mutations in protooncogenes and tumor-suppressor genes. Protooncogenes contain DNA sequences that, when altered by a mutational event into an oncogene, stimulate transformation and proliferation of an altered potentially neoplastic cell. There are a number of protooncogenes in human and animal cells that are responsible for normal cellular differentiation and maturation. In contrast, tumor-suppressor genes function as negative regulators of cell growth. A genetic change in one or more tumor-suppressor genes, which results in inactivation of a specific gene, allows unregulated growth of the altered cell. The observation that tumors develop only after activation of one or more oncogenes and inactivation of one or more tumor-suppressor genes provides a mechanistic explanation for the multistep model of carcinogenesis.

There are a number of mechanisms that result in genetic alterations, including point mutations, chromosome translocation or rearrangement, gene amplification, and the induction of numerical chromosome changes (aneuploidy), each of which theoretically could be induced by a chemical exposure. For example, point mutations in *ras* protooncogenes (so called because they were identified originally in rat sarcomas) have been observed in human and rodent tumors. The *ras* gene codes for a protein product known as p21, differing by only one amino acid from the normal protein. This protein may function as a direct cell-transforming agent, conferring malignant potential to the cell.

For most toxic effects, the persistence or progression of damage requires the continued presence of the offending chemical agent. For cancer initiators, however, a single exposure may induce genetic damage in the cell sufficient to result in tumor development years after exposure has ceased. An example of this is the development of mesothelioma more than 20 years after a single or brief exposure to asbestos.

Induction-Latency Period

In both experimental animal models of cancer and human cancers with known causes, a significant interval of time is required from first exposure to the responsible agent to the development of malignancy. This interval is referred to as the *induction-latency (latency)* or *incubation period.* The requirement for multiple heritable changes in the cell may be at least partly responsible for prolonged latency intervals.

For humans, the length of the induction-latency period varies from 3–5 years for radiation or toxin-induced leukemias to perhaps 40 or more years for some cases of asbestos-induced mesothelioma. For most tumors, however, the latency interval is approximately 12–25 years. Obviously, this long period of time may obscure the relationship between a remote exposure and a newly found tumor.

THE QUESTION OF THRESHOLDS

Many toxic agents result in known adverse effects only when the exposure is above a certain threshold dose or duration. If this threshold dose is not exceeded, there are no demonstrable consequences to the health of the animal or human. With carcinogens, it is much more difficult to determine if such a threshold exists. If no threshold exists, there is no dose (other than zero) at which the risk of cancer is nonexistent.

There is controversy about the existence of threshold doses for carcinogenic agents. An understanding of the arguments on both sides is useful, particularly when trying to comprehend the basis for policies and regulations regarding exposures both within and outside the workplace.

Given that a single alteration (mutation) in DNA in one cell may set the stage for tumor development, it is possible that exposure of the cell to only one molecule of a carcinogen ultimately could lead to tumor formation. Although the probability of tumor formation may increase with increasing frequency and magnitude of exposure to the carcinogen, a single small exposure may be sufficient. For example, in the mouse skin tumor model described earlier, a single exposure to a PAH is capable of inducing a tumor.

On the other hand, there are arguments that support the concept of a threshold dose for carcinogens. Although exposure to a single molecule of a particular offending agent may induce a tumorigenic change in a cell, the likelihood that the molecule will reach its target cell is lowered with exposure to smaller doses. Mechanisms that support the concept of threshold dose include the "first pass" effect, DNA repair, immunologic surveillance, and cellular damage–induced cancers. If the carcinogen is subject to rapid metabolic deactivation, as in a "first pass" effect in the liver after ingestion, the ability of a small or single dose to contact the susceptible cell would be reduced. DNA repair mechanisms (e.g., excision of altered DNA nucleotides) may allow repair of an induced mutation before a clone of tumor cells results, and immunologic mechanisms may be capable of destroying transformed cells before a tumor develops. Finally, some cancers are induced by prior tissue damage. For example, alcohol and probably some chlorinated hydrocarbon solvents can induce liver inflammation with subsequent cirrhosis, following which there is a higher risk of liver tumor development. Because there is a threshold for the initial toxic effects below which no damage occurs, there is also a threshold for the secondary tumor formation. If any of these phenomena pertain for a given carcinogen, there will be a threshold dose below which no carcinogenic effect will occur. Unfortunately, this theory fails to take into account the concept of individual susceptibility, which may drastically alter the exposure limit at which damage to specific organs occurs. Widely variable exposures to alcohol result in hepatic damage; this appears to be, at least in part, a result of differences in metabolism.

Although the more conventional viewpoint is that there are no demonstrable thresholds or safe levels for carcinogens, the controversy regarding thresholds persists in large part to identify "safe" exposures both within and outside the workplace. Some researchers note that the high rate of spontaneous mutation in human and animal cells induced by endogenous oxidants often may be eliminated by DNA repair mechanisms. One then might conclude that the impact of low levels of exogenous mutagens or toxins would be minimal in relation to the high rate of spontaneous endogenous mutations and as a result of effective DNA repair mechanisms. In addition, some researchers argue that the findings of animal bioassays at very high doses may well be a result of mitogenesis leading to mutagenesis (i.e., cellular proliferation stimulated by injury ultimately leads to carcinogenicity). Historical outbreaks of occupational cancer have often occurred with exposures at particularly high levels, where mitogenesis might occur. Because mitogenesis does not occur at the much lower doses to which humans generally are exposed, the carcinogenic stimulus will not be present. On the other hand, there is a poor correlation between toxicity and carcinogenicity for known carcinogens, suggesting that carcinogenicity is not simply caused by the secondary effects of cytotoxicity. Cell proliferation and cell turnover occur constantly in various organs and tissues. However, it is difficult to verify or refute the threshold hypothesis for individual carcinogens owing to the inherent limitations of animal and human studies. Efforts may be better spent identifying new carcinogens.

Dose-Response Relationships

Although thresholds may or may not exist, there is strong evidence for a dose-response effect for most of the carcinogens that have been studied adequately. In other words, exposure to larger doses of a specific agent results in a higher risk of developing cancer than do smaller doses. Both animal studies and human epidemiologic reports support this concept.

There are very large differences—10 million-fold or more—in the relative "potency" of carcinogens. For example, in long-term animal studies, a daily dose of less than 1 mg/d of aflatoxin versus greater than 1 g/d of trichloroethylene induces tumors in 50% of exposed animals.

Although dose-response curves for some carcinogens are known, data points generally represent relatively higher doses of exposure and may not reflect the behavior of the curve in the range of typical human exposures. At low doses, the curve may be linear, concave, or convex. Does a threshold exist? Figure 16–1 illustrates some possible models for low-dose extrapolation. Without additional information about the behavior of a particular toxin, the conventional public health view is that there is linearity at low doses. Although the concepts described earlier are helpful tools in understanding carcinogenic mechanisms and risk, they are still relatively static. In other words, these models generally are designed to assess the effects of a single exposure rather than the effects of repeated exposure to a low dose of carcinogen over a long period of time. In addition, it is difficult to take into account the additive or synergistic effects of other lifestyle and carcinogenic factors.

INVESTIGATIVE METHODS IN THE ASSESSMENT OF CHEMICAL CARCINOGENICITY

Evidence to support the carcinogenicity of a chemical for humans may be derived from four types of studies: human epidemiologic studies, experimental studies in animals, a variety of short-term tests, and analysis of structural similarities to known carcinogens. Epidemiologic studies provide the strongest evidence for human carcinogenicity; they are conducted on human subjects and involve a large number of individuals. However, such studies are subject to a number of limitations and confounding risks that may limit their ability to detect and confirm carcinogenic effects. Well-conducted animal bioassays can provide strong support for carcinogenicity in the animal species tested. However, the implications for humans may be less clear than with epidemiologic studies. The role of short-term assays (e.g., for bacterial mutation) is not fully defined because the significance of positive results for humans is unknown. In addition, short-term assays may miss potential carcinogens that require specific metabolism for their mutational effects.

Structural similarity of a chemical to known carcinogens also may suggest the need for further study in short-term or animal tests. Although the presence of such similarity has, in fact, predicted the carcinogenicity of previously untested compounds, the overall utility of structural analysis has not been established.

EPIDEMIOLOGIC STUDIES

Evidence for causality of an association can only be derived from analytic epidemiologic studies or, in other words, cohort or case-control studies, although case reports and descriptive epidemiologic studies may provide suggestive evidence for human carcinogenicity. Well-conducted epidemiologic studies with positive results provide strong evidence in support of carcinogenicity. Epidemiologic studies are difficult to conduct and often are not feasible because of a number of factors, including high cost, the need to study a large number of individuals, and the long duration of observation periods. A major disadvantage of these studies is that they are primarily retrospective.

A number of criteria are used to help decide whether a positive association in epidemiologic studies indicates causality. The most important are strength, consistency, biologic gradient, biologic plausibility, and temporality.

1. The *strength* of an association is the magnitude of the relative risk in the exposed group compared with that in the control group. Strong associations are more likely to be causal because it is less likely that biases (e.g., the confounding effects of smoking) would account for the association without being very obvious.

2. *Consistency* of an association is the extent to which it is reported from multiple studies conducted under different circumstances.

3. The *biologic gradient* of an association is the degree to which it exhibits a dose-response relationship (i.e., the observation that higher doses result in a higher frequency of adverse effects).

4. The *biologic plausibility* of a study is based on the assessment that it makes sense in light of what is known about the mechanism of production of the adverse effect.

5. A study's *temporality* rests on the conclusion or observation that the cause (i.e., exposure) preceded the effect in time.

Despite the utility of these criteria in making assessments of causality, only temporality is absolutely required. A weak association not consistently reported that does not exhibit a dose-response effect and does not (as yet) fully make sense nevertheless may be causal. Furthermore, fulfillment of some of the criteria may occur when the association is in fact a result of chance or bias.

If most of these criteria are met, the likelihood that an association is causal is high. The International Agency for Research on Cancer (IARC) has established similar criteria for the designation of an agent as a carcinogen.

Limitations of Epidemiologic Studies

Failure to demonstrate a positive association in an epidemiologic study does not always indicate that there is no association between the agent and the effect studied. In some cases, a false-negative epidemiologic study may result because of a variety of shortcomings. Some of these limitations include difficulties in identifying exposures and effects, difficulties in choosing appropriate study (exposed) and control populations, inadequate duration of follow-up given long induction-latency periods, and the relative lack of sensitivity of epidemiologic methods.

The existence of all these limitations accounts for the consensus among scientists that negative epidemiologic studies do not provide proof of noncarcinogenicity of an agent. Such negative data generally are outweighed by the finding of positive results in animal experimental studies. Greater credence may be given to a negative study if the subjects studied had a sufficiently long period of exposure (an average of 15 or more years), if they were followed long enough to observe an effect (25 or more years), and if the number of exposed subjects was large enough so that a small excess risk for a particular cancer could be detected.

ANIMAL BIOASSAYS

Design

Experimental studies in animals involve the administration of a test chemical to a group of animals followed by observation for the development of tumors. Procedures for such studies are now standardized and accepted by most of the sponsoring or evaluating institutions [e.g., the National Toxicology Program (NTP) and IARC]; Table 16–2 lists the basic requirements. In brief, protocols include at least 50–60 or more animals of each sex with two species in each of two to four dosage groups and incorporate thorough pathologic examination and proper statistical analysis of results. Animals most often are dosed for two years, about two-thirds of

Table 16–2. IARC requirements for animal bioassays.

---

1. Two species of animals (generally mice and rats), both males and females.
2. Sufficient numbers of animals in each test group and concurrent control group (at least 50 per sex).
3. Duration of dose administration and observation must extend over most of the animal's life expectancy (typically 2 years for rats and mice).
4. Treated groups tested at two or ideally three different doses—at a higher dose (near the maximum tolerated dose) and at a lower dose.
5. Outcome determined from adequate pathologic examination of animals.
6. Proper statistical analysis of data.

their lifetimes, at the maximal tolerated dose (MTD) and one-half the MTD and lower doses.

Interpretation

Results from well-conducted animal bioassays can yield clear evidence to support the carcinogenicity of a compound in a particular animal species and can be extrapolated to humans. The IARC, an independent scientific institution within the World Health Organization (WHO), in 2003 redefined carcinogenicity in experimental animals.

The evidence relevant to carcinogenicity in experimental animals is classified into one of the following categories:

Sufficient evidence of carcinogenicity. A causal relationship has been established between the agent or mixture and an increased incidence of malignant neoplasms or of an appropriate combination of benign and malignant neoplasms in (1) two or more species of animals or (2) in two or more independent studies in one species carried out at different times or in different laboratories or under different protocols. Exceptionally, a single study in one species might be considered to provide sufficient evidence of carcinogenicity when malignant neoplasms occur to an unusual degree with regard to incidence, site, type of tumor, or age at onset.

Limited evidence of carcinogenicity. The data suggest a carcinogenic effect but are limited for making a definitive evaluation because, for example, (1) the evidence of carcinogenicity is restricted to a single experiment, or (2) there are unresolved questions regarding the adequacy of the design, conduct, or interpretation of the study, or (3) the agent or mixture increases the incidence only of benign neoplasms or lesions of uncertain neoplastic potential or of certain neoplasms that may occur spontaneously in high incidences in certain strains.

Inadequate evidence of carcinogenicity. The studies cannot be interpreted as showing either the presence or absence of a carcinogenic effect because of major qualitative or quantitative limitations, or no data on cancer in experimental animals are available.

Evidence suggesting lack of carcinogenicity. Adequate studies involving at least two species are available that show that, within the limits of the tests used, the agent or mixture is not carcinogenic. A conclusion of evidence suggesting lack of carcinogenicity is inevitably limited to the species, tumor sites, and levels of exposure studied.

Correlation with Human Effects

Results from animal bioassays have served as good predictors of human carcinogenicity. Nearly one-third of

agents now known to be human carcinogens were first discovered to be carcinogenic in animals. In attempting to extrapolate data from animal research to conclusions about cancer risks in humans, the two important issues to be considered are (1) whether all chemicals that have been shown to cause cancer in animals are also capable of causing cancer in humans and vice versa and (2) from a quantitative viewpoint whether humans are equally susceptible to the carcinogenic effects of equivalent doses of known animal carcinogens.

Available evidence suggests that there is good correlation between animal and human results. Until recently, it had not been possible to demonstrate carcinogenicity of arsenic in animals, although it is a known skin, lung, liver, kidney, and bladder carcinogen in humans. This discrepancy between human and animal studies raised a question about the adequacy of animal bioassays to be sensitive predictors of human carcinogenicity. Subsequent studies of intracheal instillation of arsenic compounds (arsenic trioxide, calcium arsenate) in rats and hamsters did result in considerable evidence of carcinogenicity in the view of the IARC. Thus all known human carcinogens for which adequate animal studies have been conducted have shown sufficient evidence of carcinogenicity in tested animals.

The issue of the specificity of animal testing as a predictor of human carcinogenicity is more difficult to resolve. Because of limitations inherent in epidemiologic studies (discussed earlier), it is unlikely that clear-cut evidence for human carcinogenicity can be derived for many chemicals proved to be carcinogenic in animals. Nevertheless, for the limited number of compounds for which there are adequate data in both humans and animals, there are no substances proved to be carcinogenic in animals that have been proved to be noncarcinogenic in humans.

Although there appears to be a good qualitative correlation between animal and human carcinogenicity, the target site at which cancers develop may be quite different for rodents and humans. For example, benzidine produces liver tumors in rats, hamsters, and mice but produces bladder tumors in humans and dogs. Nevertheless, for all known human carcinogens, at least one site of cancer in humans matched a site in at least one animal species tested.

The second major issue in the use of animal bioassays is the degree to which the susceptibility of humans to carcinogenic effects parallels the dose-response patterns in animals. There is no database that allows comparison of sensitivity between species. For the limited numbers of substances for which there are quantitative data in both humans and animals, it appears that the sensitivity of humans, on a total dose per body weight basis, is roughly similar to that of animals.

Limitations of Animal Bioassays

There are a number of difficult issues in the analysis of animal experimental studies that may limit their utility in human cancer risk assessment. Because of the small number of animals studied, the bioassays are relatively insensitive. The agent under study must cause at least a 15% increase in the incidence of tumors in order for a statistically significant excess of tumors to be detected in a bioassay of standard size. A lower excess risk will not be demonstrable, particularly if there is any background rate of tumor development in untreated animals.

To increase the sensitivity of animal experiments, high-dose levels approaching the MTD are chosen. Depending on the agent studied, these dose levels sometimes may be above the human exposure levels in occupational or environmental settings. In some cases, an increased incidence of types of tumors not commonly observed in humans is found. Risk quantification based on animal studies conducted at high doses is difficult because predictions are based on extrapolation to the lower dose exposures experienced by humans. The mathematical models used for extrapolation are controversial and difficult to prove, thus more often adding uncertainty to risk estimates.

Certain factors affect the likelihood that animal bioassay results will be a good predictor of human response. False-positive results may result from a variety of factors if carcinogenicity occurs only secondary to primary toxic alteration or if high doses overwhelm the metabolic detoxifying mechanisms that normally would prevent damage to a susceptible organ. If a carcinogenic metabolite is produced only in the animal or only in humans, either false-negative or false-positive results could be obtained. Genetic differences in species or mechanism of metabolism in humans may determine individual susceptibility to at least some carcinogens; this may not be apparent in animal models. For most chemicals, evidence regarding comparative pharmacodynamics in humans and animals does not exist.

Because agents often are administered to animals by a route that is different from the one reported for human exposures, such as ingestion or intraperitoneal injection, it is possible that the outcome in the animal will differ from the effect in humans. However, there is no evidence to suggest that a significant discrepancy in outcome exists based on differences in route of administration. Finally, there is some controversy about the classification of an agent as a potential carcinogen in the rare circumstance where experimental results indicate an increased frequency of benign tumors only. However, both the NTP and the IARC endorse the use and significance of chemically induced benign tumors.

SHORT-TERM TESTS

Types of Assays

A number of assays have been designed that provide evidence of mutagenicity, or the ability to induce chromosomal damage by chemicals, without the long period of observation or follow-up required for epidemiologic studies or animal bioassays. These short-term tests therefore are much quicker and less expensive to perform. Assessed endpoints include gene mutation, induction of DNA damage and repair, DNA binding, chromosomal aberrations, sister chromatid exchange, and neoplastic transformation of mammalian cells and other endpoints. The tests rely on the fact that most carcinogens covalently bind to DNA and thereby induce DNA damage.

The best-studied and most commonly performed short-term test is the Ames test, which uses a mutant strain of *Salmonella typhimurium* that is deficient in the enzymes required to synthesize histidine and which will not grow unless histidine is added to the growth medium. The chemical to be tested, along with a liver microsomal enzyme fraction from rodents or humans that can metabolically activate "procarcinogens," is added to the bacterial culture. Bacterial colonies that subsequently grow and can be counted indicate the occurrence of a reversion mutation to the wild strain, reflecting the mutagenic activity of the agent studied. Similar mutagenic testing is possible in cultured mammalian cells in vitro.

Tests for DNA repair can demonstrate that DNA damage has occurred following exposure to a chemical. Chromosomal aberrations in mammalian cells are detected by cytogenetic tests that assess changes in the morphologic structure of chromosomes. Such tests can be performed on animal or human cells, including human lymphocytes. Morphologic changes that may occur include chromosomal translocations and the formation of micronuclei.

Testing for sister chromatid exchange (SCE) is a more sophisticated form of cytogenetic investigation based on differential staining of sister chromatids, allowing for detection of the interchange of genetic material between chromatids. SCEs are more subtle than gross structural chromosomal aberrations. Tests for SCEs may be performed on animal or human cells.

Tests for neoplastic transformation of mammalian cells in culture assess the ability of chemicals to induce neoplastic growth. The treated cells are injected into animals to assess the ability of the cells to form tumors. A number of other short-term tests are being or have been developed.

Interpretation & Limitations

The predictive value of short-term tests to assess human carcinogenicity of a chemical is unclear. The correlation between results in short-term assays and human or animal studies is imperfect. No single short-term test is capable of detecting all chemicals positive in animal bioassays. As a result, a battery of tests is performed routinely on a specific chemical. Interestingly, a recent study comparing the results of a battery of four commonly used short-term tests to the Ames test used alone failed to demonstrate any advantage of the battery in predicting results of animal bioassays for approximately 80 chemicals. The concordance of any of the in vitro tests with the animal bioassay results was approximately 60%. A number of compounds were identified as mutagenic in the short-term tests that were noncarcinogenic in animal bioassays. Conversely, a large number of chemicals that were nonmutagenic in the Ames test were carcinogenic to animals, and some also in humans, for example, DES and benzene. The low specificity of the Ames test for detecting carcinogenicity (i.e., the high number of false-positive results among noncarcinogens) demonstrates the difficulty in predicting animal carcinogenicity on the basis of short-term test results alone. In contrast, while most genotoxic carcinogens are positive in short-term tests, these in vitro tests generally are not able to permit detection of chemicals that induce cancers by nongenotoxic or epigenetic mechanisms (i.e., they are not sensitive to the effects of promoting agents).

Some of these tests (e.g., tests for SCEs and measurement of DNA adducts) can be performed on cells (typically lymphocytes) taken from humans exposed occupationally or environmentally to suspected carcinogens. Testing for SCEs has been performed on workers exposed to ethylene oxide. An increased frequency of SCEs has been found in some of these workers. Although this merits further study, the clinical significance of these findings for the workers is unknown. SCEs are increased by other factors, including cigarette smoking, and an increase in SCEs is not predictive of specific cancer risk. At this time, it is not possible to make predictions based on results of this type of testing in workers. Consequently, use of cellular testing should be limited to well-designed prospective research studies.

Given the current state of knowledge, most authorities state that positive results in short-term tests on previously untested materials warrant further study in animal bioassays and further scrutiny in human-exposure situations. Similarly, positive results on these tests provide corroboration for positive findings in animal bioassays, particularly when the animal results provide only limited or suggestive evidence of carcinogenicity. On the other hand, isolated positive short-term assay results generally do not constitute sufficient evidence to force immediate regulatory action.

THE ROLE OF MOLECULAR BIOLOGY IN THE STUDY OF OCCUPATIONAL CANCER

Advances in biochemistry and molecular biology have opened the door to the study of pharmacogenomics, or genetic variability in the metabolism of different drugs or toxins. Understanding these variations will lead to the ability to detect differences in individual susceptibility to chemically induced cancers and help to understand the mechanisms and etiology of occupational cancer. The term *molecular epidemiology* is applied to this development because of the combination of epidemiologic study and molecular biology methodology. Application of this field of study typically allows assessment of exposure as well as possible early health effects.

Most carcinogenic chemicals are metabolized to the active carcinogenic metabolite by phase I enzymes, primarily multiple enzymes in the cytochrome P450 monooxygenase class. Variations in the activity of these enzymes (polymorphisms), which may be genetically or environmentally determined, can result in differences in susceptibility to chemical carcinogenesis. For example, an isoform of one enzyme, CYP1A1, has been associated with an increased risk for lung cancer in smokers. This enzyme catalyzes the oxidation of PAHs to reactive metabolites such as epoxides. Other genetically determined variants in phase II enzymes, such as glutathione S-transferase (GST) and N-acetyltransferase (NAT), appear to play a role in lung cancer associated with PAHs and bladder cancer associated with exposure to aromatic amines. Polymorphisms in NAT result in delayed metabolism of aromatic amines ("slow acetylators"), presumably increasing risk by increasing duration of exposure. The relationship between isoenzyme patterns, exposure to specific chemicals or toxins, and risk for cancer induction is not well-enough defined to predict individual cancer risk associated with chemical exposure. In addition, many factors contribute to chemical carcinogenesis and may confound possible associations. Use of genetic polymorphisms to determine individual risk also could be employed to discriminate against individuals or racial groups, raising important ethical issues.

Another promising tool is the measurement of levels of specific carcinogens covalently bound to DNA or proteins, referred to as *DNA* or *protein adducts.* Binding to DNA may lead to DNA damage. Protein adducts (to albumin or hemoglobin) serve as a surrogate for DNA binding and have the advantage of representing an internalized dose. Adducts present a better potential method of quantifying dose than older available methods, such as air monitoring or measuring blood levels of an agent. Application of these methods has included measurement of PAH–DNA adducts in smokers and lung cancer patients and of hemoglobin adducts of aromatic amines in smokers and occupationally exposed groups. Epidemiologic studies ultimately may show that adduct levels are a good predictor of cancer risk, possibly allowing classification of cohorts into high- and low-risk groups.

The abnormal protein products coded for by oncogenes or altered tumor suppressor genes occasionally may be identified in the serum and urine. For example, p53 protein accumulates in the lung cancers of patients exposed to cigarette smoke and asbestos. Accumulation occurred more often in those exposed to asbestos compared with individuals who were unexposed. Moreover, there was a significant association between p53 accumulation and the measured asbestos content of the lung tissue. Similarly, patients with strongly p53-positive tumors were heavier smokers. In a study of radon-exposed uranium miners who had developed lung cancers, more than half the patients had an identical G-to-T transversion at codon 249 of the *p53* gene. It is possible that further analysis of altered proteins may be useful as preclinical response indicators in premalignant and early malignant lesions in occupationally exposed cohorts, with a role in early detection. To the extent that exposure-specific mutations can be identified, these mutations and the resulting protein products could serve as a marker for exposure as well as specific occupationally induced cancers. Considerable additional information from epidemiologic and serum studies will be necessary before these measurements can be readily applied in clinical situations.

IMPLICATIONS FOR REGULATORY ACTION & PREVENTIVE MEDICINE

When a sufficient body of evidence supporting carcinogenicity exists, corrective action to protect public and worker health must proceed, even if there is some remaining uncertainty in the conclusions. Convincingly positive results from a well-conducted epidemiologic study merit immediate action. Sufficient evidence of carcinogenicity in animal bioassays, as defined by IARC and NTP, also should prompt immediate attempts to reduce worker exposure as much as possible. The finding of limited evidence in animal bioassays or positive results in short-term tests should, at the very least, serve as a stimulus for further study of the suspect chemical. When the results in different tests are contradictory, results suggesting carcinogenicity generally outweigh the negative evidence. Given the limited sensitivity of epidemiologic methods, this axiom seems particularly applicable when positive animal studies are analyzed alongside negative epidemiologic studies.

Based on analysis of epidemiologic and animal studies then available, the IARC issued, in 1987, several lists of chemicals with different degrees of evidence for human carcinogenicity. Since that time, additional agents have been added to the lists based on new evidence.

In the first 82 volumes of the IARC monograph series, some 885 agents (chemicals, groups of chemicals, complex mixtures, occupational exposures, cultural habits, and biologic or physical agents) have been evaluated.

Group 1. The agent (mixture) is carcinogenic to humans. The exposure circumstance entails exposures that are carcinogenic to humans.

Group 2A. The agent (mixture) is probably carcinogenic to humans. The exposure circumstance entails exposures that are probably carcinogenic to humans.

Group 2B. The agent (mixture) is possibly carcinogenic to humans. The exposure circumstance entails exposures that are possibly carcinogenic to humans.

Group 3. The agent (mixture or exposure circumstance) is not classifiable as to carcinogenicity in humans.

Groups 4. The agent (mixture or exposure circumstance) is probably not carcinogenic to humans.

Table 16–3 lists some of the 88 group 1 carcinogens, along with several additional carcinogenic hazards not reviewed by IARC or that are known environmental hazards.

IARC group 1: 88 (including 12 mixtures, e.g., alcoholic beverages, and 13 exposure circumstances, e.g., the rubber industry).

IARC group 2A: 64 (with 5 mixtures, e.g., diesel engine exhaust, and 4 exposure circumstances, e.g., petroleum refining).

IARC group 2B: 236 (12 mixtures, e.g., gasoline, and 4 exposure circumstances, e.g., dry cleaning occupational exposures).

IARC Group 3: 496

IARC Group 4: 1

Table 16–4 lists some of the industrial processes that have been causally associated with cancer in humans. Table 16–5 lists some of the 64 industrial or environmental chemicals in group 2A, for which there is sufficient animal evidence but limited or inadequate human evidence of carcinogenicity (probably carcinogenic to humans). There are more than 200 agents in group 2B, for which there is less compelling evidence to suggest possible human carcinogenicity. Table 16–6 lists some of these agents. Individual data about specific agents, as well as associated occupations, can be found in the *10th Report on Carcinogens* by the National Toxicology Program of the Department of Health and Human Safety (available at http://ehp.niehs.nih.gov/roc/tocio.html).

There is a concordance between results indicating genotoxicity in short-term tests and the human and animal carcinogenicity data. The short-term tests measured DNA damage, mutations, and/or chromosomal effects; sufficient evidence of genotoxicity required effects in mammalian cells in vitro or in vivo. Overall, roughly 80–90% of the agents in each group (1, 2A, and 2B) showed sufficient or limited evidence of genotoxicity. The authors conclude that it is likely that genotoxic carcinogens and perhaps other genotoxic compounds contribute

Table 16–3. Selected occupational exposures causally associated with human cancer (group 1).[1]

Occupational Exposure	Cancer Site
4-Aminobiphenyl	Bladder
Arsenic and arsenic compounds[2]	Lung, skin, liver(?), angiosarcoma
Asbestos	Pleura and peritoneum (mesothelioma), lung, larynx(?), gastrointestinal tract, kidney
Benzene	Leukemia, multiple myeloma, lung
Benzidine	Bladder
Beryllium	Lung
Bis(chloromethyl) ether[3]	Lung (mainly oat cell)
Cadmium and cadmium compounds	Lung
Chromium compounds, hexavalent[2]	Lung
Coal tar pitches	Skin, scrotum, lung, bladder
Coal tars	Skin, scrotum, lung, bladder(?)
Ethylene oxide	Leukemia
Ionizing radiation	Leukemia, skin, other
Mineral oils, untreated and mildly treated	Skin, scrotum, lung(?)
Mustard gas	Lung
β-Naphthalamine	Bladder
Nickel and nickel compounds [oxide(?), sulfide]	Lung, nasal sinuses
Radium	Bone (sarcomas)
Radon	Lung
Shale oils	Skin, scrotum
Solar radiation	Skin
Soots, tars, and oils[2]	Skin, lung, bladder(?)
Strong inorganic acids containing sulfuric acid	Lung
Talc containing asbestiform fibers	Lung, mesothelioma(?)
Vinyl chloride	Liver (angiosarcoma), brain(?), lung

[1]Sources: International Agency for Research on Cancer http://www.iarc.fr/.
[2]The compounds responsible for the carcinogenic effect in humans cannot be specified.
[3]And technical grade chloromethyl methyl ether, which contains 1–8% bis(chloromethyl) ether.

more to the burden of cancer in humans than do nongenotoxic carcinogens, suggesting that a reduction in exposure to these agents should be a high public health/occupational health priority.

The nature of the appropriate response by government to evidence for carcinogenicity of a chemical is controversial. Given the uncertainty about the existence of thresholds and the shape of the dose-response curve at low doses, it is not possible to establish clearly "safe" doses for carcinogens. Ideally, human exposure to known carcinogens should be reduced to nil. In practice, political, economic, social, and technical factors constrain the power of regulators to adopt such stringent standards.

REFERENCES

Boffetta P: Epidemiology of environmental and occupational cancer. Oncogene 2004;23:6392 [PMID: 15322513].

Table 16–4. Selected industrial processes causally associated with human cancer.

Industrial Process	Possible or Probable Agent	Cancer Site
Aluminum production	Polycyclic aromatic hydrocarbons	Lung, bladder
Auramine manufacture	Auramine	Bladder
Boot and shoe manufacture and repair (certain occupations)	Benzene	Leukemia
Coal gasification	Polycyclic aromatic hydrocarbons	Lung, bladder, skin, scrotum
Coke production	Polycyclic aromatic hydrocarbons	Lung, kidney(?)
Furniture manufacture	Wood dust	Nasal cavity (mainly adenocarcinoma)
Iron and steel founding	Polycyclic aromatic hydrocarbons(?), silica, metal fumes	Lung
Isopropyl alcohol manufacture (strong acid process)	Diisopropyl sulfate, isopropyl oils	Paranasal sinuses, larynx(?)
Magenta, manufacture of	Magenta(?), precursors(?) (e.g., orthotoluidine)	Bladder
Nickel refining	Nickel oxides, nickel subsulfide	Nasal cavity, lung, larynx(?)
Rubber industry	Aromatic amines, solvents(?)	Bladder, leukemia (lymphatic), stomach(?), lung, skin, colon, prostate, lymphoma
Underground hematite mining (with exposure to radon)	Radon(?)	Lung

Colditz GA et al: Epidemiology: Identifying the causes and preventability of cancer. Nature Rev Cancer 2006;6:75 [PMID: 16372016].

Driscoll T et al: The global burden of disease due to occupational carcinogens. Am J Indust Med 2005;48:419 [PMID: 16299703].

Luch A: Nature and nurture: Lessons from chemical carcinogenesis. Nature Rev Cancer 2005;5:113 [PMID: 15660110].

Siemiatycki J et al: Listing occupational carcinogens. Environ Health Perspect 2004;112:1447 [PMID: 15531427].

Wei M, Wei P: Occupational risk factors for selected cancers. Am J Public Health 2004;94:1078 [PMID: 15226121].

Of course, industry health and safety staff and managers have the opportunity to go further than the regulations require in using information regarding carcinogenicity in order to make decisions about chemical use and control. For example, choosing to avoid the use of chemicals in IARC groups 1 and 2A (or those with evidence that might place them in these categories) and to use agents in group 2B only with very tight controls when there are no viable alternatives would lead to reductions in the actual rate of occupational cancers. Alternatively, use of these agents only with very tight controls (enclosure, local exhaust ventilation, etc.) that completely prevent exposure would have a similar beneficial effect. Obviously, factors that affect the likelihood of exposure (e.g., volatility or potential for skin absorption) would influence the ease with which these

materials could be controlled safely. Pressure of chemical users on chemical manufacturers to study suspect chemicals and to develop safe alternatives to potential carcinogens could be another effective approach. Additionally, proper hazard communication should inform workers of potential carcinogens and provide them with the training and tools to prevent or substantially reduce exposure.

Some assistance in policy development can be derived from quantitative risk-assessment methodology. Mathematical models have been designed that allow for the extrapolation from high-dose studies to lower-dose exposures, providing an estimate of the excess risk or excess number of cases of a specific cancer that might be seen in a given population as a result of a particular exposure.

Despite considerable uncertainty, calculated risks can provide an approximate upper limit to the excess risk attributable to specific exposures. Developments in the use of physiologically based pharmacokinetic models for the estimation of dose at the target site (through the use of pharmacokinetic data regarding absorption, distribution, and metabolism of agents) may improve the accuracy of quantitative risk assessments for cancer. Such risk assessments can help to place hazards from various chemicals in the occupational environment into perspective by allowing comparison of the risk estimate against the risk from other known hazards. The use of risk comparisons may allow

Table 16–5. Selected probable occupational carcinogens (group 2A)—limited evidence of human carcinogenicity.[1]

Occupational Exposure	Suspected Human Cancer Site
Acrylonitrile	Lung
2-Amino-3-methylimidazo (4,5-*f*)quinoline (IQ)	
Benz(*a*)anthracene	
Benzidine-based dyes	Bladder(?)
Benzo(*a*)pyrene	Lung, skin, bladder
1,3-Butadiene	Leukemia, lymphoma
p-Chloro-*o*-toluidine	Bladder
Creosotes	Skin, scrotum
Dibenz(*a,h*)anthracene	
Diesel engine exhaust	
Diethyl sulfate	Larynx
Dimethylcarbamoyl chloride	
Dimethyl sulfate	Lung(?)
Epichlorhydrin	Respiratory tract
Ethylene dibromide	
Formaldehyde	Nasopharynx
4,4'-Methylene-bis-(2-chloro-aniline) (MOCA)	Bladder
N-Nitrosodimethylamine	
Polychlorinated biphenyls	Liver
Silica (crystalline)	Lung
Styrene oxide	
Tetrachloroethylene	Esophagus, lymphoma
Trichloroethylene	Liver, lymphoma
1,2,3-Trichloropropane	
Tris(2,3-dibromopropyl) phosphate	
Vinyl bromide	
Vinyl fluoride	

[1]Source: International Agency for Research on Cancer http://www.iarc.fr/.

regulators or decision makers to prioritize exposure problems for the purpose of allocating resources for cleanup or problem resolution, although obviously this is a highly charged issue.

Ames developed an approach for risk comparisons called the *human exposure/rodent potency* (HERP) *percentage*. The HERP percentage compares the human exposure (daily lifetime dose in milligrams per kilogram) to the rodent median toxic dose (TD_{50}), the daily dose in milligrams per kilogram to halve the percentage of tumor-free animals by the end of a standard lifetime (as determined from animal bioassays). The lower the HERP percentage, the lower is the possible hazard from average human exposures. By using this index, it is possible to compare the hazard of a variety of natural and synthetic carcinogens. Such comparisons may demonstrate a greater apparent hazard from natural carcinogens (e.g., aflatoxin as a contaminant in peanut butter or hydrazines in raw mushrooms) than from nonoccupational exposures to chemical contaminants such as polychlorinated biphenyls (PCBs) in the diet or trichloroethylene in contaminated well water, although clearly the validity of such an approach is limited. The priority setting that such an index facilitates may permit policymakers to focus attention and regulation on the most significant exposure problems.

While exposure to known or suspected carcinogens clearly has declined in the United States and other economically developed countries as a result of both regulations that control exposure and changes in methods of production and chemicals produced, it is likely that exposures to workers in developing countries are increasing in frequency and intensity. When measurements exist and are reported for workers in developing countries, exposure levels in given industries to carcinogens tend to be considerably higher than in developed countries and generally are above regulatory standards in developed countries. The transfer of hazardous industries to developing countries likely will further increase carcinogen exposure for workers. There are little health data with regard to the consequences of these exposures. Recognizing the inability of many developing countries to regulate these hazards effectively, it is incumbent on industrial concerns from developed nations to attempt to control these hazards for their workers in developing countries.

Medical Surveillance

The proper role of medical surveillance in workers currently or previously exposed to known or suspected carcinogens is unclear. Surveillance of populations at high risk of cancer is only effective if the screening test is sensitive and easy to perform, if it detects premalignant abnormalities or tumors at an early stage in their development, and if there is an effective intervention that reduces morbidity and mortality when applied to such "early" tumors. For certain tumors not as yet associated with chemical exposures (e.g., cervical cancer), screening techniques and effective therapy for early lesions have had a significant impact on the disease. There is some evidence that a small group of workers at high risk of bladder tumors as a result of prior expo-

Table 16–6. Selected possible occupational carcinogens (group 2B)—inadequate evidence of human carcinogenicity.[1]

Occupational Exposure	Cancer Site	
	Animal	Human
Acetaldehyde	Nasal mucosa, larynx	
Acrylamide	Thyroid, adrenal, mammary gland, skin	
Antimony trioxide	Lung	
β-Butyrolactone		
Carbon tetrachloride	Liver	
Ceramic fibers	Lung	
Chloroform	Liver, kidney	
Chlorophenols and phenoxyacetic acid herbicides		Soft-tissue sarcoma(?) and lymphoma(?)
Chlorophenothane (DDT)	Liver, lung, lymphoma	
1,2-Dibromo-3-chloropropane (DBCP)	Nasal cavity, lung, stomach	
p-Dichlorobenzene	Liver, kidney	
1,2-Dichloroethane		
Dichloromethane	Lung, liver	
Diesel fuel, marine		
Di(2-ethylhoxyl)phthalate		
Dimethylformamide		Testicular(?)
1,4-Dioxane	Liver, nasal cavity	
Ethyl acrylate	Forestomach	
Ethylene thiourea	Thyroid	
Gasoline	Kidney	Leukemia(?) [related to benzene(?)]
Glasswool	Lung	
Hexachlorocyclohexanes	Liver	Leukemia(?)
Hydrazine	Lung, liver, mammary gland, nose	
Lead compounds, inorganic	Kidney	
Nickel, metallic		
Phenylglycidyl ether		
Polybrominated biphenyls (PBBs)	Liver	
Rockwool	Lung	Lung
Slagwool		Lung
Styrene	Lung	
2,3,7,8-Tetrachlorodibenzo-p-dioxin (TCDD)	Liver, lung, other	Soft-tissue sarcoma(?), lymphoma(?)
Tetrachloroethylene	Liver, leukemias	
Toluene diisocyanates		

(continued)

Table 16–6. Selected possible occupational carcinogens (group 2B)—inadequate evidence of human carcinogenicity.[1] (continued)

	Cancer Site	
Occupational Exposure	**Animal**	**Human**
o-Toluidine	Vascular tumors	Bladder tumors(?)
Welding fumes		Lung(?), [related to nickel, chromium(?)]

[1]Source: International Agency for Research on Cancer; http://www.iarc.fr/.

sure to aromatic amines used in dyestuff manufacturing can benefit from early detection by the use of urine cytology and cystoscopy as screening tools. For the remainder of occupational cancers, including asbestos-associated bronchogenic carcinoma, there is virtually no evidence that screening and early detection reduce mortality rates. Newer data using sensitive radiographic procedures to screen for lung cancer in high-risk populations are intriguing and suggest that judicious use of these tests may be warranted in specific situations.

Nevertheless, properly collected medical surveillance data combined with industrial hygiene data collection will prove useful in future epidemiologic studies and in the refinement of our knowledge regarding human dose-response phenomena. If medical surveillance is to be performed, the protocol should be designed for each agent of concern based on the presumed target site from prior human and animal studies and the availability of screening tools. In practice, some form of medical surveillance is required by Occupational Safety and Health Administration (OSHA) standards for asbestos, arsenic, benzene, and a variety of other carcinogens as listed in Table 16–7.

Implications for Clinical Practice

The practice of occupational medicine often requires an assessment as to whether a cancer in an exposed worker is causally related to work or to exposure. Such an assessment may occur informally in discussion with a concerned affected employee or more formally in the setting of a workers' compensation claim or toxic tort case. Unfortunately, neither the principles of carcinogenesis nor the investigative methods for assessing the carcinogenicity of a particular chemical were designed to be used in and cannot be directly applied to the assessment of an individual case.

Some of the same factors used in the assessment of the work-relatedness of any illness, largely derived from the medical and occupational history and medical, employment, and exposure records, are important in the assessment of a possible occupational cancer. Obtaining such information may be complicated by the long time elapsed since exposures began and the absence of industrial

hygiene or exposure records. Nevertheless, it is critical to assess to the best of one's ability the nature of the agents involved and the intensity, setting, control, and timing and duration of the exposures. Trends in cancer incidence in colleagues may be very useful. Potential sources for this information include the individual, coworkers and managers, material safety data sheets or other sources of chemical

Table 16–7. Carcinogens for which medical surveillance is required.[1]

2-Acetylaminofluorene
Acrylonitrille
4-Aminodiphenyl
Arsenic (inorganic)
Asbestos
Benzene
Benzidine (and its salts)
Bis (chloromethyl) ether
1,3-Butadiene
Cadmium
Coke oven emissions
1,2-Dibromo-3-chloropropane
3,3'-Dichlorobenzidine (and its salts)
4-Dimethylaminoazobenzene Ethyleneimine
Ethylene dibromide
Ethylene oxide
Formaldehyde
Lead
4,4'-Methylelene-bis(2-chloroanilline)
Methylene chloride
Methyl chloromethyl ether
Methylene dianaline
α-Naphthylamine
β-Naphthylamine
4-Nitroblphenyl
N-Nitrosodimethylamine
β-Proplolactone
Vinyl chloride

[1]Source: Subchapter 7, General Industry Safety Orders, of title B, Industrial Relations, California Administrative Code, 2006.

use information, and if available, industrial hygiene data. Knowledge of the presence or absence of other symptoms that may be due to exposure, used in conjunction with dose-response information, also can be helpful. For some industries, there may be published exposure-assessment information. From these sources it is usually possible to derive a qualitative sense of the intensity, timing, and duration of the exposures.

The medical history and medical records provide information about the cancer site and cell type and the presence of any other risk factors for the cancer. Physical examination may be helpful, by demonstrating physical findings suggestive of other conditions associated with the exposure or other risk factors.

Literature review can provide the descriptive epidemiology of the tumor type, including age, sex, and racial patterns of incidence, as well as information regarding nonoccupational risk factors for the tumor type. Literature searches can identify any relevant epidemiologic studies, which may be chemical-specific or job- or process-specific. In addition, there are a number of published occupational mortality studies that can provide some information about mortality as a consequence of cancers at certain organ sites in specific occupational groups. It is important to view these data with caution because they do not represent formal epidemiologic studies and do not correct for confounding factors. Literature searches also can identify animal experimental studies of specific chemicals that will help to identify potential tumor site, type, frequency, and dose response. Synthesis of this information first involves assessment of the quality of the epidemiologic and animal experimental evidence using the criteria discussed earlier. For example, less weight would be given to a small excess of a particular cancer in an occupational group if the number of observed cases of a common cancer was small and information regarding potential confounders was unavailable. However, these findings must not be ignored, and it would be important in such a setting to be sure that an excess of the cancer had not been observed in other studies and to assess the quality of data regarding other nonoccupational risk factors. An evaluation of the overall significance of the exposure relative to exposure-response information in the literature also should be considered. For example, one-time exposures are much less likely to be of etiologic importance than are regular, long-term exposures.

Assessing the duration of a presumed latency period can be helpful in determining possible cause and effect. Exposure-related solid tumors in humans appear to require a minimum of 10–12 years and often longer latency from exposure to clinical evidence of cancer. Therefore, it is unlikely, but not certain, that tumors that develop within a few years of initial exposure to the suspect agent are causally related to that exposure.

Cohort studies of workers exposed to known carcinogens occasionally demonstrate the occurrence of some cancers following a shorter interval since first exposure. It is possible that some of these cases, particularly for common cancers, are related to the background incidence in the general population. Although no statistically significant excess of tumors is demonstrated in the exposed group as compared with the reference population with less than about 10 years' latency, individual susceptibility may vary widely and could be represented in these cases. In contrast to the prolonged latency required for solid tumors, cancers of the blood (e.g., leukemia) and lymphatic system (e.g., lymphoma) generally are seen within 3–7 years following exposure. Slower-growing hematologic cancers (e.g., myelodysplasia or low-grade lymphomas) may be more delayed in appearance.

If an individual with cancer experienced low-level or short-duration exposures to a known or suspect carcinogen relative to high doses in cohorts demonstrated to have an increased risk for cancer, the cancer may be, but not certainly, less likely to be exposure-related. Again, individual susceptibility may play a role in increasing risk with minimal exposure in particular populations or workers. With the rare exception of tumors such as mesotheliomas, which almost universally stem from asbestos exposure, there is generally nothing about the appearance or behavior of a particular cancer that allows differentiation between work-related and spontaneous etiologies. If the dose is low and the incidence of the tumor in the general unexposed population is relatively high, it is more likely that the occurrence of the tumor reflects the background incidence of the tumor or the effect of a more prevalent risk factor present in the general population (e.g., smoking). In contrast, data regarding human carcinogenicity from chemical exposures uniformly implicate high-dose exposures. There are exceptions to this so-called high-exposure paradigm. Butadiene and benzene are carcinogenic to humans at exposures of less than 1 ppm. The no-threshold model or the "one molecule" or "one fiber" theory has been used to attribute a cancer in an individual to low-level exposures; however, these models were designed to predict for risk in exposed populations at low doses rather than for individuals. Alternatively, information indicating exposure to "one molecule," or, in other words, a very low dose, could be used to explore a connection between the exposure and the observed cancer rather than to prove causal connection. In workers' compensation and toxic tort cases, the standard of proof generally is reasonable medical probability (i.e., that the exposure or employment more likely than not caused the medical condition); possible connections may not be sufficient to establish causation.

One logical method to establish causation involves the use of the epidemiologic concept of *attributable proportion,* or the rate in the exposed population minus the rate in the unexposed population divided by the rate in the exposed population. Using epidemiologic data that establish an index of mortality (e.g., standard mortality rate) for groups exposed to different cumulative doses of a carcinogen relative to an unexposed reference population and information regarding cumulative dose for the affected individual, it is possible to estimate a relative risk for the individual related to the individual's exposure. For a relative-risk estimate of 2, 50% of the cancers observed likely would be caused by the exposure, leaving the other 50% likely to be caused by the background incidence of the tumor. This also means that those exposed have a doubling of risk of developing that particular cancer. When the relative risk estimate exceeds 2 and there is a high degree of confidence in the epidemiologic data, as well as the comparability of the individual's exposures, an observed case of cancer in that individual is more likely than not related to exposure. Conversely, when the relative-risk estimate is less than or equal to 2, it is less likely that the cancer is exposure-related. Consider a hypothetical population of service station workers who have been exposed to benzene in gasoline for a working lifetime at a time-weighted average concentration of 0.1 ppm. For example, by using epidemiologic data and risk-assessment methodology, the odds ratio for leukemia at this cumulative exposure level is 1.05. At this level of exposure, it is unlikely that a leukemia occurring in a member of this population is work-related. In fact, fewer than 5% of leukemias in this population would be exposure-related, the remainder being a result of the background incidence of leukemia in the general population. Proper use of this approach requires that the individual be roughly comparable with an exposed group in the epidemiologic study in terms of exposure level and confounding factors. Furthermore, the assessment is only as good as the quality of the epidemiologic data used and the exposure data. Demographic features, latency period, nonoccupational risk factors in the affected individual, and the scientific evidenced for a causal association between the exposure or occupation and the cancer need to be factored into the assessment of causation.

Possible clusters of cancer in a working population pose somewhat different challenges to the occupational physician in terms of investigating causation and risk communication. *Clusters* are defined as groups of like or similar illnesses aggregated in space and time within a group of individuals with the same occupation; the first challenge is to confirm that there is indeed a cluster. A commonly encountered scenario involves the recognition by a group of workers that several individuals have had cancer. The first approach is to investigate the data further by interview of the affected individuals or by review of medical records. Individuals may have distinctly different types of tumors that are etiologically unrelated (e.g., breast cancer, Hodgkin disease, and lung cancer), the individuals may not have shared the same space for very long, or one may have had cancer prior to joining the group. If initial investigation does reveal that a true cluster might exist, the next step is to confirm that the observed incidence exceeds what would have been expected in a population of comparable size and demographics (i.e., that the apparent clustering did not occur by chance). One also must take into account the "healthy-worker effect" (see Appendix). This assessment requires appropriate statistical methods and cancer incidence data. It is also important to assess exposure in the work area and to look for potential sources of exposure to carcinogens or other hazardous chemical or physical agents. There are several published investigations of clusters where no plausible responsible environmental factor could be identified; failure to determine an environmental cause after a thorough investigation should not be surprising. Better reporting of exposures with more accurate record keeping might help to identify possibly etiologies in the future. In the absence of known causes for observed clusters of cancer, careful and accurate presentation of the investigation results may help to ease concerns in the work force.

REFERENCES

Norppa H: Cytogenetic biomarkers and genetic polymorphisms. Toxicol Lett 2004;149:309 [PMID: 15093278].

Phillips DH: DNA adducts as markers of exposure and risk. Mutat Res 2005;577:284 [PMID: 15922369].

Pukkala E et al: National job-exposure matrix in analyses of Census-based estimates of occupational cancer risk. Scand J Work Environ Health 2005;31:97 [PMID: 15864903].

Watson WP, Mutti A: Role of biomarkers in monitoring exposures to chemicals: Present position, future prospects. Biomarkers 2004;9:211 [PMID: 15764289].

Wogan GN et al: Environmental and chemical carcinogenesis. Semin Cancer Biol 2004;14:473 [PMID: 15489140].

■ CLINICAL PRESENTATIONS

LUNG CANCER

Essentials of Diagnosis

- Asbestos, radon, chloromethyl ether, polycyclic aromatic hydrocarbons, chromium, nickel, inorganic arsenic exposure
- Cigarette smoking or exposure to cigarette smoke
- Cough, hemoptysis, dyspnea, weight loss
- Mass lesion, pulmonary infiltrate, hilar or mediastinal adenopathy on chest radiograph

- Diagnosis usually made with one or more of the following: sputum cytology, bronchoscopy with brushings and biopsy, transthoracic needle biopsy; thoracotomy rarely required

Occupations at Risk

- Asbestos
  - Asbestos miners
  - Insulation and filter material production
  - Shipyard workers
  - Textile manufacturing
- Radon
  - Domestic exposure
  - Uranium mining
- Chloromethyl ethers
  - Chemical production workers
- Polycyclic aromatic hydrocarbons
  - Aluminum reduction workers
  - Coke oven workers
  - Roofers
  - Rubber workers
- Chromium
  - Chromate production
- Nickel
  - Nickel mining, refining
- Arsenic
  - Arsenical pesticide production and use
  - Copper, lead, zinc smelting

General Considerations

Lung cancer is the leading cause of cancer deaths in the United States, and its incidence continues to rise, particularly in women, more of whom began smoking tobacco over the last 10–15 years. Lung cancers account for 33% of new cases and 25–30% of deaths. It is estimated that for 2003, 91,800 men and 80,100 women will develop lung cancer and that 157,200 (88,400 men and 68,800 women) will die of this disease. Fatality rates remain high; lung cancer currently accounts for almost 30% of all cancer deaths. When the number of new cases equals or comes close to the number of deaths, it is an indication that the success of treatment is not good.

Etiology

Cigarette smoking is the most important and most preventable risk factor for cancer of the lung. More than 80% of lung cancer deaths are attributable to cigarette smoking. Although its relative importance may decline if recent trends toward reduced cigarette consumption and the use of cigarettes with decreased tar and nicotine continue, the increasing incidence of lung cancer in women correlates with an increase in the smoking habit. The proportion of risks attributable to exposures in the workplace is significant; however, estimates vary widely, ranging from 4–40%. The association of lung cancer with exposure to asbestos, radon, chloromethyl ethers, PAHs, nickel, chromium, and inorganic arsenic appears to be independent of cigarette smoking. However, the effects of some known occupational carcinogens are greatly enhanced by smoking (e.g., asbestos, radon). Occupations with a high smoking prevalence have an increased risk of cancer. This includes restaurant wait staff, cashiers, orderlies, drivers, construction workers, watchmen, and others where smoking prevalence may be higher than 40%. In addition, it appears that high levels of environmental tobacco smoke, such as is found in restaurants and bars, may increase the risk of lung cancer in employees significantly.

A. ASBESTOS

Asbestos is the substance generally considered to pose the greatest carcinogenic threat in the workplace. Asbestos-related lung cancer was first reported in 1934, but perhaps the most striking data were presented in 1947 when Britain's Chief Factory Inspector reported that lung cancer was found in 31 (13.2%) of 235 men with asbestosis who died between 1924 and 1946. However, it was not until separate epidemiologic studies were published in 1955 by Doll and by Breslow that asbestos exposure indeed was recognized as being associated with cancer of the lung. Since then, many studies have documented the increase in lung cancer in workers with previous asbestos exposure, including a landmark study by Selikoff in which he followed 17,800 asbestos workers from 1967 to 1976 and found 486 deaths as a consequence of lung cancer (against an expected 105.6 deaths).

Asbestos is a fibrous silicate composed of various types. The minerals are divided into two classes: serpentine (chrysotile) and amphiboles (amosite, crocidolite, anthophyllite, and tremolite). The three most common commercial forms are chrysotile, amosite, and crocidolite; however, 90% of the asbestos used in the United States is chrysotile. All three commonly used forms of asbestos are associated with an increased risk of cancer. On a per-fiber basis, the highest risks of lung cancer have been shown for chrysotile. Some of the highest rates of lung cancer are found in the textile industry. This is thought to be a result of the higher carcinogenic potential of the very long chrysotile fibers used in the textile industry. Long, thin fibers are more likely to be inhaled and therefore result in pulmonary disease. Exposures are usually to mixed forms of asbestos.

Lung cancer is a major asbestos-related disease, accounting for 20% of all deaths in asbestos-exposed cohorts, and up to 7% of all lung cancer is attributable to asbestos exposure. Worldwide, there are over 100,000 deaths per year resulting from asbestos exposure. A latency period of approximately 20 years has been noted before the majority of lung cancer cases are seen. Although a dose-response relationship between asbestos exposure and lung cancer has now been established, increased risk is seen even after short but intense exposures. In Selikoff's study, asbestos exposure was shown to increase the risk of lung cancer fivefold in nonsmokers. Several studies show evidence that cigarette smokers who were also exposed to asbestos have a much greater risk of developing cancer of the lung, suggesting an initiator effect of cigarette smoke followed by a promoter effect from asbestos exposure.

B. Radon

Radon exposure is known to increase the risk of lung cancer. This carcinogenic effect was discovered when increased mortality rates from lung cancer were identified in uranium miners. Excesses in pulmonary disease were noted as early as 1879 in the uranium mining towns of Europe, with some cases of tuberculosis and silicosis, but much of it lung cancer. Large-scale mining of uranium began in the United States in 1948 because of the need for uranium to make nuclear weapons. By the 1960s, 20% of deaths in uranium miners in the United States were a result of lung disease. Excessive lung cancer in uranium miners is independent of cigarette smoking, although exposure to both is synergistic.

Ores containing uranium include all its decay products, which form a series of radionuclides, of which one is the inert gas radon. Radon diffuses out of the rock into the mine atmosphere, where it decays into radioisotopes of polonium, bismuth, and lead—termed *radon daughters*. These radionuclides are found in the air and then are inhaled as free ions or as attachments to dust particles. Epidemiologic studies of workers in U.S. uranium mines demonstrate that the risk of lung cancer is proportionate to the cumulative radon daughter exposure. Increased risk of lung cancer also has been found in fluorspar miners, iron ore (hematite) miners, and hard-rock miners. Data from animal models support the carcinogenic effect of radon; respiratory tumors can be induced by inhaled radon daughter products.

Data from animal models support the carcinogenic effects of radon; respiratory tumors can be induced by inhaled radon daughter products. Domestic radon exposure has been an issue of concern since 1984, when high radon levels were discovered in homes built on the Reading Prong geologic formation in Pennsylvania. The risk of lung cancer from low-level radon exposure has been extrapolated from studies of mine workers to the general population but appears to be very low.

C. Chloromethyl Ethers

Exposure to multiple chemical substances can cause an increase in lung cancers in exposed workers. Among the most important of these are the chloromethyl ethers, which include chloromethylmethyl ether (CMME) and bischloromethyl ether (BCME). Chloromethyl ethers are produced in order to chloromethylate other organic chemicals in the manufacture of ion-exchange resins, bactericides, pesticides, dispersing agents, water repellents, solvents for industrial polymerization reactions, and flameproofing agents. The potential for chloromethyl ethers to cause cancer was first suspected in humans in 1962. In Philadelphia, a cluster of three cases of small-cell lung cancer occurred among approximately 45 men working in a single building of a large chemical plant. A large proportion of tumors occurred in young men and nonsmokers. Numerous other studies confirm these findings, with increased risk seen in workers with prolonged or intense exposure. Unlike other chemical carcinogens, which can cause a variety of cancers, the chloromethyl ethers are associated primarily with the induction of small-cell lung cancer. Inhalation studies in animals show that the chloromethyl ethers produce bronchial epithelial metaplasia and atypia, and both carcinogens are active alkylating agents. BCME is a more potent carcinogen than CMME.

D. Polycyclic Aromatic Hydrocarbons

PAHs, formed from the incomplete combustion of coal tar, pitch, oil, and coke, have long been recognized as carcinogens. The first description implicating PAHs in the induction of cancer was in 1775, when Sir Percival Pott reported an increased risk of scrotal cancer in chimney sweeps as a consequence of dermal exposure to soot. Epidemiologic evidence linking PAHs to lung cancer was provided in 1936, when a study of exposed workers in a coal carbonization plant in Japan revealed a marked increase in the rate of lung cancer.

Exposures to PAHs linked to an increased risk of lung cancer have been found in coke oven workers, roofers, printers, and truckers. Rubber plant workers and those employed in asphalt production, coal gasification, and aluminum reduction facilities are also at risk. The best-described occupational group is coke oven workers, where direct exposure to the coke ovens results in increased rates of lung cancer. A clear dose-response relationship has been described based on proximity of work to the ovens.

E. Other Chemicals

1. Arsenic—Exposure to inorganic arsenic increases the risk of lung cancer; the first cases of arsenic-induced lung cancer were reported in 1930. Arsenic exposure in copper smelting, fur handling, sheep-dip compound manufacturing, and arsenical pesticide production and use has resulted in increased rates of lung cancer. Long latency periods of approximately 25 years are seen after exposure before the development of cancer. Arsenic is thought to act as a late-stage promoter of cancer and may interfere with DNA repair mechanisms. A dose-response relationship in exposed workers has been described, as has an increase in the risk of arsenic-induced lung cancer in cigarette smokers.

2. Chromium—Increased rates of lung cancer have been reported in industries that use chromate, including chromate production, chrome plating, chrome-alloy production, and others. Other lung carcinogens used in the electroplating industry, such as nickel and PAHs, may confound this relationship. The greatest risk of lung cancer appears to be present in occupations involving chromate production, in which all lung cancer types are increased.

3. Nickel—Exposure to nickel in mining, refining, and subsulfide roasting facilities is associated with increased rates of lung and nasal cancer. Soluble forms of nickel appear to be more potent carcinogens, with no increased risk seen after exposure to nickel alloys and pure nickel dust.

4. Mustard Gas—Studies of Japanese and German workers in factories that manufactured mustard gas during World War II show an excess of respiratory cancers. This is consistent with finding that mustard gas can produce lung tumors in laboratory animals. There may be a higher rate of squamous cell cancer of the lung in humans.

5. Probable Lung Carcinogens—Incomplete data exist regarding the risk of lung cancer associated with exposure to acrylonitrile (textile fiber, rubber workers), beryllium (production of beryllium alloys, aerospace industry), cadmium (cadmium and other metal smelters, manufacturers of batteries, plastics, dyes, and pigments), vinyl chloride (plastics production), formaldehyde (production of formaldehyde resins, molding, apparel), and inorganic acid mists containing sulfuric acid (metal production/processing).

Pathology

The four major types of lung cancer are squamous cell (epidermoid) carcinoma, adenocarcinoma, large-cell carcinoma, and small-cell (oat-cell) carcinoma. All histologic types of lung cancer are linked to cigarette smoking. There is no one cell type that is pathognomonic of an occupationally related lung cancer. A notable exception is workers exposed to CMME or BCME, who are much more likely to develop the relatively uncommon small-cell histology. Although early work suggested that the peripheral distribution of asbestos fibers was associated with a higher incidence of adeno-

carcinomas in this region, this has not been found in recent, more thorough studies. It appears that lung cancers in asbestos-exposed persons occur equally throughout the lung, and all pathologic types are seen.

Clinical Findings

A. SYMPTOMS & SIGNS

The findings in patients with lung cancer may arise secondary to local tumor growth, invasion of nearby structures, regional growth of nodal metastases, or paraneoplastic syndromes. The primary tumor often causes cough, hemoptysis, wheezing, dyspnea, or pneumonitis secondary to obstruction. Tumor spread may cause tracheal obstruction or esophageal compression, and superior vena cava syndrome may result from compression of vascular structures. The peripheral nervous system may be involved, with recurrent laryngeal nerve paralysis (causing hoarseness), sympathetic nerve involvement (Horner syndrome), or phrenic nerve paralysis. Nonspecific symptoms, such as weight loss, anorexia, and fatigue, may be evident.

B. LABORATORY FINDINGS

In approximately 60% of cases, a positive diagnosis can be made on the basis of sputum cytologic examination. By using flexible fiberoptic bronchoscopy, it is possible to visualize approximately 65% of lesions in lung cancer patients, with biopsy and brushings being true-positive in approximately 90% of these lesions. Transthoracic fine-needle aspiration biopsy with fluoroscopic guidance is useful for peripheral lesions that cannot be reached with the bronchoscope. If these less invasive diagnostic procedures fail to lead to diagnosis, exploratory thoracotomy may be required.

C. IMAGING

The chest radiograph is the most important tool for the diagnosis of lung cancer. Findings are related to the tumor cell type, with variation as to central or peripheral location of tumor mass, and existence of regional spread. Squamous cell cancers more often are located centrally, with associated hilar adenopathy. Adenocarcinoma presents more commonly as a peripheral nodule with pleural and chest wall involvement, and large-cell carcinoma is seen as a large peripheral mass with associated pneumonitis. A central lesion with atelectasis and both hilar and mediastinal adenopathy are common features of small-cell carcinoma. The extent of disease may be defined more accurately by computed tomographic (CT) imaging of the chest.

Prevention

Complete avoidance of exposure to the carcinogen is the ultimate goal, but this is not always possible. The most effective method of reducing the mortality rate for lung cancer is primary prevention. This includes identification of etiologic agents in the workplace, adherence to strict workplace standards, and worker education. Because tobacco use is known to increase the incidence of lung cancer in occupationally exposed groups, aggressive antismoking campaigns in the workplace are critically important.

Medical monitoring in the workplace has been attempted as a method of secondary prevention to aid in early detection. Serial chest radiographs and sputum cytologic examinations are now recommended by the National Institute for Occupational Safety and Health (NIOSH) and OSHA in high-risk occupational groups. The main problem with this approach is that there is no evidence that early detection improves the prognosis for persons with lung cancer. Thus far serial chest radiographs have been more useful than sputum cytologic examinations in detecting lung cancer. However, sputum cytology may reveal signs of mucosal damage, such as atypia, that could identify individuals at increased risk and lead to decreased exposure. Chemoprevention of lung cancer is under investigation, with only preliminary results available.

Treatment & Prognosis

Therapy of occupational lung cancers is no different from treatment for each of the specific cell types of lung cancer that may be seen. Surgical resection is currently the best hope for cure in non-small-cell cancer. Unfortunately, most patients do not qualify for a curative surgical procedure, and these patients are treated with palliative chemotherapy or radiotherapy in an attempt to improve survival because cures at this stage are rare. Survival is related to both cell type and stage of disease, with squamous cell cancers having the best prognosis. In general, even in patients with localized disease, long-term survival is the exception rather than the rule. Overall, 5-year survival ranges from 10–13%. Small-cell carcinoma traditionally has had the worst prognosis, with early and widespread metastases, although there have been some encouraging results with chemotherapy in limited disease.

MESOTHELIOMA

Essentials of Diagnosis

- Asbestos exposure, including trivial contact
- Persistent gnawing chest pain, dyspnea, dry cough, weight loss
- Findings consistent with pleural effusion, pleural friction rub on physical examination
- Chest radiograph and CT scan showing extensive pleural effusions, thick pleural rind lining the chest wall
- Diagnosis by open thoracotomy with multiple biopsies

Occupations at Risk

- Asbestos
  - Asbestos miners
  - Construction workers
  - Insulation and filter material production
  - Roofers
  - Shipyard workers
  - Textile manufacturing
  - Welders, plumbers, electricians

General Considerations

Mesothelioma was not accepted as a pathologic entity until about 50 years ago, when Klemperer and Rahn advocated general use of the term *mesothelioma* for primary pleural tumors originating from the surface-lining cells, or the mesothelium. This tumor is uncommon, accounting for only a small fraction of deaths caused by cancer, but it and other asbestos-related diseases have been of great interest to occupational health physicians, public health professionals, biomedical researchers, and personal injury attorneys.

The first case reports of mesothelioma associated with asbestos were published in the 1940s, but the problem received scant attention until 1960, when diffuse pleural mesothelioma were associated with asbestos exposure in the Cape Province of South Africa. The incidence of mesothelioma is increasing, with an annual incidence for adults in North America of approximately 12 cases per million for white men and 2–3 cases per million for women. In Canada, England, and Italy, areas of heavy occupational asbestos use, rates vary from 2.3 to 21.4 cases per million.

Etiology

Diffuse mesotheliomas of the peritoneum and pleura are considered "signal tumors," or pathognomonic of exposure to asbestos. Since the early report of Wagner, many additional reports and cohort mortality studies have clearly implicated asbestos as the etiologic factor in occupational mesothelioma. Evidence is lacking for any causal relationship between asbestos exposure and the development of solitary or localized mesothelioma.

The most convincing evidence of an association between asbestos and mesothelioma was brought out in Selikoff's report, which indicated that 8% of 17,800 asbestos insulation workers in the United States and Canada followed from 1967 to 1976 died from malignant mesothelioma. Selikoff and others have shown that a dose-response relationship exists between the risk of developing mesothelioma and the intensity and length of asbestos exposure.

The latency period from asbestos exposure to the diagnosis of mesothelioma is 30 years or more. Higher quantitative asbestos fiber content of dried lung has been found in patients with mesothelioma. Further evidence of the etiologic role of asbestos has been shown in experimental animals, in which intrapleural injection with asbestos fibers causes mesothelioma that is histologically identical to human tumors.

Epidemiologic data show that variable levels of exposure to asbestos can result in mesothelioma, despite the known dose-response relationship. In a study of 168 patients with mesothelioma in England and South Africa, one-third of cases were associated with occupational exposure intensive enough to cause asbestosis or lung cancer. Another third were asbestos-related only by trivial contact at work or in the home environment (e.g., exposure of wives washing their husbands' contaminated work clothes). The remaining third had no history of contact with asbestos.

The major value of studies done to date has been to identify segments of the population at risk, but reports of patients with mesothelioma who do not have a history of occupational or paraoccupational exposure to asbestos raise other questions. The proportion of patients with no exposure history ranges from 0–87% in various studies. The long latency period from exposure to disease results in problems with forgotten or unknown exposures. In addition, the variety of occupations associated with asbestos exposure leads to problems with overlooked exposures. Exposure occurs in the milling, mining, and transportation of raw asbestos and in the manufacture of asbestos cement pipe, friction materials, textiles, and roofing materials. Construction workers, plumbers, welders, and electricians are all exposed, and shipyard tradesmen can be "innocent bystanders" when they are exposed to airborne asbestos fibers. There is also evidence that nonasbestos agents can induce malignant mesotheliomas, and substances such as nickel, beryllium, silica dust, and zeolite fibers have been studied in this regard. Cigarette smoking does not increase the risk of malignant mesothelioma. Unlike lung cancer, there is no evidence for synergy between cigarette smoking and asbestos exposure in the development of this tumor.

Pathogenesis

All types of asbestos are capable of causing mesothelioma, although there is some evidence that crocidolite may be the most potent carcinogen. Very few mesotheliomas are associated with the chrysotile fiber alone. The mechanisms of induction are unknown. Cancer development is apparently related not to chemical composition but to physical properties (i.e., fiber size and dimension). In work done in rats, long, thin fibers of a variety of types have proved carcinogenic, whereas short fibers and those with a relatively broad diameter have failed to produce mesothelioma. Inhaled fibers are expectorated or swallowed. Short fibers are cleared more readily than long fibers. Fibers that remain accumulate in the lower lung, adjacent to the pleura. These findings are consistent with epidemiologic observations documenting the relatively common occurrence of tumors in populations exposed to grades of crocidolite consisting chiefly of long, thin fibers and the rarity of tumors in persons exposed to amosite and anthophyllite. The location of mesothelioma is related to the type of asbestos fiber as well. Chrysotile is associated with pleural, but not peritoneal, tumors in Canadian miners, although this association may be related at least in part to contamination of the asbestos with tremolite, an uncommon fiber, rather than the chrysotile. Peritoneal mesothelioma occurs only in individuals exposed to amphibole asbestos, and the pathogenesis is thought to be similar to tumor in the pleural cavity. Fibers of asbestos are transported in lymphatics to the abdomen, and asbestos is also transported across the mucosa of the gut after ingestion.

The mechanism of malignant transformation of mesothelial tissue is obscure. Mesothelial cells phagocytose asbestos and proliferate when exposed to asbestos in vitro. The activated mesothelial cells then release cytokines, which mediate an inflammatory and fibrotic reaction. Protooncogenes, such as platelet-derived growth factor, are unregulated in alveolar macrophages and result in mesothelial cell proliferation. It is of interest that malignant transformation has not been documented after exposure of cultured mesothelial cells to asbestos.

Pathology

A major area of difficulty in the study of mesothelioma has been distinguishing its pathologic features. Many tumors metastasize and spread to the mesothelial lining of the chest and abdomen. This has led to misdiagnosis of mesothelioma as a metastatic tumor. Confusion also exists because of the tumor's diverse microscopic appearance.

Two types of mesothelioma have been described: benign solitary and diffuse malignant. The benign solitary type remains localized, although it may become large and compress neighboring thoracic structures. This tumor has not been associated with asbestos exposure; it is a benign tumor arising from fibroblasts and other connective-tissue elements in the areolar submesothelial cell layers of the pleura and is not occupational in origin. By contrast, diffuse malignant mesothelioma arises from either the pluripotential mesenchymal cell or the primitive submesothelial mesenchymal cell, which retains the ability to form epithelial or connective-tissue elements.

Malignant mesothelioma is a diffuse lesion that spreads widely in the pleural space and usually is associated with extensive pleural effusion and direct invasion of thoracic structures. On gross examination, numerous tumor nodules may be noted, and in advanced cases, the tumor has a hard, woody consistency. Microscopically, malignant mesotheliomas consist of three histologic types: an epithelial type that may resemble metastatic adenocarcinoma, a mesenchymal type, and a mixed type. Histochemical techniques that use acid mucopolysaccharide with colloidal iron or Alcian blue stains can detect epithelial cells. This staining can be removed from the tissue with hyaluronidase, a helpful finding characteristic of mesothelioma that can help distinguish it from adenocarcinoma. Studies with the electron microscope have defined certain characteristic features that are also helpful in differentiating the tumor from metastatic disease.

Clinical Findings

A. SYMPTOMS

Symptoms in diffuse mesothelioma may be entirely absent or minimal at the time of onset of the disease. Disease progression results in the most common symptom of a persistent gnawing chest pain on the involved side, which may radiate to the shoulder and arm. In most patients, pain becomes the most incapacitating symptom. Dyspnea on exertion, dry cough (occasionally hemoptysis), and increasing weight loss are frequent accompanying symptoms. Some patients have low-grade fever, which can result in an incorrect diagnosis of chronic infection. A minority of patients have paraneoplastic syndromes such as hypertrophic pulmonary osteoarthropathy, syncopal attacks from hypoglycemia, or generalized anasarca from massive involvement of the pericardium or obstruction of the inferior and superior venae cavae.

B. SIGNS

Physical findings vary with the stage of disease. Most patients present with pleural effusion. Local tumor growth may depress the diaphragm and displace the liver or spleen, giving the impression of hepatomegaly or splenomegaly. In advanced disease, there may be obvious enlargement of the affected hemithorax, with bulging of the intercostal spaces and displacement of the trachea and mediastinum to the unaffected side. After removal of pleural fluid, a pericardial or pleuro-pericardial rub may be heard. Advanced signs also may include fever, arthralgias, supraclavicular and axillary node enlargement, subcutaneous nodules in the chest wall, and clubbing. Encroachment on the mediastinal structures may lead to neuropathic signs such as vocal cord paralysis or Horner syndrome. Congestion and edema may develop in the upper trunk or lower limbs secondary to compression of the superior or inferior venae cavae.

C. LABORATORY FINDINGS

Although patients may have the syndrome of inappropriate antidiuretic hormone secretion with hyponatremia,

most have normal blood chemistries. Elevation of lactate dehydrogenase may occur as a nonspecific finding.

D. IMAGING

Radiographic studies of the chest most commonly show unilateral pleural effusion. After thoracentesis, the pleura may show thickening or nodularity, seen usually at the bases. CT scanning, which is the most sensitive test for evaluating the pleural surface, may show thickened tumor along the chest wall, and late in the disease, tomograms or an overpenetrated film will show compressed lung surrounded on all sides by a tumor 2–3 cm thick. Extrapleural extension can result in soft-tissue masses or radiologic evidence of rib destruction. Signs of asbestos such as interstitial pulmonary fibrosis, pleural plaques, and calcification are valuable findings when present.

E. SPECIAL EXAMINATION

1. Sputum Cytology—Microscopic examination of sputum rarely shows malignant cells unless the tumor has invaded lung parenchyma. Asbestos bodies may be seen.

2. Thoracentesis—The considerable force necessary to enter the pleural space with a thoracentesis needle may be a clue to the presence of pleural mesothelioma. Pleural fluid is serosanguineous or hemorrhagic in 30–50% of cases but is commonly straw-colored. Cytologic examination of pleural fluid is useful in one-half to two-thirds of cases; however, distinguishing malignant mesothelioma from metastatic adenocarcinoma or benign inflammatory conditions is often difficult. The pleural fluid often contains a mixture of normal mesothelial cells, differentiated and undifferentiated malignant mesothelial cells, and a varying number of lymphocytes, histiocytes, and polymorphonuclear leukocytes. The diagnostic value of cytologic tests is limited. Mesothelial hyperplasia is not uncommon in benign pleural effusions and easily can be mistaken for malignant cells.

3. Thoracotomy and Thoracoscopy—Because of the limitations of pleural fluid cytologic examination, biopsy confirmation is required. An open thoracotomy with multiple biopsies from different pleural areas generally is required for diagnosis. Thoracoscopy with biopsy of pleural masses also can be a less invasive and effective technique.

Differential Diagnosis

The major disorders that must be differentiated from mesothelioma are inflammatory pleurisy, primary lung cancer, and metastatic adenocarcinoma or sarcoma. Inflammatory pleurisy is suggested by the associated clinical picture and by typical findings in the analysis of sputum and pleural fluid. In primary lung cancer, the more prominent symptom of cough, the less common presence of severe chest pain, the presence of parenchymal tumors, and the absence of pleural abnormalities after thoracentesis help to differentiate between these two types of cancer. Primary tumors of the pancreas, gastrointestinal tract, or ovary should be excluded because these tumors can metastasize to the pleural or peritoneal space and mimic mesothelioma.

Prevention

Regulations governing asbestos exposure have been difficult to develop. Morbidity and mortality data have been used to look retrospectively at members of occupational groups with varying exposures in the remote past or over a lifetime. The difficulties are compounded by the long latency period of asbestosis and asbestos-related cancers, especially mesothelioma. Setting permissible limits requires establishment of dose-response relationships, with subsequent determination of an acceptable level of risk. The difficulty is that all industrial processes, fiber types, and asbestos-related diseases have dissimilar dose-response relationships. Although the exposures to asbestos that lead to mesothelioma are less intense and of shorter duration than the exposures that lead to asbestosis or lung cancer, most standards are now based on preventing asbestosis.

Control of asbestos dust in industry has become progressively more rigorous over the last 40 years. Recommendations for levels of asbestos in the air of occupational settings were first established in the 1940s, but it was not until 1970 that federal regulations began as a result of the passage of the Occupational Safety and Health Act and the Clean Air Act. Initial standards were based on the light microscopic count of fibers of a length of 5 μm collected by mechanical means. A concentration of 5 fibers/mL of air averaged over an 8-hour period was considered acceptable, with stipulation for transient excesses above that concentration. In 1986, the exposure standard of 2 fibers/mL was lowered by OSHA to 0.2 fibers/mL. Allowable exposure varies with the different mineral fibers.

Treatment

A. SURGICAL MEASURES

Surgery has been used with some success as the primary method of treatment in pleural mesotheliomas. Even with tumors with extensive infiltration of adjoining viscera, partial surgical resection has led to an apparent increase in longevity. Subtotal pleurectomy with decortication is the accepted procedure. More radical surgeries such as pleuropneumonectomy may be appropriate for selected patients. Postoperative adjuvant chemotherapy and radiation therapy sometimes are used, but there are no studies to support their use. Surgical resection of all visible disease is believed to be the treatment of choice. Surgical excision has no role in the management of peritoneal mesothelioma unless the tumor is localized.

B. EXTERNAL RADIOTHERAPY

Radiation therapy clearly has been shown to be of benefit in controlling pain and pleural effusion in mesothelioma. Although antitumor efficacy has been noted using high-dose radiation, this modality is relatively ineffective in altering the dismal survival statistics for this disease.

C. INSTILLATION OF RADIOACTIVE COMPOUNDS

Because colloidal gold has an affinity for serosal lining cells, instillation of radioactive colloidal gold into the pleural space has been attempted. Responses with apparent long-term survival have been reported, with no significant toxicity. Therapy must be given early in the disease, before the pleural cavity is obliterated by tumor. Radioactive phosphate in conjunction with abdominal irradiation has been used for peritoneal mesothelioma, and the small number of patients treated in this fashion have had increased lengths of survival.

D. CHEMOTHERAPY

There has been no systematic study of the role of cytotoxic drugs in mesothelioma, but there are well-documented reports of definite antitumor effects in some patients. Doxorubicin has been demonstrated to induce tumor regression and perhaps to prolong the survival of responding patients. Single-agent doxorubicin therapy therefore has become the standard therapy for patients with unresectable disease, but no patient has been cured with chemotherapy.

Other reported active antitumor agents include methotrexate and alkylating agents such as cyclophosphamide, mechlorethamine, and thiotepa. There are few studies using combination chemotherapy, but regimens containing doxorubicin appear to be most effective.

Course & Prognosis

Approximately 75% of patients die within 1 year after diagnosis, with an average survival after diagnosis of 8–10 months. Several factors correlate with improved survival in mesothelioma. Patients whose tumors are in the pleura survive twice as long as those with peritoneal tumors; survival is longer for patients with epithelial types than for those with mixed or fibrosarcomatous types; and survival is longer for patients younger than age 65 years, those who respond well to chemotherapy, and those able to undergo surgical resection.

REFERENCES

Armstrong B et al: Lung cancer risk after exposure to polycyclic aromatic hydrocarbons: A review and meta-analysis. Environ Health Perspect 2004;112:970–978. [PMID: 15198916].

Favo V et al: Occupational and environmental exposures and lung cancer in an industrialised area in Italy. Occup Environ Med 2004;61:757 [PMID: 15317916].

Lemen RA: Chrysotile asbestos as a cause of mesothelioma: application of the Hill causation model. Int J Occup Environ Health 2004;10:233 [PMID: 15281385].

Park RM et al: Hexavalent chromium and lung cancer in the chromate industry: A quantitative risk assessment. Risk Anal 2004;24:1099 [PMID: 15563281].

Sorahan T, Esmen NA: Lung cancer mortality in UK nickel-cadmium battery workers, 1947–2000. Occup Environ Med 2004;61:108 [PMID: 14739376].

Yiin JH et al: Risk of lung cancer and leukemia from exposure to ionizing radiation and potential confounders among workers at the Portsmouth Naval Shipyard. Radiat Res 2005;163:603 [PMID: 15913392].

CANCER OF THE NASAL CAVITY & SINUSES

Essentials of Diagnosis

- Presenting symptoms are unilateral nasal obstruction, nonhealing ulcer, and occasional bleeding.
- More frequent in men than in women (2:1)
- Usually squamous cell histology

Occupations at Risk

- Wood and other dusts
  - Boot and shoe manufacturing
  - Furniture workers
  - Textile manufacturing
- Nickel
  - Nickel refinery workers
- Chromium
  - Chromate pigment manufacturing
  - Metal plating workers
- Isopropyl alcohol, formaldehyde
  - Laboratory workers
  - Other industries

Cancers of the nasal cavity and sinuses are relatively rare and account for fewer than 10 cases per million in the United States per year. This disease is very uncommon in workers under 50 years of age, and rates increase with age. Evidence suggests a fairly steady or slightly declining incidence over the years. Approximately 50% of all sinonasal tumors are squamous cell and 10% are adenocarcinomas. Both these histologies are linked to occupational exposures. Other histologic types include lymphoma, adenoid cystic carcinoma, and melanoma.

Etiology

Many different occupational exposures are linked to cancer of the nasal cavity and paranasal sinuses. These include wood dust, nickel, chromium, mustard gas, and cutting oils. Employment in several industries also has been associated with these cancers, including furniture and shoe manufacturing and coal mining. Furnace workers in the gas, coke, and chemical industries and foundries and textile workers are also at increased risk. The process of manufacturing isopropyl alcohol is associated with this form of cancer and is considered to be a consequence of the dimethyl sulfate used during the process.

A. WOOD AND OTHER ORGANIC DUSTS

The earliest report that linked cancer of the nose to exposure to wood dust was in 1965, when a laryngologist in England observed an unusually high incidence of cancer of the nasal cavity and sinuses among workers in the furniture industry. Fifteen of the 20 reported cases were involved in the production of wooden chairs. Woodworkers without carcinoma also were examined, and many exhibited chronic hypertrophic rhinitis, dry atrophic nasal mucosa, or nasal polyps. Since this first report, many studies have shown an increased incidence of carcinoma of the sinonasal area in persons exposed to wood dust. Adenocarcinoma of the ethmoids and middle turbinates is the most frequent cell type encountered in these workers. The exact substance in wood dust responsible for carcinogenesis has not been identified.

An excess of both adenocarcinomas and squamous cell carcinomas of the nasal sinuses also has been observed among workers in the boot and shoe industry. As in the case of woodworkers, the specific etiologic agent in boot and shoe manufacture is unknown. Dusts involved in the textile industry and flour dusts in bakeries and flour mills also have been associated with the development of sinonasal cancers.

B. NICKEL

Both nasal cancer and lung cancer are linked to occupational nickel exposure. Most studies have been done on nickel refinery workers exposed to complex particulates (insoluble nickel sulfide dust, nickel oxides, and soluble nickel sulfate, nitrate, or chloride) and gaseous nickel carbonyl. The mean latency period between exposure and diagnosis of cancer in refinery workers is 20–30 years.

The earliest report of an increased risk of sinonasal carcinoma in nickel refinery workers was in 1932, when 10 cases were described in Wales, where a nickel carbonyl process was employed. Studies confirming these findings were done subsequently in Canada, Norway, Germany, Japan, and the former Soviet Union. Clearly, nickel and nickel carbonyl are carcinogenic under experimental conditions, yet epidemiologic evidence points away from the nickel carbonyl process and incriminates exposure to dust from the preliminary processes. Neoplasms in nickel workers occur most frequently in the nose and ethmoid sinuses and are usually of the squamous or anaplastic cell type.

C. OTHER OCCUPATIONAL EXPOSURES

Tumors of the nasal epithelium and mastoid air cells have been noted in women exposed to radium used for painting dials of watches and in radon chemists. Workers involved in the manufacture of hydrocarbon gas are noted to have excess cases of cancer of the paranasal sinuses. Chromium is known to cause ulceration and perforation of the nasal septum, and there is an excess risk of sinonasal cancer in workers involved in manufacturing chromate pigments. Mustard gas, isopropyl alcohol, cutting oils, and formaldehyde are also linked to excess cancers of the nasal cavity and paranasal sinuses.

Clinical Findings

The earliest symptoms of nasal cavity neoplasms are a low-grade chronic infection associated with discharge, obstruction, and minor intermittent bleeding. The patient often complains of "sinus trouble" and may have been treated inappropriately with antibiotics for prolonged periods before the true diagnosis was known. Subsequent symptoms depend on the pattern of local growth. Maxillary sinus tumors develop silently when they are confined to the sinus, producing symptoms only with extension outside the walls. With extension into the oral cavity, pain may be referred to the upper teeth. Nasal obstruction and bleeding are common complaints, along with "sinus pain" or "fullness" of the involved antrum. Observation and palpation of the face may reveal a mass. Ethmoid sinus carcinoma presents initially with mild to moderate sinus aching or pain. A painless mass may present along the inner canthus, and with invasion of the medial orbit, diplopia develops.

Diagnosis & Treatment

In all cases, the patient should receive careful inspection and palpation of the facial structures, with attention to the eye and especially the extraocular movements. The nasal and orbital cavities should be examined closely. A fiberoptic nasoscope is a useful aid in visualizing the posterior and superior nasal cavities and the nasopharynx. Sinoscopy of the maxillary antrum also may be required. Helpful radiologic studies include facial bone or sinus radiograph series and CT scan of the involved areas. Identification of the site of tumor origin is important in determining the treatment plan.

Tumor in the nasal cavity is usually biopsied with a punch forceps. Biopsy of tumor in the maxillary antrum usually is approached with a Caldwell-Luc procedure, which is an incision through the gingivobuccal sulcus opposite the premolars. Biopsy of ethmoid tumors usually is taken from the extension into the nasal cavity. An undiagnosed orbital mass also may be biopsied secondary to incomplete examination of other areas. Frontal sinuses are approached by supraorbital incision and osteotomy.

Surgical therapy usually is indicated because of the frequency of osseous involvement; it involves resection of all gross disease. Any desire for wide margins is tempered by the reluctance to mutilate, and reconstructive and cosmetic surgery using prosthetic devices is often necessary. Radiation therapy nearly always is necessary because the resection margins are often narrow and the neoplasm is frequently of high grade. Chemotherapy is reserved for advanced disease. The prognosis is better for nasal cavity cancers because they tend to be diagnosed at an early stage. The 5-year survival rate is approximately 30–40% for tumors of the maxillary and ethmoid sinuses and dismal for frontal and sphenoid sinus carcinomas.

REFERENCES

Bimbi G et al: Adenocarcinoma of ethmoid sinus: An occupational disease. Acta Otorhinolaryngol Ital 2004;24:199 [PMID: 15688904].

Hauptmann M et al: Mortality from solid cancers among workers in formaldehyde industries. Am J Epidemiol 2004;159:1117 [PMID: 15191929].

Hemelt M et al: Occupational risks for nasal cancer in Sweden. J Occup Environ Med 2004;46:1033 [PMID: 15602177].

CANCER OF THE LARYNX

Essentials of Diagnosis

- Hoarseness is an early presenting symptom.
- Cigarette smoking and alcohol abuse are the primary etiologic factors.
- Much more frequent in men than in women (4.5:1), usually middle aged or older
- Usually squamous cell histology

Occupations at Risk

- Asbestos
  - Asbestos miners
  - Insulation and filter material production
  - Shipyard workers
  - Textile manufacturing

Cancer of the larynx is much more common than sinonasal cancer, representing about 2% of the total cancer risk in the United States. In most areas of the world, there is evidence that cancer of the larynx is increasing in men and, in more developed countries, also among women. In the United States in 2003, there were 7100 new cases of cancer of the larynx for men and 2400 for women; 3000 men and 800 women will die of this cancer.

Etiology

Cancer of the larynx appears to be related primarily to cigarette smoking. Alcohol is less important in the causation of laryngeal cancer than in other tumors of the head and neck. Occupational exposure to asbestos has been suggested as a risk factor for development of this disease, with one retrospective study finding asbestos to be a more important risk factor than either tobacco or alcohol. Most other studies do not support this contention, however. Asbestos exposure in miners, shipyard workers, asbestos product manufacturers, and insulators is associated with high rates of laryngeal cancers. Epidemiologic studies also link laryngeal cancer to "strong acid" manufacturing of ethanol and isopropanol, as well as to workplace exposures to wood dust, mustard gas, nickel, and cutting oils. The risk from these agents has not been clearly established.

Laryngeal cancer is primarily a disease of older workers; the median age is usually in the sixth or seventh decade. At the time of diagnosis, approximately 60% are localized, 30% show regional spread, and 10% have distant metastases. Laryngeal tumors in the United States are classified into three groups according to anatomic site of origin, with 40% supraglottic, 59% glottic, and 1% subglottic cancers. Nearly all are squamous cell carcinomas.

Clinical Findings

Symptoms of laryngeal carcinoma vary depending on the site of involvement. Any patient who complains of persistent hoarseness, difficulty in swallowing, pain on swallowing, a "lump in the throat," or a change in voice quality should be examined promptly by indirect laryngoscopy. Any limitation of motion or rigidity should be noted, and direct laryngoscopy with biopsy of suspicious lesions is necessary. Lateral soft-tissue radiographs of the neck and CT scanning are also useful, especially to delineate extent of disease.

Treatment

The treatment plan must include preservation of the patient's life and voice. There has been an increasing tendency to use more limited surgical procedures plus radiation therapy or radiation therapy alone. For failures of conservative therapy or deeply infiltrative tumors, total laryngectomy is required, necessitating tracheostomy and loss of normal voice. Because of the early symptom of hoarseness, true vocal cord tumors are detected early and carry the best prognosis; localized disease in this area has a 90% 5-year survival rate.

REFERENCES

Becher H et al: Occupation, exposure to polycyclic aromatic hydrocarbons and laryngeal cancer risk. Int J Cancer 2005;116:451 [PMID: 15810012].

Dietz A et al: Exposure to cement dust, related occupational groups and laryngeal cancer risk: Results of a population-based case-control study. Int J Cancer 2004;108:907 [PMID: 14712496].

Menvielle G et al: Smoking, alcohol drinking, occupational exposures and social inequalities in hypopharyngeal and laryngeal cancer. Int J Epidemiol 2004;33:799 [PMID: 15155704].

BLADDER CANCER

Essentials of Diagnosis

- Cigarette smoking is the most important etiologic factor.
- Naphthylamine, benzidine exposure
- Presenting complaints of hematuria and vesical irritability
- Diagnosis by urine cytologic examination and cystoscopy

Occupations at Risk

- Naphthylamine
  - Textile workers (dye/pigment manufacturing)
  - 4-Aminobiphenyl
  - Tire and rubber manufacturing
- Benzidine
  - Dye/pigment manufacturing
- Chlornaphazine
  - Leather workers
- 4-Chloro-*o*-toluidine
  - Bootblacks
  - Textile workers
- *o*-Toluidine
  - Painters
- 4,4′-Methylene bis(2-chloroaniline)
  - Rubber manufacturing
  - Truck drivers
- Methylene dianiline
  - Drill press operators
- Benzidine-derived azo dyes
  - Chemical workers
- Phenacetin-containing compounds
  - Hairdressers
  - Petroleum workers

General Considerations

Bladder cancer accounts for approximately 5% of all malignant tumors. In the United States, approximately 38,000 men and 15,000 women are diagnosed with the disease each year. Bladder cancer is the fourth most common type of cancer in men and the eighth most common type in women. The highest incidence of bladder cancer occurs in industrialized countries such as the United States, Canada, and France. In less developed countries, the incidence is about 70% lower than in the United States. The increased incidence in men is probably because more men work in potentially hazardous occupations (e.g., petroleum and chemical industries) than do women, although this trend seems to be shifting slightly. The increase in cancer of the bladder is also considered secondary to the relationship between bladder cancer and smoking. As with most cancers, the incidence of bladder cancer increases with age, with a peak incidence in the seventh decade. The incidence of urinary tract neoplasms is higher in industrialized countries than in the underdeveloped regions and higher in rural than in urban areas. Whether this has something to do with greater pollution is not clear.

Etiology

Cigarette smoking is the most important known preventable cause of bladder cancer, with as many as 60% of cases attributed to this common habit. The roles of coffee drinking and the use of artificial sweeteners also have been the objects of scrutiny. Occupations have long been suspect, and it is believed that 20% of all bladder cancers are a result of work exposures. The increasing incidence of bladder cancer despite a decrease in smoking in the United States suggests an important role for other environmental factors. Exposure to water contaminated with pesticides and other chemicals may increase the risk of bladder cancer.

As early as 1895, Rehn, a Swiss urologist, described a high incidence of bladder tumors among aniline dye workers. Large-scale production of aromatic amines as dye intermediates was started in the United States during World War I, and by 1934, the first occupational bladder cancers in the United States were described. Twenty-five cases of bladder tumor were reported in workers exposed to β-naphthylamine or benzidine and two cases in workers exposed to α-naphthylamine. Several years later, 58 additional cases were reported from the same plant. In addition, β-naphthylamine was reported to induce urinary bladder tumors in dogs, and subcutaneous injections of benzidine were shown to induce carcinomas in rats. During the next three decades, several studies in the United States and Great Britain showed an increase in urinary bladder tumors in workers exposed to these chemicals. The latency period between exposure and cancer was quite variable, with a mean of 20 years.

Occupational categories with a confirmed or strongly suspected increased risk for bladder cancer are dyestuff and chemical manufacturing, pigment and paint manufacturing, cable manufacturing, textile manufacturing (dyeing), leather working, roofing and other activities involving handling of coal tar, the coal tar industry, electrical workers, hairdressers, mechanics, metal workers, cobblers, and rubber workers. Recently, benzidine-derived dyes—Direct Blue 6, Direct Black 38, and Direct Brown 95—have been reported to cause cancers resulting from occupational exposures. NIOSH concluded that all benzidine-derived dyes should be recognized as potential human carcinogens, and since then, virtually all companies in the United States have stopped or reduced their manufacture.

Pathogenesis

Most occupation-related urinary tract tumors are thought to be caused by contact of the bladder epithelium with carcinogens in the urine. Because of the concentrating ability of the kidney, the bladder is exposed to higher concentrations of these materials than other body tissues. In addition, this exposure occurs over prolonged periods of time in certain areas of the urinary tract, most notably the bladder trigone area. Most of the proved urinary carcinogens are aromatic amines, which may be inhaled, ingested, or absorbed through the skin. Aromatic amines must be conjugated to sulfates or glucuronic acid in the liver before they can exert their carcinogenic effects. After transport to the kidneys, the conjugated amines are exposed in the urine to the enzyme β-glucuronidase and the optimal pH for its activity, with the result that there is enhanced splitting of the conjugated form and heavy exposure of urinary tract epithelium to hydroxylated carcinogens. Recent data indicate that hereditary polymorphisms of the arylamine N-acetyltransferase gene may play a role in the etiology of bladder cancer by modulating the effect of as well as the interaction between carcinogens, including cigarette smoke. The risk of cancer appears to be the highest in slow acetylators, suggesting that individual mechanisms of detoxification play an important role in the risk of toxin induced bladder cancer.

Pathology

Other less common work-related urologic neoplasms include tumors of the renal pelvis, ureter, and urethra—all with the same histologic and etiologic features as bladder tumors. Thus all four types usually are considered together as "lower urinary tract cancers" for epidemiologic purposes. More than 90% of urothelial tumors are of the transitional-cell type, approximately 6–8% are squamous cell, and 2% are adenocarcinoma. The tumors may be papillary or flat, in situ or invasive, and are graded according to degree of cellular atypia, nuclear abnormalities, and number of mitotic figures.

Multiple genetic changes have been associated with bladder cancer, such as expression of the *ras* and *myc* protooncogenes. Mutation of the tumor-suppressor gene *p53* is correlated with an increased risk of disease progression. Mutation of the retinoblastoma gene with resulting decreased expression of the retinoblastoma protein is associated with higher-grade tumors invading muscle.

Clinical Findings

The most common presenting symptom of bladder cancer is hematuria, which occurs in 80% of patients and usually is painless, gross, and intermittent. More than 20% of patients have vesical irritability alone, with increased frequency, dysuria, urgency, and nocturia. In advanced cases, patients present with symptoms secondary to lymphatic or venous occlusion, such as leg edema.

Urinalysis generally shows red blood cells, and bleeding can be severe enough to cause anemia. Uremia can occur if the bladder tumor has obstructed the ureters as they enter the bladder.

The diagnosis of bladder cancer may be made on the basis of urinary cytologic examination, which has been proposed as a screening tool. Up to 75% of patients with bladder cancer have abnormal urine cytology. Most patients undergo excretory urography, which is useful in ruling out upper tract disease and may show a filling defect in the bladder. Definitive diagnosis relies on cystoscopy and transurethral biopsy of the suspicious areas.

Bladder carcinoma that has invaded the muscular wall is potentially lethal and may metastasize even before urinary symptoms bring the patient to a physician. Bladder cancer generally spreads by local extension, through lymphatics, or by hematogenous dissemination. Clinical sites of metastatic disease include the pelvic lymph nodes, lungs, bones, and liver (in decreasing order of occurrence). Once the diagnosis has been confirmed by biopsy, a chest radiograph, radionuclide bone scan, and liver and renal function studies should be done. CT scans are extremely useful in staging. Current staging depends on depth of involvement, nodal involvement, and the presence or absence of distant metastases.

Prevention

Prevention of exposure to known carcinogens is the most effective means of preventing occupational urinary tract cancer. On an immediate basis, personal protective equipment can be used, and ultimately, the recommended means of control is by engineering methods aimed at zero exposure levels.

One appealing means of control is screening, and the use of urinary cytologic examinations has been suggested for this purpose in addition to urinalysis to look for microscopic hematuria. Estimates are of 75% sensitivity and 99.9% specificity for the urine cytology test, which would be used to screen only certain occupations at risk.

Immunocytology is under investigation and may improve the sensitivity of urine cytology. Screening of high-risk patients may result in a significant reduction in the stage of disease at diagnosis, with improved long-term survival. In addition, early detection of disease may be an indicator of inadequate primary prevention and could result in the incorporation of better local control measures.

Treatment

Therapy varies with the stage of cancer, although initial treatment for nonmetastatic disease is surgical. Carcinoma in situ is treated with transurethral resection of the malignant areas, occasionally followed by intravesical immunotherapy or chemotherapy. Superficial disease is managed by transurethral resection and fulguration but is associated with a high incidence of recurrence. This high-risk disease may be treated with intravesical therapy with improved recurrence rates. Bacille Calmette-Guérin (BCG) is used as immunotherapy, and thiotepa, mitomycin C, and doxorubicin are all effective agents when instilled intravesically in the postoperative setting.

Carefully selected patients with bladder carcinoma may undergo partial cystectomy, but invasive disease usually requires radical cystectomy. The current role of preoperative radiation therapy is controversial. Chemotherapy is reserved for metastatic disease, with cisplatin and methotrexate being the most efficacious single agents. Doxorubicin and vinblastine also demonstrate antitumor activity. Combination chemotherapy is more efficacious but also more toxic than treatment with single agents.

Prognosis

Prognosis varies with the stage of the disease. Patients with superficial disease who are treated appropriately should have excellent 5-year survival because disease becomes invasive in only one-third of these patients. The 5-year survival rate in patients with documented muscle invasion ranges from 40–50%. With local spread of disease in the pelvis, 10–17% of patients survive 5 years, and there are few long-term survivors once visceral metastases have occurred.

REFERENCES

Drdyson E et al: Occupational bladder cancer in New Zealand: A 1-year review of cases notified to the New Zealand Cancer Registry. Intern Med J 2005;35:343 [PMID: 15892763].

Gaertner RR: A case-control study of occupational risk factors for bladder cancer in Canada. Cancer Causes Control 2004;15:1007 [PMID: 15801485].

Kyam BM et al: Cancer in the Norwegian printing industry. Scand J Work Environ Health 2005;31:36 [PMID: 15751617].

Liu CS et al: Occupational bladder cancer in a 4,4′-methylene bis(2-chloroaniline) (MBOCA)–exposed worker. Environ Health Perspect 2005;113:771 [PMID: 15929884].

LIVER CANCER: HEPATIC ANGIOSARCOMA

Essentials of Diagnosis

- Major exposure to vinyl chloride
- Right upper quadrant abdominal pain, weight loss

- Hepatomegaly on physical examination
- Diagnosis by hepatic arteriogram and open liver biopsy

Occupations at Risk

- Vinyl chloride
  – Polyvinyl chloride production
- Arsenic
  – Arsenical pesticide production and use
- Copper, lead, zinc smelting
  – Wine makers (contamination of drinking water)

General Considerations

Angiosarcoma of the liver is a rare tumor with strong epidemiologic links to vinyl chloride and arsenic exposures. Thorotrast (thorium dioxide) exposure was the main nonoccupational risk factor when this agent was used as a radiographic contrast agent from about 1930 to 1955. This cancer occurs most commonly in middle-aged men, with a male-to-female ratio of 4:1. The mean age at presentation is 53 years. Characteristic features of the disease include a long period of asymptomatic laboratory abnormalities, difficulty in diagnosis, and poor response to treatment.

Etiology

Vinyl chloride is the raw material with which the common plastic polyvinyl chloride is made and, as is true of many other industrial products, was thought initially to be harmless. In 1974, a cluster of cases of angiosarcoma of the liver in men was reported by an alert physician in Louisville, Kentucky. The men were all workers at a local industrial plant that polymerized vinyl chloride. By 1981, 10 cases of hepatic angiosarcoma were identified among 1855 employees older than 35 years of age, with no other cases of angiosarcoma identified in the Louisville area. In one review of 20 patients with angiosarcoma of the liver after vinyl chloride exposure, the mean time from first exposure to development of tumor was 19 years, with a range of 11–37 years. In addition to the Louisville experience, cancer in other patients from plants elsewhere producing vinyl chloride has been noted. Similar hepatic lesions in experimental animals exposed to high concentrations of vinyl chloride also have been observed.

The carcinogenicity of the vinyl chloride monomer was first observed in laboratory animals, and a major lesion was angiosarcoma of the liver. Considerable evidence also associates exposure to vinyl chloride with other cancers, hepatocellular carcinoma, and soft-tissue sarcoma and increased mortality from lung and brain cancers and from lymphatic and hematopoietic neoplasms. A nested case-control study in the VCM/PVC industry showed an increased risk of lung cancer associated with exposure to PVC dust. Previous cohort studies failed to recognize such excess cancers probably because they used VCM exposure as the risk indicator.

Although the evidence is not as striking, angiosarcoma of the liver is also associated with arsenical pesticides, arsenic-contaminated wine, and Fowler solution used medicinally. Methylhydrazine, urethan, diethylnitrosamine, and dimethylnitrosamine induce angiosarcoma in laboratory animals, but there is no evidence to date that any of these cause human angiosarcomas.

Pathophysiology

The carcinogenicity of the vinyl chloride monomer is related to the metabolic formation of reactive metabolites. There is an enhanced positive mutagenic response in certain strains of *Salmonella typhimurium* exposed to the vinyl chloride monomer metabolized by microsomal enzymes or liver homogenates. Vinyl chloride is deactivated by conjugation with the hepatic nonprotein sulfhydryl compounds glutathione and cystine. It is hoped that further knowledge of the metabolism and pharmacokinetics of the vinyl chloride molecule will provide a scientific basis for guidelines concerning tolerable levels of exposure.

The two distinctive hepatic lesions seen after exposure to vinyl chloride are a peculiar hepatic fibrosis and angiosarcoma. The hepatic fibrosis is characterized by three features: a nonspecific portal fibrosis, capsular and subcapsular fibrosis in a nodular form (the most characteristic lesion), and focal intralobular accumulation of connective tissue fibers. In addition to this pattern of fibrosis apparent in all specimens, a focal irregular sinusoidal dilatation is also seen. A spectrum of changes occurs with increasing degrees of atypia and proliferation of sinusoidal cells, culminating in progressive multicentric, infiltrative angiosarcoma. The neoplasm is hemorrhagic and cystic and replaces most of the normal tissue. Microscopic examination shows that the angiosarcoma is multicentric, with several structural patterns, including sinusoidal, papillary, and cavernous. Hepatic angiosarcomas caused by Thorotrast and inorganic arsenicals show many of the histologic features observed in the evolution of the hepatic angiosarcoma in the vinyl chloride workers.

Clinical Findings

A. SYMPTOMS AND SIGNS

The symptoms of hepatic angiosarcoma are nonspecific, and some patients may be asymptomatic. Abdominal pain is the most common symptom, usually in the right upper quadrant. Fatigue, weakness, and weight loss are seen in 25–50% of patients. Physical examination reveals hepatomegaly with ascites, jaundice, and splenomegaly, which is seen less often. Other less-common physical findings include abdominal mass, tenderness, spider angiomas, and cachexia.

B. LABORATORY FINDINGS

A mild anemia is commonly present in these patients, and target cells and schistocytes are seen occasionally. Leukocytosis and thrombocytopenia are seen in about half of patients. Other abnormalities include prolonged prothrombin time, elevated fibrin split products, and hypofibrinogenemia.

Almost all patients have some abnormality of liver function testing. Most common is elevation of serum alkaline phosphatase. Many patients also exhibit elevated serum aspartate transaminase (serum glutamic-oxaloacetic transaminase), total serum bilirubin, serum lactic acid dehydrogenase (LDH), and serum alanine aminotransferase (serum glutamic-pyruvic transaminase), with decreased serum albumin. Tests for α-fetoprotein, carcinoembryonic antigen, and hepatitis B antigen are negative.

C. IMAGING

Routine abdominal radiographs and gastrointestinal contrast studies usually are normal. Occasionally, a mass lesion can be seen pushing aside the stomach; esophageal varices are common. Chest radiographs often will show abnormalities at or near the right hemidiaphragm, including elevation of the diaphragm, a right pleural effusion, atelectasis, or pleural masses. Radionuclide liver scans are abnormal in most patients, but the findings can range from distinct filling defects to nonspecific nonhomogeneous uptake (which can be confused with cirrhosis and splenomegaly). Hepatic arteriograms are the most helpful diagnostic tool, usually demonstrating normal-sized hepatic arteries that may be displaced by tumor, peripheral tumor stain, puddling during the middle of the arterial phase, and a central area of hypovascularity. Hepatic ultrasonography also may demonstrate a hepatic mass.

D. SPECIAL EXAMINATIONS

Definitive diagnosis of angiosarcoma is best made by thoracoscopic liver biopsy. Closed biopsy can be complicated by hemorrhage from this vascular tumor. Because of the difficulty in making the diagnosis and rapid clinical deterioration, more than 50% of hepatic angiosarcomas are diagnosed only after death.

E. SCREENING TESTS

Employees at risk of exposure should receive periodic testing consisting of history and physical examination, complete blood count, liver function tests, and liver-spleen scan. Patients with hepatomegaly or splenomeg-

aly should be evaluated with upper gastrointestinal radiographs, hepatic angiography, and liver biopsy. Those with abnormal liver scans or liver function test abnormalities that persist on retesting at 3 weeks should undergo a full workup with hepatic angiography and liver biopsy.

These tests generally are accepted in high-risk populations, but of note are serious drawbacks in using biochemical screening with liver function tests. The principal anatomic lesion in vinyl chloride–associated liver disease is fibrosis with relative sparing of the hepatocyte, so tests of hepatocellular function may be normal. Indocyanine green hepatic uptake is discussed in Chapter 22.

Prevention

Preventive measures for angiosarcoma include stringent limitations for employee exposure to vinyl chloride. The current U.S. occupational standard is 1 ppm averaged over any 8-hour period or 5 ppm averaged over 15 minutes or less. Tighter seals on polymerization vats and protective respirators for workers cleaning the vats are also recommended.

Treatment

Partial hepatectomy with intent to cure is possible in only a very limited number of patients because of extensive fibrosis in the uninvolved liver. Hepatic radiation has not been evaluated in a controlled trial. Chemotherapy with doxorubicin, cyclophosphamide, and fluorouracil have resulted in some temporary tumor regression. Recent studies suggest that liver transplantation early in the course of the disease may be curative.

Course & Progress

Major complications occurring prior to terminal events are common in these patients and include congestive heart failure secondary to arteriovenous shunts, hemolytic anemia, peripheral platelet destruction, hepatic failure, and hemoperitoneum. The major cause of death is irreversible, rapidly progressive hepatic failure. Overall survival usually is measured in months, with the median survival approximately 6 months and only a small percentage of patients surviving 2 years.

REFERENCES

Mastrangelo G et al: Increased risk of hepatocellular carcinoma and liver cirrhosis in vinyl chloride workers: Synergistic effect of occupational exposure with alcohol intake. Environ Health Perspect 2004;112:1188 [PMID: 15289165].

Wong RH et al: Interaction of vinyl chloride monomer exposure and hepatitis B viral infection on liver cancer. J Occup Environ Med 2003;45:379 [PMID: 12708141].

SKIN CANCER (NONMELANOMATOUS)

Essentials of Diagnosis

- Major risk is ultraviolet radiation.
- Skin findings: crusting, ulceration, easy bleeding, changing pigmented lesion
- Fair complexion increases risk.

Occupations at Risk

- Ultraviolet radiation
  – Outdoor workers
- PAHs
  – Coal tar workers (fuel production)
  – Electrode production
  – Pigment industry workers
  – Roofers
  – Shale oil workers, tool setters, etc. (mineral oils)
- Arsenic
  – Arsenical pesticide production and use
  – Copper, lead, zinc smelting
  – Sheep-dip manufacturers (contamination of drinking water)
- Ionizing radiation
  – Uranium miners
  – Health workers

General Considerations

Neoplastic diseases of the skin are commonly divided into melanoma and nonmelanomatous skin cancer, which consists mainly of basal cell and squamous cell carcinoma. Nonmelanomatous skin cancer (NMSC) is currently the most common form of cancer in the white population of the United States, accounting for one-third of all diagnosed cases of cancer. Although the dominant risk factor for NMSC (ultraviolet light) has been established, epidemiologic study of skin cancer has been limited. Nonmelanomatous skin cancer has an excellent prognosis, with 96–99% cure rates, making death certificate reviews useless.

There is an incorrect perception that skin cancer other than melanoma is a trivial disease. In addition, patients are rarely hospitalized, with the result that they are commonly not included in cancer registries. Because of failure to register or record skin cancers, much of the data on incidence are from surveys conducted many years ago. It is projected that more than 80,000 Americans will develop NMSC each year. Basal cell cancer is more than three times as common as squamous cell cancer.

Globally, NMSC is the most common form of cancer, more common than all other cancers combined.

Most of these cancers are due to solar (ultraviolet) radiation and occur at high rates in people who work or play in the sunlight or use tanning booths and tanning lights.

Etiology

The primary causes of skin cancer in industry include ultraviolet radiation (UV), PAHs, arsenic, and ionizing radiation. The information presented below refers primarily to NMSC. An increased risk of melanoma is associated with UV light exposure. Limited evidence exists linking melanomatous skin cancer to exposures to chemicals such as PAHs.

A. UV Radiation

Clearly, the major risk factor for skin cancer in lightly pigmented persons is radiation from the sun. The experiment of nature in which different intensities of UV radiation occur at different global latitudes has provided the opportunity for many epidemiologic studies to show an increased incidence of NMSC in whites at latitudes closer to the equator. The earliest realization that excess sun exposure leads to skin cancer was made on the basis of occupation in 1890, when Unna described changes of the skin of sailors, including skin cancer that resulted from prolonged exposure to the weather.

There are approximately 4.8 million outdoor workers in the United States, with certain occupations at greater risk, such as those in agriculture and professional sports. Another estimated 300,000 workers are exposed to industrial radiation sources (e.g., welding arcs, germicides, and printing processors). The carcinogenic hazard of industrial radiation, which includes wavelengths shorter than that of the sun, is not yet understood. In experimental animals, the most carcinogenic wavelength is in the range of 290–300 nm (sunlight does not include wavelengths lower than 290 nm); 254 nm is less carcinogenic, but wavelengths as low as 230 nm still will produce skin cancers.

The actual carcinogenic spectrum for humans is unknown. It is also notable that in experimental animals, a variety of foreign substances, including phototoxic chemicals (e.g., coal tar), chemical carcinogens (e.g., benzo[*a*]pyrene), and nonspecific irritants (e.g., xylene), under suitable conditions augment UV carcinogenesis.

B. PAHs

Although chemical carcinogenesis of the skin does not seem to be nearly as frequent a cause of NMSC as UV radiation, it was described more than a century earlier. Percival Pott described the increased incidence of scrotal cancer in chimney sweeps in 1775, but it was not until the 1940s that a PAH, benzo[*a*]pyrene, was shown to be a constituent of soot. These hydrocarbons have the ability to induce skin cancers in laboratory animals, and mixtures of them are found in coal tar, pitch, asphalt, soot, creosotes, anthracenes, paraffin waxes, and lubricating and cutting oils. Exposures to mineral oil have been linked to skin and scrotal cancers among shale oil workers, jute processors, tool setters, mule spinners, wax pressmen, metal workers exposed to poorly refined cutting oils, and machine operators using lubricating oils. Latent periods between exposure to polycyclic aromatic hydrocarbons and skin cancer vary from about 20 years (coal tar) to 50 years or more (mineral oil).

C. ARSENIC

Arsenic causes cancer in experimental animals and is a well-recognized human carcinogen. Skin tumors associated with arsenic occur following ingestion, injection, or inhalation, as well as from skin contact. Medicinal inorganic arsenicals and arsenic in drinking water are the sources most commonly implicated. Recent detailed studies in Taiwan established that use of well water with high arsenic concentrations resulted in skin cancer, with a dose-response relationship. An estimated 1.5 million workers in the United States are exposed to inorganic arsenic in such diverse trades as copper and lead smelting, the metallurgical industry, sheep-dip manufacturing, and the production and use of pesticides; however, skin tumors attributed to occupational arsenic exposure are very uncommon. It is thought that some of the cases cited in the literature of agricultural workers with arsenic-induced skin cancers may be the result of other carcinogenic influences, such as sunlight and tars. The simultaneous presence of arsenical hyperkeratoses or hyperpigmentation, which occurs at lower exposure levels, strongly implicates arsenic as the etiologic agent in an individual with NMSC. In addition, cancers tend to be multiple and occur in younger patients than those attributable to UV light.

D. IONIZING RADIATION

Ionizing radiation is as carcinogenic for skin as it is for many other tissues. Roentgen radiation–induced skin carcinoma was first reported in 1902, shortly after the discovery of x-rays, in those who worked the machines. There was a definite excess in skin cancer deaths among radiologists in the period 1920–1939, and an excess risk also has been found for uranium miners. Patients receiving radiation for acne, tinea capitis, and facial hair in the past had an increased risk of invasive skin cancers. The latent period for radiation-induced skin cancers varies inversely with the dose, with the overall range from 7 weeks to 56 years (average 25–30 years), and the skin cancers often occur in areas with chronic radiation dermatitis. Although epidemiologic studies do not give reliable data on dose-response relationships, the risk from exposures under 1000 cGy appears to be small, and skin cancer may be induced by dose equivalents of 3000 cGy. There are now strict controls on industrial and occupational exposure to ionizing radiation, and currently, it appears that ionizing radiation is not responsible for much cutaneous carcinogenesis.

E. OTHER FACTORS

Other risk factors for the development of NMSC include chewing tobacco or betel nuts, where squamous cell cancer of the lip and oral cavity have been described. Chronic irritation or inflammation is thought to induce these cancers. Patients with either primary or secondary (long-term immunosuppressive therapy) immunodeficiencies are at increased risk for skin cancer. Several genetically inherited syndromes such as xeroderma pigmentosum and albinism are associated with increased susceptibility to skin cancers.

Pathophysiology

Early studies elucidated the two-stage theory of carcinogenesis. They found that a single application of a potent carcinogen such as benzo[a]pyrene applied in a quantity insufficient to cause tumors allowed tumor development after subsequent application of croton oil, which by itself produced no tumors at all. The authors theorized that the production of a tumor was initiated by the carcinogen but that its subsequent development could be promoted nonspecifically. It appears that initiation is permanent and irreversible, but promotion, up to a point, is reversible.

UV light fits into this theory of chemical carcinogenesis in that it appears to be both an initiator and a promoter for carcinoma of the skin. Two major effects of UV radiation on the skin that seem likely to be responsible for the carcinogenic effects are photochemical alteration of the DNA and alterations in immunity. Certain immunologic defects, both in skin and in lymphocytes, can be induced by UV radiation. Exposure to UV light depletes the dermis of Langerhans cells and renders it unable to be sensitized to potent allergens. Alterations at the level of DNA are also thought to be responsible for ionizing radiation–induced skin cancers.

Pathology

The histologic types of skin lesions associated with sun exposure include solar keratoses, basal cell epitheliomas, squamous cell carcinomas, keratoacanthomas, and malignant melanomas. Solar keratoses contain morphologically cancerous cells, but they are considered premalignant because invasion is limited to the most superficial part of the dermis. Approximately 13% of all solar keratoses develop into squamous cell carcinomas, but these are rarely aggressive. The estimated incidence of metastases from all sun-induced squamous cell carcinomas is 0.5% or less. Almost all squamous cell carcinomas in whites occur in highly sun-exposed areas, but 40% of basal cell epitheliomas occur on shaded areas of the head and neck.

Regardless of the source of exposure, certain features are common in all cases of arsenic-induced skin cancers. Punctate keratoses of the palms and soles and hyperpigmentation are seen frequently. The skin tumors are of several types. Squamous cell carcinomas arise either from normal skin or from keratoses. Basal cell epitheliomas, including multiple superficial squamous cell and basal cell epitheliomas, as well as areas of intraepidermal carcinoma (Bowen disease), have been described. Multiple tumors are the rule, most of which are found on unexposed areas. Cancer of the scrotum, which is seen following topical exposure to PAHs, is rare.

Early radiation workers with heavy exposure from uncalibrated machines developed predominantly squamous cell carcinomas, found mainly on the hands and feet and occasionally on the face. More recently, basal cell cancers have been described following repeated occupational exposures.

Radiation-related tumors usually arise in areas of chronic radiation dermatitis, and whether they can occur on clinically normal skin is a matter of dispute. Radiation-induced malignant melanoma and sweat gland tumors have been described rarely.

Clinical Findings

Basal cell epithelioma frequently presents as a nodular or nodular-ulcerative lesion on the skin of the head and neck and only 10% of the time on the skin of the trunk. It is much less common on the upper extremities and very uncommon on the lower extremities. The lesion generally is smooth, shiny, and translucent, with telangiectatic vessels just beneath the surface. It is usually not painful or tender, even with ulceration, except when crusting or bleeding is seen with minor trauma. Basal cell carcinomas rarely metastasize, but they can invade widely and deeply, extending through the subcutaneous tissue to involve neurovascular structures and occasionally erode into bone.

Squamous cell carcinoma presents first in a premalignant stage characterized by actinic keratosis, a rough, reddened plaque on sun-exposed skin. There is then an in situ stage, which appears as a well-demarcated, slightly raised erythematous plaque with more substance and scaling than actinic keratosis. Squamous cell cancers arising in sun-exposed areas of the body tend to be on the most highly irradiated areas, such as the tip of the nose, the forehead, the tips of the helices of the ears, the lower lip, or the backs of the hands. Metastases are more common than from basal cell cancer, and squamous cell cancers on mucosal membranes metastasize more frequently than do those found on the skin surface.

Prevention

The most important step in prevention of occupation-related skin cancers is avoidance of UV light. This is especially true for workers who are more susceptible to UV light, such as those with fair complexions or with certain hereditary diseases (e.g., albinism and xeroderma pigmentosum).

Protective clothing, such as wide-brimmed hats and long sleeves, is the most effective barrier to UV radiation exposure in outdoor workers. Sunscreens that provide protection in the UVA and UVB spectrum should be used daily. The effectiveness of sunscreens in preventing carcinoma is unknown, though their effectiveness for avoidance of erythema has been proved. Periodic examinations are recommended to detect the presence of malignant and premalignant skin lesions.

The incidence of scrotal cancer is now rare because of preventive measures. If possible, a noncarcinogenic material should be substituted for a carcinogenic one. The efficacy of this approach was demonstrated clearly in Great Britain in 1953, when noncarcinogenic oil use became obligatory in the mule-spinning industry, with a steady fall in the number of reported cases of scrotal carcinoma. Good personal hygiene should include compulsory showering and changing of clothes when entering and leaving the plant, as well as washing of exposed skin after leaving contaminated areas. Isolated or closed-system operations, protective clothing, and employee education are also critical in avoidance of skin cancer induced by PAHs.

Currently, the maximum allowable dose equivalent of ionizing radiation for occupational exposure to the skin is 30 rems in any year, except that forearms and hands are allowed 75 rems in any year (because there is little red marrow in the forearms and hands). These recommendations are based mainly on avoidance of hematologic disease and may need to be revised in order to prevent skin cancer. Exposure can be limited further by the use of shielding devices such as lead gloves and aprons.

Treatment

Biopsy is necessary in all cases of suspected skin carcinoma. For small skin cancers not located in areas where primary closure would be difficult, excisional biopsy should be done. If an incisional biopsy is done, it is imperative that an adequate amount of tissue be obtained from the involved area.

Actinic keratoses may be excised or removed superficially with a scalpel, followed by cautery or fulguration. Also, 1–5% fluorouracil may be used topically, followed by excision of persistent lesions.

Squamous cell carcinoma should be treated with excision, but radiation is an alternative. The Mohs technique of micrographic surgery to remove skin carcinomas results in the highest cure rate. Basal cell carcinoma is treated with excision, curettage, and electrodesiccation; irradiation; or the Mohs technique. Cryosurgery may be used but is associated with a large number of recurrences.

REFERENCES

Gawkrodger DJ: Occupational skin cancers. Occup Med (Lond) 2004;54:458 [PMID: 15486177].

Puntoni R et al: Increased incidence of cutaneous malignant melanoma among longshoremen in Genoa, Italy: The role of sunlight and occupational exposure. Occup Environ Med 2005; 62:270 [PMID: 15778261].

Ramirez CC et al: Skin cancer as an occupational disease: The effect of ultraviolet and other forms of radiation. Int J Dermatol 2005;44:95 [PMID: 15689204].

HEMATOLOGIC CANCERS

Essentials of Diagnosis

- Radiation, benzene exposure
- Presenting complaints of weakness, malaise, anorexia, fever, and easy bruisability
- Pallor, hepatosplenomegaly, lymph node enlargement on physical examination
- Leukocytosis or leukopenia, with immature white cells in peripheral blood and bone marrow
- Anemia, thrombocytopenia

Occupations at Risk

- Radiation
  – Health workers
  – Military personnel
  – Nuclear power plant workers
- Benzene
  – Petrochemical and refinery workers
  – Rubber workers

General Considerations

The two major forms of leukemia that have been linked to occupation are acute nonlymphocytic leukemia (ANLL), including myelodysplasia or preleukemia, and chronic myelogenous leukemia (CML). Multiple myeloma is covered in Chapter 15. The acute leukemias are malignant diseases of the blood-forming organs characterized by a proliferation of immature blood cell progenitors in the bone marrow and other tissues. Together with replacement of the normal marrow with leukemic cells, there is a diminished production of normal erythrocytes, granulocytes, and platelets. Acute leukemias are classified morphologically by reference to the predominant cell line involved as lymphocytic and nonlymphocytic forms. Nonlympho-

cytic leukemias are further classified as de novo (no underlying cause known and without preexisting myelodysplasia) or secondary (known cause such as chemical exposure or preexisting myelodysplasia or chronic leukemia). In 2003, total leukemias accounted for 30,000 new cases (male 17,900, female 12,700) and 21,900 deaths (male 12,100, female 9800). The acute leukemias, taken collectively, are relatively common diseases, with a projected incidence in the United States of 14,100 new cases in 1996. The annual incidence of ANLL is constant from birth throughout the first 10 years at about 10 cases per million. The incidence peaks in late adolescence, remains at 15 per million to age 55 years, and then rises to 50 per million at age 75 years. Eighty percent of all adult acute leukemias are of the nonlymphocytic variety, and unlike acute lymphoblastic leukemia, ANLL has been reported as a complication of chemical exposures and irradiation.

Chronic leukemias are classified as lymphocytic and myelogenous; only chronic myelogenous leukemia has been reported as an industrial disease. Chronic myelogenous leukemia is a neoplastic disease resulting from the development of an abnormal hematopoietic stem cell. There is excessive growth of the blood cell progenitors in the marrow, which initially function as normal hematopoietic cells. The leukemic cells gradually undergo further malignant transformation, with loss of the ability to differentiate in the later stages of the disease, with the resulting development of acute leukemia and death. In the early stages of the disease, large numbers of mature and immature granulocytic cells accumulate in the blood, and extramedullary hematopoiesis produces gross enlargement of the liver and spleen. Chronic myelogenous leukemia accounts for approximately 20% of all deaths from leukemia in the Western world, with an incidence that, unlike other forms of leukemia, has not been increasing recently. Although rare cases are reported in infants, most patients with CML are age 25–60 years, with a median age of about 45 years.

Etiology

The cause of human leukemia is unknown. As in the case of most other cancers, it is probable that no single factor is responsible. Most cases are thought to result from the interaction of host susceptibility factors, chemical or physical injury to chromosomes, and in animals and presumably in humans, incorporation of genetic information of viral origin into susceptible stem cells.

A. RADIATION

Radiation remains the most conclusively identified leukemogenic factor in human beings. The earliest evidence began to accumulate soon after the discovery of x-rays, which were used mainly in the medical workplace; thus radiologists, radiation therapists, and radiation technicians were all at risk. Several studies showed an excess risk of leukemia among radiologists (approximately nine times that of other physicians) during the years 1930–1950, with a latency period of about 18 years. With the institution of dose limits, careful monitoring, and adequate shielding since that time, this excess risk has decreased significantly and should be eliminated.

The data from Hiroshima and Nagasaki atomic bomb survivors leave little doubt that the incidence of leukemia is increased following exposure to mixed gamma and neutron radiation and that the response is dose-dependent. The risk of leukemia is increased in populations exposed to ionizing radiation at doses as low as 50–100 cGy. Between 100 and 500 cGy, there is a linear correlation between dose and leukemia incidence. The data suggest that the risk of leukemia is increased at a rate of 1–2 cases per million population per year per centigray. Maximal risk occurs approximately 4–7 years after exposure, and an increased risk has been seen in Japanese people as long as 14 years after exposure.

Whole-body exposure to radiation in single doses results in suppression of marrow growth, and a single whole-body dose of more than 400 cGy usually is fatal in humans. In sublethal exposure, cytopenias may occur, which gradually recover but indicate significant damage to the marrow precursor elements. Patients are then at risk to develop leukemia with a delay between exposure and disease of 8–18 years. Following radiation exposure, both acute and chronic myelogenous leukemia may occur. In the atomic bomb survivors, chronic lymphocytic leukemia has not been seen. The specific rates per 100,000 for people within 1500 m (4921 ft) of the hypocenter are 8.1 for acute nonlymphocytic leukemia, 25.6 for chronic myelogenous leukemia, and 21.7 for acute lymphocytic leukemia.

Workers at risk secondary to exposure to ionizing radiation include military personnel in the vicinity of nuclear tests, uranium miners, and workers in nuclear power plants. Approximately 250,000 troops are estimated to have been present at multiple detonations of nuclear devices carried out by the United States from 1945 to 1976. In 1976, more than 3000 men exposed at the 1957 nuclear test explosion "Smoky" were studied, and a significant excess of leukemia was discovered. A review of death certificates of former workers at the Portsmouth Naval Shipyard in Portsmouth, New Hampshire (where nuclear submarines are repaired and refueled), revealed an observed-to-expected ratio of leukemia deaths of 5.62 among former nuclear workers.

B. BENZENE

Certain chemicals (e.g., chemotherapeutic agents) are known to be toxic to marrow cells, and many of these also possess leukemogenic potential. Occupational evidence of leukemogenicity is strongest for benzene, where recent epidemiologic studies have shown significant increases in leukemia in workers with past exposure to benzene. Benzene has been known for almost a century to be a powerful bone marrow poison, leading to aplastic or hypoplastic anemia. It is now widely believed that any chemical capable of inducing bone marrow damage must be assumed to be a potential leukemogen. Over the past few decades, evidence has been accumulating that benzene produces not only aplastic anemia but also leukemia and that the fatal cases of leukemia outnumber those of true aplastic anemia. In 1928, the first case of acute leukemia in a worker from a plant with such heavy exposure to benzene that none of the employees could work for more than 2 months without becoming ill was reported. In 1932, leukemia was induced in white rats given benzene in olive oil, but many subsequent animal studies were inconclusive. Only in the last few years have investigators shown that benzene can systematically induce cancers in rats.

Benzene is a cyclic hydrocarbon obtained in the distillation of petroleum and coal tar. It is used widely in chemical synthesis in many industries, in the manufacture of explosives, and in the production of cosmetics, soaps, perfumes, drugs, and dyes. Benzene once was used in the dry-cleaning industry, but that is no longer the case. In addition, nearly 2% of unleaded gasoline is benzene.

An estimated 2 million workers in the United States have exposure to benzene. One of the most recent studies in workers exposed to benzene in the manufacture of rubber showed a nearly sixfold greater incidence of death from leukemia than would be expected. Workers exposed for 5 years or more had a 21-fold increased risk of death from leukemia. Many other studies, including several undertaken in the shoe manufacturing industry, have shown an increase in the risk of leukemia in workers with exposure to benzene. Although many studies have suggested a link between benzene exposure and an increased risk of CML, no definitive data exist.

C. OTHER CHEMICALS

Chemicals other than benzene are suspected of causing leukemia, but the epidemiologic data in this area are incomplete. Ethylene oxide exposure has been associated with an increased risk of leukemia. This chemical is used as a sterilant and in chemical processing. An increase in leukemia in chemists in Norway has been described, and an increase in marrow chromosome breakage has been noted in patients with leukemia who have histories suggesting occupational exposure to carcinogens. Indirect evidence of leukemogenicity of organic hydrocarbons comes from a study that showed an increased incidence of leukemia in Nebraska farmers, thought to be secondary to exposure to chemicals used on the farm. The data linking exposure to electromagnetic fields with an increased risk of leukemia remain unclear. Treatment with a variety of chemotherapeutic agents has been associated with an increased risk of leukemia within 2–5 years of initiation of chemotherapy. This can occur after very short-term exposure. There is a known synergistic interaction of radiation therapy and treatment with alkylating chemotherapeutic drugs for underlying malignancies such as Hodgkin disease, resulting in a significant increase in the risk of subsequent leukemia. 1,3-Butadiene is another occupational chemical known to cause cancers of the hematopoietic and lymphatic systems.

Pathophysiology

A. Ionizing Radiation

The effects of radiation on human tissue depend on multiple factors, such as type of radiation, dose of radiation, length of exposure, body part exposed, and oxygen content of the exposed tissue. Damage secondary to radiation is greatest in rapidly dividing cells such as bone marrow stem cells, epithelial cells, and gamete-forming cells. The mechanism of radiation-induced injury at the cellular level involves direct and indirect damage to nucleic acids and proteins. DNA is a radiosensitive target, with even minor molecular damage resulting in profound effects on the cell and the organism. Radiation-induced molecular damage may be so severe that the cell no longer functions, and cell death results. Cells exposed to radiation may survive with no effects (if only a small number of nonessential molecules are affected) or may survive with altered structure and function. If the alteration is within the DNA, clinical disease may not appear until after a latency period. Cancer induction appears to depend on an interaction of defective cellular repair and damage to the cell's regulator genes.

B. Benzene

Benzene toxicity may present as an acute illness or as a chronic disease developing up to 30 years after exposure. Chronic or recurrent exposure to concentrations of benzene exceeding 100 ppm (320 mg/m^3) leads to a very high incidence of cytopenias. When the exposure ends, there is usually spontaneous remission. Among workers who have been exposed to atmospheric concentrations of benzene in excess of 300 ppm for at least 1 year, as many as 20% will acquire pancytopenia or aplastic anemia. The chronic form of illness is related to the effect of benzene on the bone marrow, where benzene appears to exert a colchicine-like effect, blocking mitosis of the marrow proliferative cells. This then results in mutagenic effects that play a role in the subsequent development of leukemia. Aplastic anemia generally occurs in subjects while they are still exposed to high concentrations of benzene; leukemia may occur at the same time or shortly after cessation of exposure.

Leukemia often develops in subjects with benzene-induced hyporegenerative anemia or long-standing pancytopenia and represents the acute terminal stage of the disease. Approximately 1 patient in 60 with benzene-induced pancytopenia or aplastic anemia and 1 patient in 10 with unremitting, progressive marrow failure who survive beyond 1 year will develop acute nonlymphocytic leukemia.

Clinical Findings

A. Symptoms and Signs

1. Radiation—As noted earlier, 300–400 cGy of whole-body radiation is lethal in humans. Sublethal exposures will cause symptoms of nausea and vomiting, after which bone marrow suppression occurs. Thrombocytopenia, anemia, and neutropenia will develop, with their attendant symptoms. The development of leukemia occurs after a delay of 8–18 years after the onset of exposure. Most patients with early-stage CML are asymptomatic. Occasionally, patients will present with fatigue, fevers, anorexia caused by massive splenomegaly, or retinal hemorrhages. When the disease progresses, symptoms are identical to acute leukemia. Physical examination reveals splenomegaly in the majority of cases. The symptoms of acute leukemia, which also may develop after radiation exposure, are described below.

2. Benzene—Acute exposure to benzene may result in headache, dizziness, and vertigo. Chronically, there is inhibition of marrow cell proliferation, and symptoms appear as pancytopenia develops. A decrease in hematocrit results in pallor, shortness of breath, and weakness. Thrombocytopenia leads to the appearance of petechiae and purpura. Infections and painful mouth sores can occur secondary to a decrease in the number of neutrophils. Leukemia may present with general complaints such as fever, weakness, malaise, anorexia, bone pain, and easy bruisability. Physical findings such as hepatosplenomegaly, enlarged lymph nodes, swollen gums, skin nodules, and ecchymoses are seen. Occasionally, gum bleeding after dental procedures or major ecchymoses after minor trauma may be the major presenting complaint.

B. Laboratory Findings

Most cases of CML present with the well-recognized hematologic characteristics of peripheral myeloid leukocytosis, thrombocytosis, anemia, and basophilia. Granulocytic leukocytosis is the fundamental abnormality, averaging 200,000/µL, with a range of 15,000–600,000/µL at diagnosis. The bone marrow is hypercellular, with granulocytic hyperplasia and, often, increased numbers of megakaryocytes. The presence of the Philadelphia chromosome [t(9;22)] on chromosomal analysis or the *bcr/abl* translocation on polymerase chain reaction is diagnostic.

Patients with benzene toxicity usually present with pancytopenia, but any combination of anemia, thrombocytopenia, or leukopenia may occur. The anemia usually is normochromic and normocytic, with normal red cell morphology. The reticulocyte count is inappropriately low, and parameters of hemolysis such as bilirubin and LDH will be normal. White cell morphology is also normal initially, with a decrease in neutrophils and an increase in the percentage of lymphocytes.

Evaluation of the blood counts in acute leukemia usually reveals a marked decrease in at least two cell lines. Leukocytosis with circulating blasts found on evaluation of the peripheral blood smear is common, but leukopenia also may be seen. Circulating blast cells may contain Auer rods or peroxidase stain–positive granules. The bone marrow may be hyper- or hypocellular, with more than 30% leukemic blast forms. Secondary leukemias may develop slowly, beginning as myelodysplasia, with a gradually increasing blast count in the bone marrow and markedly abnormal growth of the myeloid, erythroid, and platelet precursor cells. Secondary leukemias often are associated with chromosomal abnormalities such as loss of all or part of chromosome 5 or 7, which is unusual in de novo disease.

Prevention

A. RADIATION

X-rays were discovered by Roentgen in 1895, and by 1902, the basic principles of radiation protection already had been elaborated: to minimize dose by reducing the time of exposure and by using shielding and distance. Since 1928, the International Council on Radiation Protection (ICRP) and the National Council on Radiation Protection have defined acceptable levels of radiation exposure for workers. The concept of dose equivalent or rem (Roentgen-equivalent man) is used because the same amounts of absorbed radiation energy can produce different levels of damage depending on the type of radiation present. Acceptable exposures for different organs vary, with a maximum permissible dose ranging from 5 rems of whole-body exposure to 30 rems of skin or bone exposure.

B. BENZENE

Regulated standards of benzene began in 1926, and in 1974, NIOSH published a recommended standard based on the evidence for hematologic changes: 10 ppm as an 8-hour time-weighted average (TWA), with a ceiling limit of 25 ppm. In 1977, OSHA issued an emergency standard decreasing the acceptable 8-hour TWA exposure to 1 ppm after a study showing excess deaths as a result of leukemia in benzene-exposed workers, but these recommendations as a permanent standard were not upheld. Subsequently, OSHA promulgated a ppm

workplace standard. Even this "acceptable" level remains an area of controversy, in that with current allowable levels the lifetime incidence of excess leukemia for exposed workers is estimated to be from 1.4–15.2%. Periodic hematologic screening is believed to be mandatory in populations exposed to increased atmospheric levels of benzene, with both removal from the work environment and further hematologic testing indicated for any aberrations found.

Treatment & Prognosis

With excess exposure or signs of toxicity in workers exposed to either radiation or benzene, removal from the offending environment is the first priority. Benzene-induced aplastic anemia is treated like any pancytopenia (i.e., with supportive care in the form of transfusions, infection precautions, etc.). The outcome is similar to that of other aplastic anemias, with a 5-year survival rate of 30%. One-half of deaths occur in the first 6 months. Bone marrow transplantation is the only known cure for severe aplastic anemia. Immunosuppressive therapy is not effective for toxin-induced aplasia.

There have been recent major advances in the treatment of acute leukemias with the use of combination chemotherapy and bone marrow transplantation. ANLL is treated most successfully with an induction protocol consisting of daunorubicin and cytarabine, resulting in a 60% complete response in adults. This is followed by repeated courses of consolidation chemotherapy or bone marrow transplantation. For de novo ANLL, a 45–60% long-term disease-free survival is seen following aggressive therapy. Unfortunately, secondary ANLL has a poor prognosis, with median survivals of 1–2 years and no cures obtained from chemotherapy alone. Bone marrow transplantation is the only curative option and is limited by patient age and donor availability. Lighter preparative regimens are now being used to reduce immediate toxicity from and broaden applicability for allogeneic transplantation. There are insufficient long-term data to know how effective this approach will be for aggressive leukemias. The median survival for CML is 3–5 years from the date of diagnosis. Treatment is aimed initially at controlling leukocytosis and thrombocytosis and results in improved symptoms. Hydroxyurea is the initial agent of choice. Treatment with the oral medication imatinib mesylate (Gleevec, an inhibitor of the activated enzyme thought to be responsible for malignant transformation in CML) results in prolonged cytogenetic remissions (loss of the Philadelphia chromosome), although long-term survival data are not yet available. Although some patients may have prolonged and durable remissions with this novel therapy, bone marrow transplantation is still the only known cure for CML and, like ANLL, is limited by patient age, donor availability, and mortality from complications. The transformation of CML to acute leukemia (blast-phase CML) is associated with survivals of 6 months or less.

REFERENCES

Bloemen LJ et al: Lymphohaematopoietic cancer risk among chemical workers exposed to benzene. Occup Environ Med 2004; 61:270 [PMID: 14985523].

Boffetta P: Risk of acute myeloid leukemia after exposure to diesel exhaust: A review of the epidemiologic evidence. J Occup Environ Med 2004;46:1076 [PMID: 15602182].

Cartwright RA, Watkins G: Epidemiology of Hodgkin's disease: A review. Hematol Oncol 2004;22:11 [PMID: 15152367].

Collins JJ: Formaldehyde exposure and leukaemia. Occup Environ Med 2004;61:875 [PMID: 15477279].

Goldstein B: Benzene exposure and leukemia. Epidemiology 2004; 15:509 [PMID: 15232416].

Jaga K, Dharmanni C: The epidemiology of pesticide exposure and cancer: A review. Rev Environ Health 2005;20:15 [PMID: 15835496].

Muller AM et al: Epidemiology of non-Hodgkin's lymphoma (NHL): Trends, geographic distribution, and etiology. Ann Hematol 2005;84:1 [PMID: 15480663].

Pyatt D: Benzene and hematopoietic malignancies. Clin Occup Environ Med 2004;4:529 [PMID: 15325320].

Sorahan T et al: Cancer risks in a historical UK cohort of benzene exposed workers. Occup Environ Med 2005;62:231 [PMID: 15778255].

OTHER CANCERS

Many other cancers are reported to be associated with specific occupational or environmental exposures. However, the majority of these associations is casual and is not yet supported with sufficient epidemiologic or animal data. An increased incidence of renal cell cancer has been reported in some workers. PAHs, and other organic solvents, asbestos, cadmium, and lead salts all have been investigated as possible etiologic agents. Cancers of the gastrointestinal tract may be increased in workers exposed to asbestos (gastric, colon) and coal dust (gastric). Cancer of the thyroid has been definitely associated with exposure to ionizing radiation, as has cancer of the salivary glands. Outdoor workers have an increased risk of cancer of the lip resulting from exposure to ultraviolet radiation. The association of exposure to electromagnetic fields with brain and other neoplasms remains unclear. Recent data suggest a possible increase in brain cancer in radar workers. The explosion of the semiconductor industry and an enormous work force worldwide have brought the risks of these workers into concern. Recent studies have shown that length of employment in the semiconductor industry is associated positively with brain cancer. Other cancers with increased relative risks are leukemia, non-Hodgkin lymphoma, lung, breast, ovarian, and prostate cancer. Additional cancer studies among workers in the semiconductor industry should be performed.

REFERENCES

Beall C et al: Mortality among semiconductor and storage device-manufacturing workers. J Occup Environ Med 2005;47:996 [PMID: 16217241].

Bonner MR et al: Breast cancer risk and exposure in early life to polycyclic aromatic hydrocarbons using total suspended particulates as a proxy measure. Cancer Epidemiol Biomarkers Prev 2005;14:53 [PMID: 15668476].

Boers D et al: The influence of occupational exposure to pesticides, polycyclic aromatic hydrocarbons, diesel exhaust, metal dust, metal fumes, and mineral oil on prostate cancer: A prospective cohort study. Occup Environ Med 2005;62:531 [PMID: 16046605].

Borak J et al: Risks of brain tumors in rubber workers: A meta-analysis. J Occup Environ Med 2005;47:294 [PMID: 15761326].

Carreon T et al: Gliomas and farm pesticide exposure in women: The Upper Midwest Health Study. Environ Health Perspect 2005;113:546 [PMID: 15866761].

Forssen UM et al: Occupational magnetic fields and female breast cancer: A case-control study using Swedish population registers and new exposure data. Am J Epidemiol 2005;161:250 [PMID: 15671257].

Guo J et al: Testicular cancer, occupation and exposure to chemical agents among Finnish men in 1971–1995. Cancer Causes Control 2005;16:97 [PMID: 15868451].

Kaerlev L et al: Colon cancer controls versus population controls in case-control studies of occupational risk factors. BMC Cancer 2004;4:15 [PMID: 15102323].

Lee WJ et al: Agricultural pesticide use and adenocarcinomas of the stomach and oesophagus. Occup Environ Med 2004;61:743 [PMID: 15317914].

Sahmoun AE et al: Cadmium and prostate cancer: A critical epidemiologic analysis. Cancer Invest 2005;23(3):256.

Schlehofer B et al: Occupational risk factors for low grade and high grade glioma: Results from an international case control study of adult brain tumours. Int J Cancer 2005;113:116 [PMID: 15386358].

Zhang Y et al: A population-based case-control study of occupation and renal cell carcinoma risk in Iowa. J Occup Environ Med 2004;46:235 [PMID: 15091286].

Occupational Infections

17

Ken Takahashi, MD, PhD, MPH, & Gary Fujimoto, MD

Occupational infections are human diseases caused by work-associated exposure to microbial agents, including bacteria, viruses, fungi, and parasites. An infection is distinguished as occupational by some aspect of the work that involves contact with a biologically active organism. Occupational infection can occur following contact with infected persons or surfaces, as in the case of health care workers; with infected animal or human tissue, secretions, or excretions, as in laboratory workers; with asymptomatic or unknown contagious humans, as happens during business travel; or with infected animals, as in agriculture.

The etiology, pathogenesis, clinical findings, diagnosis, and treatment of occupational, nonoccupational, and bioterrorism infections are essentially the same except for practical differences related to identification of the source of exposure, epidemiologic control, and prevention. This chapter focuses on the occupational aspects of microbial exposures and relevant strategies for prevention.

NEWLY EMERGING INFECTIOUS DISEASES

SEVERE ACUTE RESPIRATORY SYNDROME (SARS)

The worldwide SARS epidemic peaked in the spring of 2003 and was traced back to the first case of an unidentified "atypical pneumonia" in Guangdong, China, in November 2002. By the end of the epidemic, health care workers accounted for 21% of SARS cases, which demonstrated the vulnerability of health care workers to occupational infections. It also was a reminder of the critical societal responsibility of health care workers to respond to the needs of contagious patients. This chapter highlights SARS and avian flu, tuberculosis, hepatitis B and C, acquired immunodeficiency syndrome (AIDS), travel-related infections, and work-related bioterrorism as examples of different types of exposure.

SARS is a viral respiratory illness caused by the SARS-associated coronavirus (SARS-CoV). A worldwide epidemic was triggered in late February 2003 when an ill physician from Guangdong, China, infected several other guests at a hotel in Hong Kong. The infected guests traveled and became index patients for subsequent large outbreaks in Hong Kong, Vietnam, Singapore, and Canada. Over the next few months, the epidemic spread to 29 countries in Asia, North and South America, and Europe. A global alert for SARS was issued and maintained by the World Health Organization (WHO) from March through July 2003. During this outbreak, 8098 people were infected, and 774 people died of the disease (fatality rate approximately 10%). Significant economic losses were incurred as well, especially in the aviation and tourist industries. As of August 2005, there is no known SARS transmission in the world. The most recent cases were reported in China in April 2004 in an outbreak resulting from laboratory-acquired infections, which raised biosafety concerns.

The 2003 SARS epidemic evoked a global public health emergency response as the disease, in the absence of control measures, spread rapidly on a global scale. SARS is clearly an occupational health hazard because health care workers who cared for patients accounted for 21% of all cases (>50% in some settings). Here health care workers were not only affected but also propagated the outbreaks in hospitals and into the community. Other groups of workers at risk include wildlife traders, food handlers, laboratory workers, traveling workers, and flight attendants. Another important feature is the age predilection, children being remarkably spared from the infection in general and persons over 60 years of age incurring case-fatality rates of greater than 50%.

SARS-CoV is significantly different from previously known human coronaviruses and has common features with coronaviruses found in some wildlife species indigenous to China. It is transmitted primarily by respiratory droplets from coughing and sneezing. Droplets can be propelled up to 3 ft and deposited on mouth, nose, and eyes (hence the need for masks and goggles). Droplets also can contaminate surfaces, which become fomites. Another possible mode of transmission is airborne spread, that is, viruses spreading broadly through the air and being inhaled. The incubation period for SARS is approximately 4–6 days. Symptoms begin with high fever (>38.0° C). Other initial symptoms include headache, discomfort, body ache, sore throat, and runny nose, but they all may not be present. Dry nonproductive cough may develop after 2–7 days of initial symptoms, during and after which

262

the risk of transmission increases. Almost all patients with laboratory evidence of SARS-CoV eventually develop pneumonia, which may be accompanied by hypoxia requiring mechanical ventilation. Lymphopenia is likely to accompany pneumonia. Diarrhea occurs in 10–20% of patients.

Laboratory confirmation involves detection of SARS-CoV in blood, stool, and nasal secretions by reverse-transcription polymerase chain reaction (RT-PCR) and less frequently by viral culture. SARS-CoV antibodies also can be detected with serologic testing. It should be noted that although these laboratory tests are sensitive and specific, they do not reliably detect SARS-CoV early in the course of disease. Although many different treatments were used during the outbreak, none was implemented in a controlled manner. The Centers for Disease Control and Prevention (CDC) recommend that medical treatment for SARS should be the same as for any serious, community-acquired atypical pneumonia. The development of vaccines is under way, and the inactivated SARS-CoV vaccine may be the first one available for clinical use.

Response in Health Care Facilities

In health care facilities, owing to the high transmissibility of SARS-CoV, all potential SARS patients should be identified and isolated rapidly (triaged and cohorted if warranted) with the implementation of a wide range of infection-control practices, for example, basic hygiene measures incorporating respiratory hygiene/cough etiquette, use of personal protective equipment (PPE), in particular N95 masks, use of airborne infection isolation rooms (AIIR), and procedural protocols for the use of ventilators, nebulizers, endotracheal intubation, and other droplet- and aerosol-generating devices and procedures. The level of response in health care facilities, which would vary from "no alert" to "mass-casualty response," depends on the extent of SARS activity in the community and the world. In a situation requiring high alert, certain hospitals may be designated to be the primary providers of SARS patient care or alternative "overflow" facilities.

Social Issues

Among the lessons learned from the worldwide SARS epidemic was "the power of traditional public health measures" to contain and control an outbreak. Some key public health measures include surveillance, infection control, isolation (of patients), and quarantine (of healthy contacts). Isolation and quarantine are warranted to prevent further transmission but call for ethical considerations with respect for human dignity and, hence, optimally should be performed on a voluntary basis. However, there is consensus that if it is deemed necessary to protect public health, governments should exert legal authority to compel man-

datory isolation and quarantine. Also at the international level, if a passenger is identified as having possible SARS, quarantine officials should arrange for appropriate medical assistance, including isolation, to be available on arrival. In terms of occupational health, some health care workers may be placed on "working quarantine (allowed to travel only between home and health care facility)" to ensure sufficient staffing levels. In relation to the corporate setting, "snow day" measures may be warranted involving closure of businesses and cancelation of public gatherings. The International Labour Office (ILO) documented a working paper on practical and administrative responses to SARS in the workplace in relation to preexisting ILO standards.

It is not possible to predict whether SARS-CoV will reappear, but it could from the natural reservoir, persistent infection in humans, or the laboratory. To the extent that such possibility cannot be ruled out, there are grounds to maintain a high level of preparedness. The exercise also can be extended to cover other public health emergencies such as pandemic influenza and bioterrorism.

REFERENCES

Department of Health and Human Services, Centers for Disease Control and Prevention: Severe acute respiratory syndrome (SARS), www.cdc.gov/ncidod/sars/.

Groneberg DA et al: Treatment and vaccines for severe acute respiratory syndrome. Lancet Infect Dis 2005;5:147 [PMID: 15766649].

International Labour Office. SARS—Practical and administrative responses to an infectious disease in the workplace, www.ilo.org/public/english/protection/safework/index.htm.

Jiang S et al: SARS vaccine development. Emerg Infect Dis 2005; 11:1016 [PMID: 16022774].

Sepkowitz KA, Eisenberg L: Occupational deaths among health care workers. Emerg Infect Dis 2005;11:1003 [PMID:16022771].

World Health Organization: Severe acute respiratory syndrome (SARS). www.who.int/csr/sars/en/.

AVIAN INFLUENZA ("BIRD FLU")

Bird flu is an infectious disease of birds caused by avian influenza (bird flu) viruses belonging to the type A group of influenza viruses (flu viruses). In general, bird flu viruses infect only birds and less commonly pigs and do not infect humans. But as of August 2005, there have been 112 (57 fatal) documented cases of human infection in Southeast Asia (90 in Vietnam and 17 in Thailand) caused by a certain subtype (H5N1) of type A bird flu (flu A) virus. Investigation revealed that human infection was caused by close contact with live infected poultry during an outbreak of bird flu. Studies at the genetic level further determined that the virus had jumped directly from birds to humans.

Flu A viruses are divided into subtypes based on two proteins on the surface of the virus, that is, hemagglutinin (H; 15 subtypes: H1–H15) and neuraminidase

(N; 9 subtypes: N1–N9). Wild birds are the primary natural reservoir for all subtypes of flu A viruses. Wild birds worldwide carry the viruses in their intestines, and while shedding the virus in saliva, nasal secretions, and feces, they mostly remain healthy hosts. But when domesticated birds (i.e., chickens, ducks, turkeys, etc.) become infected, the infection spreads quickly and widely and leads to a bird flu outbreak in poultry. If the virus is of a highly pathogenic type, the epidemic is highly lethal. Viruses can be transmitted from farm to farm by contaminated equipment, vehicles, feed, cages, or clothing. Thus, the standard control measures in poultry are quarantine and depopulation (or culling) and surveillance around affected flocks. Although the risk of infection to humans from bird flu is generally low, people should avoid contact with infected birds or contaminated surfaces and should be careful when handling and cooking poultry.

Flu A viruses genetically are labile and well adapted to escape host defenses because they lack mechanisms for repair of errors during replication. Consequently, small changes constantly occur in the antigenic composition (*antigenic drift*). Alternatively, an abrupt major change (*antigenic shift*) may occur if viruses from two different species infect the same host (human or animal) and mix together. The new virus may acquire most genes from a human virus, but a hemagglutinin and/or neuraminidase from an avian virus, and as such likely will become capable of efficient spread from person to person.

Influenza Pandemics

In the twentieth century, the great influenza pandemic of 1918–1919 ("Spanish flu" [A(H1N1)]) caused an estimated 40–50 million deaths worldwide and was followed by pandemics in 1957–1958 ("Asian flu" [A(H2N2)]) and 1968–1969 ("Hong Kong flu" [A(H3N2)]). Although the origin of the 1918–1919 pandemic virus is not clear, the latter two pandemics were caused by viruses containing a combination of genes from a human flu virus and an avian flu virus. Influenza pandemics may occur when new virus subtypes emerge and are readily transmitted from person to person. WHO asserts that another influenza pandemic is inevitable but unpredictable. Influenza pandemics are distinct from the more usual and smaller-scale influenza epidemics occurring almost every winter caused by type A or B flu viruses (the only other type of flu virus, type C, causes mild respiratory illness and does not cause epidemics).

The CDC and WHO have large surveillance programs to monitor influenza activity around the world, including the emergence of possible pandemic strains of influenza virus. Coordinated efforts also have been called on for the development of a vaccine against a potential pandemic strain of flu virus. Currently, the U.S. Food and Drug Administration (FDA) approves four different flu antiviral medications (amantadine, rimantadine, oseltamivir, and zanamivir) for the treatment and/or prevention of influenza. However, some flu virus strains become resistant to drugs, as was the case for human infection by the A(H5N1) virus. Because health care workers and first responders will be at high risk of infection in a pandemic situation, preparedness strategies with a strong occupational health component are highly warranted.

REFERENCES

Department of Health and Human Services: Checklist to help businesses prepare for a pandemic, www.hhs.gov/news/press/2005pres/20051207a.html.

Department of Health and Human Services, Centers for Disease Control and Prevention: Avian influenza (bird flu); influenza (flu), www.cdc.gov/flu/avian/, www.cdc.gov/flu/.

Fleming D: Influenza pandemics and avian flu. BMJ 2005;331:1066 [PMID: 16269494].

World Health Organization: Avian influenza, www.who.int/mediacentre/factsheets/avian_influenza/en/.

■ INFECTIONS CAUSED BY EXPOSURE TO INFECTED HUMANS OR THEIR TISSUES

Health care and clinical laboratory workers are also at increased risk of infection by organisms whose natural hosts are humans, as in the case of hepatitis, rubella, AIDS, tuberculosis, and staphylococcal disease. Some infections may be transmitted through close personal contact with infected patients. Exposure and infection caused by almost any of the viruses, bacteria, fungi, and parasites pathogenic for humans can result from direct contact with the organism in culture or in human tissue. Tuberculosis is an example of a relatively common occupational infection resulting from repeated close contact with infected patients, and hepatitis B exemplifies a serious and relatively frequent infection resulting from manipulation of infected human blood and inoculation by infectious virus particles.

TUBERCULOSIS

Mycobacterium tuberculosis can cause disseminated disease but is associated most frequently with pulmonary infections. The bacilli are transmitted by airborne route and, depending on host factors, may lead to latent tuberculosis infection (LTBI) or tuberculosis disease (TB). Only people who are ill with TB of the lungs are infectious, whereas people with LTBI are not.

Globally, it is estimated that TB caused 8.8 million incident cases and 1.75 million deaths in 2003. A breakdown by region for 2003 shows that Southeast Asia ranks first for the estimated number of incident cases (3.1 million, 35% of world population) and number of deaths (617,000), with Africa ranking second for the corresponding numbers (2.4 million incident cases, 27% of world population, and 538,000 deaths) but ranking first for the estimated incidence rate at 345 per 100,000 population (compare with Southeast Asia at 190 per 100,000 population). WHO in August 2005 declared TB an emergency in Africa in response to the growing epidemic in the region. In the United States, a total of 14,874 incident cases (5.1 per 100,000 population) was reported in 2003, and 802 deaths were reported in 2002. The U.S. 2003 number of incident cases decreased 44.2% from 1992, when the number of cases and incidence rate most recently peaked during a resurgence of the disease. Recently, the proportion of total cases occurring in non-U.S.-born persons exceeds 50%.

Medical house staffs have two to three times the tuberculosis infection rate of nonmedical personnel, and laboratory workers exposed to *M. tuberculosis* have three times the incidence of nonexposed workers. Staffs of laboratories and necropsy rooms are estimated to be between 100 and 200 times more likely than the general public to develop tuberculosis. Other high-prevalence work environments include most health care settings (especially hospitals, long-term care facilities, and dialysis centers), refugee/immigration centers, homeless shelters, substance abuse treatment centers, and correctional institutions.

Tubercle bacilli may be present in gastric fluid, cerebrospinal fluid, urine, sputum, and tissue specimens harboring active lesions. Infectious patients disseminate the organism when coughing, sneezing, or talking by expelling small infectious droplets that may remain suspended in the air for several hours and then be inhaled by susceptible persons. After an incubation period of 4–12 weeks, infection usually remains subclinical and dormant without development of active disease, but the purified protein derivative (PPD) skin test will become positive. However, the organism may be activated at any time, resulting in acute severe pulmonary or other systemic disease. The risk of development of clinical disease following infection is higher in selected age groups (infancy, 16–21 years of age), in states of undernutrition, in certain immunopathologic states (e.g., AIDS), in certain genetic groups (persons with HLA-Bw15 histocompatibility antigen), and in persons with some coexisting diseases (silicosis, end-stage renal disease, malnutrition, leukemia, lymphoma, upper gastrointestinal tract carcinoma, diabetes).

PPD is a chemical fractionation product of tubercle bacilli culture filtrate. Intradermal injection of 5 tuberculin units of PPD in a patient with subclinical or clinical tuberculous infection results in a delayed hypersensitivity reaction manifested by induration at the site of injection within 48–72 hours. A minimum of 5 mm of induration is required for a test to be positive or reactive in close contacts of infectious patients, immunosuppressed patients, organ recipients, or persons with known or suspected human immunodeficiency infection (HIV) infection. A reaction of 10 mm or more is considered positive in other high-prevalence (>5%), high-risk occupational groups (above) or high-risk groups such as immigrants from high-prevalence areas, alcoholics, intravenous drug users, and those with the other disease states just mentioned. In persons with no risk factors in areas of low prevalence, induration of 15 mm or more is required for a positive reaction. The PPD test may be negative in the presence of overwhelming tuberculosis, measles, Hodgkin disease, sarcoidosis, or immunosuppressive states. The test usually will revert to negative following elimination of viable tubercle bacilli. If the initial test is negative in individuals with suspected reduced immune response or in those who will be screened annually because of occupational or other risk, it should be repeated.

PPD skin testing is an accepted method for screening high-risk populations for primary infection. Persons having a reactive test are at risk of developing active clinical infection at any time (lifelong) following the primary infection owing to reactivation of the primary infection as long as viable tubercle bacilli remain in the body.

Recently, the QuantiFERON-TB Gold test has been approved for use in place of the PPD skin test for diagnosing both LTBI and TB infections in the United States. This new test uses freshly heparinized whole blood to detect the release of interferon-γ from individuals sensitized to tuberculin proteins. It has been found to be more sensitive than the PPD test with approximately the same specificity. This provides the additional benefit of needing only one visit for testing and eliminating the two-step PPD for those staff needing yearly testing and with more than one year since their last PPD.

Control & Treatment

PPD testing can identify persons whose tests are reactive, indicating primary infection. Serial testing (biennially or more frequently) can identify recently infected individuals whose tests have become reactive (*converters*) within the past 2 years. Occupational candidates for periodic PPD testing include those having contact with suspected or known infected patients, persons working with potentially infected primates or cattle (e.g., veterinarians, zoo keepers, primate handlers), and all others working in the higher-risk environments mentioned earlier.

Recent asymptomatic converters or others recently discovered to be tuberculin-reactive (reactors) whose date of conversion is unknown and who are least likely to develop complications as a consequence of antibiotic therapy should receive drug treatment according to protocols recommended by the CDC or local health departments.

Prophylaxis is recommended for persons found to have a positive PPD who fall into any of the following categories: newly infected persons, including recent converters (within 2 years); household contacts of active cases; persons with an abnormal chest radiograph consistent with clinical tuberculosis and inadequate past antituberculous therapy or prior active disease with inadequate past therapy; persons whose reactivation may have public health consequences (e.g., school teachers); patients with AIDS (or persons with antibodies to HIV), silicosis, insulin-dependent diabetes mellitus, hematologic or reticuloendothelial cancer, prior gastrectomy, chronic undernutrition, ileal bypass, renal failure requiring dialysis, or a history of prolonged use of glucocorticoid or immunosuppressive therapy, as well as intravenous drug users; and all reactors younger than 35 years of age who have none of the preceding risk factors.

Before starting prophylaxis, a chest radiograph should be taken on all skin test reactors. Any abnormalities found should be thoroughly evaluated for evidence of clinically active disease. If adequate prior prophylaxis or therapy for active disease has been completed, prophylaxis should not be given.

Current treatment regimens recommended by the American Thoracic Society (ATS)/CDC are based on evidence from clinical trials and are rated by a system using a letter (A, B, C, D, or E) that indicates strength of the recommendation and a roman numeral (I, II, or III) that indicates the quality of evidence supporting the recommendation. There are four recommended regimens for patients with tuberculosis caused by drug-susceptible organisms. Each regimen has an initial phase of 2 months followed by a choice of several options for the continuation phase of either 4 or 7 months. Isoniazid and rifampicin are the two most powerful anti-TB drugs included in the regimen in most circumstances. Because of rapidly changing drug resistance patterns, the reader should refer to current recommendations regarding prophylaxis or therapy of active disease.

Bacilli in lungs of patients may develop resistance to anti-TB medicines when the patient fails to complete standard treatment regimens or is given the wrong treatment regimen. A particularly dangerous form of drug-resistant TB is multidrug-resistant TB (MDR-TB), which is defined as the disease caused by TB bacilli resistant to at least isoniazid and rifampicin. High rates of MDR-TB are known in some countries and threaten TB control efforts. For a cost-effective control of TB, WHO and other international organizations advocate DOT, a comprehensive strategy centered on direct observed therapy (DOT). Health and community workers or trained volunteers observe patients swallowing the full course of the correct dosage of anti-TB medicines. By doing so, DOT prevents the development of drug resistance.

Persons for whom prophylactic antibiotic therapy is contraindicated should receive surveillance chest radiographs if they become symptomatic. Persons having known contact with an infectious patient for whom PPD status is not previously documented should be PPD tested immediately and then retested 8–12 weeks after the infectious contact. If conversion occurs, physical examination and chest radiography should occur to rule out acute clinical infection.

Attenuated tubercle bacilli—particularly bacille Calmette-Guérin (BCG)—have been used in many countries as a vaccine. However, BCG has variable efficacy in preventing the adult forms of TB and interferes with testing for latent TB infection. Thus, it is not recommended routinely for use in the United States.

REFERENCES

Taylor Z et al: Controlling tuberculosis in the United States: Recommendations from the American Thoracic Society, CDC, and the Infectious Diseases Society of America. MMWR Recomm Rep 2005;54:1 [PMID: 16267499].

WHO: Tuberculosis fact sheet no. 104, April 2005, www.who.int/mediacentre/factsheets/fs104/en/print.html.

HEPATITIS B

Prior to the introduction of the hepatitis B vaccine in 1981, hepatitis B infections constituted the most frequent occupational infection among health care, laboratory, and public safety workers following human blood or body fluid exposures in the United States. Hepatitis B virus (HBV) can cause fulminant hepatitis and also can lead to chronic carrier states in up to 10% of those following acute infection. Chronic carriers suffer higher rates of cirrhosis and liver failure as well as liver cancer. The prevalence of HBV infection among health care personnel was 10 times higher than the general population in the decade preceding the HBV vaccine's release.

Blood contains the highest titers of virus in infected individuals, with lower levels in various other body fluids, including cerebrospinal, synovial, pleural, peritoneal, pericardial, and amniotic fluids, as well as semen and vaginal secretions. Viral titers in urine, feces, tears, and saliva are low enough that these are not felt to be routes of transmission except in cases of human bites that usually involve some blood transmission. Sexual and maternal-child transmissions are alternative modes of contracting HBV in the general population.

The risk for transmission of HBV through needlestick injuries is approximately 30%. However, over 50% of acute infections in adults are asymptomatic. Given that 10% of acute HBV infections lead to chronic infections, a significant number of those with occupational infections become chronic asymptomatic carriers.

HBV can remain viable for at least 1 month on dried surfaces at room temperature. This poses additional opportunities to acquire occupational HBV infections when individuals with open cuts or abraded skin or mucous membranes contact contaminated surfaces. In fact, most occupational infections have no clear percutaneous injury leading to HBV transmission.

Prescreening serologic testing prior to vaccination generally is not recommended because the prevalence of HBV-infected individuals in the United States is low. Some groups have instituted prescreening of all potential vaccine recipients with hepatitis B core antibodies when a high percentage of potential vaccinees come from endemic countries. Positive core antibodies indicate past or present HBV infections and should prompt testing for surface antigens to identify chronic carriers and for surface antibodies to identify those with resolved past infections.

While the original hepatitis B vaccine was plasma-derived, studies showed no transmission of infectious agents with this vaccine. The development of a recombinant DNA vaccine in 1986 provided an even more acceptable and highly safe method for mass vaccination of health care personnel. Since 1991, it has been recommended to vaccinate newborn infants at birth even though the prevalence of chronic hepatitis B is less than 0.5% of the populace. That same year, the Bloodborne Pathogens Act was passed, mandating employer-funded vaccination for at-risk health care workers. Since that time, a dramatic reduction in occupational HBV transmission has occurred. However, there are still some workers who have not completed or have refused vaccination and remain vulnerable to infection. There is an additional subset of those vaccinated who do not develop antibodies and who remain susceptible to infection.

Known exposures to HBV-infected blood or blood products in those who were not vaccinated or where antibody protection did not develop require the use of hepatitis B immune globulin (HBIG), which is expensive and needs a second dose 1 month later unless hepatitis B vaccination is administered concomitantly.

The usual schedule for HBV vaccination is 0, 1, and 6 months. Those who have received only one or two doses do not need to restart the series: They only need to complete the doses they did not receive (as with most other vaccines requiring multiple dosing). Since only 50–60% of those vaccinated with two doses get immunity, some institutions will consider an accelerated series for those who will be actively working with blood or blood products, giving doses at 0, 1, 2, and 12 months with the Engerix-B vaccine (which has twice as much antigen as the Recombivax vaccine and is the only one approved by the FDA for this series). Since this still leaves a window of time before antibody protection is achieved in high-risk workers, an extremely accelerated schedule with doses at 0, 1, and 3 weeks and a final dose at 12 months is used in some cases. This schedule provides up to 83% protection by week 4 (and this continues to rise without additional doses of vaccine) and is used in over 15 European countries. The final dose, given at 6–12 months depending on the schedule, is critical because this provides long-term protection. Once the three- to four-dose initial series is given, no further doses are necessary assuming that hepatitis B surface antibodies are produced.

In 1997, the Advisory Committee on Immunization Practices began recommending testing for hepatitis B surface antibodies in those with ongoing exposures to blood or blood products. While the committee did not recommend testing those vaccinated prior to December 1997, there are several reasons to verify antibody responses in this population (with positive surface antibodies defined as levels greater than 10 mIU/mL). While the vaccine is highly protective in infants vaccinated at birth, the degree of protection declines with advancing age, with 90% responding to a three-dose series by 40 years of age and 75% by 60 years of age. Moreover, those who develop antibodies lose them over time, although they remain protected. If a positive antibody response is never verified, it will not be possible to differentiate the responder who lost antibodies (who is protected) from the nonresponder who never developed antibodies (who is not protected). Therefore, documenting the development of surface antibody protection at any time following the vaccination series significantly improves postexposure management for hepatitis B.

The current recommendations are to check for surface antibodies 4 weeks to 6 months following the primary series. If the person tests negative for antibodies, the data show that one additional dose of vaccine will induce antibody protection in 15–25% of nonresponders and that three additional doses (for a total of six doses) will induce antibodies in 30–50% of nonresponders. The official recommendation for additional doses is to follow the 0-, 1-, and 6-month schedule. This can be shortened effectively to 0, 1, and 2 months because a 6-month spacing from first to last dose (important for long-term immunity) already has been achieved with the primary vaccination series. Those who do not develop antibodies after six total doses should consider changing positions at work not involving blood or blood products. In cases where this is not possible or feasible, consideration of a three-dose series with 40 µg of antigen with either the Merck Recombivax HB formulated for hemodialysis patients (*Note:* Routine Recombivax HB contains only 10 µg of antigen) or two doses of the Engerix-B vaccine containing 20 µg of antigen per dose can be attempted. If more than 6 months have elapsed since vaccination and the individual tests negative for surface antibodies, giving one additional dose of vaccine and retesting for antibodies 4 weeks later is warranted because 50% of patients lose antibodies after 7 years.

REFERENCE

CDC: Recommendations and reports, www.cdc.gov/mmwr/preview/mmwrhtml/rr5011a1.htm.

HEPATITIS C

Hepatitis C is a viral infection of the liver caused by the hepatitis C virus (HCV) and now known to be responsible for more than 75% of what was previously termed *posttransfusion non-A, non-B hepatitis.* In the United States, HCV is more frequently associated with a history of blood transfusion (prior to the introduction of enzyme immunoassays in the late 1980s), parenteral drug use, sexual or household exposures, and in some instances, bloodborne pathogen transmission. Worldwide there are six major genotypes of HCV, with type 1 the most frequent in the United States.

The current estimate for transmission of HCV following a needlestick injury from a positive carrier of HCV is approximately 1.8%. Transmission following mucous membrane exposure is rare, with no apparent transfer following exposures to intact skin.

With the current third-generation enzyme immunoassay (EIA), sensitivity is estimated to be approximately 97% within 6–8 weeks of exposure. However, the presence of antibodies does not correlate with protection because 70–90% of those infected become chronic carriers despite positive antibodies. Chronic carriers have a 20% chance of developing cirrhosis and an increased risk for developing hepatocellular carcinomas. Positive EIA tests usually warrant confirmatory testing with highly sensitive RT-PCR assays for HCV RNA. The recombinant immunoblot assay (RIBA) still can be used in cases where the EIA is positive with a negative HCV RNA to determine whether the EIA is a false-positive result.

Major advances in the treatment of chronic carriers have occurred recently with the introduction of parenteral peg-interferon-alfa combined with oral ribavirin. *Sustained virologic response* (SVR) is defined as no measurable virus 6 months following completion of treatment. Unfortunately, type 1 genotypes (most frequent in the United States), are less responsive to this regimen (42–46% SVR) and require 12 months of treatment, unlike other genotypes (76–82% SVR) that usually respond after 6 months.

Following exposures to known HCV-positive blood or blood products, HCV RNA testing is often considered 2–4 weeks after exposure as a sensitive diagnostic tool to detect early disease. The issues of postexposure prophylaxis are currently less clear. However, some studies now seem to indicate that treatment of early seroconversions with interferon-alfa possibly with ribavirin may prevent chronic carrier states. There is no indication for the use of immune globulin in postexposure management of these cases.

HUMAN IMMUNODEFICIENCY VIRUS

The advent of the human immunodeficiency virus (HIV) has lead to devastating effects in the world, particularly affecting the poorest countries least equipped to handle this infectious disease. The symptomatic phase of HIV, manifest with opportunistic infections and Kaposi's sarcoma, is the acquired immunodeficiency syndrome (AIDS). With the evolution of highly active antiretroviral therapy (HAART), greater control of the HIV-infected populations in the United States and other nations able to afford such treatment has led to a marked drop in the numbers of deaths attributable to this disease.

HIV transmission occurs via blood and sexual contact. Fortunately, occupationally acquired infection has been a relatively infrequent (albeit serious) occurrence. The body fluids other than blood that are considered higher risk for HIV transmission include semen and vaginal secretions and cerebrospinal, synovial, pleural, peritoneal, pericardial, and amniotic fluids. Nasal secretions, saliva, sputum, sweat, tears, urine, and vomitus are not considered potentially infectious unless they are visibly bloody.

The established rate of transmission following a positive HIV exposure from a needlestick injury is approximately 0.3%, making it approximately 10-fold less transmissible as HCV and 100-fold less transmissible as HBV. Moreover, the incidence of occupational HIV transmission appears to have declined substantially in recent years. There are several factors that may account for this including the widespread use of antiretroviral agents in HIV-infected individuals leading to lower viral loads as well as broader use of antiretroviral treatment following HIV exposures.

However, the growing number of HIV-resistant strains has required a greater understanding of the various treatment options available when these high-risk injuries occur. Similarly, the problems encountered with drug toxicity make it imperative that postexposure prophylaxis be used only in high-risk injuries.

Postexposure antiretroviral medications now include reverse-transcriptase inhibitors, nonnucleoside reverse-transcriptase inhibitors, protease inhibitors, and the newest class of agents, the fusion inhibitors. Two or three drug regimens are now considered following HIV exposures, with multiple drugs used when injuries involve larger amounts of HIV-infected blood (e.g., large-bore needles, deep punctures, and visible blood on devices or needles that were used in patients' arteries or veins) or when higher concentrations of virus are suspected (e.g., AIDS patients, acute seroconversions, high viral loads, and concentrated virus in special laboratory situations).

It is important to understand that in situations where the source is unknown or has an unknown HIV status, postexposure prophylaxis generally is not warranted. Expert advice on the need and choice of antiretroviral agents can be obtained 24/7 by calling the University of California, San Francisco National Clinician's Hotline at (888) 448-4911.

HIV postexposure prophylaxis usually constitutes a 4-week course of treatment. Close monitoring for drug side effects should be conducted within the first 3 days. Monitoring throughout the 4-week course of treatment is highly advisable because many people on these regimens experience side effects that lead to discontinuation of treatment. Close follow-up monitors for potential side effects and ensures a complete course of treatment. Baseline testing for preexisting infection at the time of the exposure always should be established, with follow-up testing at 6 weeks and 3 and 6 months. Prolonged testing up to 12 months can be considered for situations where source patients are coinfected with HIV and HCV or where the exposed individual is HCV-positive.

Counseling and support of the exposed individual (and partner) are imperative because these injuries are psychologically traumatic and include recommendations for sexual abstinence or the use of condoms if postexposure prophylaxis is warranted.

New guidelines for managing these injuries were published in the *Morbidity and Mortality Weekly Report* (CDC publication) on September 30, 2005. It is imperative that all clinicians regard these types of occupational exposures as urgent issues because early initiation of treatment can prevent occupational transmission.

REFERENCE

CDC: MMWR: Recommendations and reports, www.cdc.gov/mmwr/pdf/rr/rr5409.pdf.

▇ TRAVEL

The ever-expanding global marketplace has continued to have an impact on the need for international business travel. Travel to areas of the world with suboptimal public health systems and/or tropical diseases warrant special considerations because there are many vaccine- or medication-preventable diseases that can have significant morbidity and mortality in healthy adults. Moreover, illnesses contracted during travel that are specific to the destination,

such as malaria or hepatitis A, are covered under workers' compensation. Even more significant is the loss of productivity when an employee becomes ill and cannot function in activities that warranted the trip. Unfortunately, many businesses and physicians fail to prepare traveling employees adequately with proper vaccinations and pretravel preparations.

Few vaccinations are currently required for entry into some countries. What is often not recognized is the larger number of vaccine-preventable diseases for which vaccinations are not required but where their administration could prevent significant illness, such as hepatitis A. Another area often ignored is the repeat business traveler returning multiple times to a foreign subsidiary where multiple trips will add up to many months of travel. In light of this, vaccinations considered for longer durations of travel, such as hepatitis B, Japanese encephalitis, and in some cases, preexposure rabies need to be considered. These and other vaccines also should be considered when preparing families for long-term foreign assignments.

Useful guidelines for determining which vaccines would be appropriate for a particular country can be found on the CDC Web site under "travel" or by referring to the CDC's *Health Information for International Travel* (also known as the "Yellow Book"). However, these sources list all recommended vaccines and do not differentiate between short- or long-term or urban or rural travel, which are important factors when deciding which vaccines should be used.

ROUTINE VACCINATIONS

The vaccinations for tetanus-diphtheria (Td); measles, mumps, and rubella (MMR); and polio (IPV) all have been administered routinely to most working adults in the United States. There are some special considerations that should be undertaken when preparing for foreign travel to certain destinations.

The current recommendation for Td boosters (assuming primary immunization has been completed) is every 10 years, and this should be checked prior to travel. Recently, a vaccine for tetanus-diphtheria that includes acellular pertussis (whooping cough–Tdap) has been released for distribution in the United States. Acellular pertussis is a significant addition because pertussis has been found to be grossly underdiagnosed in adults and is responsible for illnesses manifest with multiple weeks of cough.

The presence of measles in countries where children are not vaccinated routinely poses issues for travelers who have not received two doses of MMR and who were born after 1956 (those born in 1956 or earlier generally are felt to have immunity owing to natural exposure).

Polio is still present in parts of Africa, India, and more recently, Indonesia. Adult travelers visiting these areas are advised to receive one additional booster dose of injectable polio vaccine after 18 years of age if traveling to areas where polio is still present.

REQUIRED TRAVEL VACCINATIONS

As stated previously, required vaccinations are those that certain countries require proof of in order to enter the country. Often they do not include the many diseases that are endemic to that country that can be contracted by travelers from nonendemic locations.

Yellow Fever

Yellow fever is an acute viral hemorrhagic disease transmitted through mosquitoes that occurs in tropical areas of Africa, South America, and parts of Panama. Yellow fever vaccination may be required when entering a country (even if only in transit) when travel has occurred through another country where yellow fever is known or thought to be present. It is also recommended when travel into endemic zones occurs.

Vaccination must be obtained from a certified yellow fever vaccination center where the International Certificate of Vaccination (or "yellow card" as it is commonly referred to) is stamped and signed. These centers can be located by checking the CDC Web site (www2.ncid.cdc.gov/travel/yellowfever/). The Certificate of Vaccination must be presented at customs in order to enter and is valid 10 days following vaccination and for the next 10 years (the duration of protection from vaccination).

Since yellow fever vaccine is a live-virus vaccination, it should not be given to immunosuppressed individuals and is relatively contraindicated in pregnancy (although it can be given if travel to high-risk areas is unavoidable). It is contraindicated in those with severe allergies to eggs or when a severe allergic reaction has occurred with previous doses. There have been rare cases of yellow fever vaccine–associated neurotropic disease (YEL-AND) with encephalitis, primarily in infants but also in a few adults along with autoimmune neurologic disease (e.g., Guillain-Barré syndrome), estimated to occur in 4–6 persons per million. Since 1996, cases of vaccine-associated viscerotropic disease (YEL-AVD) with febrile multiorgan-system failure have been reported in 26 individuals in the world (3–5 cases per million doses administered). This seems to occur slightly more frequently in those over 60 years of age (19 cases per million doses). Recent studies have shown a high association among those with thymic disorders (e.g., myasthenia gravis), which now are a contraindication to vaccination. Both YEL-AND and YEL-AVD have occurred with primary vaccination and do not appear to be problems for those needing booster doses.

It is also important to remember that live-virus vaccines (yellow fever, MMR, and varicella) must be given simultaneously or be separated by at least 4 weeks.

RECOMMENDED TRAVEL VACCINATIONS

Hepatitis A

Hepatitis A is a viral hepatitis transmitted through the fecal-oral route and is the most frequent vaccine-preventable disease in travelers. Children younger than 6 years of age usually have little to no clinical symptoms, although transmission to others can occur. However, adults who contract hepatitis A can be ill with fever, malaise, nausea, abdominal pain, and jaundice, with symptoms lasting weeks to months (adults lose an average of 27 days of work with an estimated 1.8% mortality over 40 years of age). Many of the western states in the United States have twice the national average of hepatitis A, which has warranted vaccination of children in those areas. Given this perspective, it is clear why vaccination prior to travel to Mexico, the Caribbean, and all the other countries where food and water are less than optimal is important.

The vaccine for hepatitis A is both safe and effective, inducing protection rates of 80–96% by 2 weeks and almost 100% protection by week 4. A second dose is recommended 6–12 months after the first, which provides long-term protection. As with the other injectable vaccines, if the interval is longer than recommended, there is no need to restart the vaccination series, only to complete the remaining doses. The vaccine is well tolerated in most individuals with few serious adverse reactions. One manufacturer has combined hepatitis A and B in a single injection, although this formulation has half the usual dose of hepatitis A antigen and requires a three-dose vaccination series at 0, 1, and 6 months. Immune globulin can be used in cases where hepatitis A vaccination is contraindicated or where travel is imminent, but it is less protective and only for short periods of time.

Typhoid Fever

Typhoid fever is a bacterial infection caused by *Salmonella typhii*. While this is less common than hepatitis A, typhoid fever is a disseminated lymphatic or bloodstream infection that can be fatal if not treated. Initial symptoms can be either diarrhea or constipation followed by high fever, myalgias, abdominal pain, and headache and often are similar to those seen with malaria.

Two vaccines are available for typhoid fever: an injectable and an oral vaccine. The injectable vaccine is both safe and effective following a single dose with only occasional symptoms of soreness and fever following vaccination and provides protection for two years. The oral vaccine is a live-bacteria vaccine that is administered with four enteric-coated capsules taken on alternate days (0, 2, 4, and 6 days). The capsules have to be kept refrigerated, swallowed intact with cool liquids, and cannot be taken with any antibiotics or during an active gastrointestinal disorder. The oral vaccine is protective for 5 years and occasionally has side effects that can include nausea, vomiting, and abdominal discomfort.

Hepatitis B Virus (HBV)

Hepatitis B virus (HBV) can be a significant risk for certain long-term or repeat travelers to countries where the disease is endemic and where chronic carriers constitute 8–15% of the population (as opposed to the United States, where carriers constitute fewer than 0.5%) (see above). These areas include parts of Asia, Southeast Asia, Africa, and the Caribbean. Slightly lower-risk areas include southern Asia, Japan, Israel, eastern and southern Europe, the former Soviet republics, and parts of Central and South America. Since HBV can remain viable on dried surfaces for weeks, railings, doorknobs, and medical facilities pose potential sources of infection if contact with nonintact skin occurs. Groups at risk include all health care workers, those living in endemic countries for over 6 months, those anticipating close contact or sexual contact with local populations, or those in whom medical/dental care is anticipated.

Japanese Encephalitis

Japanese encephalitis (JE) is a disease spread by an evening-biting mosquito in various parts of Asia, Southeast Asia, India, and the Philippines. While this is often an asymptomatic infection, it can cause death in approximately 30% and residual neurologic or psychological damage in approximately 50% of survivors. Vaccination is recommended when travel to rural areas where JE is endemic during the summer or autumn months exceeds 4 weeks. The vaccine is given in a series of three doses given at 0, 7, and 14–30 days. Delayed side effects, although rare, can include anaphylaxis that can occur up to 10 days after a dose of vaccine.

Rabies

Rabies poses a hazard in countries where animals are not vaccinated routinely and where dogs are the most frequent hazard. Usually young children, hikers, and long-term travelers are the groups where preexposure vaccination should be considered (as opposed to the postexposure prophylaxis with rabies immune globulin and the five-dose vaccination series). The three-dose preexposure vaccination series is administered at 0, 7,

and 21–28 days. Once completed, this provides two significant advantages by eliminating the need for rabies immune globulin (from human blood products) and by providing additional time to get the final two doses of vaccine at 0 and 3 days. This is important in situations where an individual cannot readily access care where the safe and appropriate immune globulin and vaccine can be obtained.

Meningococcal Disease

Meningococcal meningitis and bacteremia caused by *Neisseria meningitidis* is endemic in parts of sub-Saharan Africa during the dry season (generally from December to June). Vaccination for travelers to these regions where close contact with the local population is anticipated is recommended and required for those traveling to Saudi Arabia for the Hajj. Two vaccines are used currently in the United States. The older polysaccharide vaccine protects for only 3 years. The newer conjugate vaccine provides longer immunity and is used currently for adolescents, in whom protection through the college years is anticipated.

Malaria

Malaria is a significant protozoal disease transmitted by infected female *Anopheles* mosquitoes, which bite in the evening hours. Malaria infects up to 300 million people around the world each year. Moreover, those coming from nonendemic countries such as the United States have a greater chance for developing severe illness or developing symptoms many months after returning from malarious regions when the diagnosis is more likely to be missed. There are four types of malaria that infect humans: *Plasmodium falciparum, P. vivax, P. ovale,* and *P. malariae. P. falciparum* is the most serious form and has developed resistance in many areas of the world.

In nonresistant areas for *P. falciparum* and other forms (generally in Central America and the Middle East), chloroquine or hydroxychloroquine can be used. This is taken weekly beginning 1 week before entering, weekly during travel, and for 4 weeks after leaving the malarious area.

In areas of chloroquine resistance (Asia, Southeast Asia, India, Africa, and South America), other forms of malaria prophylaxis must be used. These include mefloquine, doxycycline, and atovaquone-proguanil. Mefloquine has been associated with bad dreams, anxiety, depression, psychosis, a lowered seizure threshold, and cardiac conduction abnormalities. This drug is taken once a week in a schedule similar to chloroquine. Doxycycline, as a form of tetracycline, has been associated with photosensitivity, gastrointestinal disorders, rash, and diarrhea. This is taken once a day 1–2 days before entering and daily continuing up to 4 weeks after leaving the malarious area. Atovaquone-proguanil is the most recent addition to the antimalarial agents and has relatively few adverse effects that include abdominal pain, nausea, vomiting, diarrhea, headache, elevated transaminases, and pruritus. This medication is taken daily 1 day before entering and continuing up to 7 days after leaving the malarious region.

Since antimalarial medications are highly but not completely protective, additional measures to reduce mosquito bites are important. These should include the use of an effective DEET-containing repellent on exposed skin (avoiding the eyes and mouth), use of mosquito netting if sleeping in nonprotected areas, treatment of clothing and mosquito netting with permethrin, and avoidance of outdoor activity during the evening hours.

Traveler's Diarrhea (TD)

Traveler's diarrhea (TD) is a common problem for travel to areas where food and sanitation are less than optimal. This problem affects up to 30–70% of traveler's during the first 2 weeks of travel. While TD can be due to noninfectious causes such as jet lag and changes in diet, the infectious causes can include a host of organisms, such as enterotoxigenic *Escherichia coli* (ETEC), *Campylobacter, Salmonella, Shigella,* enteroaggregative *E. coli,* and many other bacterial agents. Viral agents include norovirus (affecting many cruise ships) as well as rotaviruses. Protozoal infections are less likely, although they often lead to more chronic diarrheal states.

Prevention by eating piping-hot foods, avoiding foods handled by hand and not thoroughly cooked, and avoiding contaminated water (including ice) can be useful, although often difficult to adhere to. Standby treatment with quinolone antibiotics (given as single dose of 750–1000 mg for uncomplicated diarrhea or as a 3-day course for more severe forms) or rifaximin (a nonabsorbable antibiotic given 200 mg tid for 3 days) can be used often in conjunction with loperamide as long as fever or bloody diarrhea is absent. With the advent of quinolone-resistant *Campylobacter* in Thailand and India, use of azithromycin as a backup should be considered.

REFERENCES

Callahan MV, Hamer DH: On the medical edge: Preparation of expatriates, refugee and disaster relief workers, and Peace Corps volunteers. Infect Dis Clin North Am 2005;19:85 [PMID: 15701548].

CDC: MMWR: Travelers' health, www.cdc.gov/travel/.

CDC: *Health Information for International Travel 2005–2006.* Atlanta: USDHHS, 2005 (www.cdc.gov/travel/destinat.ht).

■ INFECTIONS TRANSMITTED FROM ANIMALS TO HUMANS: ZOONOSES

Zoonoses are defined as any disease and/or infection that is naturally transmissible from vertebrate animals to humans. Occupations involving contact with infected animals and/or their infected secretions or tissues or contact with arthropod vectors from infected animals can result in work-related zoonotic disease (Table 17–1). Zoonoses involve different types of agents: bacteria (e.g., salmonellosis and campylobacteriosis), parasites (e.g., cysticercosis/taeniasis), *Rickettsia* (e.g., Q-fever), viruses (e.g., rabies and avian influenza), and unconventional agents [e.g., bovine spongiform encephalopathy (BSE) as a cause of variant Creutzfeldt-Jakob disease]. Avian flu, BSE and Nipah virus are examples of "emerging" zoonoses, defined by WHO/FAO/OIE in 2004.

REFERENCES

O'Brien SJ: Foodborne zoonoses. BMJ 2005;331:1217 [PMID: 16308359].

WHO: Zoonoses and veterinary public health. www.who.int/zoonoses/en/.

BRUCELLOSIS

Brucellosis is an infectious disease caused by the bacteria of the genus *Brucella*. The species varies with the animal host as follows: *Brucella abortus,* cattle; *B. melitensis,* goats and sheep; *B. suis,* swine; and *B. canis,* dogs. U.S. cattle herds had nearly been rid of *B. abortus* infection by 2003. The CDC asserts that the risk of contracting brucellosis through occupational exposure to livestock in the United States or consumption of domestically produced dairy products is minimal. The majority of U.S. cases of bru-

Table 17–1. Occupations at risk for zoonoses.

Veterinarian	Laboratory worker
Farmer	Breeder
Dairy worker	Hunter
Wildlife worker	Hide and wool handler
Slaughterhouse (abattoir) worker	Rancher
Rendering plant worker	Pet shop worker
Taxidermist	Zoo attendant
Sewer worker	Miner
Military personnel	Butcher

cellosis occur among returned travelers or recent immigrants from endemic areas.

Pathogenesis & Clinical Findings

Occupational brucellosis occurs as a result of mucous membrane or skin contact with infected animal tissues. Aborted placental and fetal membrane tissues from cattle, swine, sheep, and goats are well-documented sources of human exposure. The incubation period is from 1–6 weeks. The onset is insidious, with fever, sweats, malaise, aches, and weakness. The fever has a characteristic pattern, often rising in the afternoon and falling during the night (*undulant fever*). The infection is systemic and may result in gastric, intestinal, neurologic, hepatic, or musculoskeletal involvement. There is usually an initial septicemic phase, following which a more chronic stage may develop characterized by low-grade fever, malaise, and in some cases, psychoneurotic symptoms.

Diagnosis & Treatment

Brucellosis is diagnosed by finding *Brucella* organisms in samples of blood or bone marrow or by detecting antibodies. Treatment will vary with organism sensitivity, but brucellae are often sensitive to tetracyclines or ampicillin. More resistant species may require combined therapy with streptomycin and trimethoprim-sulfamethoxazole. Prolonged treatment often is necessary.

Prevention

Identification and treatment or slaughter of infected animals combined with effective immunization of susceptible animals can eliminate disease in livestock populations. Personal hygiene and protective precautions should be observed in handling potentially infected animal tissues or secretions, particularly those resulting from abortion. Immunization of humans is still experimental.

REFERENCES

Cutler SJ et al: Brucellosis: New aspects of an old disease. J Appl Microbiol 2005;98:1270 [PMID: 15916641].

Hopkins RS et al: Summary of notifiable diseases—United States, 2003. MMWR 2005;52:1 [PMID: 15889005].

■ OCCUPATIONAL IMMUNIZATION, PROPHYLAXIS, & BIOLOGIC SURVEILLANCE

Laboratory workers at risk of contact with live organisms and travelers to areas of endemic infection should be considered for appropriate immunization, prophylaxis, or surveillance if the technology is available. Preparations are available for protection against diphtheria, pertussis, tetanus, measles, mumps, rubella, smallpox, yellow fever, poliomyelitis, hepatitis A, hepatitis B, influenza, rabies, cholera, pneumococcal pneumonia, meningococcal disease (certain serotypes), plague, typhoid fever, tuberculosis, Q fever, adenovirus infection, anthrax, pertussis, and *Hemophilus influenzae* infection. In addition, many unlicensed or experimental vaccines are available through the CDC (e.g., for various arthropod-borne viruses).

Skin testing can be useful in surveillance of tuberculosis and some mycoses (e.g., coccidioidomycosis, histoplasmosis, and blastomycosis). Skin tests also may detect prior infection with mumps and vaccinia. Serologic testing for evidence of subclinical infection in selected high-risk populations should be considered carefully but may be of value for the following diseases: brucellosis, chlamydial infections, leptospirosis, plague, tularemia, salmonellosis, toxoplasmosis, some parasitic diseases (amebiasis, trichinosis), most occupational viral diseases (hepatitis A and B, herpes simplex, influenza, rabies, infectious mononucleosis), mycoplasmal pneumonia, and some rickettsioses.

As with the administration of any surveillance test or therapeutic agent, disease prevalence, occupational exposure risk, contraindications, and side effects from the prophylactic agent all should be considered before administration of any immunologic agent or use of any biologic surveillance test. Measles-mumps-rubella (MMR) vaccine, for example, should not be given within 3 months before or during pregnancy. Yellow fever and oral polio vaccines should not be given during pregnancy unless there is a substantial risk of exposure.

Exposure Evaluation

Serologic or other clinical microbiologic techniques can be used to investigate human or animal sources of infectious agents. Environmental exposure evaluation associated with inanimate sources such as contaminated ventilation systems or centrifuges is more esoteric. However, technologies exist for collection and measurement of airborne bacteria and viruses. A knowledgeable industrial hygienist can select the appropriate instrumentation and sampling strategy based on the presumed biologic characteristics of the organism, air velocity, sampler efficiency, anticipated concentration, "particle" size, sampler physical requirements, and the study objective.

REFERENCE

CDC, ACIP: National Immunization Program, www.cdc.gov/nip/publications/ACIP-list.htm.

■ BIOTERRORISM

The 2001 anthrax release in the United States served to alert the medical community that such acts of bioterrorism can and will occur. However, the ever-present issues of emerging infectious agents such as HIV, SARS, avian influenza, and Marburg virus clearly demonstrate the broader need for constant vigilance for new or unusual outbreaks that can occur in any region of the world. Unlike chemical terrorism, where first responders will be the front line of defense, the victims of biologic agents will present at medical facilities. These potential and real threats necessitate that all physicians be observant for patterns or unusual presentations that may herald future outbreaks.

Table 17–2 provides a rapid way to evaluate the biologic agents that have been deemed most likely to be used in a bioterrorism attack. This provides a list of the salient clinical and diagnostic findings for some of the biologic agents that have been identified as more likely agents in future attacks. The table provides information on the various categories of clinical syndromes, such as the severe pulmonary syndromes, that these agents would present. The table also provides information regarding the diagnostic tests needed to confirm the presence of such agents, the treatment options (if any), and the levels of infectious precautions that should be exercised. In several instances, the prompt diagnosis and identification to national databases of affected cases will be the first line of defense in the case of a biologic attack.

The following are some early considerations that would be useful when evaluating potential victims of a

Table 17–2. Biologic agents in a terrorist attack.

Presentation	Findings	Diagnosis	Treatment	Infection Control
Anthrax (Bacillus anthracis)				
Severe febrile respiratory illness with dyspnea, **without** rhinorrhea or pharyngitis + widened mediastinum on CXR following inhalation exposure Incubation: Usually <1 week, up to 2 months	Abrupt high fever, severe dyspnea, shock, death within 24–36 hours, occasional meningeal signs	CXR with widened mediastinum, often with pleural effusioLns, rare infiltrates Gm (–) bacilli on Gram stain Diagnosis: Positive culLtures from blood, pleural, and CSF **Obtain cultures before initiating antibiotics**	**Inhalation anthrax:** Doxycycline 100 mg bid or ciprofloxacin 500 mg bid (or other quinolone) and 1 or 2 additional antibiotics **Cutaneous anthrax:** Doxycycline (as above) or ciprofloxacin (as above) **PEP:** Doxycycline (as above) or ciprofloxacin (as above) for 60 days or more	Standard precautions No person-to-person transmission
Pneumonic plague (Yersinia pestis)				
Severe febrile respiratory illness with dyspnea, CXR pneumonia Incubation: 1–6 days for pneumonic plague	High fever with severe respiratory illness, often with hemoptysis, cyanosis, and pulmonary infiltrates, occasionally with gastrointestinal signs and shock	Culture sputum, blood, or lymph node aspirate. Check for organisms on blood smear or bronchial/tracheal washings Gm (–) bacilli or coccobacilli with "safety pin" appearance Diagnosis: Serum sent to public health or CDC with positive antigen dilution, IgM immunoassay, immunostaining and/or PCR	**With limited number of patients:** Streptomycin 1 g IM bid or gentamicin 5 mg/kg IM or IV qd or 2 mg/kg load f/b 1.7 mg/kg IM or IV tid times 10 days **With mass casualties or PEP:** Doxycycline 100 mg PO bid (times 10 days for treatment and 7 days for PEP) Alternative: Chloramphenicol 25 mg/kg PO qid	Standard and droplet precautions Person-to-person transmission occurs

(continued)

Table 17–2. Biologic agents in a terrorist attack. (continued)

Presentation	Findings	Diagnosis	Treatment	Infection Control
Tularemia (*Francisella tularensis*)				
Abrupt onset fever (temp 100°–104°F), chills, headache, myalgias with hemorrhagic inflammation of airways (postinhalation exposure), and bronchopneumonia; possible eye and skin ulceroglandular or glandular disease Incubation: 1–14 days	Pneumonic tularemia: Hemorrhagic inflammation of airways or bronchopneumonia CXR: Peribronchial cuffing or lobar consolidation possibly with pleural effusion and/or hilar adenopathy Typhoidal tularemia; signs of sepsis with skin or lymph node involvement frequently with pulse-temperature dissociation Can persist for months	Tiny intra- and extracellular Gm (–) coccobacilli Sputum, pharyngeal washings, or gastric aspirate with special testing for tularemia and notation for laboratory precautions (infectious precautions) Microscopic fluorescent antibody testing through public health Diagnosis: Positive cultures or fluorescent antibody testing	**With limited number of infected patients:** Parenteral streptomycin 1 g IM q12h × 10 days or gentamicin 5 mg/kg IM or IV qd × 10 days **With mass casualties and PEP:** Doxycycline 100 mg IV or PO bid × 14 days or ciprofloxacin 400 mg IV bid or 500 mg PO bid × 14 days	Standard precautions, no human-to-human spread
Smallpox (*Variola major*)				

Asymptomatic incubation period (7–17 days) followed by **febrile prodrome:** Fever > 101°F + one of the following:
  1. Headache
  2. Prostration
  3. Backache
  4. Chills
  5. Vomiting
  6. Severe abdominal pain
Febrile prodrome followed in 1–4 days with deep-seated vesicular or pustular rash on face and distal extremities with spread centrally with lesions in same stage in given body part. Palms and soles frequently involved
	Deep-seated, firm vesicular/pustular lesions over face and distal extremities in same stage in given body part in toxic/moribund patient	Evaluate patients preferably by vaccinia (smallpox) vaccinated staff
		Follow public health directives to analyze virus from active skin lesions
		Specimen collection guidelines found at http://www.bt.cdc.gov/agent/smallpox/response-plan/index.asp#guided CDC Risk Algorithm for Suspected Smallpox cases; www.bt.cdc.gov/agent/smallpox/diagnosis/riskalgorithm/index.asp.
			Possible use of cidofovir (consult public health, nephrotoxic)
			PEP: Ring or mass vaccination with vaccinia (smallpox) vaccination within 4 days of exposure. Vaccinia immune globulin (VIG) potentially useful for those at increased risk for vaccination (pregnant, chronic dermatitis, or immunosuppressed) but limited supplies
				Standard, contact, and airborne precautions

(continued)

Table 17–2. Biologic agents in a terrorist attack. (continued)

Presentation	Findings	Diagnosis	Treatment	Infection Control
Botulism (*Clostridium botulinum* toxins A, B, E + F)				
Dysphagia, blurred vision, ptosis, and other bulbar symptoms followed by a descending symmetric pure motor paralysis (visual symptoms due to extraocular and pupillary muscle paralysis) **without** fever in responsive patient; toxin inhibits acetylcholine release Exposure by inhalation or ingestion most likely with bioterrorism. Incubation: 12–72 hours (range 2 hours–8 days)	Descending symmetric motor paralysis with intact sensorium; may require several months of ventilatory support in cases with respiratory muscle paralysis	Clinical diagnosis essential because tests will not be available before need to initiate treatment—Contact public health immediately Collect serum, stool, gastric aspirate, and vomitus for analysis at select labs (or CDC)	Equine antitoxin A, B, +E available through CDC (limited quantities) that requires skin testing for equine hypersensitivity prior to administration; prompt administration important to prevent further paralysis; antibiotics **not** indicated for inhalation exposure to toxin only for wound botulism (penicillin)	Standard precautions, no human-to-human spread
Ricin (noninfectious toxin from castor beans)				
Cough, dyspnea followed by noncardiogenic pulmonary edema, hypotension, respiratory and multiorgan failure with death occurring within 36–72 hours.	Respiratory and multiorgan failure, death within 36–72 hours	Urinary ricinine (through public health – CDC) or environmental sampling for ricin by PCR or other tests	None	Standard precautions
Viral hemorrhagic fever (VHF) (Marburg, Ebola, lassa fever, and others)				
Initial flulike illness followed by severe hemorrhage from multiple sites Not likely as bioterrorism agent Suspect if: 1. Travel in a country where VHF has recently occurred 2. Unprotected contact with blood or body fluids from patient or animal with VHF 3. Possible lab exposure where VHF is handled Incubation; 2 days–3 weeks depending on agent Must consider other diagnoses, including malaria and typhoid fever with foreign travel	Chest and abdominal pain, shock, petechiae, and severe hemorrhage from multiple sites with high mortality	Contact public health prior to sending specimens to CDC with alert for high infectious precautions	Supportive only; use high infectious precautions for most VHF. Ribavirin may be effective for Rift Valley fever, hantavirus, and Crimean-Congo hemorrhagic fever 30 mg/kg loading then 15 mg/kg q6h × 4 days then 7.5 mg/kg q8h × 6 days	Standard, contact, and droplet precautions and consider airborne precautions in suspected VHF cases with severe respiratory symptoms or with procedures that generate aerosols

(continued)

Table 17–2. Biologic agents in a terrorist attack. (continued)

Presentation	Findings	Diagnosis	Treatment	Infection Control
Brucellosis (*Brucella* species—multiple animal hosts)				
Nonspecific flulike illness	Undulant form: < 1 year from illness onset; undulant fever, arthritis, epididymoorchitis (in males) Chronic form: > 1 year from illness onset; chronic fatigue, depression, arthritis, and possible endocarditis, hepatitis, arthritis, and meningitis	Culture blood/bone marrow aspirate Diagnosis through isolation of *Brucella* species from clinical specimens or 4-fold increase in acute convalescent sera ≥ 2 weeks apart or positive *Brucella* immunofluorescent tests on clinical specimens	Combination Rx with doxycycline 100 mg bid and rifampin 600–900 mg qd Postexposure prophylaxis: doxycycline 100 mg bid possible with rifampin 600-900 mg qd	Standard precautions, rare sexual and breast-feeding transmission
Q fever (*Coxiella burnetii*)				
Only half show signs of clinical infection; high fever >104°F, myalgias, severe headache, nonproductive cough, sore throat, nausea, vomiting, diarrhea, abdominal or chest pain, elevated transaminases, possible pulmonary infiltrates, or confusion Late symptoms of endocarditis and hepatitis may appear Incubation: 14–39 days	Endocarditis, hepatitis, osteomyelitis, encephalitis, aseptic meningitis, and/or dementia	*Coxiella burnetii* serologies with 4 times increase in acute/convalescent titers; two antigenic phases, I and II; acute infections: phase II > phase I; chronic infections phase I > phase II	**Q fever without endocarditis:** Doxycycline 100 mg bid (if sensitive) or rifampin, TMP-SMX **Endocarditis:** Combination therapy with doxycycline and a quinolone or doxycycline and hydroxychloroquine (needs prolonged treatment)	

biologic attack or with the presentation of an emerging infectious disease:

- Does the patient present with a rare or unusual disease?
- Does an otherwise healthy individual present with a severe disorder?
- Are there an unusual number of cases of an uncommon or severe disease?
- Is there an unusual geographic clustering of cases?
- Is there a common area (e.g., building or housing unit) where cases are arising?
- Is there a common association (e.g., friends and family or coworkers) developing a disease?
- Is there an unusual age distribution of cases?

- Are there an unusual number of deaths occurring, particularly with an unusual or severe disease?

While these are only guidelines, astute clinical acumen and observation are the real first lines of defense. There should be a general understanding throughout the medical community that any observation of an unusual disease or presentation should be shared with the laboratories where samples are processed, the emergency responders, and the public health authorities where the most rapid recognition of a new disease entity could be assessed. This information also should be passed on to the larger public health organizations such as the CDC or the WHO, where a more global understanding of an outbreak could occur. This lends significant importance to the newer modalities of electronic communication regarding these outbreaks through groups such as ProMed (www.promedmail.org).

The other issue that should be addressed by all medical professionals is the question of proper disaster planning, whether it be for biologic, chemical, or radiologic exposures. Methods to contain the spread of an infectious disease were employed only slowly during the SARS outbreak described earlier in this chapter. However, such plans should be considered for even larger outbreaks that potentially would paralyze even larger medical facilities and warrant dedicating special areas, such as hotels or other housing units, where patients could be quarantined appropriately. It should be noted that quarantine has seldom been an effective mode to limit the spread of an infectious outbreak. However, there could be situations, arising from agents such as pandemic influenza with a highly resistant organism, where this would be the most appropriate response. Such an outbreak would be managed more optimally by medical staff, from custodians to technicians and physicians, trained on higher levels of respiratory protection in order to respond to the needs of such an outbreak.

There also will be a need for flexibility and adaptation in order to use potentially untested or new medications and techniques to respond to situations where known therapeutic options do not currently exist. The medical community also should strongly encourage the development of a system for rapid deployment of targeted medical supplies and medications to areas where suspected infectious outbreaks occur. Finally, the challenge to avoid panic and overreaction to a new infectious disease or outbreak is paramount. This type of response was seen with the airport screening for nail files and other potentially threatening objects following the September 11, 2001 attacks, where the appropriate response was securing airplane cockpits from such assaults.

FIRST RESPONDERS

In responding to bioterrorism events, it is helpful to distinguish the nature of the postexposure time course of signs and symptoms of biological agents. Figure 17–1 shows the time course following a bioterrorist event. The delay between exposure to biological agents and their effect means that unlike traditional first responders such as emergency medical services or hazardous materials personnel, the first responders to biological events will likely be traditional health care providers in hospitals, urgent care clinics, and private practice offices. This means that health care providers need to be trained to recognize the signs and symptoms of bioterrorism agents and be knowledgeable in the appropriate response channels to report these observations. Because of the nature of their training in surveillance, epidemiology, chemical toxicology, radiation health effects, and infectious diseases, OEM medical providers will be called upon to serve as experts in establishing programs to deal with the threats of terrorism in the workplace. This is especially true for the coordination of crisis intervention

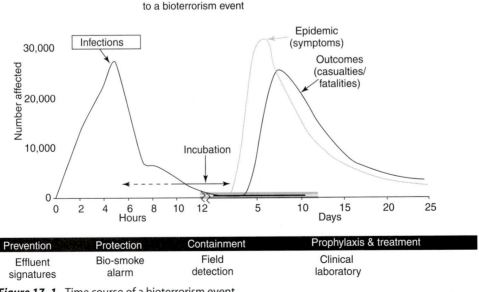

Figure 17–1. Time course of a bioterrorism event.

and subsequent medical response to acts directly affecting workers (as in the case of the anthrax-contaminated letters). Routine medical surveillance in the workplace, treatment for work-related illness or injury, removal from and the return to work of affected individuals are within the purview of OEM medical providers. Issues of privacy for medical information and the psychological evaluation of individuals working with select agents, toxic chemicals, or radiologic substances for fitness for duty are complex, requiring appropriate training in these areas.

REFERENCES

CDC: Emergency Preparedness and Response Site. www.bt.cdc.gov

Kamoie B: The National Response Plan and legal issues in public health emergency preparedness. Public Health Rep 2005;120: 571 [PMID: 1622499].

Occupational Skin Disorders

18

Mahbub M.U. Chowdhury, MBChB, FRCP, & Howard I. Maibach, MD

Although human skin can withstand many of the assaults of a hostile environment, the skin is the most commonly injured organ in industry. Skin disorders comprise more than 35% of all occupationally related diseases, affecting annually approximately one worker per thousand. Reporting remains highly incomplete, however, and the hardship and financial loss to workers and employers alike are substantial. Most occupational skin disease results from contact with a chemical substance, of which there are more than 90,000 in the environment today. Under certain conditions, all of them can irritate the skin, and approximately 2000 substances are now recognized as contact allergens. In addition, workers bring to their work preexisting diseases, which can be aggravated by their work.

REFERENCE

Centers for Disease Control and Prevention: Skin exposures and effects: www.cdc.gov/niosh/topics/skin/skinpg.html.

CONTACT DERMATITIS

1. Irritant Contact Dermatitis Syndrome

Irritant contact dermatitis (ICD) is a spectrum of disease processes with a complex pathophysiology, a varied natural history, and divergent clinical appearance. This contrasts with allergic contact dermatitis (ACD), in which a specific chemical is the central cause. Many factors can induce irritant reactions, either in isolation or in combination. These include the intrinsic nature of the substance (i.e., pH, solubility, physical state, and concentration), environmental factors (i.e., temperature, humidity, and pressure), and predisposing individual characteristics (i.e., age, gender, ethnicity, concurrent and preexisting skin disease, and the skin region exposed). Irritant contact dermatitis is a common form of occupational skin disease and, in the United States, accounts for nearly 80% of all occupational dermatitis. Statistics from other countries, where patch testing is performed more routinely, report irritant dermatitis at rates of approximately 50%, but reliable data are still limited.

Acute (primary) irritation was a common phenomenon in industry in the early twentieth century. As knowledge of dealing with primary irritants improved, less acute irritant dermatitis began to receive more attention. Today we recognize at least 14 biologic entities within the irritant dermatitis syndrome.

Acute (primary) irritation and/or corrosion. This refers to a single exposure of a material that is so irritant that damage is seen within hours to a day or so. Typically, this is best exemplified by strong acids and bases (Table 18–1). Many other chemicals produce similar exaggerated effects. The likelihood of a mixture producing such acute irritation frequently can be estimated by high concentrations of chemicals with extremes of pH.

Irritant reaction. This refers to a slowly developing redness and chapping of the skin that, with prompt cessation, usually leads to prompt amelioration without therapy. The prototypic situation is the hairdresser trainee who becomes the shampoo person, washing heads many times a day for weeks and months. The erythema and chapping frequently start on the dorsal hand. When discontinued, resolution is rapid. Many (but not all) moisturizers will inhibit the response. Some individuals will go on, with repeated exposure, to a cumulative irritant dermatitis, which may become severe.

Delayed acute irritant dermatitis. Typically, acute (primary) irritant dermatitis develops within hours to a day or so. Another form exists in which a single exposure produces irritation as late as 2 and 3 days. This form of irritant dermatitis can be confused with allergic contact dermatitis responses.

Subjective/sensory irritation. This is a form of irritation that consists of burn, sting, itch, and other discomfort but without visible signs to observe. The same symptoms can occur with visible dermatitis, but this is not then called subjective/sensory irritation. The syndrome is readily confused with low-dose chemicals that also produce burn, sting, and itch but which, with higher doses, will produce contact urticaria. This must be ruled out in order for the symptoms to be defined as subjective/sensory irritation. Although visible damage does not occur, some individuals are highly annoyed by the symptoms. A classic chemical class that induces this is the pyrethroids.

Suberythematous irritation. This is defined as skin discomfort in which there is no visible erythema, induration, or scaling. However, careful examination of the skin with a stratum corneum assay (squamome-

Table 18–1. Examples of contact irritants and allergens.

Irritants
  Soaps/detergents
  Water
  Acids/alkalis
  Organic solvents
  Metalworking fluids

Allergens
  Chromate
  Epoxy resins
  Biocides
  Fragrances
  Formaldehyde
  Rubber chemicals
  Methacrylates

Table 18–2. Examples of acne in the workplace.

Type	Occupation
Cosmetic acne	Actors, models, cosmetologists
Acne mechanica	Auto and truck mechanics, athletes, telephone operators
Ultraviolet acne	Models, lifeguards
Oil acne	Machinists, auto mechanics, fry cooks, roofers, petroleum refinery workers, rubber workers, highway pavers

try) reveals changes in the protein conformation of the stratum corneum. This nonvisible clinical problem is well worth noting by the occupational health care professional because it can be the first sign of early clinical (visible) irritant dermatitis.

Cumulative irritation. This is often confused with allergic contact dermatitis. This biologic entity refers to the fact that some chemicals (frequently at appropriately low doses) may not produce irritation on multiple exposures until weeks, months, or years of exposure. It is essential, when a visible dermatitis develops after a prolonged period of time, to exclude allergic contact dermatitis on the basis of appropriate diagnostic patch testing. If the worker is patch-test-negative, the clinical dermatitis in fact may be cumulative irritation. Discontinuing the irritant and allowing healing eventually may allow the chemical to be used without clinical difficulty.

Traumative irritant dermatitis. This refers to an uncommon and little understood clinical phenomenon where a small area of dermatitis heals and then exacerbates. The subsequent dermatitis may be long lasting (weeks to years). Triggering factors include acute irritant dermatitis, occasionally allergic contact dermatitis, and trauma such as cuts.

Pustular and acneiform irritant dermatitis. Some individuals can develop, on exposure to irritants such as oils, greases, and tars, acne-like lesions such as comedones (Tables 18–2 and 18–3). They also develop pustules, which the individual frequently identifies, if on the face, as acne.

Exsiccation eczematoid dermatitis. This refers to a chronic low-humidity dermatitis leading to an eczematous morphology. The trigger is low humidity and often frequent changes of air. This is nonim-

munologic, and management consists of raising the relative humidity.

Friction. Many industries deal with repetitive exposures of the skin leading to friction. Friction has been studied extensively and can be measured readily with various bioengineering instruments. This form of irritation is not chemically induced.

Nonimmunologic contact urticaria (NICU). NICU is a common event but fortunately is typically of minimal clinical significance. An appropriate dose of a chemical such as sorbic acid or dimethyl sulfoxide (DMSO) will produce at low doses burn, sting, and itch, at higher doses will produce erythema, and at still higher doses will produce a frank wheal. Involution is rapid.

Airborne irritant dermatitis. This refers to irritation (with appropriate negative patch tests and a photopatch test) in a photoexposed area. Lachapelle and Dooms-Goosens have provided tables of the irritants that can produce this clinical phenotype.

Photoirritation (phototoxicity). This refers to chemical irritation that requires typically ultraviolet light A to elicit it. It would not occur in the dark. The prototype chemical that has been most studied is bergaptene. Predictive tests to identify chemicals that produce photoirritation are well developed and highly predictive. Management generally consists of removing the chemical from the environment.

Tandem irritant dermatitis. In this case, one irritant may not produce clinical disease; two irritants may

Table 18–3. Chloracne-producing chemicals.

Polyhalogenated naphthalenes
Polyhalogenated biphenyls
Polyhalogenated dibenzofurans
Contaminants of polychlorophenol compounds: herbicide 4, 5-T
Contaminants of 3, 4-dichloroaniline and related herbicides
Dichlorodiphenyltrichloroethane (DDT) (crude trichlorobenzene)

do so. However, this is not a ubiquitous phenomenon, and some combinations do not produce tandem irritation.

Other general clinical patterns include repeated rubbing and friction in many individuals producing a thickened, sharply demarcated, scaly plaque resembling psoriasis known as *lichen simplex.* Excessive sweating, especially under occlusion, and ultraviolet and infrared radiation may cause miliaria. Irritation also may result in hyperpigmentation or hypopigmentation, alopecia, urticaria, and granulomas.

Anatomic differences in exposure site are important. Irritation usually is greater in areas where the skin is thin, such as dorsa of the hands, between the fingers, volar forearms, inner thighs, and dorsum of the feet. Irritant dermatitis from airborne substances such as dusts and volatile chemicals develops most commonly on regions most heavily exposed, such as the face, hands, and arms.

The diagnosis of ICD is often made by exclusion of allergic contact dermatitis. Patch testing is necessary to rule out allergic contact dermatitis, but it should be emphasized that testing should be avoided with irritants unless in nonirritating concentrations.

The most common predisposing factor for the development of ICD in the workplace is atopy, occurring in 15–20% of the population. Dry skin and advancing age are also important predisposing factors. Self-induced lesions are seen occasionally and can be recognized by their bizarre shapes and locations with an inconsistent and suspicious history of occurrence.

REFERENCES

Chew AL, Maibach HI: Occupational issues of irritant contact dermatitis. Int Arch Occup Environ Health 2003;76:339 [PMID: 12827369].

Jungbauer FH et al: Irritant hand dermatitis: Severity of disease, occupational exposure to skin irritants and preventive measures 5 years after initial diagnosis. Contact Dermatitis 2004; 50:245 [PMID: 15186383].

Lushniak BD: Occupational contact dermatitis. Dermatol Ther 2004;17:272 [PMID: 15186373].

2. Phototoxic (Photoirritation) Reactions

A nonimmunologic phototoxic eruption may result from contact with certain chemicals, such as the juice of a plant, with simultaneous exposure to natural or artificial light. Vesicle and bullae formation are characteristic, with minimal erythema, followed by hyperpigmentation. The most common causes are the polycyclic aromatic hydrocarbons in tar and creosote and furocoumarins (psoralens) found in certain plants (Table 18–4). Numerous systemic drugs also can cause these reactions.

Table 18–4. Causes of phototoxic (photoirritant) reactions.

Coal tars
Furocoumarins: Psoralen; 8-methoxypsoralen; 4,5,8-trimethylpsoralen
Aminobenzoic acid derivative: Amyl-ortho-dimethyl-aminobenzoic acid
Dyes: Disperse blue 35
Drugs: Sulfonamides; phenothiazines; tetracyclines; thiazides

SPECIFIC TYPES OF CUTANEOUS IRRITATION

1. Hydrofluoric Acid Burns

Hydrofluoric acid readily penetrates intact skin, dissociating into free hydrogen and free fluoride ions, causing tissue destruction. The typical signs and symptoms of an acute hydrofluoric acid injury usually are delayed for several hours after contact. If the concentration of the hydrofluoric acid is 50–70%, there may be immediate burning, giving a warning of exposure. However, the concentrations of hydrofluoric acid employed are usually much lower at between 15% and 20%, and the typical signs and symptoms of injury after exposure can be delayed for several hours. There is usually a deep, throbbing, excruciating pain. At this stage, however, there may be an absence of visible signs of injury. The area becomes erythematous and swollen, and as the tissue injury progresses, pallor and blistering of the skin occur, followed by tissue necrosis. Fluoride ions have a marked affinity for bone, and extensive demineralization can occur. Hydrofluoric acid burns can cause marked tissue destruction, including the loss of entire digits. Management of hydrofluoric acid burns is covered in Chapter 28.

REFERENCE

Wedler V et al: Extensive hydrofluoric acid injuries: A serious problem. J Trauma 2005;58:852 [PMID: 15824669].

2. Cement Burns

Severe burns can result from contact with wet cement because of its high alkalinity resulting from the presence of calcium oxide and hydroxide. The burns usually result from workers kneeling in wet cement or spilling it into their boots or gloves. Workers frequently delay removing contaminated boots and gloves in order to finish a job before the concrete hardens. Initially, there is burning and erythema, with ulceration delayed for several hours and followed by deep necrosis. Healing is slow, requiring several weeks and leaving disfiguring scars.

REFERENCE

Lewis PM et al: Wet cement remains a poorly recognized cause of full-thickness skin burns. Injury 2004;35:982 [PMID: 15351662].

3. Fiberglass Dermatitis

Commercially produced since the 1930s, fiberglass is available in two forms: wool fiberglass and textile fiberglass. The former is used chiefly for insulation, acoustic panels, and ceiling boards in construction. Textile fiberglass is made into yarns or processed into short fibers for reinforcement of plastics, rubber, and paper. Binders are used on wool fiberglass, such as thermosetting phenolformaldehyde-type resins. The sizing agent for textile fiberglass varies, but once the sizing agent is cured, the risk of allergic contact dermatitis is diminished. Almost all fiberglass manufactured has a diameter of more than 4.5 μm, which can readily penetrate the sweat glands and cause irritation.

Contact with fiberglass produces irritation, with itching and prickling of the skin, especially in skin folds and areas where clothing rubs. A maculopapular rash may be present, usually obscured by excoriations. When widespread, the rash can be diagnosed incorrectly as scabies. Application of a piece of cellophane tape to the skin and then to a microscopic slide will disclose the uniform, rodlike fibers of glass (readily visualized with polarization).

The symptoms usually subside after a few days. Allergic sensitization has not been proven, and many workers develop "hardening" and thus are able to return to work and continue without recurrence.

REFERENCE

Patiwael JA et al: Airborne irritant contact dermatitis due to synthetic fibers from an air-conditioning filter. Contact Dermatitis 2005;52:126 [PMID: 15811024].

4. Pigmentary Changes

Chemical agents may induce either increased or decreased pigmentation and sometimes both in the same patient. *Melanosis* denotes hyperpigmentation, whereas *leukoderma* refers to loss of pigment. Inflammation usually precedes the color change. Repeated trauma, friction, chemical and thermal burns, and exposure to ultraviolet (UV) light can increase pigmentation, especially in dark-skinned persons. Coal tar, pitch, asphalt, creosote, and other tar and petroleum derivatives can induce skin darkening. Psoralens, found in certain plants, induce phytophotodermatitis with contact followed by sun exposure, which can cause hyperpigmentation.

Occupational leukoderma resembles idiopathic vitiligo, and differentiation can be difficult. However, to be considered work-induced, the initial site of leukoderma, usually the hands and forearms, should be the

Table 18–5. Chemicals causing leukoderma.

Hydroquinone
Monobenzylether of hydroquinone
Monomethylether of hydroquinone
para-Tertiary-butylphenol
para-Tertiary-butylcatechol
para-Tertiary-amylphenol
para-Isopropylcatechol

site of repeated contact with a known depigmenting chemical (Table 18–5). With continued contact, depigmentation may spread to distant body sites not in direct contact with the chemical.

Chemical leukoderma is reversible if exposure is discontinued soon after onset. If continued exposure occurs, it may be permanent. Topical and oral psoralen and ultraviolet A (PUVA) therapy has been used to induce repigmentation, but acral lesions, especially on the hands, often are refractory to treatment.

REFERENCES

Mahendran R et al: Contact leukoderma secondary to occupational toluene diamine sulfate exposure. Contact Dermatitis 2002; 47:109 [PMID: 12423410].

Watson K, Rycroft R: Unintended cutaneous reactions to CS spray. Contact Dermatitis 2005;53:9 [PMID: 15982225].

5. Allergic Contact Dermatitis

Although reportedly occurring less often than irritant contact dermatitis, allergic contact dermatitis (ACD) is of great importance because ordinary protective measures can be ineffective, and many workers have to change jobs or learn a new trade. By contrast, workers with irritant dermatitis often can return to work, provided they use adequate personal protective measures, such as gloves, and if the workplace is made less hazardous.

ACD is an immunologic reaction classified as a delayed type IV or cell-mediated hypersensitivity. This distinguishes it from type I reactions, which are immediate and antibody-mediated. Although most contact allergens produce sensitization in only a small percentage of exposed persons, there is great variation among individuals depending on numerous factors such as the nature of the allergen itself. The allergen in poison ivy or poison oak will sensitize nearly 70% of exposed persons, whereas *p*-phenylenediamine, the allergen in permanent hair dyes, sensitizes a relatively small percentage of persons who repeatedly come into contact with it.

Sensitization requires at least 4 days to develop. Many workers, however, contact an allergen repeatedly in their work for months and even years before developing clinical sensitivity. The precipitating cause of sensitization can be a minor episode of irritant dermatitis or even increased frequency of contact with greater pressure and sweating at the site. Once allergic sensitization has occurred, the dermatitis begins within 24–48 hours after contact. A pruritic, erythematous rash develops rapidly, followed by papule formation, vesicles, or blistering. Itching usually is prominent. The dermatitis originates at the site of contact with the allergen, but new lesions may appear at distant, seemingly unrelated sites, usually because of inadvertent transfer of the allergen by the hands. A subacute and chronic stage can evolve, characterized by thickened, fissured skin that occasionally erupts into more acute dermatitis on reexposure to the allergen or with aggravation by contact with irritating substances.

There is considerable variation in the intensity of reaction depending on the body area affected. The mucous membranes usually are not affected, and the hair-bearing scalp usually is much less involved than the adjacent skin. The palms and soles may be less affected than the dorsal and interdigital areas. The eyelids and periorbital skin are especially sensitive, whereas involvement of the vault of the axillae is rare.

ACD must be differentiated from atopic dermatitis, psoriasis, pustular eruptions of the palms and soles, herpes simplex and zoster, idiopathic vesicular reactions secondary to *Trichophyton* infections of the feet, dyshidrotic and nummular eczemas, drug eruptions, and irritant contact dermatitis. Examples of occupational contact allergens include epoxy resins, biocides, chromate, and formaldehyde (see Table 18–1).

REFERENCES

Lushniak BD: Occupational contact dermatitis. Dermatol Ther 2004;17:272 [PMID: 15186373].

Uter W et al: Clinical update on contact allergy. Curr Opin Allergy Clin Immunol 2005;5:429 [PMID: 16131919].

Epoxy Resin Dermatitis

Epoxy resins are used commonly as adhesives and can be found in paints, cement, and electrical insulation. Most epoxy resins are based on diglycidyl ether of bisphenol A. Epichlorohydrin combined with bisphenol A produces an epoxy resin of varying molecular weights from 340 to larger polymers, which are less sensitizing. However, there are other potential allergens, including pigments, fillers, reactive diluents, and solvents, that are mixed with a curing or hardening agent to polymerize the resin. Once hardened, the sensitizing potential is reduced.

Patch testing to epoxy resins must be thorough because there may be unknown compounds, and testing with the patient's own resins is essential. Irritant reactions and sensitization on patch testing may occur, particularly to the amine epoxy hardeners. Facial dermatitis may suggest allergy to hardener rather than to the epoxy resin itself because the latter has low volatility. Detection of epoxy resin can be undertaken by a spot test with sulfuric acid or thin-layer chromatography.

Epoxy resin dermatitis can be prevented with exclusion or low concentrations of molecular weight 340 and 624 epoxy oligomers, high-molecular-weight (>1000) reactive diluents, and hardeners that exclude aliphatic amines.

REFERENCES

Cahill J et al: Prognosis of contact dermatitis in epoxy resin workers. Contact Dermatitis 2005;52:147 [PMID: 15811030].

Guin JD: Airborne contact dermatitis from a polymercaptan hardener in a finished epoxy resin. Contact Dermatitis 2005;52:45 [PMID: 15701131].

Kaukiainen A et al: Chemical exposure and symptoms of hand dermatitis in construction painters. Contact Dermatitis 2005; 53:14 [PMID: 15982226].

Photoallergic Reactions

Photoallergic reactions are immunologically based. They are more uncommon than phototoxic reactions and develop only in individuals previously sensitized by simultaneous exposure to a photosensitizing chemical and appropriate UV radiation. The biologic process is similar to ACD, except that UV converts the chemical to a complete allergen. The radiation is usually in the UVA spectrum, although it may extend into the UVB.

Photoallergic reactions appear suddenly with an acute eczematous eruption, later becoming lichenoid and thickened, on the face, neck, dorsum of the hands, and exposed arms, often extending to other areas. The diagnosis is suggested by the distribution and character of the eruption, but confirmation requires careful questioning and photopatch testing. Sparing of skin under the chin and upper eyelids is strongly suggestive of a photo eruption. Table 18–6 lists some causes of photoallergic reactions.

REFERENCE

Lankerani L, Baron ED: Photosensitivity to exogenous agents. J Cutan Med Surg 2005 [PMID: 15988550].

Table 18–6. Causes of photoallergic reactions.

Halogenated salicylanilides
Tetrachlorosalicylanilide
3,4,5-tribromosalicylanilide
4,5-dibromosalicylanilide
Phenothiazines: Chlorpromazine, promethazine
Fragrances: Musk ambrette
Optical brighteners (stilbenes)
Sunscreens: PABA esters
***Compositae* plants**

A. DIAGNOSIS

The key to diagnosis of allergic contact dermatitis is diagnostic patch testing. The opportunity to select the site of application and the ability to use only a minute concentration of test substance, confining it to a small area, are important features. The organ tested is the same as that affected by the disease and the same mechanism for production of the disease is used; hence the patch test remains one of the most direct and valuable of all methods of medical testing.

Standardized procedures in patch testing are important, especially the concentration of the allergen and the type and characteristics of the vehicle. During recent decades, attempts to standardize patch testing have occurred.

Two methods are currently in use worldwide. The older method is the Finn chamber, which employs an aluminum cup, 8 mm in diameter, fixed to a strip of Scanpor tape, a finely meshed paper tape with a polyacrylate adhesive. The allergens are applied to the cups, covering more than half the diameter of each cup, and fixed to the skin with Scanpor tape. A newer method, the T.R.U.E. Test, manufactured in Denmark, is a convenient, ready-to-use strip of tape on which a measured amount of allergen is incorporated in a thin hydrophilic gel film printed on a polyester patch measuring 9×9 mm. The patches contain 24 different allergens, are mounted on strips of acrylic tape protected by a plastic sheet, and are packaged in airtight envelopes. The thin sheet of plastic is removed, and the strips are placed on the skin. On contact with skin moisture, the dry film dissolves into the gel, and the allergen is released onto the skin. This method permits rapid application and avoids the hazard of mistakes in preparation of the application. The T.R.U.E. Test system was not designed for occupational use and is now out of date in terms of current knowledge.

The upper back is the favored site for patch testing. Any hair must be removed using an electric rather than a safety razor to minimize damage to the keratin layer. The patches are left on the skin for 48 hours and then removed, and the sites are identified with a fluorescent-inked pen. Reading is done at 72 or 96 hours after application and occasionally at 1 week. When a fluorescent pen has been used to delineate the allergens, a hand-held black light will identify the sites. A single reading at 48 hours misses approximately 35% of positive results. Table 18–7 lists patch test interpretation codes.

Clinical interpretation is the most difficult aspect of patch testing. Irritant reactions show varied patterns such as fine wrinkling, erythematous follicular papules, petechiae, pustules, and sometimes large bullae. A classic positive patch test reaction consists of erythema, mild edema, and small, closely set vesicles.

Table 18–8 describes the allergens present in the T.R.U.E. Test and additional allergens for detecting

Table 18–7. Patch test interpretation codes.

1 +	= Weak reaction, nonvesicular, erythema, mild infiltration
2 +	= Strong reaction, erythema, edema, vesicles
3 +	= Extreme reaction, spreading, bullous, ulcerative
4	= Doubtful, faint erythema only
5	= Irritant reaction
6	= Negative
7	= Excited skin reaction
8	= Not tested

vehicle and preservative allergy. Table 18–9 lists other additional occupational series available for patch testing.

Adverse reactions can occur but are rare. The most common are increased pigmentation at the site of a positive reaction, persistence of a reaction (especially with a positive reaction to gold), mild flare of the original dermatitis with brisk reactions, the development of psoriasis in a positive test site (rare), active sensitization (very rare), and anaphylactoid reactions (exceedingly rare).

Keep in mind that the test is a template of allergic contact sensitization developed over a person's lifetime. Therefore, clinical relevance of each positive reaction must be determined. This can be accomplished only with extensive knowledge of commercial and industrial materials and their ingredients. Information can be obtained from numerous sources, including standard textbooks, manufacturers, and material safety data sheets. A review of the patient's clinical history, a workplace visit, chemical analysis of other allergens or cross-reacting substances, and further patch testing may be required.

Operational Definition of Occupational ACD

There are many steps in the full assessment and operational definition or final diagnosis of occupational ACD. A history of occupational exposure and a definite time relationship between exposure and onset of dermatitis is essential. Other factors required are a consistent morphology of the dermatitis and positive diagnostic testing with appropriate vehicle and concentration such as patch testing. Clinical relevance needs to be defined, and this may require a provocative use test (PUT) or a repeat open application test (ROAT) with the suspected allergens. This involves application of the substance onto the inner forearm twice daily for 7–28 days until a red, itchy patch appears, confirming ACD. Serial dilutions of the chemicals tested may be needed to confirm initial findings and suspicions. Control subject testing is essential to confirm nonirritating concentrations. Finally, clearing of the dermatitis once the allergen is removed or exposure is reduced significantly provides further information regarding the relevance of the allergen.

Table 18–8. Allergens tested in various standard series: Main uses (European, International, British).

1. Potassium dichromate 0.5% petrolatum (pet)	Tanning leather, cement
2. 4-Phenylenediamine base 1% pet	Azo dye intermediate, hair dye
3. Thiuram mix 1% pet	Rubber accelerator, fungicides
4. Neomycin sulfate 20% pet	Antibiotic in creams
5. Cobalt(II) chloride hexahydrate 1% pet	Metal
6. Benzocaine 5% pet	Local anesthetic in creams
7. Nickelsulfate hexahydrate 5% pet	Metal
8. Clioquinol 5% pet	Synthetic anti-infective agent
9. Colophony 20% pet	Pine resin, adhesives, printing ink
10. Paraben mix 16% pet	Preservatives in creams
11. N-Isopropyl-N-phenyl-4-phenylenediamine (IPPD)	Black rubber chemical
12. Wool alcohols 30% pet	Ointment base in creams
13. Mercapto mix 2% pet	Rubber additives
14. Epoxy resin 1% pet	Resin in adhesives, paint, insulation
15. Balsam of Peru 25% pet	Fragrance and flavoring agent
16. 4-tert-Butylphenoformaldehyde resin (PTBP) 1% pet	Resin in adhesives
17. 2-Mercaptobenzothiazole 2% pet	Rubber chemical
18. Formaldehyde 1% aqueous (aq)	Disinfectants, cosmetic preservatives
19. Fragrance mix 8% pet	Fragrances
20. Sesquiterpene lactone mix 0.1% pet	Plants
21. Quaternium 15 1% pet	Formaldehyde releaser
22. Primin 0.01% pet	Main allergen in primula dermatitis
23. 5-Chloro-2-methyl-4-isothiazolin-3-one 0.01% aq	Preservative in oils and creams
24. Budesonide 0.01% pet	Nonhalogenated steroid
25. Tixocortol-21-pivalate 0.1% pet	Topical steroids (hydrocortisone)

REFERENCES

Krob HA et al: Prevalence and relevance of contact dermatitis allergens: A meta-analysis of 15 years of published T.R.U.E. Test data. J Am Acad Dermatol 2004;51:349 [PMID: 15337975].

Pratt MD et al: North American Contact Dermatitis Group patch test results, 2001–2002 study period. Dermatitis 2004;15:176 [PMID: 15842061].

Templet JT et al: Etiology of hand dermatitis among patients referred for patch testing. Dermatitis 2004;15:25 [PMID: 15573645].

Wetter DA et al: Patch test results from the Mayo Clinic Contact Dermatitis Group, 1998–2000. J Am Acad Dermatol 2005;53:416 [PMID: 16112346].

B. TREATMENT

Treatment of contact dermatitis depends on the stage of the disease. Acute vesicular eruptions are treated with wet dressings for the first 24–36 hours using Burow's solution, followed by a topical corticosteroid; only the most potent topical corticoids (classes 1 and 2) are effective in the acute phase. When the eruption begins to dry, corticosteroid creams can be used, accompanied by oral sedating antihistamines for itching. Oral antibiotic therapy is indicated only when secondary infection is suspected. Topical antibiotic and antihistamine preparations should be avoided, however, because of risk of sensitization. In addition, based on current evidence, cold compresses have been shown to decrease inflammation in contact dermatitis. High-potency topical corticosteroids decrease mild to moderate, but not severe, ACD. Topical corticosteroids are possibly not significantly effective with some irritants such as sodium lauryl sulfate. There are no controlled studies, but oral corticosteroids are effective in severe ACD.

REFERENCE

Saary J et al: A systematic review of contact dermatitis treatment and prevention. J Am Acad Dermatol 2005;53:845 [PMID: 16243136].

Table 18–9. Additional occupational series for patch testing.

Hairdressing
Bakery
Dental
Epoxy
Fragrance
Isocyanate
Oils and cooling fluid
Methacrylates: dental, nails, printers
Photographic chemicals
Plant
Plastics and glues
Rubber additives
Textile colors and finish

6. Contact Urticaria

Contact urticaria develops within minutes to an hour following contact with a substance. Interest in and knowledge of this reaction have increased greatly during the past 15 years, particularly with natural rubber latex allergy. The two main types are nonallergic and allergic.

Nonimmunologic (Nonallergic) Contact Urticaria

With sufficient provocation, nearly all exposed individuals will develop a reaction. Previous sensitization is not necessary. Gardeners may develop reactions from contact with nettles and other plants, caterpillar hair, moths, and other insects; cooks from cinnamic acid and aldehyde, sodium benzoate, sorbic acid, fruits, vegetables, fish, and meat; and medical personnel from alcohols, balsam of Peru, and dimethyl sulfoxide.

Immunologic (Allergic) Contact Urticaria

Immunologic (allergic) contact urticaria is caused most commonly by latex in natural rubber, especially gloves, which is a problem for medical and dental personnel, kitchen and dairy workers, pharmacists, semiconductor workers, and others who must wear gloves throughout the workday. The reactions range from mild erythema with itching at the site of contact to severe anaphylactic reactions, sometimes resulting in death. They are immunoglobulin (Ig) E–mediated type I immediate hypersensitivity reactions and appear to be more common in atopics. The cause is natural latex from the sap of the tree *Hevea brasiliensis*, a *cis*-1,4-polyisoprene, the precursor of the rubber molecule. It is estimated that there are 50 or 60 different proteins in latex that provoke the allergic response. The chief symptoms are itching, redness, and wheal-and-flare reaction at the site of contact. The symptoms usually appear 10–60 minutes after contact and, when mild, disappear without treatment in 2–3 hours. Severe reactions progress rapidly and include generalized urticaria, swelling of the face and lips, asthma, collapse, and death. Natural rubber latex gloves most commonly cause these reactions, but condoms, urinary catheters, elastic bandages, adhesive tape, wound drains, dental dams, hemodialysis equipment, balloons, pacifiers, barium enema tips, and many other latex-based rubber products are implicated. Cross-reactions can occur to foods such as avocados, water chestnuts, kiwi, papaya, and bananas, provoking reactions in sensitive persons. Airborne contamination by rubber glove powder also may induce symptoms in very sensitive patients.

Open testing on intact skin and skin prick testing are the most common diagnostic methods for this condition. A standardized test material should be used, and testing should be performed only if resuscitation measures are readily available. "Use tests" with a glove or a single finger of a glove should be performed with special care in patients who have a history of anaphylaxis or when the results of skin prick test or the latex radioallergosorbent test (RAST; Pharmacia, Sweden) are positive. Note that the RAST is only 60–65% sensitive.

The Food and Drug Administration (FDA) prohibits the labeling of latex-containing medical products as "hypoallergenic" and requires the statement: "This product contains natural rubber latex" on all latex-containing products that are directly or indirectly in contact with the body.

REFERENCES

Taylor JS, Erkek E: Latex allergy: diagnosis and management. Dermatol Ther 2004;17:289 [PMID: 15327474].

Valks R et al: Allergic contact urticaria from natural rubber latex in healthcare and non healthcare workers. Contact Dermatitis 2004;50:222 [PMID: 15186377].

BIOLOGIC CAUSES

1. Bacterial Diseases

Staphylococcal and Streptococcal Infections

Infection of minor lacerations, abrasions, burns, and puncture wounds accounts for most staphylococcal and streptococcal infections. A work relationship is not always easy to establish, however, and many cases are unreported. Nevertheless, these infections are common in certain occupations, especially agricultural and construction workers, butchers, meat packers, and slaughterhouse workers. The history should clarify whether a work relationship is likely, although frequently in workers' compensation cases the patient's statements must be accepted as valid.

Furunculosis is common among automobile and truck repair persons, especially in dirty jobs, such as tire repair. Paronychia may be seen in occupations such as nurses, hairdressers, and manicurists.

Atopic dermatitis patients are especially likely to experience skin colonization with staphylococci. In a high percentage of atopics, *Staphylococcus aureus* can be cultured from their eczematous skin, which often has been made worse by heavy and prolonged application of corticosteroid creams and ointments. Daily oral antibiotics should be part of the long-term treatment of these patients. Employment of persons with active atopic dermatitis in food service industries and hospital patient care may need to be restricted.

Cutaneous Mycobacterial Infections

Infection with tubercle bacilli is covered in Chapter 17. A classic example of tuberculosis of the skin acquired through inoculation of *Mycobacterium tuberculosis hominis* is seen in pathologists (*prosector's wart*) and morgue attendants (*necrogenic wart* or *anatomic tubercle*). Surgeons are also at risk for such granulomatous infections. Veterinarians, farmers, and butchers may acquire infection with *M. tuberculosis* var. *bovis,* which at one time was a common cause of disease in livestock in the United States, but bovine tuberculosis has declined since the middle 1930s. In some countries, however, the disease is still common. In the United States and other parts of the world, as a result of population movement and the increasing prevalence of human immunodeficiency virus (HIV) infection, the incidence of infection with human strains of tuberculosis has increased greatly. Between 1985 and 1991, 39,000 more cases occurred in the United States than expected, and drug resistance, especially in those with HIV infection, has seriously compounded the problem.

The typical skin lesions are slowly progressive, warty, hyperkeratotic plaques, which, if left untreated, eventually regress after many months or years, leaving disfiguring scars. Demonstration of organisms either directly or from cultures is often difficult.

Atypical Mycobacterial Infections

Atypical mycobacterial infections are caused most commonly by infection with *M. marinum.* This infection usually is acquired from exposure to infected fish, especially in aquariums and fish tanks by persons who clean these tanks. Swimming pools have become contaminated with this organism, and pool attendants and cleaners are also at risk. Treatment with rifampin or ethambutol is usually effective.

As in other mycobacterial skin infections, the clinical picture consists of granulomatous papules and nodules that ulcerate and exude a clear, thin serum. Sometimes a pattern resembling sporotrichosis develops, with nodules and papules ascending the arm (or leg) along the course of regional lymphatics. Persons with AIDS are at special risk for developing these infections. Other atypical mycobacteria include *M. ulcerans, M. fortuitum, M. avium, M. intracellulare, M. kansasii,* and *M. chelonae.*

Brucellosis (Malta Fever, Undulant Fever)

Brucellosis is caused by one of several *Brucella* organisms and is still observed in some rural areas, affecting farmers, veterinarians, slaughterhouse workers, meat packers and inspectors, and livestock workers. The disease has an abrupt onset with chills, fever, headache, and extreme weakness. A maculopapular rash occurs that may become petechial. A chronic form of the disease was common in the past with a recalcitrant ulcer at the site of inoculation and abscesses in internal organs.

Treatment with tetracycline, when started early, is curative. Streptomycin is useful for more serious cases.

Anthrax

Anthrax is caused by the spore-forming bacterium *Bacillus anthracis* and produces a "malignant" pustule at the site of inoculation and elaborates a highly toxic endotoxin that is lethal to infected animals. A vegetative form of the organism may remain dormant in soil for many years. Infection in humans is usually through the skin but also has resulted from ingestion of contaminated meat. A pulmonary form of the disease caused by inhalation of the spores is often rapidly fatal if not promptly treated.

Occupational infection usually is caused by importation of contaminated animal products and occurs chiefly in agricultural workers, stock farmers, slaughterhouse workers, butchers, and those employed in bone and bone meal processing. Workers handling imported goat hair, wool, and hides from endemic regions are at special risk. These include longshoremen, freight handlers, warehouse workers, and employees of processing industries where the hides are treated for sale. Anthrax responds to treatment with intravenous penicillin. Tetracycline and erythromycin are alternatives.

Erysipeloid

This acute, slowly evolving skin infection is almost always occupational in origin. Caused by inoculation of the gram-positive bacillus *Erysipelothrix rhusiopathiae,* usually through a penetrating hand wound, the disease begins with a characteristic raised, purplish red, indurated maculopapular lesion, with burning and itching. Regional lymphadenopathy does not occur. The disease is self-limiting, usually clearing within 3–4 weeks.

Butchers and fish handlers are at most risk (*fish-handlers' disease*). Turkeys and chickens also may carry the organism. Penicillin, ciprofloxacin, and erythromycin are curative.

2. Viral Diseases

Herpes Simplex

This is the most frequent viral infection of occupational origin, affecting dentists and dental assistants, physicians and nurses, and respiratory technicians. This is caused by the herpes simplex virus (HSV). Transmission is by contaminated saliva or pharyngeal or laryngotracheal secretions. Wearing disposable gloves, masks, and safety glasses reduces the risk of infection in these workers.

Viral Warts

Meat handlers, especially butchers and slaughterhouse workers, are at greatest risk for development of the common wart, caused by the human papilloma virus (HPV), of which there are at least 35 types. These warts are most numerous on the hands and fingers of these workers, and minor cuts and abrasions inoculate the virus. Molluscum contagiosum occurs in wrestlers, boxers, and other sportsmen.

Orf

Endemic in sheep and goats, orf is caused by infection with a parapox virus, usually involving the mouth and nose of infected animals. Mostly farmers and veterinarians are affected with this relatively mild, self-limited disease. Only one or two lesions may be present, almost always on fingers, and are associated with mild fever, lymphangitis, and regional lymphadenopathy. An erythema multiforme–like rash occurs 10–14 days after onset. Treatment is symptomatic, with antibiotics given only for complications such as secondary infection.

3. Fungal Infections

Candida

Infection with *Candida,* mainly *Candida albicans,* is the most common occupationally related fungal disease. The organism is ubiquitous, and proliferation is favored by moisture, occlusion, and irritation. Most occupationally acquired candidal infections are on the hands, especially in the paronychial areas and interdigital spaces. Occupations in which prolonged wearing of rubber gloves is required, such as dentistry, medicine, and technical work in clean rooms in the semiconductor industry, show the highest incidence of this condition. Diabetics and neutropenic, immunocompromised patients are especially at risk.

Dermatophytes

Dermatophytic infections are common. *Trichophyton verrucosum* is an animal fungus that readily infects farmers and cattle tenders. The lesions are often quite inflammatory and may resemble pyoderma. Farmers, milkers, cattle tenders, veterinarians, and tannery workers, especially hide sorters, are at risk. *T. rubrum* and *T. mentagrophytes* are examples of fungi that cause tinea infections in the general population, especially tinea manuum and tinea pedis. *Microsporum canis* frequently infects small animals and causes infection in pet shop workers, veterinarians, and personnel in contact with laboratory animals. *M. gypseum* is a rare fungus found in soil, causing occasional infection in agricultural workers.

Physicians are often requested to decide whether a *Trichophyton* infection is work-related, especially *T. rubrum* and *T. mentagrophytes* infections of the hands and nails. Onychomycosis is extremely common, and most of those affected do not seek medical attention. Workers engaged in repetitive hand activities, especially where there is sweating and pressure or repetitive nail trauma in the case of onychomycosis, may believe their work to be the primary cause of the infection. Each case must be studied individually, but most often the work cannot be considered a primary cause.

Sporotrichosis

This fungal disease is acquired most often by persons who work with soil, such as nursery, agricultural, and forestry workers, veterinarians, and miners. The etiologic agent is the dimorphic fungus *Sporothrix schenckii,* which has a worldwide distribution. There are two clinical manifestations. A fixed type restricted to the site of inoculation may be nodular, ulcerative, or verrucous. The more common, and classic form, of the disease is a relatively nontender subcutaneous nodule that appears at the site of inoculation of the fungus. The nodule enlarges slowly and later ulcerates, followed by the appearance of secondary lesions (*nodular lymphangitis*) along the lymphatics draining the initial site. The cutaneous forms of the disease are chronic, indolent, and rarely fatal. Treatment with potassium iodide solution for a prolonged period of time is effective. In disseminated disease, which is fatal in approximately 30% of cases, intravenous administration of amphotericin B is indicated. Itraconazole also has been recommended for treatment of both forms. Other possible causes of nodular lymphangitis should be kept in mind. These include *M. marinum, Nocardia brasiliensis, Leishmania brasiliensis, C. immitis,* and *F. tularensis.*

4. Parasitic Diseases

Protozoa

A. Cutaneous Leishmaniasis

Most parasitic diseases, such as amebiasis, giardiasis, and malaria, present with general rather than cutaneous health problems. An exception is cutaneous leishmaniasis, caused by *Leishmania tropica* (Oriental sore, bouton d'orient), found in the Middle East, and *L. braziliensis* (American leishmaniasis, uta), found in Central and South America. The disease is transmitted by sandflies that thrive in warm climates and is endemic in persons working in tropical forests in southeastern Mexico, Colombia, and Venezuela. The disease manifests as cutaneous ulcers with metastatic mucocutaneous lesions known as *espundia.* Pentavalent antimonials, such as sodium stibogluconate, are the treatment of choice. Pentamidine and liposomal or conventional amphotericin are alternatives.

B. Helminths

Penetration of the cercariae of schistosomes into the papillary dermis induces a highly pruritic papular eruption termed *swimmer's itch.* Urticaria may accompany the rash and be widespread. Migratory birds usually are the definitive hosts, with saltwater mollusks serving as intermediate hosts. The condition lasts for 2–3 weeks, often with secondary infection of excoriated lesions. Skin divers, lifeguards, dock workers, and workers who maintain lakes and ponds may be affected. Treatment is symptomatic.

Larva migrans (creeping eruption) occurs in subtropical and tropical regions where people work on moist soil infected with hookworm larvae. Dogs, cats, cattle, and human feces carry the larvae, and humans are the final host. A threadlike, red or flesh-colored, circuitous, slightly raised line occurs often on the feet, legs, back, or buttocks caused by movement of the larva in the epidermis. Humans are infected with the larvae of *Ancylostoma braziliense* and *Necator americanus,* the ova of which are deposited in the soil. Topical application of 10% suspension of thiabendazole to affected areas four times daily for 7–10 days is usually curative. Agricultural workers, lifeguards, shoreline fishermen, ditch diggers, and sewer workers are at greatest risk.

Other nematode diseases that are occasionally occupational include trichinosis, dracunculosis, filariasis, loiasis, enterobiasis, strongyloidiasis, and toxocariasis.

Arthropods

Bees, wasps, ants, moths, flies, mosquitoes, fleas, and blister beetles are among the most common causes of occupation-related arthropod diseases. Mites, ticks, spiders, and scorpions are also included in this group. Millipedes and centipedes can induce severe skin reactions caused by their toxins or allergenic products. Outdoor workers, food handlers, and entomologists are affected most frequently. Chicken farmers are exposed to chicken mites. Mites infect grain in food-processing plants, and dock workers and restaurant workers also are affected.

A. Scabies

Epidemics of scabies have occurred in nursing homes, hospitals, and residential facilities for the aged. The disease is highly contagious and spreads rapidly, especially in the immunosuppressed. It is often initiated by an infected employee who transmits the mite to patients. They then spread the disease to other personnel. The scabicide of choice is permethrin, but treatment of the more severe types of scabies (e.g., crusted scabies) can be difficult and may require repeated treatments with other scabicides such as lindane, permethrin, precipitated sulfur, and oral ivermectin.

B. Lyme Disease

Lyme disease is an important inflammatory disease that follows tick-induced erythema chronicum migrans (ECM) weeks or months after inoculation. ECM begins with a small erythematous macule, usually on an extremity, that enlarges with central clearing. The lesion sometimes reaches a diameter of 50 cm, and smaller satellite lesions often are present. In nearly half the patients, a type of arthritis occurs within weeks or months of the ECM, and there may be associated neurologic abnormalities, as well as myocardial conduction alterations, serum cryoprecipitates, elevated serum immunoglobulin M (IgM) levels, and an increased sedimentation rate. Elevated serum IgM and later IgG appear within weeks of infection with circulating cryoprecipitates and other immune complexes. Erythema chronicum migrans is an important diagnostic marker for this disease. The ticks *Ixodes dammini, I. pacificus* (in the United States), and *I. ricinus* (in Europe) transmit the spirochete *Borrelia burgdorferi* that is responsible for the disease. In some cases, localized scleroderma appears to be linked to *Borrelia* infection. Tick bites are common in outdoor workers, loggers, wilderness construction workers, guides, and ranchers. Other major tick-borne diseases in the United States are relapsing fever, tularemia, Rocky Mountain spotted fever, ehrlichiosis, Colorado tick fever, babesiosis, and tick paralysis.

REFERENCE

Harries MJ, Lear JT: Occupational skin infections. Occup Med 2004;54:441 [PMID: 15486175].

PHYSICAL CAUSES

1. Mechanical Trauma

Intermittent friction of low intensity will induce lichenification (thickening) of the skin. With greater pressure, corns and calluses appear. After minor trauma, calluses frequently develop painful fissures, which may become infected. After years of repeated frictional hand trauma during work, permanent calluses may result, leading to disability and early retirement. With increasing automation, less frequent manual operation of tools, and better protective clothing, occupational marks are less frequent and have almost disappeared from many industries.

2. Heat

Burns

Burns arising from the occupation are common and exhibit characteristic occupational patterns. The resulting scarring and pigmentary changes are of chief concern to dermatologists, who rarely treat acute burns. Hypopigmentation is especially susceptible to actinic damage, and scars and the hyperpigmentation often are disfiguring.

Miliaria

Miliaria is caused by sweat retention and often is seen in the work environment. The eruption can be extensive, accompanied by burning and itching. The most superficial form, miliaria crystallina, is caused by poral closure and rupture of the ducts within the upper level of the epidermis. The condition commonly occurs on the palms and in intertriginous areas, with asymptomatic desquamation of the surface. When the closure occurs deeper in the epidermis, vesiculation with marked pruritus results. Miliaria rubra, or prickly heat, is the type most likely to be confused with contact dermatitis. If poral obstruction extends deeper in the epidermis and into the upper dermis, the condition is known as *miliaria profunda,* resulting in deep-seated, asymptomatic vesicles. This condition is caused by prolonged exposure to a hot environment and often follows an extended period of miliaria rubra. Heat exhaustion and collapse may be sequelae.

Intertrigo

A macerated, erythematous eruption in body folds, intertrigo results from excessive sweating, especially in obese workers. Secondary bacterial and candidal infections are common. The interdigital space between the third and fourth fingers is a common site in workers whose hands are continuously wet, especially from rubber gloves. Medical and dental personnel, bartenders, cannery workers, cooks, swimming instructors, and housekeepers are especially predisposed to this condition.

Overheating, especially in conjunction with physical exercise, may result in heat-induced urticaria and, rarely, in anaphylaxis. Acne vulgaris and rosacea are aggravated by prolonged exposure to heat, especially from ovens, steam, open furnaces, and heat torches. Herpes simplex may be triggered by intense heat, especially with sunburn and UVB exposure.

3. Cold

Frostbite

In frostbite, there is progressive vasoconstriction causing impairment of circulation. In superficial frostbite, only the skin and superficial dermis are involved. Redness, transient anesthesia, and superficial bullae are seen. In more severe cases, deep tissue destruction occurs, often with gangrene and loss of a limb. As the temperature falls, the affected area becomes numb, and the initial redness is replaced by a white, waxy appearance with blistering and later areas of necrosis. The area ultimately becomes pain-free, and the cold discomfort disappears. At this stage it is impossible to estimate future tissue loss accurately; several weeks may be necessary. Long-term effects include Raynaud-like changes with paresthesia and hyperhidrosis. Squamous cell carcinoma may develop in old, healed scars.

Treatment consists of slow rewarming in a whirlpool or waterbath, a painful procedure requiring adequate relief. Infection must be treated vigorously.

Persons at greatest risk are military personnel, utility maintenance personnel, sailors, fishermen, firefighters, mail delivery persons, rescue personnel, and arctic laboratory workers.

Chilblains (Perniosis)

This mild form of cold injury, although an abnormal reaction to cold, is less common in very cold climates where homes are usually well heated and warm clothing is worn. The northern United States and Europe are areas where this condition is seen frequently. The lesions are reddish blue, swollen, boggy discolorations with bullae and ulcerations. The fingers, toes, heels, lower legs, nose, and ears are especially affected. Genetic factors with vasomotor instability often are found to be important background features. Treatment is symptomatic with calcium channel blockers such as nifedipine.

4. Vibration Syndrome

Vibration of hand-held tools and Raynaud phenomenon have been known to be associated since the early twentieth century. Popular names include *dead fingers* and *white fingers;* clinically, the condition is a type of Raynaud phenomenon. Operation of heavy vibrating tools such as jackhammers, especially in cold weather, produces vasospasm of the digital arteries, causing episodic pallor, cyanosis, and erythema of fingers. Chain saws, hand-held grinders, riveting hammers, and other pneumatic tools also are associated with this condition. Tingling and numbness, blanching of the tips of one or more fingers, and clumsiness of the fingers and hands occur. The symptoms may be indistinguishable from other forms of Raynaud phenomenon, but asymmetry usually is observed. Occupational disability seldom results, and most workers continue at their jobs. Vibration frequencies between 30 and 300 Hz are most likely to be responsible.

Acroosteolysis (Vinyl Chloride Disease)

A serious form of Raynaud phenomenon occurs from exposure to vinyl chloride monomer in workers cleaning reactor tanks used for polymerization. Lytic lesions also occur in bones, especially the fingers; hence the name *acroosteolysis.* Sclerodermatous skin changes can occur. With engineering modifications during manufacture and better protective measures, the condition has nearly disappeared.

5. Ionizing Radiation

Numerous industrial processes use ionizing radiation, including the curing of plastics, sterilization of food and drugs, testing of metals and other materials, medical and dental radiography, therapy with radioisotopes, and operation of high-powered electronic equipment. Exposure is much less now than it was several decades ago mainly as a consequence of better construction and shielding of the radiographic equipment.

Occupational exposure to ionizing radiation may be acute or chronic and usually is localized. Acute radiodermatitis often results from a single accidental exposure to around 1000 R and presents with rapid onset of erythema, edema, and blanching of the skin, reaching a peak at about 48 hours. Anorexia, nausea, vomiting, and other systemic symptoms also occur. There follows a latent period of apparent recovery lasting a few days, after which the skin again becomes erythematous, with purplish ecchymotic areas that become vesicular and bullous. Pain is intense, usually requiring narcotics. A repair stage follows, and as reepithelialization takes place, the skin becomes atrophic, hairless, and lacks functioning sebaceous glands. With large single doses, ulceration usually follows but often is delayed for 2–3 months. Healing is very slow, and an atrophic, disfiguring scar is left.

Chronic radiodermatitis results from exposures to smaller doses of ionizing radiation (300–800 R) received daily or weekly over a long period of time to a total dose of 5000–6000 R. The skin becomes red and eczematous with burning and hyperesthesia. Often the epidermis sloughs, and regrowth occurs slowly over a period of 4–6 weeks. Hair is also lost, often permanently, and the sebaceous glands cease activity. The skin becomes hypopigmented and atrophic with multiple telangiectasias. The systemic effects of irradiation are described in Chapter 12.

Video Display Terminals

Measurements of radiation emissions from video display terminals have consistently shown nondetectable or background levels. As with many electrical devices, there is an increase in static magnetic energy very close to the terminal, but these levels have never been associated with adverse health effects. The ergonomics of the work are important, however, because tendonitis of the hands and forearms, neck strain, and back pain are work-related disorders that may result from disharmony between the position of the operator and the workstation.

REFERENCE

McMullen E, Gawkrodger DJ: Physical friction is under-recognized as an irritant that can cause or contribute to contact dermatitis. Br J Dermatol 2006;154:154 [PMID: 16403110].

OCCUPATIONAL ACNE

Oil Acne (Folliculitis)

Oil acne, or oil folliculitis, is a common condition resulting from heavy exposure to oil, especially under oil-soaked clothing. The arms and thighs usually are affected with numerous, often black comedones, pustules, furuncles, and sometimes carbuncles. This condition was once very common, especially in oil fields and refineries, but with improved engineering and less heavy contact with oils, it is seen much less often today. Many cases are never reported because most workers know that with better hygiene the condition improves. The most common sources are insoluble cutting oils in machinists and greases and lubricating oils in mechanics. Melanosis and photosensitivity also occur. Workers handling heavy tar distillates and coal tar pitch, roofers, oil well drillers, coke oven workers, petroleum refiners, rubber workers, textile mill workers, and road pavers are affected commonly.

Another form of environmental acne is acne cosmetica, occurring in actors and cosmetologists. Acne mechanica secondary to local pressure, friction, rubbing, squeezing, and stretching can occur in the wearers of heavy clothing and helmets. Tropical acne is common in hot, moist climates. During World War II, thousands of military personnel were evacuated from the South Pacific because of this condition. The so-called McDonald's acne results from contact with the grease and fat of frying hamburgers (see Table 18–2). Nonoccupational sources of environmental acne also should be considered, including acne from medications such as corticosteroids, testosterone, progesterone, isoniazid, and iodides and bromides.

Treatment of oil folliculitis consists of oil-impervious aprons and environmental measures to limit exposure. Gloves usually cannot be worn by machinists and mechanics because of the danger of catching them in the machinery. Modernization of cutting machines with automation and special guards decreases skin contact.

Chloracne

Chloracne is a rare condition with multiple closed comedones and pale-yellow cysts on the skin from cutaneous and systemic exposure to certain halogenated chemicals (see Table 18–3). Body areas affected are the cheeks, forehead, and neck. The shoulders, chest, back, buttocks, and abdomen also may be involved. The genitalia are especially affected, whereas the nose often is spared, except in systemic exposure. In addition, there may be hypertrichosis, hyperpigmentation, and increased skin fragility suggesting porphyria cutanea tarda. Conjunctivitis, swelling, and discharge from swollen meibomian glands of the eyelids can be seen, as well as a brownish pigmentation of the nails. Peripheral neuritis and hepatotoxicity may occur, suggesting systemic toxicity.

Although treatment of chloracne is often unsatisfactory, oral antibiotics, oral isotretinoin, acne surgery, and occasionally dermabrasion may be helpful. The majority of cases clear within 1–2 years following cessation of exposure.

REFERENCE

Violante FS et al: Chloracne due to *o*-dichlorobenzene in a laboratory worker. Contact Dermatitis 2005;52:108 [PMID: 15725291].

OCCUPATIONAL SKIN CANCER

Approximately 400,000 new cases of nonmelanoma skin cancer occur in the United States each year, comprising approximately 30–40% of all cancers reported annually. Malignant melanoma accounts for another 18,000 cases. The exact number of skin cancers induced by the workplace is disputed, but most observers agree that it is a significant proportion. The most common causes of skin cancers in the work environment are ultraviolet light, polycyclic aromatic hydrocarbons, arsenic, ionizing radiation, and trauma. (For more information on occupational cancers, see Chapter 16.)

Ultraviolet Light

Sunlight is the most common cause of skin cancer, but workers seldom consider sunlight from the workplace as contributing to their actinically damaged skin and skin cancer. The most common skin cancers are squamous cell and basal cell carcinomas. These are related to prolonged exposure to sunlight but also may be initiated by tar and oils, mechanical trauma, and burns. The primary carcinogenic action spectrum of sunlight is in the UVB range (290–320 nm), but UVC (100–290 nm) and UVA (320–400 nm) rays also are photocarcinogenic. UVA rays accelerate UVB-induced malignancy, and even though UVC rays are not present in sunlight, there is exposure from welding arcs and germicidal lamps.

The evidence for the skin carcinogenicity of UVB and UVA is overwhelming. Such cancers occur much more frequently in outdoor workers and in persons with fair skin and light hair and eye color and in those who tan poorly and burn easily. In addition to the time spent in sunlight, the ultraviolet radiation received by an outdoor worker depends on the latitude, season, time of day, altitude, and weather. Artificial sources of carcinogenic UV radiation include welding arcs; germicidal lamps; devices for curing and drying printing ink, plastics, and paint; UV lasers; mercury vapor lamps; and medical UV therapy machines. Radiometers are available that can measure the amount of UV radiation a worker is receiving.

Epidemiologic studies in countries where there is a large blond, fair-skinned population, as in Australia, show a higher incidence of melanomas of the head, face, and neck in outdoor workers, which contrasts with office workers, who have melanomas more commonly on the covered parts of the trunk and limbs. Lentigo maligna is almost always present on exposed, sun-damaged skin and becomes invasive after a variable period of time. Persons with xeroderma pigmentosa, a hereditary disease, are extremely sensitive to the carcinogenic effects of sunlight. A frequent cause of death in these individuals is malignant melanoma, often occurring at a young age.

Polycyclic Aromatic Hydrocarbons

For 250 years, coal tar products and certain petroleum oils were considered potential causes of cutaneous cancers in individuals who work in certain industries. In the twentieth century, the relationship became firmly established not only from experimental animal studies but also from numerous epidemiologic surveys. Polycyclic aromatic hydrocarbons, such as those found in soot and carbon black, coal tar, pitch and tarry products, creosote oil, and certain oils, account for the majority of cutaneous tumors. Photosensitization develops initially, with recurring erythema and intense burning of the exposed skin. After repeated episodes, poikilodermatous changes appear, especially on the exposed skin of the face, neck, and hands. Keratotic papillomas (tar warts) then develop, which later may become squamous cell carcinomas, basal cell carcinomas, and keratoacanthomas. Polycyclic aromatic hydrocarbons and UVB appear to act synergistically to induce malignant change.

Arsenic

Since the late 1940s, epidemiologic studies have strongly linked inorganic arsenic exposure to squamous cell cancers of skin and lungs. Arsenic keratoses, characteristic of chronic arsenicalism, are multiple yellow, punctate keratoses distributed symmetrically on the palms and soles. Squamous cell carcinomas and multiple lesions of intraepidermal squamous cell carcinoma (Bowen disease) may develop from these keratoses. Basal cell carcinomas also occur from arsenic exposure, and they are often multiple, superficial, and pigmented.

Occupational arsenic exposure occurs in ceramic enamel workers, copper smelters, fireworks makers, gold refiners, hide preservers, carpenters (removing old wallpaper), semiconductor workers, and taxidermists. Arsenic is rarely used as an insecticide today but is still employed as a rodenticide.

Trauma

Malignancies resulting from burn scars and other trauma, such as the Kangri cancers in India and the Kairo cancers in Japan, have been reported since early in the nineteenth century. In 1863, Virchow proposed a theory for carcinogenesis based on repeated trauma; however, cancer arising from a single trauma has remained a controversial subject. Litigation alleging that malignant tumors were caused by a single injury has been increasing in the United States since the 1950s, especially in workers' compensation hearings. The courts generally have accepted a relationship with trauma if the evidence shows a greater than 50% probability that a cancer was caused by a specific trauma.

REFERENCES

Almahroos M, Kurban AK: Ultraviolet carcinogenesis in nonmelanoma skin cancer: II. Review and update on epidemiologic correlations. Skinmed 2004;3:132 [PMID: 15133392].

Lens MB, Dawes M: Global perspectives of contemporary epidemiological trends of cutaneous malignant melanoma. Br J Dermatol 2004;150:179 [PMID: 14996086].

WORKUP & DIAGNOSIS OF PATIENTS

The workup and diagnosis of patients with work-related skin disease requires considerably more time than does a general dermatologic workup. Making a premature diagnosis before studying all the evidence should be resisted because an incorrect diagnosis can have long-lasting and severely detrimental effects. Review of the medical records, patch testing, fungal and bacterial cultures, biopsy, and plant visits often are necessary to reach a correct diagnosis. Diagnosis of an endogenous or constitutional eczema or dermatitis as primary cause can be difficult for many workers to accept. Atopic eczema, although inherited, often has onset for the first time in adult life when precipitated by work activities, and aggravation often is considered work-related. Many other constitutional diseases can be considered similarly.

Table 18–10 outlines a typical evaluation of a work-related illness. The following headings can serve as a form for recording the results of the workup. The text under each heading details the information that should be gathered and recorded.

History of Injury & Current Complaints

Learn exactly which anatomic skin site was first affected. With a diagnosis of contact dermatitis, the

Table 18–10. Outline for dermatologic examinations for workers' compensation patients.

1. History	12. Support for diagnosis
2. Job description	13. Discussion
3. Current treatment	14. Disability status
4. Present complaints	15. Factors of disability
5. Medical history	Subjective
6. Family history	Objective
7. Social history	16. Apportionment
8. Personal data	17. Future medical care
9. Medical record review	18. Vocational rehabilitation
10. Physical examination	Work restrictions
11. Diagnosis	

eruption should begin at the site of contact with the offending agents. Spreading then occurs, especially in the case of allergic sensitization. The date of the initial appearance of the dermatitis is important because often a change in workplace ergonomics, contact with new substances, or increased contact with long-used substances can precipitate dermatitis. Itching is important because irritant contact dermatitis, and especially allergic contact dermatitis, is almost always pruritic. If improvement occurs away from work and aggravation regularly takes place on resumption of the same work, a work relationship is almost always found, and workers' compensation courts often will accept this, even without other evidence. Over-the-counter medicines and home remedies often contain contact allergens that sometimes can be the sole cause.

A. JOB HISTORY

A description of the job as provided by the patient is often more accurate than the official job title. Often the worker has performed the same job for a long period of time before onset of dermatitis. This suggests a new process or contactant introduced into the workplace or home environment.

B. PRIOR EMPLOYMENT

The nature of previous jobs and dermatitis, as well as previous exposure to irritants and potential sensitizers, is important.

C. OFF-WORK ACTIVITIES

The 40-hour work week leaves sufficient opportunity for other part-time jobs, hobbies, and house and garden work.

D. PAST MEDICAL HISTORY

Although 15–20% of the population has a family or personal history of atopy, it is an often-overlooked cause of recurrent dermatitis, especially among hairdressers, kitchen helpers, medical and dental personnel, and automobile repair workers. Even persons with mild atopy may develop a major work-related hand dermatitis at the time of first employment, following repeated contact with irritants. Psoriasis also can be precipitated by trauma, especially repeated intense friction and pressure on the hands.

E. FAMILY HISTORY

A family history of atopy is most important. Psoriasis (type 1) also may be a relevant family condition.

F. HOBBIES/HABITS

Hobbies and nonwork activities should be explored during the history taking, including habitual traumatic activities such as picking and digging the skin, especially with wooden or metal articles used for scratching and rubbing.

G. REVIEW OF SYSTEMS

A general review of body systems should be done.

Review of Medical Records

The medical records must be examined thoroughly to supplement the history as provided by the patient.

Examination

Examination should not be limited to the part affected because the presence of dermatitis elsewhere and other skin conditions can change an initial impression. This is especially true when psoriasis, tinea infections, and lichen planus are found.

A. SPECIAL INVESTIGATIONS

Patch testing is the most important special investigation and should include not only suspected specific allergens but also a standard series of common allergens.

B. DIAGNOSIS

The specific diagnosis should be recorded with an opinion regarding a work relationship.

C. SUMMARY

This should be a brief summary of the findings with an explanation of the conclusions. Nonmedical terms should be used as much as possible.

REFERENCE

Van Wendel de Joode B et al: Assessment of dermal exposure. Occup Environ Med 2005;62:633 [PMID: 16109820].

Temporary & Total Disability

The disability status, total or partial, is described here. In most cases of hand dermatitis, the disability is temporary, but because of the manual nature of most work, total disability is also possible.

Permanent & Stationary Status

Once the dermatitis has reached a plateau and no further improvement is anticipated, permanent and stationary (P&S) status is reported. This does not mean, however, that treatment cannot be resumed should a recurrence cause a worsening of symptoms.

Objective Findings

A brief review of the objective findings is recorded here.

Subjective Findings

A review of the patient's complaints and a description of any impairment are provided here.

Work Restrictions

Work restrictions, if any, can be recorded here.

Loss of Preinjury Capacity

For purposes of permanent disability rating, one should describe any loss of preinjury capacity, such as may occur with contact allergy.

Causation & Apportionment

If any aspect of the impairment is related to a previous employment or any preexisting disability, this is explained here, estimating the percentage of impairment associated with each.

Future Medical Treatment

An estimation of the type and duration of future medical treatment is given here.

Vocational Rehabilitation

Once a permanent and stationary state is reached, vocational rehabilitation must be considered. It is important to offer guidance to vocational rehabilitation personnel in job selection for disabled workers.

Patch Testing

The most important diagnostic test for occupational skin disease is the patch test. This is especially true because nearly 90% of occupational disease is contact dermatitis. Since irritant and allergic dermatitis can be similar clinically, differentiation can be done only by patch testing, which not only will reveal the specific cause of a work-related dermatitis but also when negative after testing all possible allergens in the patient's work will effectively rule out allergic contact dermatitis as a cause. Unfortunately, the test is often performed inadequately or incompletely, if at all. Patch testing should be done by experienced physicians according to accepted methods with nonirritating concentrations of test substances, preferably chemicals obtained commercially from manufacturers of patch test materials. Table 18–8 lists and describes common contact allergens.

Additional Diagnostic Tests

Fungal, bacterial, and viral smears and cultures, biopsies, and prick testing, if contact urticaria is suspected, sometimes are required. Plant visits are an essential and integral part of the evaluation, often providing information vastly different from that learned during the patient's evaluation.

TREATMENT

In many occupations, avoidance of irritants and allergens is not always possible. Prophylactic measures are necessary in industry to avoid the risk of developing irritant and allergic contact dermatitis. The specific treatment of occupational skin disease depends on the cause and does not differ from treatment of nonoccupational skin disease. Protective measures include moisturizers, barrier creams, and appropriate gloves and clothing. In many cases, a specific cause is not found, and recurrences may continue to affect the patient; hence treatment with topical or oral corticosteroids often continues for prolonged period of time, leading to atrophy of skin and systemic complications. Although recovery may occur rapidly following treatment, the skin retains a nonspecific hypersensitivity for several weeks, and hence work should not be resumed too early, even when the patient and/or employer are pressuring the physician.

PREVENTION

Measures to lower the incidence of dermatitis in the workplace include (1) identification of potential irritants and allergens in the workplace (use of the MSDS), (2) chemical substitution or removal to prevent recurrence, (3) personal protective measures, (4) personal and environmental hygiene, (5) education to promote awareness of potential irritants and allergens both at work and at home, (6) preemployment and periodic health screening, and (7) engineering controls with automated, closed systems.

Skin Cleaners

These should be readily available and designed for the use intended, for example, heavy-duty cleansers for mechanics and others working with grease and oils and mild bar or liquid soaps for workers in less dirty occupations. Industrial cleansers often contain harsh abrasives and potentially allergenic antibacterial agents.

Waterless hand cleaners remove industrial dirt without water and can be of value in work sites without convenient washing facilities. Most are based on relatively nonirritating detergents and are removed from the skin with towels, waste papers, or rags. When used repeatedly, rags may contain a large number of irritants from the work site.

Protective Clothing and Gloves

Protective clothing is available for most work situations and exposures. It must be selected with specific consideration of the type of work and exposure and must be inspected regularly for holes and tears. Remember that certain allergens, such as methyl and ethyl methacrylate, glyceryl monothioglycolate, and paraphenylenediamine, pass readily through rubber gloves. Workers may wear gloves to protect an active dermatitis, but the occlusion can aggravate an existing eruption, and contact with rubber can lead to allergic sensitization to ingredients of the gloves.

REFERENCES

Centers for Disease Control and Prevention: Skin exposures and effects, www.cdc.gov/niosh/topics/skin/skinpg.html.

Semple S: Dermal exposure to chemicals in the workplace: Just how important is skin absorption? Occup Environ Med 2004;61:376 [PMID: 15031402].

Barrier Creams

Barrier creams are popularly termed "invisible gloves." Although the benefit of this physical barrier to penetration is debated widely, barrier creams have reduced allergic and irritant contact dermatitis in both experimental and clinical studies. Barrier creams should be applied to intact skin only and prior to contact with irritants, including application after breaks. High frequency of application with adequate amounts is essential. Barrier creams may induce irritant or allergic contact dermatitis caused by various preservatives, lanolin, and fragrances. Workers should not become lax in other protective measures because of this "invisible glove" provides a sense of false security.

REFERENCE

Drexler H: Skin protection and percutaneous absorption of chemical hazards. Int Arch Occup Environ Health 2003;76:359 [PMID: 12761626].

Emollients

Emollients and moisturizers are designed to increase the water content of the skin and can be used on irritated skin. They play an important role in treating and preventing irritant contact dermatitis, but further assessment is required in both animal and human models in the workplace.

Plant Surveys

An essential, often neglected feature of assessing patients with occupational skin disorders is a survey of the conditions at the work plant. The visit should not focus only on the patient's work site but attempt to include other areas. The various work sites can be walked through with a knowledgeable person as a guide. The incidence of dermatitis in the past, the presence of engineering controls and protective measures such as protective clothing, and the general environment of the plant should be checked, including the temperature and relative humidity. Material safety data sheets (MSDS) should be available to the workers, and if there is a research and development section, further information can be obtained as necessary. Examination of workers should be conducted in private, giving the worker an opportunity to discuss the working conditions openly, including perceived attitudes of management. A detailed written report is required after the visit.

Upper Respiratory Tract Disorders

19

Dennis Shusterman, MD, MPH

The respiratory tract, with its limited defense mechanisms and high degree of exposure to the environment, is vulnerable to chemical pollutants. As the initial portal of entry for airborne contaminants, the upper airway, including the nasal cavity, pharynx, and larynx, is the first line of defense—as well as target—for these pollutants. In addition to toxicologic agents, the upper respiratory tract can react to antigenic stimuli, allergic rhinitis occurring with (or without) asthma in some individuals. This chapter describes the spectrum of upper respiratory tract health effects associated with workplace (and environmental) chemical exposures, as well as allergic syndromes unique to workplace settings.

ANATOMY & PHYSIOLOGY

Functions of the Upper Airway

The upper respiratory tract, extending from the nares to the larynx, performs several essential physiologic functions, including air conditioning, filtering, microbial defense, sensation, and phonation. During the fraction of a second that inspired air travels through the upper airway, its temperature is raised (or, occasionally, lowered) to near body temperature, and its relative humidity is brought to between 75% and 80%. Particulate matter larger than 5–10 µm in diameter is captured on the surface of the nasal turbinates by a mechanism known as *impaction*. The majority of impacted material—captured in the mucous blanket—is transported via ciliary action until it empties into the nasopharynx and then is swallowed (a smaller fraction being transported anteriorly to the nasal vestibule). The high surface area of the turbinates and the high water content of nasal mucus further provide a "scrubbing" mechanism for water-soluble air pollutants. In terms of microbial defense, nasal secretions contain both nonspecific antimicrobial factors (lysozyme and lactoferrin) and specific factors [secretory and nonsecretory immunoglobulin A (IgA)]; these substances are important in the host defense against viral and bacterial infections carried by the airborne route.

The sensory functions of the upper airway are twofold: odor and irritant perception. Odor perception, mediated by cranial nerve I, the olfactory nerve, both conveys quality to life—augmenting the primary tastes in the appreciation of food, for example—and has a safety function. Individuals lacking odor perception (anosmics) cannot distinguish fresh from spoiled food, tell that a gas pilot light has gone out in their kitchen, or sense that a respirator filter has become saturated with a vapor against which they were to be protected. Upper respiratory tract irritant perception (conveyed by cranial nerve V, the trigeminal nerve) is also protective in that nose and throat, as well as eye, irritation will trigger escape behavior during an industrial mishap, thus helping the exposed individual protect the lower respiratory tract against serious chemical injury. With lower-level exposures, however, eye, nose, and throat irritation may be the primary health endpoints of concern and, as noted below, may be difficult to distinguish from allergy symptoms in some individuals.

Acute Response Mechanisms in the Upper Airway

A. ALLERGY

Like all mucous membranes, the mucosa of the upper respiratory tract is invested with mast cells, bearing on their surface receptors for the Fc fragments of immunoglobulin (Ig) E molecules. In sensitized individuals, IgE molecules encountering the proper antigen can cross-link at adjacent Fc receptor sites and initiate mast cell degranulation. (In addition to antigen-mediated activation, mast cells can degranulate in response to plant lectins, bee venom, and systemically administered opiates.) Mast cell degranulation immediately releases such preformed mediators as histamine, heparin, tryptase, and leukocyte chemotactic factors; leukotrienes, prostaglandins, and cytokines are released on a delayed basis. The effects of these mediators include glandular secretion (rhinorrhea), chemotaxis (inflammation), and vasodilation (congestion). Unlike in the lower respiratory tract, airflow limitation occurs in the upper respiratory tract as a result of venous engorgement and/or extravasation of plasma, not via smooth-muscle contraction. This produces swelling of the nasal mucosa and thereby encroaches on the airway.

B. NEUROGENIC REFLEXES

Of perhaps equal importance with reference to occupational and environmental exposures are the various neurogenic reflexes that can be triggered by chemical irritant exposures. Stimulation of trigeminal nerve afferents—

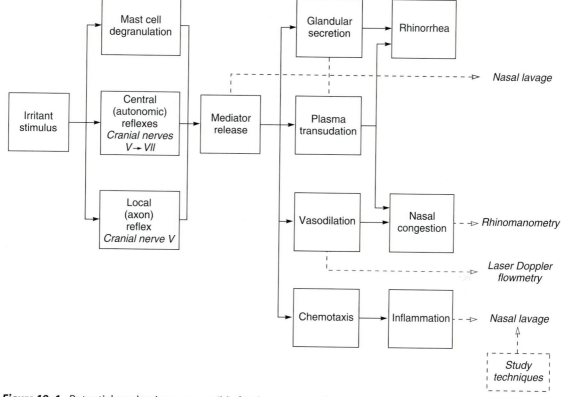

Figure 19–1. Potential mechanisms responsible for the acute nasal response to irritants. Applicable study techniques appear on the right.

which are sensitive to low pH, some endogenous inflammatory mediators (such as bradykinin), and chemical irritants (the prototype being capsaicin)—results in two major types of reflex response: (1) parasympathetic reflexes, carried by the facial nerve (cranial nerve VII), and (2) axon reflexes, consisting of neuropeptides released from afferent branches of the trigeminal nerve. A familiar example of a parasympathetic response is so-called gustatory rhinitis, a copious, watery rhinorrhea that occurs with the ingestion of spicy foods. The axon reflex, on the other hand, is of more theoretical than proven importance in the upper airway response to chemical irritants. Figure 19–1 shows a postulated pathophysiologic scheme including both allergic and neurogenic mechanisms.

REFERENCES

Davis SS, Eccles R: Nasal congestion: Mechanisms, measurement and medications. Clin Otolaryngol Allied Sci 2004;29:659 [PMID 15533155].

Fodil R et al: Inspiratory flow in the nose: A model coupling flow and vasoerectile tissue distensibility. J Appl Physiol 2005;98: 288 [PMID 15333615].

OCCUPATIONAL/ENVIRONMENTAL CONDITIONS

Occupational Allergic Rhinitis

An estimated 20% of the population suffers from allergic rhinitis, and another 5% suffers from various forms of nonallergic rhinitis. Typically, these individuals experience either seasonal pollinosis or, if allergic to common indoor allergens, perennial symptoms of sneezing, rhinorrhea, and nasal congestion. Workplace allergens producing allergic rhinoconjunctivitis may be either commonly encountered allergens, exposure to which may be incidental to the work environment (e.g., grass pollen exposure in a landscaper), or unusual agents encountered only in industrial environments (e.g., trimellitic anhydride exposure in a plastics worker). Initial sensitization may occur either in the workplace or outside, with the latter scenario being more likely with common environmental allergens. Thus, as is the case with asthma, occupational allergic rhinitis may either be work-induced or work-exacerbated. Table 19–1 lists representative agents producing occupational allergic rhinitis; the reader will recognize immediately that these same

Table 19–1. Agents associated with occupational allergic rhinitis.

High-molecular-weight compounds (proteins)

Animal antigens (animal handlers, farmers, veterinarians)
Green coffee beans and castor beans (dock workers)
Proteolytic enzymes (detergent workers, cosmetologists)
Grains/contaminants (bakers, farmers, grain handlers)
Insect antigens (various occupations)
Gum arabic/gum acacia (printers)
Psyllium (health care workers)
Natural rubber latex (health care workers)

Low-molecular-weight compounds

Diisocyanates (polyurethanes → painters, boat builders, etc.)
Acid anhydrides (plastics → painters, fabricators, etc.)
Colophony (rosin core solder → electronics workers)
Plicatic acid (western red cedar → sawmill workers)
Antibiotics (health care workers)

agents can produce occupational asthma (and, indeed, many sensitized individuals suffer from both conditions).

Additional—and unanticipated—consequences may accrue from the diagnosis of allergic rhinitis. Limited data link nasal congestion and rhinitis to obstructive sleep apnea symptoms. In addition, high-grade nasal obstruction predisposes to oral breathing, thus bypassing some of the microbial defenses normally operative during nasal breathing, potentially, in some occupational contexts, making the worker more susceptible to selected airborne pathogens.

A. DIAGNOSIS AND MANAGEMENT

Allergic rhinitis is characterized by sneezing, itching, rhinorrhea, and congestion, with or without associated eye and chest symptoms. Nonoccupational symptoms occurring during a portion of the year (typically from pollens) characterize *seasonal allergic rhinitis,* in contrast to *perennial allergic rhinitis* (with symptoms occurring year-round in response to such indoor allergens as dust mites, cat dander, cockroaches, or mold spores). Occupational allergic rhinitis may exhibit either of the preceding temporal features, although perennial is somewhat more common. Superimposed on variations across the calendar year may be variation across the work week, with "ratcheting" of symptoms on successive workdays and improvement on weekends and vacations. Importantly, individuals with occupational allergic rhinitis may be sensitized to both workplace and nonworkplace antigens and also may react to irritants, further complicating the diagnostic picture.

The diagnosis of occupational allergic rhinitis is based on the history, physical examination (a pale, boggy nasal mucosa being typical), and laboratory testing, which might include a complete blood count and/or nasal smear demonstrating eosinophilia and increased serum total IgE and the in vitro radioallergosorbent testing (RAST) or enzyme-linked immunosorbent assay (ELISA) finding of work antigen-specific IgE. Skin prick testing, with saline and histamine controls, is considered by many clinicians to be the "gold standard" of allergy testing. If neither an in vitro system nor an allergy-testing extract is available for a suspected occupational allergen, response to allergen avoidance or workplace challenge may provide the best clue to the specific diagnosis. Nasal inspiratory peak-flow measurements (see below) may provide objective validation of cross-shift symptoms and can be employed during adjacent periods of allergen avoidance and normal work routine to help establish an occupational etiology.

Allergen avoidance should be an important component of therapy both for the control of nasal symptoms and to prevent the progression of incipient occupational asthma. Whether engineering controls or personal protective equipment can control antigen exposure levels sufficiently must be answered on a case-by-case basis; some individuals may require reassignment, particularly if chest symptoms are coincident. A particularly frustrating situation presents itself in health care settings, where latex-sensitive individuals with respiratory allergies are not only prevented from wearing latex gloves but also frequently cannot work near others wearing such gloves (the powder on the gloves serves as a carrier for the latex antigen).

Mainstays of medical therapy for allergic rhinitis include systemic antihistamines, nasal steroids, and the mast cell stabilizer cromolyn sodium; newer medications include a topical antihistamine (azelastine) and a topical cholinergic blocker (ipratropium bromide). Of the systemic antihistamines, fexofenadine, loratadine, and desloratadine are nonsedating alternatives that may enable one to control symptoms while simultaneously staying productive and alert. Of the nasal topical steroids, aqueous-based formulations tend to be less irritating than alcohol-based formulations. Patients should be instructed that as much as 2 weeks of therapy may be necessary before an optimal response is observed from either topical steroids or cromolyn sodium. Nasal topical decongestants are to be avoided except for very brief control of acute symptoms, the possibility of tachyphylaxis and rebound (*rhinitis medicamentosa*) being ever present. For patients complaining of prominent "vasomotor" symptoms (e.g., nasal congestion and/or rhinorrhea in response to cold, dry air or exercise), a trial of ipratropium bromide nasal spray may be indicated. The efficacy of desensitization ("allergy shots") has been better evaluated for common aeroallergens than for specific occupational sensitizers.

REFERENCES

Casale TB, Dykewicz MS: Clinical implications of the allergic rhinitis-asthma link. Am J Med Sci 2004;327:127 [PMID: 15090751].

Gautrin D et al: Occupational rhinitis. Curr Opin Allergy Clin Immunol 2006;6:77 [PMID: 16520669].

Storaas T et al: Occupational rhinitis: diagnostic criteria, relation to lower airway symptoms and IgE sensitization in bakery workers. Acta Otolaryngol 2005;125:1211 [PMID: 16353405].

Occupational Irritant Rhinitis

The eyes, nose, and throat are sensitive to chemical irritants (including gases, vapors, dusts, and smokes), with mucous membrane irritation giving rise to the most commonly reported symptoms in problem work environments. Subtypes of chemical irritants in the office or home air include combustion products (from tobacco smoke and malfunctioning appliances) and volatile organic compounds (VOCs; from cleaning products, office supplies and machines, and building materials and furnishings). Industrial environments may present workers with an even wider range of airborne irritants, with the majority of both threshold limit values (TLVs) and permissible exposure levels (PELs) being based on the irritancy of the compound in question. Extreme forms of industrial irritant rhinitis occur in electroplaters and others exposed to chromic acid, who may develop nasal mucosal ulcerations and even septal perforation. Finally, exposure to photochemical air pollution also can produce objective inflammatory changes in the upper airway. Pathophysiologically, it is believed that the most important determinant of a compound's initial site of irritancy is its water solubility (see Chapter 30).

Persistent rhinitis symptoms and signs after a one-time high-level irritant exposure are termed *reactive upper airways dysfunction syndrome* (RUDS). This diagnosis was meant to be analogous to the lower airway condition referred to as *irritant-induced asthma* or *reactive airways dysfunction syndrome* (RADS). However, in contradistinction to RADS, RUDS lacks strict diagnostic criteria (e.g., absence of preexisting symptoms, objective physiologic changes), and hence its utility has yet to be fully established.

A. DIAGNOSIS AND MANAGEMENT

Because irritant-associated symptoms, such as nasal congestion and rhinorrhea, may mimic an allergic response, the treating health professional may be faced with a diagnostic challenge in determining responsible etiologic agents and pathophysiologic processes. The report of predominantly irritant symptoms rather than itching or sneezing, a high symptom prevalence rate among coworkers, and dramatic improvement at night and on weekends supports a diagnosis of irritant rhinitis. Similarly, erythema of the mucous membranes, particularly punctate erosion of the nasal mucosa, supports an irritant process, although the finding is neither sensitive nor specific. In irritant rhinitis, the laboratory workup is essentially "negative," including a lack of systemic eosinophilia, a normal total serum IgE level, the predominance of neutrophils on nasal smear, and when applicable, a lack of skin test (or in vitro) reactivity to identified workplace allergens. Air-monitoring data may be of assistance in industrial settings but more often are a source of frustration in the investigation of so-called problem buildings because symptoms may be reported in settings in which levels of VOCs are low relative to current occupational exposure limits. The role of complex mixtures in explaining such discrepancies is explored below, under "Research Studies."

Treatment for occupational irritant rhinitis consists of reduction of exposure, nonspecific supportive measures (e.g., saline nasal lavage), and occasionally, topical steroids. Patients troubled by prominent reflex symptoms (particularly rhinorrhea) may benefit from the topical cholinergic blocker ipratropium bromide. In atopic patients, control of intercurrent allergic rhinitis—whether occupational or nonoccupational—also may decrease reactivity to chemical irritants, although this issue has not been well studied.

REFERENCES

Moscato G et al: Occupational asthma and occupational rhinitis in hairdressers. Chest 2005;128:3590 [PMID: 16304318].

Slavin RG: The allergist and the workplace: occupational asthma and rhinitis. Allergy Asthma Proc 2005;26:255 [PMID: 16270717].

Occupational Nonallergic Rhinitis

Vasomotor rhinitis, a subcategory of nonallergic rhinitis, is a term that is used sometimes to describe augmented nasal reactivity to nonspecific physical stimuli. Symptoms of rhinorrhea and/or congestion tend to predominate. Relevant physical stimuli include low humidity, extremes in or rapid changes of temperature, and excessive air motion. Possibly linked to this diagnosis are *gustatory rhinitis* (rhinorrhea in response to the ingestion of spicy foods) and *bright-light rhinitis* (self-explanatory). The American Society of Heating, Refrigerating, and Air-Conditioning Engineers (ASHRAE) and the Occupational Safety and Health Administration (OSHA) have promulgated guidelines for temperature and humidity control in indoor air; these parameters should be assessed as part of any "problem building" investigation.

A. DIAGNOSIS AND MANAGEMENT

Although no routine diagnostic tests characterize this condition, methacholine or histamine sometimes have been used, in titrated doses, to document nonspecific nasal reactivity in this and other rhinitis syndromes (see "Diagnostic Techniques" below). Treatment of vasomotor rhinitis may include environmental intervention, nonspecific topical measures (e.g., saline lavage), or use of the topical anticholinergic agent ipratropium bromide. Decongestant nasal sprays should be used with caution because of potential tachyphylaxis and rebound.

REFERENCES

Brandt D, Bernstein JA: Questionnaire evaluation and risk factor identification for nonallergic vasomotor rhinitis. Ann Allergy Asthma Immunol 2006;96:526 [PMID: 16680922].

Staevska M, Baraniuk JN: Persistent nonallergic rhinosinusitis. Curr Allergy Asthma Rep 2005;5:233 [PMID: 15842962].

Wheeler PW, Wheeler SF: Vasomotor rhinitis. Am Fam Physician 2005;72:1057 [PMID: 16190503].

Other (Nonoccupational) Rhinitis Syndromes

Along with the rhinitis syndromes reviewed earlier, which may have occupational, nonoccupational, or mixed inciting factors, there are a number of other rhinitides that have not been linked with environmental exposures. These diagnoses are listed here for the sake of completeness in differential diagnosis.

• Nonallergic rhinitis with eosinophilia (NARES) syndrome
• Endocrine rhinitis (including rhinitis of pregnancy)
• Wegener granulomatosis
• Nasal polyposis
• Immotile cilia/Kartagener syndrome
• Cystic fibrosis

Paranasal Sinus Disease

Active smokers are at higher risk for developing acute (and chronic) sinusitis than are nonsmokers. Evidence for a link between sinusitis and environmental tobacco smoke exposure, on the other hand, is equivocal at this time. Relatively few studies have examined the endpoint of sinusitis and occupational exposures. Surveys of furriers, spice workers, vegetable picklers, hemp workers, and grain and flour workers all include increased prevalence rates for sinusitis, but these studies are based on self-reports only and should be viewed as preliminary. Pathophysiologically, the causal sequence for an occupationally induced (or exacerbated) sinusitis may include initial allergic or irritant rhinitis, ciliostasis (with impaired clearance of pathogenic organisms), mucous membrane swelling (with occlusion of sinus ostia and impaired drainage), and finally, infection. Clinically, a worker who recounts a story of apparent occupational rhinitis followed by sinusitis may well be describing a work-related condition. Cases refractory to antibiotic treatment should be revisited from the standpoint of allergen avoidance, irritant avoidance, or both.

Inflammation in the upper and lower respiratory tracts appears to be linked, in that active sinusitis apparently augments nonspecific bronchial reactivity in asthmatics. Postulated mechanisms include upregulation of neurogenic responses and aspiration of biochemical-mediator-laden nasal secretions into the lower respiratory tract. Another link between the upper and lower respiratory tracts occurs in the clinical triad of nasal polyposis, asthma, and aspirin sensitivity, although no occupational connection is known to exist with this syndrome.

A number of occupations and imputed exposures have been linked with the development of malignant neoplasms of the paranasal sinuses; these appear in Table 19–2. The strongest (and most consistent) findings pertain to leather- and woodworkers, although some studies also have found nickel refining, chrome refining and plating, and formaldehyde-exposed workers to be at risk.

Table 19–2. Agents and processes associated with sinonasal cancer.

Wood dust
Leather dust
Nickel refining
Chromates (Cr^{6+})
Cigarette smoking
Formaldehyde (?)
Mustard gas manufacturing
Isopropanol manufacturing (strong acid method)
Welding, flame cutting, and brazing(?)

? = possible association.

REFERENCES

Becher H et al: Occupation, exposure to polycyclic aromatic hydrocarbons and laryngeal cancer risk. Int J Cancer 2005;116:451 [PMID: 15810012].

Jansson C et al: Airborne occupational exposures and risk of oesophageal and cardia adenocarcinoma. Occup Environ Med 2006; 63:107 [PMID: 16421388].

Luc D et al: Sinonasal cancer and occupational exposures: A pooled analysis of 12 case-control studies. Cancer Causes Control 2002;13:147 [PMID: 11936821].

Laryngeal Pathology

Symptoms referable to phonation, typically, hoarseness, also can occur in work settings. Temporary and reversible hoarseness may occur either from exposure to inhaled chemical irritants or from overuse of the voice. Although overuse is most widely recognized in lecturers and singers, it also occurs among industrial employees who need to communicate (shout) in noisy environments. The most ominous condition heralded by hoarseness—squamous cell carcinoma of the larynx—is associated with a

Table 19–3. Agents and processes associated with laryngeal cancer.

Asbestos
Cigarette smoking
Ethanol consumption
Leather and textile workers(?)
Gasoline, diesel oil, mineral oil(?)

? = possible association.

number of occupations/exposures, which are listed in Table 19–3.

In terms of anatomically apparent lesions, two other occupational/environmental conditions deserve mention. Laryngeal strictures may occur after a smoke inhalation injury, resulting either from the initial chemical/thermal insult or secondary to prolonged intubation. In addition, laryngeal papillomatosis has been described in a physician whose apparent exposure was human papillomavirus aerosolized during laser surgery; this occurred despite the use of a conventional smoke extractor and paper mask during the procedure.

A final condition of note is so-called vocal cord dysfunction (VCD). VCD involves episodic stridor, hoarseness, shortness of breath, and globus (a pressure sensation in the glottic region). Because of overlapping symptoms and signs, VCD may be confused with asthma. In the occupational setting, VCD has been documented after acute irritant exposures in some individuals, giving rise to the diagnosis of irritant-associated VCD. Diagnosis of VCD involves documentation of paradoxical vocal cord motion (adduction during inspiration) on direct inspection (e.g., during flexible rhinolaryngoscopy). After ruling out more serious conditions (e.g., neoplasms, vocal cord paralysis, and spasmodic dysphonia), treatment consists of voice rest, hydration, and biofeedback/voice training under the supervision of a qualified speech pathologist.

REFERENCE

Williams NR. Occupational groups at risk of voice disorders: A review of the literature. Occup Med (Lond) 2003;53:456 [PMID: 14581643].

Otitis Media in Children

An increased incidence of otitis media with effusion has been reported among children exposed to environmental tobacco smoke, typically in the home. The highest risk appears to occur at approximately 18 months of age, although measurable excesses occur from at least ages 6 months to 3 years. Postulated mechanisms center on eustachian tube dysfunction, with environmental tobacco smoke–associated irritants producing ciliostasis and mucous membrane congestion, resulting in impaired pressure equalization, middle ear effusion, reduced drainage of middle ear secretions, and finally, infection. Because of the strength and consistency of this finding, the workup of recurrent otitis media in young children always should include questions about parental smoking.

REFERENCE

Heinrich J, Raghuyamshi VS: Air pollution and otitis media: A review of evidence from epidemiologic studies. Curr Allergy Asthma Rep 2004;4:302 [PMID: 15175145].

Sensory (Olfactory) Alterations

Both temporary and long-lasting alterations in olfactory function have been reported among workers exposed to a variety of industrial chemicals. Chemically induced olfactory dysfunction may include (1) quantitative defects, including hyposmia (reduced odor acuity) and anosmia (absent odor perception), and (2) qualitative defects, including olfactory agnosia (decreased ability to identify odors) and various dysosmias (distorted odor perception), including aliosmias (unpleasant sensations from normally pleasant odorants) and parosmias (phantom odors). Occupational groups and exposures for which defects in odor detection or identification have been identified include alkaline battery workers and braziers (cadmium ± nickel exposure), tank cleaners (hydrocarbon exposure), paint formulators (solvent ± acrylic acid exposure), and chemical plant workers (ammonia and sulfuric acid exposures); other groups have been studied less systematically. Toxicologically, hydrogen sulfide is well known to produce acute and reversible "olfactory paralysis" on exposure at levels in excess of approximately 50 ppm; the various mercaptans may share this property. Among patients with hyposmia or anosmia as a group, nasal obstruction is the most common etiology. Chemical irritant exposures may cause hyposmia via inflammation and consequent nasal obstruction or may produce direct damage to the olfactory epithelium itself.

Experimentally, at least one study has shown the olfactory equivalent of a *temporary threshold shift* (reversible olfactory deficit) after several hours of controlled exposure to either toluene or xylene; subjects recovered olfactory acuity within about 2 hours of cessation of exposure. Because the deficit was evident for the test odorant closely related to the experimental exposure (toluene) but not for a test compound unrelated to the exposure (phenyl-methyl carbinol), this phenomenon might be thought of as an extension of the familiar process of adaptation, in which odors lose their intensity during continuous exposure.

Of importance in the differential diagnosis, causes of olfactory impairment not directly related to chemical exposures include head trauma, chronic nasal obstruction (of whatever etiology), postinfectious inflammation, neurodegenerative and endocrine disorders, hepatic and renal disease, neoplasms, various drugs, ionizing radiation, congenital defects (e.g., Kallmann syndrome), and selected psychiatric conditions.

REFERENCES

Cheng SF et al: Olfactory loss in poly (acrylonitrile-butadiene-styrene) plastic injection-moulding workers. Occup Med (Lond) 2004;54:469 [PMID: 15486179].

Dalton P et al: Olfactory function in workers exposed to styrene in the reinforced-plastics industry. Am J Ind Med 2003;44:1 [PMID: 12822130].

Mascagni P et al: Olfactory function in workers exposed to moderate airborne cadmium levels. Neurotoxicology 2003;24:717 [PMID: 12900085].

DIAGNOSTIC TECHNIQUES

A number of different diagnostic techniques may be useful in the study of nasal responses to environmental agents; these have been classified here as routine, semiroutine, and experimental methods.

Routine Methods

Several techniques that are routine in otolaryngologic and allergy practice may contribute to the diagnostic workup of patients with upper airway conditions of suspected occupational or environmental origin.

A. ALLERGY SKIN TESTING

Often called *skin prick testing*, allergy skin testing is the most commonly applied diagnostic test in allergy specialty practices. In vitro allergy tests (RAST and ELISA) provide analogous (but not necessarily equivalent) data to skin testing and require less time and technical expertise on the part of the treating physician. Both techniques are used to identify antigen-specific IgE in clinically significant concentrations. Skin prick testing results in an acute skin reaction, with the size of a wheal being compared with saline and histamine controls, whereas the in vitro assays provide a quantitative estimate of allergen-specific IgE. Because of limited numbers of affected individuals, some occupational allergens may not be readily available as either skin test antigens or in vitro reagents.

B. NASAL CYTOLOGY

Nasal smears for cytologic analysis are used to provide information regarding the inflammatory cells in nasal mucus and/or the superficial mucosal layers. Various staining techniques are used to distinguish among cell types.

Typically, eosinophils predominate in allergic inflammation, whereas lymphocytes and neutrophils predominate with viral and bacterial infections, respectively. Based on both experimental and field studies of air pollutant effects, one would expect neutrophils to predominate in nasal smears taken from individuals with irritant rhinitis.

C. IMPEDANCE TYMPANOMETRY

This test is used to document middle ear pathology, including eustachian tube dysfunction and middle ear effusions. The technique is based on the premise that tympanic membrane impedance is increased (and sound energy conduction is decreased) if tympanic membrane mobility is restricted in any way and that the changes in sound conduction that occur with changes in externally applied pressure reveal the state of pressurization of the middle ear. Functionally, impedance tympanograms are classified as types A (normal), B (otitis media with effusion), and C (eustachian tube dysfunction). Impedance tympanometry is a valuable screening tool in children because it is objective, minimally invasive, and does not require a high degree of cooperation by the child being tested.

D. NASAL ENDOSCOPY

Nasal endoscopy—particularly that using a flexible scope—is a procedure that can be mastered by most primary care (including occupational medicine) clinicians. With an external diameter of less than 3.5 mm, the flexible nasopharyngoscope is generally well tolerated and permits the examiner to directly visualize nasal, pharyngeal, and glottic structures with relative ease. Identification of nasal polyps, purulent secretions per sinus ostia, lymphoid hyperplasia, neoplasms, vocal cord pathology, and other pathologic conditions becomes relatively straightforward using the flexible nasopharyngoscope. The examination requires use of both a topical anesthetic and a vasoconstrictor for optimal visualization and patient comfort. Some otolaryngologists prefer the use of rigid nasal endoscopes because of their superior optics; multiple instruments (with varying view angles) then may be needed in order to provide an adequate field of view.

Semiroutine Methods

In addition to routine techniques, there are several study methods that, in experienced hands, may prove valuable in diagnosing occupational or environmental upper airway conditions. These methods include

- Nasal peak-flow measurement
- Rhinomanometry
- Acoustic rhinometry
- Psychophysical testing
- Mucociliary clearance tests

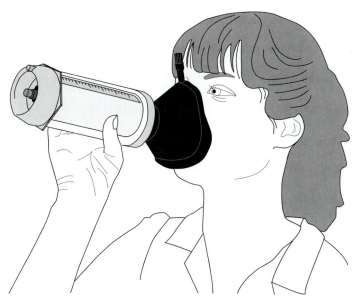

Figure 19–2. Commercial nasal inspiratory flow meter. (Courtesy of Clement-Clark International, Columbus, OH.)

A. NASAL PEAK-FLOW MEASUREMENT

Nasal inspiratory peak-flow measurement is not considered routine because the technique and equipment are not well known, not because of any technical difficulty involved. One readily available commercial unit consists of a Wright mini peak-flow meter mounted "backwards" within a transparent plastic cylinder, with an anesthesia mask mounted at the outlet of the flow meter (Figure 19–2). A stainless steel rod allows patients to reset the sliding pointer, which otherwise would be inaccessible within the plastic sleeve. To take a measurement, the patient breathes out maximally (to residual volume), places the mask over his or her nose and mouth, and then inhales forcefully through the nose to total lung capacity. Three replicate measures usually are taken, with the highest value being "counted." A diary of nasal peak-flow measurements (along with nasal symptom ratings) can be kept, with the patient recording peak flow before, during, and after a work shift, preferably over at least 1 work week and adjacent weekends (Figure 19–3). Interpretation of these data is very similar to the process of interpreting peak expiratory flow data in the diagnosis of occupational asthma, although no consensus standards exist for "significant" work-related decrements in peak flow. Inevitably, issues of trust arise in cases involving medical/legal issues; instructions consequently should be explicit with respect to technique but not with respect to expected data patterns.

B. RHINOMANOMETRY

Rhinomanometry, the measurement of nasal airway resistance, was first described using modified pulmo-nary function equipment in the mid-1960s. Basically, the technique involves measuring two pressure differentials—one across a precision flow resistor, or pneumotachometer (flow), and the other between the nasopharynx and anterior nares (pressure). Usually, the individual being tested wears a face mask (e.g., anesthesia mask) during testing, and the pressure within the mask is taken as anterior nasal pressure. Nasopharyngeal pressure, in turn, is measured in one of two ways. In anterior rhinomanometry, one nostril at a time is occluded with a pressure tap, and the subject breathes slowly through the opposite nostril. In posterior rhinomanometry, the subject holds a flexible tube between the tongue and hard palate and breathes slowly through both nostrils.

The two approaches to rhinomanometry have different strengths, weaknesses, and anatomic/patient cooperation requirements. Anterior rhinomanometry is particularly useful for documenting fixed anatomic pathology that may be unilateral in distribution (e.g., deviated septum or polyposis). Posterior rhinomanometry gives a more stable estimate of total nasal airway resistance than does the anterior technique and is therefore of particular utility in documenting the response of the nose to challenge agents (allergens or irritants). In anterior rhinomanometry, the pressure at the anterior nares on the occluded side can be taken as equal to nasopharyngeal pressure as long as flow is zero between the two points (the nares is indeed sealed), the nasal cavity on the occluded side is at least partially patent, and there is no septal perforation. The zero-flow requirement is also relevant in posterior rhinomanometry (i.e., the oral pressure

Name _____   ID No. _____

		Nasal Peak Flow			Please rate any symptoms (0–5)*					Notes
Date	Time	1	2	3	Nasal Con-gestion	Nasal Irritation	Runny Nose	Post-nasal Drip	Head-ache	

* Symptom rating: 0=None; 1=Slight; 2=Moderate; 3=Strong; 4=Very strong; 5=Overpowering.

Figure 19–3. Sample format for nasal symptom/nasal peak inspiratory flow rate diary.

tap is taken to be at the same pressure as the nasopharynx as long as the lips are tightly sealed). Although the other anatomic requirements do not pertain to the posterior technique, patient cooperation is sometimes problematic, with an estimated 10–15% of subjects being unable to produce usable curves without extensive coaching. Anterior rhinomanometry, on the other hand, requires minimal subject preparation.

Measurement conventions for rhinomanometry specify a location from which a line is drawn to the graphic origin (0 pressure, 0 flow) in order to estimate a slope that defines nasal airway resistance (NAR = pressure/flow). Alternatives include (1) the intersection of the pressure-flow tracing with a line of constant pressure (normally 150 Pa for anterior rhinomanometry and 75 Pa for posterior rhinomanometry), (2) the intersection of the pressure-flow tracing with an ellipse connecting specified pressure and flow intercepts (the Broms method), and (3) the point at which the pressure-flow tracing crosses a line of constant flow (e.g., 150 mL/s). Of these, the first two conventions have been favored. Figure 19–4 illustrates a single posterior rhinomanometry tracing that is interpreted by using different measurement conventions.

Factors influencing nasal airway resistance include chronic anatomic changes (see above), short-term physiologic changes (the so-called nasal cycle, in which the two sides of the nose alternately congest and decongest during the day), and reversible pathophysiologic processes (allergen- or irritant-induced vasodilatation or plasma extravasation, producing engorgement of the turbinates and encroachment on the airway). Other factors known to influence NAR include exercise (decreases) and recumbency (increases). NAR has been used as the endpoint for various pharmacologic challenge protocols, notably the use of serially increasing concentrations of histamine or methacholine designed to specify the concentration necessary to induce a predetermined percentage increase in NAR. Using this method, allergic rhinitis sufferers studied in and out of season show systematic differences in nonspecific nasal reactivity (greater during allergy season). This information is analogous to that provided by a bronchial methacholine challenge test and may be of equal utility in diagnosing occupational allergic or irritant rhinitis.

C. Acoustic Rhinometry

Acoustic rhinometry is another technique designed to measure nasal airway patency. The apparatus consists of a tube with an acoustic pulse generator (and microphone) at one end and a nasal speculum at the other; the instrument alternately sends and receives sound pulses. By measuring the intensity of reflected sound waves at various time intervals from the initial pulse, an acoustic rhinometer produces a map of total nasal cross-

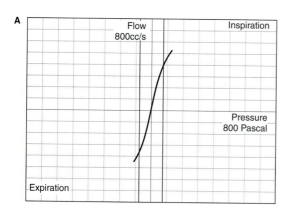

NAR = 211 Pa / L / sec

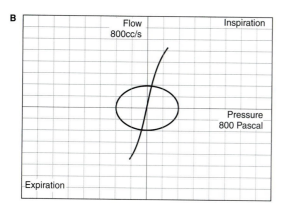

NAR = 190 Pa / L / sec

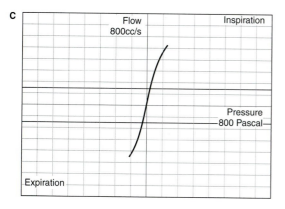

NAR = 143 Pa / L / sec

Figure 19–4. A single posterior rhinomanometry tracing interpreted using (*A*) the pressure-cutoff method (75 Pa), (*B*) the Broms method (200 units), and (*C*) the flow-cutoff method (150 mL/s). Note that the different methods yield different nasal airway resistance (NAR) values.

sectional area as a function of distance from the nares. The relationship between cross-sectional area and nasal airway resistance, however, is a complex one, rendering the physiologic and symptomatic interpretation of acoustic rhinometry even more difficult than is the case with rhinomanometry.

D. PSYCHOPHYSICAL TESTING

Psychophysical testing of olfaction focuses on one endpoint. Qualitative odor testing uses panels of test odorants to assess odor identification ability. Typically, such tests are administered as a multiple-choice task in order to prevent the patient's personal experiential background from having undue influence on testing results. One commercially available qualitative test, the University of Pennsylvania Smell Identification Test (UPSIT), takes the form of scratch-and-sniff panels on a paper or cardboard base for ease of administration; the test has been well standardized with adequate population norms. Quantitative odor testing takes two general forms: threshold and suprathreshold. Threshold testing usually involves a forced-choice discrimination task using an ascending (or, occasionally, descending) series of squeeze bottles with matching blanks. The concentration of the test odorant (usually dissolved in water or mineral oil) varies geometrically rather than arithmetically in accordance with the so-called Weber-Fechner law, which states that the perceived intensity of a stimulus varies with the log of its intensity. A threshold so obtained is an olfactory detection threshold. At least one commercial vendor (Sensonics, Haddon Heights, NJ) markets test odorants in prediluted bottles; again, the clinical utility of these test sets is predicated on their population standardization. A hybrid qualitative-quantitative test is the determination of the so-called olfactory identification threshold of a familiar odorant. Olfactory stimuli above threshold also can be rated quantitatively using a variety of systems, some of which allow for comparisons of the so-called psychophysical function (steepness of the rating response versus stimulus strength curve) between subjects.

E. MUCOCILIARY CLEARANCE TESTS

Mucociliary clearance tests include both invasive and noninvasive procedures. Perhaps the best standardized test is the observation of ciliary beat frequency in vitro. This method is often employed as a screening step (prior to electron microscopic examination of biopsy specimens) in the diagnosis of disorders involving ultrastructural abnormalities in epithelial cilia (e.g., primary ciliary dyskinesia, with or without full-blown Kartagener syndrome). Specimens typically are obtained either by scraping or biopsy of the inferior turbinate; ciliary beat frequency is normally in the range of 9–15 Hz. In addition to frequency, trained observers can note the degree of spatial coordination of adjacent ciliary units, an important component of intact function. Although ciliary beat frequency is a relatively objective and reproducible measure, its relationship to particle clearance and clinical symptoms is less constant, as noted below.

Another method of documenting mucociliary clearance involves tracking—radiographically—the movement of objects placed in the nasal cavity, typically on the superior surface of the inferior turbinate. The object in question may be a radiopaque disk or spherule (in which case imaging is by serial plain films) or a radiotagged particle that is tracked with a gamma camera. An obvious drawback of this technique is the exposure of patients (or experimental subjects) to small doses of ionizing radiation.

The so-called saccharine test is the least intrusive measure of nasal mucociliary dysfunction currently in use. In this procedure, a small grain of saccharine is placed on the anterior portion of the inferior turbinate, and the time interval before the subject tastes the saccharine is recorded. A prolonged test—defined as greater than 30 minutes—indicates impaired mucociliary function. The major drawback of the saccharine test lies in its lack of cross-test correlation with other mucociliary clearance measures.

Mucociliary clearance is important because of its essential function in microbial defense. Patients with impaired mucus formation (cystic fibrosis) or impaired ciliary function (primary ciliary dyskinesia) experience repeated episodes of bronchitis, otitis, and sinusitis, with ultimate cardiopulmonary complications (bronchiectasis and cor pulmonale) being a distinct likelihood. Environmental factors that have been noted to impair mucociliary clearance include viral infection, antigen challenge, cigarette smoke, and sulfur dioxide (see below).

Experimental Methods

A. Nasal Mucosal Blood Flow

Nasal mucosal blood flow is significant physiologically because engorgement of submucosal venous sinusoids produces reversible thickening of the nasal mucosa and a consequent decrease in airway cross-sectional area and increase in airway resistance. This parameter can be documented noninvasively by the use of laser Doppler flowmetry, enabling investigators to measure flow rate (per unit volume of tissue), mean red blood cell velocity, and tissue blood volume percent. The technique works on the principle that coherent light reflected from moving blood elements is shifted in frequency relative to incident (and reflected) light. A drawback of this technique is the requirement that a fiberoptic probe remain in relatively constant approximation to the mucosa, severely restricting an experimental sub-

ject's movement during provocation testing. Consistent with this limitation, provocation tests to date have focused on rapidly acting (pharmacologic or antigenic) stimuli. Notwithstanding these limitations, this technique could be adapted for irritant inhalation challenge tests in the future, particularly with such rapidly acting agents as environmental tobacco smoke.

B. Nasal Lavage

Nasal lavage is a technique used in experimental studies for examining the effect of allergens (or irritants) on inflammatory cell recruitment and biochemical mediators. Several specific techniques have been developed, including the use of aerosol sprays with either forced expulsion of lavage fluid or drainage under suction. Another set of techniques involves the introduction of several milliliters centimeters of warmed physiologic saline via syringe and nasal olive (plug), with subsequent withdrawal of the lavage fluid directly into the syringe. Potential parameters examined in nasal lavage fluid include (1) cell count and differential and (2) concentrations of biochemical mediators (e.g., histamine, tryptase, neuropeptides, cytokines, and leukotrienes) and markers of plasma transudation, glandular secretion (e.g., albumin, lactoferrin, and lysozyme), or both. Depending on the response patterns of these various markers, it may be possible to distinguish between allergic (mast cell–mediated) and neurogenic (parasympathetic and/or neuropeptide-mediated) response mechanisms to various provocation stimuli.

C. Chemosensory Evoked Responses

Chemosensory evoked responses include responses to olfactory nerve stimulation (olfactory evoked potentials) and responses to trigeminal nerve stimulation (chemosomatosensory evoked potentials). As is the case with other sensory evoked responses, special stimulus-delivery devices must be constructed to allow sharply demarcated pulsed stimuli to be presented to the target site (the nose). Electroencephalographic differentiation of these stimuli involves differing spatial patterns of recording potentials, with olfactory evoked potentials being more apparent in the parietocentral area and chemosomatosensory (or trigeminal) evoked potentials being stronger in the vertex. These techniques are of considerable theoretical importance, although, to date, their clinical applications have been explored to only a limited degree.

D. Irritant-Induced Mucosal Potentials

Irritant-induced mucosal potentials consist of negative voltage spikes that occur transiently with the onset of nasal irritant stimuli. Recording of these potentials requires the placement of an electrode in contact with the nasal septum, with the placement of a reference

Table 19–4. Controlled exposure studies of upper respiratory tract irritants.

Pollutant	Rhinomanometry	Nasal Lavage	Mucociliary Clearance	Mucosal Blood Flow
Ozone	Blocks exercise decongestion of nonallergics	↑ PMNs (+ eosinophils in allergic rhinitis)		
Sulfur dioxide	↑/nc NAR		↓ Clearance	
Environmental tobacco smoke (ETS)	↑ NAR*	nc histamine albumin, kinins	↓ Clearance	
Volatile organic compounds		↑ PMNs		
Carbonless copy paper	↑ NAR			
Ammonia, Cl₂, acetic acid	↑ NAR			
Capsaicin	nc NAR	nc histamine albumin, kinins; sl. ↑ TAME		Blood flow

↑ = Increased   NAR = Nasal airway resistance
↓ = Decreased   TAME = (tosyl-L-arginine methyl ester) esterase activity
"nc" = No change   * = Historically ETS-sensitive subjects only

electrode in a remote location. Interestingly, capsaicin desensitization, a method of reducing one's symptomatic response to irritant stimuli, simultaneously decreases this electrophysiologic response. This technique represents an important advance in recording technology, although its invasiveness may limit its use to research applications.

Controlled Exposure Studies of Upper Airway Irritants

A number of study techniques, listed earlier as either semiroutine or experimental, have been applied to the study of the upper airway response to chemical irritants under controlled circumstances. These studies appear in condensed form in Table 19–4. These studies are important because of their ability to isolate the effects of single exposures, in contrast to the multiple exposures in most work situations. In addition, some of these studies were structured to elucidate response mechanisms (e.g., allergic versus neurogenic). Pathophysiologically, the most important findings to date have come from studies of environmental tobacco smoke (ETS) exposure.

1. Approximately 25–30% of the general public report reacting to ETS with nasal symptoms, including congestion, rhinorrhea, postnasal drip, and sinus headache. Individuals with a history of allergic rhinitis are more likely than those without such a history to report nasal reactivity to ETS (and other air pollutants).

2. On average, individuals reporting more pronounced nasal reactivity to ETS do, indeed, respond to ETS challenge with greater increases in nasal airway resistance than do subjects who report that ETS does not bother them.

3. Despite the similarity of ETS-induced nasal symptoms to classical allergy, neither nasal lavage studies nor allergy skin testing supports the notion that the acute response to ETS in most individuals is allergically mediated.

4. Alternative response mechanisms to nasal irritants may include the two neurogenic pathways: central (parasympathetic) and local (axon) reflexes. The clinical implications of these pathways in air pollution situations have been largely unexplored.

REFERENCES

Illum L: Nasal clearance in health and disease. J Aerosol Med 2006; 19:92 [PMID: 16551220].

Kim JK et al: The effect of allergen provocation on the nasal cycle estimated by acoustic rhinometry. Acta Otolaryngol 2006; 126:390 [PMID: 16608791].

Occupational Lung Diseases

John R. Balmes, MD

The respiratory tract is often the site of injury from occupational exposures. The widespread use of potentially toxic materials in the environment poses a major threat to both the airways and lung parenchyma. The respiratory tract has a limited number of ways to respond to injury. Acute responses include rhinosinusitis, laryngitis, upper airway obstruction, bronchitis, bronchoconstriction, alveolitis, and pulmonary edema. Chronic responses include asthma, bronchitis, bronchiolitis, parenchymal fibrosis, pleural fibrosis, and cancer. Early recognition and appropriate treatment of occupational lung diseases by physicians can reduce both morbidity and mortality significantly and greatly affect patient outcome. This chapter focuses on common occupational lung diseases and on how to diagnose and manage them.

The site of deposition of inhaled materials depends on water solubility for gases and particle size for solids (Table 20–1). Water-soluble gases and particles with a diameter in excess of 10 μm tend to get deposited in the upper airways, whereas insoluble gases and smaller particles penetrate to the lower airways. Subsequent respiratory injury depends on both the site of toxin deposition and the type of cell/structure damaged.

EVALUATION OF PATIENTS WITH OCCUPATIONAL LUNG DISEASE

A careful evaluation can identify and diagnose occupational lung disease successfully in most cases. The following four approaches are recommended: (1) detailed history, including occupational and environmental exposures, (2) thorough physical examination, (3) appropriate imaging studies, and (4) pulmonary function testing.

History

A detailed history of both the patient's complaints and environmental/occupational exposures is essential. Work practices should be explored extensively with attention to types and durations of exposures, whether appropriate environmental controls are present, and if respiratory protective gear is used. If available, material safety data sheets (MSDS) should be reviewed. These documents profile the important health, safety, and toxicologic properties of the product's ingredients and under federal law must be fur-

nished by the employer to the worker or to the worker's health care provider on request.

If available, actual industrial hygiene data on the level of exposure and the agent to which the patient was exposed should be obtained. The history should include the condition of the patient's home, any hobbies, and social habits because exposures outside the workplace that contribute to or cause the lung injury may be discovered.

Physical Examination

Occupational lung diseases do not present with specific clinical findings. It is difficult, for example, to distinguish asbestosis from idiopathic pulmonary fibrosis or chronic beryllium disease from sarcoidosis. Only in the context of the exposure history will the correct diagnosis be made. A physician who suspects the presence of an occupational lung disease should, nonetheless, perform a complete physical examination rather than focus narrowly on findings suggested by the exposure history. Relevant nonoccupational disease otherwise may be missed.

The physical examination may be helpful if abnormal, but it is, in general, insensitive for detection of mild respiratory tract injury. The vital signs and the level of respiratory distress, if any, should be assessed. The presence of cyanosis and finger clubbing should be noted. Examination of the skin and eyes can yield signs of irritation and inflammation. Oropharyngeal and nasal areas should be inspected for inflammation, ulcers, and polyps. The presence of wheezing, rhonchi, or both is evidence of airways disease, and crackles are suggestive of the presence of parenchymal disease. Examination of the cardiovascular system for evidence of left ventricular failure is important when crackles are heard. The presence of isolated right ventricular failure suggests the possibility of cor pulmonale as a result of chronic severe lung disease with hypoxemia.

Imaging Studies

A chest radiograph should be part of the workup when lung disease is suspected. However, normal radiographic findings do not exclude significant damage to the lung. Immediately after toxic inhalational injury, the chest radiograph frequently is normal. On the other hand, dramati-

Table 20–1. Site of respiratory tract deposition and effect.

Water Solubility	Examples	Site of Injury
High	Ammonia, formaldehyde	Upper airway
Moderate	Chlorine, sulfur dioxide	Lower airways
Low	Nitrogen oxides, phosgene	Lung parenchyma
Particle Size (Aerodynamic Diameter)		
>10 μm	Dust from Earth's crust	Upper airway
2.5-6 μm	Some fire smoke particles	Lower airways
<2.5 μm	Metal fumes, asbestos fibers	Lung parenchyma

cally abnormal chest radiographs can be seen in individuals without significant lung injury who are exposed chronically to iron oxide or tin oxide. Abnormalities on the chest radiograph do not necessarily correlate with the degree of pulmonary impairment or disability. These are better assessed by pulmonary function testing and arterial blood gas determination.

With dust-exposed persons, chest films should be interpreted according to the International Labour Organization (ILO) classification for pneumoconiosis, in addition to the routine interpretation. The purpose of the ILO classification is to provide a standardized, descriptive coding system for the appearance and extent of radiographic change caused by pneumoconiosis. The classification scheme consists of a glossary of terms and a set of standard radiographs that demonstrate various degrees of pleural and parenchymal change caused by pneumoconiosis. The worker's posteroanterior chest film is scored in comparison with the standard films. In the United States, a certification process for readers using the ILO classification was developed under the auspices of the National Institute for Occupational Safety and Health (NIOSH). By NIOSH parlance, an "A reader" has taken the American College of Radiology (ACR) pneumoconiosis course but has not passed the certification examination. A "B reader" has taken the ACR course and passed the examination.

Computed tomographic (CT) scanning is a radiographic technique that scans axial cross sections and produces tomographic slices of the organ(s) scanned. Conventional CT scanning of the chest is better able to detect abnormalities of the pleura and the mediastinal structures than is plain chest radiography in large part because it is more sensitive to differences in density. When performed after the administration of intravenous contrast medium, CT scanning is considered to be the imaging study of choice for evaluation of the pulmonary hila.

High-resolution CT (HRCT) scanning incorporates thin collimation (1–2 mm as opposed to 10 mm in conventional CT) with high spatial-frequency reconstruction algorithms that sharpen interfaces between adjacent structures. Studies suggest that HRCT scanning is more sensitive than either conventional CT scanning or chest radiography for assessing the presence, character, and severity of a number of diffuse lung processes such as emphysema and interstitial lung disease.

Pulmonary Function Testing

Pulmonary function testing is used to detect and quantitate abnormal lung function. Measurement of lung volumes and diffusing capacity, gas exchange analysis, and exercise testing need to be performed in a well-equipped pulmonary function laboratory, but spirometry can and should be done in most evaluating centers. There are two different types of spirometers: volume- and flow-sensing devices. Modern computerized versions of both types of spirometers can produce exhaled volume-time and expiratory flow-volume curves. There are advantages and disadvantages to each type of spirometer. Whether a volume- or flow-sensing device is chosen, the best spirometers have comparable accuracy and precision. Performance requirements for spirometers of either type were described in a 1994 American Thoracic Society (ATS) statement.

The most valuable of all pulmonary function parameters are those obtained from spirometry, namely, forced expiratory volume in 1 second (FEV_1), forced vital capacity (FVC), and the FEV_1/FVC ratio. These parameters provide the best method of detecting the presence and severity of airway obstruction, as well as the most reliable assessment of overall respiratory impairment. The forced expiratory flow from 25–75% of vital capacity (FEF_{25-75}) and the shape of the expiratory flow-volume curve are more sensitive indicators of mild airway obstruction. A simple portable spirometer can be used to obtain the necessary measurements. Lack of patient cooperation, poor testing methods, and unreliable equipment can produce misleading results. The

1994 ATS statement contains criteria for the performance of spirometry, and NIOSH oversees courses for spirometry technicians that lead to their certification. Results of spirometry can be compared with predicted values from reference populations (adjusted for age, height, and sex) and expressed as a percentage of the predicted value. The presence of obstructive, restrictive, or mixed ventilatory impairment then can be determined from the comparison of observed with predicted values. Because the commonly used reference populations consist entirely of whites, there can be problems using predicted values to evaluate patients of nonwhite background. Typically, a 10–15% lowering of the predicted value is done to correct for the generally smaller lungs of nonwhites. A recent NIOSH study produced separate reference-value equations for whites, African Americans, and Mexican Americans.

Another commonly used single-breath test that reflects the degree of airway obstruction is the peak expiratory flow rate (PEFR). Portable instruments such as the mini-Wright peak-flow meter can be used for its measurement. The major limitation of the PEFR is that patient self-recording of measurements usually is done, and thus there is a potential for malingering. Despite this limitation, the test is useful in detecting changes in airway obstruction over time. In addition, the use of computerized instruments, although more expensive than simple mechanical peak-flow meters, avoids the problems of patient self-recording. Serial peak-flow measurements are especially valuable in the diagnosis of occupational asthma to document delayed responses after the work shift is over.

Because FVC can be reduced as a consequence of disease processes that either restrict airflow into or obstruct airflow from the lungs, differentiation of restrictive from obstructive processes often requires measurement of static lung volumes, that is, total lung capacity (TLC), functional residual capacity (FRC), and residual volume (RV). These lung volumes are measured by inert gas dilution or body plethysmography. Restrictive lung diseases cause a reduction in TLC and other lung volumes, whereas obstructive diseases may result in hyperinflation and air trapping, that is, increased TLC and RV:TLC ratio.

The diffusing capacity of the lung for carbon monoxide (DL_{CO}) is a test of gas exchange in which the amount of inhaled carbon monoxide absorbed per unit time is measured. The DL_{CO} is closely correlated with the capacity of the lungs to absorb oxygen. A reduced DL_{CO} is a nonspecific finding; obstructive, restrictive, or vascular diseases all can cause reductions. Nevertheless, the DL_{CO} is used often in combination with other clinical evidence to support a specific diagnosis or to assess respiratory impairment.

Bronchoprovocation Tests

Bronchoprovocation tests are useful in the diagnosis of occupational asthma. Pulmonary function responses to inhaled histamine and methacholine are relatively easy to measure and give an indication of the presence and degree of nonspecific hyperresponsiveness of the airways. A measure of airway obstruction, such as FEV_1, is obtained repeatedly after progressively increasing doses of histamine or methacholine so as to generate a dose-response curve. The test is usually terminated after a 20% fall in FEV_1. Patients with asthma typically respond with such a change in lung function after a relatively low cumulative dose of methacholine. Nonspecific challenge testing as described earlier is relatively inexpensive and can be performed on an outpatient basis. A recent ATS statement provides guidelines for the proper conduct of methacholine challenge.

Inhalation challenge testing with specific allergens thought to be causing occupational asthma also can be performed. Bronchoconstriction may occur early (within 30 minutes), late (in 4–8 hours), or in with a dual response (Figure 20–1). The occurrence of any of these responses after inhaled allergen is specific and diagnostic of occupational asthma. Unfortunately, specific inhalation challenge tests are both expensive and potentially hazardous. These tests should be performed only at specialized centers.

REFERENCES

Cockcroft DW et al: Methacholine challenge: Comparison of two methods. Chest 2005;127:839 [PMID: 15764765].

Miller MR et al: Standardization of spirometry. Eur Respir J 2005;26;319 [PMID: 16055882].

NIOSH: B reader certification: www.cdc.gov/niosh/pamphlet.html.

TOXIC INHALATION INJURY

Short-term exposures to high concentrations of noxious gases, fumes, or mists generally are a result of industrial or transportation accidents or fires. Inhalation injury from high-intensity exposures can result in severe respiratory impairment or death. The effects of inhaled irritants are also discussed in Chapter 30.

The site of injury depends on the physical and chemical properties of the inhaled agent. As discussed earlier, the site of deposition of an inhaled gas is determined primarily by water solubility. Other important factors are the duration of exposure and the minute ventilation of the victim. The concentration of an inhaled water-soluble gas such as ammonia is greatly reduced by the time it reaches the trachea because of the efficient scrubbing mechanisms of the moist surfaces of the nose and throat. In contrast, a relatively water-insoluble gas, such as phosgene, is not well-absorbed by the upper airways and thus may penetrate to the alveoli. The effects of inhalational exposure to toxic materials can range from transient, mild irritation of the mucous membranes of the upper airways to fatal adult respiratory distress syndrome (ARDS) (Table 20–2).

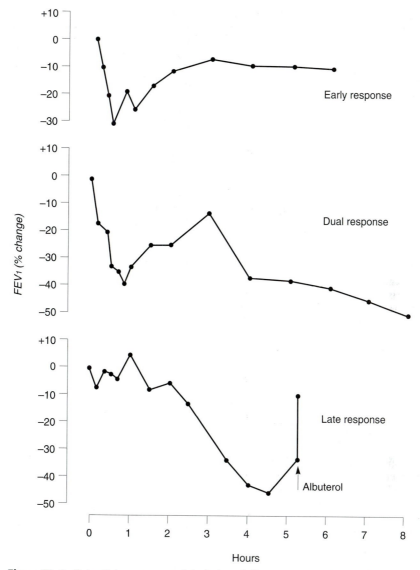

Figure 20–1. Potential responses to inhalation of allergen in sensitized workers with asthma.

The adverse respiratory effects depend on the concentration of the substances inhaled. Low-dose exposure to a water-soluble agent such as ammonia or chlorine usually produces local irritation of conjunctival membranes and the upper airway. Moderate exposure to such an agent can result in hoarseness, cough, and bronchospasm. Acute high-level exposure can cause ARDS. Because of poor water solubility, certain agents, such as phosgene and oxides of nitrogen, are only mildly irritating to the upper respiratory tract. Once inhaled and deposited in the lower respiratory tract, however, these agents are highly irritating

to the pulmonary parenchyma and may cause tissue necrosis. Long-term sequelae from toxic inhalation injury include bronchiectasis, bronchiolitis obliterans, and persistent asthma (see the discussion of irritant-induced asthma below).

Evaluation

Details about the exposure in most cases should establish the causative chemical. The more serious exposures generally occur after major spills from industrial or

Table 20–2. Potential effects of inhaled irritants.

Site of Injury	Acute Effects	Chronic Effects
Eye, nose, sinuses, oropharynx	Irritation, inflammation	Corneal scarring, nasal polyps
Upper airway	Laryngeal edema, upper airway obstruction	Laryngeal polyps
Lower airways	Tracheobronchitis, bronchorrhea, decreased mucociliary clearance	Asthma, bronchiectasis
Lung parenchyma	Pneumonitis, pulmonary edema/adult respiratory distress syndrome	Pulmonary fibrosis, bronchiolitis obliterans

transportation accidents or fires. Early effects depend on the level of exposure and may range from mild conjunctival and upper respiratory membrane irritation in low-dose exposures to life-threatening laryngeal or pulmonary edema in high-dose exposures.

The initial focus of the physical examination must be on the airway. If the nose and throat are badly burned, or if there is hoarseness or stridor, chemical laryngitis should be suspected. The presence of early wheezing suggests that the exposure was relatively heavy. Spirometry or peak-flow measurements may demonstrate airway obstruction relatively early after exposure.

The chest radiograph usually will be normal immediately postexposure. Chemical pneumonitis and pulmonary edema (ARDS) may develop within 4–8 hours of heavy exposure. Arterial blood gas measurements may show hypoxemia prior to radiographic evidence of parenchymal injury. Because of the relative lack of immediate signs and frequent delayed reactions to poorly water-soluble agents such as phosgene and oxides of nitrogen, patients exposed to significant concentrations of these agents should be observed for a minimum of 24 hours.

Management

Management of toxic inhalation injury should include immediate decontamination of exposed cutaneous and conjunctival areas by irrigation with water. If facial cutaneous burns are noted, direct laryngoscopy or fiberoptic bronchoscopy is recommended by some to assess for the presence of laryngeal edema. If present, endotracheal intubation should be considered. However, it is by no means clear as to who will develop life-threatening upper airway obstruction. A conservative approach of careful clinical monitoring of the victim in an intensive-care unit may be appropriate. If bronchoscopy is performed, evidence of significant inhalation injury includes erythema, edema, ulceration, and/or hemorrhage of the airway mucosa. If particulate material was inhaled, it may be visualized on the airway mucosa.

Simple spirometry or peak expiratory flow measurements to detect early airway obstruction are often quite useful. Flow-volume loops have been used both to diagnose upper airway obstruction and as a more sensitive detector of early lower airway obstruction and they do so better than simple spirometry or peak expiratory flow rates. Supplemental oxygen should be administered if there is any sign of respiratory distress. Wheezing should be treated with inhaled bronchodilator. Serial periodic clinical examinations, spirometry or peak-flow measurements, chest radiographs, and arterial blood gases are useful in monitoring progression of disease. There is no evidence to support the use of prophylactic antibiotics or the immediate use of corticosteroids in exposed patients.

Vigorous bronchial hygiene measures are required in those who develop severe tracheobronchitis. Drainage of mucus plugs and respiratory secretions should be encouraged by postural drainage, chest physical therapy, deep inspiratory maneuvers, and adequate hydration. If intubated, frequent suctioning of the airways should be performed to remove any adherent soot that may contain irritant and corrosive chemicals. Some authors recommend fiberoptic bronchoscopy to lavage off this adherent material.

Patients who develop pulmonary edema/ARDS require intensive-care-unit management, including mechanical ventilatory assistance. However, if such patients can be supported through the acute phase of the disease process, they may recover with no significant loss of lung function.

Controversy exists, however, about the potential for long-term pulmonary sequelae after toxic inhalation injury. For example, there are well-documented reports of persisting airway obstruction, nonspecific airway hyperresponsiveness, and sequential reduction in residual volume following acute chlorine gas exposure. Until this controversy is resolved, it would seem prudent to follow exposed individuals with periodic clinical examinations and pulmonary function testing for the development of any persistent respiratory impairment. Although there is no controlled experimental evidence to support the practice, a trial of corticosteroids can be considered in a patient who is not recovering promptly. Such a trial may be especially beneficial in a patient with bronchiolitis obliterans following inhalation injury.

OCCUPATIONAL ASTHMA

Asthma is characterized by airway obstruction that is reversible (but not completely so in some patients), either spontaneously or with treatment, airway inflammation, and increased airway responsiveness to a variety of stimuli. In occupational asthma, there is variable airway obstruction and/or airway hyperresponsiveness as a consequence of workplace exposure(s). Work-related variable airway obstruction can be caused by several mechanisms, including type I immune (immediate hypersensitivity) reactions, pharmacologic effects, inflammatory processes, and direct airway irritation. More than 250 agents in the workplace cause asthma, and the list is growing as new materials and processes are introduced. Work-aggravated asthma occurs when workplace exposures lead to exacerbations of preexisting nonoccupational asthma. In the United States, asthma occurs in approximately 5% of the general population. Work-related asthma (i.e., both occupational asthma and work-aggravated asthma) has been estimated to be 15–20% of all adult asthma.

There are two major types of occupational asthma. Sensitizer-induced asthma is characterized by a variable time during which *sensitization* to an agent present in the work site takes place. Irritant-induced asthma occurs without a latent period after substantial exposure to an irritating dust, mist, vapor, or fume. *Reactive airways dysfunction syndrome* (RADS) is a term used by some to describe irritant-induced asthma caused by a short-term, high-intensity exposure. Sensitizing agents known to cause occupational asthma can be divided into high-molecular weight (>1000 Da) and low-molecular-weight compounds (Table 20–3). High-molecular-weight compounds tend to cause occupational asthma via type I immunoglobulin E (IgE)–mediated reactions, whereas the mechanism(s) of low-molecular-weight compounds is (are)

unknown. Sensitizer-induced asthma is characterized by specific responsiveness to the etiologic agent. The mechanism of irritant-induced asthma is also unknown, but there is no clinical evidence of sensitization. Irritant-induced asthma involves persistent nonspecific airway hyperresponsiveness but not specific responsiveness to an etiologic agent. While there is no doubt that irritant-induced asthma can be caused by a single intense exposure (e.g., RADS), it appears that lower-level exposure over a longer duration of time (months to years) also can cause the disease.

Pathophysiology

Airway inflammation is now recognized as the paramount feature of asthma. Asthmatic airways are characterized by (1) infiltration with inflammatory cells, especially eosinophils, (2) edema, and (3) loss of epithelial integrity. Airway obstruction in asthma is believed to be the result of changes associated with airway inflammation. Airway inflammation is also believed to play an important role in the genesis of airway hyperresponsiveness.

Most of the research on mechanisms that mediate airway inflammation in asthma has focused on high-molecular-weight allergen-induced responses. In a previously sensitized individual, inhalation of a specific allergen allows interaction of the allergen with airway cells (mast cells and alveolar macrophages) that have specific antibodies (usually IgE) on the cell surface. This interaction initiates a series of redundant amplifying events that lead to airway inflammation. These events include mast-cell secretion of mediators, macrophage and lymphocyte activation, and eosinophil recruitment to the airways. The generation and release of various cytokines from alveolar macrophages, mast cells, sensitized lymphocytes, and bronchial epithelial

Table 20–3. Some agents causing occupational asthma.

Mechanism	Examples
Without "sensitization"	
Anticholinesterase effect	Organophosphate pesticide (agricultural workers)
Endotoxin effects	Cotton dust (textile workers)
Airway inflammation	Acids, ammonia, chlorine (custodial workers, paper manufacturing workers)
Airway irritation	Dusts, fumes, mists, vapors, cold (construction workers, chemical workers)
With "sensitization"	
High-molecular-weight agents	
IgE-mediated (complete allergens)	Animal and plant proteins (laboratory workers, bakers)
Low-molecular-weight agents	
IgE-mediated (haptens)	Antibiotics, metals (pharmaceutical workers, metal plating workers)
Mechanism undefined	Acid anhydrides, diisocyanates, plicatic acid (epoxy plastics and paints, polyurethane foams and paints, western red cedar products)

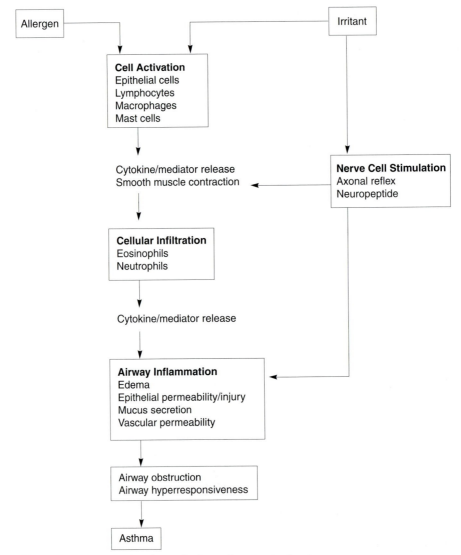

Figure 20–2. Proposed pathways in the pathogenesis of asthma.

cells are central to the inflammatory process (Figure 20–2). Cytokine networking, with both enhancing and inhibitory feedback loops, is responsible for inflammatory-cell targeting to the bronchial epithelium, activation of infiltrating cells, and potential amplification of epithelial injury. Adhesion molecules also play critical roles in the amplification of the inflammatory process. The expression of various adhesion molecules is upregulated during the inflammatory cascade, and these molecules are essential for cell movement, cell attachment to the extracellular matrix and other cells, and possibly cell activation. As noted earlier, the mechanism of low-molecular-weight sensitizer-induced asthma is not well

understood, although bronchial biopsy studies of affected workers clearly have demonstrated that airway inflammation is present.

Inhalation of the specific etiologic agent in a worker with sensitizer-induced asthma often will trigger rapid-onset but self-limited bronchoconstriction, called the *early response* (see Figure 20–1). In many sensitized workers, a delayed reaction will occur 4–8 hours later, called the *late response*. The late response is characterized by airway inflammation, persistent airway obstruction, and airway hyperresponsiveness. In some workers, there is a dual response, and in others, only an isolated late response (see Figure 20–1). Mast-cell degranulation and release of mediators such as histamine are believed to be responsible for the early response. The role of the mast cell in the genesis of the late response is more controversial, but the release of chemoattractant substances such as leuko-trienes, chemokines [e.g., regulated on activation, normal T-cell expressed, and secreted (RANTES) and interleukin-8 (IL-8)] and cytokines (e.g., IL-4, IL-5, and IL-13) may be involved in the influx of neutrophils and eosinophils into the airway epithelium. The eosinophil can release pro-teins (e.g., major basic protein, eosinophilic cationic pro-tein, eosinophil-derived neurotoxin, and enzymes), lipid mediators, and oxygen radicals that can cause epithelial injury. There is increasing evidence that lymphocytes, especially a CD4+ subset known as T-helper 2 (TH$_2$) cells, are involved in the release of cytokines that may activate both mast cells and eosinophils. In IgE-mediated allergic asthma, TH$_2$ cells may be responsible for the maintenance of chronic airway inflammation.

Although the mechanisms by which airway inflam-mation occurs in irritant-induced asthma are not well understood, neurogenic pathways may be involved (see Figure 20–2). The axonal reflex involving C-fiber stim-ulation and the release of neuropeptides have been implicated in models of irritant-induced airway inflam-mation. With high-level irritant exposure, direct chemi-cal injury can lead to an inflammatory response. The important unanswered question is what causes this response to persist in certain individuals.

As the sensitizer- or irritant-induced airway inflam-matory process proceeds, mucosal edema, mucus secre-tion, and vascular and epithelial permeability all increase, leading to a reduction of the caliber of the air-way lumen and resulting airflow obstruction (Figure 20–3). The level of airway obstruction in patients with asthma is a marker of the severity of disease. With mild asthma, there may be no evidence of obstruction between acute exacerbations, but nonspecific airway hyperresponsiveness is likely to be present. With more severe asthma, there is increased airway hyperrespon-siveness, and airway obstruction is present between attacks.

Two other mechanisms by which variable airway obstruction owing to workplace exposure can occur are reflex and pharmacologic bronchoconstriction. In reflex bronchoconstriction, neuroreceptors in the airway are stimulated by agents such as cold air, dusts, mists, vapors, and fumes. The reaction does not involve immunologic mechanisms and does not lead to airway inflammation. In most cases, the patient has a history of preexisting nonoccupational asthma with nonspecific airway hyper-responsiveness so that this is the primary mechanism of work-aggravated asthma. Pharmacologic bronchocon-striction occurs when an agent in the workplace causes the direct release of mediators (e.g., cotton dust in textile mills) or a direct effect on the autonomic regulation of

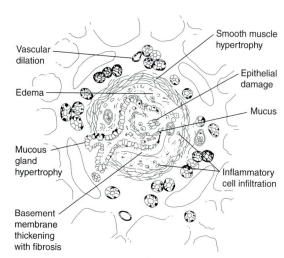

Figure 20–3. Morphologic changes in asthma.

bronchomotor tone (e.g., organophosphate pesticides inhibit cholinesterase).

Diagnosis

The diagnosis of occupational asthma is made by con-firming the diagnosis of asthma and by establishing a rela-tionship between asthma and the work environment. The diagnosis of asthma should be made only when both intermittent respiratory symptoms and physiologic evi-dence of reversible or variable airways obstruction are present. The relationship between asthma and workplace exposure may fit any of the following patterns: (1) symp-toms occur only at work, (2) symptoms improve on week-ends or vacations, (3) symptoms occur regularly after the work shift, (4) symptoms increase progressively over the course of the work week, and (5) symptoms improve after a change in the work environment.

At least one of the symptoms of wheezing, shortness of breath, cough, and chest tightness should occur while the worker is at or within 4–8 hours of leaving the work-place. Often the worker's symptoms improve during days off work or while away from the worker's usual job. With persistent exposure, the symptoms may become chronic and lose an obvious relationship to the workplace. Con-comitant eye and upper respiratory tract symptoms also may be noted. The diagnosis of occupational asthma also should be considered when there is a history of recurrent episodes of work-related "bronchitis" characterized by cough and sputum production in an otherwise healthy individual. While high-molecular-weight sensitizers typi-cally cause early or dual responses, the low-molecular-weight sensitizers tend to induce isolated late responses that may occur hours after the work shift is over.

The evaluation for possible occupational asthma requires a detailed history of the work environment (Figure 20–4). As noted earlier, attention should be given to the agents to which the worker is exposed, the type of ventilation in the workplace, whether respiratory protective equipment is used, and if possible, the level of exposure (i.e., whether it is high or low or if accidental exposure through spills ever occurs). A helpful clue to a significant problem in a workplace is the presence of other workers with episodic respiratory symptoms.

The detection of wheezing on chest auscultation is helpful, but the physical examination is frequently normal in asthmatic patients not currently suffering from an exacerbation. Chest radiographs are normal in most individuals with asthma because the disease involves the airways rather than the lung parenchyma. Hyperinflation and flattening of the diaphragms, indicating air trapping, may be seen during exacerbations. Fleeting infiltrates indicating mucus plugging and bronchial wall thickening reflecting chronic inflammation also may be noted.

As noted previously, spirometry for measurement of FEV_1 and FVC is the most reliable method for assessing airway obstruction. However, because asthmatic patients typically have reversible airway obstruction, they may have normal lung function during intervals between acute attacks. The response to inhaled bronchodilator administration has been used as a measure of airway hyperresponsiveness. A 12% improvement in FEV_1 of at least 200 mL after inhaled bronchodilator is how the American Thoracic Society (ATS) defines a significant improvement indicative of hyperresponsive airways. Across-work-shift spirometry, when available, can provide objective evidence of occupational asthma. A greater than 10% fall in FEV_1 across a work shift is suggestive of an asthmatic response.

Serial recording of PEFR over a period of weeks to months is often the best way to document the work-relatedness of asthma. The worker records his or her PEFR at least four times while awake, as well as respiratory symptoms and medication use. When interpreting the worker's log, attention should be given to any work-related pattern of change. A 20% or greater diurnal variability in PEFR is considered evidence of an asthmatic response (Figure 20–5). The major advantage of serial PEFR measurement over spirometry is the ability to detect late responses that occur after the work shift ends.

Methacholine or histamine challenge can demonstrate the presence of nonspecific airway hyperresponsiveness in a worker suspected of having occupational asthma who has normal spirometry. Such testing can be particularly valuable if it demonstrates an increase in airway responsiveness on returning to work or a decrease when away from work. Specific inhalational challenge testing, that is, challenging the patient with the suspected agent at levels and under conditions that mimic workplace conditions, can be done for medicolegal purposes or to determine the precise etiology in a complex exposure scenario. However, specific challenge testing is time-consuming, potentially dangerous, and usually should be reserved for evaluation of patients in whom there is diagnostic uncertainty.

Allergy skin tests with common aeroallergens can be used to establish whether or not the worker is atopic.

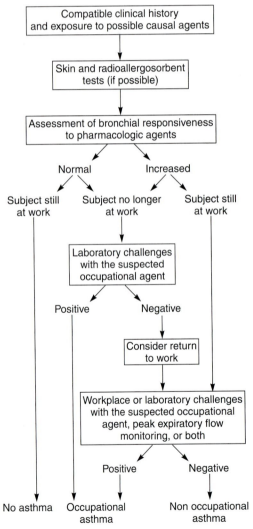

Figure 20–4. Algorithm for the clinical investigation of occupational asthma.

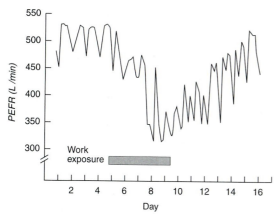

Figure 20–5. Serial peak expiratory flow rates (PEFRs) during a 16-day period in a worker with occupational asthma before, during, and after 1 week of exposure to the inciting agent.

Atopy is a risk factor for high-molecular-weight sensitizer-induced asthma. When high-molecular-weight compounds are responsible for occupational asthma, skin tests with the appropriate extracts may help to identify the etiologic agent. Extracts of materials such as flour, animal proteins, and coffee will give positive skin tests in specifically sensitized individuals. Skin testing also may be helpful for a few low-molecular-weight compounds such as platinum salts. IgE antibodies assayed by the radioallergosorbent test (RAST) or by enzyme-linked immunoabsorbent assay (ELISA) may confirm exposure to allergens such as flour, animal proteins, acid anhydrides, plicatic acid, or isocyanates. However, the presence of positive skin reactions and/or specific antibodies is not always correlated with the presence of occupational asthma.

Treatment

Acute asthma attacks requiring emergency management should be treated with supplemental oxygen, beta-agonists, corticosteroids, and if infection is suspected, antibiotics. Hospitalization should be considered in the more severe cases because of the potential for respiratory failure.

Once the diagnosis of occupational asthma is made, the primary intervention is to reduce or eliminate the worker's exposure to the offending agent. This may be achieved through modifications in the workplace. It may be possible to substitute the offending agent with another safer one. Improved local exhaust ventilation and enclosure of specific processes also may be helpful. With irritant-induced asthma, the use of personal protective equipment may lower exposures to levels that do not induce broncho-

spasm. Workers who are allowed to continue in the job should have regular follow-up visits, including monitoring of their lung function and nonspecific airway responsiveness. With sensitizer-induced asthma, however, the worker should be precluded from further exposure to the sensitizing agent. It may be necessary to completely remove the worker from the workplace because exposure to even minute quantities of the offending agent may induce bronchospasm. If a worker is required to leave the workplace (e.g., a baker with flour-induced asthma), the worker should be considered 100% impaired on a permanent basis for the job that caused the illness and for other jobs with exposure to the same causative agent.

In addition to reduction or elimination of exposure to any specific offending agent, the worker also should avoid exposure to other materials/processes that may exacerbate the worker's asthma, such as irritating dusts, mists, and vapors. Cessation of smoking and avoidance of exposure to environmental tobacco smoke are also essential.

Prevention

Prevention of further occupational asthma should be considered in all workplaces where cases are diagnosed. This can be achieved primarily through environmental control of processes known to involve exposure to potential sensitizers and irritants. Protection of workers by the use of appropriate ventilation systems, respiratory protective equipment, and worker education about appropriate procedures should be recommended. Avoidance of high-intensity exposures from leaks and spills that may initiate the development of occupational asthma is essential. Medical surveillance for early detection of cases also can contribute to reducing the burden of impairment/disability owing to occupational asthma.

Severity of Disease

Once occupational asthma has been diagnosed, an attempt should be made to classify the degree of impairment/disability. An approach to the evaluation of impairment in patients with asthma was developed by the ATS and has been adopted by the American Medical Association. Asthma is a dynamic disease that does not generally result in a static level of impairment. The criteria used for impairment rating are degree of postbronchodilator airway obstruction by spirometry, measurement of airway responsiveness, and medication requirements. Assessment of impairment/disability should be done only after optimization of therapy and whenever the worker's condition changes substantially, whether for better or worse.

Natural History

Multiple follow-up studies of workers with occupational asthma caused by such diverse agents as diisocyanates, snow crab, and western red cedar showed persistence of symptoms and the presence of nonspecific airway hyperresponsiveness for periods up to 6 years after removal from the offending agent. Factors that affect the long-term prognosis of the patient with occupational asthma are the total duration of exposure, the duration of exposure after the onset of symptoms, and the severity of asthma at the time of diagnosis. Those who do poorly have a delayed diagnosis, lower lung function values, and greater nonspecific airway hyperresponsiveness, hence the importance of early diagnosis and early removal from future exposure to the etiologic agent. Treatment with inhaled corticosteroid medications has been shown to improve prognosis for sensitizer-induced occupational asthma.

Specific Agents

A. DIISOCYANATES

Chemicals of the diisocyanate group are used widely in the manufacture of polyurethane surface coatings, insulation materials, car upholstery, and furniture. The most commonly used diisocyanate is toluene diisocyanate (TDI). Because of its high vapor pressure, the less volatile agent methylene diphenyl diisocyanate (MDI) is used in some production processes. Other diisocyanates, such as hexamethylene diisocyanate (HDI), naphthalene diisocyanate (NDI), and isophorone diisocyanate (IPDI), also have commercial uses. These chemicals are all highly reactive because of the presence of –N–C–O groups, which easily react with biologic molecules and are potent irritants to the respiratory tract. Upper respiratory tract inflammation occurs in almost everyone exposed to TDI levels of 0.5 ppm or more.

Five major patterns of airway response to TDI have been described in humans: (1) occupational asthma of the sensitizer-type, which occurs in 5–10% of exposed workers weeks to months after the onset of exposure, (2) chemical bronchitis, (3) acute but asymptomatic deterioration of respiratory function during a work shift, (4) chronic deterioration of respiratory function associated with chronic exposure to low doses, and (5) persistent asthma or RADS after exposure to high doses.

B. VEGETABLE DUSTS, INCLUDING COTTON (BYSSINOSIS), FLAX, HEMP, AND JUTE

Byssinosis occurs in certain workers in the cotton textile industry. The characteristic symptoms are chest tightness, cough, and dyspnea 1–2 hours after the patient returns to work after several days off. The symptoms usually resolve overnight and on subsequent days become milder until by the end of the work week the worker may become asymptomatic. The prevalence of byssinosis is higher in workers with longer duration of exposure and with greater respirable dust exposure, such as during opening bales and carding, and lowest in those with a shorter exposure history and with lesser dust exposure. The mechanism underlying byssinosis remains unclear. Cotton-dust extracts are capable of causing direct release of histamine and contain endotoxins that can induce a number of inflammatory responses.

C. METAL SALTS

Complex salts of platinum used in electroplating, platinum refinery operations, manufacture of fluorescent screens, and jewelry making are known to cause occupational asthma. Specific IgE antibodies to platinum salts conjugated to human serum albumin have been found in sensitized workers by RAST. Rhinitis and urticaria frequently accompany asthma, and this triad is sometimes called *platinosis*. Nickel, vanadium, chromium, and cobalt are other metals known to cause occupational asthma.

D. ACID ANHYDRIDES

Epoxy resins often contain acid anhydrides as curing or hardening agents. Phthalic anhydride, trimellitic anhydride (TMA), and tetrachlorophthalic anhydride (TCPA) are several of the more commonly used acid anhydrides. Occupational asthma occurs in a small percentage of exposed workers. The serum of affected workers typically contains specific IgE antibodies against acid anhydride–protein conjugates. Trimellitic anhydride exposure can give rise to four clinical syndromes: (1) symptoms of immediate airway irritation, (2) immediate rhinitis and asthma, (3) late asthma with systemic symptoms of fever and malaise, and (4) infiltrative lung disease (hemorrhagic alveolitis) with hemoptysis and anemia.

E. WOOD DUSTS

A large number of wood dusts are known to cause rhinitis and asthma. Western red cedar is the best studied. This wood contains the low-molecular-weight compound plicatic acid, which is believed to be responsible for causing asthma through an unclear mechanism. Western red cedar asthma falls under the category of low-molecular-weight sensitizer-induced asthma and clinically is much like diisocyanate asthma. There is often a long period between onset of exposure and onset of symptoms, and asthma only develops in a small proportion of exposed subjects. A small dose of plicatic acid can induce a severe asthmatic attack in a sensitized individual, and many workers continue to have persistent asthma years after cessation of exposure.

REFERENCES

Le Moual N et al. Asthma severity and exposure to occupational asthmogens. Am J Respir Crit Care Med 2005;172:440 [PMID: 15961697].

Mapp CE et al: Occupational asthma. Am J Respir Crit Care Med 2005;172:280 [PMID: 15860754].

HYPERSENSITIVITY PNEUMONITIS

Hypersensitivity pneumonitis, also known as *extrinsic allergic alveolitis,* refers to an immunologically mediated inflammatory disease of the lung parenchyma that is induced by inhalation of organic dusts that contain a variety of etiologic agents (e.g., bacteria, fungi, amebae, animal proteins, and several low-molecular-weight chemicals). Although many different antigens are capable of causing hypersensitivity pneumonitis (Table 20–4), the basic clinical and pathologic findings are similar regardless of the nature of the inhaled dust. The nature of the inhaled antigen, the exposure conditions, and the nature of the host immune response all contribute to the risk for the disease. Hypersensitivity pneumonitis is characterized initially by a lymphocytic alveolitis and granulomatous pneumonitis, with improvement or complete resolution if antigen exposure is terminated early. Continued antigen exposure may lead to progressive interstitial fibrosis.

The pathogenesis of hypersensitivity pneumonitis involves repeated inhalational exposure to the antigen, sensitization of the exposed individual, and immunologically mediated damage to the lung. The inflammatory response that results in hypersensitivity pneumonitis appears to involve a combination of humoral, immune complex–mediated (type III), and cell-mediated (type IV) immune reactions to the inhaled antigen. In the presence of excess antigen, immune complexes may be deposited in the lungs. These complexes activate complement, leading to an influx of neutrophils. The local immune response later shifts to a T-lymphocyte-predominant alveolitis, with a differential cell count in bronchoalveolar lavage (BAL) fluid of up to 70% lymphocytes. Examination of BAL lymphocyte subpopulations in patients with hypersensitivity pneumonitis often has revealed a predominance of CD8+ suppressor/cytoxic cells. The periph-

Table 20–4. Some agents causing hypersensitivity pneumonitis.

Antigen	Exposure	Syndrome
Bacteria		
Faenia rectivirgula	Moldy hay	Farmer's lung
Thermoactinomycetes vulgaris	Moldy grain, compost	Grain worker's lung, mushroom worker's lung
Thermoactinomycetes sacchari	Moldy sugar cane fiber	Bagassosis
Thermoactinomycetes candidus	Heated water reservoirs	Humidifier lung
Bacillus subtilus	Detergent	Detergent worker's lung
Fungi		
Aspergillus clavatus	Moldy malt	Malt worker's lung
Penicillium casei	Moldy cheese	Cheese worker's lung
Penicillium frequentans	Moldy cork dust	Suberosis
Cryptostroma corticale	Moldy maple bark	Maple bark stripper's lung
Aureobasidium pullulans	Moldy redwood dust	Sequoiosis
Graphium spp.		
Amoebae		
Naegleria gruberi	Contaminated water	Humidifier lung
Acanthamoeba castellani		
Animal proteins		
Avian proteins	Bird droppings, feathers	Bird breeder's lung
Rodent proteins	Urine, sera, pelts	Animal handler's lung
Wheat weevil	Infested flour	Wheat weevil lung
Chemicals		
Toluene diisocyanate	Paints, coatings	Isocyanate lung
Hexamethylene diisocyanate		
Diphenylmethane diisocyanate	Polyurethane foam	
Trimellitic anhydride	Epoxy resins, paints	Trimellitic anhydride pulmonary hemorrhage-anemia syndrome

eral blood and BAL T lymphocytes from patients with hypersensitivity pneumonitis will proliferate and undergo blastogenic transformation with cytokine generation when exposed in vitro to antigen. Animal models also support the role of cell-mediated immunity in the disease. Passive transfer of lymphocytes from sensitized animals to unexposed, nonsensitized animals results in a hypersensitivity pneumonitis–like disease when the latter animals subsequently are exposed to the specific antigen by inhalation. Alveolar macrophages also may play an important role in the pathogenesis of the disease by processing and presenting inhaled antigen to T-helper lymphocytes, as well as by releasing cytokines, which may help to amplify the inflammatory response.

Because only a small number of exposed persons ever develop hypersensitivity pneumonitis, the underlying mechanism of the disease may be a form of immune dysfunction in which a normal host defense response cannot be appropriately downregulated. This immune dysfunction may be, at least in part, genetically mediated. Other environmental factors also may be involved because a number of studies show that hypersensitivity pneumonitis occurs more frequently in nonsmokers than in smokers.

Diagnosis

Inhalational exposure to antigen in a sensitized individual may result in either an acute or chronic presentation of hypersensitivity pneumonitis depending on the exposure conditions. The acute and more common form of presentation of hypersensitivity pneumonitis usually occurs within 4–6 hours of an intense exposure to the offending antigen. Symptoms of chills, fever, malaise, myalgia, cough, headache, and dyspnea are noted commonly. Physical examination may reveal a relatively ill-appearing patient with bibasilar inspiratory crackles on chest auscultation. Frequently, acute hypersensitivity pneumonitis is misdiagnosed as an acute viral syndrome or pneumonia because it tends to closely mimic these conditions. Laboratory findings include peripheral blood leukocytosis with increased neutrophils and a relatively decreased lymphopenia. Arterial blood gas values may show hypoxemia.

Chest radiographic findings may be completely normal even in symptomatic individuals. Typically, however, the acute phase is associated with the presence of a reticulonodular pattern. Patchy densities that tend to coalesce also may be seen. These infiltrates usually are bilaterally distributed, but a more focal presentation sometimes occurs.

Pulmonary function testing may reveal a decrease in the FEV_1 and FVC with an unchanged FEV_1/FVC ratio consistent with a restrictive impairment. A decrease in the DL_{CO} reflecting impaired gas exchange also is typical

of the acute presentation. The acute form generally progresses for up to 18–24 hours and then begins to resolve. Recurrence of the syndrome may be seen subsequently with reexposure to the antigen.

Recurrent low-level exposure to an appropriate antigen may result in the insidious onset of chronic interstitial lung disease with fibrosis. Progressive respiratory impairment with symptoms of dyspnea, cough, excessive fatigue, and weight loss may develop without acute episodes. Physical examination may reveal cyanosis, clubbing, and inspiratory crackles. Chest radiographic findings include diffusely increased linear markings and reduced lung size. Findings on HRCT scanning of the chest include centrilobular micronodules, ground-glass opacification, patchy airspace consolidation, and linear densities. Chest CT findings can be suggestive of the diagnosis of hypersensitivity pneumonitis but are not always pathognomonic. Pulmonary function testing usually will show a restrictive impairment with a decreased DL_{CO}, although some patients may be seen with a mixed or obstructive pattern.

The diagnosis of hypersensitivity pneumonitis should be suspected in patients with episodic respiratory symptoms and evidence of fleeting infiltrates on chest radiographs or restrictive impairment on pulmonary function testing. A careful history may elicit the onset of respiratory symptoms with exposure to the offending antigen. The temporal relationship of symptom development after exposure is crucial to the diagnosis. Additional supporting evidence is provided by the remission of symptoms and signs after cessation of exposure to the antigen and their reappearance on reexposure. The home environment also can be a source of the offending antigen. Workplace and home inspections may provide information supportive of the diagnosis (e.g., evidence of mold or water damage).

Serologic studies demonstrating specific IgG precipitating antibodies by the traditional double-immuno-diffusion technique will be positive in most patients with hypersensitivity pneumonitis if the correct antigen is used, although such antibodies are also detected frequently in exposed individuals who are healthy. False-positive results may be obtained with the use of more sensitive assays for IgG, such as ELISA. False-negative results frequently are a result of the failure to test for the correct antigen. Most commercially available hypersensitivity pneumonitis panels involve only a limited number of common antigens. Inhalational challenge studies with the suspected antigen may assist in the diagnosis of hypersensitivity pneumonitis. Antigen extracts may be administered in an aerosolized form followed by serial pulmonary function testing. Specific challenge testing should be conducted only by a laboratory experienced in the technique. While such challenges provide the "gold standard" method of confirming a direct relationship between a suspected offending antigen and the disease process, workplace studies involving the actual conditions of patient exposure are safer and usually easier to conduct.

As noted earlier, analysis of BAL fluid obtained by fiberoptic bronchoscopy in patients with hypersensitivity pneumonitis often demonstrates an increased percentage of T lymphocytes that are primarily CD8+ suppressor cells. In sarcoidosis, another condition characterized by increased T lymphocytes in BAL, the predominant cells are of the CD4+ helper subtype.

Lung biopsy may be necessary to make the diagnosis in difficult cases, such as those with the chronic form and an insidious presentation of dyspnea. Video-assisted thoracoscopic surgery (VATS) or open lung biopsy is preferred because transbronchial biopsy may not provide adequate tissue for pathologic differentiation of hypersensitivity pneumonitis from other diseases such as sarcoidosis. In acute or early chronic (subacute) hypersensitivity pneumonitis, there is patchy infiltration of predominantly lymphocytes in a bronchocentric distribution, usually with accompanying epithelioid (i.e., noncaseating) granulomas. The granulomas are likely what appear as centrilobular micronodules on HRCT scanning. In chronic hypersensitivity pneumonitis, peribronchiolar inflammation remains prominent, and bronchiolitis obliterans is common. Large histiocytes with foamy cytoplasm may be seen in the alveoli and interstitium. Interstitial fibrosis with honeycombing occurs in advanced disease, by which time granulomas no longer may be evident.

Treatment

The key to successful treatment of hypersensitivity pneumonitis is avoidance of the offending antigen. As described for occupational asthma, this may be achieved by product substitution or institution of effective engineering controls. Respiratory protective equipment also may be appropriate in situations where possible exposure is only occasional. If persistence of symptoms occurs despite engineering control measures and respiratory protective equipment, complete removal of the worker from exposure is necessary.

Corticosteroids remain the mainstay of treatment of patients with severe or progressive hypersensitivity pneumonitis, despite the lack of controlled data regarding the effect of these agents on the disease process. An empirical trial of prednisone (1 mg/kg per day), with monitoring of chest radiographic and pulmonary function changes 1 month after starting the trial, is a reasonable approach. Therapy should be continued until there is significant clinical improvement. If bronchospasm is present, beta-agonists should be administered. Supplemental oxygen should be given to patients with hypox-

emia, and intensive-care-unit support may be needed in particularly severe acute cases.

Workers with a diagnosis of hypersensitivity pneumonitis should have frequent follow-up, especially if continued exposure to antigen is possible. Significant pulmonary morbidity may occur if persistent exposure is allowed.

REFERENCES

Jacobs RL et al: Hypersensitivity pneumonitis. Ann Allergy Asthma Immunol 2005;95;115 [PMID: 16136760].

Mohr LC: Hypersensitivity pneumonitis. Curr Opin Pulm Med 2004;10:401 [PMID: 1531644].

INHALATION FEVERS

Inhalation fever refers to several syndromes that are characterized by short-term but debilitating flulike symptoms after exposure to organic dusts, polymer fumes, and metal fumes (Table 20–5). In addition to fever, the symptoms include chills, myalgia, headache, malaise, cough, and chest discomfort. In contrast to occupational asthma and hypersensitivity pneumonitis, which require susceptibility and/or sensitization, the attack rate for the inhalation fevers is high; that is, most people will experience symptoms as a result of high-level exposure to the etiologic agents.

Metal Fume Fever

Inhalation of certain freshly formed metal oxides can cause metal fume fever, an acute self-limiting flulike ill-

Table 20–5. Some agents causing inhalation fever.

Agent	Syndrome
Metals Zinc Copper Magnesium	Metal fume fever
Teflon pyrolysis products Polytetrafluoroethylene	Polymer fume fever
Bioaerosols Contaminated water	Humidifier fever
Moldy silage, compost, wood chips	Organic dust toxic syndrome
Sewage sludge	
Cotton, jute, hemp, flax dust	Mill fever
Grain dust	Grain fever

ness. The most common cause of this syndrome is the inhalation of zinc oxide, which is generated from molten bronze or welding galvanized steel. The oxides of only two other metals, copper and magnesium, have been proven to cause metal fume fever. When zinc is heated to its melting point, zinc oxide fumes are generated. The particle size of the generated fumes ranges from 0.1–1.0 μm in diameter, although aggregation with the formation of larger particles occurs readily. The underlying pathogenesis of metal fume fever is incompletely understood. However, there is evidence from controlled human exposure studies that zinc oxide fume inhalation induces a leukocyte recruitment to the lungs with an associated release of cytokines, which causes systemic symptoms.

It is estimated that more than 700,000 workers in the United States are involved in welding operations, so the potential for inhalational exposure and metal fume fever is great. The clinical syndrome begins 3–10 hours after exposure to zinc oxide. The initial symptom may be a metallic taste associated with throat irritation and followed within several hours by the onset of fever, chills, myalgia, malaise, and a nonproductive cough. Occasionally, nausea, vomiting, and headache are noted. Physical examination during the episode may reveal a febrile patient with crackles on auscultation of the chest. Laboratory evaluation frequently reveals a leukocytosis with a left shift and an elevated serum lactate dehydrogenase level. The chest radiograph, pulmonary function tests, and arterial blood gas measurements usually are normal. Transient chest radiographic infiltrates and reduced lung volumes and DL_{CO} have been reported in severe cases. Signs and symptoms generally peak at 18 hours and resolve spontaneously with complete resolution of abnormalities within 1–2 days.

Treatment of metal fume fever is entirely symptomatic. Control of elevated body temperature by antipyretics and oxygen therapy for hypoxemia may be required. There is no evidence that steroid therapy is of any benefit. Prevention relies on appropriate engineering controls and/or personal protective equipment to reduce exposure. There are no good data on the long-term sequelae of repeated exposures.

Polymer Fume Fever

A syndrome similar to metal fume fever may occur after inhalation of combustion products of polytetrafluoroethylene (Teflon) resins. The properties of Teflon—strength, thermal stability, and chemical inertness—make it a widely used product in the manufacture of cooking utensils, electric appliances, and insulating material. When Teflon is heated to temperatures greater than 300°C (572°F), numerous degradation products are formed that appear to cause the syndrome. Exposure to such combustion prod-

ucts can occur during welding of metal coated with Teflon, during the operation of molding machines, and while smoking cigarettes contaminated with the polymer.

Exposure to a high concentration of polymer fumes causes a fever to develop within several hours. Often this occurs toward the end of the work shift or in the evening after work. The symptoms, signs, and laboratory findings of polymer fume fever are essentially the same as those of metal fume fever. The syndrome is self-limiting and resolves within 12–48 hours. Exposure to very high concentrations of polymer fumes may lead to the development of severe chemical pneumonitis with pulmonary edema. In such cases, the symptoms, signs, and laboratory features are similar to pulmonary edema from other causes.

Organic Dust Toxic Syndrome

Inhalation of various bioaerosols contaminated with fungi, bacteria, and/or endotoxins can cause an acute febrile syndrome known as *organic dust toxic syndrome* (ODTS). Exposures to moldy silage, moldy wood chips, compost, sewage sludge, grain dust (grain fever), cotton dust (mill fever), animal confinement building environments, and contaminated humidifier mist (humidifier fever) are associated with the development of inhalation fever. The clinical syndrome of ODTS is essentially identical to that described earlier for metal or polymer fume fever. Severe pulmonary inflammatory reactions have been described with massive exposures, but these are rare.

REFERENCES

El-Zein M et al: Is metal fume fever a determinant of welding related respiratory symptoms and/or increased bronchial responsiveness? Occup Environ Med 2005;62:688 [PMID: 16169914].

Seifert SA et al: Organic dust toxic syndrome. J Toxicol Clin Toxicol 2003;41:185 [PMID: 12733858].

METAL-INDUCED LUNG DISEASE

Hard Metal

Hard metal is a cemented alloy of tungsten carbide with cobalt, although other metals, such as titanium, tantalum, chromium, molybdenum, or nickel, also may be added. These cemented carbides have found wide industrial use because of their properties of extreme hardness, strength, and heat resistance. Their major use is in the manufacture of cutting tools and drill-tip surfaces.

Workers exposed to hard metal are at risk for developing interstitial lung disease, so-called hard-metal disease, and occupational asthma. The putative cause of both these disease processes is cobalt. Some workers may present with features of both hard metal–induced airway and parenchymal diseases. Workers at risk for these diseases are those engaged in the manufacture of the alloy, grinders and sharpeners of hard metal tools, and diamond polishers and others who use disks containing cobalt and metal coaters who use powdered hard metal. Occupational asthma caused by cobalt in hard-metal workers is similar to that caused by other low-molecular-weight sensitizer agents.

Workers with hard-metal disease typically complain of symptoms of dyspnea on exertion, cough, sputum production, chest tightness, and fatigue. Physical examination may reveal evidence of crackles on chest auscultation, reduced chest expansion, clubbing, and in advanced cases, cyanosis. Chest radiographs may show bilateral rounded and/or irregular opacities with no pathognomonic features. Pulmonary function tests tend to show both a restrictive ventilatory impairment and a decreased DL_{CO}. The diagnosis of hard-metal disease often is made on the basis of pathologic examination of lung tissue rather than by clinical evaluation. The histologic findings are those of interstitial pneumonitis, frequently of the giant-cell type (e.g., giant-cell interstitial pneumonia), and interstitial fibrosis. Characteristic multinucleated giant histiocytes may be seen in BAL fluid as well.

The primary treatment of hard-metal disease is removal of the affected worker from further exposure. Relatively rapid progression to impairment is not infrequent, and resolution after cessation of exposure may not occur. Complete removal from cobalt exposure is advisable because a case has been reported of a worker who developed rapidly fatal lung disease with continued exposure. Because hard-metal disease is often progressive, empirical therapy with corticosteroids may be required.

Beryllium

Beryllium is a light-weight, tensile metal that has a high melting point and good alloying properties. It has a wide range of applications in modern industrial processes. Although beryllium is no longer used in the manufacture of fluorescent light tubes, it is used commonly in the ceramics, electronics, aerospace, and nuclear weapons/power industries. Workers at risk are those involved in processes that generate airborne beryllium, including melting, casting, grinding, drilling, extracting, and smelting of beryllium. Acute beryllium-induced pneumonitis can occur after high-intensity exposure but has largely disappeared owing to improved workplace control of exposures. Chronic beryllium disease, which involves sensitization to the metal through a cell-mediated (type IV) mechanism, still occurs after lower-level exposures in susceptible workers. Beryllium can be phagocytosed by macrophages that present beryllium antigen to lymphocytes, resulting in sensitization and proliferation of beryl-

lium-specific CD4+ T cells. Beryllium-activated T cells may release various cytokines and other inflammatory mediators, resulting in granuloma formation. Latency from time of initial beryllium exposure to the development of clinically manifest disease ranges from months to many years.

Why only a small percentage of an exposed population becomes sensitized to beryllium is not well understood. Recent studies have found a genetic marker of risk for beryllium sensitization, a glutamic acid substitution in residue 69 of the beta chain of the major histocompatibility complex molecule HLA-DP.

Chronic beryllium disease is a granulomatous inflammatory disorder that is very similar to sarcoidosis. In fact, the histologic findings in chronic beryllium disease are identical to those of sarcoidosis; that is, epithelioid (noncaseating) granulomas with mononuclear cell infiltrates and varying degrees of interstitial fibrosis. Chronic beryllium disease usually affects only the lungs, but involvement of skin, liver, spleen, salivary glands, kidney, and bone may occur. Extrapulmonary involvement is less common than in sarcoidosis.

Workers with chronic beryllium disease commonly present with insidious onset of dyspnea on exertion, cough, and fatigue. Anorexia, weight loss, fever, chest pain, and arthralgias also may occur. Physical examination findings usually are confined to the lungs, with crackles being the most common, but they may be absent with mild disease.

Chest radiographic findings are ill-defined nodular or irregular opacities and hilar adenopathy. The latter is seen somewhat less frequently (up to 40% of patients) than in sarcoidosis and rarely occurs in the absence of parenchymal changes. The small nodular opacities sometimes are more prominent in the upper lung zones and may coalesce into more conglomerate masses. High-resolution CT scanning is more sensitive than plain chest radiography, but histologically confirmed cases occur with normal scans.

Pulmonary function testing may be normal with mild disease, but there is usually a restrictive, obstructive, or mixed pattern of impairment and a reduced DL_{CO}. Resting arterial hypoxemia and further desaturation with exercise are common with more severe disease.

Often a meticulously obtained occupational history is required to suggest beryllium as the causative agent. Because of the similarity between chronic beryllium disease and sarcoidosis, demonstration of beryllium sensitization is necessary to confirm the diagnosis. A relatively specific blood lymphocyte proliferation test (LPT) is available in which the beryllium-specific uptake of radiolabeled DNA precursors by the patient's lymphocytes cultured in vitro is quantitated. The sensitivity of the LPT for chronic beryllium disease is greater than 90% when using peripheral blood lymphocytes and can be increased if lung lymphocytes obtained from BAL are used. The blood LPT also can be used to screen for sensitization among beryllium-exposed workers.

The current criteria for the diagnosis of chronic beryllium disease are (1) a history of beryllium exposure, (2) a positive peripheral blood or BAL LPT, and (3) the presence of epithelioid granulomas and mononuclear infiltrates, in the absence of infection, in lung tissue. This approach relies on the LPT to confirm sensitization to beryllium and transbronchial biopsy of lung tissue to confirm the presence of disease.

Because the disease process involves a type of hypersensitivity, a worker with chronic beryllium disease should be completely removed from further beryllium exposure. A trial of corticosteroids is warranted in symptomatic workers with documented pulmonary physiologic abnormalities because this may induce a remission in some. If steroid therapy is initiated, objective parameters of response such as chest radiographs and pulmonary function test results should be monitored serially in order to adjust appropriately the dose and duration of treatment. Chronic beryllium disease has the propensity to develop into chronic irreversible pulmonary fibrosis, so careful monitoring of affected workers is necessary.

Other Metals

Inhalation of relatively high concentrations of cadmium, chromium, or nickel fumes or mercury vapor can cause toxic pneumonitis. Occupational exposure to certain metals (e.g., antimony, barium, iron, and tin) can lead to deposition of sufficient radiodense dust that chest radiographs demonstrate opacities in the absence of lung parenchymal inflammation and fibrosis.

REFERENCES

McCanlies EC et al: The association between HLA-DPB1Glu69 and chronic beryllium disease and beryllium sensitization. Am J Indust Med 2004;46:95 [PMID: 15273960].

Newman L et al: Beryllium sensitization progresses to chronic beryllium disease: A longitudinal study of disease risk. Am J Respir Crit Care Med 2005;171:54 [PMID: 15374840].

Stange AW et al: The beryllium lymphocyte proliferation test: Relevant issues in beryllium health surveillance. Am J Indust Med 2004;46:453 [PMID: 15490468].

PNEUMOCONIOSES

The pneumoconioses are a group of conditions resulting from the deposition of mineral dust in the lung and the subsequent lung tissue reaction to the dust.

Silicosis

Silicosis is a parenchymal lung disease that results from the inhalation of silicon dioxide, or silica, in crystalline form. Silica is a major component of rock and sand. Workers with potential for exposure are miners, sandblasters, foundry workers, tunnel drillers, quarry workers, stone carvers, ceramic workers, and silica flour production workers.

Exposure to silica can lead to one of three disease patterns: (1) chronic simple silicosis, which usually follows more than 10 years of exposure to respirable dust with less than 30% quartz, (2) subacute/accelerated silicosis, which generally follows shorter, heavier exposures (i.e., 2–5 years), and (3) acute silicosis, which is seen often following intense exposure to fine dust of high silica content over a several-month period.

Chronic silicosis is characterized by the formation of silicotic nodules in the pulmonary parenchyma and the hilar lymph nodes (Figure 20–6). The lesions in the hilar lymph nodes may calcify in an "egg shell" pattern that, while only occurring in a small proportion of cases, is virtually pathognomonic for silicosis. Lung parenchymal involvement tends to have a predilection for the upper lobes. The coalescence of small silicotic nodules into larger fibrotic masses, called *progressive massive fibrosis* (PMF), may complicate a minority of cases. PMF tends to occur in the upper lung fields, may obliterate blood vessels and bronchioles, causes gross distortion of lung architecture, and leads to respiratory insufficiency.

Accelerated silicosis is similar to chronic silicosis except that the time span is shorter and the complication of PMF is seen more frequently. Acute silicosis is a rare condition seen in workers who are exposed to very high concentrations of free silica dust with fine particle size. Such exposures occur frequently in the absence of

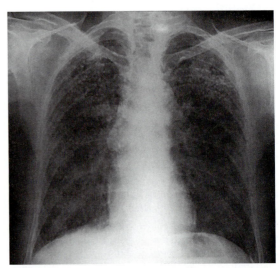

Figure 20–6. Radiographic changes of simple silicosis.

adequate respiratory protection. The characteristic findings differ from chronic silicosis in that the lungs show consolidation without silicotic nodules, and the alveolar spaces are filled with fluid similar to that found in pulmonary alveolar proteinosis. Acute silicosis leads to death in most cases.

Alveolar macrophages play an important role in the pathogenesis of silicosis because these cells ingest inhaled silica and then release cytokines that recruit and/or stimulate other cells. Although crystalline silica can be cytotoxic secondary to direct chemical damage to cellular membranes, the primary effect of inhaled silica on macrophages is activation. The silica-activated macrophages recruit and activate T lymphocytes, which, in turn, recruit and activate a secondary population of monocytes-macrophages. The activated macrophages produce cytokines, which stimulate fibroblasts to proliferate and produce increased amounts of collagen.

There are few symptoms and signs of chronic simple silicosis. The diagnosis usually is made by chest radiographs, which frequently reveal small round opacities (<10 mm in diameter) in both lungs, with a predilection for the upper lung zones. If an adequate occupational history is obtained from the patient along with a thorough review of the chest radiographs, the diagnosis of silicosis should not present any great difficulty. Pulmonary function testing in patients with simple silicosis is usually normal but occasionally may demonstrate evidence of a mild restrictive ventilatory defect and decreased lung compliance. In addition, a mild obstructive impairment is found occasionally in patients with simple silicosis, often as a consequence of chronic bronchitis caused by nonspecific dust effects and/or smoking. With complicated silicosis involving progressive fibrosis (nodules >10 mm in diameter), increasing dyspnea is noted, initially with exertion and then progressing to dyspnea at rest. Complicated chronic silicosis is associated with greater reductions in lung volumes, decreased diffusing capacity, and hypoxemia with exercise. Progressive massive fibrosis is the end-stage of complicated chronic silicosis.

There is an increased incidence of mycobacterial disease, both typical and atypical, in silicosis. Fungal diseases (especially cryptococcosis, blastomycosis, and coccidioidomycosis) are also seen with greater frequency. The mechanism by which the immune-inflammatory responses to inhaled silica lead to the increased incidence of mycobacterial and fungal infections is not clearly understood.

Because no treatment for silicosis is currently known, management is directed toward the prevention of progression and the development of complications. Continued exposure should be avoided, and surveillance for tuberculosis should be instituted. Tuberculin-positive persons with silicosis have an approximately 30-fold greater risk for developing tuberculosis and should be treated for latent tuberculosis with a regimen proven to be efficacious. In acute silicosis, therapeutic whole-lung lavage has been employed to physically remove silica from the alveoli.

The prognosis for patients with chronic silicosis is good, especially if they are removed from exposure. Mortality remains high, however, in those who develop PMF.

Asbestosis

Asbestos is the name for the fibrous forms of a group of mineral silicates. The types of asbestos that have been used commercially are chrysotile, amosite, crocidolite, anthophyllite, tremolite, and actinolite, with chrysotile being the most commonly used. The durability, heat resistance, and ability to be woven into textiles of asbestos led to a wide variety of industrial applications. Major occupational exposures occurred with asbestos mining and milling, manufacture or installation of insulation for ships or buildings, manufacture of friction materials for brake linings and clutch facings, asbestos cement manufacture, asbestos textile manufacture, and asbestos-containing spray products for decorative, acoustical, and fireproofing purposes.

Asbestosis refers to the diffuse interstitial pulmonary fibrosis caused by inhalation of asbestos fibers. The inhaled fibers are deposited primarily at the bifurcations of conducting airways and alveoli, where they are phagocytosed by macrophages. The initial injury is characterized by damage to the alveolar epithelium, incomplete phagocytosis by and activation of alveolar and interstitial macrophages, and release of proinflammatory cytokines as well as cytotoxic oxygen radicals by activated macrophages. A peribronchiolar inflammatory response ensues involving fibroblast proliferation and stimulation, which eventually may lead to fibrosis. Many factors are felt to play a role in disease initiation and progression, including the type and size of fiber, the intensity and duration of exposure, history of cigarette smoking, and individual susceptibility. A dose-response relationship exists such that asbestosis is more common in workers with a higher exposure level. Once asbestosis begins, it may progress irrespective of removal from continued exposure. Finally, there is a considerable latency period (usually at least 20 years) between onset of exposure and development of clinically apparent disease.

The diagnosis of asbestosis is made by a thorough exposure history, clinical examination, appropriate imaging studies, and pulmonary function testing. The symptoms of asbestosis are indistinguishable from those of any other gradually progressive interstitial pulmonary fibrosing disorder, with progressive dyspnea and nonproductive cough being the most prominent. Bibasilar crackles with a "Velcro" quality can be auscultated over the posterolateral chest in the middle to late phase of inspiration. The crackles of asbestosis are unaffected by coughing.

Imaging studies that are helpful in the evaluation of asbestos-exposed patients are the chest radiograph and HRCT scan. The chest radiograph shows characteristic small, irregular or linear opacities distributed throughout the lung fields but more prominent in the lower zones. There is loss of definition of the heart border and hemidiaphragms. The most useful radiographic finding is the presence of bilateral pleural thickening, which does not occur commonly with other diseases-causing interstitial pulmonary fibroses (Figure 20–7). Diaphragmatic or pericardial calcification is almost a pathognomonic sign of asbestos exposure. The ILO classification system is often used in the United States to rate the degree of profusion of small, irregular opacities and of pleural thickening on the chest radiograph. Conventional chest CT scanning is more sensitive than chest radiography for the detection of pleural disease but not for parenchymal disease. HRCT scanning is the most sensitive imaging method for detecting early asbestosis.

Depending on the severity of disease, pulmonary function testing will show varying degrees of restrictive impairment and decreased DL_{CO}. Because asbestosis begins as a peribronchiolar process, reduced flow rates at low lung volumes, indicative of small airways obstruction, may be seen.

As for silicosis, there is no known treatment for asbestosis. Fortunately, only a minority of those exposed are likely to develop radiographically evident disease, and among these, most do not develop significant respiratory impairment. Workers with asbestosis should be removed from further asbestos exposure because the risk that parenchymal scarring will progress appears to increase with cumulative asbestos exposure. Any other factors that may contribute to respiratory disease should be reduced or eliminated. This is especially true of cigarette smoking because there is some evidence that it may contribute to the initiation and progression of asbestosis.

The substitution of other fibrous materials for asbestos and the institution of strict environmental controls where it is still present have led to a dramatic reduction in occupational exposures to asbestos. Medical surveillance of all currently exposed workers in the United States is required by Occupational Safety and Health Administration (OSHA) regulation.

Coal Workers' Pneumoconiosis

Coal workers' pneumoconiosis is the term used to describe parenchymal lung disease caused by the inhalation of coal dust. Miners who work at the coal face in underground mining and drillers in surface mines are at greatest risk of contracting this disease. A heavy coal dust burden is required to induce coal workers' pneumoconiosis, and the condition is seen rarely in those who have spent fewer than 20 years underground.

The coal macule is the primary lesion in coal workers' pneumoconiosis. It is formed when the inhaled dust burden exceeds the amount that can be removed by alveolar macrophages and mucociliary clearance. This leads to retention of coal dust in the terminal respiratory units. Prolonged retention causes lung fibroblasts to secrete a limiting layer of reticulin around the dust collection, or macule, near the respiratory bronchiole. Progressive enlargement of the macule may weaken the bronchiole wall to create a focal area of centrilobular emphysema; coalescence of small macules into larger lesions may occur. Initially, there is a predilection for the upper lung lobes, but with progression of the disease, the lower lobes become involved. As for silicosis, coal workers' pneumoconiosis can be characterized as simple (radiographic lesions <10 mm in diameter) or complicated (lesions >10 mm in diameter). Only a small proportion of miners (<5%) develop complicated or progressive fibrotic disease. Progressive massive fibrosis, identical to that described earlier for silicosis, may occur.

The symptoms of cough and sputum production are common among coal miners and often are the result of chronic bronchitis from dust inhalation rather than coal workers' pneumoconiosis. As with silicosis, simple coal workers' pneumoconiosis is often asymptomatic. The symptoms and signs associated with complicated dis-

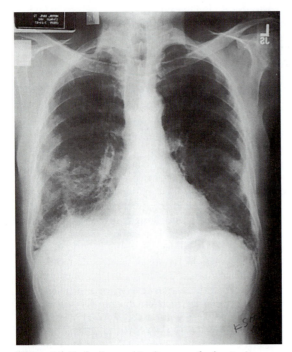

Figure 20–7. Radiographic changes of asbestosis.

ease are the same as those described earlier for silicosis. Progressive massive fibrosis almost invariably leads to respiratory insufficiency and death.

The chest radiograph in simple coal workers' pneumoconiosis shows the presence of small, rounded opacities in the lung parenchyma. Often seen first in the upper lung zones, these opacities may involve the lower zones in the later stage of the disease. Calcification of the hilar lymph nodes is not seen unless there is concomitant silica exposure. Complicated coal workers' pneumococcosis/PMF is diagnosed when large parenchymal opacities are present.

Caplan's syndrome may occur in coal miners with rheumatoid arthritis and is characterized by the appearance of rapidly evolving rounded densities on chest radiographs. These have a propensity to cavitate and histologically are composed of layers of necrotic collagen and coal dust. The pulmonary manifestations of Caplan's syndrome may precede or coincide with the onset of arthritis.

Pulmonary function findings vary with the stage of disease in a manner similar to that described for silicosis. In simple disease, there are usually no significant pulmonary function abnormalities. In complicated disease, either a restrictive or mixed restrictive and obstructive pattern may occur with a decreased diffusing capacity and abnormal arterial blood gases. It is important to remember that an obstructive ventilatory impairment in a coal miner may be a result of chronic bronchitis, coal workers' pneumoconiosis, or both.

Simple coal workers' pneumoconiosis usually follows a benign course. Unlike silicosis, no increase is seen in either pulmonary tuberculosis or fungal infections of the lung. In complicated disease, the affected worker may have mild to severe respiratory symptoms and significant impairment. In such cases, depending on the degree of impairment, the worker should be removed from continued dust exposure. In the United States, underground miners are able to participate in a federally run medical surveillance program that provides free periodic chest radiographs. If coal workers' pneumoconiosis is evident on the chest radiograph, the affected miner has the right to work in a low-dust job in the mine without loss of pay. In addition, personal dust exposure is monitored to confirm that exposures remain low.

Prevention of coal mine dust-related respiratory disease depends primarily on effective control of exposure to coal mine dust. In the United States, good progress has been made in reducing the incidence and prevalence of coal workers' pneumoconiosis since the passage in 1969 of the Coal Mine Health and Safety Act, which established programs to monitor dust levels in mines and to provide radiographic surveillance of miners.

Other Pneumoconioses

Other mineral dusts capable of causing pulmonary parenchymal fibrosis include graphite (which causes

disease similar to coal workers' pneumoconiosis), kaolin and diatomaceous earth (which cause silicosis-like disease), and talc and mica (which cause disease that has features of both silicosis and asbestosis). A metal dust that can cause pneumoconiosis is aluminum oxide, which can form fibers under certain conditions.

A new cause of interstitial lung disease (ILD) was reported recently. A series of cases of ILD was reported from a single nylon flock manufacturing plant. Finely cut nylon, called *flock*, is used to make fabric for upholstery, clothing, and automobiles. Nylon flock fibers are 10–15 μm in diameter, but respirable-size particles are generated during cutting operations. Lung biopsies from patients with nylon flock–related ILD have shown lymphocytic bronchiolitis and peribronchiolitis with lymphoid hyperplasia.

REFERENCES

Taylor Z et al: Controlling tuberculosis in the United States. MMWR Recomm Rep 2005;54:1 [PMID: 16267499].

Weill D, Weill H: Diagnosis and initial management of nonmalignant diseases related to asbestos. Am J. Respir Crit Care Med 2005;171:527 [PMID: 15722420].

CHRONIC OBSTRUCTIVE PULMONARY DISEASE

Chronic Bronchitis

Chronic bronchitis is characterized by inflammation of the bronchial tree and is manifested by persistent cough productive of sputum on most days for at least 3 months of the year for at least 2 successive years. The inhalation of irritant dusts, fumes, and gases can cause chronic simple bronchitis, that is, persistent sputum production without airflow obstruction (Table 20–6). Whether workers with chronic simple bronchitis are at risk for the development of chronic airflow obstruction and permanent respiratory impairment is an area of controversy that has yet to be completely resolved. The development of permanent respiratory impairment may depend on a variety of host factors such as preexisting nonspecific airway hyperresponsiveness, protease-antiprotease activity, and whether there is concomitant cigarette smoking. The ATS recently published an official statement that supports a population attributable risk of approximately 15% for occupational factors in the etiology of chronic obstructive pulmonary disease (COPD).

A. DIAGNOSIS

The diagnosis of chronic bronchitis is straightforward and based entirely on whether the worker's history is consistent with the definition given earlier. Once chronic bronchitis has been diagnosed, establishing a causal role for an occupational exposure is also based on the history obtained from the worker. Symptoms of cough and spu-

Table 20–6. Some agents causing chronic bronchitis.

Minerals
Coal
Oil mist
Silica
Silicates
Synthetic vitreous fibers
Portland cement
Metals
Osmium
Vanadium
Welding fumes
Organic dusts
Cotton
Grain
Wood
Smoke
Tobacco smoke
Fire smoke
Engine exhaust

tum production that are temporally associated with workplace exposure should suggest the diagnosis. Smoking workers are at greater risk of developing respiratory symptoms with exposure to other irritants, and a work-related contribution to their symptoms should be considered. Upper respiratory tract inflammatory symptoms, eye irritation, and an increased incidence of symptoms among coworkers all are features that support a work-related problem. Physical examination may demonstrate no evidence of pulmonary abnormality. Spirometry and expiratory flow-volume curves may or may not show evidence of airway obstruction. A nonsmoking worker exposed to high concentrations of an irritant at the workplace who has evidence of airway obstruction and no history of asthma should be suspected of having occupationally induced chronic bronchitis.

B. TREATMENT

Because chronic bronchitis often has a multifactorial etiology, a multifocal approach to management should be taken. If the worker smokes, cessation should be encouraged. Work exposure to the suspected agent should be reduced or eliminated. Pharmacologic agents of benefit are the beta$_2$-agonists, inhaled steroids, and inhaled anticholinergic agents. Periodic follow-up with particular attention to symptoms and worsening airway obstruction on serial spirometry is warranted.

The prognosis of workers with chronic irritant-induced bronchitis has not been well described. Some data, however, suggest that accelerated loss of ventilatory function can occur. In light of this, it may be prudent to assume that all workers with chronic work-related bronchitis are at risk of developing permanent respiratory impairment. Those with worsening symptoms or lung function abnormalities should be considered for removal from further exposure. Reduction of exposure to conditions capable of causing chronic bronchitis through engineering controls or respiratory protective equipment is necessary to prevent further cases.

Bronchiolitis Obliterans

Bronchiolitis is inflammation of the small airways, and when the inflammatory response leads to obstruction of bronchiolar lumens, the term *bronchiolitis obliterans* is used. The bronchiolar obstruction is caused by intraluminal polyps of organizing connective tissue (proliferative-type) and/or airway remodeling and smooth-muscle hypertrophy (constrictive-type). The most common occupational cause is irritant gas inhalation (e.g., oxides of nitrogen, chlorine, phosgene, ozone, hydrogen sulfide, and sulfur dioxide) (see discussion of toxic gas inhalation above). Bronchiolitis obliterans also has been reported in nylon-flock workers, battery workers (exposed to thionyl chloride), and textile workers exposed to polyamide-amine dyes. A new cause of bronchiolitis obliterans was reported recently in a group of workers from a single microwave popcorn plant, exposure to buttery flavoring (putative agent, diacetyl). A NIOSH survey of other workers in the plant found a high prevalence of obstructive-type spirometric abnormalities with a diacetyl exposure-response relationship.

REFERENCES

Balmes JR: Occupational contribution to the burden of chronic obstructive pulmonary disease. J Occup Environ Med 2005;47:154 [PMID: 15706175].

Matheson MC et al: Biological dust exposure in the workplace is a risk factor for chronic obstructive pulmonary disease. Thorax 2005;60:645 [PMID: 16061705].

PLEURAL DISORDERS

The pleura is the serous membrane that lines the lungs, the mediastinum, the diaphragm, and the rib cage. It is divided into the *visceral pleura,* which lines the lung surface, and the *parietal pleura,* which lines the remaining structures. The primary cause of occupationally induced pleural disease is asbestos, although talc and mica can cause benign pleural disease and zeolite can cause mesothelioma.

Benign Pleural Effusions

Pleural effusions resulting from asbestos exposure may occur in up to 3% of exposed workers. The risk of developing an effusion is greater in those with heavy exposure. Benign asbestos effusions tend to develop within 5–20 years of the onset of exposure.

A pleural effusion can be attributed to asbestos if the following criteria are met: (1) a significant history of occupational exposure with an appropriate latent period since onset of exposure, (2) exclusion of other known causes of pleural effusion, and (3) a repeat evaluation of the effusion within a minimum of 2 years confirms that it is benign.

The majority of workers who have pleural effusions from asbestos exposure are asymptomatic. Physical examination in those with large effusions may show diminished rib cage expansion, dullness to percussion, and decreased breath sounds on the side of the effusion. Chest radiographs typically show small to moderately large, unilateral pleural effusions. Bilateral involvement occurs in approximately 10% of cases of benign asbestos effusions. Pleural thickening may be noted, although often the effusion is the first manifestation of asbestos-induced disease. Diffuse pleural thickening involving both pleural surfaces and obliteration of the costophrenic angle may develop in the wake of benign asbestos effusions. Thoracentesis will obtain pleural liquid that is a sterile exudate with no specific findings, although increased eosinophils are suggestive of an asbestos etiology.

It is essential to exclude other etiologies of pleural effusion, especially tuberculosis and malignancy. Regular follow-up with repeat thoracentesis if pleural fluid persists is essential. There is no known treatment. Recurrences occur, but in most cases the effusion clears spontaneously within a year without any obvious residual pleural disease.

Pleural Plaques

Pleural plaques are circumscribed areas of pleural thickening that are the most common radiographic findings as a result of chronic asbestos exposure. Plaques usually involve the parietal pleural surface and tend to occur over the central portions of the hemidiaphragm and along the inferior posterolateral aspect of the lower ribs.

Bilateral pleural plaques almost invariably are a result of past asbestos exposure, and their prevalence is related to both the intensity of exposure and the duration since onset of exposure. Workers with a greater exposure have a higher chance of developing plaques. In workers without asbestosis, plaques rarely cause signs and symptoms. The diagnosis usually is made from a routine chest radiograph. When plaques lie parallel to the beam, they appear as slightly to moderately protuberant linear or ovoid opacities along the costal or diaphragmatic margins. If calcified, they have an irregular, unevenly dense appearance. Although oblique radiographic views are recommended by some, chest CT scanning provides the most sensitive and specific technique for confirming the pres-

ence of plaques. Pathologically, the plaques are composed mainly of collagen with little accompanying inflammation. Asbestos fibers can be demonstrated in plaque tissue by electron microscopy, although this is not required for routine clinical diagnosis.

A worker with a past history of asbestos exposure and pleural plaques on chest radiograph should be evaluated for the presence of asbestosis. Even if no evidence of parenchymal disease is found, the worker should be monitored periodically for the possible development of this condition. Although workers with pleural plaques and no parenchymal disease typically do not develop respiratory impairment, there is evidence that heavily exposed workers with radiographic evidence of plaques, but no asbestosis, tend to have decreased lung function in comparison with workers with similar exposure histories whose chest radiographs are normal.

Because of the risk of development of bronchogenic carcinoma with asbestos exposure, cigarette smoking should be discouraged. The increased risk of lung cancer is not due to the plaques but to the cumulative dose of asbestos, the plaques merely acting as a marker of exposure.

Diffuse pleural thickening involving both visceral and parietal pleura also can result from past asbestos exposure. Such thickening occasionally is associated with a restrictive-type respiratory impairment even in the absence of asbestosis. Neither circumscribed plaques nor diffuse pleural thickening is believed to undergo malignant transformation to mesothelioma.

Mesothelioma

Malignant mesotheliomas are rare pleural tumors of which up to 80% occur in asbestos-exposed individuals. The exposure to asbestos may be relatively light, and the latent period between exposure and onset of disease is in the range of 30–40 years. Crocidolite and amosite appear to be the asbestos fiber types with the highest potential for inducing mesotheliomas. Exposure to the fibrous mineral zeolite and thoracic radiation are other risk factors for mesothelioma.

Mesotheliomas generally present with the symptoms of chest pain and dyspnea. The chest pain is often nonpleuritic and may be referred to the upper abdomen or the shoulder when there is diaphragmatic involvement. Other common symptoms are fatigue, decreased appetite, and weight loss. The clinical findings are influenced by the histologic type of the tumor. Epithelial and mixed mesotheliomas are associated more commonly with large pleural effusions, whereas mesenchymal tumors rarely have an associated effusion. Patients with the epithelial type are more likely to have supraclavicular or axillary lymph node involvement and extension to the pericardium. Those with the mesenchymal type have a higher incidence of extrapulmonary metastases.

Chest radiographic findings may be suggestive of a pleural effusion but without either a meniscus or a contralateral shift of the mediastinal structures. In advanced cases, tumor is noted to encase the lung, the mediastinum is shifted toward the side of the tumor, and the involved hemithorax is contracted. Chest CT scans are especially helpful in the diagnosis of mesothelioma and often show a thickened pleura with a distinctive irregular or nodular internal margin.

Pleural fluid analysis shows a serosanguineous exudate that is often quite viscid. The cellular content is a mixture of mesothelial cells, differentiated and undifferentiated malignant mesothelial cells, and varying numbers of lymphocytes and polymorphonuclear leukocytes. While cytologic examination of the fluid may be suggestive of malignant mesothelioma, it is rarely diagnostic. An open thoracotomy or VATS with multiple biopsies usually is required to confirm the diagnosis. Even with adequate tissue for pathologic examination, distinguishing mesothelioma from metastatic adenocarcinoma may be difficult. Special stains and/or electron microscopy usually are required. A recent report provided evidence that the level of osteopontin (a phosphorylated cell-attachment glycoprotein) in serum could be useful to distinguish patients with mesothelioma from those with asbestos exposure without the disease.

The treatment of malignant mesothelioma is palliative. Death from wasting or respiratory failure usually occurs within months of diagnosis. Radiotherapy, chemotherapy, and surgical treatments have been tried, but there are no good data to show that these prolong survival or improve quality of life.

REFERENCES

O'Regan AW et al: Asbestos exposure and serum osteopontin. N Engl J Med 2006;354:304 [PMID: 16421377].

Pass HI et al: Asbestos exposure, pleural mesothelioma, and serum osteopontin levels. N Engl J Med 2005;353:1564 [PMID: 16221779].

Piirila P et al: Impairment of lung function in asbestos exposed workers in relation to high-resolution computed tomography. Scand J Work Environ Health 2005;31:44 [PMID: 15751618].

Reid A et al: The effect of asbestosis on lung cancer risk beyond the dose related effect of asbestos alone. Occup Environ Med 2005;62:885 [PMID: 16299098].

LUNG CANCER

Although cigarette smoking is the most important preventable cause of lung cancer, occupational exposures to respiratory tract carcinogens are also preventable. Estimates of the percentage of lung cancers attributable to occupational factors range from 3–17%. Table 20–7 lists agents both known and suspected to cause lung cancer. In addition, workers in several industries, including foundries, welding, printing, and rubber manufacturing, are at increased risk

Table 20–7. Known and suspected lung carcinogens.

Known
  Asbestos
  Arsenic
  Chloromethyl ethers (e.g., BCME)
  Chromium (hexavalent)
  Environmental tobacco smoke
  Mustard gas
  Nickel
  Polyaromatic hydrocarbons [e.g., benzo(a)pyrene]
  Radon
Suspected
  Acrylonitrile
  Beryllium
  Cadmium
  Formaldehyde
  Silica
  Synthetic vitreous fibers
  Vinyl chloride monomer

of lung cancer without identification of specific carcinogenic agents.

The evaluation of any patient with lung cancer should include a careful occupational and environmental exposure history. The determination of whether a given exposure caused a cancer involves assessment of dose and latency, as well as consideration of the smoking history. When exposure to more than one carcinogen has occurred (e.g., an occupational agent and tobacco smoke), both exposures may have contributed to the development of lung cancer. The management of a patient with work-related lung cancer is similar to that of any patient with lung cancer, with the exception that an effort should be made to prevent the exposure of other workers to the responsible agent at the patient's workplace.

Specific Agents

A. ASBESTOS

Lung cancer is a more common cause of death as a consequence of asbestos exposure than mesothelioma. The effects of asbestos and cigarette smoke are believed to interact positively to increase the risk of lung cancer, but the magnitude of the interaction (additive or multiplicative) remains somewhat controversial and probably is dose-related. It is rare to see a lung cancer in an asbestos-exposed worker who does not smoke. Therefore, cessation of both smoking and exposure to asbestos is necessary to prevent lung cancer among asbestos-exposed workers. Data from epidemiologic studies of heavily exposed workers support a linear relationship between level of asbestos exposure and lung cancer mortality. The nature of the dose-response relationship at lower levels of exposure is more controversial, with some data suggesting a threshold and other data suggesting that there is no "safe" level of exposure.

The mechanism of asbestos-related carcinogenesis is unclear, but it is likely that asbestos acts more as a promoting than an initiating agent. Both the physical and chemical characteristics of asbestos fibers appear to be factors in determining carcinogenic potential. Long, thin fibers are the most carcinogenic, but fibers that are cleared from the lungs more slowly (probably related to chemical characteristics) also appear to be more carcinogenic than those with a shorter residence time.

There are no distinctive features of asbestos-related lung cancer, although asbestos-related tumors occur somewhat more frequently in the lower lobes. Contrary to earlier reports, the distribution of histologic types of lung cancer is similar among asbestos-exposed workers to that of the general population. The risk of lung cancer is highest among workers with the greatest cumulative exposure to asbestos, and the latency since onset of exposure ranges from 15–30 years. The presence of asbestosis or asbestos-related pleural disease on the chest radiograph of a patient with lung cancer confirms a history of significant occupational or environmental exposure.

B. Chloromethyl Ethers

These compounds are alkylating agents capable of causing damage to DNA and are highly carcinogenic. In particular, occupational exposure to bischloromethyl ether (BCME) is associated with an increased risk of small-cell carcinomas at a relatively young age. Smoking does not appear to further increase the risk among BCME-exposed workers. Some animal toxicologic data support the carcinogenicity of BCME.

C. Metals

Occupational exposure to several metals has been associated with an increased risk of lung cancer. Workers exposed to arsenic in the smelting, pesticide manufacturing, and other industries have been shown to have a dose-related increased risk, although there is no animal model of arsenic-induced carcinogenesis. Exposure to hexavalent, but not trivalent, chromium is another risk factor for lung cancer. Exposure to intermediate compounds in nickel refining, but not exposure to metallic nickel, also has been associated with increased relative risk for lung cancer.

D. Radon

Radon is an inert gas that is a decay product of uranium-235; radon itself decays with emission of alpha particles. Uranium miners as well as other underground miners exposed to radon have a strikingly elevated risk of lung cancer. Exposure to radon and cigarette smoke appear to act synergistically to increase the risk of lung cancer. Small-cell carcinomas are increased disproportionately among uranium miners when compared with the distribution of cell types in the general population. Although usually at much lower levels than in uranium mines, exposure to radon in homes has been estimated to be an important environmental risk factor for lung cancer in the United States.

E. Environmental Tobacco Smoke

Environmental tobacco smoke is made up of both mainstream smoke exhaled by smokers and sidestream smoke released by burning cigarettes. There are now abundant data from epidemiologic studies to support an increased risk of lung cancer from environmental tobacco smoke. The workplace environment can be an important source of exposure to environmental tobacco smoke.

F. Other Potential Lung Carcinogens

Table 20–7 lists several agents for which either animal or epidemiologic data suggest an increased risk of lung cancer. These agents are listed as suspect lung carcinogens by the U.S. National Toxicology Program's 11th Report on Carcinogens (RoC). Further research is needed to confirm the carcinogenic risk of exposure to these agents for humans.

REFERENCES

Cullen MR et al: Predictors of lung cancer among asbestos-exposed men in the β-carotene and retinol efficacy trial. Am J Epidemiol 2005;161:260 [PMID: 15671258].

National Toxicology Program: 11th Report on Carcinogens, http://ntp.niehs.nih.gov/ntp/roc/eleventh/intro.pdf.

Cardiovascular Toxicology

21

Neal L. Benowitz, MD

Heart disease and stroke cause the majority of deaths in the United States. The major risk factors for coronary heart disease—family history, hypertension, diabetes, lipid abnormalities, and cigarette smoking—explain only a minority of the cases. Other factors, such as stress and exposure to occupational or environmental toxic agents, are believed to contribute to the development of heart disease, although the magnitude of the risk is unknown. This chapter focuses on cardiovascular disease caused by occupational toxic substances.

CAUSATION IN TOXIC CARDIOVASCULAR DISEASE

Table 21–1 lists the types and possible toxic causes of cardiovascular disease. Massive exposure may occur (e.g., in acute carbon monoxide poisoning), but toxic cardiovascular disease usually is the result of chronic low-level exposures.

Problems in establishing the cause of cardiovascular disease include the following:

1. Cardiovascular disease is common even in the absence of toxic exposures.
2. There is usually nothing specific, either clinically or pathologically, to point to toxic cardiovascular disease.
3. It is rarely possible to document high tissue levels of suspected toxic substances.
4. It is difficult to establish occupational exposure levels over the 20 or more years it may take to develop cardiovascular disease.
5. Cardiovascular toxic substances are likely to interact with other risk factors in causing or manifesting cardiovascular disease.

With these limitations in mind, this chapter discusses current information concerning toxic cardiovascular disease.

EVALUATION OF PATIENTS

Evaluation of patients with suspected toxic cardiovascular disease should include the following steps:

1. Take a detailed occupational history (see Chapter 2), with attention to the temporal relationship between cardiovascular symptoms and exposure to toxic substances in the workplace.
2. Attempt to document exposure to suspected toxic substances by obtaining industrial hygiene data and, if possible, monitoring worker exposure directly.
3. Evaluate other cardiovascular risk factors.
4. Perform a complete physical examination.
5. Perform appropriate diagnostic studies such as exercise stress testing and coronary angiography to establish the presence and extent of coronary artery disease; echocardiography or radionuclide angiography to establish myocardial disease and the presence of cardiomyopathy; and ambulatory electrocardiographic recordings taken on workdays and at other times to document work-related arrhythmias.

CARDIOVASCULAR ABNORMALITIES CAUSED BY CARBON DISULFIDE

Chronic exposure to carbon disulfide appears to accelerate atherosclerosis and/or precipitate acute coronary ischemic events. Carbon disulfide is a widely used solvent, especially in the rubber and viscose rayon industries, in the manufacture of carbon tetrachloride and ammonium salts, and as a degreasing solvent. Early epidemiologic studies indicated that there is a 2.5- to 5-fold increase in the risk of death from coronary heart disease in workers exposed to carbon disulfide. However, more recent analyses of the results of multiple studies found the association between carbon disulfide exposure and circulatory disease to be weaker and inconsistent. For a complete discussion of the systemic effects of carbon disulfide, see Chapter 28.

Pathogenesis

The mechanism of accelerated atherogenesis caused by carbon disulfide has not been proved. One theory is that carbon disulfide reacts with amino- and thiol-containing compounds in the body to produce thiocarbamates, which are capable of complexing trace metals and inhibiting many enzyme systems. This causes metabolic abnormalities such as disturbances of lipid metabolism and thyroid function and can lead to elevations of low-density lipoprotein/cholesterol concentrations and hypothyroidism, which are risk factors for atherosclerosis. Aldehyde dehydrogenase may be inhibited, resulting in a disulfiram-like reaction

Table 21–1. Classification of cardiovascular diseases and possible toxic causes.

Condition	Toxic Agent
Cardiac arrhythmia	Arsenic
	Chlorofluorocarbon propellants
	Hydrocarbon solvents (e.g., 1,1,1-trichloroethane and trichloroethylene)
	Organophosphate and carbamate insecticides
Coronary artery disease	Air pollution
	Carbon disulfide
	Carbon monoxide
	Lead(?)
Hypertension	Cadmium
	Carbon disulfide
	Lead
Myocardial asphyxiation	Carbon monoxide
	Cyanide
	Hydrogen sulfide
Myocardial injury	Antimony
	Arsenic
	Arsine
	Cobalt
	Lead
Nonatheromatous ischemic heart disease	Organic nitrates (e.g., nitroglycerin and ethylene glycol dinitrate)
Peripheral arterial occlusive disease	Arsenic
	Cadmium
	Lead

after alcohol ingestion. Other possible contributors to ischemic heart disease in workers exposed to carbon disulfide are increased vascular permeability, which may lead to greater lipid deposition; interference with normal inhibition of elastase activity, resulting in excess elastase activity with disruption of blood vessel walls and formation of aneurysms; depressed fibrinolytic activity, resulting in a greater tendency to thrombosis; and hypertension.

Pathology

The findings are those of accelerated atherosclerotic vascular disease involving the coronary, cerebral, and peripheral arteries. Renovascular hypertension also has been reported.

Clinical Findings

A. SYMPTOMS AND SIGNS

Acute intoxication may produce symptoms and signs of encephalopathy or polyneuropathy, including fatigue,

headaches, dizziness, disorientation, paresthesias, psychosis, and delirium. In cases of chronic exposure, patients may present with hypertension or manifestations of atherosclerotic vascular disease such as angina or myocardial infarction. An early sign of chronic carbon disulfide poisoning is abnormal ocular microcirculation, characterized by microaneurysms and hemorrhages resembling those of diabetic retinopathy. Disturbed color vision may be reported. Presenile dementia, stroke, and sudden death have been reported in patients with chronic poisoning.

B. LABORATORY FINDINGS

Findings may include a decrease in serum thyroxine levels and an increase in serum cholesterol levels, particularly those of the very-low-density lipoproteins. There are no practical methods for measuring carbon disulfide levels in biologic fluids.

C. CARDIOVASCULAR STUDIES

Delayed filling of the retinal arteries, as measured by fluorescein angiography, may be an early sign of vascular disease. The electrocardiogram sometimes shows evidence of ischemia or previous myocardial infarction. The presence of coronary artery disease may be confirmed by exercise stress testing and coronary angiography.

Differential Diagnosis

The vascular findings in patients with chronic carbon disulfide poisoning are the same as those seen in any patient with atherosclerotic vascular disease. The most specific finding is abnormal ocular microcirculation in the absence of diabetes. The diagnosis is based on a clinical picture of premature vascular disease and a history of exposure to excessive levels of carbon disulfide for more than 5 or 10 years.

Prevention

Carbon disulfide exposure is primarily by inhalation. The Occupational Safety and Health Administration (OSHA) recommends that workplace exposure be limited to 4 ppm (time-weighted average for a 40-hour workweek). Periodic examination of the ocular fundi may help to detect early signs of vascular disease.

Treatment

Treatment consists of removing the worker from sources of carbon disulfide exposure and providing medical measures for atherosclerotic vascular disease.

Course & Prognosis

The course of the disease is similar to that of any atherosclerotic vascular disease. There is evidence of reversibility—at least of ocular changes—after exposure to carbon disulfide is discontinued.

REFERENCES

Luo JC et al: Elevated triglyceride and decreased high density lipoprotein level in carbon disulfide workers in Taiwan. J Occup Environ Med 2003;45:73 [PMID: 12553181].

Takebayashi T et al: A six-year follow-up study of the subclinical effects of carbon disulphide exposure on the cardiovascular system. Occup Environ Med 2004;61:127 [PMID: 14739378].

Tan X et al: Cross-sectional study of cardiovascular effects of carbon disulfide among Chinese workers of a viscose factory. Int J Hyg Environ Health 2004;207:217 [PMID: 15330389].

CARDIOVASCULAR ABNORMALITIES CAUSED BY CARBON MONOXIDE

Excessive carbon monoxide exposure can reduce maximal exercise capacity in healthy workers; aggravate angina pectoris, intermittent claudication, and chronic obstructive lung disease; and aggravate or induce cardiac arrhythmias. Acute intoxications can cause myocardial infarction or sudden death. Chronic high-level carbon monoxide exposure may result in congestive cardiomyopathy.

Carbon monoxide is the most widely distributed of all industrial toxic agents and accounts for the greatest number of intoxications and deaths. It is formed wherever combustion engines or other types of combustion are present. Workers at high risk include forklift operators, foundry workers, miners, mechanics, garage attendants, and firefighters. Carbon monoxide poisoning also may occur with the use of faulty furnaces or heaters, particularly improperly vented kerosene or charcoal heaters. Cigarette smoking is an important source of carbon monoxide, and occupational sources may be additive to exposure from cigarettes. The solvent methylene chloride is metabolized within the body to carbon monoxide. For a complete discussion of carbon monoxide, see Chapter 30.

Pathogenesis

The affinity of carbon monoxide for hemoglobin is more than 200 times that of oxygen. The binding of carbon monoxide and hemoglobin to form carboxyhemoglobin reduces the delivery of oxygen to body tissues because the oxygen-carrying capacity of hemoglobin is decreased and because less oxygen is released to tissues at any given oxygen tension (i.e., there is a shift in the oxygen dissociation curve). Thus a carboxyhemoglobin concentration of 20% represents a greater reduction in oxygen delivery than a 20% reduction in erythrocyte count. Other heme-containing proteins (e.g., myoglobin, cytochrome oxidase, and cytochrome P450) bind 10–15% of the total-body carbon monoxide, but the medical significance of their binding at usual levels of exposure to carbon monoxide is unclear.

In healthy individuals exposed to carbon monoxide, the decrease in delivery of oxygen to tissues causes the cardiac output and coronary blood flow to increase to meet the metabolic demands of the heart. Although these compensatory responses enable healthy individuals to perform at normal work levels, their maximal exercise capacity is decreased. If, on the other hand, compensatory responses are limited, as in patients with coronary artery disease, carbon monoxide exposure may cause angina or myocardial infarction (Figure 21–1). Reduced exercise thresholds for the development of angina have been reported when carboxyhemoglobin concentrations are as low as 2.7% (Table 21–2). Carbon monoxide decreases the ventricular fibrillation threshold in experimental animals and may do the same in humans. This would explain why sudden death occurs in people who have coronary artery disease and are exposed to carbon monoxide, as has been reported to occur on smoggy days in large cities. Severe carbon monoxide poisoning (carboxyhemoglobin concentrations > 50%) can cause severe hypoxic injury, including cardiovascular collapse.

Chronic exposure to carbon monoxide is thought to accelerate atherogenesis. Cigarette smokers demonstrate advanced coronary and peripheral atherosclerosis, and carbon monoxide is believed to contribute. Several animal studies have tested the effects of chronic high-level carbon monoxide exposure combined with feeding of atherogenic diets; the results of some of these studies showed increased severity of atherosclerosis. Possible mechanisms include abnormal vascular permeability, increased vascular uptake of lipids, and increased platelet adhesiveness. Whether atherosclerosis is accelerated at levels of carbon monoxide commonly encountered in the workplace is unclear.

Chronic exposure to carbon monoxide results in increased red blood cell mass in response to chronic tissue hypoxia and in increased blood viscosity, which could contribute to acute cardiac events.

Pathology

Cardiac necrosis is observed often in cases of fatal carbon monoxide poisoning and presumably is due to severe hypoxia. Myocardial infarction may occur in workers who have coronary artery disease and are exposed to high levels of carbon monoxide, particularly while performing strenuous work or exercise. Cardiomyopathy with cardiac enlargement and congestive heart failure has been described in workers with chronic high-level exposure to carbon monoxide (carboxyhemoglobin concentrations > 30%).

Clinical Findings

A. SYMPTOMS & SIGNS

Headache is typically the first symptom of carbon monoxide poisoning and may occur at carboxyhemoglobin

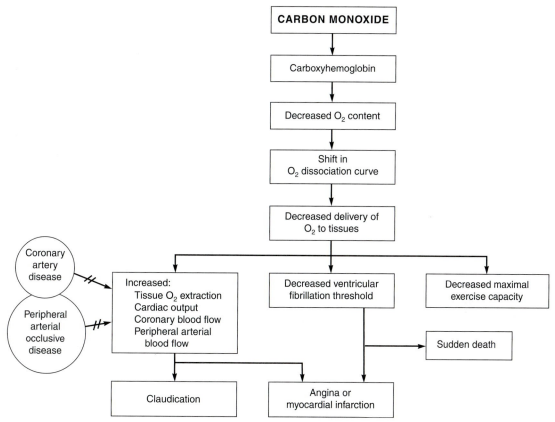

Figure 21–1. Cardiovascular consequences of exposure to carbon monoxide. The presence of coronary artery disease or peripheral arterial occlusive disease prevents (//) the usual compensatory increase in coronary or peripheral arterial blood flow, which results in symptoms of arterial insufficiency.

concentrations as low as 10%. At higher concentrations, nausea, dizziness, fatigue, and dimmed vision are reported commonly.

In patients with angina pectoris or peripheral arterial occlusive disease, carbon monoxide exposure may reduce exercise capacity to the point of angina or claudication (see Table 21–2). All workers experience a reduction in maximal exercise capacity.

In neuropsychiatric tests, findings such as increased reaction time and decreased manual dexterity may be

Table 21–2. Effects of carbon monoxide on exercise capacity.

Group	Baseline Exercise Duration (s)	Level of Exposure to Carbon Monoxide	Increase in Concentration of Carboxyhemoglobin	Exercise Duration after Exposure (s)	Exercise Endpoint
Healthy individuals	698	100 ppm for 1 h	1.7% → 4%	662	Exhaustion
Patients with angina pectoris	224	50 ppm for 2 h	1% → 2.7%	188	Angina
Patients with intermittent claudication	174	50 ppm for 2 h	1.1% → 2.8%	144	Claudication
Patients with chronic lung disease	219	100 ppm for 1 h	1.4% → 4.1%	147	Dyspnea

seen at carboxyhemoglobin concentrations between 5% and 10%. At concentrations of 25%, there may be decreased visual acuity and impaired cognitive function; at 35%, ataxia; at 50%, vomiting, tachypnea, tachycardia, and hypertension; and at higher levels, coma, convulsions, and cardiovascular and respiratory depression. Myocardial ischemia may be evident at any carboxyhemoglobin concentration in susceptible individuals.

B. LABORATORY FINDINGS

The only finding specific for carbon monoxide intoxication is elevation of the carboxyhemoglobin concentration. Table 21–3 lists normal carboxyhemoglobin concentrations and provides examples of concentrations resulting from exposure to carbon monoxide in the environment and the workplace.

When arterial blood gases are measured, they usually show a normal or a slightly reduced arterial oxygen tension, with substantial reductions in venous P_{O2} and oxygen content. Although respiratory alkalosis caused by hyperventilation is observed commonly, there is respiratory failure in the most severe poisonings. When there is marked tissue hypoxia, lactic acidosis develops.

Table 21–3. Normal carboxyhemoglobin concentrations and examples of concentrations resulting from exposure to carbon monoxide in the environment and the workplace.

Source of Carbon Monoxide	Carboxyhemoglobin Concentration	
	Average (%)	Range (%)
Endogenous metabolism (normal level[1])	0.5	—
Environmental exposure		
Air pollution	2	1.5–2.5
Cigarette smoking	6	3–15
Occupational exposure (nonsmokers)		
Foundry workers	4	2–9
Mechanics	5	—
Garage attendants	7	—

[1]Carbon monoxide is normally formed as a product of metabolism of hemoglobin. Endogenous levels may be higher if there is increased hemoglobin turnover.

C. CARDIOVASCULAR STUDIES

The electrocardiograph (ECG) may show ischemic changes or myocardial infarction. Various types of arrhythmias, including atrial fibrillation and premature atrial and ventricular contractions, are observed. Abnormalities seen on the ECG usually are transient, although ST-T-wave abnormalities may persist for days or weeks.

Differential Diagnosis

The most important clue to carbon monoxide poisoning is the occupational or environmental exposure history. A typical symptom, such as headache, confusion, or sudden collapse, with findings of myocardial ischemia or metabolic acidosis should suggest the diagnosis, and carboxyhemoglobin concentrations should be measured.

Prevention

Levels of carbon monoxide should be monitored if there are sources of combustion such as combustion engines or furnaces in the workplace. The current 8-hour threshold limit value is 25 ppm, which at the end of an 8-hour workday results in a carboxyhemoglobin concentration of 2–3%. This concentration is tolerated well by healthy individuals but may impair function in people with cardiovascular or chronic lung disease. Workplace monitoring is done easily with a portable carbon monoxide meter. Biologic monitoring of workers involves measuring either the carboxyhemoglobin concentration in blood or the level of expired carbon monoxide, which is directly proportional to the carboxyhemoglobin concentration. Elevated carbon monoxide levels should be anticipated in cigarette smokers.

Treatment

Carbon monoxide is eliminated from the body by respiration, and the rate of elimination depends on ventilation, pulmonary blood flow, and inspired oxygen concentration. The half-life of carbon monoxide in a sedentary adult breathing air is 4–5 hours. The half-life can be reduced to 80 minutes by giving 100% oxygen by face mask or to 25 minutes by giving hyperbaric oxygen (3 atm) in a hyperbaric chamber.

Course & Prognosis

Recovery usually is complete after mild to moderate carbon monoxide intoxication in the absence of a cardiac complication such as myocardial infarction. With severe carbon monoxide poisoning, particularly if coma has occurred, there may be permanent neurologic abnormalities ranging from subtle neuropsychiatric disturbances to gross motor or cognitive dysfunction to vegetative states. Abnormal findings on a computed

CARDIOVASCULAR TOXICOLOGY / **339**

tomographic (CT) scan of the brain (e.g., lesions in the basal ganglia or the periventricular white matter) predict a poor neurologic outcome.

REFERENCES

Henry CR et al: Myocardial injury and long-term mortality following moderate to severe carbon monoxide poisoning. JAMA 2006;295:398 [PMID: 16434630].
Satran D et al: Cardiovascular manifestations of moderate to severe carbon monoxide poisoning. J Am Coll Cardiol 2005;45:1513 [PMID: 15862427].

CARDIOVASCULAR ABNORMALITIES CAUSED BY ORGANIC NITRATES

In the 1950s, an epidemic of sudden death in young munitions workers who hand-packed cartridges was observed. It was discovered subsequently that abrupt withdrawal from excessive exposure to organic nitrates, particularly nitroglycerin and ethylene glycol dinitrate, may result in myocardial ischemia even in the absence of coronary artery disease. Occupations in which workers may be exposed to organic nitrates include explosives manufacturing, construction work involving blasting, weapons handling in the armed forces, and pharmaceutical manufacturing of nitrates.

Pathogenesis

Nitrates directly dilate blood vessels, including those of the coronary circulation. With prolonged exposure (usually 1–4 years), compensatory vasoconstriction develops that is believed to be mediated by sympathetic neural responses, activation of the rennin-angiotensin system, or both. When exposure to nitrates is stopped, the compensatory vasoconstriction becomes unopposed (Figure 21–2). Coronary vasospasm with angina, myocardial infarction, or sudden death may result.

Chest pain occurring during nitrate withdrawal has been termed *Monday morning angina* because it typically occurs 2–3 days after the last day of nitrate exposure. Case-control studies suggest a 2.5- to 4-fold increase in the risk of cardiovascular death in workers handling explosives.

Pathology

In patients who have died following withdrawal from nitrates, there is often no or minimal coronary atherosclerosis. In one patient, coronary vasospasm was observed during angiography, and the spasm was reversed promptly with sublingual nitroglycerin.

Clinical Findings

A. SYMPTOMS & SIGNS

Workers exposed to excessive levels of nitrates typically experience headaches and have hypotension, tachycardia, and warm, flushed skin. With continued exposure, the symptoms and signs become less prominent. After 1–2 days without exposure to nitrates—generally on weekends—there may be signs of acute coronary ischemia ranging from mild angina at rest to manifestations of myocardial infarction (e.g., nausea, diaphoresis, pallor, and palpitations associated with severe chest pain), or sudden death may occur.

B. LABORATORY FINDINGS & CARDIOVASCULAR STUDIES

During episodes of pain, the ECG may show evidence of acute ischemia: ST-segment elevation or depression with or without T-wave abnormalities. At other times, in the absence of pain, the ECG may be perfectly normal. Typical findings of myocardial infarction include development of a pathologic Q wave on ECG and elevation of serum troponin and other cardiac enzymes.

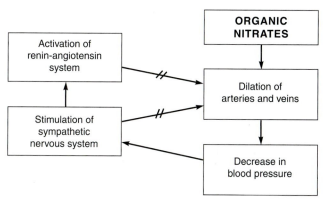

Figure 21–2. Mechanism of vasospasm after withdrawal from chronic exposure to nitrates. Vasoconstrictor forces antagonize (//) nitrate-induced vasodilation. Withdrawal from exposure to nitrates results in unopposed vasoconstriction and in coronary vasospasm.

Results of exercise stress testing and coronary angiography may be normal.

Differential Diagnosis

Workers chronically exposed to nitrates also may have organic coronary artery disease, which must be identified.

Prevention

Nitrates are extremely volatile and are absorbed readily through the lungs and skin. They can permeate the wrapping material of dynamite sticks, so workers who handle dynamite should be advised to wear cotton gloves. Natural rubber gloves should not be used because they tend to become permeated with nitrates and may enhance absorption.

With current automated processes in explosives manufacturing, direct handling of nitrates by employees is minimized. However, levels of nitrates in the workplace environment must be controlled by adequate ventilation and by air conditioning during periods of hot weather. The current OSHA exposure limit is 0.05 ppm for nitroglycerin, but even at lower levels (0.02 ppm), personal protective gear is recommended to avoid headache. Although there are no readily available biochemical measures to detect excessive nitrate exposure, findings of progressively decreasing blood pressure and increasing heart rate during the workday are suggestive of excessive exposure. Monitoring for these signs in employees also may help to prevent adverse effects of exposure to nitrates.

Treatment

Treatment of myocardial ischemia caused by nitrate withdrawal includes cardiac nitrates (e.g., nitroglycerin or isosorbide dinitrate) or calcium entry-blocking agents. Case reports indicate that ischemic symptoms may recur for weeks or months, indicating a persistent tendency to coronary spasm, so long-term cardiac nitrate or calcium blocker therapy may be needed. The worker should be removed from sources of organic nitrate exposure.

Course & Prognosis

In the absence of myocardial infarction or sudden death, anginal symptoms resolve fully after exposure to nitrate is stopped.

REFERENCE

Ward MH et al: Drinking-water nitrate and health—recent findings and research needs. Environ Health Perspect 2005;113:1607 [PMID: 16263519].

CARDIOVASCULAR ABNORMALITIES CAUSED BY HYDROCARBON SOLVENTS & CHLOROFLUOROCARBONS

Exposure to various solvents and propellants may result in cardiac arrhythmia, syncope with resulting accidents at work, or sudden death. Most serious cases of arrhythmia are associated with abuse of or industrial exposure to halogenated hydrocarbon solvents (e.g., 1,1,1-trichloroethane and trichloroethylene) or exposure to chlorofluorocarbon (Freon) propellants. Nonhalogenated solvents and even ethanol present similar risks. Dilated cardiomyopathy, with or without histologic evidence of myocarditis, associated with severe cardiac failure has been reported in several people with occupational exposures to solvents, although causation is still unproven.

Exposure to solvents is widespread in industrial settings such as dry cleaning, degreasing, painting, and chemical manufacturing. Chlorofluorocarbons are used extensively as refrigerants and as propellants in a wide variety of products and processes. For example, a pathology resident developed various arrhythmias after exposure to chlorofluorocarbon aerosols used for freezing samples and cleaning slides in a surgical pathology laboratory.

Pathogenesis

Figure 21–3 illustrates two ways in which halogenated hydrocarbons and other solvents are thought to induce cardiac arrhythmia or sudden death. First, at low levels of exposure, these solvents "sensitize" the heart to actions of catecholamines. For example, experimental studies show that the amount of epinephrine required to produce ventricular tachycardia or fibrillation is reduced after the solvents are inhaled. Catecholamine release is potentiated by euphoria and excitement as a consequence of inhalation of the solvent, as well as by exercise. This, in combination with asphyxia and hypoxia, causes arrhythmia, which can result in death. Second, at higher levels of exposure, solvents may depress sinus node activity, thereby causing sinus bradycardia or arrest, or they may depress atrioventricular nodal conduction, thereby causing atrioventricular block. In some cases, they do both. Bradyarrhythmia then predisposes to escape ventricular arrhythmia or, in cases of more severe intoxication, to asystole. The arrhythmogenic action of solvents also may be enhanced by alcohol or caffeine.

Pathology

Most cardiovascular deaths following exposure to hydrocarbons are sudden deaths. Autopsies usually reveal no specific pathologic findings in sudden death cases but may reveal myocarditis in cases of dilated cardiomyopa-

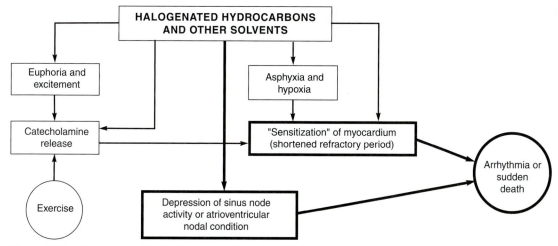

Figure 21–3. Mechanisms of arrhythmia or sudden death following low-level exposure (*light arrows*) or high-level exposure (*heavy arrows*) to halogenated hydrocarbons and other solvents.

thy. The finding of a fatty liver suggests chronic exposure to high levels of halogenated solvents or to ethanol.

Clinical Findings

A. Symptoms & Signs

Symptoms of intoxication with hydrocarbon solvents or chlorofluorocarbons include dizziness, light-headedness, headaches, nausea, drowsiness, lethargy, palpitations, and syncope. Physical examination may reveal ataxia, nystagmus, and slurred speech. The heart rate and blood pressure usually are normal, except at the time of arrhythmias, when a rapid or irregular heartbeat sometimes is accompanied by hypotension.

Convulsions, coma, or cardiac arrest may occur in severe cases of exposure to solvents. Workers who have heart disease or chronic lung disease with hypoxemia may be more susceptible to the arrhythmogenic actions of solvents.

B. Laboratory Findings

The concentrations of some hydrocarbons can be measured in expired air or in the blood (see Chapters 29 and 36).

C. Cardiovascular Studies

Arrhythmias induced by solvents or chlorofluorocarbons are expected to occur only at work, while the worker is exposed to these agents. The diagnosis is based on abnormalities observed during ambulatory electrocardiographic monitoring, which consist of one or more of the following: premature atrial or ventricular contractions, recurrent supraventricular tachycardia, and recurrent

ventricular tachycardia. It is essential to monitor patients on both workdays and off days and to request a log of times of exposure to solvents or chlorofluorocarbons as well as a log of symptoms of palpitations or dizzy spells. A 12-lead ECG and an exercise stress test can help to determine the presence of coronary artery disease, which might increase sensitivity to hydrocarbon- or chlorofluorocarbon-induced arrhythmia.

Differential Diagnosis

The diagnosis of solvent- or chlorofluorocarbon-induced arrhythmia is based on exclusion of other causes of arrhythmias at work (e.g., the presence of a cardiac disease, metabolic disturbance, or drug abuse) and demonstration of a temporal relationship between episodes of arrhythmia and exposures to the toxic agent. The diagnosis is supported by industrial hygiene measurements documenting the level of exposure in the workplace and by objective and subjective evidence that the worker was intoxicated following exposure.

Prevention

Preventive measures include proper handling of solvents and propellants, adequate ventilation in the workplace, and in some cases, the use of protective respiratory equipment. Workers with heart disease—especially those with chronic arrhythmia—should be advised to avoid exposure to potentially arrhythmogenic chemicals.

Treatment

β-Adrenergic blocking agents may be useful in managing solvent- or chlorofluorocarbon-induced arrhythmias. In cases of episodic arrhythmia, the worker should be removed from excessive exposure or advised to use protective respiratory equipment. If a worker collapses and resuscitation is required, use of epinephrine and other sympathomimetic drugs should be avoided, if possible, because they may precipitate further arrhythmia.

Course & Prognosis

Arrhythmias are expected to resolve fully after exposure to hydrocarbons is stopped.

REFERENCES

Armstrong SR, Green LC: Chlorinated hydrocarbon solvents. Clin Occup Environ Med 2004;4:481 [PMID: 15325317].

Hardin BD et al: Trichloroethylene and cardiac malformations. Environ Health Perspect 2004;112:607 [PMID: 15289177].

Tsai WT: An overview of environmental hazards and exposure risk of hydrofluorocarbons (HFCs). Chemosphere 2005;61:1539 [PMID: 15936055].

CARDIOVASCULAR ABNORMALITIES CAUSED BY ORGANOPHOSPHATE & CARBAMATE INSECTICIDES

Intoxication with organophosphate and carbamate insecticides can produce diverse cardiovascular disturbances, including tachycardia and hypertension, bradycardia and hypotension, heart block, and ventricular tachycardia. Organophosphate and carbamate insecticides are used widely in agriculture and can be applied to crops by aerial spraying or by hand. Agricultural workers thus may absorb the insecticides by inhalation of mist or via cutaneous absorption. Acute insecticide poisoning affects the circulatory system and may be fatal. Chronic poisoning may cause neuropsychiatric disturbances, as described in Chapter 31.

Pathogenesis

Organophosphates and carbamates inhibit acetylcholinesterase, and this causes accumulation of acetylcholine at cholinergic synapses and myoneural junctions. The cardiovascular effects may vary over the time course of poisoning. Early in acute poisoning, acetylcholine stimulates nicotinic receptors at sympathetic ganglia and causes tachycardia and mild hypertension. Later, when acetylcholine acts at muscarinic receptors or blocks ganglionic transmission by hyperpolarization, it causes bradycardia and hypotension. As a consequence of autonomic imbalance and asynchronous repolarization of different parts of the heart, there may be QT-interval prolongation and polymorphous ventricular tachycardia (torsade de pointes).

The excess of acetylcholine at the myoneural junctions initially causes muscle fasciculations and later causes muscle paralysis, including paralysis of the diaphragm, which results in respiratory failure or respiratory arrest. Other consequences are described below.

Pathology

Since organophosphates act on autonomic neurotransmitters, there are no specific pathologic findings.

Clinical Findings

A. Symptoms & Signs

Typical symptoms of mild organophosphate or carbamate poisoning include weakness, headache, sweating, nausea, vomiting, abdominal cramps, and diarrhea. Moderate poisoning may be associated with chest discomfort, dyspnea, inability to walk, and blurred vision.

The signs are those of cholinergic excess and include small pupils, diaphoresis, salivation, lacrimation, an increase in bronchial secretions (which may resemble pulmonary edema), and muscle fasciculations. Early cardiovascular manifestations may include tachycardia and hypertension. Later, there may be bradycardia and hypotension. There is sometimes frank muscular weakness or, in severe poisoning, paralysis accompanied by respiratory failure, convulsions, or coma. The failure of usual doses of atropine to reverse cholinergic signs is highly suggestive of the diagnosis of organophosphate or carbamate poisoning.

B. Laboratory Findings

The diagnosis is confirmed by the finding of markedly depressed cholinesterase activity in red blood cells. Depression to below 50% of normal usually is required for patients to have any symptoms, and depression to less than 10% of normal usually is seen in patients with severe poisoning. Plasma cholinesterase activity also is usually depressed, but this correlates less well with clinical manifestations. Arterial blood gases may show carbon dioxide retention, hypoxia, or both.

The presence of a particular type of organophosphate may be detected in the blood or gastric fluids. Some organophosphates (e.g., parathion) have metabolites that can be measured in the urine.

C. Cardiovascular Studies

Delayed repolarization with QT-interval prolongation and episodes of ventricular tachycardia may be seen for up to 5–7 days after acute intoxication. The ECG also commonly shows nonspecific ST- and T-wave changes. A number of arrhythmias, including premature ventricular contractions, ventricular tachycardia and fibrillation, and heart block and asystole, have been observed.

D. Imaging

Chest radiography may show a pattern similar to that of pulmonary edema.

Differential Diagnosis

The signs and symptoms of cholinergic excess are fairly specific for poisoning with cholinesterase-inhibiting insecticides. However, similar findings may be seen in people treated with cholinesterase inhibitors, such as pyridostigmine, for myasthenia gravis. Small pupils also may be seen following ingestion of narcotics, clonidine, phenothiazines, and sedative drugs and in patients with pontine brain infarction or hemorrhage.

Prevention

Most organophosphate and carbamate insecticides are absorbed rapidly following ingestion, inhalation, or contact with the skin or eyes. Continuing exposure may occur from contact with contaminated clothing or hair. Prevention requires the use of protective clothing and respirators and monitoring of red blood cell cholinesterase levels on a regular basis.

Treatment

General measures include decontamination (removal of clothing and thorough cleaning of skin and hair), support of respiration (including mechanical ventilation in patients with respiratory failure), and support of the circulation. Specific measures include the use of pralidoxime to reverse muscular paralysis and other manifestations of excess acetylcholine and the use of atropine to reverse bronchorrhea and bradycardia.

Intensive cardiac and respiratory monitoring of patients for several days after exposure is recommended, with particular attention to the possible late development of arrhythmia or respiratory failure. High-degree heart block and polymorphous ventricular tachycardia with a prolonged QT interval are treated optimally with cardiac pacing. The use of antiarrhythmic drugs that depress conduction (e.g., quinidine, procainamide, and disopyramide) and calcium channel blockers should be avoided.

Course & Prognosis

Recovery from acute intoxication is usually complete. Chronic intoxication may be associated with neuropsychiatric consequences (see Chapters 24 and 31).

REFERENCES

Asari Y et al: Changes in the hemodynamic state of patients with acute lethal organophosphate poisoning. Vet Hum Toxicol 2004;46:5 [PMID: 14748407].

Kamanyire R, Karalliedde L: Organophosphate toxicity and occupational exposure. Occup Med (Lond) 2004;54:69 [PMID: 15020723].

Karki P et al: Cardiac and electrocardiographical manifestations of acute organophosphate poisoning. Singapore Med J 2004; 45:385 [PMID: 15284933].

CARDIOVASCULAR ABNORMALITIES CAUSED BY HEAVY METALS

Several metals are associated with disturbances in cardiovascular function, but their causative role is not fully established.

Antimony

Therapeutic use of antimonial compounds for the treatment of parasitic infections produces electrocardiographic abnormalities—primarily T-wave changes and QT-interval prolongation—and has caused sudden death in some patients. Electrocardiographic changes also have been observed in workers exposed to antimony. Although these changes usually resolve after removal from exposure, a few studies report increased cardiovascular mortality rates in exposed workers. Studies in animals confirm that chronic exposure to antimony can produce myocardial disease.

Arsenic

Subacute arsenic poisoning caused by ingestion of arsenic-contaminated beer is associated with cardiomyopathy and cardiac failure. Chronic arsenic poisoning has been reported to produce "blackfoot disease," which is characterized by claudication and gangrene, presumably secondary to spasms of the large blood vessels in the extremities. Arsenic exposure in drinking water is associated with an increased prevalence of hypertension. Acute arsenic poisoning can cause electrocardiographic abnormalities, and in one case it was reported to cause recurrent ventricular arrhythmia of the torsade de pointes type. A mortality study of copper smelters exposed to arsenic indicated that these workers have an increased risk of death as a result of ischemic heart disease.

Arsine

Arsine gas causes red blood cell hemolysis. Massive hemolysis produces hyperkalemia, which can result in cardiac arrest. Electrocardiographic manifestations progress from high, peaked T waves to conduction disturbances and various degrees of heart block and then to asystole. Arsine also may directly affect the myocardium, causing a greater magnitude of cardiac failure than would be expected from the degree of anemia.

Cadmium

Some earlier epidemiologic and experimental animal studies linked high-level cadmium exposure with hypertension, but recent epidemiologic studies do not support the association. Environmental exposure to cadmium, as assessed by blood or urine levels, is associated with an increased risk of peripheral arterial disease.

Cobalt

In Quebec City, Canada, in 1965 and 1966, an epidemic of cardiomyopathy occurred in heavy drinkers of beer to which cobalt sulfate had been added as a foam stabilizer. The mortality rate in affected patients was 22%, and a major pathologic finding in those who died was myocardial necrosis with thrombi in the heart and major blood vessels. Other clinical features in affected patients included polycythemia, pericardial effusion, and thyroid hyperplasia. Cobalt is known to depress oxygen uptake by the mitochondria of the heart and to interfere with energy metabolism in a manner biochemically similar to the effects of thiamine deficiency. Because individuals receiving higher doses of cobalt for therapeutic reasons have not developed cardiomyopathy, it is possible that cobalt, excessive alcohol consumption, and nutritional deprivation acted synergistically to produce cardiomyopathy in this epidemic. Occupational exposure to cobalt has been associated with diastolic dysfunction on echocardiography. Several cases of cardiomyopathy in workers exposed to cobalt have been reported.

Lead

Exposure to excessive levels of lead causes chronic renal diseases, and epidemiologic studies suggest that it also contributes to hypertension in the absence of renal disease. Some of the workplace studies of exposure to lead report an increased incidence of ischemic electrocardiographic changes and an increased risk of hypertensive or coronary artery disease and cerebrovascular disease in exposed workers. Nonspecific electrocardiographic changes and fatal myocarditis in the absence of hypertension have been observed in children with lead poisoning. Cardiomyopathy in moonshine drinkers is also attributed to lead exposure. Studies in animals indicate that lead may have direct toxic effects on the myocardium.

REFERENCES

Linna A et al: Exposure to cobalt in the production of cobalt and cobalt compounds and its effect on the heart. Occup Environ Med 2004;61:877 [PMID: 15477280].

Navas-Acien A et al: Metals in urine and peripheral arterial disease. Environ Health Perspect 2005;113:164 [PMID: 15687053].

Navas-Acien A et al: Arsenic exposure and cardiovascular disease: A systematic review of the epidemiologic evidence. Am J Epidemiol 2005;162:1037 [PMID: 16269585].

Navas-Acien A et al: Lead, cadmium, smoking, and increased risk of peripheral arterial disease. Circulation 2004;109:3196 [PMID: 15184277].

Palda VA: Is foundry work a risk for cardiovascular disease? A systematic review. Occup Med (Lond) 2003;53:179 [PMID: 12724552].

Simeonova PP, Luster MI: Arsenic and atherosclerosis. Toxicol Appl Pharmacol 2004;198:444 [PMID: 15276425].

Selvin E, Erlinger TP: Prevalence of and risk factors for peripheral arterial disease in the United States. Circulation 2004;110:738 [PMID: 15262830].

CARDIOVASCULAR ABNORMALITIES CAUSED BY AIR POLLUTION

Epidemiologic studies, by using time-series analysis, have demonstrated an association between the level of exposure to air pollution and increased mortality, including increased mortality from cardiovascular disease and stroke. Higher levels of air pollution are associated with more hospital admissions for cardiovascular disease. Furthermore, several case-control studies of welders have reported increased risk of myocardial infarction and cardiovascular mortality. Welders inhale fumes containing gases and respirable particles (as well as metals such as zinc).

Inhalation of particulates has been shown to alter heart rate variability, with an increase in average heart rate, and to increase plasma viscosity. Gaseous pollutants include oxidizing gases that generate free radicals, which may result in generalized inflammatory responses, endothelial dysfunction, and enhanced blood coagulation. Hemodynamic stress, inflammation, and hypercoagulability are the suspected mechanisms for the link between air pollution and acute cardiovascular events.

REFERENCES

Filleul L et al: Twenty-five-year mortality and air pollution: Results from the French PAARC survey. Occup Environ Med 2005;62:453 [PMID: 15961621].

Goodman PG et al: Cause-specific mortality and the extended effects of particulate pollution and temperature exposure. Environ Health Perspect 2004;112:179 [PMID: 14754572].

Harrabi I et al: Effects of particulate air pollution on systolic blood pressure: A population-based approach. Environ Res 2006;101:89 [PMID: 16563371].

Ibald-Mulli A et al: Effects of particulate air pollution on blood pressure and heart rate in subjects with cardiovascular disease. Environ Health Perspect 2004;112:369 [PMID: 14998755].

Nafstad P et al: Urban air pollution and mortality in a cohort of Norwegian men. Environ Health Perspect 2004;112:610 [PMID: 15064169].

Liver Toxicology

22

Robert J. Harrison, MD, MPH

The liver is the target organ of many occupational and environmental chemicals and plays a central role in their detoxification and elimination. Bacterial and viral infections and certain chemical and physical agents encountered in the workplace also involve the liver. Tables 22–1, 22–4, and 22–5 present the main causes of occupational liver disease.

DETECTION OF OCCUPATIONAL LIVER DISEASE

With the exception of a few chemicals that cause specific lesions (Table 22–1), hepatic injury as a consequence of industrial exposure does not differ clinically or morphologically from drug-induced damage (including damage caused by ethanol). Thus it may be difficult to differentiate occupational from nonoccupational causes on the basis of screening tests.

Occupational liver disease may be of secondary importance to damage that occurs to other organs or may occur only at high doses after accidental exposure or ingestion. While acute toxic liver injury does occur, concern is focused increasingly on chronic liver disease resulting from prolonged low-level toxic exposure. In this respect, cancer is of central concern. Because chemical studies frequently are done on animals first, the occupational health practitioner must be able to evaluate—without the assistance of adequate human studies—the results of positive carcinogenesis studies in light of actual workplace exposures (e.g., methylene chloride; see Chapter 29).

In individual cases, the clinician usually is first alerted to the presence of hepatic disease by routine enzyme tests and then must make a determination about whether the cause is occupational or nonoccupational. The occupational history and result of personal or workroom air sampling are crucial to formulation of a presumptive diagnosis. It is occasionally necessary to remove the patient from exposure to the suspected workplace toxic substance to establish the workplace relationship.

LIMITATIONS OF DETECTION

Unfortunately, the detection of preclinical disease is made difficult by the lack of sufficiently sensitive and specific tests. It is common practice to measure liver enzymes periodically in workers exposed to a known hepatotoxin. This surveillance technique is complicated, however, by the problems of false-positive results (i.e., elevated enzyme levels as a result of nonoccupational causes) and false-negative results (i.e., normal values in the presence of biochemical dysfunction). In addition, little is known about the effects of multiple hepatotoxic exposures common to many occupations (e.g., painters, printers, and laboratory technicians). (For a detailed discussion of these limitations, see "Medical Surveillance and Detection of Occupational Hepatotoxicity" below.)

EPIDEMIOLOGIC EVIDENCE OF LIVER DISEASE

Epidemiologic studies have been performed on many groups of workers exposed to hepatotoxic agents. However, relatively few workplace hepatotoxic substances have been studied in humans. Epidemiologic studies, where available, generally provide the best evidence of toxicity; however, they may be limited by inadequate study design and other confounding factors, such as body mass index, alcohol ingestion, and medication use.

Serum Aminotransferase

Cross-sectional studies that include biochemical liver tests have been conducted among many groups of workers exposed to hepatotoxic agents. Serum aminotransferase elevations have been found in workers exposed to polychlorinated and polybrominated biphenyls (PCBs, PBBs) and polychlorinated naphthalenes. Hepatocellular liver enzyme abnormalities have been found among microelectronics equipment maintenance technicians, pharmaceutical industry workers exposed to mixed solvents, dry-cleaning operators, and petrochemical workers exposed to mixed aliphatic and aromatic hydrocarbons. Increased levels of liver enzymes have been found among chemical plant operators exposed to carbon tetrachloride. Hepatocellular damage with increased liver enzymes has been seen among coke oven workers exposed to coke oven emissions, with a greater risk among those with the cytochrome P450 MspI polymorphism. Solvent-exposed

Table 22-1. Chemical agents associated with occupational liver disease.

Compound	Type of Injury	Occupation or Use
Arsenic	Cirrhosis, hepatocellular carcinoma, angiosarcoma	Pesticides
Beryllium	Granulomatous disease	Ceramics workers
Carbon tetrachloride	Acute hepatocellular injury, cirrhosis	Chemical manufacturing
Dimethylformamide	Acute hepatocellular injury	Solvent, chemical manufacturing
Dimethylnitrosamine	Hepatocellular carcinoma	Rocket manufacturing
Dioxin	Porphyria cutanea tarda	Pesticides
Halothane	Acute hepatocellular injury	Anesthesiology
Hydrazine	Steatosis	Rocket manufacturing
Methylene dianiline (MDA)	Cholestasis	MDA production workers
2-Nitropropane	Acute hepatocellular injury	Painters
Phosphorus	Acute hepatocellular injury	Munitions workers
Polychlorinated biphenyls	Subacute liver injury	Production, electrical utility
Tetrachloroethane	Acute or subacute hepatocellular injury	Aircraft manufacturing
Trichloroethylene	Acute hepatocellular injury	Cleaning solvent sniffing
Trinitrotoluene	Acute or subacute hepatocellular injury	Munitions workers
Vinyl chloride	Angiosarcoma	Rubber workers

painters and paint makers have lifetime and peak solvent dose-related increases in serum transaminase and alkaline phosphatase activity, with a significant interaction with concurrent alcohol and hepatotoxic medication use. Increased levels of liver enzymes have been reported after occupational exposure to methylene chloride, polychlorinated naphthalenes, ethylene dichloride, hydrazine, and 2,3,7,8-tetrachlorodibenzo-*p*-dioxin (dioxin).

Microsomal Enzyme Induction

By using the noninvasive antipyrine clearance test, induction of the microsomal enzyme system has been demonstrated in workers exposed to various pesticides [chlordecone, phenoxy acids, dichlorodiphenyltrichloroethane (DDT), lindane], halothane, PCBs, and various solvents. Functional abnormalities of liver metabolism, measured by antipyrine clearance or other noninvasive tests of liver function, are not accompanied by other clinical or laboratory signs of toxicity and so may provide a sensitive index of biologic change.

Mortality Studies

Cohort mortality studies show an increased mortality rate from liver cirrhosis among newspaper pressmen, spray painters, chlorinated naphthalene workers, and oil refinery workers and from liver cancer among vinyl chloride, rubber, dye, and shoe factory workers. Case-control studies show a statistically significant association between primary liver cancer and exposure to chlorinated solvents, particularly among laundry workers, dry cleaners, gasoline service station attendants, printing industry workers, asphalt workers, automobile workers, and bartenders.

CHEMICAL AGENTS THAT CAUSE LIVER TOXICITY

Pathogenesis & Epidemiology

Occupational hepatotoxicity caused by chemicals is most frequently part of systemic toxicity involving other organ systems of primary clinical importance (e.g., central nervous system depression, following exposure to hydrocarbon solvents). Occasionally, the liver toxicity is responsible for the major clinical findings (e.g., carbon tetrachloride intoxication associated with renal and central nervous system damage); rarely is liver disease the sole manifestation of toxicity.

The study of hepatotoxic potential in animals is an important first step for newly introduced chemicals. Differences among species, circumstances of exposure, and the difficulty in performing human studies may limit detection of experimental observations in the workplace. For example, while ingestion of arsenicals causes severe acute hepatic damage in both experimental animals and humans, there are reports of liver disease in humans in vintners exposed to arsenical pesticides.

There is no comprehensive repository of data on animal and human hepatotoxic agents. Identification of chemicals that may produce liver damage in humans has come about through a combination of experimental animal data, clinical observation, and epidemiologic studies. Some agents, such as trinitrotoluene (TNT), dimethylnitrosamine (DMA), tetrachloroethane, PCBs, and vinyl chloride, led to serious industrial hepatotoxicity before their effects on experimental animals were fully investigated. In the case of chlordecone (Kepone), human hepatotoxicity was found several years after experimental animal studies demonstrated clear evidence of liver damage following exposure.

Routes of Exposure

Inhalation, ingestion, and percutaneous absorption are the routes by which toxic chemicals can gain entry to the body. Inhalation is probably the most important route for hepatotoxic material, particularly for the volatile solvents. Several chemicals are lipophilic and may be absorbed through the skin in sufficient quantities to contribute to hepatotoxicity (e.g., TNT, 4,4-diaminodiphenylmethane, tetrachloroethylene, PCBs, and dimethylformamide). In cases of liver damage by industrial agents that are not airborne, it is often difficult to distinguish between contamination of ingested material, absorption from mucous membranes, and absorption through the skin. Oral intake of hepatotoxic agents is usually of importance only in the rare case of accidental ingestion, although mouth breathing and gum and tobacco chewing can increase the amount of gaseous substances absorbed during the workday.

Mechanisms of Toxicity

As Table 22–2 illustrates, chemical agents that cause hepatic injury may be classified into two major categories.

A. INTRINSICALLY TOXIC AGENTS

Agents intrinsically toxic to the liver—directly or indirectly—cause a high incidence of dose-dependent hepatic injury in exposed persons and similar lesions in experimental animals. Furthermore, the interval between exposure (under specified conditions) and onset of disease is consistent and usually short.

1. Direct hepatotoxins—Direct hepatotoxins or their metabolic products injure the hepatocyte and its organelles by a direct physicochemical effect, such as peroxidation of membrane lipids, denaturation of proteins, or other chemical changes that lead to destruction or distortion of cell membranes.

Carbon tetrachloride is the prototype and the best-studied example of the direct hepatotoxins, producing centrilobular necrosis and steatosis in humans and experimental animals. This agent appears to exert its hepatotoxic effects by the binding of reactive metabolites to a number of critical cellular molecules that interfere with vital cell function or cause lipid peroxidation of cell membranes. The toxicity of carbon tetrachloride is mediated by metabolism to the toxic trichloromethyl radical catalyzed by cytochrome P450 2EI. Damage to cellular membranes results in leakage of intracellular enzymes and electrolytes, leading to calcium shifts and lipid peroxidation.

Chloroform likewise may cause direct hepatic necrosis. A large number of haloalkanes (e.g., trichloroethylene, carbon tetrabromide, tetrachloroethane, 1,1,1-trichloroethane, 1,1,2-trichloroethane, and hydrochlorofluorocarbons) produce hepatic injury ranging from steatosis to trivial or nondemonstrable liver damage. Their hepatotoxic potential is inversely proportional to chain length

Table 22–2. Mechanisms of toxicity of chemicals causing hepatic injury.

Category of Agent	Incidence	Experimental Reproducibility	Dose Dependent	Example
Intrinsic toxin				
Direct	High	Yes	Yes	Carbon tetrachloride
Indirect				
Cytotoxic	High	Yes	Yes	Dimethylnitrosamine
Cholestatic	High	Yes	Yes	Methylene dianiline
Host idiosyncrasy				
Hypersensitivity	Low	No	No	Phenytoin
Metabolic abnormality	Low	No	No	Isoniazid

and bond energy and directly proportional to the number of halogen atoms in the molecule and to the atomic number of the halogen.

Most aromatic hydrocarbons are relatively low in hepatotoxic potential, with some evidence for acute hepatic injury caused by benzene, toluene, xylene, and styrene.

2. Indirect hepatotoxins—Indirect hepatotoxins are antimetabolites and related compounds that produce hepatic injury by interference with metabolic pathways. This may result in cytotoxic damage (degeneration or necrosis of hepatocytes) by interfering with pathways necessary for the structural integrity of the hepatocyte (morphologically seen as steatosis or necrosis) or may cause cholestasis (arrested bile flow) by interfering with the bile secretory process.

The cytotoxic indirect hepatotoxins include compounds of experimental interest (e.g., ethionine and galactosamine), drugs (e.g., tetracycline, asparaginase, methotrexate, and mercaptopurine), and botanicals (e.g., aflatoxin, cycasin, mushroom alkaloids, and tannic acid). Ethanol belongs to this category by virtue of a number of selective biochemical lesions that lead to steatosis. Only one industrial chemical, 4,4-diaminodiphenylmethane [commonly known as *methylene dianiline* (MDA)], has been categorized as a cholestatic indirect hepatotoxin. Used as a plastic hardener—most commonly for epoxy resins—this agent has caused a number of epidemics (see "Acute Cholestatic Jaundice" below).

B. AGENTS CAUSING LIVER INJURY BY VIRTUE OF HOST IDIOSYNCRASY

Chemically induced hepatic injury may be a result of some special vulnerability of the individual and not the intrinsic toxicity of the agent. In such cases, liver damage occurs sporadically and unpredictably, has low experimental reproducibility, and is not dose-dependent. The injury may be a result of allergy (hypersensitivity) or of production of hepatotoxic metabolites. A well-established example is halothane, which causes acute hepatitis in a small percentage of individuals with a hypersensitivity immune response. The mechanism for halothane-induced hepatitis is thought to be a hypersensitivity reaction to liver neoantigens produced by the halothane metabolite 2-chloro-1,1,1-trifluoroethane. There appears to be a role for inherited susceptibility in halothane hepatitis.

Hepatic Metabolism of Xenobiotics

The liver is especially vulnerable to chemical injury by virtue of its role in the metabolism of foreign compounds, or xenobiotics. The metabolism of xenobiotics is thus of central clinical interest. These chemicals, taken up by the body but not incorporated into the normal metabolic economy of the cell, are metabolized chiefly by the liver. Xenobiotic lipid-soluble compounds are well absorbed through membrane barriers and poorly excreted by the kidney as a result of protein binding and tubular reabsorption. Increasing polarity of nonpolar molecules by hepatic metabolism increases water solubility and urinary excretion. In this way, hepatic metabolism prevents the accumulation of drugs and other toxic chemicals in the body.

The strategic role of the liver as the primary defense against xenobiotics depends largely on cellular enzyme systems [mixed-function oxidases (MFOs)]. The enzyme systems responsible for the metabolism of xenobiotics are attached to the membrane layers of the smooth endoplasmic reticulum. Although enzymes that catalyze the metabolism of nonpolar xenobiotics are present in the intestines, lungs, kidneys, and skin, the vast majority of metabolic conversions occur in the liver. Most xenobiotics that are toxic by the oral route are also hepatotoxic parenterally or by inhalation.

Xenobiotic Agents Activated by the MFO System

Many hepatotoxic agents and hepatocarcinogens must be activated first by the MFO system to a toxic or carcinogenic metabolite. Examples include carbon tetrachloride, vinyl chloride, PCBs, bromobenzene, azo dyes, DMA, and allyl compounds. Electrophilic intermediates react with enzymes and regulatory or structural proteins and lead to cell death.

Many drugs, insecticides, organic solvents, carcinogens, and other environmental contaminants are known experimentally to stimulate some type of microsomal activity that is associated with the metabolism of xenobiotics. The administration of ethanol concomitantly with carbon tetrachloride enhances the toxicity of the latter, presumably via induction of the MFO system. Clinically, this may explain the well-documented synergistic effect between ethanol abuse and carbon tetrachloride toxicity in humans. Ethanol pretreatment in experimental human studies enhances the metabolic clearance of *m*-xylene and antipyrine by microsomal enzyme induction, and studies show that workers with prior alcohol consumption may be more likely to develop acute hepatotoxicity after occupational exposure to isopropyl alcohol, xylene, and toluene.

Other mechanisms may be at work as well because a single dose of alcohol given to animals several hours prior to administration of carbon tetrachloride potentiates toxicity. Experiments show that many other factors may affect the metabolism of xenobiotics: diet, age, sex, cigarette smoking, endocrine status, genetic factors, diurnal variations, underlying liver disease, and stress. There is considerable inter- and intraindividual variation in xenobiotic metabolism, and the relative importance of these factors in the occupational setting is not currently known. There is increasing evidence that tissue repair increases in a dose-dependent manner up to a threshold dose but that this threshold can be lowered when one or more components of the mixture inhibit cell division and tissue repair. Enhanced microsomal enzyme function has been demonstrated in industrial workers exposed to hepatotoxins at levels below those shown to result in hepatic necrosis. Increasing attention has been directed to the use of noninvasive measurements of MFOs in the preclinical detection of liver disease (see below).

DISEASE PATTERNS & MORPHOLOGY OF HEPATIC INJURY

As Table 22–3 shows, occupational exposure to xenobiotics can lead to acute, subacute, or chronic liver disease. The clinical syndromes can be associated with several types of morphologic changes, as seen by light microscopy. Hepatic injury may be clinically overt or may be discovered only as a functional or histologic abnormality. Clinical evaluation of individuals with chronic liver dis-

Table 22–3. Morphologic patterns of liver injury.

Type of Injury	Examples of Causes
Acute	
Cytotoxic	
Necrosis	
Zonal	Carbon tetrachloride, chloroform
Massive	Trinitrotoluene
Steatosis	Carbon tetrachloride, chloroform, phosphorus, dimethyl formamide, hydrazine
Cholestatic	Methylene dianiline, rapeseed oil
Subacute	Trinitrotoluene
Chronic	
Cirrhosis	Trinitrotoluene, polychlorinated biphenyls, tetrachloroethane
Sclerosis	Arsenic, vinyl chloride
Porphyria	Dioxin
Neoplasia	Arsenic, vinyl chloride
Steatosis	Dimethylformamide, carbon tetrachloride
Granuloma	Beryllium, copper

Table 22–4. Agents causing acute hepatic injury (partial list).

Anesthetic gases (halothane, methoxyflurane)
Bromobenzene
Carbon tetrabromide
Carbon tetrachloride
Chlorinated naphthalenes
Chloroform
Dichlorohydrin
Dimethylformamide
Elemental phosphorus
2-Nitropropane
Tetrachloroethane
Trichloroethane
Trichloroethylene
Trinitrotoluene

ease caused by subtle repeated injury owing to workplace exposures has been of growing concern.

ACUTE HEPATIC INJURY

Acute liver disease was a cause of serious occupational liver disease in the first part of the twentieth century and may be still encountered. Acute hepatic injury has been reported as a result of exposure to agents listed in Table 22–4.

Clinical Findings

Occupational exposure to xenobiotics may lead to degeneration or necrosis of hepatocytes (cytotoxic injury) or to arrested bile flow (cholestatic injury). The latency period is relatively short (24–48 hours), and clinical symptoms are often of extrahepatic origin. Anorexia, nausea, vomiting, jaundice, and hepatomegaly are often present. Severely exposed individuals who have sustained massive necrosis may have coffee-ground emesis, abdominal pain, reduction in liver size on examination, rapid development of ascites, edema, and hemorrhagic diathesis. This is often followed within 24–28 hours by somnolence and coma.

Morphologically, hepatic necrosis may be zonal, massive, or diffuse. Centrizonal necrosis is the characteristic lesion produced by the agents listed in Table 22–4, as well as by the toxins of *Amanita phalloides* and acetaminophen. Periportal or peripheral necrosis is produced by elemental phosphorus. TNT, PCBs, and chloronaphthalenes can produce massive rather than zonal necrosis.

Various degrees of fatty change or steatosis also may be seen morphologically in association with toxicity owing to carbon tetrachloride, chloroform, tetrachloroethane, dimethylformamide, trichloroethane, styrene, hydrazine, and elemental phosphorus.

CARBON TETRACHLORIDE–INDUCED ACUTE HEPATIC INJURY

Carbon tetrachloride presents the classic example of an acute hepatotoxin. It was first recognized as such in the 1920s, when it was in common use as a liquid solvent, dry-cleaning agent, and fire extinguisher. Since then, hundreds of poisonings and fatalities have been reported, mostly from inhalation in confined spaces.

Clinical Findings

Clinically, immediate nervous system symptoms of dizziness, headache, visual disturbances, and confusion are observed as a result of the anesthetic properties of carbon tetrachloride. This is followed by nausea, vomiting, abdominal pain, and diarrhea during the first 24 hours. Evidence of hepatic disease usually follows after 2–4 days but may appear within 24 hours. The liver and spleen become palpable, and jaundice develops, accompanied by elevated serum transaminase concentrations and prolonged prothrombin time. Renal failure may ensue a few days after the hepatic damage becomes manifest and in fact has been the cause of death in most fatal cases. Sequelae of hepatic failure such as hypoglycemia, encephalopathy, and hemorrhage may be complications. Some instances of carbon tetrachloride toxicity have occurred with accompanying ethanol intake, which may be a potentiating factor in hepatotoxicity.

Treatment with *N*-acetyl-L-cysteine (NAC) is effective in cases of massive carbon tetrachloride ingestion. Animal studies suggest that NAC may decrease the covalent binding of carbon tetrachloride–reactive metabolites, decrease the amount of carbon tetrachloride reaching the liver, or partially block lipid peroxidation.

ACUTE HEPATIC INJURY INDUCED BY OTHER XENOBIOTICS

Tetrachloroethylene causes acute hepatotoxicity when used as a dry-cleaning agent and causes acute centrilobular necrosis following recreational "solvent sniffing" of cleaning fluids. This may have been a result of contamination with dichloroacetylene rather than a consequence of tetrachloroethylene itself.

Both trichloroethylene and trichloroethane have been reported to cause acute, reversible hepatitis with fatty infiltration in several workers. A liver biopsy specimen from one trichloroethane-exposed printer showed focal bridging fibrosis and nodule formation with evidence of marked portal tract fibrosis, a pattern suggestive of macronodular or early cirrhosis.

Carbon tetrabromide caused a syndrome in chemists that is similar to acute carbon tetrachloride hepatotoxicity. Dimethylacetamide caused acute, reversible hepatitis in one worker with severe inhalational and dermal exposure. Intentional nonoccupational exposure to the herbicide 2,4-dichlorophenoxyacetic acid (2,4-D) was reported to result in acute hepatitis with pronounced cholestasis, portal inflammation, and periportal edema. 2-Nitropropane, a nitroparaffin used as a solvent in epoxy-resin paints and coatings, has caused several cases of acute fulminant hepatitis following exposure in confined spaces.

Hydrochlorofluorocarbons, increasingly used in industry as substitutes for ozone-depleting chlorofluorocarbons, have been reported to cause hepatocellular necrosis in workers after repeated exposure. The formation of trifluoroacetyl-adducted proteins may result in direct toxicity. The aromatic nitro amino compound 5-nitro-*o*-toluidine was reported recently to cause acute, reversible hepatitis among 15 hospitalized workers.

The solvent dimethylformamide (DMF) has been reported to acutely cause increased levels of liver enzymes among workers involved in synthetic textile production and synthetic leather workers. In the study of synthetic leather workers, accidental skin contact with DMF led to significant DMF uptake. Liver biopsy specimens in acutely DMF-exposed workers showed focal hepatocellular necrosis with microvesicular steatosis. Liver biopsy specimens from workers with longer exposures showed macrovesicular steatosis without persisting acute injury or fibrosis. Abnormal liver function and chronic liver disease were associated with the glutathione *S*-transferase (GSTT-1) polymorphism. Progression to cirrhosis was not demonstrated up to 22 months following exposure. Workers with concomitant alcohol use and infection with hepatitis B virus had a greater risk of liver disease.

Fulminant hepatic failure has been reported in a recreational solvent abuser exposed to a mixture of isopropyl alcohol, methyl amyl alcohol, and butylated hydroxytoluene and in a worker following exposure to dichlorohydrin during tank cleaning.

ACUTE CHOLESTATIC JAUNDICE

This is a rare manifestation of occupational toxicity. MDA was responsible for an epidemic of cholestatic jaundice observed in Epping, England (*Epping jaundice*), in 1965. This compound, used as a hardener for epoxy resin, had spilled from a plastic container onto the floor of a van that was carrying both flour and the chemical. Acute cholestatic injury was found subsequently in 84 persons who had eaten bread made from the contaminated flour. Onset was abrupt—with abdominal pain—in 60% of cases and was insidious in one-third. Histologic evidence of bile stasis with only slight parenchymal injury was seen in most cases, and all victims recovered without evidence of persistent hepatic injury. An analysis 38 years later found no deaths from liver cancer or non-malignant liver disease. Similar cases have been reported subsequently for industrial exposure during the manufacture and application of epoxy resins. Cholestatic liver injury has been reported after accidental ingestion of denatured rapeseed oil and after ingestion of moldy grain and nuts contaminated with aflatoxin.

SUBACUTE HEPATIC NECROSIS

This form of hepatic injury is characterized by a smoldering illness with delayed onset of jaundice. It usually follows repeated exposure to relatively small doses of a hepatotoxin. The onset of anorexia, nausea, and vomiting accompanied by hepatomegaly and jaundice may occur after several weeks to months of exposure and may lead variably to recovery or to fulminant hepatic failure. A few patients are reported to have developed macronodular cirrhosis, although clinical data are limited.

The histologic features of subacute hepatic necrosis consist of various degrees of necrosis, fibrosis, and regeneration. In cases where the clinical course is relatively brief (2–3 weeks), necrotic features predominate. In patients with a prolonged course of several months or more, postnecrotic scarring with subacute hepatic necrosis is seen. In the past, trinitrotoluene caused many cases of both acute and subacute hepatic necrosis. Fortunately, subacute hepatic necrosis caused by occupational exposure is rare today.

■ CHRONIC HEPATIC INJURY

Several forms of chronic liver damage can result from continuing or repeated injury caused by prolonged exposure: cirrhosis and fibrosis, hepatoportal sclerosis, hepatic porphyria, and neoplasia.

CIRRHOSIS & FIBROSIS

The histologic pattern of progressive necrosis accompanied by regenerating nodules, fibrosis, and architectural distortion of the liver (*toxic cirrhosis*) is well described as part of the syndrome of subacute hepatic necrosis caused by TNT, tetrachloroethane, and the PCBs and chloronaphthalenes. Additionally, some survivors of trinitrotoluene-induced injury were found to have macronodular cirrhosis.

Cirrhosis may occur after prolonged, repeated low-level exposure to carbon tetrachloride in dry-cleaning plants and to inorganic arsenical insecticides among vintners and from drinking arsenic-contaminated well water. Micronodular cirrhosis was described in a worker with repeated exposure to a degreasing solvent containing a mixture of trichloroethylene and 1,1,1-trichloroethane, and chronic active hepatitis was reported in a worker exposed to 1,1,1-trichloroethane.

Thirteen painters with no history of drug or alcohol ingestion exposed over 6–39 years to a variety of organic solvents had persistent biopsy-verified histologic changes of steatosis, focal necrosis, and enlarged portal tracts with fibrosis. Three nurses were reported to have irreversible liver injury after years of handling cytostatic drugs, with liver biopsies showing piecemeal necrosis in one and steatosis with fibrosis in the other two. The anesthetic agent halothane has been reported to cause cirrhosis and chronic active hepatitis after acute exposure.

A few studies of occupational cohorts exposed to acute hepatotoxins (e.g., carbon tetrachloride and chlorinated naphthalenes) have demonstrated increased cirrhosis mortality, suggesting persistent subclinical injury after high exposures. Increased mortality as a consequence of cirrhosis has been observed among pressman, shipyard workers, metal fabrication employees, marine inspectors, and anesthesiologists. In some of these studies, limited data were available on the role of confounding factors such as ethanol consumption or viral hepatitis.

HEPATOPORTAL SCLEROSIS & HEPATIC PORPHYRIA

Portal and periportal fibrosis leading to portal hypertension (*noncirrhotic portal hypertension*) can be caused by exposure to inorganic arsenicals, thorium, and vinyl chloride. A few cases of porphyria cutanea tarda as a consequence of occupational exposure to the herbicide 2,4,5-trichlorophenoxyacetic acid, probably caused by contamination by dioxin, have been recorded. Turkish peasants developed liver disease and hepatic porphyria after ingesting wheat contaminated with the fungicide hexachlorobenzene.

GRANULOMATOUS DISEASE

Beryllium and copper exposure can result in granulomatous liver disease, with hepatic granulomas located near or within the portal tracts. Clinical liver disease usually is not significant, but granulomas occasionally result in hepatomegaly, necrosis, or fibrosis.

STEATOSIS

Steatosis is characterized morphologically by microvesicular or macrovesicular intracellular lipid formation. Steatosis may occur as a result of acute occupational exposure to elemental phosphorus, TNT, arsenical pesticides, dimethylformamide, and certain chlorinated hydrocarbons (e.g., carbon tetrachloride, methyl chloroform, and tetrachloroethane). Nonoccupational causes include diabetes, hypertriglyceridemia, and obesity. Intracellular hepatic lipid formation results from xenobiotic effects on fat metabolism. Minimal to moderate elevation in transaminase levels is seen after acute occupational exposure, with resolution in several weeks after removal. Steatosis also may occur after chronic exposure to carbon tetrachloride or dimethylformamide. Progression from steatosis to fibrosis or cirrhosis has not been documented.

NEOPLASIA

While many occupationally encountered chemical agents are known to cause hepatocellular carcinoma in experimental animals, only a relatively few studies have been performed in humans. Vinyl chloride, a halogenated aliphatic compound used since the 1940s in the production of polyvinyl chloride, was known to be an animal hepatotoxin in the early 1960s. Acroosteolysis was reported in humans in 1966 (see Chapter 28). In 1974, three cases of angiosarcoma, a rare liver tumor, were found in employees who had been exposed to vinyl chloride for up to 20 years. Subsequent reports and surveillance activities through the end of 1998 have recorded more than 190 cases of vinyl chloride–associated hepatic angiosarcoma. Epidemiologic studies confirm a strong relationship between cumulative vinyl chloride exposure and occurrence of liver and biliary cancer and hepatic angiosarcoma. Pathologically, hepatic damage in association with vinyl chloride exposure appears to progress sequentially from focal hepatocyte hyperplasia to sinusoidal dilatation to peliosis hepatis and sarcomatous transformation of the lining of the cells of sinusoids and portal capillaries. Recent studies indicate that vinyl chloride acts as a genotoxic carcinogen, with transformation of vinyl chloride into chloroethylene oxide (CEO) by cytochrome P450 isozyme 2E1. CEO can alkylate nucleic acid bases, with adducts leading to base-pair substitutions. Some evidence suggests that the *K-ras*-2 mutation pattern or other genetic polymorphisms may increase the risk of developing hepatic angiosarcoma and hepatocellular carcinoma. Underlying hepatitis B virus infection and alcohol intake appear to increase the risk of developing hepatocellular carcinoma owing to VCM exposure. In the past, liver disease usually was unrecognized until the late stages of histologic damage and with the victim only a few months from death. Recently, persistent serum transaminase elevations have been observed among workers previously exposed to vinyl chloride, with liver biopsies showing nonspecific fatty changes. Medical surveillance of vinyl chloride–exposed workers by using liver ultrasonography shows that workers exposed to 200 ppm for at least 1 year have a fourfold increased risk of developing periportal liver fibrosis.

Hepatic angiosarcoma also has developed in vintners with long exposure to inorganic arsenic, in patients with psoriasis treated with inorganic potassium arsenite (Fowler solution) in the 1940s and 1950s, and in patients injected with a colloidal suspension of thorium dioxide (Thorotrast), used for carotid angiography and liver-spleen scans from 1930 to 1955. Excess liver cancer incidence has been shown among occupational cohorts exposed to trichloroethylene.

Case-control studies show elevated odds ratios for the development of liver cancer among workers in a variety of occupations such as chemical, clerical, automobile repair, and food service workers; transport equipment operators; and workers exposed to welding fumes. While some of these studies were not able to evaluate the significance of confounding factors such as alcohol and hepatitis B and C virus infection, taken as a whole, these studies indicate prolonged exposure to organic solvents represents a risk factor for liver cancer.

REFERENCES

AOEC Peer-Reviewed Modules: Occupational and environmental liver disease, www.aoec.org/resources.htm.

ATSDR: Trichloroethylene: A review of the literature in view of the results of the trichloroethylene subregistry results, www.atsdr.cdc.gov/NER/TCE/a6rev.html.

Cotrim HP et al: Clinical and histopathological features of NASH in workers exposed to chemicals with or without associated metabolic conditions. Liver Int 2004;24:131 [PMID: 15078477].

Malhi H et al: Apoptosis and necrosis in the liver: A tale of two deaths? Hepatology 2006;43:31 [PMID: 16447272].

Maroni M, Fanetti AC: Liver function assessment in workers exposed to vinyl chloride. Int Arch Occup Environ Health 2006;79:57 [PMID: 16091976].

McCullough AJ: The clinical features, diagnosis and natural history of nonalcoholic fatty liver disease. Clin Liver Dis 2004;8:521 [PMID: 15331061].

■ INFECTIOUS AGENTS CAUSING LIVER TOXICITY

Infectious hepatotoxic agents (Table 22–5) may be of importance in the pathogenesis of both acute and chronic liver disease. In 2000, an estimated 16,000 hepatitis A virus (HAV), 66,000 hepatitis B virus (HBV), and 1000 hepatitis C virus (HCV) infections may have occurred worldwide among health care workers owing to occupa-

Table 22–5. Infectious agents associated with occupational liver disease.

Hepatitis A virus	Nursery and kindergarten staff, sewer workers
Hepatitis B and C viruses	Health care workers with blood and body fluid contact
Cytomegalovirus	Pediatric health care workers
Coxiella burnetii	Animal care workers, farm workers, slaughterhouse workers
Leptospira icterohaemorrhagiae	Sewer workers, farm workers

tional exposure to percutaneous injuries. Occupational exposure to infectious hepatotoxic agents also may occur among sewer workers; emergency health care personnel; animal-care, slaughterhouse, and farm workers; and laboratory workers. Additional information can be found in Chapter 17.

HEPATITIS A

Exposure

The cause of hepatitis A is the HAV, a 27-nm RNA agent that is a member of the picornavirus family. Outbreaks of hepatitis A infection have been reported among personnel working with nonhuman primates and in neonatal intensive-care units. Serologic surveys suggest a higher prevalence of HAV antibodies among health care workers working in emergency rooms, surgery, laundry rooms, and children's psychiatry and among day-care workers and dentists. There are several case reports of HAV infection among waste water treatment plant workers, and some serologic studies have confirmed an increased risk in this population. Although day-care centers can be the source of outbreaks of occupationally acquired hepatitis A infection within some communities, disease within day-care centers more commonly reflects extended transmission within the community. There are no reports of hepatitis A outbreaks in correctional settings. While contaminated food and water are common epidemic sources, hepatitis A is transmitted primarily by person-to-person contact, generally through fecal contamination. Transmission of HAV is facilitated by poor personal hygiene and intimate household or sexual contact. Transmission by blood transfusion has occurred but is rare. Transmission in saliva has not been demonstrated.

Clinical Findings & Diagnosis

The incubation period for hepatitis A is 15–50 days (average: 28–30 days). The illness caused by HAV char-

acteristically has an abrupt onset, with fever, malaise, anorexia, nausea, abdominal discomfort, and jaundice. High concentrations of HAV (10 particles/g) are found in stools of infected persons. Fecal virus excretion reaches its highest concentration during the incubation period and early in the prodromal phase; it diminishes rapidly once jaundice appears. Greatest infectivity is seen in the 2-week period immediately before the onset of jaundice or elevation of liver enzymes.

A chronic carrier state with HAV in blood or feces has not been demonstrated. The fatality rate among reported cases is approximately 0.3%. The diagnosis of acute hepatitis A is confirmed by the presence of immunoglobulin (Ig) M class anti-HAV in serum collected during the acute or early convalescent phase of the disease. IgG antibodies appear in the convalescent phase and remain positive for life, apparently conferring enduring protection against disease.

Treatment

Treatment for hepatitis A is symptomatic, with rest, analgesics, and fluid replacement where necessary. Fulminant hepatic failure occasionally follows acute HAV infection. Orthotopic liver transplantation is well established as the appropriate treatment for severe cases.

Prevention

Numerous studies show that a single intramuscular dose of 0.02 mL/kg of immune globulin (immune serum globulin, gamma globulin) given before exposure or during the incubation period of hepatitis A is protective against clinical illness. The prophylactic value is greatest (80–90%) when immune globulin is given early in the incubation period and declines thereafter. Since hepatitis A cannot be diagnosed reliably on clinical presentation alone, serologic confirmation of hepatitis A in the index case is recommended before treatment of contacts. Once the diagnosis of acute infection is made, close contacts should be given immune globulin promptly to prevent development of secondary cases. Such close contacts may include staff of day-care facilities and institutions for custodial care—or hospital staff if an unsuspected patient has been fecally incontinent.

Routine immune globulin administration is not recommended under the usual office or factory conditions for persons exposed to a fellow worker with hepatitis A or for teachers with schoolroom contact. Food handlers should receive immune globulin when a common-source exposure is recognized and restaurant patrons when the infected person is involved directly in handling uncooked foods without gloves. This is especially the case when the patrons can be identified within 2 weeks of exposure and the food handler's hygienic practices are known to be deficient. Serologic screening of contacts for anti-HAV antibodies to the hepatitis A virus before giving immune globulin is not recommended because screening is more costly than immune globulin and would delay administration. Pregnancy or lactation is not a contraindication to immune globulin administration.

The inactivated hepatitis A vaccine is currently recommended for persons traveling to or working in countries with intermediate or high HAV endemicity, for laboratory workers with exposure to live virus, or for animal handlers with exposure to HAV-infected primates. Prevaccination testing should be considered depending on the cost of the vaccine and age of the person being immunized. Immunogenicity studies show that virtually 100% of children, adolescents, and adults develop protective levels of antibody to hepatitis A virus (anti-HAV) after completing a two-dose vaccine series (each given as an intramuscular injection of 1 mL of 1440 enzyme-linked immunosorbent assay units). Protective antibodies remain for as long as 4 years, with kinetic models suggesting that protective levels of anti-HAV persist for at least 20 years. Routine hepatitis A vaccination is not recommended for child-care workers, hospital workers, teachers, sewage treatment employees, correctional workers, or staff in institutions for the developmentally disabled. When outbreaks are recognized in these settings, use of immune globulin for persons in close contact with infected patients or students is recommended. Routine hepatitis A vaccination among restaurant employees is not recommended given the incidence of infection and present cost of the vaccine, even during epidemics.

An employee with symptoms and confirmed HAV infection should be restricted from work until symptoms subside or for 1 week after the onset of jaundice.

HEPATITIS B

Exposure & Epidemiology

Hepatitis B infection (see also Chapter 17) is caused by the HBV, a major cause of acute and chronic hepatitis, cirrhosis, and primary hepatocellular carcinoma worldwide. Health care workers with primary blood and body fluid contact are the primary group at risk. This includes workers with significant contact with blood, blood products, or body secretions: surgeons, oral surgeons, dental hygienists, pathologists, anesthesiologists, phlebotomists, medical technologists, respiratory therapists, emergency room personnel, and medical and surgical house staff.

In serologic studies in the United States in the 1970s, the annual rate of clinically manifest hepatitis B infection in hospital workers was approximately 0.1%, or about 10 times that of control populations. Hospital staff with frequent blood contact had a prevalence rate of hepatitis B surface antigen (HBsAg) of 1–2% and a prevalence rate of anti-HBV antibody (anti-HBs) of 15–30% compared with healthy controls, who had rates of 0.3% and 3–5%, respectively. Since the advent of standard precautions to prevent exposure to blood and other potentially infectious body fluids, along with preexposure vaccination against HBV, there has been a sharp decline in the incidence of HBV infection among health care workers.

The risk of infection with HBV depends on the titer of virions in the infectious fluid and correlates with the presence or absence of hepatitis e antigen in the source patient. The risk of infection following percutaneous injury with both HBsAg- and HBeAg-positive blood is 22–31%; the risk of developing serologic evidence of HBV infection is 37–62%. Percutaneous injuries are the most efficient mode of HBV transmission, although in many nosocomial outbreaks health care workers cannot recall this history. Some HBV infections may result from indirect blood or body fluid exposures onto cutaneous scratches, abrasions, or burns or on mucosal surfaces. HBV survives in dried blood at room temperature on environmental surfaces for at least 1 week. Blood contains the highest titer of HBV, but HBsAg may be found in breast milk, bile, cerebrospinal fluid, feces, nasopharyngeal washings, saliva, semen, sweat, and synovial fluid. Employment in a hospital without blood exposure carries no greater risk than that for the general population.

Most hospital workers experience accidental blood contact by needlestick injuries, usually during disposal of needles, administration of parenteral injections or infusion therapy, drawing blood, and handling linens and trash containing uncapped needles. To minimize the risk of blood-borne pathogen transmission, all health care workers should adhere to standard precautions, including the appropriate use of handwashing, protective barriers, and care in the use and disposal of needles and other sharp instruments. U.S. regulations require the use of safety-engineered devices where available, and this has resulted in a significant decline in percutaneous injuries among health care workers.

Forms of Illness & Transmission

Three forms of hepatitis B are encountered in clinical practice: acute hepatitis B, inapparent sporadic episodes of unknown origin, and the chronic carrier state—detected by screening for HBsAg—in apparently healthy persons. Transmission occurs via percutaneous or permucosal routes when exposure to blood or potentially infectious body fluids occurs; HBV is not transmitted via the fecal-oral route or by contamination of food or water.

Course of Illness

The onset of acute hepatitis B is generally insidious, with anorexia, malaise, nausea, vomiting, abdominal pain, and jaundice. Skin rash, arthralgia, and arthritis also can occur. The incubation period ranges from 45–

60 days after exposure to HBV. HBsAg can be detected in serum 30–60 days after exposure to HBV and persists for variable periods. Antibody to hepatitis B surface antigen (anti-HBs) develops after a resolved infection and indicates long-term immunity. The antibody to the core antigen (anti-HBc) develops in all HBV infections and persists indefinitely. Overall fatality rates for acute infection do not exceed 2%.

The chronic carrier state is defined as the presence of HBsAg-positive serum on at least two occasions at least 6 months apart and is characterized by high levels of HBsAg and anti-HBc and various levels of serum transaminases, reflecting liver disease activity. The natural course of HBsAg-positive chronic active hepatitis is progressive, frequently evolving to cirrhosis, hepatocellular carcinoma, and death owing to hepatic failure or bleeding esophageal varices.

Depending on the country, the estimated relative risk for developing hepatocellular carcinoma after chronic HBV infection ranges from 6- to 100-fold. Hepatocellular carcinoma usually develops after 20–30 years of persistent HBV infection accompanied by hepatocellular necrosis, inflammation, and regenerative hyperplasia. Chronic hepatitis and liver cirrhosis are important endogenous factors in the development of hepatocellular carcinoma.

Treatment

Therapeutic agents such as the interferons that have been approved for treatment of chronic hepatitis B can result in sustained suppression of HBV replication and remission of liver disease in selected individuals. Periodic screening with a-fetoprotein or imaging studies can enhance early detection of hepatocellular carcinoma (HCC). Chronically infected persons with HCC who have undergone such screening have been reported to experience long-term survival after resection or ablation of small HCCs.

Prevention

Postexposure prophylaxis should be based on the hepatitis vaccination status of the exposed person and whether the source of blood and the HBsAg status of the source are known or unknown. Multiple doses of hepatitis B immune globulin provides approximately 75% protection from HBV infection. Guidelines for hepatitis B prophylaxis following percutaneous exposure are given in Chapter 17.

Routine vaccination of infants, young children, and adolescents is expected to eliminate transmission of HBV eventually among adults in the United States. For individuals who have not been vaccinated previously and who are at risk for blood-borne pathogen exposure, vaccination should be done with the HBV vaccine, administered as a three-dose series via the intramuscular route in the deltoid muscle. For those workers who may at risk for both hepatitis A and B infection, administration of the combination hepatitis A-B vaccine may be cost-effective. Protective immunity is conferred in more than 95% of vaccine recipients. The availability of recombinant hepatitis B vaccines has eliminated previous, albeit unwarranted, concerns regarding the risk of blood-borne infections transmitted by plasma-derived vaccines. Nearly 90% of vaccine recipients have protective levels of anti-HBs 5 years after vaccination. Loss of detectable anti-HB levels after immunization does not imply loss of protection because studies show that exposure to HBV leads to an amnestic rise in anti-HB levels after natural infection. Therefore, routine booster doses of hepatitis B vaccine are not recommended.

Measurement of prevaccination anti-HB levels generally is not recommended but may be performed depending on the cost of screening and the prevalence of antibody in the group to be vaccinated. Approximately 5% of immunocompetent adults fail to respond to the hepatitis B vaccine, with vaccine nonresponsiveness increasing with age greater than 40 years, obesity, and smoking. Postvaccination anti-HB testing may be useful in establishing immune status for postexposure treatment or for administering booster doses to vaccine nonresponders. Nonresponders to the primary series have a 30–50% chance of responding to a second three-dose series. Revaccinated persons should be retested at completion of the second vaccine series. Nonresponders to vaccination who are HBsAg-negative should be counseled regarding the need to obtain hepatitis B immune globulin prophylaxis for known or probable parenteral exposure to HBsAg-positive blood. Screening by ultrasonography and serum α-fetoprotein measurement are indicated for patients at high risk for developing hepatocellular carcinoma.

The employee with HBV infection and liver disease should be advised to avoid exposure to other potentially hepatotoxic agents such as ethanol or workplace solvents.

HEPATITIS C

Exposure & Epidemiology

HCV is a single-stranded RNA virus of the family Flaviviridae. The virus has a striking ability to persist in the host after infection, with chronic hepatitis occurring in approximately 70% of infected individuals. Viral persistence appears to be related to rapid mutation under immune pressure, with coexistence within the host as related but immunologically distinct strains. The high rate of mutation appears to be the primary mechanism underlying the absence of effective neutralization and the development of persistent infection. In the United States alone, approximately 3.5 million people are infected with HCV, with nearly 150,000 new infections annually.

HCV is spread primarily through parenteral exposures from blood transfusions or intravenous drug abuse. Up to 40% of cases in the United States have no identified exposure source. There is minimal evidence for sexual transmission or mother-to-infant transmission of HCV.

In contrast to HBV, the epidemiologic data for HCV suggest that environmental contamination with blood containing HCV is not a significant risk for transmission in the health care setting, with the possible exception of the hemodialysis setting, where HCV transmission related to environmental contamination and poor infection-control practices has been implicated. The risk of infection following occupational percutaneous exposure averages 1.8% (range: 0–7%) and is increased following deep injury or injury from a hollow-bore needle. Transmission rarely occurs from mucous membrane exposures (including conjunctivae) to blood, and no transmission in health care workers has been documented from intact or nonintact skin exposures to blood. Environmental contamination with blood containing HCV is not a significant risk for transmission. The risk of transmission from tissues or other body fluids is not well characterized but is expected to be low.

Clinical Findings & Diagnosis

Acute hepatitis C is usually a benign illness, with up to 80% of cases being anicteric and asymptomatic. The mean incubation period following transfusion-associated hepatitis C is 6–8 weeks. Mild elevations of transaminase levels occur in the acute phase; fulminant hepatic failure is rare. Persistent infection leads to liver cell destruction, possibly via direct cytopathic or immune-mediated mechanisms, with fluctuating levels of serum transaminases. Serum transaminase levels are a relatively poor indicator of the severity of disease as measured histologically.

Chronic active hepatitis or cirrhosis occurs in 3–20% of individuals with acute infection. Progression to cirrhosis appears to correlate with age at exposure, duration of infection, and degree of liver damage on biopsy. HCV is a major agent in the etiology of hepatocellular carcinoma throughout the world, with almost all cases occurring in the setting of cirrhosis. Alcohol appears to be an important cofactor in the development of complications from chronic HCV infection.

Diagnosis of HCV infection usually is based on detection of elevated serum transaminase or anti-HCV antibody levels. Anti-HCV antibodies become detectable an average of 12 weeks following exposure but may take as long as 6 months. First-generation anti-HCV assays used the c100-3 antigen and were highly effective

in identifying HCV-positive blood donors. The anti–c100-3 assay failed to detect HCV-infected patients for several weeks after exposure, and some HCV-infected patients never developed anti-HCV antibody. Second-generation assays added two epitopes (c22-3 and c33c) to both the enzyme-linked immunosorbent assay (ELISA) and the confirmatory recombinant immunoblot assay (RIBA-2). Antibodies to these epitopes develop much earlier after infection than do antibodies to c100-3. The second-generation assay is highly sensitive but relatively nonspecific for the detection of HCV. Nonspecificity is associated with aged sera, hypergammaglobulinemia, rheumatoid factor–positive sera, and sera from persons recently vaccinated for influenza. Because of the nonspecificity, ELISA reactivity should be confirmed with a supplemental RIBA-2 assay.

The most sensitive method to detect HCV is measurement of HCV RNA by the polymerase chain reaction (PCR). HCV RNA is detectable by PCR in almost all patients within 1–2 weeks of exposure. In approximately 80% of individuals, HCV RNA persists with fluctuating serum transaminase levels.

Liver biopsy specimens from patients with chronic HCV infection may show portal inflammation, focal piecemeal necrosis, bile ductular proliferation, and characteristic lymphoid follicles within the portal tracts. Chronic HCV infection is associated with polyarteritis nodosa, membranous glomerulonephritis, and idiopathic Sjögren syndrome.

Treatment

Studies assessing the effectiveness of immune globulin following HCV exposure are inconclusive, and immune globulin is not recommended for postexposure prophylaxis for HCV. No clinical trials have been performed to determine the efficacy of antiviral agents (interferon with or without ribavirin) after HCV exposure. No evidence currently supports the use of immediate postexposure prophylaxis with immune globulin, immune modulators, or antiviral agents. Existing data suggest that established HCV infection is needed before antiviral treatment can be effective. Some studies suggest that a short course of interferon early in the course of acute hepatitis C may be more effective in resolving infection than if antiviral treatment is initiated after chronic hepatitis C has been established. Among patients with chronic HCV infection, antivirals have been less effective in those with genotype 1 than those with genotypes 2 or 3. Therapeutic trials have shown that combinations of interferons and ribavirin are more effective than monotherapy. Data on which to base recommendations regarding the use of antivirals in acute infection are insufficient because 15–25% of patients with acute HCV infection resolve their infection spontaneously, and antiviral treatment early in the course of chronic HCV infection may be as effective as acute treatment. Following percutaneous or mucosal occupational exposure to HCV, baseline and follow-up HCV antibody measurements should be performed to assess the risk of seroconversion (6 weeks, 3 months, and 6 months). During this follow-up period, the health care worker should refrain from donating blood, plasma, organs, tissue, or semen. The exposed person does not need to modify sexual practices or refrain from becoming pregnant, and women may continue breast-feeding.

Prevention

No vaccine is currently available for HCV. Prospects for vaccine development are challenging because of the transient efficacy of neutralizing antibodies, the high frequency of mutation in critical envelope protein regions, the high rate of persistent infection, and the possibility of reinfection with both homologous and heterologous strains.

OTHER INFECTIOUS AGENTS

Seroprevalence studies are inconsistent in demonstrating an increased risk of cytomegalovirus infection among potentially high-risk health care workers (pediatric and immunosuppressed adult units), kindergarten teachers, and child-care workers. Cytomegalovirus may cause hepatitis, but the more serious consequence of infection for the pregnant worker may be a neonate with a congenital malformation. Nevertheless, hospital employers may consider that prudent policy is to reassign seronegative employees who wish to become pregnant to jobs where there is no contact with infected patients or their biologic fluids.

Coxiella burnetii, the agent of Q fever, may cause acute infection among personnel exposed to infected sheep and goats. Persons at risk include animal-care technicians, laboratory research personnel, abattoir workers, and farmers. Acute hepatitis occurs in up to 50% of cases and usually is self-limited. The clinical picture of leptospirosis among farm and sewer workers because of exposure to *Leptospira icterohaemorrhagiae* also may be dominated by hepatic injury. Other causes of infectious hepatitis include yellow fever among forest workers (arbovirus) and schistosomiasis among agricultural workers (*Schistosoma mansoni, S. japonicum*).

REFERENCES

Chen CJ et al: Risk of hepatocellular carcinoma across a biological gradient of serum hepatitis B virus DNA level. JAMA 2006;295:65 [PMID: 16391218].

Herrine SK et al: Management of patients with chronic hepatitis C infection. Clin Exp Med 2006;6:20 [PMID: 16550340].

Yim HJ, Lok AS: Natural history of chronic hepatitis B virus infection. Hepatology 2006;43:173 [PMID: 16447285].

▪ MEDICAL SURVEILLANCE & DETECTION OF OCCUPATIONAL HEPATOTOXICITY

MEDICAL SURVEILLANCE FOR OCCUPATIONAL LIVER DISEASE

The choice of a surveillance test or tests to detect chemical liver disease in a working population exposed to potential hepatotoxins is determined by its specificity, sensitivity, and positive predictive value (see "Diagnostic Tests for Liver Dysfunction" below). In an occupational setting, a screening test with high sensitivity (to correctly identify all those with disease) and specificity (to correctly identify all those without disease) is needed. Indocyanine green clearance and serum alkaline phosphatase have been suggested as the initial tests of choice for the surveillance of vinyl chloride workers (to reduce the number of false-positive results), followed by a test of high sensitivity such as serum γ-glutamyl transpeptidase (to reduce the number of false-negative results).

For most hepatoxins, it is currently justified to base the choice of tests on practical criteria such as noninvasiveness, simplicity of test performance, availability, and adequacy of test analysis and cost. Although serum transaminases have a relatively high sensitivity for detection of liver disease, their low specificity limits the practical utility of periodic measurement in a worker population exposed to potential hepatotoxins. Nevertheless, serum transaminases remain the test of choice for routine surveillance of such populations.

Clearance tests have been used successfully in research settings but are not recommended for daily clinical or surveillance practice until further prospective studies in well-defined groups are completed. It is not known whether changes in microsomal enzyme activity in workers exposed to hepatotoxins may result in long-term liver damage.

So-called preemployment baseline measurement of serum transaminases may be helpful in establishing causality for purposes of workers' compensation where a claim is made alleging industrial liver disease. Routine medical surveillance involving measurement of serum transaminase levels should be conducted only when exposure assessment suggests a potential for hepatic injury. When the prevalence of liver disease in the population is low, the poor predictive value of an abnormal serum transaminase level after routine screening may lead to many costly diagnostic evaluations for nonoccupational liver disease.

Gray-scale ultrasonography of the liver has been used in surveillance of vinyl chloride–exposed workers but has not been applied routinely in other workplace settings for surveillance of hepatic disease. Hepatic parenchymal imaging by ultrasonography has been suggested as a sensitive marker for preclinical effects among solvent-exposed dry cleaners. The use of this technique as a routine tool for medical surveillance for hepatotoxin exposure remains to be determined.

Individuals with chronic elevations of serum transaminase levels may continue to work if exposure to potential hepatotoxins is minimized through appropriate workplace controls and exposure assessment.

DIAGNOSTIC TESTS FOR LIVER DYSFUNCTION

The ideal test for detection of liver dysfunction would be sensitive enough to detect minimal liver disease, specific enough to point to a particular derangement of liver function, and capable of reflecting the severity of the underlying pathophysiologic problem. Unfortunately, no such laboratory test is available, and "liver function tests" are used instead (Table 22–6).

Broadly speaking, these tests encompass tests of biochemical evidence of cell death and hepatic synthesis, as well as actual physiologic liver dysfunction. In addition, radiologic and morphologic evaluations are used often to delineate the nature of liver disease and, as such, may be viewed as tests of liver function. Biochemical tests and tests of synthetic function are indicated commonly for routine use; clearance tests are not widely available and are not indicated for routine use.

Epidemiologic studies in which measurement of serum enzyme levels is used to determine the hepatotox-

Table 22–6. Tests for evaluation of liver disease.

Biochemical tests
  Serum enzyme activity
    Serum alkaline phosphatase
    Serum lactate dehydrogenase
  Serum bilirubin
  Urine bilirubin
Tests of synthetic liver function
  Serum albumin
  Prothrombin time
  α-Fetoprotein
  Serum ferritin
Clearance tests
  Exogenous clearance tests
    Sulfobromophthalein
    Indocyanine green
    Antipyrine test
    Aminopyrine breath test
    Caffeine breath test
  Endogenous clearance tests
    Serum bile acid
    Urinary D-glucaric acid

icity of solvents have not included long-term outcomes such as chronic liver disease. Bile acids and other tests of metabolic function generally are more sensitive indicators of hepatic effect from organic solvents at levels of exposure below those expected to cause elevation of serum enzyme levels. It is not known if these more sensitive measures of hepatic function can predict subsequent disease in workers exposed to hepatotoxins.

Biochemical Tests for Liver Disease

A. SERUM ENZYME ACTIVITY

The tests used most commonly to detect liver disease are aspartate aminotransferase (AST) and alanine aminotransferase (ALT) determinations. Transaminase release is a consequence of release of enzyme protein from liver cells as a result of cell injury. Elevations of serum aminotransferase levels may occur with minor cell injury, making such determinations useful in the early detection and monitoring of liver disease of drug or chemical origin. However, transaminase levels may be elevated in viral, alcoholic, or ischemic hepatitis, as well as in extrahepatic obstruction, limiting the specificity of these tests. In addition, elevations of transaminase levels are found in obese individuals, and false-positive results have been reported in patients receiving erythromycin and aminosalicylic acid and during diabetic ketoacidosis. Conversely, significant liver damage may be present in individuals with normal levels of transaminases. There is some evidence that a serum AST:ALT ratio of greater than 1 may indicate occupational liver disease. The height of transaminase elevation in liver disease does not correlate with the extent of liver cell necrosis on biopsy and therefore has little prognostic value.

B. ALKALINE PHOSPHATASE

Serum alkaline phosphatase activity may originate from liver, bone, intestine, or placenta. Measurement of serum 5-nucleotidase may be used to determine the tissue origin of an elevated alkaline phosphatase; if elevated, it generally implies that the source of alkaline phosphatase is hepatobiliary, not bony. Toxic liver injury that results in disturbances in the transport function of the hepatocyte or of the biliary tree may cause elevation of serum alkaline phosphatase activity. Increased serum alkaline phosphatase levels also may be noted in the third trimester of pregnancy, as well as normally in persons older than age 50 years and in patients with osteoblastic bone disorders and both intrahepatic and extrahepatic cholestatic disease.

Assay of alkaline phosphatase enzymatic activity in serum in anicteric individuals is particularly useful in detecting and monitoring suspected drug- or chemical-induced cholestasis; it is not helpful in screening individuals for toxic liver injury except when there is primary involvement of the biliary network.

C. Serum Bilirubin

Hyperbilirubinemia may be classified as conjugated or unconjugated. Conjugated hyperbilirubinemia indicates dysfunction of the liver parenchyma or bile ducts and may be found in Dubin-Johnson syndrome and Rotor syndrome and in viral hepatitis, drug- or toxin-induced hepatitis, shock liver, and metastatic disease of the liver. Unconjugated hyperbilirubinemia may be seen in Gilbert disease, uncomplicated hemolytic disorders, and congestive heart failure.

Serum bilirubin is of some value in detecting toxic cholestatic liver injury but is frequently normal in the presence of more common cytotoxic damage. It is probably most useful in the presence of severe acute liver damage; although patients with fulminant hepatitis may be anicteric, the level of serum bilirubin is of prognostic importance in chemical and alcoholic hepatitis, primary biliary cirrhosis, and halothane hepatitis.

D. Urine Bilirubin

Bilirubin in the urine is direct bilirubin because indirect bilirubin is tightly bound to albumin and not filtered by the normal kidney. A positive urine bilirubin test can confirm clinically suspected hyperbilirubinemia of hepatobiliary origin or may predate the appearance of overt icterus and thus serve as a useful screening test. Quantitative analysis of urine bilirubin is of no diagnostic significance.

E. Other Biochemical Tests

1. Serum γ-glutamyl transferase (SGGT)—SGGT is considered a more sensitive indicator than aminotransferases of drug-, virus-, chemical-, and alcohol-induced hepatocellular damage. Because of its lack of specificity, however, one must interpret abnormalities in conjunction with other tests.

2. Liver-specific enzymes—Liver enzymes, such as ornithine carbamyl dehydrogenase, phosphofructose aldolase, sorbitol dehydrogenase, and alcohol dehydrogenase, are less useful clinically than the aminotransferases, glutamyl transferases, or alkaline phosphatases.

3. Serum lactate dehydrogenase (LDH)—Serum LDH may originate from myocardium, liver, skeletal muscle, brain or kidney tissue, and red blood cells. Isoenzyme fractionation may determine the hepatic origin (lactate dehydrogenase 5) but generally is too nonspecific for purposes of evaluating toxic chemical liver injury.

Tests of Synthetic Liver Function

Measurement of serum albumin concentrations may be a useful index of cellular dysfunction in liver disease. It is of little value in differential diagnosis.

Because all the clotting factors are synthesized by the liver, acute liver injury can result in prolongation of the prothrombin time, which depends on the activities of factors II, V, VII, and X. Measurement of prothrombin time is useful chiefly in fulminant hepatic failure, where a markedly elevated prothrombin time has prognostic significance, or in advanced chronic liver disease. It is a relatively insensitive indicator of liver damage and of little value in the differential diagnosis.

High serum concentrations of α-fetoprotein are present in 70% of patients with primary hepatocellular carcinoma in the United States, and serial determinations may aid in monitoring the response to therapy or in detecting early recurrence. α-Fetoprotein has no utility for surveillance in the occupational setting.

Serum ferritin levels accurately reflect hepatic and total-body iron stores. Serum ferritin is useful in screening for idiopathic genetic hemochromatosis as a cause of liver disease but has no utility for surveillance in the occupational setting.

Clearance Tests

Tests that measure the clearance of substances by the liver provide the most sensitive, specific, and reliable means of detecting the early phase of liver disease. Clearance tests may be used to determine the specificity of increased enzyme activity, to detect liver disease not reflected in abnormalities of serum enzymes, and to determine when recovery has occurred in reversible liver disease. This is especially the case when decreases in the functional state of the liver occur in patients with liver disease without active necrosis, including fatty liver, and in active cirrhosis in the absence of clinical abnormalities or abnormal enzymes.

In the occupational setting, measures of hepatic functional capacity have been used epidemiologically to demonstrate liver dysfunction in the absence of clinical or serologic abnormalities. The clinical utility of clearance tests in screening for chemical liver injury—or in confirming occupational etiology of disease in workers with known liver dysfunction—has not been demonstrated.

A. Exogenous Clearance Tests

Exogenous clearance tests are given to detect liver function by the administration of various test substances to the individual.

1. Bromsulfalein (BSP)—Practical use of hepatic clearance as a diagnostic measure began with BSP. Its use has been discontinued because of side effects of phlebitis, severe local skin reactions, and occasionally fatal anaphylactic reactions.

2. Indocyanine green—Hepatic uptake of indocyanine green, a tricarbocyanine anionic dye, is an active process depending on sinusoidal perfusion, membrane transport, and secretory capacity. The dye is not metabolized or conjugated by the liver and is excreted directly into the bile. After a single intravenous injection of indocyanine green, clearance is calculated from serial dye levels at 3, 5, 7, 9, 12, and 14 minutes or by ear densitometry. Unlike BSP, indocyanine green causes negligible toxicity or allergic reactions.

Studies of workers exposed to vinyl chloride show that indocyanine green clearance after a dose of 0.5 mg/kg is the most sensitive test for subclinical liver injury and has a specificity exceeded only by serum alkaline phosphatase. There is also a dose-response relationship between cumulative exposure to vinyl chloride and indocyanine green clearance. This has not been demonstrated in other groups of workers exposed to occupational hepatotoxins, and indocyanine green for detection of subclinical liver disease cannot be recommended for routine use.

3. Antipyrine test—This is the most widely used in vivo index of hepatic microsomal enzyme activity. Antipyrine is completely and rapidly absorbed from the gastrointestinal tract, distributed in total-body water, and almost completely metabolized by the liver via three major oxidative pathways. The rate of elimination is virtually independent of hepatic blood flow, with first-order kinetics of elimination and a half-life of approximately 10 hours in normal subjects. At 24–48 hours after an orally administered dose of 1 g, antipyrine clearance can be calculated by serial plasma or salivary measurements. Clearance can be calculated from a single salivary sample collected at least 18 hours after dosing, permitting a simpler, more convenient method of study. Repeat tests cannot be done less than 3 days apart, and to avoid the induction of antipyrine metabolism in the individual, an interval of 1 week is recommended.

The antipyrine test has undergone the most extensive study of all clearance tests in the detection of subclinical liver disease in occupational settings. It has been used to detect mean differences in hepatic enzyme activity between workers exposed to solvent mixtures and unexposed controls. Asymptomatic chlordecone-exposed workers had increased antipyrine clearance and biopsy-proved liver disease that normalized after exposure was terminated.

4. Aminopyrine breath test—The aminopyrine breath test has the advantage of being simple, noninvasive, safe, and relatively cheap. Clinical studies have documented the use of aminopyrine breath tests in patients with chronic advanced liver disease, but the sensitivity and specificity of the test for detection of subclinical chemical liver injury in asymptomatic populations have not been assessed.

After oral administration of about 2 μCi of [^{14}C]aminopyrine, the labeled methyl group is oxidized by the microsomal enzyme system and ultimately excreted as $^{14}CO_2$. Breath samples are collected 2 hours after administration, and the specific activity of $^{14}CO_2$ is measured in a liquid scintillation counter. The test requires physical rest from dose to breath sampling. For example, this test has been employed as a sensitive measure of increased microsomal enzyme activity among coke oven workers.

5. Caffeine breath test—Inhaled ^{14}C-labeled caffeine, labeled at one or all three methyl groups, followed by exhaled breath $^{14}CO_2$ measurement, was introduced recently as a noninvasive means of studying hepatic microsomal enzyme function. It has not undergone evaluation in asymptomatic worker populations.

B. ENDOGENOUS CLEARANCE TESTS

1. Serum bile acids—Serum bile acid measurement has been used to detect subclinical liver dysfunction following halogenated hydrocarbon exposure and also may be useful in further medical workup for the individual with persistent enzyme abnormalities. Bile acids are synthesized by the liver and undergo enterohepatic circulation. Serum levels of bile acids are normally low in a fasting state (<6 μmol/L) and reflect only hepatic excretory function and not synthesis rate or volume distribution. Fasting bile acid levels are increased in relation to the degree of liver disease and impairment in excretion.

Depending on the population screened, the positive predictive value of an abnormal (>8.4 μmol/L) serum bile acid test ranges from 10% (general population) to 94% (hospitalized population with biopsy-proved hepatobiliary disease). In a large workplace study of vinyl chloride–exposed workers, measurement of serum bile acids had a sensitivity of 78%, a specificity of 93%, and a positive predictive value of 10%.

Serum bile acids have been suggested as a more sensitive indicator of hepatic dysfunction than biochemical tests for liver toxicity. Many animal studies have shown increased serum bile acids after exposure to aliphatic hydrocarbon solvents and the nonchlorinated aromatic hydrocarbon solvent toluene. A dose-dependent increase in the concentration of serum bile acids has been observed in workers exposed to hexachlorobutadiene and trichloroethylene. Other standard tests of liver function were normal in these workers. The serum concentration and odds of abnormal total serum bile acids were increased among paint manufacturing workers directly exposed to solvent mixtures. The risk of increased bile acids in this study was influenced by gender, hepatitis B infection, alcohol consumption, and body mass index. The significance of these findings and their clinical correlation with disease outcome have yet to be determined.

2. Urinary D-glucaric acid—Urinary D-glucaric acid (UDGA) has been used as an indirect measure of liver induction. D-Glucaric acid, a product of carbohydrate metabolism, is produced via the glucuronic acid pathway after initial xenobiotic metabolism. The mechanism for UDGA induction has not been elucidated, but UDGA excretion is correlated with microsomal enzyme content. Operating room personnel exposed to isoflurane and nitrous oxide have increased UDGA excretion.

CLINICAL MANAGEMENT OF OCCUPATIONAL LIVER DISEASE

OCCUPATIONAL & MEDICAL HISTORY

A careful occupational history of exposure to known human hepatotoxins should be obtained in every case of suspected occupational liver disease. The past medical history of liver disease should be noted. The review of symptoms should include those of acute central nervous system toxicity, such as headache, dizziness, and light-headedness, because the presence of these symptoms may indicate excessive solvent exposure.

Nonoccupational causes of liver disease should be evaluated carefully. Steroid use, glue sniffing, or other recreational solvent use should be determined. Travel to areas with endemic parasitic or viral diseases may be a significant risk for infectious hepatitis. A history of hobbies involving exposure to hepatotoxins should be taken. Previous blood transfusions, percutaneous exposures (e.g., tattoos, needlesticks, ear piercing, or acupuncture), and intravenous drug use may be risk factors for viral hepatitis. A relationship between obesity and elevated liver enzyme levels has been well documented. Numerous medications may be hepatotoxic.

Use of protective work practices (such as respiratory protection, gloves, and work clothes) should be described because this may indicate the extent of pulmonary and skin absorption. Material data safety sheets (see Chapter 2) should be obtained on the relevant products used. Airborne contaminant monitoring data (see Chapter 36) should be requested and reviewed for excessive exposure. Inquiry should be made of the employer about other employees with possible liver disease.

PHYSICAL EXAMINATION

Acute liver disease owing to occupational exposure may present with right upper quadrant tenderness, hepatosplenomegaly, or jaundice. Mild hepatotoxicity may cause few physical findings. Examination of the respiratory tract or skin should be performed depending on the route of exposure. Chronic liver disease may result in stigmata such as spider angiomata, palmar erythema, testicular atrophy, ascites, and gynecomastia.

DIFFERENTIAL DIAGNOSIS

Other causes of liver disease should be ruled out, particularly infectious and alcohol- and drug-induced hepatitis. The most common causes of elevated serum transaminase are ingestion of ethanol and obesity. If a history of excessive ethanol ingestion is elicited, the serum transaminase measurement should be repeated after 3–4 weeks of abstinence. If serum transaminase levels are normal on follow-up, ethanol should be suspected as the probable cause. Persistent serum transaminase elevation may represent chronic alcoholic hepatitis or continued occupational exposure.

The onset of liver transaminase elevations after exposure to a known or suspected hepatotoxin is suggestive of occupational liver disease, particularly if normal liver tests before exposure can be documented. Even if preexposure tests are normal, liver disease may develop coincidentally without relation to workplace exposure.

MANAGEMENT OF ACUTE LIVER DISEASE

The most common clinical problem is the individual with elevated serum transaminase levels on routine screening who may have occupational exposure to a known hepatotoxin. Nonoccupational causes of liver disease should be ruled out carefully and the workplace inspected for the presence of hepatotoxic exposures. If an occupational cause is suspected, the individual should be removed immediately from exposure for 3–4 weeks. The serum transaminase measurement then should be repeated; with few exceptions, serum transaminase concentrations will normalize following removal from exposure. A persistently elevated serum transaminase concentration suggests a nonoccupational cause of liver disease or, rarely, chronic occupational liver disease.

Although there is little evidence that individuals with nonoccupational liver disease are more susceptible to further liver damage as a consequence of occupational exposure, it is prudent to monitor these workers carefully for evidence of worsening liver damage. Appropriate engineering controls and personal protective equipment should be made available to reduce potential hepatotoxic exposures. If there is evidence of worsening liver disease, or if exposure cannot be reduced satisfactorily, the individual should be reassigned. In one study of workers exposed to hydrocarbon solvents at a petrochemical plant, most workers with biopsy-proven nonalcoholic steatohepatitis improved after removal from the work environment. Aside from removing the individual from exposure to the offending agent, there is no specific treatment for acute occupational liver disease.

MANAGEMENT OF CHRONIC LIVER DISEASE

Persistent abnormalities in liver function tests after removal from exposure have been reported rarely, and a thorough search for other causes always should be conducted. Occasionally, chronic liver disease may follow acute chemical hepatitis or years of low-dose exposure.

Hepatic ultrasonography may show hepatic steatosis or periportal fibrosis. A recent study found that liver ultrasonography is a useful tool for the medical surveillance of vinyl chloride monomer workers, particularly among those exposed to VCM above 200 ppm for at least 1 year. Liver biopsy usually is not helpful in differentiating occupational from nonoccupational liver disease and is rarely indicated.

Treatment of hepatocellular carcinoma caused by occupational exposure does not differ from that of disease that is a result of other causes.

REFERENCES

Beekmann SE, Henderson DK: Protection of health care workers from blood-borne pathogens. Curr Opin Infect Dis 2005;18: 331 [PMID: 15985830].

Keeffe EB: Occupational risk for hepatitis A: A literature-based analysis. J Clin Gastroenterol 2004;38:440 [PMID: 15100525].

Pruss-Ustun A et al: Estimation of the global burden of disease attributable to contaminated sharps injuries among health care workers. Am J Indust Med 2005;48:482 [PMID: 16299710].

Smellie MK et al: Hospital transmission of hepatitis B virus in the absence of exposure prone procedures. Epidemiol Infect 2006;134:259 [PMID: 16490128].

U.S. Department of Labor: Safety and health topics; Blood-borne pathogens and needlestick prevention, www.osha.gov/SLTC/bloodbornepathogens/index.html.

U.S. Public Health Service: Prevention and control of infections with hepatitis viruses in correctional settings, www.cdc.gov/mmwr/preview/mmwrhtml/rr5201a1.htm.

U.S. Public Health Service: A comprehensive immunization strategy to eliminate transmission of hepatitis B virus infection in the United States: Recommendations of the Advisory Committee on Immunization Practices (ACIP): 1. Immunization of infants, children, and adolescents, www.cdc.gov/mmwr/preview/mmwrhtml/rr5416a1.htm.

U.S. Public Health Service: Updated U.S. Public Health Service guidelines for the management of occupational exposures to HBV, HCV, and HIV and recommendations for postexposure prophylaxis, www.cdc.gov/mmwr/preview/mmwrhtml/rr5011a1.htm.

U.S. Public Health Service: Workbook for designing, implementing, and evaluating a sharps injury prevention program, www.cdc.gov/sharpssafety/index.html.

U.S. Public Health Service: NIOSH safety and health topic: Blood-borne infectious diseases: HIV/AIDS, hepatitis B virus, and hepatitis C virus, www.cdc.gov/niosh/topics/bbp/.

Yazdanpanah Y et al: Risk factors for hepatitis C virus transmission to health care workers after occupational exposure. Clin Infect Dis 2005;41:1423 [PMID: 16231252].

Renal Toxicology

23

Rudolph A. Rodriguez, MD, & German T. Hernandez, MD, FASN

In the United States, 431,284 patients were treated for end-stage renal disease (ESRD) in the year 2002 at a cost of well over $25 billion a year. Both the number of patients and the associated costs are expected to double over the next 10 years. The etiology of the renal failure in a significant percentage of these patients is never fully elucidated, and the diagnosis of renal disease of occupational origin is rarely considered. The true incidence of chronic kidney disease secondary to occupational and environmental exposures in the United States is unknown. However, these exposures represent potentially preventable causes of chronic kidney disease. Even if occupational and · environmental exposures account for only a small percentage of the causes of ESRD in the United States, the significant morbidity, mortality, and costs associated with renal replacement therapy potentially could be prevented.

The kidney is especially vulnerable to occupational and environmental exposures. Approximately 20% of the cardiac output goes to the kidneys, and a fraction of this then is filtered; this is represented by the glomerular filtration rate (GFR). The GFR is normally 125 mL/min, or 180 L/d. Along the nephron, this filtrate is largely reabsorbed and then concentrated and acidified. Thus occupational and environmental toxins can be highly concentrated in the kidney, and as the pH of the filtrate changes, some toxins can exist in certain ionic forms. These factors help to explain the pathophysiologic mechanisms involved in certain toxins. For example, lead and cadmium cause much of their renal ultrastructural damage in the proximal tubule, where two-thirds of the filtered load is reabsorbed.

Following relatively high-dose exposure to certain organic solvents, metals, or pesticides, acute renal failure may develop within hours to days. The renal lesion usually is acute tubular necrosis. The clinical picture usually is dominated by the extrarenal manifestations of these exposures, and if the other organ systems recover, renal recovery is the rule. Chronic kidney disease or ESRD also may develop after certain exposures. The renal lesion in these cases usually is chronic interstitial nephritis, and lead nephropathy is a prime example. However, glomerular lesions are also seen after selected exposures such as to organic solvents or silicosis; in general, glomerular lesions after occupational or environmental exposures are very uncommon.

The renal evaluation of patients thought to have renal disease associated with an environmental or occupational exposure should be guided by the history, physical examination, and clinical presentation of the renal disease. The time course will separate acute from chronic kidney disease. In acute renal failure, the urine sediment usually is diagnostic of acute tubular necrosis. Most chronic kidney diseases associated with exposure to agents such as lead or cadmium present with chronic interstitial nephritis characterized by tubular proteinuria (usually less than 2 g/24 h) and a urinary sediment usually lacking any cellular elements. A nephritic sediment is suggestive of a proliferative renal lesion and has been associated only with a few exposures, such as to organic solvents. The nephrotic syndrome, characterized by more than 3.5 g protein per 24 hours, edema, and hypercholesterolemia, is also associated with exposure to some heavy metals, including mercury.

Monitoring workers for the possible renal effects of occupational exposures is very difficult because of the lack of sensitive and specific tests of renal injury. Serial measurement of traditional tests such as creatinine or blood urea nitrogen (BUN) is inadequate because these tests do not become abnormal until significant renal damage has occurred. The currently recommended core groups of tests for use in adult studies recommended by the U.S. Department of Health correlate with site of possible damage. Some of these tests detect possible glomerular injury (e.g., urine albumin), proximal tubule damage (e.g., retinol-binding protein, N-acetyl-β-D-glucosaminidase, and alanine amino peptidase), and distal tubule injury (e.g., osmolality). Most of these tests were designed to detect early renal tubular damage. Unfortunately, their use is limited by many factors; for instance, some are unstable at certain urine pHs, others return to normal levels within a few days of the exposure despite renal damage, and others exhibit large interindividual variations. Most important, unlike microalbuminuria, which is able to predict future nephropathy in insulin-dependent diabetics, the predictive value of these newer tests has not been validated. More long-term studies are needed before these newer renal tests can be used routinely to monitor renal injury in the workplace.

The National Kidney Foundation publishes practice guidelines for the evaluation, classification, and stratification of chronic kidney disease. These guidelines suggest classifying patients with chronic kidney disease into five stages according to the calculated GFR, with stage 5 representing kidney failure with a GFR of less than 15 mL/min and stage 1 representing a normal GFR of greater than 90 mL/min but with kidney damage such as proteinuria. In addition, the guidelines give evidence-based recommendations on the best approach to estimate total urinary protein excretion and GFR. The Web site has a useful GFR calculator that uses the modification of diet in renal disease formula for GFR estimation.

REFERENCES

National Kidney Foundation: www.kidney.org/professionals/kdoqi/guidelines.cfm.

United States Renal Data System: www.usrds.org/.

ACUTE RENAL DYSFUNCTION

A large number of occupational and environmental toxins can cause acute renal failure, usually after high-dose exposure. Although the extrarenal manifestations of the particular toxic exposure usually dominate the clinical presentation and course, the characteristics and time course of the acute renal failure are very similar in all exposures. In the vast majority of cases, acute tubular necrosis is the renal lesion that develops. Hours to days after the exposure, the acute tubular necrosis is manifested by decreased urine output, usually in the oliguric range of less than 500 mL/d. The urinalysis typically is diagnostic of acute tubular necrosis, with renal tubular cells, muddy brown granular casts, and little or no protein. Red blood cells, white blood cells, or casts of either cell type are not typically seen with acute tubular necrosis and suggest the presence of a glomerulonephritis. Increases in BUN and creatinine and in electrolyte abnormalities develop as expected in acute renal failure, and patients may require dialysis until the renal function recovers. After 1–2 weeks, recovery from acute tubular necrosis usually is heralded by the onset of a diuresis.

Hemodialysis and/or hemoperfusion have almost no role in accelerating the clearance of occupational and environmental toxins. For these techniques to be effective, toxins must have a low apparent volume of distribution and molecular weight, a low affinity for plasma proteins, and low tissue-binding properties. For example, charcoal

hemoperfusion can result in almost complete removal of circulating paraquat, but because of high tissue binding, only small amounts of total-body paraquat are removed. Consequently, hemoperfusion does not affect the prognosis in paraquat poisoning. These extracorporeal techniques are effective only after a few intoxications, which include certain alcohols, salicylate, lithium, and theophylline.

ACUTE RENAL DYSFUNCTION CAUSED BY HEAVY METALS

Significant exposure to any of the divalent metals—chromium, cadmium, mercury, and vanadium—is capable of producing acute tubular necrosis. Of these metals, the only one encountered in industrial settings in high enough concentrations to produce acute tubular necrosis with notable frequency is cadmium. Exposure to cadmium in toxic amounts is usually through inhalation, and the classic history of exposure is that of workers welding cadmium-plated metals. Welders exposed to cadmium fumes present with coughing and progressive pulmonary distress leading to adult respiratory distress syndrome. Renal failure occurs rapidly in the form of acute tubular necrosis. Severe exposure is capable of producing bilateral cortical necrosis.

ACUTE RENAL DYSFUNCTION CAUSED BY ORGANIC SOLVENTS

In the occupational setting, the lungs are the most common route of absorption of hydrocarbons. Inhaled hydrocarbons then quickly pass into the pulmonary circulation. Transcutaneous absorption is also an important route of absorption for solvents. Organic solvents are lipophilic and therefore are distributed in highest concentration in the fat, liver, bone marrow, blood, brain, and kidneys.

1. Halogenated Hydrocarbons

Carbon Tetrachloride

Carbon tetrachloride (CCl_4) is used as an industrial solvent and as the basis for manufacture of fluorinated hydrocarbons. It was once used as a household cleaning agent and as a component of fire extinguisher fluid under the brand name Pyrene.

After acute exposure, patients typically present with confusion, somnolence, nausea, and vomiting. Mucous membrane irritant effects, such as burning eyes, may occur, although some workers may be symptom-free for several days following exposure and then present with complaints of vomiting, abdominal pain, constipation, diarrhea, and in some cases fever. Physical findings may be compatible with the acute abdomen at this stage of illness, and many patients have been improperly subjected to laparotomy for that reason.

After 7–10 days of illness, there may be a decline in urine output even to the point of anuria. Patients with carbon tetrachloride intoxication usually show signs of prerenal azotemia, as demonstrated by a low urinary sodium excretion, and if ischemic acute tubular necrosis does not supervene, the prerenal azotemia may improve after volume repletion. If the hepatotoxicity is severe, patients also may develop hepatorenal syndrome.

Other Aliphatic Halogenated Hydrocarbons

Other aliphatic halogenated hydrocarbons are nephrotoxic, some to a greater and some to a lesser degree than carbon tetrachloride. Ethylene dichloride ($C_2H_4Cl_2$) is used as a solvent for oils, fats, waxes, turpentine, rubber, and some resins; as an insecticide and fumigant; and in fire extinguishers and household cleaning fluids. It is slightly less potent than carbon tetrachloride as a renal toxicant but causes far greater central nervous system toxicity. Ingestion or heavy inhalation may produce acute tubular necrosis similar to that encountered with mercury poisoning.

Chloroform (CCl_3H) is more nephrotoxic than carbon tetrachloride and produces proximal tubule cell damage in animal models. Trichloroethylene (C_2HCl_3) has a number of industrial uses and also has been used as an anesthetic agent. Acute renal failure has followed inhalation of this agent and has occurred in persons using it as a solvent for cleaning. Although it is partially unsaturated, it has toxic effects comparable with those of carbon tetrachloride and chloroform.

Tetrachloroethane (1,1,2,2,-tetrachloroethane, $C_2H_2Cl_4$) is an excellent solvent for cellulose acetate and is by far the most toxic of the halogenated hydrocarbons. Vinylidene chloride (1,1-dichloroethylene, $C_2H_2Cl_2$) is a monomer used in the manufacture of plastics and is not used as a solvent. Its toxicology is similar to that of carbon tetrachloride.

Ethylene chlorohydrin (2-chloroethyl alcohol, C_2H_4ClOH) is used as a solvent and as a chemical intermediate. It is far more toxic than any of the other aliphatic halogenated hydrocarbons. Unlike the others, it penetrates the skin readily and is absorbed through rubber gloves. Its mechanism of toxicity is not well understood.

2. Nonhalogenated Hydrocarbons as a Cause of Acute Renal Failure

Dioxane

Dioxane is a cyclic diether; it is colorless, has only a faint odor, and is freely soluble in water. The vapor pressure of dioxane is quite low, so respiratory overexposure is rare. Although dioxane is less toxic than the halogenated hydrocarbons, toxicity can be insidious, and large amounts can be inhaled without warning. Injury may become apparent hours after exposure.

Clinically, patients present with anorexia, nausea, and vomiting. Jaundice is uncommon. In fatal cases, clinical presentation may resemble an acute abdominal emergency. Urine output decreases on about the third day of illness.

Toluene

There are several reports of acute renal failure occurring with toluene inhalation (glue sniffing); most case reports describe reversible acute tubular necrosis, with a few reports documenting acute interstitial nephritis. However, metabolic acidosis associated with toluene abuse has been well documented. The two mechanisms involved are overproduction of hippuric acid and reduction of excretion of net acid (primarily NH^{4+}) in some abusers. Sodium and potassium depletion also occurs commonly in these patients.

Alkyl Derivatives of Ethylene Glycol

The principal derivatives of ethylene glycol used commercially are the monoethyl ether (Cellosolve), the monomethyl ether (methyl Cellosolve), and the butyl ether (butyl Cellosolve). The three compounds are similar pharmacologically, with increasing toxicity in the order listed above. All can be absorbed through the skin or lungs, as well as through the gastrointestinal tract. These agents are irritants of skin and mucous membranes and act as central nervous system depressants, with resulting symptoms of headache, drowsiness, weakness, slurred speech, staggering gait, and blurred vision. The renal injury caused by these ethers is not related to the oxalic aciduria caused by the parent compounds, which are dialcohols.

Phenol

Phenol (carbolic acid) causes local burns and may be absorbed both through the lungs and transdermally. Although phenol causes severe local burns, systemic symptoms also may occur. These include headache, vertigo, salivation, nausea and vomiting, and diarrhea. In severe intoxication, urinary albumin excretion may be increased. Red cells and casts are found in the urine. The potentially disastrous consequences of transdermal absorption should not be underestimated.

Patients may present with hypothermia, which is followed by convulsions. The urine may be dark, and oliguria may develop. Phenol is metabolized to hydroquinone, which, when excreted in the urine, may be oxidized to colored substances, causing the urine to change to green or brown (carboluria). Prolonged exposure has been reported to result in proteinuria.

Pentachlorophenol

Pentachlorophenol is used as a preservative for timber and as an insecticide, herbicide, and defoliant. It is readily absorbed through the skin. In addition to causing acute renal failure, pentachlorophenol causes a hypermetabolic state, with hyperpyrexia and vascular collapse. Workers exposed to pentachlorophenol in clearly subtoxic doses may present with reversible decreased proximal tubular function as manifested by reduced tubular resorption of phosphorus. When these workers are reexamined after a 21-day vacation, renal function—both GFR and proximal tubular function—has returned to normal.

Dinitriphenols & Dinitro-o-Cresols

These agents have been used as pesticides and herbicides. After absorption, they uncouple oxidative phosphorylation. Fatal hyperpyrexia has been reported. Although patients develop acute renal failure, it is not known whether this is a direct effect of the agents or secondary to the metabolic consequences, such as myoglobinuria.

ACUTE RENAL DYSFUNCTION CAUSED BY UNIDENTIFIED PESTICIDES

Exposure, Pathogenesis, & Clinical Findings

A reduction in GFR, as well as tubular reabsorption of phosphate suggestive of mild proximal tubular dysfunction, has occurred in some agricultural workers. Changes in tubular function and in GFR rate occur in conjunction with depression of serum cholinesterase, suggesting that organophosphates may be responsible for these changes in renal function.

In an ethically questionable study, prisoners in a New York State prison were fed carbaryl. This pesticide is similar in action to the organophosphates, and the prisoners likewise demonstrated a decrease in GFR and tubular resorption of phosphate. There is no evidence that structural damage occurs after exposure to any of these agents.

Organic mercurials are used as fungicides. Absorption of these agents in agricultural workers has been reported to lead to nephrotic syndrome in the case of methoxymethyl mercury silicate, and a dose-dependent increase in the urinary excretion of γ-glutamyl transpeptidase has been reported in the case of phenyl mercury, indicating a direct nephrotoxic effect of this class of compounds.

ACUTE RENAL DYSFUNCTION CAUSED BY ARSINE

Exposure

Arsine (AsH_3) is a heavy gas and is the most nephrotoxic form of arsenic. It is produced by the action of acids on arsenicals, usually during coal or metal-processing operations. Exposure to arsine may be insidious

because even as simple an operation as spraying water on metal dross may liberate arsine. Arsine is also used in the semiconductor industry. It may be shipped over long distances with a potential for public health disasters because arsine is an extremely toxic gas.

Clinical Findings

Arsine is primarily hemotoxic and is a potent hemolytic agent after acute or chronic exposure. The first signs of poisoning are malaise, abdominal cramps, nausea, and vomiting. This may take place immediately or after a delay of up to 24 hours. Renal failure results from acute tubular necrosis secondary to hemoglobinuria.

Treatment & Prognosis

Acute tubular necrosis may be delayed by treatment with hydration and mannitol. However, exchange transfusion is necessary to prevent further hemolysis. Recovery from acute tubular necrosis induced by arsine may not be complete, and there is evidence that residual interstitial nephritis may result.

ACUTE RENAL DYSFUNCTION CAUSED BY PHOSPHORUS

Ingestion of only a few milligrams of elemental yellow phosphorus may produce acute hepatic and acute renal necrosis. Chronic exposure may result in proteinuria, although the kidney is not the primary organ affected by phosphorus.

REFERENCES

Barbier O et al: Effect of heavy metals on, and handling by, the kidney. Nephron Physiol 2005;99:105 [PMID: 15722646].

Brautbar N: Industrial solvents and kidney disease: A review. Int J Occup Environ Health 2004;10:79 [PMID: 15070029].

Voss JU et al: Nephrotoxicity of organic solvents: Biomarkers for early detection. Int Arch Occup Environ Health 2005;78:475 [PMID: 15895243].

BALKAN-ENDEMIC NEPHROPATHY

The prototypical renal disease associated with an environmental exposure is Balkan-endemic nephropathy (BEN). BEN highlights the difficulties involved in identifying specific toxins that may cause renal disease. In the late 1950s, BEN was first described as an interstitial nephropathy associated with urinary tract tumors. It is endemic to rural areas along the Sava, Danube, and Morava rivers in Serbia, Croatia, Bosnia-Herzegovina, Bulgaria, and Romania. It strikes predominantly farm workers in the fifth to sixth decades. Most victims have resided for at least 20 years in villages where the disease is endemic, and children are not affected.

Patients present with abnormalities of tubular function, including renal tubular acidosis, glycosuria, and hyperuricosuria with hypouricemia. Proteinuria is usually less than 1 g/d, which is consistent with the absence of glomerular disease. Not all patients with chronic kidney disease will progress to ESRD. Renal pathology includes interstitial fibrosis and periglomerular fibrosis; there is no inflammatory component, and glomeruli are normal. Papillary transitional-cell cancer is seen in 30–40% of patients with BEN. Anemia seems to be disproportionate to the degree of renal failure in these patients.

Many etiologies have been proposed to account for BEN. Both lead and cadmium have been excluded as possibilities. Aristolochic acid is a known renal toxin and has been found in flour obtained from wheat contaminated with the seeds of *Aristolochia clematis* in areas of endemicity. In addition, aristolochic acid DNA adducts have been found in the kidney tissue of patients from endemic regions. The true cause of BEN remains unknown, but aristolochic acid exposure is an intriguing theory (see "Herbal Nephropathy/Analgesic Nephropathy" below).

REFERENCES

Andonova IE et al: Balkan endemic nephropathy and genetic variants of glutathione *S*-transferases. J Nephrol 2004;17:390 [PMID: 15365959].

Atanasova SY et al: Genetic polymorphisms of cytochrome P450 among patients with Balkan endemic nephropathy. Clin Biochem 2005;38:223 [PMID: 15708542].

HERBAL NEPHROPATHY/ANALGESIC NEPHROPATHY

When evaluating patients suspected of having renal disease associated with environmental or occupational exposures, it is very important to exclude herbal and analgesic nephropathy. Both commonly present with chronic interstitial nephritis, as do most occupationally related renal disease. Chinese herb nephropathy was first described in 1991; physicians in Belgium noted an increasing number of young women presenting with ESRD following exposure to Chinese herbs at a weight-reduction clinic. The renal pathology and the association with papillary transitional-cell cancer are very similar to the renal findings in BEN. In fact, aristolochic acid was the common denominator found in the weight-reduction formulas and thought to be the cause of Chinese herb nephropathy. Cases of Chinese herb nephropathy now have been reported worldwide, and aristolochic acid exposure in rat models has produced similar renal lesions as in humans. Aristolochic acid DNA adducts also have been demonstrated in the kidney tissue of patients with Chinese herb nephropathy. *Aristolochic acid nephropathy* should replace the term *Chinese herb nephropathy*.

Most other herbal remedies are safe, but adulteration of these herbal remedies is fairly common. The common contaminants that may cause renal disease include botanicals (e.g., aristolochic acid), synthetic drugs [e.g., nonsteroidal anti-inflammatory drugs (NSAIDs), and diazepam], and heavy metals (e.g., lead and cadmium). Renal dysfunction as a consequence of NSAIDs and selective cyclooxygenase-2 inhibitors may present in three different forms. The most common form is hemodynamic renal failure after the loss of prostaglandin-mediated afferent arteriolar vasodilatation. This then leads to afferent arteriolar vasoconstriction in patients with preexisting volume depletion. Both classes of drugs also can cause acute renal failure secondary to acute interstitial nephritis, which usually is accompanied by nephrotic-range proteinuria. Both forms of renal failure are reversible after discontinuation of the offending drug, although the renal failure as a consequence of interstitial nephritis is usually more severe and may require dialysis support. The third form of renal dysfunction is papillary necrosis, which is not reversible and which occurs after many years of high doses of NSAIDs. Papillary necrosis occurs more commonly after chronic phenacetin use. Phenacetin is no longer available in the United States. It is controversial whether chronic acetaminophen use causes papillary necrosis.

In addition to NSAIDs and aristolochic acid, herbal remedies may contain heavy metals, such as lead, cadmium, or mercury; the renal disease associated with these metals is discussed in the following sections.

REFERENCES

Cheng HF, Harris RC: Renal effects of nonsteroidal anti-inflammatory drugs and selective cyclooxygenase-2 inhibitors. Curr Pharm Des 2005;11:1795 [PMID: 15892676].

Isnard Bagnis C et al: Herbs and the kidney. Am J Kidney Dis 2004;44:1 [PMID: 15211432].

Szeto CC, Chow KM: Nephrotoxicity related to new therapeutic compounds. Renal Failure 2005;27:329 [PMID: 15957551].

CHRONIC KIDNEY DISEASE

CHRONIC KIDNEY DISEASE CAUSED BY LEAD

Although organic lead, which is used as an additive to gasoline, is not nephrotoxic, its combustion products are. At one time, lead was released into the environment at a rate of approximately 60 million kg/year as inorganic lead through the combustion of gasoline. Its environmental fate is unknown. Lead can be absorbed from the gastrointestinal tract or the lungs. Gastrointestinal absorption is approximately 10% in adults and 50% in children. Within 1 hour of absorption by the gut, lead is concentrated in bone (90%) and kidneys. The biologic half-life ranges from 7 years to several decades.

Although the link between lead exposure and small, contracted kidneys was noted by Lancereaux in 1863, the modern awareness of lead nephropathy originated with the Australian experience. Acute lead poisoning in childhood was very common in Queensland between 1870 and 1920, when lead paint was still being used. Twenty years later, a follow-up study of children hospitalized for acute lead poisoning found that more than 30% of these children had chronic nephritis, hypertension, or proteinuria. Gouty arthritis was noted in approximately 50% of patients. Epidemiologic data in the United States also confirm the link between overt lead exposure and chronic kidney disease, hypertension, and gout.

Experimental models of lead nephropathy found that administration of continuous high-dose lead to rats over a 1-year period resulted in a significant reduction in GFR, and the renal pathology revealed the characteristic proximal tubule intranuclear inclusions that are prominent early in human lead nephropathy. After 6 months of lead exposure, focal tubular atrophy and interstitial fibrosis appeared, and after 12 months, enlarged, dilated tubules were noted. Chelation of lead with dimercaptosuccinic acid (DMSA) resulted in an increase in GFR in rats, but the tubulointerstitial disease did not reverse. Continuous low-level lead exposure in rats did not produce significant changes in renal function and produced only mild alterations in renal morphology after 12 months.

Many studies have noted an approximate incidence of gout of 50% among subjects with lead nephropathy. The possible mechanisms of saturnine gout include decreased renal clearance of uric acid, crystallization at low urate concentrations, and lead-induced formation of guanine crystals. Human studies have found that patients with gout and renal insufficiency have significantly higher urinary lead excretion after chelation than do either subjects with gout and normal renal function or subjects with no gout and renal insufficiency. These findings implicate lead as the cause of both the gout and the renal insufficiency in these patients.

Hypertension is associated with acute lead intoxication, but the relationship between chronic lead exposure and hypertension remains controversial in the setting of mounting evidence. Despite the continued decline in lead exposure in the U.S. population, Muntner recently reported (2005) a significant association between relatively low blood lead levels and hypertension among Mexican Americans and African Americans. Many large population studies have found a direct correlation between blood lead levels and zinc protoporphyrin and blood pressure. The possible mechanisms linking lead and hypertension include increased intracellular calcium, inhibition of the Na^+,K^+-adenosine triphosphatase (ATPase) system, direct vasoconstriction, and alterations in the rennin-angiotensin-aldosterone axis.

Human studies also have investigated the role that lead plays in the association of hypertension and renal failure. Early studies in patients with overt lead exposure, hypertension, and renal insufficiency have implicated lead as a cause of both the renal insufficiency and hypertension. However, these studies included patients with high-level lead exposure, including those with moonshine consumption. There is growing evidence that low-level lead exposure is associated with chronic kidney disease among certain populations. Data from the Normative Aging Study suggest that low-level lead exposure may be associated with impaired renal function among veterans in Boston. Also, small studies from Taiwan recently have reported low-level environmental lead exposure as an independent risk factor for renal disease progression among nondiabetics with chronic kidney disease. Furthermore, intravenous chelation therapy with ethylenediaminetetraacetic acid (EDTA) seems to ameliorate the decline in renal function when compared with placebo in the same Taiwanese patient population.

Presentation

The classic presentation for lead nephropathy is chronic kidney disease accompanied by a history of hypertension and gout. However, the diagnosis of lead nephropathy also should be considered in patients with chronic kidney disease and low-grade proteinuria, even without gout or significant hypertension. The urinalysis usually reveals 1+ to 2+ proteinuria but is otherwise normal, without cells or cellular casts. Twenty-four-hour urine collection usually has non-nephrotic-range proteinuria in the range of 1–2 g, and renal ultrasonography typically shows small, contracted kidneys. Renal biopsy reveals nonspecific tubular atrophy, interstitial fibrosis, and minimal inflammatory infiltrates, and the arteriolar changes are indistinguishable from nephrosclerosis and appear even in patients with lead exposure and no history of hypertension. Electron microscopy shows mitochondrial swelling and increased numbers of lysosomal dense bodies within proximal tubule cells; intranuclear inclusion bodies usually are present in the early stages of lead exposure but often are absent after chronic exposure or after lead chelation.

Diagnosis

The diagnosis is considered after documenting significant lead exposure. Blood lead levels are not useful unless elevated because low serum levels do not exclude chronic lead exposure. The EDTA lead mobilization test correlates well with bone lead levels. One gram of EDTA is given intravenously or two grams of EDTA with lidocaine are given intramuscularly in two divided doses 8–12 hours apart, and urine is then collected for 72 hours in patients with chronic kidney disease or for 24 hours in patients with normal renal function. Early studies in patients with overt lead exposure demonstrated that a total excretion greater than 600 µg lead chelate over 3 days was indicative of significant lead exposure. The recent studies of patients with low-level exposure raise the possibility that total lead chelate excretion of 80–599 µg may be significant. Tibial K x-ray fluorescence measurements also correlate well with bone lead levels and, if available, should replace the EDTA mobilization test.

Treatment

Overt lead nephropathy is one of the few preventable renal diseases. Whether renal function improves with treatment is controversial, but in some patients treatment has resulted in a modest improvement in GFR or, at the minimum, a slowing of the progression of the renal insufficiency even with low-level exposure. In addition, lead chelation treatment has led to increased urate excretion, which might have an impact on the management of gout in these patients. For patients with overt lead nephropathy, treatment consists of continued EDTA injections thrice weekly, with the goal of normalizing the urinary lead chelate.

Among patients with nondiabetic chronic kidney disease and low-level lead exposure (urine lead chelate excretion between 80 and 599 µg), treatment is continued with weekly intravenous infusions of 1 g EDTA until the urine lead chelate decreases to below 60 µg. The oral lead chelator DMSA is currently being studied and should replace EDTA as the treatment of choice for lead exposure. However, the safety and efficacy of chronic DMSA and EDTA in patients with moderate to severe renal insufficiency have not been well studied, and these agents should be used with caution in these patients.

REFERENCES

Lin JL et al: Environmental exposure to lead and progressive diabetic nephropathy in patients with type II diabetes. Kidney Int 2006;69:2049 [PMID: 16641918].

Yu CC et al: Environmental exposure to lead and progression of chronic renal diseases: A four-year prospective longitudinal study. J Am Soc Nephrol 2004;15:1016 [PMID: 15034104].

CHRONIC KIDNEY DISEASE CAUSED BY CADMIUM

Cadmium, which is found primarily as cadmium sulfide in ores of zinc, lead, and copper, accumulates with age, having a biologic half-life in humans in excess of 10 years. In the United States, the use of cadmium doubled every decade in the twentieth century because it is used commonly in the manufacture of nickel-cadmium batteries, pigments, glass, metal alloys, and electrical equipment.

Between 40% and 80% of accumulated cadmium is stored in the liver and kidneys, with one-third in the kidneys alone. Cadmium is also a contaminant of tobacco smoke, and in the absence of occupational exposure, accumulation is substantially greater in smokers than in nonsmokers. Nonindustrial exposure is primarily via food; only approximately 25% of ingested cadmium is absorbed. "Normal" daily dietary intake varies between 15 and 75 mg/d in different parts of the world, although only a small fraction of this amount (0.5–2.5 mg/d) is absorbed. The cadmium body burden of a 45-year-old nonsmoker in the United States is approximately 9 mg, whereas in Japan the total is approximately 21 mg. Although clinical disease has been recognized among the general population in Japan, this has not been the case in the United States, where cadmium generally has been regarded as an exclusively industrial hazard. This may represent a failure to assign the correct cause to conditions commonly regarded as the result of aging.

After exposure to cadmium, the blood concentration rises sharply but falls after a matter of hours as the cadmium is taken up by the liver. In red blood cells and soft tissues, cadmium is bound to metallothionein, which is a low-molecular-weight polypeptide. This cadmium-metallothionein complex is filtered at the glomerulus, undergoes endocytosis in the proximal tubule, and is later degraded in the lysosomes. The adverse effects of cadmium on the proximal tubule are probably mediated by unbound cadmium, which can interfere with zinc-dependent enzymes.

The principal target organs for cadmium toxicity after chronic low-dose exposure are the kidneys and lungs. Once a critical concentration of 200 µg/g of renal cortex is achieved, the renal effects, such as Fanconi syndrome, become evident. Hypercalciuria with normocalcemia, hyperphosphaturia, and distal renal tubular acidosis all contribute to the osteomalacia, pseudofractures, and nephrolithiasis seen in certain patients. Many of the symptoms usually originate from the increased calcium excretion that accompanies the renal tubular dysfunction. Ureteral colic from calculi is seen in up to 40% of patients subjected to industrial exposure. Itai-Itai ("ouch-ouch") disease is a painful bone disease associated with pseudofractures in Japan, and it is attributed to local cadmium contamination of food staples by polluted river water. The possible causes of osteomalacia include a direct effect of cadmium on bone, diminished renal tubular reabsorption of calcium and phosphate, and increased parathyroid hormone and the subsequent decreased hydroxylation of vitamin D.

The role of cadmium in the induction of chronic interstitial nephritis is controversial. A study of 1021 workers with low-level cadmium toxicity found that early kidney damage evidenced by tubular proteinuria was evident at levels thought to be safe by World Health Organization health-based limits. Although some studies demonstrate subtle declines in GFR or an increase in odds ratios of ESRD in cross-sectional studies, few studies demonstrate an increase incidence of severe chronic kidney disease.

However, workers should be monitored closely. Renal cadmium toxicity should be suspected in patients with low-molecular-weight proteinuria, urinary calculi, multiple tubular abnormalities, and a urine cadmium concentration greater than 10 µg/g of urine creatinine. There is no definitive treatment except removal from the exposure and treatment of osteomalacia, if present.

REFERENCES

Akesson A et al: Tubular and glomerular kidney effects in Swedish women with low environmental cadmium exposure. Environ Health Perspect 2005;113:1627 [PMID: 16263522].

Trzcinka-Ochocka M et al: The effects of environmental cadmium exposure on kidney function. Environ Res 2004;95:143 [PMID: 15147919].

CHRONIC KIDNEY DISEASE CAUSED BY MERCURY

Exposure

Occupational mercury poisoning usually results from inhalation of metal fumes or vapor, although toxicity has been reported after exposure to oxides of mercury, mercurous or mercuric chloride, phenylmercuric acetate, mercuric oxide, and mercury-containing pesticides. Divalent mercury is quite nephrotoxic when ingested, accumulates in the proximal tubule, and can produce acute renal failure in doses as low as 1 mg/kg. Although acute tubular necrosis will result after administration of mercuric chloride ($HgCl_2$), such exposures occur either rarely or not at all as occupational hazards.

The two forms of renal disease resulting from mercury toxicity are acute tubular necrosis and nephrotic syndrome. In humans, acute tubular necrosis develops after ingestion of 0.5 g $HgCl_2$, and in rats, $HgCl_2$ is used routinely to produce an experimental model of acute tubular necrosis. There also have been sporadic case reports of nephrotic syndrome after mercury exposure. These may be idiosyncratic reactions, and accordingly, occupational studies have not been able to find an association between mercury exposure and proteinuria. Membranous nephropathy, minimal-change disease, and anti–glomerular basement membrane antibody deposition all have been reported following mercury exposure.

Mercuric chloride can induce membranous nephropathy in certain rat strains. Before the development of the basement membrane immune deposits seen in membranous nephropathy, an autoimmune glomerulonephritis with linear immunoglobulin (Ig) G deposits along the glomerular capillary wall is first seen, but no pulmonary findings are seen as in Goodpasture syndrome. A T-cell-dependent polyclonal B-cell activation is responsible for the IgG deposits. As in humans, removal from mercury exposure, which can be in vapor or injections, results in reversal of the proteinuria in these rat models.

Diagnosis

The clinical presentation in patients with acute renal failure from acute tubular necrosis usually is dominated by the extrarenal manifestations of mercury toxicity. When the history of mercury exposure is available, the diagnosis of acute tubular necrosis from mercury toxicity is not difficult. On the other hand, it is more difficult to attribute glomerular disease such as membranous nephropathy to mercury exposure. Although elevated blood and urine mercury concentrations are consistent with significant exposure, these concentrations do not correlate with renal disease. Spontaneous resolution of the proteinuria following removal from the source of mercury exposure is consistent with mercury-mediated glomerular disease.

Treatment

The mainstay of treatment is removal from the source of mercury exposure and chelation with British anti-Lewisite (dimercaprol BAL). BAL is given intramuscularly. Following an initial dose of up to 5 mg/kg, 2.5 mg/kg is given twice daily for 10 days. DMSA is an oral chelating agent that has been used successfully in isolated human cases; in studies in rats, it successfully decreased mercury levels in the kidneys. In severe cases of mercury toxicity with anuric renal failure, the use of hemodialysis with the prefilter infusion of DMSA has been reported to increase the removal of inorganic mercury.

REFERENCES

Bhan A, Sarkar NN: Mercury in the environment: Effect on health and reproduction. Rev Environ Health 2005;20:39 [PMID: 15835497].

Block LS: The toxicology of mercury. N Engl J Med 2004;350:945 [PMID: 14985496].

Booth S, Zeller D: Mercury, food webs, and marine mammals: Implications of diet and climate change for human health. Environ Health Perspect 2005;113:521 [PMID: 15866757].

CHRONIC KIDNEY DISEASE CAUSED BY BERYLLIUM

Exposure

Beryllium is encountered in the manufacture of electronic tubes, ceramics, and fluorescent light bulbs, as well as in metal foundries. Because its absorption through the gut is very poor, beryllium's principal route of entry into the body is by inhalation.

Clinical Findings

The main manifestation of berylliosis is as a systemic granulomatous disease involving primarily the lungs, as well as the bone and bone marrow, the liver, the lymph nodes, and many other organs. Kidney damage occurs not as an isolated finding but only in conjunction with other forms of toxicity. In the kidneys, berylliosis can produce granulomas and interstitial fibrosis. Beryllium nephropathy is associated with hypercalciuria and urinary tract stones. Renal stone disease is common in berylliosis and may occur in up to 30% of patients. Parathyroid hormone levels are depressed, and the presumed mechanism of hypercalciuria is increased calcium absorption through the gut similar to that encountered in sarcoidosis. Hyperuricemia is also characteristic of beryllium nephropathy.

REFERENCE

Infante PF, Newman LS: Beryllium exposure and chronic beryllium disease. Lancet 2004;366:415 [PMID: 14962519].

CHRONIC KIDNEY DISEASE CAUSED BY URANIUM

It is unclear whether uranium is responsible for significant occupationally related renal disease in humans. Uranium can cause acute renal failure in experimental models, and the pathologic changes are consistent with acute tubular necrosis. During the Manhattan Project, acute tubular necrosis occurred in men working on the atomic bomb. Whether uranium can cause chronic kidney disease remains controversial. Although a previous study of workers in a uranium-refining plant revealed an increase in urinary β_2-microglobulin excretion, the study did not document decreased renal function, and the urinary β_2-microglobulin level still was in the normal range.

REFERENCE

Kurttio P et al: Kidney toxicity of ingested uranium from drinking water. Am J Kidney Dis 2006;47:972 [PMID: 16731292].

CHRONIC KIDNEY DISEASE CAUSED BY SILICOSIS

Silicosis is a form of pneumoconiosis associated with pulmonary exposure to silica. Heavy exposure can result in a generalized systemic disease resembling collagen-vascular disease, such as systemic lupus erythematosus. Inhalation of silica may trigger an autoimmune response in sensitive individuals; in fact, the occurrence of positive antinuclear antibody and antineutrophil cytoplasmic autoantibodies is increased in patients with silicosis.

The possible association of silica and glomerulonephritis is suggested by animal studies, case-control studies, and multiple case reports. Animals experimentally exposed to silica developed acute interstitial nephritis with deposition of silica in the kidney. This fact led to speculation that silica may contribute to analgesic nephropathy as a result of the widespread use of silicates in analgesic preparations. Certain studies have found that patients with silicosis have a high prevalence of albuminuria, impaired renal function, and glomerular abnormalities at autopsy. The reported

cases of possible silica-associated glomerular disease include glomerular proliferation with occasional crescents, subendothelial and membranous deposits, and tubular degeneration. The renal silica content was elevated in most of the patients in whom it was measured. Interestingly, not all patients reported to have possible silica-associated nephropathy had pulmonary disease.

REFERENCES

McDonald JC et al: Mortality from lung and kidney disease in a cohort of North American industrial sand workers: An update. Ann Occup Hyg 2005;49:367 [PMID: 15728107].

Steenland K: One agent, many diseases: Exposure-response data and comparative risks of different outcomes following silica exposure. Am J Ind Med 2005;48:16 [PMID: 15940719].

CHRONIC KIDNEY DISEASE CAUSED BY ORGANIC SOLVENTS

Solvent exposure may occur in many industries where there is use of paints, degreasers, and fuels, including the petrochemical and aerospace industries. There have been a number of intriguing case reports over the last 20 years of anti–glomerular basement membrane antibody–mediated glomerulonephritis occurring after solvent exposure. However, it remains unclear whether the solvent exposure is truly causal in these cases. Membranous nephropathy also has been reported after long exposure to mixed organic solvents. Twenty-five case-control studies have investigated hydrocarbon exposure and renal disease, and although most of these studies have major limitations, 20 found an increased odds ratio between solvent exposure and a variety of renal diseases. Animal studies show that solvents can cause acute renal damage at high doses, and only mild chronic renal changes have been produced with chronic low-dose exposure. There are no animal models for immunologic renal disease caused by solvents.

It is clear that solvent exposure at high doses may lead to acute renal failure as a consequence of acute tubular necrosis, and substantial evidence supports that solvent exposure is associated with glomerulonephritis. However, solvent exposure is common, and glomerulonephritis is rare, which suggests that if the association does exist, certain host factors are necessary for this idiosyncratic reaction to develop.

CHRONIC KIDNEY DISEASE CAUSED BY CARBON DISULFIDE
Exposure History & Clinical Findings

Carbon disulfide is used in the manufacture of rayon and neoprene tires. A number of renal disorders are reported, along with accelerated atherosclerosis. The latter may affect the renal circulation and lead to renal dysfunction, hypertension, proteinuria, and renal insufficiency. The renal effects of carbon disulfide probably are a direct result of its atherogenic effect and not related to direct nephrotoxicity. However, there is a case report of a worker with long-term high-level exposure who did develop ESRD and focal segmental glomerular sclerosis.

REFERENCES

Brautbar N: Industrial solvents and kidney disease. Int J Occup Environ Health 2004;10:79 [PMID: 15070029].

Voss JU et al: Nephrotoxicity of organic solvents: Biomarkers for early detection. Int Arch Occup Environ Health 2005;78:475 [PMID: 15895243].

END-STAGE RENAL DYSFUNCTION CAUSED BY AGENTS THAT ALTER RENAL METABOLISM (XENOBIOTIC SUBSTANCES)

EXPOSURE HISTORY

Certain individuals are more likely than others to develop renal damage from exposure to toxic materials. Contact with occupational or environmental hazards may reduce the threshold for the appearance of overt renal damage after exposure to a generally subtoxic dose of a second substance. For example, recent work demonstrates that oxidative stress conditions such as exposure to xenobiotics may lead to an excess of free heme, which, in turn, interferes with the defenses against oxidative tissue injuries such as those that occur with ischemic acute renal failure.

Experiments suggest that response to a toxic agent may be predetermined by prior exposure to chemicals capable of inducing enzyme synthesis (e.g., P450 and aryl hydrocarbon hydrolase), which results in increased metabolism of xenobiotics. These agents permanently—albeit imperceptibly—predispose the individual to react unfavorably when challenged by a second toxic chemical. Identification of the potential role of these substances in modulating the course of a renal disease—long after exposure—will be difficult both clinically and epidemiologically.

REFERENCE

Zoccali C: Biomarkers in chronic kidney disease: Utility and issues towards better understanding. Curr Opin Nephrol Hypertens 2005;14:532 [PMID: 16205471].

Neurotoxicology

24

Yuen T. So, MD, PhD

The nervous system is vulnerable to a wide range of insults from environmental or occupational toxins. Despite the presence of selective permeability barriers separating the systemic circulation from the brain and peripheral nerves, metals, gases, solvents, and other chemicals penetrate sufficiently to cause deleterious effects. There are many historical descriptions of neurotoxicity, for example, lead poisoning described by Greek physicians before the birth of Christ, homicidal use of arsenic by Nero, and the more recent accounts of the Minamata Bay epidemic (organic mercury) and glue-sniffer's neuropathy (hexacarbons).

Disorders of the nervous system manifest in a diverse manner. Each region of the neuraxis—brain, spinal cord, peripheral nerve, or muscle—responds differently to toxic injuries. Within any given region, different cell populations also react differently. This "selective vulnerability" is important because toxic exposure leads to different clinical syndromes, depending on the locations and cell types affected. Clinical presentations may include some combination of headache, pain, cognitive and psychiatric disturbances, visual changes, seizures, ataxia, tremors, rigidity, weakness, and sensory loss.

The extent and severity of neurologic deficits are difficult to assess with precision. Despite advances in neuroimaging techniques over the past two decades, commonly used tools such as computed tomography (CT) and magnetic resonance imaging (MRI) provide only visualization of macroscopic structural changes. While they are invaluable in detecting neoplastic, inflammatory, and infectious disorders of the nervous system, they are less helpful in documenting neurotoxic injuries. Imaging of cerebral function, such as positron-emission tomography (PET), MR spectroscopy, and functional MRI, hold promise but are still in their infancy and not in widespread clinical use.

Neurologic evaluation of patients largely depends on bedside history and physical examination, supplemented by traditional diagnostic tests such as electroencephalography (EEG), nerve-conduction study, electromyography (EMG), lumbar puncture, and neuropsychological testing.

With few exceptions, the pathophysiology of most neurotoxic injuries is not well understood. Animal models of toxin exposure provide at best a rough guide to human disease. Moreover, it is nearly impossible to

study the effects of toxins under controlled conditions in humans. Much of our current knowledge is gained from clinical observations of intense exposures during accidents or chronic heavy occupational exposures. Extrapolation of these classic observations to other situations is problematic. For instance, for many compounds, there is considerable uncertainty concerning the exposure level and duration necessary to cause neurologic injury. It has been especially difficult to ascertain the sequelae of chronic low-level exposure, a situation particularly likely to be encountered by today's physicians.

GENERAL PRINCIPLES

Despite our incomplete understanding in many of these diseases, several generalizations have been useful in the clinical approach to these disorders.

1. A dose-toxicity relationship exists in the majority of neurotoxic exposures. In general, neurologic symptoms appear only after a cumulative exposure reaches a threshold level. Individual susceptibility varies over a limited range, but idiosyncratic reactions seldom occur.

2. Toxins typically cause a nonfocal or symmetric neurologic syndrome. Significant asymmetry such as weakness or sensory loss of one limb or one side of the body with complete sparing of the contralateral side should suggest an alternate cause.

3. There is usually a strong temporal relationship between exposure and the onset of symptoms. Immediate symptoms after acute exposure are often a consequence of the physiologic effects of the chemical (e.g., the cholinergic effects of organophosphates). These symptoms subside quickly with elimination of the chemical from the body. Delayed or persistent neurologic deficits that occur after toxic exposures (e.g., delayed neuropathy after organophosphate poisoning) generally are a result of pathologic changes in the nervous system. Recovery is still possible, but it tends to be slow and incomplete.

4. The nervous system has a limited capability to regenerate; some recovery is possible after removal of the insulting agent. By contrast, worsening neuro-

373

logic deficits more than a few months after cessation of exposure to a toxin generally argue for a direct causative role of the toxin.

5. Multiple neurologic syndromes are possible from a single toxin. Different neuron populations and different areas of the nervous system react differently to the neurotoxin. Furthermore, the level and duration of exposure, as well as physiologic variables such as the subject's age, influence the clinical manifestations. A well-known example is lead toxicity, which may lead to an acute confusional state, chronic mental slowing, or a peripheral neuropathy.

6. Few toxins present with a pathognomonic neurologic syndrome. Symptoms and signs may be mimicked by many psychiatric, metabolic, inflammatory, neoplastic, and degenerative diseases of the nervous system. It is therefore important to exclude other neurologic diseases with appropriate clinical examination and laboratory investigations.

A noteworthy caveat is the phenomenon of *coasting*—the continuing deterioration sometimes seen for up to a few weeks after discontinuation of toxic exposure. Coasting has been well documented in toxic neuropathies caused by pyridoxine (vitamin B_6) abuse, *n*-hexane toxicity, and vincristine chemotherapy. The delay reflects the time necessary for the pathophysiologic steps to evolve to neuronal injury and death.

Another qualification is illustrated by a hypothesis used to explain the pathogenesis of chronic degenerative diseases such as Parkinson's disease, amyotrophic lateral sclerosis, and Alzheimer dementia. It has been postulated that an environmental or toxic exposure may reduce the functional reserve of the brain. The patient, however, remains asymptomatic until aging or other biologic events further deplete the neuronal pool over many more years. Symptoms appear only when neuronal attrition reaches a threshold level. The hypothesis predicts a long latent period between toxic exposure and symptom manifestation. Although present evidence does not totally support an environmental cause, age-related neuronal attrition is an important concept in our understanding of neurodegenerative diseases. The prevalence and severity of these disorders increase with age. Attrition may explain the occasional observation of continuing deterioration for many years after cessation of a toxic exposure (e.g., extrapyramidal dysfunction after manganese poisoning and worsening many years after mercury poisoning in the Minamata Bay epidemic).

APPROACH TO PATIENTS

A confident diagnosis of a neurotoxic disorder can be made only after the documentation of all the following: (1) a sufficiently intense or prolonged exposure to the toxin, (2) an appropriate neurologic syndrome based on knowledge about the putative toxin, (3) evolution of symptoms and signs over a compatible temporal course, and (4) exclusion of other neurologic disorders that may account for a similar syndrome.

A detailed history of the nature, duration, and intensity of the exposure is essential in every evaluation. What are the potential toxins? What is the mode of exposure? How long and how intense are the exposures? Are there other confounding factors such as alcoholism, psychosocial issues, and possibility of secondary gains? Chronic exposures are especially difficult to assess. Not only is it essential to assess the average intensity and total duration of exposure, but intermittent peak exposures also are important to quantify because they may play a vital role in the pathogenesis of neurologic dysfunction.

The toxicology history should be followed by a detailed characterization of the neurologic complaints. Patients frequently use descriptors such as *weakness, dizziness, forgetfulness, pain,* and *numbness* to refer to vastly different personal experience. Dizziness may mean vertigo from vestibular dysfunction, gait imbalance from sensory loss, or simply a nonspecific sense of ill feeling. Fatigue or asthenia may be referred to as weakness. Fatigue implies reduced endurance or a disinclination for physical activity rather than true weakness. Fatigue may be seen in association with depression, various systemic illnesses, and a wide range of neurologic diseases. Only weakness specifically implies motor system dysfunction. Each patient's complaints therefore should not be accepted at face value. It is especially useful to inquire about the functional consequences of the neurologic deficits. Questioning about activities of daily living is particularly useful both to better understand the nature of the complaints and to provide a reasonably objective measure of severity.

Documentation of the temporal course of the disease is very important. Symptoms may appear acutely (minutes or days), subacutely (weeks or months), or chronically (years). Fluctuating symptoms may suggest recurrent exposures or unrelated superimposed factors. Recovery after discontinuation of exposure helps to implicate the exposure. By contrast, a continuing progression of deficits beyond the "coasting" period argues against an etiologic role of the exposure.

Central Nervous System

Symptoms and deficits depend on which groups of brain or spinal cord neurons are affected primarily (Table 24–1). A common syndrome is an encephalopathy from diffuse dysfunction of cortical or subcortical structures. Acutely, the encephalopathy may be associated with alteration in the level of consciousness. Chronically, the primary symptoms may be cognitive and psychiatric. Some toxins cause relatively selective injury to the vestibular system or the cerebellum, resulting in dysequilibrium, vertigo, and gait or limb ataxia. Basal ganglia involvement may lead to an

Table 24–1. Neurologic symptoms and signs.

Syndrome	Neuroanatomy	Symptoms and Signs	Examples
Acute encephalopathy	Diffuse; cerebral hemi-spheres	Varying combination of head-ache, irritability, disorientation, convulsions, amnesia, psycho-sis, lethargy, stupor and coma	Acute exposure to many toxins at sufficient doses
Chronic encephalopathy	Diffuse; cerebral hemi-spheres	Cognitive and psychiatric dis-turbances	Chronic or low-dose exposure to many toxins
Parkinsonism	Basal ganglia and other extra-pyramidal motor pathways	Tremor, rigidity, bradykinesia, gait instability	Manganese, carbon monoxide, methanol
Motor neuron disease	Spinal cord motor neurons	Muscle atrophy, weakness	Lead, manganese
Myeloneuropathy (myelopathy and polyneuropathy)	Spinal cord and peripheral nerves	Paresthesias, sensory loss, hy-perreflexia, Babinski sign, gait ataxia	Nitrous oxide, organophos-phates, *n*-hexane
Polyneuropathy	Peripheral sensory, motor and autonomic nerve fibers	Paresthesias, numbness, weak-ness, loss of deep tendon re-flexes, more rarely, auto-nomic failure	Many toxins at sufficient doses (see Table 24–2)

extrapyramidal syndrome of bradykinesia, tremors, and rigidity. This may resemble idiopathic Parkinson disease for all practical purposes.

Evaluation of cognitive complaints should include at least a mini–mental state examination. Referral to neuro-psychological testing may be needed in patients with prominent cognitive complaints to better understand the pattern and severity of the cognitive deficits. Good patient cooperation and an experienced interpreter are necessary for meaningful neuropsychological testing. Patients with gait unsteadiness, dizziness, or vertigo should be examined for cranial nerve or cerebellar deficits. The evaluation should include testing of gait, tandem walk, and Romberg sign. The examiner also should note extraocular move-ments and the presence or absence of nystagmus, hearing deficits, limb ataxia, and sensory deficits. Tremors, if present, should be characterized with the outstretched hands, with the hands at rest, and with the hands perform-ing pointing maneuvers (e.g., the finger-to-nose test). Muscle tone should be tested for rigidity. Rapid tapping of the fingers, hands, or feet is a useful test of the motor sys-tem. Along with formal strength testing, they should be part of the routine neurologic examination.

Laboratory tests, such as brain or spinal cord imaging studies (e.g., MRI), lumbar puncture, electroencephalo-gram (EEG), and evoked potentials, often are needed to detect unrelated neurologic diseases that mimic neuro-toxic disorders.

Peripheral Nervous System

Peripheral nervous system disorders lead to sensory disturbances and weakness, often accompanied by impairment of the deep tendon reflexes on physical examination (see Table 24–1). Of the various compo-nents of the peripheral nervous system, the peripheral nerve is by far the most vulnerable to exogenous tox-ins. Because toxins reach the nerves systemically and affect all nerves simultaneously, the resulting syndrome is a symmetric peripheral neuropathy. This is often also referred to as a *polyneuropathy,* in contrast to the mononeuropathy that is more frequently the result of local mechanical injury (see Chapter 7). With the exception of the myopathy caused by alcoholism and medical use of the statins (e.g., hydroxymethyl glutaryl coenzyme A reductase inhibitors), toxic myopathy is uncommon.

The hallmark of most polyneuropathies is the distal distribution of the clinical symptoms and signs. The most common syndrome is subacute onset of tingling or numbness experienced in a symmetric stocking-and-glove distribution. Neuropathic pain is sometimes present and is described variously as burning, deep ach-ing, or lancinating. Pain may be evoked by normally innocuous stimuli such as touching or stroking of the skin, a phenomenon known as *hyperpathia* or *allodynia.* Involvement of the motor nerve fibers manifests as muscle atrophy and weakness. These deficits may appear first in the distal-most muscles (i.e., the intrinsic foot and hand muscles). More severe cases may involve muscles of the lower legs and forearms, leading to bilat-eral foot drop or wrist drop.

Physical examination of patients with peripheral nervous system disorders should include testing of mus-cle strength, sensation, and tendon reflexes of all four extremities. Are the sensory and motor deficits relatively symmetric? Are the feet more affected than the hands? Because the longest axons are the most vulnerable, neurologic deficits frequently are more severe in the feet than in the hands. Prominent sensory impairment in the hands without signs of neuropathy in the feet is more likely to be caused by carpal tunnel syndrome than by a systemic polyneuropathy. Most polyneuropathies are accompanied by diminished or absent stretch reflexes of the Achilles tendons and demonstrable sensory impairment in the toes. Testing of these functions therefore should be included in any screening examination of the peripheral nervous system.

The clinical pattern of sensory and motor nerve involvement is useful in the differential diagnosis of peripheral neuropathy (Table 24–2). The most nonspecific syndrome is a distal symmetric sensorimotor polyneuropathy. This is indistinguishable from the neuropathies caused by common systemic diseases such as alcoholism, uremia, diabetes mellitus, and vitamin B_{12} deficiency. Some toxins, such as lead, cause a neuropathy with prominent weakness. The differential diagnosis of such a neuropathy is relatively narrow and encompasses a few hereditary and immunologic neuropathies.

There are literally hundreds of causes of peripheral neuropathies. Nontoxic causes of neuropathy, such as those caused by systemic diseases, should be investigated and excluded. Approximately one-half to two-thirds of all polyneuropathies remain undiagnosed despite thorough investigation. Thus the absence of an alternate etiology does not necessarily implicate a toxin. Aside from the presence of sufficient exposure and a compatible syndrome, the diagnosis quite frequently depends on the documentation of progressive sensory or motor deficits during exposure and recovery of function months or years after cessation of exposure.

Nerve-conduction studies and EMG are the primary tools in the laboratory evaluation of neuromuscular disorders. These two tests are often performed together, and the term *EMG* is often used loosely to refer to both tests. (These tests are described in detail in Chapter 7.) Nerve-conduction and EMG studies, occasionally supplemented by nerve biopsy, are important in the pathophysiologic characterization of peripheral neuropathies. A fundamental categorization subdivides neuropathies into those with primary degeneration of nerve axons (axonal neuropathy) and those with significant myelin breakdown (demyelinative neuropathy). Discussion of classification of polyneuropathies is beyond the scope of this chapter. Diagnostic management is best left to experienced specialists.

Quantitative sensory testing (QST) makes use of special equipment to deliver precisely calibrated sensory stimuli. The test provides quantitative parameters of sensory function and reduces interexaminer variability (see Chapter 7). The result may be used for longitudinal follow-up of patients to document progression or recovery from toxic exposures.

Table 24–2. Toxic polyneuropathies.

Mostly sensory or sensorimotor polyneuropathy (little or no weakness)
    Acrylamide
    Carbon disulfide
    Ethylene oxide
    Metals: arsenic, lead, mercury, thallium
    Methyl bromide
    Polychlorinated biphenyls (PCBs)
    Thallium
Predominantly motor polyneuropathy or sensorimotor polyneuropathy with significant weakness
    Hexacarbons: *n*-hexane, methyl *n*-butyl ketone
    Metals: lead, arsenic, mercury
    Organophosphates
"Purely" sensory neuropathy (disabling sensory loss with no weakness)
    cis-Platinum
    Pyridoxine abuse
Cranial neuropathy
    Thallium
    Trichloroethylene (trigeminal neuropathy)
Prominent autonomic dysfunction
    Acrylamide
    n-Hexane (glue-sniffer)
    Thallium
    Vacor (PNU)
Possible association with neuropathies (mostly anecdotal)
    Benzene
    Carbon monoxide
    Dioxin
    Methyl methacrylate
    Pyrethrins

REFERENCES

Albers JW et al: The effects of occupational exposure to chlorpyrifos on the neurologic examination of central nervous system function: A prospective cohort study. J Occup Environ Med 2004;46:367 [PMID: 15076655].

Pogge A, Slikker W Jr: Neuroimaging: new approaches for neurotoxicology. Neurotoxicology 2004;25:525 [PMID: 12428721].

Schaumburg HH, Albers JW: Pseudoneurotoxic disease. Neurology 2005;65:22 [PMID: 16009881].

NEUROLOGIC DISORDERS CAUSED BY SPECIFIC TOXINS

It is impossible to review all the major neurotoxic disorders in this chapter. The reader is referred to the corresponding chapters on specific toxins for more detailed discussion on general toxicology and health effects. The discussions below are restricted to neurologic complications.

Acrylamide

The population most at risk of developing neurologic toxicity consists workers who handle monomeric acrylamide in the production of polyacrylamides and those exposed to monomeric acrylamide used in grouting. Intoxication occurs by inhalation or skin absorption. Features of poisoning include local skin irritation, weight loss, lassitude, and neurologic symptoms of central and peripheral nervous system involvement.

Acute exposure typically causes a confusional state, manifesting as disorientation, memory loss, and gait ataxia. These symptoms are largely reversible, although irreversible dysfunction does occur, albeit rarely, after very intense exposure. Chronic lower-dose exposure sometimes leads to dizziness, increased irritability, emotional changes, and sleep disturbances. The primary site of action of acrylamide, however, is the peripheral nerve. A neuropathy may develop as a delayed manifestation a few weeks after acute exposure or insidiously after chronic exposure. Both sensory and motor nerves are affected, leading to sensory loss, weakness, ataxia, and loss of tendon reflexes. The loss of reflexes especially may be generalized, unlike other toxic neuropathies, in which only distal reflexes are lost. Autonomic involvement, such as hyperhidrosis and urinary retention, is common.

Acrylamide causes abnormal accumulation of neurofilaments in axons. In this respect, its action is similar to that of organic solvents, notably the hexacarbons. Unlike hexacarbons, secondary demyelination does not occur. Nerve-conduction studies typically show a neuropathy accompanied by little or no slowing of nerve-conduction velocities, that is, a neuropathy predominantly with features of axonal degeneration.

REFERENCES

Comblath DR: Neuropathy in grout workers. Scand J Work Environ Health 2004;30:253 [PMID: 15250655].

Lopachin RM: The changing view of acrylamide neurotoxicity. Neurotoxicology 2004;25:617 [PMID: 15183015].

Lopachin RM, Decaprio AP: Protein adduct formation as a molecular mechanism in neurotoxicity. Toxicol Sci 2005;86:214 [PMID: 15901921].

Arsenic

Arsenic was once used in Fowler solution for the treatment of psoriasis and asthma in the nineteenth and twentieth centuries. It was popular as a homicidal poison in medieval times. In developed countries, arsenic compounds are used as wood preservatives, as gallium arsenide in the semiconductor industry, and as defoliant and desiccant in agriculture. Contamination of well water may result from leaching of arsenic by-products in smelting or heavy agricultural use of arsenicals. Acute intoxication by arsenical compounds leads to nausea, vomiting, abdominal pain, and diarrhea. Dermatologic lesions, such as hyperkeratosis, skin pigmentation, skin exfoliation, and Mees lines, occur in many patients 1–6 weeks after onset of disease.

Peripheral neuropathy is the most common neurologic manifestation of toxicity and may occur after either acute or chronic exposure. After a single massive dose, an acute polyneuropathy develops within 1–3 weeks. This neuropathy mimics Guillain-Barré syndrome in many ways, and respiratory failure may occur rarely. Symmetric paresthesias and pain may occur in isolation or may be accompanied by distal weakness. With progression of neuropathy, sensory and motor deficits spread proximally. Shoulder and pelvic girdle weakness, as well as gait ataxia, are common in severe cases. Chronic exposure leads to a more insidious sensorimotor polyneuropathy, although there is no agreement for a threshold limit.

Intense exposure to arsenic may lead to mental confusion, psychosis, anxiety, seizure, or coma. Chronic low-level exposure to arsenic, often from environmental or occupational sources, has been associated with more subtle impairment of memory and concentration. In exposed children, there are also reports of lower verbal performance and hearing impairment.

The diagnosis of arsenic toxicity is difficult. EMG and nerve-conduction studies provide evidence of a nonspecific axonal neuropathy. Blood arsenic level returns to normal in about 12 hours, and urine arsenic clears within 48–72 hours after exposure. Arsenic remains detectable in hair and nails for months after exposure. Thus hair or nail analysis can be useful. However, external arsenic contamination may give false-positive results. Pubic hair is preferable to scalp hair for its lesser susceptibility to contamination.

In the treatment of arsenic toxicity, *meso*-dimercaptosuccinic acid (DMSA) and 2,3-dimercapto-1-propanesulfonic acid (DMPS) can control the systemic toxicity and prevent development of neuropathy if given sufficiently early. They are preferred over the previously used chelating agent, dimercaprol [British anti-Lewisite (BAL)]. There is no evidence that treatment speeds up recovery of neuropathy. Even without treatment, peripheral neuropathy improves slowly after cessation of exposure.

REFERENCES

Ratnaike RN: Acute and chronic arsenic toxicity. Postgrad Med J 2003;79:391 [PMID: 12897217].

Rodriguez VM et al: The effects of arsenic exposure on the nervous system. Toxicol Lett 2003;145:1 [PMID: 12962969].

Tchounwou PB et al: Arsenic toxicity, mutagenesis, and carcinogenesis: A health risk assessment and management approach. Mol Cell Biochem 2004;255:47 [PMID: 14971645].

Carbon Disulfide

Carbon disulfide is employed as a solvent in perfume production and varnishes, in soil fumigants and insecticides, and in industrial manufacturing. Relatively brief inhalation exposure to a toxic level (300 ppm or above) of carbon disulfide causes dizziness and headache, followed by delirium, mania, or mental dulling. Concentrations above 400 ppm have a narcotizing effect and may lead to convulsion, coma, and respiratory failure.

Chronic exposure has been associated with both central nervous system abnormalities and peripheral neuropathy. The peripheral neuropathy presents with paresthesias and pain in the distal legs, loss of Achilles reflexes, and evidence of involvement of sensory and motor axons on nerve-conduction study. A nonspecific syndrome of fatigue, headache, and sleep disturbances is attributable to chronic low-level exposure to carbon disulfide. On MRI of the brain, some exposed patients have scattered abnormal foci in the subcortical white matter. The radiologic picture resembles that seen in patients with small-vessel disease and multiple subcortical strokes, although pathologic confirmation is not available.

REFERENCES

Bartholomaeus AR, Haritos VS: Review of the toxicology of carbonyl sulfide, a new grain fumigant. Food Chem Toxicol 2005; 43:1687 [PMID: 16139940].

Krstev S et al: Neuropsychiatric effects in workers with occupational exposure to carbon disulfide. J Occup Health 2003;45:81 [PMID: 14646298].

Nishiwaki Y et al: Six-year observational cohort study of the effect of carbon disulphide on brain MRI in rayon manufacturing workers. Occup Environ Med 2004;61:225 [PMID: 14985517].

Carbon Monoxide

Carbon monoxide binds to hemoglobin to form carboxyhemoglobin and causes neuronal hypoxia. Inhaling low concentrations (0.01–0.02%) of carbon monoxide causes headache and mild confusion. A higher concentration of 0.1–0.2% may result in somnolence or stupor, and inhalation of 1% for more than 30 minutes can be fatal. Early on, symptoms include headache, dizziness, and disorientation. More prolonged or severe hypoxia is accompanied by a varying combination of tremor, chorea, spasticity, dystonia, rigidity, and bradykinesia. Recovery from the hypoxia may be incomplete. Residual dementia, spasticity, cortical blindness, and parkinsonian features are relatively common.

Occasional patients recover completely after acute exposure only to worsen again 1–6 weeks later with acute disorientation, apathy, or psychosis. Neurologic examination often reveals an encephalopathy with prominent signs of frontal lobe and extrapyramidal dysfunction. Physical findings include bradykinesia, retropulsion, frontal release signs, spasticity, and limb rigidity. Risk factors for developing this delayed encephalopathy are a significant period of unconsciousness and an advanced age. CT or MRI most commonly shows abnormalities in bilateral subcortical white matter. Some patients also have involvement of the basal ganglia, especially the globus pallidus and the thalamus. Rarely, hemorrhagic infarction of the white matter or basal ganglia may be seen. Partial recovery is possible but may take one or more years. Some residual memory deficits and parkinsonism are common.

The effect of long-term exposure to low levels of carbon monoxide is unclear. A number of nonspecific symptoms—anorexia, headache, personality changes, and memory disturbances—are attributed to carbon monoxide, but a causal relationship has not been proven.

REFERENCES

Lassinger BK et al: Atypical parkinsonism and motor neuron syndrome: A possible complication of chronic hypoxia and carbon monoxide toxicity? Mov Disord 2004;19:465 [PMID: 15077246].

Prockop LD: Carbon monoxide brain toxicity: Clinical, magnetic resonance imaging, magnetic resonance spectroscopy, and neuropsychological effects in 9 people. J Neuroimaging 2005;15:144 [PMID: 15746226].

Hexacarbons (*n*-Hexane and Methyl *n*-Butyl Ketone)

n-Hexane and methyl *n*-butyl ketone represent a group of widely used volatile organic compounds employed in homes and industries as solvents and adhesives. Human disease is a result of a toxic intermediary metabolite g-diketone 2,5-hexanedione. Toxic exposure results from inhalation, especially in poorly ventilated spaces, or excessive skin contact. Another solvent used in paints and adhesives, methyl ethyl ketone, may potentiate the neurotoxicity.

Like other organic solvents, the hexacarbons can induce an acute encephalopathy characterized by euphoria, hallucination, and confusion. The acute euphoric effect of hexacarbons leads to their abuse as a recreational drug. The most well-known syndrome is a distal symmetric sensorimotor polyneuropathy, the so-called glue-sniffer's neuropathy. Early symptoms are paresthesias and sensory loss. Weakness follows and involves distal muscles initially. Proximal musculatures are affected in more severe cases. Patients complain of easy tripping because of ankle weakness. Optic neuropathy and facial numbness may be present. Autonomic symptoms are uncommon and are present only in very severe cases. Nonspecific central nervous system (CNS) symptoms, such as insomnia and irritability, may be present. On examination, sensory loss and weakness are readily demonstrable. Achilles stretch reflexes are lost early in the disease. Recovery begins after a few months of abstinence and may be incomplete. In some instances, spasticity and hyperreflexia appear paradoxically during the recovery stage. In these cases, there is probably degeneration of central axons, and the CNS signs are masked initially by the severe neuropathy.

A less dramatic polyneuropathy was recognized in the 1960s in workers in the shoe and adhesive industries, well before the recognition of glue-sniffer's neuropathy. The exposure to *n*-hexane was less intense and more chronic than that of glue sniffers. The clinical features are essentially similar, although the syndrome evolves more slowly and results in less severe deficits.

n-Hexane neuropathy has a distinctive neuropathology. Multiple foci of neurofilament accumulations form inside the nerve axons. Demyelination is common, but it is probably secondary to the axonal pathology. Because of this demyelination, nerve-conduction studies show slowing of motor nerve-conduction velocities. Cerebrospinal fluid (CSF) protein content is typically normal, in contrast to most other demyelinating neuropathies, which are associated with elevated CSF protein.

REFERENCES

Pastore C et al: Partial conduction blocks in *n*-hexane neuropathy. Muscle Nerve 2002;26:132 [PMID: 12115958].

Spencer PS et al: Aromatic as well as aliphatic hydrocarbon solvent axonopathy. Int J Hyg Environ Health 2002;205:131 [PMID: 12018006].

Lead

Lead is present in paint, batteries, pipes, solder, ammunition, and cables. Nonindustrial sources include pottery, bullet fragments, and traditional folk remedies. Acute high-level exposure typically comes from accidental ingestion, inhalation, or industrial exposure. It results in a syndrome of abdominal colic and intermittent vomiting, accompanied by neurologic symptoms such as headache, tremor, apathy, and lethargy. Massive intoxication can lead to convulsions, cerebral edema, stupor, or coma and eventually to transtentorial herniation. Lead encephalopathy typically appears in adults at blood levels of 50–70 µg/dL or higher. Children are more vulnerable than adults probably because of the immaturity of the blood-brain barrier. Behavioral disturbances and neuropsychologic impairment may be present at blood levels as low as 10 µg/dL, although the exact threshold is debatable. Chronic low-level exposure to lead is responsible for impaired intellectual development in children. Studies link chronic exposure to decreased global IQ, as well as a wide range of behavioral disturbances, such as poor self-confidence, impulsive behavior, and shortened attention span.

Emerging data suggest that adults with past industrial exposure may have a faster rate of cognitive decline than that expected from normal aging. These subjects typically have normal blood lead levels but elevated lead levels in bone, as measured by x-ray fluorescence. The lead storage in bone potentially can be mobilized throughout life, particularly with bony fractures. It remains to be seen whether the accelerated decline in cognition is a result of continuing exposure to lead or from accelerated aging or attrition of neuronal reserves.

Peripheral neuropathy is a well-recognized complication of chronic lead poisoning in adults. Asymptomatic nerve-conduction-study abnormalities are detectable at lead levels greater than 40 µg/dL. The best-known clinical syndrome is a predominantly motor neuropathy with little, if any, sensory symptoms. It mimics in many ways motor neuron diseases such as amyotrophic lateral sclerosis (Lou Gehrig disease). The classic description emphasizes bilateral wrist drop and foot drop. Toxicity also may manifest as a generalized proximal and distal weakness and loss of the tendon reflexes. In addition to the classic syndrome of motor neuropathy, some patients may present with distal limb paresthesias and no weakness. This is especially likely in patients with long-term low-level lead exposure.

In patients with acute lead-induced encephalopathy, brain CT or MRI may show focal areas of edema, most commonly in bilateral thalami and basal ganglia. Imaging studies, and sometimes autopsy, may detect intracranial calcification in patients with chronic lead toxicity. The radiologic findings are not specific to lead, and the differential diagnosis may include other causes of calcification, inflammation, and demyelination.

REFERENCES

Gidlow DA: Lead toxicity. Occup Med (Lond) 2004;54:76 [PMID: 15020724].

Lindgren KN et al: Pattern of blood lead levels over working lifetime and neuropsychological performance. Arch Environ Health 2003;58:373 [PMID: 14992313].

Needleman H: Lead poisoning. Annu Rev Med 2004;55:209 [PMID: 14746518].

Seeber A, Meyer-Baron M: Neurobehavioural testing in workers occupationally exposed to lead. Occup Environ Med 2003; 60:145 [PMID: 12554847].

Manganese

Manganese is used widely in the manufacture of steel, alloys, and welding. Manganese is also found in alkaline batteries and various fungicides. Poisoning occurs most commonly in the mining, smelting, milling, and battery-manufacturing industries, although there are occasional reports of environmental contamination. Of recent interest is the potential risk of organic manganese in the form of methylcyclopentadienyl manganese tricarbonyl (MMT), an additive used in gasoline.

The classic syndrome of manganese poisoning, or manganism, is the appearance of an extrapyramidal disorder that resembles idiopathic Parkinson disease. Tremor, rigidity, masked facies, and bradykinesias develop slowly. The appearance of these extrapyramidal signs may be preceded by a period of malaise and mild encephalopathy that often goes unnoticed. Dystonia, an uncommon finding in idiopathic Parkinson disease, has been reported in some patients. Compared with idiopathic Parkinson disease, the extrapyramidal symptoms of manganism are less responsive to dopaminergic therapy. Also, neurologic deficits often continue to progress for many years after cessation of exposure.

Manganese preferentially accumulates in the globus pallidus and selectively damages neurons in globus pallidus and the striatum. On brain MRI, manganese accumulation can be visualized as increased signal on T_1-weighted images in the globus pallidus, a distinctive finding not seen in Parkinson disease and other forms of parkinsonism. A variable syndrome of parkinsonism, cognitive impairment, and gait ataxia has been seen in patients with chronic liver failure. These patients also may have an abnormal T_1 signal in the globus pallidus and a mildly elevated blood manganese level. The liver is responsible for clearance of dietary manganese. It is likely that the neurologic abnormalities of these patients are also due to manganese toxicity.

REFERENCES

Cersosimo MG, Koller WC: The diagnosis of manganese-induced parkinsonism. Neurotoxicology 2006;27:340 [PMID: 16325915].

Finley BL, Santamaria AB: Current evidence and research needs regarding the risk of manganese-induced neurological effects in welders. Neurotoxicology 2005;26:285 [PMID: 15713349].

Josephs KA et al: Neurologic manifestations in welders with pallidal MRI T_1 hyperintensity. Neurology 2005;64:2033 [PMID: 15888601].

Mercury

Mercury poisoning results from exposure to methyl mercury or other alkyl-mercury compounds, elemental mercury (mercury vapor), and inorganic mercuric salts. Mercury is used in batteries, fungicides, electronics, and other industries. Mercury in sludges and waterways is methylated by microbes into methyl mercury that is readily absorbed by humans. Several large endemics resulted from methyl mercury contamination in Minamata Bay (Japan) in the 1950s and 1960s, in Iraq in the 1970s, and in the Amazon River basin in the 1990s. Exposure occurred primarily through ingestion of contaminated fish. Despite several anecdotal claims, there is no convincing evidence that the widely used mercury dental amalgam poses a significant health hazard.

Like many other toxins, mercury poisoning causes a diffuse encephalopathy. In its early stage, the encephalopathy is characterized by euphoria, irritability, anxiety, and emotional lability. More severe exposure leads to confusion and an altered level of consciousness. Patients may develop tremor and cerebellar ataxia. Hearing loss, visual field constriction, hyperreflexia, and Babinski sign may be present. All the preceding symptoms may be encountered in intoxication from organic mercury, metallic mercury, mercury vapor, or inorganic salts. Organic mercury poisoning typically presents with prominent CNS disturbances, with little or no peripheral nervous system involvement. Neuropathy is associated primarily with inorganic mercury. A subacute predominantly motor neuropathy has been reported after metallic mercury or mercury vapor exposure. If acute, the syndrome resembles Guillain-Barré syndrome, whereas a more subacute syndrome may mimic amyotrophic lateral sclerosis. Nerve-conduction study and nerve biopsy suggest a primary axonal loss.

There is considerable uncertainty concerning the neurologic effect of low-level mercury exposures such as that from dental amalgam and dietary fish consumption. Overall, there is no strong evidence to associate low-level exposure with significant neurologic disease.

REFERENCES

Kingman A et al: Amalgam exposure and neurological function. Neurotoxicology 2005;26:241 [PMID: 15713345].

Weil M et al: Blood mercury levels and neurobehavioral function. JAMA 2005;293:1875 [PMID: 15840862].

Methanol

The neurotoxicity of methanol is caused largely by formaldehyde and formate, the end products of alcohol dehydrogenase and aldehyde dehydrogenase. Most cases result from accidental ingestion or occupational exposure. Neurologic symptoms usually appear after a latent period of 12–24 hours after intoxication. Patients suffer from headache, nausea, vomiting, and abdominal pain. Tachypnea, if present, indicates significant metabolic acidosis. Visual symptoms appear early and range from blurring to complete blindness. These are accompanied by an encephalopathy, from mild disorientation to convulsion, stupor, or coma. In severely affected individuals, bilateral upper motor neuron signs, such as hyperreflexia, weakness, and Babinski sign, are present. Brain CT or MRI often reveals characteristic infarction or hemorrhage localized in bilateral putamina, often accompanied by similar involvement of subcortical white matter.

Treatment of acute poisoning depends on control of the metabolic acidosis with sodium bicarbonate, competitive inhibition of the conversion of methanol to formaldehyde (by administration of fomepizole or ethanol), and swift removal of methanol by gastric lavage or hemodialysis.

The neurologic effect of chronic low-level methanol is less clear. There are case reports of parkinsonism developing after exposure, although a causal relationship has not been confirmed.

REFERENCES

Hovda KE et al: Methanol outbreak in Norway 2002–2004: Epidemiology, clinical features and prognostic signs. J Intern Med 2005;258:181 [PMID: 16018795].

Koaarix M, Dart RC: Rethinking the toxic methanol level. J Toxicol Clin Toxicol 2003;41:793 [PMID: 14677789].

Megarbane B et al: Current recommendations for treatment of severe toxic alcohol poisonings. Intensive Care Med 2005;31:189 [PMID: 15627163].

Nitrous Oxide

Excessive exposure to nitrous oxide, usually in the setting of substance abuse, causes a myeloneuropathy indistinguishable from vitamin B_{12} (cobalamin) deficiency. Patients present with paresthesias in the hands and feet. Gait ataxia, sensory loss, Romberg sign, and leg weakness may be present. Tendon reflexes may be diminished or lost (peripheral neuropathy) or may be pathologically brisk (spinal cord involvement; i.e., myelopathy). Nitrous oxide inactivates vitamin B_{12} and interferes with B_{12}-dependent conversion of homocysteine to methionine. Serum vitamin B_{12} and the Schilling test often are normal, whereas the serum homocysteine level may be elevated. Repeated exposures are necessary to cause symptoms in normal individuals. Of interest is the observation that a brief exposure to nitrous oxide, for example during anesthesia, is sufficient to precipitate symptoms in patients with presymptomatic B_{12} deficiency.

REFERENCE

Doran M et al: Toxicity after intermittent inhalation of nitrous oxide for analgesia. BMJ 2004;328:1364 [PMID: 15178617].

Organophosphates

Organophosphates (OPs) are used commonly as pesticides and herbicides and, to a lesser extent, as petroleum additives, antioxidants, and flame retardants. They are highly lipid soluble and are absorbed through skin contact or through mucous membranes via inhalation and ingestion. All the OPs share a common property of inhibiting the enzyme acetylcholinesterase.

The acute neurologic effects of OPs are those of muscarinic and nicotinic overactivity. Symptoms usually are apparent within hours of exposure. These include abdominal cramps, diarrhea, increased salivation, sweating, miosis, blurred vision, and muscle fasciculations. Convulsions, coma, muscle paralysis, and respiratory arrest occur with severe intoxication. Unless there are complications from secondary anoxia or other insults to the brain, these symptoms improve either with atropine treatment or metabolism and excretion of the OP. Recovery usually is complete within 1 week, even though the acetylcholinesterase activity level may be restored only partially.

In some patients, an intermediate syndrome may occur within 12–96 hours of exposure. This is a result of excessive cholinergic stimulation of nicotinic receptors in skeletal muscles. This leads to blockade of neuromuscular junction transmission. Weakness of proximal muscles, neck flexors, cranial muscles, and even respiratory muscles may be evident. Sensory function is spared. Electrodiagnostic testing is very useful in diagnosis. The most characteristic finding is the presence of repetitive muscle action potentials after single electrical stimulus applied to motor nerves. Another finding is a decremental motor response to repetitive nerve stimulation.

In some other patients, a delayed syndrome of peripheral neuropathy occurs 1–4 weeks after acute exposure. There is little or no correlation between its onset and the severity of acute or intermediate symptoms. OPs inhibit another enzyme, neuropathy target esterase (NTE), forming an OP-NTE complex. This inhibition becomes irreversible when the OP-NTE complex undergoes a second step known as *aging* (loss of an R group from the OP molecule). Compounds that lead to aging are neurotoxic, resulting in the delayed polyneuropathy. Paresthesias and cramping pain in the legs are often the first symptoms. Sensory loss is usually mild on physical examination. Weakness begins distally and progresses to involve proximal muscles. Weakness dominates the clinical picture and at times may be very severe. Spasticity and other upper motor neuron signs suggesting concomitant spinal cord involvement are present in some patients. Cranial neuropathy or autonomic dysfunction is unusual. Recovery is slow and incomplete and depends on the degree of motor axons loss. Those with significant spasticity tend to recover less satisfactorily.

How inhibition and aging of NTE eventually cause neuronal damage is unclear. Although NTE activity may be measured in lymphocytes, it usually normalizes by the time neuropathy appears. All the neurotoxic compounds are phosphates, phosphoramidites, or phosphonates. Important examples are tricresyl phosphates (e.g., triorthocresyl phosphate), mipafox, leptophos, trichlorphon, trichlornate, dichlorovos, and methamidophos. Of these,

Table 24-3. Neurologic manifestations of toxins not discussed in text.

Toxins	Acute Exposure	Chronic Exposure
Carbamates	Cholinergic overactivity (similar to organophosphates)	Encephalopathy, tremor, polyneuropathy
Ethylene oxide	Encephalopathy	Sensorimotor polyneuropathy
Manganese	None (symptoms take weeks or months to develop)	Parkinsonism (tremor, rigidity, gait disturbances), encephalopathy, possible motor neuron disease
Organotin	Encephalopathy, visual disturbances	Encephalopathy, visual disturbances, hearing loss, vertigo
Thallium	Subacute polyneuropathy after massive exposure, encephalopathy	Sensorimotor polyneuropathy
Toluene	Euphoria or narcosis, encephalopathy	Cerebellar ataxia, tremor, encephalopathy
Trichloroethylene	Euphoria or narcosis, encephalopathy, trigeminal neuropathy	Trigeminal neuropathy, encephalopathy

triorthocresyl phosphate probably has caused the largest number of neuropathies. The so-called jake paralysis was a result of drinking extracts of contaminated Jamaica ginger during the prohibition era. Other well-known outbreaks include contamination of cooking oil in Morocco and gingili oil in Sri Lanka.

Erythrocyte acetylcholinesterase level may be depressed because of the recent exposure. Its clinical utility is limited by the wide range of normal levels. Also, a low level does not predict development of delayed neuropathy. By the time neuropathy appears, nerve-conduction studies show an axonal polyneuropathy affecting motor greater than sensory axons. These findings are not pathognomonic for OPs but are useful to distinguish this neuropathy from other causes of acute weakness such as Guillain-Barré syndrome and neuromuscular junction disorders.

Persistent subtle neuropsychological impairment after an episode of acute poisoning may be more prevalent than previously thought. Also, chronic low-level exposure to OPs is linked to an encephalopathy with forgetfulness and other cognitive dysfunctions as chief complaints, although the clinical significance or severity of this effect is being debated.

REFERENCES

Albers JW et al: The effects of occupational exposure to chlorpyrifos on the neurologic examination of central nervous system function: A prospective cohort study. J Occup Environ Med 2004;46:367 [PMID: 15116371].

Delgado E et al. Central nervous system effects of acute organophosphate poisoning in a two-year follow-up. Scand J Work Environ Health 2004;30:362 [PMID: 15529800].

Lotti M, Moretto A: Organophosphate-induced delayed polyneuropathy. Toxicol Rev 2005;24:37 [PMID: 16042503].

Miranda J et al: Muscular strength and vibration thresholds during two years after acute poisoning with organophosphate insecticides. Occup Environ Med 2004;61:4 [PMID: 14691285].

Miscellaneous Organic Solvents

Clinically important exposure to organic solvents occurs primarily as a result of industrial contact or volitional abuse. Most organic solvents possess acute narcotizing properties. Brief exposure at high concentrations causes a reversible encephalopathy. Coma, respiratory depression, and death occur after extremely high exposures. Chronic exposure to moderate or high levels of solvent can cause a dementing syndrome, with personality changes, memory disturbances, and other nonspecific neuropsychiatric symptoms. A sensorimotor polyneuropathy also may be present either as the only manifestation or in combination with CNS dysfunction. The better known syndromes are either discussed under specific headings or are tabulated in Table 24–3.

Despite general agreement on the effects of moderate to high doses of organic solvents, the effect of chronic low-level exposure is uncertain. The sequelae of this low-level exposure have been variously termed *painters' syndrome, chronic toxic encephalopathy,* and *psycho-organic solvent syndrome.* The neurologic symptoms are diverse and nonspecific and include headache, dizziness, asthenia, mood and personality changes, inattentiveness, forgetfulness, and depression. The scientific literature regarding this syndrome consists of epidemiologic studies of exposed workers and provides conflicting results. A number of studies report a higher-than-expected incidence of cognitive and psychiatric impairment, electrophysiologic abnormalities, and cerebral atrophy in exposed subjects. The methodology of these studies has been criticized on the choice of control groups, measurement of exposures, or evaluation of dose-response relationship. Other studies have not identified significant differences between exposed subjects and controls. Confounding factors such as psychiatric illnesses and alcoholism also may explain some of the discrepancies.

The controversy remains unresolved. Some physicians make the diagnosis of psycho-organic solvent syndrome in exposed individuals whenever compatible symptoms are present and another neurologic disease is not identified by laboratory evaluations. This practice is unjustified because the syndrome is not sufficiently specific to be distinguished from depression, other affective disorders, conversion or malingering, and other injuries of the brain. Each individual case should be examined critically. Additional useful clues include the temporal relationship between symptoms and exposure, documentation of neurologic recovery after cessation of exposure, and careful neurologic examination for evidence of nonorganic neurologic signs. A confident diagnosis often cannot be made even after thorough evaluation.

REFERENCES

Jin CF et al: Industrial solvents and psychological effects. Clin Occup Environ Med 2004;4:597 [PMID: 15465471].

Louis ED et al: Essential tremor: Occupational exposures to manganese and organic solvents. Neurology 2004;63:2162 [PMID: 15596771].

Rutchik JS, Wittman RI. Neurologic issues with solvents. Clin Occup Environ Med 2004;4:621 [PMID: 15465472].

Female Reproductive Toxicology

25

Gayle C. Windham, MSPH, PhD, & Ana Maria Osorio, MD, MPH

The occurrence of adverse reproductive outcomes is of fundamental concern to the individuals and families affected. This is especially true if the individuals perceive that they are living or working in areas with potential exposure to hazardous agents over which they have little or no control. Concern has been fueled by incidents such as the contamination of fish with methyl mercury in Minamata Bay, Japan, which was caused by a release from a manufacturing plant. Consumption of the contaminated fish by pregnant women resulted in an epidemic of mental retardation, cerebral palsy, and developmental delay in their offspring. Use of polychlorinated biphenyl (PCB)–contaminated cooking oil in Taiwan resulted in intrauterine growth retardation and hyperpigmentation of the skin in infants of exposed women. Effects on that cohort continue to be uncovered today, including on offspring pubertal development. In recent years, there have been concerns about the reproductive effects of occupational exposure to solvents, pesticides, and video-display terminals or electromagnetic fields. A new area of research has sprung up to identify and study chemicals that may act to disrupt the endocrine system, affecting both wildlife and humans.

Only a few substances are known to have strong associations with adverse reproductive outcomes in humans, but relatively little research has been devoted to these outcomes until the last few decades. A larger number of agents are suspected to cause reproductive harm based on the animal literature and toxicologic assessment. In addition to the emotional stress on affected families, the societal burden of these adverse health outcomes includes high medical costs for compromised children and the increasing use of advanced technology to achieve conception and monitor pregnancy. Another reason to better understand reproductive outcomes is that they may act as sentinels for detecting occupational and environmental hazards because of the relatively short latency between exposure and clinical health event. If workers or community residents are protected from exposures that are harmful to the fetus, they usually will be protected from other health effects associated with these exposures as well. Measures that can be taken to prevent further exposure include substitution or containment of the suspect hazard. Thus, preventing exposure should be a primary goal in the health care provider's overall assessment of the patient's situation.

POPULATION AT RISK

In 2004, women aged 20–44 years old represented 51.9 million individuals in the U.S. population (Figure 25–1). The number of women in the U.S. workforce (age 16 years or older) increased dramatically in a few decades: from about 30 million in 1970, representing 43% of the workforce, to over 50 million in 1990 (58%) (Figure 25–2). This has been followed by a leveling off during the last two decades. In 2004, 35 million women within the age range of 20–44 years were employed (55.6% of all females employed in the U.S. workforce). Women in this age group have the highest birth rates, so they merit special attention with respect to potential reproductive hazards in the workplace. In the United States, females comprise greater than 70% of all employees in the following job categories: office and administrative support, education/library, health care provider or support, and personal care and service (Table 25–1). Some of the leading occupations for women have potential exposures to known reproductive toxicants (e.g., large numbers of women work in the nursing profession or health service occupations with potential exposure to chemotherapeutic agents, anesthetic gases, ionizing radiation, and biologic agents). In addition, there is an increasing number of women in occupations traditionally held by men where there is potential for exposure to reproductive hazards. For example, 2% of construction workers; 4.4% of installation, maintenance, or repair workers; 12.7% of transportation or material-moving workers; and 18.5% of farming, fishing, or forestry workers are women. When women are employed in jobs traditionally held by men, there can be difficulty in obtaining personal protective equipment that fits, accessing separate changing rooms and wash areas, and getting health and safety information that is gender-specific, where appropriate.

Women also may be exposed to reproductive hazards in the environment, which can be more difficult to detect than in the workplace. Often these environmental hazards may be local exposures, but some are of nationwide interest, such as the widespread use of pesticides that persist in the environment and food chain. In

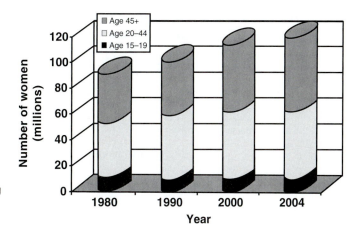

Figure 25–1. Resident female population by age for selected years, United States (excluding military overseas). (*U.S. Census: Statistical Abstract of the United States, www.census.gov/.*)

addition, exposure to fetuses or children may have lasting effects, so these represent a wider population at risk.

REPRODUCTIVE OUTCOMES & RATES

A number of adverse reproductive effects may result from exposure to chemical and physical agents either pre- or postconception. These effects range from infertility to birth defects in the infant. Several of these outcomes are quite frequent and represent a serious public health concern (Table 25–2). Accurate data on the rates of these outcomes can be difficult to obtain because of the lack of national monitoring systems and methodologic differences between individual epidemiologic studies. Approximately 10% of couples in the United States are infertile, which is defined as an inability to conceive during 12 months of unprotected intercourse. Additional couples may experience periods of subfertil-

ity or delayed conception. After conception, a continuum of reproductive loss may occur from the time of implantation to delivery. Up to 50% of embryos may be lost after implantation (the earliest time at which conception can be detected), with approximately 15–20% of pregnancies ending in clinically detected spontaneous abortion (SAB) and approximately 1% ending in fetal death (see Table 25–2). Of all liveborn infants, 7–9% are of low birth weight (LBW), approximately 11% are born prematurely, and approximately 3% will have a congenital anomaly. Whereas rates of fetal and infant death have decreased over the past few decades, rates of LBW and preterm delivery have not, and in some areas they have shown slight increases. Some of the observed risk patterns for these outcomes include (1) older maternal age associated with increased rates of infertility, SAB, and some birth defects and (2) black race associated with nearly doubled rates of LBW, pre-

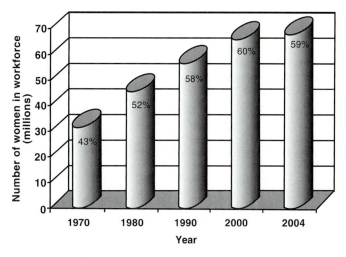

Figure 25–2. Annual female employment and labor force participation for selected years, United States. (Workforce includes civilian noninstitutional population age 16 and older, and labor force participation is indicated by percentage of all women who are in the workforce.) (*U.S. Department of Labor, Current Population Survey, www.bls.gov/cps/.*)

Table 25–1. Female employment by occupation for year 2004, United States.[1]

Occupation	No. of Females (millions)	Percent of Total Workforce
Office + administrative support	11.1	74.3
Sales + related occupations	4.4	44.3
Education/training/library	4.3	71.9
Management	4.0	39.1
Health care provider/technical	3.5	74.1
Business/finance	2.6	57.3
Production	2.5	28.9
Food prep/serving related	1.9	49.4
Health care support	1.8	88.4
Personal care + service	1.4	72.7
Building/grounds maintenance	1.2	35.2
Community/social services	1.1	58.6
Transportation/material moving	0.8	12.7
Computer/math	0.8	27.1
Art/design/entertainment/sports/media	0.6	43.3
Legal	0.6	54.3
Protective services	0.5	18.8
Life/physical/social science	0.4	39.7
Architect/engineer	0.3	13.2
Installation/maintenance/repair	0.2	4.4
Farming/fishing/forestry	0.1	18.5
Construction/extraction	0.1	2.0
Total	44.2	43.7

[1]Source: U.S. Department of Labor, Occupational Employment Statistics, www.bls.gov/oes/.

term delivery, and fetal death. Ethnic differences may reflect in part unequal access to regular or early prenatal medical care. Other reproductive endpoints that may be affected by exogenous exposures include menstrual function and age at menopause or menarche. Recent studies indicate trends to earlier onset of puberty in girls; about 12% of white girls and 28% of black girls in the United States enter puberty by age 8.

REFERENCES

Gnoth C et al: Definition and prevalence of subfertility and infertility. Human Reprod 2005;20:1144 [PMID: 15802321].

National Center for Health Statistics Web site: www.cdc.gov/nchs.

REPRODUCTIVE & DEVELOPMENTAL PHYSIOLOGY & SENSITIVE PERIODS

Germ Cell Development & Menstrual Cycle Function

The female reproductive cycle is a complex process regulated by the autonomic nervous and endocrine systems and mediated by the hypothalamic-pituitary-gonadal axis (Figure 25–3). Unlike males, the female germ cells (oogonia) develop and begin the first meiotic division in

Table 25–2. Prevalence of selected adverse pregnancy outcomes in the United States.[1]

Endpoint	Frequency per 100	Unit
Infertility	8–12	Couples
Recognized spontaneous abortion	15–20	Women or pregnancies
Birth weight < 2500 g	7–9	Livebirths
Preterm (≤ 37 wks)	11–13	Livebirths
Fetal death (or stillbirth)	0.7–1	Stillbirths and livebirths
Infant death (< 1 yr)	0.7	Livebirths
Birth defects (through 1 year of life)	3	Livebirths
Chromosomal anomalies in livebirths	0.2	Livebirths

[1]Compiled from multiple sources, but primarily from the National Center for Health Statistics (www.cdc.gov/nchs).

utero, with no new generation after birth. The oocytes remain arrested until follicular activation occurs 15–40 years later. Under gonadotropin hormone stimulation at the start of each menstrual cycle, a group of primary follicles begins to develop. Increased levels of the follicle-stimulating hormone (FSH) lead to the selection and growth of a dominant follicle, which produces estrogen to support proliferation of endometrial tissue. A midcycle release of the gonadotropins FSH and luteinizing hormone (LH) results in the release of the ovum, or ovulation. The remaining corpus luteum secretes increasing amounts of progesterone and other hormones to prepare for implantation, exerting a negative feedback on the gonadotropins (Figure 25–3). In the absence of fertilization, the corpus luteum degenerates. The subsequent decrease in ovarian steroids leads to sloughing of the endometrium, as well as to rising levels of FSH, and menstruation occurs after a 12- to 14-day luteal phase. Although this general pattern of menstrual function is known, there is much interwoman variation (Figure 25–4), and the exact mechanisms are not well understood. If a sperm successfully fertilizes an ovum, the ovum completes a second meiotic division and forms a zygote. This zygote undergoes several rapid cell divisions as it is transported down the fallopian tube to the uterus.

Endocrine control of the reproductive process might be disrupted by chemicals that, in turn, could lead to menstrual disorders and infertility. This is especially true for those chemicals with steroid-like activity (e.g.,

certain pesticides and dioxins; see below). Because the germ cells are present from birth and many exposures occur during a woman's life, there is great potential for genetic or cytotoxic harm to the oocytes. It is postulated that the cumulative effects of occupational, environmental, and other exposures may explain the increased incidence of chromosomal abnormalities and SAB that occurs as maternal age increases. But because the greatest potential for genetic damage is most likely to occur during replication and division of the genetic material, the actual sensitivity during the relatively long dormant period is unknown. Genetic damage could result in lack of fertilization or unsuccessful implantation, which can be seen clinically as infertility, or could lead to later fetal loss. Preconception mutagenesis also might result in a birth defect in an infant. Certain mutagenic chemicals are in use in industry, such as organic solvents, ethylene oxide, and metals (e.g., arsenic and nickel). Oocyte destruction by chemicals such as polyaromatic hydrocarbons (PAHs) could lead to infertility or to early menopause.

Development of the Fetus

The dividing zygote reaches the uterus approximately 1 week after fertilization, and approximately 1 week later,

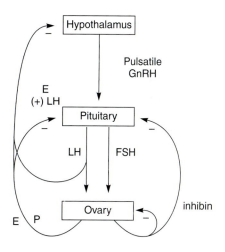

E = estrogens
P = progesterone
LH = luteinizing hormone
FSH = follicle stimulating hormone
GnRH = gonadotropin releasing hormone

Figure 25–3. Feedback regulation of the hypothalamic-pituitary-ovarian axis. Abbreviations: E = estrogens; P = progesterone; LH = luteinizing hormone; FSH = follicle-stimulating hormone; GnRH = gonadotropin-releasing hormone.

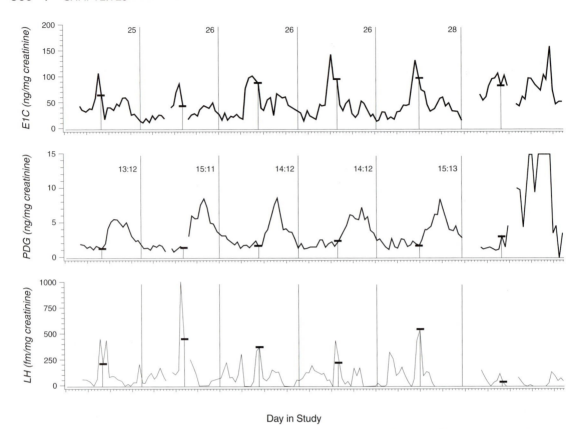

Figure 25–4. Examples of urinary sex steroid (estrogen and progesterone) and luteinizing hormone metabolite profiles. E1C = estrogen metabolite; LH = luteinizing hormone; PDG = progesterone metabolite. Long vertical lines indicate first day of bleeding during each cycle, with the numbers in row 1 indicating cycle length. Short vertical lines topped by a horizontal bar indicate probable day of ovulation in each cycle and split the cycle into the follicular phase (length indicated by first number in second row) and the luteal phase (second number). Data from six cycles of a subject in the Women's Reproductive Health Study, conducted by the California Department of Health Services.

implantation is complete. The placental villi secrete human chorionic gonadotropin (hCG), which is necessary to maintain pregnancy, and the placenta also takes over the secretion of estrogen and progesterone. The next 6 weeks are called the *embryonic period* and are the most critical for development because all the major organ systems are formed in precise sequence (Figure 25–5). During the subsequent fetal period, growth and organ maturation continue until term. In particular, the central nervous, genitourinary, and immune systems continue to develop throughout pregnancy. The period of most rapid fetal growth is considered to occur during the last trimester. Full term is typically 38 weeks after conception, with a normal fetal weight of 6.6–7.9 lb (3000–3600 g) and a length of 19–20 in (360 mm).

Exposures during weeks 1 and 2 after conception may cause early pregnancy loss if they interfere with tubal transport, implantation, or endocrine control or if they are cytotoxic to the fetus itself. Such a loss may appear only as a late or heavy menstrual flow. With increasingly sensitive laboratory assays available, women trying to conceive or being studied for pregnancy outcome can have these very early losses detected by a short rise and subsequent fall in hCG. The embryo may be less sensitive to structural damage at this time because differentiation has not yet begun, and damage is potentially correctable by the rapidly dividing cells. Thus congenital anomalies are unlikely to result from very early embryo exposures.

The greatest susceptibility to teratogenic agents occurs during the embryonic period, or organogenesis, when major morphologic abnormalities may be induced. The timing of an effect can be very specific. Although different agents administered at the same time may cause the same anomaly, the same agent given at two different times may induce different anomalies. Known or suspected human teratogens include antineoplastic drugs, diethylstilbestrol

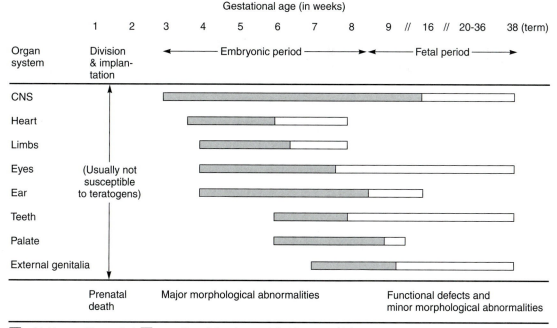

Gestational age (in weeks)

| | 1 | 2 | 3 | 4 | 5 | 6 | 7 | 8 | 9 | // | 16 | // | 20-36 | 38 (term) |

| Organ system | Division & implantation | ← Embryonic period → | ← Fetal period → |

- CNS
- Heart
- Limbs
- Eyes (Usually not susceptible to teratogens)
- Ear
- Teeth
- Palate
- External genitalia

Prenatal death   Major morphological abnormalities   Functional defects and minor morphological abnormalities

▨ = highly sensitive period; ☐ = continued development, but less sensitivity to teratogens.

Figure 25–5. Critical periods of fetal development by organ system.

(DES), lead, and ionizing radiation (Table 25–3). The embryonic period is when the highest rates of pregnancy loss occur, with approximately 60–75% of recognized losses in the first trimester. Approximately 35% of aborted conceptuses are karyotypically abnormal, and another 30% have morphologic abnormalities.

Exposure after the first trimester may induce minor morphologic abnormalities or growth deficits. Since the endocrine, central nervous, and other systems are still developing, their respective function might be affected by exposures during this time. Organic mercury, tobacco smoke, and lead are examples of substances that have adverse effects with exposure later in pregnancy (see Table 25–3). Potentially, carcinogens could cross the placenta and exert an effect at any stage of development.

Postnatal Development & Lactation

The young infant continues development after birth, with general body growth and central nervous system maturation the most obvious changes. In children, prenatal exposures may result in deficits in growth or behavior and mental function (e.g., fetal alcohol syndrome). Prenatal maternal cigarette smoking is strongly related to sudden infant death syndrome and is thought to be related to growth. In addition, prenatal exposures may exert effects manifested during reproductive maturation of the offspring, with early pubertal development

an increasing concern in industrialized countries. Prenatal exposures or conditions are also being investigated for long-term effects into adulthood.

Child development also may be affected by postnatal exposures: Environmental exposures may be present in the residence or community, and parental occupational exposures may be brought home on clothing or delivered through breast-feeding. Contamination of breast milk occurs primarily by passive diffusion. Thus low-molecular-weight lipophilic nonpolar substances can have higher concentrations in breast milk than in maternal serum. Substances with higher milk-to-plasma ratios (>3) include the polychlorinated biphenyls (PCBs) and dichlorodiphenyltrichloroethane (DDT) residues. Lactation is the main route of excretion for toxicants that bioaccumulate in maternal adipose tissue. Although acute toxicity in infants from contaminated breast milk has been reported (e.g., PCBs), the effects of low-level chronic exposures have not been well studied. Therefore, most pediatricians would continue to recommend the benefits of breast-feeding, except for unusual exposure circumstances. Details of postnatal effects are beyond the scope of this chapter.

Maternal Physiologic Changes

A number of physiologic changes and medical complications can occur in the pregnant woman that might be affected by occupational or environmental exposures.

Table 25–3. Human evidence for adverse female reproduction or developmental effects of selected agents.[1]

Agent	Human Outcomes[2]	Strength of Data[3]
Anesthetic gases	Subfertility/SAB, BDs	?/+
Antineoplastic drugs	SAB/BDs	++/+
Arsenic	SAB, LBW	+
Cadmium	LBW	+
Carbon disulfide	SAB/menstrual disorders	+/?
Carbon monoxide	SAB/LBW	+/++
Chlorination by-products	SAB, LBW, menstrual disorders	?
Dichlorodiphenyltrichloroethane (DDT)	Menstrual disorders, SAB, neurodevelopment, SGA/preterm	?/+
Dioxins	Menstrual disorders, SAB, BDs	?
Electromagnetic fields (EMF)	SAB/childhood cancer	+/+
Ethylene glycol ethers	SAB	++
Ethylene oxide	SAB/fertility	+/?
Lead	Infertility, SAB, preterm/neurobehavioral/delayed puberty	+/++/?
Mercury	Menstrual disorders, SAB, LBW/CNS malformation, cerebral palsy, neurobehavioral	+/++
Pesticides	Fertility, fetal loss/menstrual disorders, BDs	+/?
Physical stress	Preterm, LBW/SAB	+/?
Phthalates	Preterm, structural anomaly, premature thelarche	?
Polyaromatic hydrocarbons (PAHs)	LBW, SGA	?
Polychlorinated biphenyls (PCBs)	LBW, hyperpigmentation/menstrual disorders	+/?
Radiation, ionizing	Infertility, menstrual disorders, SAB, BDs, childhood cancer	++
Solvents, organic	Menstrual disorders/fertility, SAB, BDs	?/+
Tobacco smoke	Fertility, fetal loss/LBW, SIDS	+/++
Video display terminals (VDT)	SAB, BDs	–

[1]Compiled from multiple sources including original reports. See also www.oehha.ca.gov/prop65.html
[2]All have shown at least limited positive effects in animals. BDs = birth defects; CNS = central nervous system; LBW = low birthweight or decreased weight; SAB = spontaneous abortion with fetal loss, including later losses as well; SGA = small for gestational age; SIDS = sudden infant death syndrome.
[3]++ = strong evidence; + = limited evidence; ? = preliminary or conflicting evidence; – = no association.

These changes are also noteworthy to the physician for the way in which they may modify fetal exposures or require accommodation in the workplace. For example, increased tidal volume and respiratory rate of the pregnant woman may increase the absorbed dose of aerosolized chemicals. An increased metabolic rate also may lead to changes in metabolism of specific compounds, leading to a different effective dose. Pregnant women also can experience fatigue and nausea. The nausea may increase sensitivity to substances with strong odors or tastes. Thus potential changes in exposure dose and common consumption patterns (e.g., caffeinated or alcoholic beverages) could occur.

SCIENTIFIC LITERATURE

Toxicologic risk assessment is the means of characterizing health effects of hazards in the workplace or environment by combining evidence from scientific studies with likely exposure scenarios using mathematical modeling (see Chapter 45). When evaluating a patient, the clinician will identify potential exposures via a detailed environmental and occupational history. Existing databases should be consulted for information about reproductive hazards (see Chapter 2); however, many chemicals and physical hazards have not been studied adequately with respect to reproduction. Because the clinician may need to consult the original literature, this section provides an explanation of basic issues in conducting or interpreting experimental and epidemiologic studies.

As a consequence of the scarcity of human data dealing with reproductive effects, regulatory and oversight agencies often must rely on animal studies when identifying toxicants. Animal studies are applicable to humans with respect to whether there is any harm but are not necessarily predictive of specific human effects. Furthermore, animal studies generally use a range of doses extending well beyond typical human exposures that may involve different routes of exposure and examine endpoints not seen in humans (e.g., fetal resorptions). In the evaluation of the animal literature and its relevance to humans, the following aspects need to be considered: species tested; route, timing, and dose of exposure; endpoints examined; systemic or maternal toxicity; litter effects; consistency among animal studies; concordance with reproductive biology; and biologic plausibility of the mechanism of action. From the higher-quality animal studies, the dose-response relationship is assessed to set standards for exposure levels. One goal is to try to ascertain the no-observed-adverse-effect level (NOAEL), which is the highest dose level at which no biologically adverse effects occur, or alternatively, the lowest-observed-adverse-effect level (LOAEL). Then it is customary to apply uncertainty factors (or safety factors) to this level when estimating the "safe" exposure level for humans.

Epidemiologic Studies

Well-conducted epidemiologic studies should provide the best means of evaluating whether a specific agent or group of agents adversely affects human reproduction and development but are less often used for setting standards. Human studies have many limitations, so certain criteria or a weight-of-evidence type of scheme is often used in evaluating whether a substance reasonably can be considered as having an adverse effect. Besides performing qualitative comparison of consistency of results, quality of studies, and biologic plausibility, this might involve conducting a meta-analysis where results from several studies are combined statistically.

A. STUDY DESIGNS

The basic study designs used to examine the association of an exposure and possible outcomes include the cross-sectional, case-control, and cohort studies, which are discussed in the Appendix. The cross-sectional design is the simplest and has been used often in occupational and environmental reproductive studies. In these studies, there is potential selection bias because the population existing in the workplace at the time of study may not be representative of the workforce during the time of previous exposure. For example, women with live births may leave the workforce temporarily to care for their infants, whereas women experiencing SABs may continue to work and are at greater risk for subsequent SABs. On the other hand, women who experience adverse outcomes that they associate with a workplace exposure may change jobs. The case-control study is most appropriate for evaluating relatively rare diseases (e.g., birth defects or childhood cancers). Because the outcome of interest is specified at the onset, the continuum of reproductive effects that may result from a given exposure cannot be evaluated. The cohort study is the preferred study design for most reproductive outcomes. A prospective cohort study allows specific measures of an exposure and potential confounders to be ascertained at the etiologically relevant time periods, before the health endpoint is ascertained.

The cohort and case-control studies are considered hypothesis-testing studies and usually are conducted after a possible association has been suggested. For example, an acute clinician may recognize a series of cases that seem to have a factor in common. This situation is most likely to occur with a rare disease or new syndrome and was instrumental in identifying such associations as thalidomide and severe limb defects and DES and vaginal clear-cell carcinoma. A reported cluster of adverse outcomes occurring in a group of persons is a common way for environmental and occupational problems to be brought to attention, but such clusters often remain unexplained on further investigation.

Valuable data could be obtained from surveillance systems, but there are few established systems in place for adverse reproductive outcomes other than birth defects and, very recently but on a limited basis, autism and other developmental disabilities. Reasons for this include the fact that not all outcomes attract medical attention or require hospitalization (e.g., SABs and subfertility), so they are more difficult to ascertain routinely.

B. EXPOSURE ASSESSMENT

Although the methods used to measure occupational or environmental exposure are beyond the scope of this chapter, a brief overview of issues specific to evaluating exposure with respect to reproductive outcomes is presented. It should be kept in mind that the exposures of three individuals may be involved (e.g., each parent and the fetus/offspring).

To cause reproductive damage, an agent must be absorbed into the bloodstream, and to harm the fetus directly (e.g., changes in maternal hormones could affect the fetus) it also must cross the placenta. This process is affected by individual metabolism and the molecular structure of the compound. Some chemicals react with the first tissues they encounter, such as the lungs or skin, and are not absorbed into the bloodstream unless they are ingested (e.g., acids, chlorine, and asbestos). Once in the bloodstream, agents that are of low molecular weight, are lipophilic, and are in a nonionized state are most likely to cross the placenta. Maternal metabolism may result in a metabolite that is more or less toxic to the fetus than the original substance. Unless chronic exposure results in a steady-state level in the body, the rapidity with which a substance is cleared also can affect its toxicity. Often these issues are beyond the scope of epidemiologic studies but should be considered within the overall body of evidence about the toxicity of a substance. When evaluating epidemiologic studies, an association with an exposure at the critical time is more relevant to establishing causality. In addition to timing, a dose-response relationship is examined if exposure data are sufficiently detailed. However, this relationship may not be evident with reproductive outcomes because different doses may result in different outcomes (e.g., birth defect versus fetal death).

In epidemiologic studies, exposures can be ascertained from interviews, existing records, or biomarkers. If exposure history is obtained by retrospective interview, the possibility of biased recall among cases or misclassification because of a lack of records or diminished memory is of concern. Ascertainment of current exposure status for cohort studies limits possible recall bias, but women may not be aware of all their exposures, and asking one spouse about the other may not provide sufficiently accurate information.

Existing records often do not provide detailed information but rather serve to group women broadly. For example, residence on the birth certificate might be used to assign likelihood of an environmental exposure. However, residence at delivery may not reflect residence in the first trimester, nor does it account for individual behavioral differences, such as how much time is spent away from the area. Similarly, occupational registries may be used to group women by broad exposures, but specific work-site practices will be unknown. The most accurate occupational exposures are obtained by an industrial hygienist, but such studies are also more costly and often limited in sample size to allow for more detailed study.

Laboratory measurement of exposure provides a quantification of exposure that is less likely to be biased. Techniques for measuring environmental levels in air, water, and soil have been developed for many agents, including radon, electromagnetic fields, solvents, pesticides, metals, and particulate levels. Measurements on biologic samples provide an indication of internal dose, which would be more biologically relevant. For exam-

ple, cotinine (a metabolite of nicotine) is used to assess tobacco smoke exposure. Biologic monitoring requires a prospective study unless stored samples are available. A number of difficulties can arise with such studies, for example, small sample size or selection bias because of the higher costs and greater participation required of subjects. Sampling at one point in time may not reflect the critical exposure period, particularly if the substance is metabolized rapidly.

C. HEALTH ENDPOINTS & STUDY DESIGN ISSUES

Numerous endpoints have been examined in reproductive and developmental toxicity studies (see Table 25–2). Table 25–4 summarizes the definition and ascertainment of these outcomes as well as potential confounders. For a factor to be a confounder, it must be related to both the endpoint and the exposure in the study of interest. Lack of control for one of the variables in the list does not imply that the study is deficient if the investigators found that this factor did not act as a confounder in their study.

Many of the pregnancy outcomes in Table 25–4A are relatively frequent and lend themselves to a prospective study design. One design is to enroll women when they come in for a prenatal visit and then ascertain pregnancy outcomes by medical records, vital records, or both. However, the detection of SAB depends on the time at which the pregnancy is recognized. Women who have had prior losses and are worried about an exposure may seek medical attention sooner than other women, and thus more of their losses will be detected. A case-control design also can be used to study SAB, but when SABs are ascertained from medical or laboratory records, a certain percentage of early losses will be missed, which may be related to exposure status. Studies have been conducted that collect urine samples for the measurement of hCG and early pregnancy loss (or for ovulation detection). These studies are very labor-intensive, and the types of participants may represent a selected population.

In contrast to fetal loss, specific congenital anomalies are not common, and thus a case-control study design is usually used. The primary concerns with these types of studies are ascertainment of relevant cases, selection of appropriate control subjects, and possible recall bias. Classification of defects is problematic because they may have varying etiologies, but any single defect is extremely rare. Many defects are not evident at birth; therefore, additional postnatal follow-up may be necessary for identification.

Because birth weight is recorded fairly accurately and is associated with subsequent mortality and morbidity, it has been the subject of much perinatal research using a variety of study designs. Mean birth weight can be examined, or it is often categorized as low birth weight (<2500 g). However, this category includes infants who are born

Table 25–4. Developmental and reproductive outcomes, definitions, and source of ascertainment in epidemiologic studies.

Outcome	Definition	Source of Ascertainment	Possible Confounders
A. Developmental outcomes			
Clinical spontaneous abortion	Fetal loss by 20 weeks	Interview, MDs or MRs Pregnancy test	Mat. age, prior SAB, smoking, alcohol, gest. age at preg. recognition
Early, or subclinical loss	Loss by 6–8 weeks Short rise and fall in hCG level	Urinary assay (days 5–20 after ovulation)	Same as clinical (unknown)
Congenital anomalies	Varies—structural, physiologic, genetic, major & minor	Problematic—vital records incomplete; MRs, MDs, or registries	Few known—mat. age, prior hx, gender, race (defect specific)
Fetal growth	LBW: < 2500 g SGA: ≤ 10th percentile weight-for-age Preterm: < 37 weeks	Vital records (accuracy of gest. age), MRs, interview	Mat. age, race, SES, parity, mat. weight & gain, prior hx, prenatal care, gest. age, gender, multiple birth, nutrition, smoking, stress
Fetal, neonatal, or infant death	FD: 21 wks-term ND: 1st month of life ID: 1st year	Vital records (underreport FDs), MRs, interview	Vary by timing & cause: mat. age, race, SES, parity, infant gender, multiple birth, birth weight & gest. age
B. Reproductive outcomes			
Infertility	No conception in 12 mos. unprotected intercourse or specific dx (e.g., tubal disease, ovulatory factor, cervical factor, endometriosis)	Interview or survey Vital records crude	Mat. age, STD hx, IUD or OC use hx, smoking, weight (?), stress (?)
Time to conception	Continuous = mos. of unprotected intercourse, or Categorize (3, 6, 12 mos)	Interview Diary	See above, frequency of intercourse
Age at puberty	Age at menarche, breast or pubic hair development	Interview, physical exam, MRs	Race, body size, birth weight, exercise, diet (unknown)
Menstrual cycle dysfunction	Cycle length (or categorize; < 24, > 34 days), bleed characteristics, pain, anovulation, long FP or short LP	Interview, BBT or cervical mucous test, hormone measurements in serum or urine	Mat. age, obesity, alcohol abuse, smoking, stress, exertion, some drugs or medical conditions (more work needed)
Age at menopause	Cessation of menstruation: mean about 50 years, but perimenopausal many years prior	Interview, MRs, hormone levels	Smoking, age at menarche, preg. hx

Abbreviations: BBT = basal body temperature; dx = diagnosis; FD = fetal death; FP = follicular phase; hx = history; ID = infant death; IUD = intrauterine device; LBW = low birth weight; LP = luteal phase; MD = Medical Doctor, physician records; MR = medical (hospital) records; ND = neonatal death; OC = oral contraceptives; SAB = spontaneous abortion; SES = socioeconomic status; SGA = small for gestational age; STD = sexually transmitted disease.

prematurely, as well as those who are growth retarded for their age. These two groups may be etiologically different and experience different risks of mortality. To distinguish these, investigators can examine LBW among only term infants or small for gestational age infants (SGA; usually defined as births below the tenth percentile on standard-weight-for-gestational-age curves).

Perinatal deaths include a variety of causes with a number of classification schemes developed to summarize them. For occupational or environmental factors, it is useful to distinguish between prepartum and peripartum stillbirths because a toxic effect is more likely to be related to death in utero. When infant deaths are examined, neonatal deaths are found to be more likely to be related to exposures or conditions of pregnancy, whereas postnatal deaths also reflect conditions of infancy.

The reproductive endpoints in Table 26–4B are less well studied epidemiologically than are pregnancy outcomes. This is partly because the population at risk is harder to determine, and such outcomes only recently have come under more public concern. Infertility and subfertility often are studied retrospectively because it is difficult to assemble a population of women trying to become pregnant. The definition of infertility is based on waiting time and may include some people in whom no physiologic change has occurred. If cases are limited to a medically diagnosed population, the study may be biased by a differential likelihood of seeking treatment after varying waiting times, potentially dependent on suspected exposures. Often control subjects are difficult to select for these studies. Because the label of infertility ignores the potential continuum of effects, time to pregnancy is a preferred measure. Retrospectively, women who are pregnant or have delivered recently can be questioned about past use of contraception. The choice of a reference date about when exposures are determined in controls is critical. If the time of conception is used, women who had been trying unsuccessfully before that time may have changed their exposures, and the true period at risk (when contraception is stopped) will not be included. Prospective studies may be conducted by having women keep diaries of when their menstrual periods occur, when they have intercourse, and when they use contraception to identify cycles truly "at risk" of pregnancy, as well as monitoring conception by hormone tests. Menstrual cycle function is the least well investigated but is best studied prospectively with the use of diaries to record signs and symptoms. Cycle length can be used as a crude measure of function, but normal lengths may mask such problems as insufficient luteal phase and progesterone production. Studying such defects requires accurate determination of day of ovulation and measurement of hormone patterns. These types of studies have become

relatively easier to conduct in population-based groups by the recent development of cost-efficient serial-sample laboratory assays of urinary hormone metabolites. Such studies may be well suited to an occupational cohort in which a well-defined worker population is assembled and has the advantage of including more women, not just those who are pregnant. The ages at menarche and menopause define the length of natural reproductive capacity and are also related to other endpoints such as breast cancer. Age at menarche is relatively well recalled, even by adults, but other measures of puberty are determined most accurately by trained physical examiners, so prospective or cross-sectional studies would be necessary.

REFERENCES

Savitz DA et al: Methodologic issues in the design and analysis of epidemiologic studies of pregnancy outcome. Stat Methods Med Res 2006;15:93 [PMID: 16615651].

Surkan PJ et al: Previous preterm and small-for-gestational-age births and the subsequent risk of stillbirth. N Engl J Med 2004;350:777 [PMID: 14973215].

Selected Reproductive Hazards

As noted, few chemicals have been studied adequately in terms of their reproductive effects, and most exposure standards are not based on reproductive effects. Nevertheless, a number of potential reproductive or developmental hazards have been identified in humans (see Table 25–3). Details of the physical qualities and use of some of these substances can be found in other chapters (e.g., Chapter 27 for lead and Chapter 29 for solvents). Many of the toxic agents in Table 25–3 have been examined in occupational settings, where exposures tend to be higher than those encountered in the environment and relatively easier to document. However, some of these hazards are encountered environmentally from long-term use and disposal by industry, natural occurrence, or acute releases. After brief discussion of the evidence for some of these, the following section presents three more detailed examples of accumulating epidemiologic data.

The agents that have been shown conclusively to be reproductive toxicants in humans, other than medications, are few and include ionizing radiation, mercury, lead, and polychlorinated biphenyls (PCBs). Among the others listed, anesthetic gases induced fetal loss and congenital defects in animals, and early studies, although flawed, suggested effects in humans. The National Institute for Occupational Safety and Health (NIOSH) recommended exposure limits that led to reductions in exposure, making further study difficult. A meta-analysis yielded a pooled risk ratio for SAB of 1.5 in all studies or 1.9 in the best. Health care workers may be exposed to other hazards, including biologics and antineoplastic drugs, associated with increased risks of SAB. Workers involved in the manufacture of these and other pharmaceuticals also may be put at risk. Pesticides are used commonly worldwide and represent different classes, such as insecticides, herbicides, and fungicides, some of which may be endocrine disruptors (see below). A recent review particularly implicated phenoxy herbicides, pyrethroids, and organophosphates as affecting multiple reproductive endpoints. General exposure to pesticides most likely occurs via the diet or home use, but worker exposures tend to be the highest. In addition to diet, chemicals in air and water may lead to environmental exposures. Increasing evidence shows that air pollutants may be associated with adverse pregnancy outcomes on a population level, including low birth weight, preterm delivery, stillbirth, and infant death.

Reports of clusters of malformations in women working with video-display terminals (VDTs) in the early 1980s led to extensive public and scientific interest. A review of subsequent analytical studies from several countries did not generally support much association of adverse reproductive outcomes with VDT work; a meta-analysis found a pooled odds ratio of 1.0 for VDT use and SAB. However, a Finnish report released later showed an elevated risk [odds ratio (OR): 3.4] among women who used VDTs with a high level of extremely low-frequency magnetic fields. The concern shifted to electromagnetic fields (EMFs) that are present in all workplaces and homes. The next generation of EMF studies examining electric appliance use, residential wire coding, and residential spot measurements yielded inconsistent results with respect to SAB and little evidence of increased risk for birth defects. Two studies with better exposure measures (e.g., the subjects wore measuring devices for 24 hours) subsequently found increased risks of SAB (OR: 1.7–1.8) associated with various EMF metrics. These findings led the California EMF Program to conclude in their risk evaluation document that EMFs were a possible risk for miscarriage and that further research to study the nature of changing or high magnetic fields was warranted. The evidence for birth defects continues to be examined as well but was inconclusive at the time.

Whether employment per se has a harmful effect on pregnancy outcome has been evaluated, with the general consensus that it does not. Physical exertion at work has been a cause of concern because of the extreme effects seen in professional athletes and dancers. The American College of Obstetricians and Gynecologists published guidelines on exertion levels during later stages of pregnancy indicating that moderate or light exertion levels should be safe throughout pregnancy. Heavy lifting, prolonged standing, or repetitive stooping and bending are recommended to be discontinued early during the second trimester. The most consistent adverse effect of physical exertion seems to be on preterm delivery and possibly low birth weight and SAB, with less consistent results seen for fecundability and menstrual disorders. Several studies show that shift work, or working irregular hours, is associated with a moderately increased risk of SAB, with similar results for LBW and decreased fecundability or longer time to pregnancy.

REFERENCES

American College of Obstetrics and Gynecology (ACOG): Effects of pregnancy on work performance (guidelines) Web site: www.acog.org/.

California Department of Health Services: An evaluation of the possible risks from electric and magnetic fields (EMFs) from power lines, internal wiring, electrical occupations and appliances, www.dhs.ca.gov/ehib/emf/RiskEvaluation/riskeval.html.

Dugandzic R et al: The association between low level exposures to ambient air pollution and term low birth weight. Environ Health 2006;5:3 [PMID: 16503975].

Sram RJ et al: Ambient air pollution and pregnancy outcomes. Environ Health Perspect 2005;113:375 [PMID: 15811825].

Zhu JL et al: Occupational exposure to pesticides and pregnancy outcomes in gardeners and farmers. J Occup Environ Med 2006;48:347 [PMID: 16607187].

A. ENDOCRINE-DISRUPTING CHEMICALS

In the last two decades, concern has risen about a variety of compounds that may affect the endocrine system by mimicking or antagonizing endogenous hormones. Hormones act as chemical messengers, directing a wide variety of biologic functions through gene expression, and are particularly important during fetal development. Alterations were first noticed in the 1980s among various wildlife populations and later confirmed experimentally. Disruption of the hormone system by chemical contaminants now has been seen in a wide range of species from birds to fish, mollusks, frogs, alligators, and polar bears. Effects in both males and females have been observed, with one unusual but predominant finding being the development of intersex reproductive systems, with both male and female aspects. Originally focused on chemicals that interfered with estrogen receptor pathways, research from a variety of disciplines during the last 5 years has revealed a number of other actions such as antiandrogens, progesterone blockers, or interference with thyroid hormone.

These so-called endocrine-disrupting chemicals (EDCs) or hormonally active agents (HAAs) vary structurally, from persistent pesticides such as DDT/dichlorodiphenyl dichloroethylene (DDE) to PCBs and plasticizers such as phthalates and bisphenol-A. Because some of these compounds persist for years in the environment and have entered the food chain, low exposure may continue despite bans on the use of some of them in the United States. Immigrants from Southeast Asia or Latin America have higher body burdens of persistent pesticides such as DDT, as well as ongoing exposure to other pesticides in agricultural work. More recently, a group of chemicals structurally similar to PCBs, called *polybrominated diphenyl ethers* (PBDEs), has become a cause for concern because their concentration in human tissues has increased in the United States and Europe. Thyroid hormone disruption and neurodevelopmental deficits have been found in animal studies. These compounds are used widely as flame retardants in plastics used in electrical appliances, computers, building materials, and furnishings. Exposure may occur in manufacture and dismantling of these products as well as from their degradation in the environment. Another class of compounds with similar manufacturing uses owing to their chemical stability that are now being measured in the environment and wildlife are perfluorinated organic compounds (PFOCs).

Relatively few studies of health effects had been conducted in humans until a national research agenda sped up the process, providing some examples of effects, with even more data anticipated in upcoming years. Furthermore, most of these chemicals have been measured in humans by the Centers for Disease Control and Prevention and others. A number of studies now have shown effects of DDT/DDE on pregnancy loss, low birth weight, and preterm delivery but not entirely consistently. One study with daily measures of hormone metabolites found that luteal-phase progesterone levels generally were lower with higher DDE body burdens. PCBs and mercury have been associated with adverse neurodevelopmental effects in prenatally exposed children. Polybrominated biphenyl (PBB) and PCB exposure in utero also have been associated with earlier menarche, whereas lead exposure has been associated with delayed puberty. Thus a variety of effects from these ubiquitous compounds may be revealed in humans as the research progresses, including other reproductive endpoints such as infertility and tumorigenesis.

Some unique aspects of EDCs are that effects may occur not only at high doses but also lower doses, making classic high-dose experiments potentially misleading. Furthermore, the developing fetus is exquisitely sensitive to both natural hormone signals and exogenous chemical signals. Besides guiding the fetus through critical developmental pathways, these early interactions also help to set its sensitivity to subsequent hormonal signals, leading to potential lifelong consequences. These compounds also may act by creating changes that are permanent to the lineage, leading to transgenerational effects.

REFERENCES

Centers for Disease Control and Prevention (CDC): National report on human exposure to environmental chemicals, www.cdc.gov/exposurereport/.

Davis SI et al: Menstrual function among women exposed to polybrominated biphenyls. Environ Health 2005;4:1 [PMID: 16091135].

Law DC et al: Maternal serum levels of polychlorinated biphenyls and 1,1-dichloro-2,2 bis(p-chlorophenyl) ethylene (DDE) and time to pregnancy. Am J Epidemiol 2005;162:523 [PMID: 16093292].

Trubo R: Endocrine-disrupting chemicals probed as potential pathways to illness. JAMA 2005;294:291 [PMID: 16030264].

Tulane University: Environmental estrogens and other hormones, www.som.tulane.edu/ecme/eehome/.

Windham GC et al: Exposure to organochlorine compounds and effects on ovarian function. Epidemiol 2005;16:182 [PMID: 15703532].

B. SOLVENTS

Solvents may well be one of the most pervasive chemical exposures of women because they include many compounds used in the workplace and the home. In the early 1980s, solvent exposure was considered a potential reproductive hazard when increased risks for adverse outcomes were identified among laboratory workers in Scandinavia. In some industries (e.g., dry-cleaning and pharmaceutical industries), use of specific solvents, such as perchloroethylene, methylene chloride, toluene, xylene, and glycol ethers, has been associated with concurrent elevation in SAB risk. Several case-control studies show associations of solvent exposure and cardiac and other congenital anomalies. A meta-analysis that combined raw data from five studies for each outcome found that the odds for major malformations increased 64% (e.g., OR: 1.64) and for SAB increased 25% with solvent exposure. Confounding and dose-response patterns were not assessed. Suggestive study findings indicate a potential association between solvent use and fetal growth or preterm delivery. A recent study found that offspring of pregnant women occupationally exposed to organic solvents obtained lower scores on various tests of neurodevelopmental function. These results would be consistent with effects of heavy maternal alcohol consumption. Because alcohol is a type of solvent, a "fetal solvent syndrome" has been proposed. Many of the epidemiologic studies suffer from crude exposure assessment, making definitive conclusions difficult, but animal data support the findings. Some studies have examined menstrual patterns, but few consistent results have emerged. At least one study reported reduced fecundability among women with daily or high solvent exposure. Exposures in the semiconductor industry, which employs a largely female workforce, have become of increased interest. A collaborative study of 14 semiconductor companies nationwide reported rates of SAB to be slightly increased, fecundability reduced, and menstrual cycle length increased in exposed workers. The investigators implicated exposures to photoresist and developer solvents (e.g., glycol ethers and xylene) and fluoride compounds as the primary etiologic agents.

REFERENCES

Laslo-Baker D et al: Child neurodevelopmental outcome and maternal occupational exposure to solvents. Arch Pediatr Adolesc Med 2004;158:956 [PMID: 15466682].

Till C et al: Vision abnormalities in young children exposed prenatally to organic solvents. Neurotoxicology 2005;26:599 [PMID: 16054697].

Wennborg H et al: Congenital malformations related to maternal exposure to specific agents in biomedical research laboratories. J Occup Environ Med 2005;47:11 [PMID: 15643154].

C. TOBACCO SMOKE EXPOSURE

Active smoking has been causally associated with a number of developmental and reproductive endpoints; infants of women who smoke during pregnancy are estimated to have twice the risk of low birth weight or a decrement in mean birth weight of 150–200 g compared with infants of nonsmokers. Other adverse developmental outcomes associated with maternal tobacco smoking include preterm delivery, fetal and infant death, and behavioral deficits in offspring. Tobacco smoking is also associated with infertility, menstrual disorders, and earlier age at menopause. In the workplace or other environments, nonsmokers may be exposed to passive smoke, also called *environmental tobacco smoke* (ETS). Tobacco smoke contains thousands of compounds; those with potential reproductive toxicity include nicotine, carbon monoxide, PAHs, heavy metals, aromatic solvents, and others. Based on studies measuring biomarkers in the early to mid-1990s, from 40% to nearly 100% of nonsmokers may be exposed to some ETS, with working representing, on average, 35% of exposure time.

Reviewing the evidence for adverse effects of ETS exposure on reproduction, over 30 studies have examined mean birth weight, with the better studies indicating a weight decrement ranging from 25–100 g. In an earlier meta-analysis, the adequate studies conducted among nonsmoking mothers yielded a pooled weight decrement of 31 g (CL: –42, –20). Studies base on measurement of cotinine (a metabolite of nicotine) in nonsmokers, yield even greater weight decrements, particularly as assays have gotten more sensitive so that a truly not (or very low) exposed comparison group can be identified. Of the studies that examined dose-response effects, several found evidence for such trends, further strengthening the argument for causality. At least 20 studies of LBW or SGA have been conducted; the higher-quality studies of LBW yielded a pooled OR of 1.4, or a 40% increase. Some evidence suggests that specific subsets of women may be more susceptible to effects, including older women and nonwhites.

Reviews by several agencies generally conclude there is a consistent slight effect of ETS exposure on reducing mean birth weight (or slightly increasing the risk of growth retardation). There is also good evidence that ETS exposure can lead to sudden infant death syndrome in offspring and may be associated with preterm delivery, SAB, and adverse effects on cognition and behavior. There is a lack of studies of effects of ETS exposure on adult reproductive function, although a few have consistently found earlier mean age at menopause. Therefore, women who are pregnant or attempting it should be counseled to avoid areas where exposure to ETS is likely. In the workplace, other exposures, such as particulates or chemicals, may interact to magnify the effects of ETS. Exposure in other places, such as in commuting or recreation, may become more important sources of exposure as workplace restrictions on smoking are increasingly imposed.

REFERENCES

Kharrazi M et al: Environmental tobacco smoke and pregnancy outcome. Epidemiology 2004;15:660 [PMID: 15475714].

OEHHA: Proposition 65: Environmental tobacco smoke (ETS) Known to the State of California to Cause Reproductive Toxicity, http://www.oehha.ca.gov/prop65.html.

US Department of Health and Human Services: *Women and Smoking,* www.surgeongeneral.gov/library.

REPRODUCTIVE ASSESSMENT

The medical evaluation of the patient with potential exposure to a reproductive hazard follows the traditional components of history taking, physical examination, and laboratory assessment.. In addition, special consideration is needed in the evaluation, communication, and management of reproductive risk for the patient.

Medical Evaluation

In the clinical setting, infertility is defined as an inability to conceive after 12 months of unprotected intercourse. Potential causes for infertility in the female include ovulatory dysfunction, tubal or pelvic factors, and uterine or cervical factors. It is estimated that the cause of infertility is a result of male factors in 40% of affected couples, a result of female factors in 40–50% of affected couples, and of no known etiology in 10–20% of the affected couples. Therefore, for the infertility workup, the male partner needs to be assessed concurrently (see Chapter 26). Adverse pregnancy outcomes include SAB, stillbirth, prematurity, congenital birth defects, low birth weight, and developmental disorders (see Tables 25–2 and 25–4). A full discussion of the diagnosis and treatment of various obstetric/gynecologic or pediatric conditions is beyond the scope of this chapter. However, the following is a general overview of the types of evaluation techniques that can be used to assess the female reproductive system.

A. INTERVIEW

The patient interview should start with the following areas: demographic data, general medical history, and reproductive history (including age at puberty, menstrual function, past pelvic surgeries or gynecologic procedures, pregnancy and birth outcomes, sexually transmitted diseases, contraception, and familial illness). In addition, it should cover lifestyle habits (such as smoking and alcohol consumption, exercise, and stress), work history and current job tasks and exposures, and potential environmental exposures (e.g., ETS; commuting; residential proximity to industry, waste sites, or heavy traffic; and possibly hobbies or home products use; see also Chapter 2).

B. PHYSICAL EXAMINATION

This examination should assess the physical integrity of the reproductive system and rule out any extraneous mass or structural abnormality.

C. LABORATORY

A hormonal profile can be obtained for the assessment of potential fetal loss (hCG and LH), ovarian function (progesterone and estrogen metabolites), and pituitary function (LH and FSH). A wide range of tests and assays is available and needs to be selected based on the medical conditions under consideration. During field biologic monitoring studies, urine samples are relatively easy to collect for hormonal assays. Exposure burden for some hazards may be measured in biologic tissues (e.g., exhaled breath, blood, or urine), but few of these lead to diagnostic interpretation.

Risk Evaluation

The steps generally conducted in the toxicologic risk assessment may be adapted in simplified form for the clinical workup, including

1. Hazard identification of any hazardous agents the patient may be exposed to from a detailed occupational and environmental history during interview

2. Hazard evaluation to determine whether a given substance or physical agent may be a reproductive hazard by consulting databases and the literature

3. Exposure assessment, which is performed by estimating the level of exposure from patient work history, product labels, material safety data sheets, industrial hygiene data, environmental sampling, or biologic monitoring results, as well as potential routes of exposure and consistency of symptoms

4. Risk characterization with respect to effects on the reproductive system (This activity is based on information gathered in the first three steps and considers toxicity, timing and extent of exposure, potency, severity of outcome, and degree of uncertainty in animal and human studies.)

Often, not all the needed information is available, and an educated guess is necessary. It is very helpful to have established contacts for additional consultation when a more difficult risk assessment is involved. Potential contacts include local or state health departments, university medical centers, poison control centers, NIOSH, Environmental Protection Agency (EPA), Agency for Toxic Substances and Disease Registry (ATSDR), Occupational Safety and Health Administration (OSHA), and the Association of Occupational and Environmental Clinics. Access to online literature databases is very useful (e.g., REPRORISK, REPROTOX, and TERIS; see references).

REFERENCES

Centers for Disease Control and Prevention: National Center for Birth Defects and Developmental Disabilities, www.cdc.gov/ncbddd.

Center for the Evaluation of Risks to Human Reproduction (CERHR): http://cerhr.niehs.nih.gov.

Jahnke GD et al: Center for the Evaluation of Risks to Human Reproduction: The first five years. Birth Defects Res B Dev Reprod Toxicol 2005;74:1 Review [PMID: 15729732].

National Pesticide Information Center (npic.orst.eud) provides online information about pesticide safety and toxicity (also, toll-free hotline: 1-800-858-7378).

NIOSH: *The Effects of Workplace Hazards on Female Reproductive Health,* www.cdc.gov/niosh/99–104pd.html.

Office of Environmental Health Hazard Assessment (OEHHA), California Environmental Protection Agency, Oakland, CA: Web site with information on current activities, publications, and list of chemicals considered to cause reproductive toxicity by the state of California, www.oehha.ca.gov/prop65.html.

Organization of Teratology Information Services (OTIS): http://orpheus.ucsd.edu/otis/index.html.

Reproductive Toxicology Center (REPROTOX), Bethesda, MD: Computer database (or CD-ROM) dealing with reproductive and developmental hazards, www.reprotox.org/.

REPRORISK, Micromedex, Inc., 600 Grant Street, Denver, CO 80203, 303–831–1400: Computer database dealing with reproductive and developmental health effects of drugs, chemicals, and physical and environmental hazards. Fee-based, includes REPROTOX and TERIS, www.micromedex.com/products/reprorisk/.

Risk Communication

Building on the information gathered during the risk assessment process, risk communication is the logical follow-up by which the involved person or persons obtain the information needed to make informed and independent decisions about health and safety risks. In general, there is an underlying principle that needs to be acknowledged and dealt with sensitively: The threat or actual fact of adverse reproductive outcome has a profound impact on an individual's life. All questions must be answered truthfully and completely. A description of the limitations in knowledge may be needed. The timing of exposure and of the first contact with the involved person is very important. When possible, the risk communication is conducted prior to actual exposure in order to intervene at the primary prevention stage. The options available for the female worker should be presented in such a way that the medical impact and the economic consequences of decisions are understood and discussed. The clinician may need to communicate the risks to an employer as well in order to resolve the situation, but the medical confidentiality of the involved individual must be maintained.

Risk Management

It is very important that the employer, involved employee(s), and medical consultant work together in resolving a particular situation. Ideally, a general policy on reproductive hazards in the workplace that involves both genders is developed within a safety committee composed of representatives from management and labor and consultants in occupational medicine and industrial hygiene. Remediation should occur before conception (which is not always planned) to provide protection during organogenesis, as well as to prevent fertility problems. Furthermore, it may be important to extend protection postpartum during lactation. This may require a written request from the personal physician.

In order of priority, the following actions may be considered for managing the risks of a given reproductive hazard situation: (1) Exposure reduction or elimination, replacement of hazards with safer agents, improved engineering controls, safer work practices, and personal protective equipment (the latter should not be the primary mode of protection). Exposure reduction or elimination is the most desirable option and should be attempted in all situations involving a reproductive hazard. (2) Temporary job transfer: Remove individual from work environment in which reproductive hazard exists. Problems may occur when there is no nonexposed job location. Thus this option should be considered when there is a high-risk situation and exposure reduction/elimination is not possible. (3) Disability leave: Paid leave is subject to company policy, and temporary pregnancy disability leave must be treated the same as any other medical disability leave. The early embryo sensitivity period already has occurred during potential workplace exposure by the time a disability leave is granted. There is no guarantee that the medical disability will be approved, and benefits rarely are equivalent to the individual's current wage. This option should be considered when there is a high-risk situation in which the employer will not reduce exposure and a temporary transfer is not possible (see also Chapter 4 and 5). (4) Remove individual from work: This is the least desirable action. It is illegal for an employer to terminate the affected individual because of pregnancy. A woman may choose to quit work because of personal reasons, but it is important to help her evaluate all options and to understand the possible consequences. This option is to be considered only when all other options have been explored, and the woman is comfortable with the possible consequences.

If an environmental exposure is of concern, options for individual amelioration are less but generally follow the principles just outlined (e.g., substitution, safer practices, and removal). Since some exposures may act synergistically, reducing those possible for an individual in the workplace, the home, or the diet is desirable. Additionally, this points to the need to control other environmental exposures at the population level.

REFERENCE

Taylor A et al: Differences in national legislation for the implementation of lead regulations. Int Arch Occup Environ Health 2006;79:463 [PMID: 16752159].

LEGAL ISSUES & WORKPLACE STANDARDS

In the lawsuit involving International Union, UAW versus Johnson Controls, Inc., the U.S. Supreme Court held that an employer violated Title VII's ban on sex discrimination by excluding from production jobs in a lead-battery factory all women who could not prove their sterility. The Court indicated that a policy directed only at fertile women is overt discrimination on the basis of sex regardless of the scientific evidence of heightened safety concerns for mothers or potential mothers. In addition, any policies or actions taken by the employer must not violate existing laws prohibiting discrimination on the basis of pregnancy, childbirth, or related medical conditions. Employers cannot require that an individual be sterilized as a condition of employment. If an employee disabled by pregnancy, childbirth, or a related medical condition transfers to a less hazardous job, an employer must allow her to return to her original job or to a similar one when the disability has resolved.

OSHA has the mandate to promulgate standards that protect workers from adverse health effects (including reproductive effects) resulting from workplace hazards. However, only a few agents have OSHA standards that are based partially on reproductive effects. Included among these agents are dibromochloropropane (DBCP), lead, ethylene oxide, glycol ethers, and ionizing radiation. There are OSHA standards requiring reporting of employee exposure to hazardous chemicals and training of employees using these chemicals. But it should be recognized that many chemical and physical agents found in the workplace are not covered by an OSHA standard and that those standards that do exist for the most part are not based on reproductive endpoints. This is why the simplified risk evaluation process should be implemented at any worksite that has potential reproductive hazards present.

REFERENCES

Feitshans IL: Protecting posterity: The occupational physician's ethical and legal obligations to pregnant workers. Occup Med 2002;17:673 [PMID: 12225936].

NIOSH: Topics on reproductive health, http://www.cdc.gov/niosh/topics/repro.

Male Reproductive Toxicology

26

Ana María Osorio, MD, MPH, & Gayle C. Windham, MSPH, PhD

In studying male reproductive toxicants, the ultimate aim is to protect the reproductive health of men and the health of their offspring, which is fundamentally important for the health of future generations. The occurrence of adverse reproductive outcomes is of great concern to the individuals and families involved. This is especially true if the individuals perceive that they are living or working in areas with potential exposure to hazardous agents. Adverse reproductive effects can be very stressful for affected families. Existing human information on this subject is very sparse and inadequate for the reproductive assessment of most suspect compounds and physical agents.

Another reason to better understand male reproductive functions is that they may act as sentinels for detecting occupational and environmental hazards. Reproductive effects have a relatively short latency between exposure and detectable health event (such as abnormal semen profile) as compared with the long latency for cancer. If workers or community residents are protected from exposures that are harmful to reproduction, they usually will be protected from other health effects associated with these exposures as well. While the extent to which workplace and environmental hazards affect reproductive function is unknown, these hazards are potentially preventable. Measures that can be taken to prevent further exposure include substitution or containment of the suspect hazard. Thus, preventing exposure should play a primary role in the health care provider's overall assessment of the patient's situation.

REPRODUCTIVE OUTCOMES & RATES

Definitions

A number of adverse reproductive effects may result from male exposure to chemical and physical agents. These effects range from infertility to birth defects in the infant. Infertility is present when a couple has not conceived after 1 year of unprotected sexual intercourse. Male sexual dysfunction may involve changes in libido (interest in sexual activity), erectile dysfunction, or ejaculatory problems. Semen abnormalities can include azoospermia (complete absence of sperm), oligospermia (decreased sperm count), teratospermia (abnormally shaped sperm), and asthenospermia (sperm showing decreased motility). Abnormal birth outcomes include spontaneous abortion (fetal loss

prior to the twenty-eighth gestational week), stillbirth (fetal loss after the twenty-eighth week), death (infant: younger than 1 year of age; neonatal: younger than 28 days of age; or postneonatal: 28 days to 11 months of age), congenital defect (abnormal appearance or function at birth), prematurity (birth prior to the thirty-seventh week of gestation), low birth weight (weight < 2500 g at birth), and very low birth weight (weight < 1500 g at birth).

Population Rates

Precise rates for these types of pregnancy loss are difficult to obtain because of a lack of national monitoring systems and methodologic differences in individual epidemiologic studies. Nevertheless, a range of prevalence rates can be estimated (Table 26–1). Approximately 10% of couples in the United States are infertile. Additional couples may experience periods of subfertility or delayed conception. After conception, a variety of reproductive losses may occur at any time from conception up to full term. Up to 50% of embryos may be lost after implantation (the earliest time at which conception can be detected), with approximately 15% of pregnancies ending in a clinically detected spontaneous abortion (SAB). Of all liveborn infants, 7.8% are of low birth weight (LBW), and approximately 3% will have a clinically detectable congenital anomaly. The causes for most of these outcomes are unexplained. However, there are a few known risk factors for women such as older maternal age (associated with increased rates of SAB), certain infectious agents [e.g., cytomegalovirus, hepatitis B virus, human immunodeficiency virus (HIV), rubella, toxoplasmosis, varicella-zoster virus, and human parvovirus], cancer treatment (e.g., methotrexate), strenuous physical labor, and certain environmental agents (e.g., lead and ionizing radiation). A full discussion of female factors is found in Chapter 25. Possible male risk factors are discussed later in this chapter.

REFERENCES

Lawson CC et al: Implementing a national occupational reproductive research agenda. Environ Health Perspect 2006;114:435 [PMID: 16507468].

National Center for Health Statistics, *Health, United States, 2005,* www.cdc.gov/nchs/hus.htm.

National Institute for Occupational Safety and Health (NIOSH), Centers for Disease Control and Prevention (CDC), Na-

Table 26–1. Prevalence of selected adverse reproductive events.[1]

Endpoints	Rate per 1000	Unit	Reference Population
Birth defects			
Spina bifida	0.35	Live births + fetal deaths	California, 1997–2001
Anencephaly	0.26	Live births + fetal deaths	California, 1997–2001
Conotruncal heart defects	0.73	Live births + fetal deaths	California, 1997–2001
Down syndrome	1.01	Live births + fetal deaths	California, 1997–2001
Deaths			
Infant (< 1 year of age)	7.00	Live births	U.S., 2002
Neonatal (< 28 days)	4.70	Live births	U.S., 2002
Postneonatal (28 days to 11 months)	2.30	Live births	U.S., 2002
Birth weight			
Low birth weight (< 2500 g)	78.00	Live births with known birth weight	U.S., 2002
Very low birth weight (< 1500 g)	14.60	Live births with known birth weight	U.S., 2002
Other outcomes			
Recognized spontaneous abortion	100–200	Pregnancies or women	Estimated U.S.
Infertility	100–150	Couples	Estimated U.S.
Abnormal sperm morphology	40.00	Men	Estimated U.S.
Azoospermia	10.00	Men	Estimated U.S.

[1]Compiled from multiple sources including California Birth Defects Monitoring Program, Registry data; www.cbdmp.org; National Center for Health Statistics, *Health, United States, 2005*; www.cdc.gov/nchs/hus.htm; Lawson CC et al: Implementing a national occupational reproductive research agenda. Environ Health Perspect 2006;114:435 [PMID: 16507468].

tional Occupational Research Agenda: Fertility and pregnancy abnormalities, www2.cdc.gov/nora/.

REPRODUCTIVE PHYSIOLOGY

Although this section focuses on male-mediated exposure associated with reproductive and developmental abnormalities, it is important to note that maternal and fetal exposures also need to be assessed for a complete evaluation. It is recognized that more prolonged direct sources of exposure to the products of conception occur in the woman and that maternal exposure can continue postnatally during lactation. However, changes in fertility have been reported in both sexes, and genetic changes can be transmitted by either parent. An extensive discussion of fetal and postnatal development can be found in Chapter 25.

Male Reproductive System

Adequate hormonal regulation is necessary for proper functioning of the male reproductive system (Figure 26–1). For this to occur, coordinated hypothalamic,

pituitary, and gonadal interactions are critical. These include (1) hypothalamic production of gonadotropin-releasing hormone (GnRH), (2) pituitary gland production of follicle-stimulating hormone (FSH) and luteinizing hormone (LH), and (3) testis production of spermatozoa (germ cells) from the germinal epithelium, testosterone from the Leydig cell, and inhibin B from the Sertoli cell. GnRH release stimulates the pituitary gland production of FSH and LH. FSH acts on the Sertoli cell within the seminiferous tubules to stimulate spermatogenesis and produce inhibin B (which inhibits pituitary gland hormones). The action of LH is to stimulate testosterone production in the Leydig cell. Conversely, testosterone has a negative-feedback effect on the pituitary and hypothalamic hormones, as well as the production of germ cells (sperm) and Sertoli cell activity. Testosterone is found bound to sex hormone–binding globule (SHBG) or albumin and may be converted to the more potent dihydrotestosterone or estradiol in the circulatory system. In males, puberty is due to adequate testosterone levels and manifested by reproductive system maturity and development of secondary sex-

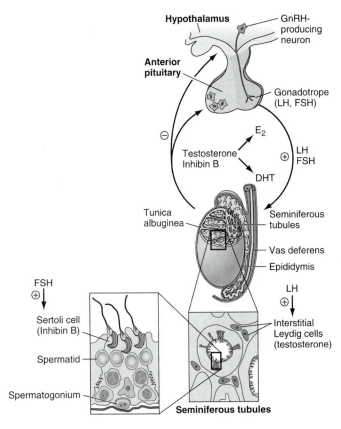

Hypothalamus

GnRH-
producing
neuron

**Anterior
pituitary**

Gonadotrope
(LH, FSH)

E_2

Testosterone
Inhibin B

LH
FSH

$\oplus$

$\ominus$

DHT

Tunica
albuginea

Seminiferous
tubules

Vas deferens

Epididymis

FSH
$\oplus$

LH
$\oplus$

Sertoli cell
(Inhibin B)

Spermatid

Spermatogonium

Interstitial
Leydig cells
(testosterone)

Seminiferous tubules

Figure 26–1. Hypothalamic, pituitary, and testicular interactions involved in hormonal homeostasis necessary for adequate male reproductive function. DHT = dihydrotestosterone; E_2 = estradiol; FSH = follicle-stimulating hormone; GnRH = gonadotropin-releasing hormone; LH = luteinizing hormone. (Reprinted with permission from Shalendar B, Jameson JL: Disorders of the testes and male reproductive systems, in Kasper D et al (eds): Harrison's Principles of Internal Medicine, 16th ed. New York: McGraw-Hill, 2005, Fig. 325-2.)

ual characteristics (e.g., increased muscle mass, beard growth, axillary and pubic hair, deepening of the voice, libido, and external genitalia growth).

In general, spermatogenesis involves two major sites within the testis (see Figure 26–1). Starting from a germ cell, it takes 74 days for development through the stages of spermatogonium, spermatocyte, and spermatid into a mature spermatozoon (or sperm) in the seminiferous tubules of the testis. During the next 12 days, the sperm travels along the epididymis for eventual ejaculation. Thus approximately 3 months are required to complete the maturation and transport of the sperm.

Teratology

There are important issues in teratology to be considered when evaluating male reproductive function. Preconception exposure may act directly on the germ cell (sperm). This condition could lead to either no fertilization or an aberration of the zygote and an eventual SAB (possibly clinically undetected) or birth defect. The reproductive toxicant may affect the embryo even when exposure occurs prior to conception either to the mother or to the father. Thus one must consider infer-

tility, SABs, and birth defects when assessing men exposed to suspect reproductive toxicants.

Another important aspect to consider is that spermatogenesis involves a continuously replicating cell population (in the billions), whereas oogenesis occurs prenatally with a finite population at birth (only approximately 400 oocytes ovulated during the reproductive years) that is depleted at around age 50 years. Therefore, chemical or physical agents whose toxicity depends on cell division will have greater effect on the male germ cell. A complete evaluation of a male exposed to a reproductive hazard should take into account the large variability in individual susceptibility to reproductive agents; the environmental, occupational, and lifestyle factors of both parents; and the possibility that a toxic effect may lead to a clinically nondetectable abnormality at the birth of the offspring.

Potential Mechanisms of Action

Most male reproductive hazards can be characterized by having one or more of the following potential mechanisms of action: central nervous system or endocrine abnormality (decreased libido and fertility as possible adverse reproductive effects), direct testicular toxicity (decreased fertility), spermatogenesis or germ cell damage in the form of morphologic change, decreased cell number, abnormal motility or chromosomal abnormality (decreased fertility, fetal loss, congenital malformations, childhood developmental disabilities, and cancers), and toxicants in the semen leading to abnormal sperm motility or direct action on the uterus or fetus (all the prior possible effects or outcomes). Although the focus of this chapter is on direct male reproductive effects, the potential for take-home exposure from the workplace leading to family member exposure needs to be assessed concurrently in the evaluation of a worker.

SCIENTIFIC LITERATURE

Human risk assessment of reproductive or other hazards in the workplace or environment involves the following components: hazard identification, dose-response assessment, exposure assessment, and risk characterization. The clinician may be involved in one or more of these steps when evaluating the health risk for a patient or worker. Although this process is covered extensively in Chapter 45, this section focuses on key aspects that deal with male reproductive health.

Informational Sources

When evaluating a patient with potential exposure to reproductive hazards, the clinician needs to identify biologic, chemical, and physical agents in the workplace or environment via the patient exposure history and any available informational material such as warning signs, product labels, material safety data sheets, and purchase orders. These documents may identify the agents to which a person is potentially exposed but usually provide very little information on reproductive hazards. In 1998, the U.S. Environmental Protection Agency (EPA) estimated that more than 84,000 chemicals were being used in industry, with only 4000 of these having been evaluated in animals (with a much smaller number studied in humans). Adding to this problem is the approximately 2000 new chemicals being introduced into the workplace each year. Many of these chemicals lack adequate pre-market reproductive assessment. Some informational sources on animal and human studies are available for those hazards that have been evaluated, such as the Registry of Toxic Effects of Chemical Substances (RTECS), REPROTOX (reproductive hazard information database), Shepard's Catalog of Teratogenic Agents, and the Teratogen Information System (TERIS). All these sources review the human and animal literature for toxic effects of environmental chemicals and, for the latter three databases, drugs. Because of the scarcity of human data dealing with reproductive effects, it is important to know where this type of information can be obtained. In addition to the research databases listed, there are govern-ment-based efforts to evaluate the existing scientific literature with respect to reproductive hazards. In California, there is a state-mandated program that evaluates chemicals known to cause cancer or reproductive toxicity. As of December 2005, there were 59 pharmaceutical or environmental compounds determined to have male reproductive toxicity by this program (Table 26–2).

REFERENCES

California Environmental Protection Agency: Proposition 65 list of chemicals known to cause cancer or reproductive toxicity, www.oehha.ca.gov/prop65.html.

NIOSH, CDC: National occupational research agenda: Fertility and pregnancy abnormalities, www2.cdc.gov/nora/.

NIOSH, CDC: Registry of Toxic Effects of Chemical Substances (RTECS), www.cdc.gov/niosh/rtecs/default.html.

REPROTOX (reproductive hazard information), http://reprotox. org/.

Shepard's Catalog of Teratogenic Agents, http://depts.washington. edu/~terisweb/teris/.

Teratogen Information System (TERIS), http://depts.washington. edu/~terisweb/teris/ (both Shepard's catalog and TERIS are accessed via a common Web site).

Epidemiologic Studies

Well-conducted epidemiologic studies should provide the best means of evaluating whether a specific agent or group of agents adversely affects *human* reproduction and development. Human studies cannot be controlled, as can animal experiments, so certain criteria or a weight-of-evidence type of scheme often is used in evaluating whether a substance reasonably can be considered as having an adverse effect.

A. STUDY DESIGNS

The basic study designs used to examine the association of an exposure and possible outcomes include the cross-sectional, case-control, and cohort studies, which are discussed thoroughly in the Appendix. The cross-sectional design is the simplest and has been used often in occupational and environmental reproductive studies. If the mechanism of action is thought to be interference with spermatogenesis, this study design is useful because there is a relatively short 3-month lag period between exposure and abnormal health outcome. However, if direct germinal epithelium damage is being considered as the mechanism of action, there is potential selection bias because the population existing in the workplace at the time of study may not be representative of the workforce during the time of prior exposure. For example, testicular biopsy among the workers exposed to chronic and high levels of dibromochloropropane (DBCP) demonstrated tissue scarring. This could result in permanent decreased sperm concentration, even after exposure has ended. The case-control study is most appropriate for evaluating relatively rare diseases in large populations (e.g., birth defects or

Table 26–2. Chemicals known to cause male reproductive toxicity.[1]

Altretamine
Amiodarone hydrochloride
Anabolic steroids
Benomyl
Benzene
Bromacil lithium salt
1- and 2-Bromopropane
1,3-Butadiene
Cadmium
Carbon disulfide
Chlorsulfuron
Cidofovir
Colchicine
Cyclophosphamide (anhydrous or hydrated)
2,4-D-butyric acid
o,p'- and p,p'-DDT
1,2-Dibromo-3-chloropropane (DBCP)
Di-n-butyl 1 phthalate (BBP)
Di-n-hexyl phthalate (DnHP)
m-, o-, and p-Dinitrobenzene
Dinitrotoluene (2,4-, 2,6- and technical grade)
Dinoseb
Doxorubicin hydrochloride
Epichlorohydrin
Ethylene dibromide
Ethylene glycol (monoethyl ether, monomethyl ether, monoethyl ether acetate, and monomethyl ether acetate)
Ganciclovir sodium
Gemfibrozil
Goserelin acetate
Hexamethylphosphoramide
Hydramethylnon
Idarubicin hydrochloride
Lead
Leuprolide acetate
Myclobutanil
Nifedipine
Nitrofurantoin
Oxydemeton methyl
Paclitaxel
Quizalofop-ethyl
Ribavirin
Sodium fluoroacetate
Streptozocin (streptozotocin)
Sulfasalazine
Thiophanate methyl
Tobacco smoke (primary exposure)
Triadimefon
Uracil mustard

---

[1]Source: California Environmental Protection Agency: Proposition 65 list of chemicals known to cause cancer or reproductive toxicity, www.oehha.ca.gov/prop65.html.

childhood cancers). Because the outcome of interest is specified at the onset, the continuum of reproductive effects that may result from a given exposure cannot be evaluated. The cohort study is the preferred study design for most reproductive outcomes. A prospective cohort study allows specific measures of an exposure and potential confounders to be ascertained at the etiologically relevant time periods. In addition, a cohort design allows repeated test measurements (e.g., semen analysis) that tend to have relatively high individual variability.

The cohort and case-control studies are considered hypothesis-testing studies and usually are conducted after a possible association has been suggested by previous observations or a documented group exposure. For example, an acute clinician may recognize a series of cases that seem to have a factor in common. This situation is most likely to occur with a rare disease or new syndrome and was instrumental in identifying associations such as thalidomide and severe limb defects and diethylstilbestrol (DES) and vaginal clear-cell carcinoma. A reported cluster of adverse outcomes occurring in a group of people is a common way for environmental and occupational problems to be brought to attention, but such clusters often remain unexplained on further investigation.

Valuable data could be obtained from surveillance systems, but there are few established systems in place for adverse reproductive outcomes other than birth defects. Reasons for this include the fact that not all outcomes attract medical attention or require hospitalization (e.g., semen abnormalities, SABs, and subfertility). As a result, these outcomes are more difficult to ascertain and are associated with a smaller financial impact for society.

B. Exposure Assessment

Although the methods used to measure occupational or environmental exposure are beyond the scope of this chapter, a brief overview with issues specific to evaluating male exposure associated with reproductive outcomes is presented. In addition, it should be kept in mind that the exposures of three individuals may be involved (i.e., each parent and the embryo/fetus/offspring).

To affect fertility or spermatogenesis, an agent must reach the appropriate organs via the bloodstream (e.g., chemical agent) or physical change (e.g., radiation or excessive heat). Some chemicals react with the first tissues they encounter, such as the lungs or skin, and are not absorbed into the bloodstream unless they are ingested (e.g., acids, chlorine, and asbestos). Unless a chronic exposure results in a steady-state level in the body, the rapidity with which a substance is cleared also can affect its toxicity. Often these issues are beyond the scope of epidemiologic studies but should be considered within the overall body of evidence about the toxicity of a substance.

In epidemiologic studies, exposures can be ascertained from interviews, existing records, or biomarkers. If exposure history is obtained by retrospective interview, there is the possibility of biased recall among cases or misclassification because of a lack of monitoring records or diminished memory. Recall may be affected by changes in exposures. Ascertainment of current exposure status for cohort studies limits possible recall bias, but men may not be aware of all their exposures. In interview studies, asking one spouse about the other may not provide sufficiently accurate information. Also, obtaining residence at time of delivery many not reflect timing of importance for sperm development.

Existing records often do not provide detailed information but rather serve to group men broadly. For example, the residence listed on a birth certificate might be used to assign the likelihood of an environmental exposure. However, residence at delivery may not reflect residence of the father, nor does it account for individual differences, such as how much time is spent out of the area at work. Similarly, occupational registries may be used to group men by broad exposures, but specific work-site practices will be unknown. The most accurate occupational exposures would be obtained by an industrial hygienist, but such studies are also likely to cost more or be limited in sample size to allow for more detailed study.

Laboratory measurement of exposure may be done in a prospective study or on stored biologic samples and provides a quantification of exposure that is less likely to be biased. Techniques for measuring environmental levels have been developed for many agents, including radon, electromagnetic fields (EMFs), solvents, pesticides, metals, and dust levels. Measurements on biologic samples provide an indication of internal dose, which would be more biologically relevant. A number of difficulties can arise with these types of studies, including small sample size or selection bias owing to the higher costs and greater participation required of subjects. Sampling at one point in time may not reflect the critical exposure period, particularly if the substance is cleared rapidly.

As noted earlier, it is important to consider the timing of exposure in an epidemiologic study. An association with an exposure at the critical time is more relevant, and such information may be useful for excluding the possibility of a particular effect if the timing is wrong. In addition to timing, a dose-response relationship usually is examined.

In summary, exposure assessment in epidemiologic studies may involve problems with unknown exposure levels, unknown biologic indicators, poor sources of information on exposure, imprecise exposure timing, and multifactorial exposure sources.

C. BIOLOGIC OUTCOMES

There is variable quality in the detection and measurement of biologic endpoints for male reproductive toxicity studies. For specific male reproductive conditions and male-mediated reproductive outcomes, the range of conditions includes sexual dysfunction, endocrine changes, semen abnormalities, chromosomal anomalies, infertility, and abnormalities in the fetus and offspring. The spectrum of birth outcome endpoints is discussed in Chapter 25. Case ascertainment methods can include the following: birth certificates, hospital records, surveillance programs (e.g., birth defects registries), medical insurance forms, reproductive history questionnaires, and semen analyses. The latter two methods tend to be the most useful type of case ascertainment because of relatively more precise male information as opposed to the usually inadequate paternal information found in birth outcome records.

D. STATISTICAL ISSUES

For selected reproductive endpoints, the necessary number of study participants for adequate statistical power is shown in Table 26–3. One advantage of conducting studies of semen analysis is that relatively fewer participants are needed, and there is a direct measurement of the abnormality being studied (e.g., abnormal number, motility, and shape of sperm). It should be noted that the general population normal ranges for these semen endpoints are unreliable because of differences in laboratory proficiency and techniques. It is preferable to test for internal trend within a given worker group or community group or to obtain an appropriate control group. Although fewer participants are needed for semen studies, there may be a problem in selecting the most appropriate comparison group.

E. CONFOUNDING FACTORS

Potential confounders need to be considered in the evaluation of men exposed to occupational or environmental reproductive hazards. For a factor to be a confounder, it must be related to both the endpoint and the exposure in the study of interest. Lack of control for a known confounder in prior studies does not imply that the study is deficient if the investigators found that this factor did not act as a confounder in their study or had reason to believe that the factor would not be associated with the exposure of interest. Potential confounding factors in male reproductive studies include personal characteristics (e.g., paternal age), medical conditions (e.g., recent infection, trauma to the gonads, impaired autoimmune status, high fever, mumps orchitis, diabetes, prostatitis, varicocele, and hydrocele), drug use (e.g., marijuana, estrogen, chlorambucil, cyclophosphamide, and nitrofurantoin), and habits (e.g., tobacco

Table 26–3. Sample sizes needed to detect a relative risk of 2.0 among exposed and unexposed groups for selected reproductive endpoints (95% confidence level and 80% power).

Outcome	Estimated Prevalence in Unexposed Group[1]	Unit	Sample Size Needed		
			Exposed Group	Nonexposed Group	Study Total
Fetal loss (recognized spontaneous abortions + stillbirths)	15.0%	Pregnancies	133	133	266
Infertility	12.5%	Couples	167	167	334
Low birth weight	7.8%	Live births with known birth weight	290	290	580
Major congenital malformation	3.0%	Live births + fetal deaths	814	814	1628
Sperm with abnormal morphology	40.0%	Men	27	27	54

[1]Prevalence rates derived from estimated general population values in Table 26–1; and Lawson C: Occupational reproductive research agenda for the 3rd millennium. Environ Health Perspect 2003;111:584 [PMID: 12732741].

use, alcohol use, and frequent sauna or hot tub use). In addition, there is the possibility of a potential synergistic health effect from two or more coexisting exposure or risk factors. In conducting occupational studies, a potential confounder may be an environmental agent such as exposure to solvents, metals, pesticides, excess heat, ionizing radiation, and neurotoxins in nonworkplace settings. Conversely, one needs to assess workplace hazards when conducting community-based reproductive studies.

Selected Examples of Reproductive Hazards

Few chemicals have been studied adequately in terms of their reproductive effects. Most exposure standards are not based on reproductive effects. More evidence is available from animal than human studies, but direct extrapolation to the human cannot always be made. Although epidemiologic studies can be more difficult to interpret because of the methodologic issues described earlier, a number of potential reproductive or developmental hazards have been identified (Table 26–4). The agents that have been shown conclusively to be reproductive toxicants in humans (other than medications) are few and include DBCP, ionizing radiation, and lead.

The majority of toxic agents in Table 26–4 have been examined in occupational settings where exposures tend to be of higher concentrations than those encountered in the environment and relatively easier to document. In the literature, most occupational events

involving high-level exposures and documented adverse reproductive effects have occurred in male workers (e.g., dibromochloropropane and exogenous estrogens). In addition, known reproductive hazards have been encountered environmentally from long-term use and disposal by industry, as well as from acute releases.

A. DECLINING SEMEN QUALITY AND ENVIRONMENTAL FACTORS

Several studies have noted a historical decrease in sperm count, with one report providing data as far back as 50 years. Over time, the method for evaluating sperm count (unlike the other semen-quality parameters) has not changed and is thought to be less susceptible to chronologic changes in laboratory technique. However, most of these retrospective trend analyses have been conducted at fertility centers that include semen donors, vasectomy candidates, or infertility clinic patients and thus may not be representative of the general male population. Furthermore, geographic differences and lack of information for known risk factors usually are associated with these older studies. Despite these limitations, various studies demonstrate decreased sperm concentrations in many European countries and in various U.S. regions. The International Study of Semen Quality in Partners of Pregnant Women found significant differences in mean sperm count between men in Copenhagen, Paris, Edinburgh, and Turku, Finland. In the United States, a four-city prenatal clinic study (Los Angeles, Minneapolis, Columbia, Missouri, and New York City) is being conducted that uses identical clinical

Table 26–4. Established or highly suspect relationships between male reproductive abnormalities and selected environmental and occupational agents or processes, based on human studies.[1]

Agent	Oligospermia	Teratospermia	Asthenospermia	Hormonal or Sexual Dysfunction	Other Effects
Alcohol	X (azoospermia)				Testicular atrophy
Boron	X				
Bromine vapor	X	X	X		
2-Bromopropane	X (azoospermia)				
Cadmium					Decreased fertility
Carbon disulfide	X	X	X	X	
Carbaryl (Sevin)		X			
Chlordecone[2]	X	X	X		
Dibromochloropropane[2]	X (azoospermia)			X	Testicular atrophy
2,4-Dichlorodiphenoxy-acetic acid (2,4-D)	X (azoospermia)	X	X		
DDT (dichlorodiphenyl-trichloroethane)[2]					Found in semen of infertile men
Estrogens	X				
Ethylene dibromide[2]	X	X	X		
Ethylene glycol ethers (e.g., 2-ethoxyethanol)	X	X			
Heat, excessive	X		X		
Lead	X	X	X	X	
Manganese				X	
Mercury, inorganic	X	X	X	X	
Perchloroethylene			X		
Radiation, ionizing	X	X	X	X	
Radiation, microwave	X	X	X		
Styrene	X				
Toluene diamine & dini-trotoluene	X				
Vinyl chloride				X	
Process					
Greenhouse work	X	X			
Nuclear power plant cleanup (Chernobyl)	X	X	X	X	
Oral contraceptive man-ufacturing				X	
Plastic production (sty-rene & acetone)		X			
Welding		X	X		

[1]Compiled from multiple sources, including NIOSH, CDC: National Occupational Research Agenda: Fertility and Pregnancy Abnormalities; www.cdc.gov/nora/; and Kumar S et al: Occupational exposures associated with reproductive dysfunction. J Occup Health 2004;46:1 [PMID: 14960825].
[2]Use banned in the United States.

evaluation, data collection, and semen analysis techniques as the European study. Preliminary findings from the U.S. study show a significantly lower sperm count among fertile men in Columbia, Missouri, in comparison with those in the other three cities. It is interesting to note that Columbia is in a more agricultural area than the other cities. Possible explanations given for the lower sperm count include estrogen exposure in utero, diet, lifestyle factors, and environmental pollution as a result of the increased worldwide use of chemicals (especially compounds with estrogen-like activity; see Chapter 37). Further follow-up of these multicenter studies will help to better explain this difference.

B. DIBROMOCHLOROPROPANE

DBCP (1,2-dibromo-3-chlorporpane) is noteworthy for its role in the first documented outbreak of a male reproductive hazard in the workplace. DBCP is a nematocide that is associated with reproductive and developmental abnormalities in animals. These animal effects include oligospermia, asthenospermia, and testicular and seminiferous tubule atrophy. Workers exposed to DBCP in chemical production facilities have shown exposure-dependent testicular toxicity. The following associations have been noted in DBCP-exposed workers: azoospermia, oligospermia, increased plasma FSH levels, and histologic abnormalities of the testicular tissue (decrease or absence of germ cells in seminiferous tubules). Decreased fertility was experienced among workers with testicular changes, and the most extreme FSH elevations were found in workers who did not recover after a period of no exposure. Thus this compound represents one of the few well-established male reproductive toxicants and provided the stimulus for subsequent increased activity in male-mediated reproductive research in the work setting.

C. LEAD

Lead is one of the most studied occupational and environmental agents and has a broad range of effects on multiple organ systems. Male reproductive effects have been found with both organic and inorganic lead exposures. Organic lead compounds, unlike the inorganic form, can be absorbed dermally. Sexual dysfunction (e.g., decreased libido, abnormal erectile function, and premature ejaculation) has been noted in case reports after ingestion of fuels containing organic lead. A case series of tetraethyl lead–intoxicated men revealed reversible semen abnormalities: oligospermia, azoospermia, asthenospermia, and teratospermia. Inorganic lead case reports have noted decreased libido (including erectile problems) and abnormal ejaculations. Endocrine changes (decreased testosterone and increased LH levels) have been observed in clinic-based case series. In men not exposed to high levels of lead, detectable lead concentrations in sperm have been reported that are less than those found in whole blood but greater than those of serum.

Epidemiologic studies have used semen analyses to better quantify male reproductive outcomes. A cross-sectional survey of 150 male lead battery workers was conducted in Romania. Blood lead levels ranged from 23–75 µg/dL, with a mean lead exposure duration of 3.5 years. Oligospermia, asthenospermia, and teratospermia were noted in a dose-response fashion. There were certain methodologic problems with this study: (1) Both masturbation and coitus interruptus were allowed in semen collection. The latter method is not normally accepted because of the potential of semen mixing with the body fluids of the partner. (2) No environmental exposure data were presented. (3) The dose-response curve was constructed allowing multiple results from the same subject. And (4) the controls included 50 plant technicians and office workers who were not assessed for comparability. This study provided the basis for the consideration of reproductive effects in establishing the Occupational Safety and Health Administration (OSHA) lead standard.

Lead exposure was evaluated among 18 battery workers and 18 cement workers in Italy. There was a statistically significant decrease in median sperm count and an increase in the prevalence of oligospermia among the battery workers. Participation rates were low, with 47% for the exposed and 22% for the comparison group. The exposed group had a mean blood lead level (BLL) of 61 µg/dL and a mean zinc protoporphyrin (ZPP) level of 208 µg/dL. In contrast, the nonexposed group had a mean BLL of 18 µg/dL and a mean ZPP of 24 µg/dL. Oligospermia was noted at a BLL as low as 40 µg/dL.

In summary, semen abnormalities (i.e., oligospermia, asthenospermia, and teratospermia) have been detected in the blood lead range of 40–139 µg/dL. Also, hormonal disturbances have been documented for men at BLLs as low as 44 µg/dL (testosterone) and 10 µg/dL (FSH and/or LH).

D. ENDOCRINE DISRUPTORS

The term *endocrine disruptor* is used to refer to a variety of manufactured chemicals that may cause health abnormalities by interfering with the normal hormonal balance of humans or animals. The most commonly studied chemicals that may fit this category are polychlorinated biphenyls (PCBs), dioxins, and persistent pesticides. The four main disease categories attracting the most attention in endocrine disruptors research are reproductive, carcinogenic, neurologic, and immunologic health outcomes. Because of the complexity of the male reproductive system, each of these diseases may have an impact on this system.

There appears to be an increased incidence for endocrine-mediated cancers such as breast, testicular, and prostate tumors. Thus far no specific chemical has been identified as the cause for the increase in these tumors.

Current studies are concentrating on several suspect chemical groups that may act via an endocrine-mediated neurotoxicity: PCBs, dioxins, DDT, and other chlorinated pesticides and metals. It should be noted that for the male reproductive system to function normally, an intact neurologic system is necessary. Thus the results of these studies may have an impact on related reproductive research.

The suggestion of possible immunosuppression comes from the fact that certain endocrine disruptors (e.g., DES, PCBs, and dioxins) alter the types of lymphocytes present in the bloodstream. Laboratory animals and wildlife have demonstrated such changes in association with exposure to DES, PCBs, carbamate, organochlorine pesticides, and organic and heavy metals. As was noted earlier, infection and associated immunologic disturbances are considered a risk factor for male infertility.

There are well-documented reports of human reproductive effects (semen abnormalities) from exposure to endocrine disruptors. For example, kepone exposure at a U.S. pesticide factory led to workers with oligospermia. DES use during pregnancy can increase the incidence of nonmalignant genital abnormalities in both male and female offspring. Also, wildlife and experimental animals with offspring showing feminization, demasculinization, and abnormalities in sexual behavior and development demonstrate endocrine-disrupting chemicals in their environment. Further studies are being conducted to better understand this situation.

Phthalates represent a newer type of chemical being considered as an endocrine disruptor. The CDC National Report on Human Exposure to Environmental Chemicals has shown that urinary phthalate metabolites are detectable in the general population at all ages and in different regions of the country. Phthalates are used in the production of hundreds of items, such as food packaging, plastic clothing, personal care products, detergents, adhesives, and vinyl flooring. More recent research looked at boys aged 2–36 months old and found that concentrations of four phthalate metabolites (prenatal urinary monoethyl, mono-*n*-butyl, monbenzyl, and monoisobutyl phthalates) were inversely related to anogenital distance. Also, the median concentrations for each of the metabolites associated with short anogenital distance and incomplete testicular descent are below the corresponding median levels seen among women in the National Exposure Survey. Animal studies support this potentially hazardous human health effect. These preliminary results may suggest that current widespread exposure to phthalates may cause human male reproductive damage at levels found in the general population.

Another endocrine disruptor with possible male reproductive effects is 2,2'4,4'5,5'-hexachlorobiphenyl (CB-153). This chemical is a persistent organochloride pollutant and has been associated with decreased sperm motility among fishermen having a diet high in fatty fish. Although the association in this study was not statistically significant, there is much interest in evaluating any possible reproductive effect from this persistent environmental contaminant, as well as other categories of endocrine disruptors.

REFERENCES

Grajewski B et al: Occupational exposures and reproductive health. Birth Defects Res B Dev Reprod Toxicol 2005;74:157 [PMID: 15834899].

Kumar S et al: Occupational exposures associated with reproductive dysfunction. J Occup Health 2004;46:1 [PMID: 14960825].

Rignell-Hydbom A et al: Exposure to CB-153 and *p,p'*-DDE and male reproductive function. Human Reprod 2004;19:2066 [PMID: 15802324].

Swan SH et al: Decrease in anogenital distance among male infants with prenatal phthalate exposure. Environ Health Perspect 2005;113:1056 [PMID: 16079079].

Swan SH et al: Geographic differences in semen quality of fertile U.S. males. Environ Health Perspect 2003;111:414 [PMID: 12676592].

REPRODUCTIVE ASSESSMENT

The medical evaluation of the patient with a potential exposure to a reproductive hazard follows the traditional components of history taking, physical examination, and laboratory assessment with an emphasis on both health and exposure parameters. In addition, special consideration is needed in the assessment, communication, and management of reproductive risk for the patient, as well as possible environmental evaluation and sampling at the work site or other location of potential exposure.

Medical Evaluation

In the clinical setting, infertility is defined as an inability to conceive after 12 months of unprotected intercourse. It is estimated that the cause of infertility is related to male factors in 40% of the affected couples, female factors in 40–50% of the affected couples, and no known etiology in 10–20% of the affected couples. For the infertility and adverse pregnancy outcome workup, the female partner needs to be assessed concurrently (see Chapter 25). A full discussion of the diagnosis and treatment of various urologic and other related medical conditions is beyond the scope of this chapter. However, the following is a general overview of the types of evaluation techniques that can be used to assess the male reproductive system.

A. MEDICAL HISTORY

The patient interview should cover the following areas: demographic data (e.g., both maternal and paternal age if birth outcome is being assessed), general medical history (e.g., febrile illnesses, trauma, infections and structural abnormalities of the genitourinary system, and past surgeries), drug use (including medications, street drugs, alcohol, and tobacco), habits (e.g., sauna and hot tub use), work history, and reproductive history (e.g., past problems of infertility and pregnancies and birth outcomes for each sexual partner). It is important to ask about potential occupational and environmental exposure to any of the known or suspected reproductive hazards cited in Table 26–4. More complete details for an environmental and occupational history can be found in Chapter 2.

B. PHYSICAL EXAMINATION

This examination should focus on the physical integrity of the genital system to rule out any extraneous mass or abnormality and the presence of secondary sex traits (e.g., hair growth pattern and possible gynecomastia). A physical abnormality may impede spermatogenesis, ejaculation, and erection (e.g., varicocele, hydrocele, hypospadias, and cryptorchism). It is important to evaluate testicular size, prostate tenderness, and the presence of any structural anomalies. Testicular size averages 4.6 cm in length (range 3.5–5.5 cm) and 12–25 mL in volume, with the seminiferous tubules accounting for 95% of the testicular volume. Hypovirilization and infertility can indicate Klinefelter syndrome (47,XYY, often associated with small testes and occurring in 0.2% of adult men) or viral orchitis.

C. HORMONAL PROFILE

A number of hormonal tests are available, and selection needs to be based on the medical conditions under consideration. A preliminary hormonal profile that can be obtained for field surveys includes FSH, LH (pituitary function), and testosterone (testicular function). For field biologic monitoring surveys, blood samples are relatively easy to collect for hormonal assays, but care must be taken to obtain samples at standardized times to avoid diurnal variability problems. The FSH is increased in individuals with azoospermia, such as the DBCP episode. With a normal testosterone level and an increased FSH level, a decrease in spermatogenesis occurs, which is usually associated with severe germinal epithelium damage. If there is a sperm abnormality with normal LH and testosterone, then an obstruction to the reproductive system can be ruled out. If both LH and testosterone are low, then a hypothalamic or pituitary abnormality is likely. In the situation where low testosterone and high LH concentrations are seen, there is the possibility of a primary defect at the testicular level. When there is a high level of testosterone and a low level of LH, an autonomous or exogenous source of testosterone needs to be considered. Finally, having both LH and testosterone elevated would suggest an autonomous LH secretion or resistance to testosterone action. One additional hormone being studied for utility in screening situations is inhibin B, which is reduced when damage to the seminiferous tubules occurs.

D. SEMEN ANALYSIS

Analysis of semen parameters can be conducted by both traditional and computer-aided semen analysis (CASA) methods. The basic parameters of interest are ejaculate volume, sperm count or concentration, motility, morphology, swim velocity (direct measurement obtainable via CASA), and the presence of any suspect toxicant. The subsequent normal ranges discussed are to be used as general guidelines for the interpretation of a semen profile. There is much variability in the quality of semen analysis by laboratory, and the CASA may not be available at all reproductive/infertility laboratories. Because the normal ranges for semen characteristics may vary by laboratory, it is important to review the ranges provided by the laboratory being used.

The sperm concentration refers to the number of sperm per milliliter of ejaculate, with a normal level of more than 20 million per milliliter. Normal ejaculate volumes are 1.5–5.5 mL. Sperm motility is the percentage of motile sperm, with a normal sample showing greater than 40% motile sperm. Morphology refers to the percentage of normal (oval) and abnormal sperm head, midpiece, and tail shapes. The 10 general categories of sperm morphology are oval/normal, microcephalic, macrocephalic, tapered head, double head, headless, no head or tail, amorphous head, immature forms, and abnormal tails. Normal morphology is greater than 50% normally shaped sperm if using the World Health Organization (WHO) classification system and greater than 14 if using the stricter Kruger classification.

When semen analyses are used for epidemiologic or screening purposes, certain aspects need to be addressed. There is a need to conduct concurrent motility and count measures because most cells are nonmotile or poorly motile. Thus sperm count alone is not recommended. For count and motility, it is important to note the time since last ejaculation (48–72 hours maximum for accurate reading). Also, all semen analyses should be conducted at the same laboratory because of the high interlaboratory variability. Optimally, a semen sample should be analyzed within 1 hour of production so that the sperm remain viable for analysis. A standardized semen collection procedure needs to be established and followed by the individual being evaluated. Masturbation is recommended (preferably with no sexual partner, condom, or lubricant use), with the collection of semen in specially provided containers. It is extremely important that the entire volume of ejaculate be collected and that the specimen not be subjected to extreme temperatures in transport to the analysis site. Multiple samples from the same individual can show much variability; therefore, serial measurements are preferred. Most infertility evaluations involve three subsequent samples on separate days. Finally, there are three potential barriers to cooperation from individuals being recruited for participation in a study. (1) Highly motivated subjects are needed for the study, yet the individual is usually asymptomatic and may not understand the usefulness of an evaluation. (2) Religious and cultural taboos may be encountered. And (3) there may be a lack of available sperm because of a preexisting medical condition such as vasectomy.

E. OTHER TESTS

Other male reproductive tests are available for further clinical evaluation but are not usually included in epidemiologic field studies. These tests include GnRH challenge, thyroid profile, testicular biopsy, postcoital test, and sperm-oocyte interaction. Some more recent evaluation methods involve sperm DNA, chromosome and maturity bioassays, and biologic markers for fertilization function (e.g., sperm antigen). In azoospermia or severe oligospermia, a testicular biopsy can assess the seminiferous tubules and Leydig cell histology for fibrosis and lack of spermatogenesis. The postcoital test involves the interaction of sperm examined in mucus following intercourse. If the index sperm penetrates a donor mucus but not the sexual partner's mucus, the mucus of the sexual partner may be a problem. The patient's sperm is considered abnormal if no penetration of either mucus occurs. The sperm-oocyte interaction test uses the zona pellucida of a hamster oocyte to evaluate if the patient's sperm is able to fuse (the capacitation and acrosomal reaction needed for eventual conception). Antisperm antibodies on the sperm surface are a form of immunologic infertility and sometimes are a result of prior surgical reversal of a vasectomy. Furthermore, a wide range of medical tests and assays may be indicated for the underlying medical conditions thought to be present. Lastly, the assessment of body burden for certain exposures may be estimated via exhaled breath, blood, urine, semen, and other biologic tissue measurements.

To allow comparison among different studies, the WHO has published two manuals on a standardized approach to evaluating infertile men. One manual deals with the investigational process, diagnosis, and management of infertile males. Included are a patient data-collection form and a diagnostic decision flow diagram to facilitate the analysis of data between different clinicians. The laboratory manual describes procedures for examining human semen and provides lower limits for the normal range of various tests. These lower limits include 2.0 mL for semen volume, 20 million sperm per milliliter for concentration, and 40 million for number of sperm per ejaculate, 50% with progressive motility and 30% with normal morphology.

REFERENCES

Nallella KP et al: Significance of sperm characteristics in the evaluation of male infertility. Fertil Steril 2006;85:629 [PMID: 16500330].

World Health Organization: *WHO Laboratory Manual for the Examination of Human Semen,* www.who.int/reproductive-health/pages_resources/listing_infertility.en.html.

World Health Organization: *WHO Manual for Standardized Investigation, Diagnosis and Management of the Infertile Male,* www.who.int/reproductive-health/pages_resources/listing_infertility.en.html.

Occupational and Environmental Health Consultation

The health risk assessment process may prove to be difficult because of inadequate exposure or a lack of toxicologic or medical information. It is very helpful to have established professional contacts with expertise in occupational or environmental health consultation when a more difficult risk assessment is involved. Potential contacts may include local or state health departments, university medical centers or schools of public health, poison control centers, National Centers for Disease Control and Prevention (CDC, including the National Institute for Occupational Safety and Health and the National Center for Environmental Health), U.S. Environmental Protection Agency, Agency for Toxic Substances and Disease Registries, Occupational Safety and Health Administration, and the Association of Occupational and Environmental Clinics. Access to online literature databases also can be very useful such as REPROTOX and TERIS (see "Informational Sources" above for more details).

Communication Regarding Reproductive Hazards

There is an underlying principle that needs to be acknowledged and sensitively dealt with: The threat or actual fact of reproductive dysfunction or adverse reproductive outcome has a profound impact on an individual's life and his or her family. All questions must be answered truthfully and completely. A description of the limitations in knowledge may be needed. The timing of exposure for the male and of the first contact with the involved female partner is very important. Whenever possible, the risk communication is conducted prior to actual exposure in order to intervene at the primary prevention stage. The options available for the male worker should be presented in such a way that the medical impact and the economic consequences of decisions are understood and discussed. The medical confidentiality of the involved individual should be maintained at all costs. If an occupational situation, it is imperative that the employer, involved employee(s), and medical consultant work together in resolving a particular exposure, as well as in developing a general policy on reproductive hazards in the workplace that involves both genders. Ideally, this policy should be developed within a health and safety committee composed of representatives from management and labor and consultants in occupational medicine and industrial hygiene.

Recommendations for Controlling Exposure

In the evaluation of the patient, a clinician can play an important consultative role in the control or elimination of exposure in the home, workplace, or other site of high risk. Working with the key health personnel or public health officials involved in this process, the following actions may be considered for a given reproductive hazard situation:

A. EXPOSURE REDUCTION OR ELIMINATION

Replace hazards with safer ones; improved engineering controls, safer work practices, and personal protective equipment (this latter item should not be the primary mode of protection—emphasis should be placed on the other actions). Exposure reduction or elimination is the most desirable option and should be attempted in all situations where a reproductive hazard exists.

B. TEMPORARY JOB TRANSFER OR REMOVAL FROM AREA OF EXPOSURE

Remove the individual from work environment, residence, or other site where the reproductive hazard exists. This option is rarely considered for men considering having children. In occupational settings, problems may occur when there is no nonexposed job location. This option should be considered when there is a high-risk situation, and exposure reduction/elimination is not possible.

C. DISABILITY LEAVE IF OCCUPATIONAL EXPOSURE

This option usually is considered by the personal physician for the pregnant woman facing reproductive hazards and to our knowledge has not been used for men.

D. PERMANENT REMOVAL OF INDIVIDUAL FROM WORK OR EXPOSURE SETTING

This is the least desirable action in the occupational setting and has been used in the past for female workers. For female workers, it is illegal for an employer to terminate an affected woman because of pregnancy. An individual may choose to quit work for personal reasons, but it is impor-

tant to help the individual to evaluate all the other options and to understand the possible consequences. In the residential setting, there have been permanent relocation of populations owing to environmental contamination, but this is a rare occurrence. The permanent removal of an individual from a residence, work setting, or other exposure site is considered after all the other options have been explored and the individual is comfortable with the possible consequences.

LEGAL ISSUES & WORKPLACE STANDARDS

In the lawsuit International Union, UAW versus Johnson Controls, Inc., the U.S. Supreme Court held that an employer violated Title VII's ban on sex discrimination by excluding from production jobs in a lead-battery factory all women who could not prove their sterility. The Court indicated that a policy directed only at fertile women is overt discrimination on the basis of sex regardless of the scientific evidence of heightened safety concerns for mothers or potential mothers. In addition, any policies or actions taken by the employer must not violate existing laws prohibiting discrimination on the basis of pregnancy, childbirth, or related medical conditions. Employers cannot require that an individual be sterilized as a condition of employment. If an employee disabled by pregnancy, childbirth, or a related medical condition transfers to a less hazardous job, an employer must allow the employee to return to the employee's original job or a similar one when the disability has resolved. Thus the workplace must be made safe, and reproductive hazard information must be provided to both men and women.

OSHA has the mandate to promulgate standards that protect workers from adverse health effects (including reproductive effects) resulting from workplace hazards. However, there are only four agents with OSHA standards that are based partially on reproductive effects: dibromochloropropane (DBCP), lead, ethylene oxide, and ionizing radiation. It should be recognized that many chemical and physical agents found in the workplace are not covered by an OSHA standard and that those standards that do exist for the most part are not based on reproductive endpoints. This is why the risk assessment process discussed earlier should be implemented at any work site that has potential reproductive hazards present.

REFERENCE

NIOSH: Topics on reproductive health, http://www.cdc.gov/niosh/topics/repro.

SECTION IV
Occupational Exposures

Metals

Richard Lewis, MD, MPH

The diverse physical properties of metals have resulted in their extensive use in industry. These naturally occurring materials have long been recognized for their ability to impart a variety of valuable characteristics to finished goods. Metals are used in the construction, automotive, aerospace, electronics, glass, and other manufacturing industries. Metals are major sources of pigments and stabilizers for paints and plastics. Metals are also used as catalysts and intermediates in the chemical and pharmaceutical industries. Metals may be emitted as contaminants or by-products from industrial operations and power generation, and these have become the major sources of ongoing environmental contamination.

Metals are used rarely in their pure form, usually being present in alloys. They also may be bound to organic materials, altering their physical characteristics and potential toxicity. Some compounds, such as hydrides and carbonyls, are highly toxic and may be formed accidentally when the parent metal reacts with acids. Metals may be altered by burning and smelting or after uptake by biologic systems. The chemical structure of the metal or organometallic compound alters absorption, distribution, and toxicity.

Metals exert biologic effects chiefly through the formation of stable complexes with sulfhydryl groups, altering the structure and function of many proteins and enzyme systems. Certain metals, such as zinc, chromium, and manganese, are essential for normal metabolism. Others, such as lead, mercury, and arsenic, serve no recognized biologic purpose, raising public health concerns owing to their ubiquitous presence in living organisms. Understanding and eliminating health risks from low-level background exposures remains a top priority in environmental health.

General population exposure to many metals is related primarily to air, water, and food contamination. Background exposures vary considerably around the world owing to natural occurrence in soil and groundwater, as well as pollution from industrial operations, automotive exhaust, and power generation. Familiarity with the potential health effects of metals in different settings is critical not only for the health and safety professional but also for the general medical practitioner.

ACUTE METAL TOXICITY

Acute toxicity usually occurs after ingestion of metal-containing compounds or inhalation of high concentrations of metal dusts or fumes. These can arise from improperly ventilated burning or welding operations or from unexpected chemical reactions. Home remodeling activities can generate dust from paint pigments, particularly lead. This and ingestion of paint chips (*pica*) are important causes of childhood poisoning. Familiarity with the symptoms of acute heavy metal poisoning, along with an awareness of the potential sources of exposure, is critical for rapid detection and treatment. The levels of most metals can be measured in blood or urine to confirm the diagnosis and guide therapy.

CHRONIC METAL TOXICITY

Research into the health effects of low-level exposure to metals indicates that physiologic alterations occur at levels that have been considered safe previously. The evidence for neurotoxicity, circulatory effects, nephrotoxicity, reproductive toxicity, and carcinogenicity at low levels of exposure continues to grow. Regulatory agencies must consider these factors as they devise exposure standards that provide adequate margins of safety in protecting long-term population health. The challenge for physicians is to differentiate global public health issues from specific clinical concerns in individual patients.

ARSENIC

Essentials of Diagnosis

A. ACUTE EFFECTS

- Nausea, vomiting, diarrhea
- Intravascular hemolysis, jaundice, oliguria (arsine)
- Cardiovascular collapse
- Delayed, ascending peripheral neuropathy

B. CHRONIC EFFECTS

- Hyperkeratosis and hyperpigmentation (melanosis)
- Peripheral neuropathy
- Anemia
- Cardiac and peripheral vascular disease
- Skin and lung cancer, hepatic angiosarcoma

Exposure Limits

Arsenic

American Conference of Governmental Hygienists (ACGIH) threshold limit value (TLV): 0.01 mg/m^3 time-weighted average (TWA)

Occupational Safety and Health Administration (OSHA) permissible exposure level (PEL): 0.01 mg/m^3 TWA

National Institute of Occupational Safety and Health (NIOSH) recommended exposure limit (REL): 2 µg/m^3 ceiling (15 minutes)

Arsine

ACGIH TLV: 0.05 ppm TWA

OSHA PEL: 0.05 ppm TWA

NIOSH REL: 2 µg/m^3 ceiling (15 minutes)

ACGIH biologic exposure index (BEI): 50 µg/g creatinine

General Considerations

Arsenic occurs in numerous ferrous and nonferrous ores and in volcanic ash. Important industrial sources of exposure include smelting operations, pesticide use, and emissions from coal-fired power plants. Arsenic is ubiquitous in living organisms, although it is not an essential trace element for humans.

Pure elemental arsenic is relatively nontoxic. More common forms encountered from industrial uses include trivalent arsenic (AsIII) and pentavalent arsenic (AsV). Most of the reports of both acute and chronic toxicity of arsenic are attributable to arsenic trioxide, a trivalent form. Organic arsenic compounds, such as arsenobetaine, are found in many seafoods and are virtually nontoxic. In contrast, arsine gas (AsH_3) is highly toxic.

Use

Arsenic is used for hardening lead in battery grids, bearings, and cable sheaths. Arsenic trioxide and arsenic pentoxide are used in the manufacture of calcium, copper, and lead arsenate pesticides. Arsenic acid (AsV) is a common pesticide used on grapes and tobacco. Arsenic compounds are used as pigments and refining agents in glass and as preservatives in tanning and taxidermy. Copper-chromated arsenate (CCA) is a widely used wood preservative that imparts a green color to treated wood. Arsenic compounds are also used as herbicides and desiccants in cotton harvesting and in sheep and cattle dips. Potassium arsenite (Fowler solution) was used as a medicinal agent until the 1940s, and arsenic compounds still may be found in some folk remedies and health foods (e.g., kushtay and kelp). Arsanilic acid is used in veterinary pharmaceuticals and feed additives. Arsine gas and other arsenic compounds are used in the microelectronics industry as a source of dopant arsenic atoms and in the manufacture of gallium arsenide substrates.

Occupational & Environmental Exposure

Exposure to arsenic occurs in the smelting of lead, copper, gold, and other nonferrous metals. Readily volatilized arsenic trioxide is concentrated in flue dust and can be condensed and recovered in a cooling chamber. Furnace and flue maintenance operations carry a high risk of exposure. Arsenic also may be found in fly ash from coal boilers.

Pesticide manufacturers and applicators have the potential for significant arsenic exposure. Forestry and farm workers may be exposed to residual arsenic compounds after their use in the field. In the microelectronics and glass industries, workers may be exposed to arsenic from source materials, finished products, or maintenance operations. Arsine is used in semiconductor manufacturing and also may be formed accidentally when water or acid reacts with metal arsenides.

Background exposure to arsenic is primarily from the diet, although intake from water can be substantial in some regions. Average daily intake ranges from 10–50 µg/d. Dietary arsenic arises from pesticide residues and feed additives, particularly in pork and poultry products. Marine organisms accumulate and metabolize arsenic to organic forms that are generally excreted unchanged after consumption. In the United States, the drinking water standard for arsenic is 10 ppb; however, background levels in various parts of the world may exceed this by several orders of magnitude.

Nonoccupational arsenic poisoning has resulted from ingestion of contaminated well water, dried milk, soy sauce, and moonshine whiskey. Arsenic compounds may be used in intentional poisonings. Other sources of exposure include burning arsenic-treated wood, smoking treated tobacco, and drinking wine made from treated grapes. Pesticides, smelting, and coal burning are the primary sources of environmental contamination.

Absorption, Metabolism, & Excretion

Arsenic compounds may be absorbed after ingestion, inhalation, or skin contact. Arsenic is readily taken up by red blood cells and then deposited in the liver, kidney, muscle, bone, skin, and hair. Trivalent arsenic (+3) avidly binds to sulfhydryl groups and interferes with enzyme systems involved in cellular respiration, glutathione metabolism, and DNA repair. This binding leads to accumulation in hair and nails. Pentavalent arsenic (+5) and arsine are converted to trivalent arsenic in vivo. The majority of the absorbed trivalent arsenic is metabolized to dimethylarsinic acid (DMA) and monomethylarsonic acid (MMA) and excreted in the urine with a half-life of 10 hours. Organic arsenic compounds are excreted unchanged in the urine.

Clinical Findings

A. Symptoms & Signs

1. Acute exposure—Symptoms of acute arsenic poisoning may develop minutes to hours after ingestion and consist of nausea, vomiting, abdominal pain, and copious blood-tinged diarrhea. Cold, clammy skin, muscle cramps, and facial edema may be present. Seizures, coma, and circulatory collapse precede death. A dose of 120 mg arsenic trioxide may be fatal. Liver enlargement and oliguria also may occur.

Persons who recover may develop delayed peripheral neuropathy, presenting after several weeks as symmetric distal sensory loss. The lower extremities usually are more affected than the upper. Motor involvement extending to total paralysis also may occur.

Acute exposure to arsine results in intravascular hemolysis. Other complaints include headache, nausea, and chest tightness. Exposure to 10 ppm rapidly causes delirium, coma, and death. The triad of abdominal pain, jaundice, and oliguria should strongly suggest arsine exposure. Physical examination may reveal bronzing of the skin and hepatosplenomegaly.

2. Chronic exposure—Distal paresthesias or anesthesia indicate arsenic-induced peripheral neuropathy. In more severe cases, motor involvement may be evident as well, with weakness and reflex loss. Chronic exposure to arsine gas has been reported to cause a syndrome similar to arsenic trioxide. Symptoms of sore throat, cough, and phlegm production may be a result of chronic exposure to irritant arsenic dusts. Complaints of asthenia and fatigue may be a result of arsenic-induced anemia. Other reported effects include cardiac failure, liver disease, and renal disease. Environmental exposures have been reported to cause peripheral vasospasms and gangrene, termed *blackfoot disease*. This has not occurred in the occupational setting.

Dermatologic manifestations of chronic exposure to arsenic compounds are common, principally after long-term ingestion of arsenic in drinking water or for medicinal purposes. Arsenical keratoses are raised punctate or verrucous lesions occurring primarily on the palms and soles. Enlarging masses or ulcerations should suggest Bowen disease, basal cell carcinoma, and squamous cell carcinoma, which are all increased in persons with chronic arsenic exposure. In some individuals, a diffuse bronze hyperpigmentation develops, characterized by interspersion of 10-mm macules of hypomelanosis. Alopecia may occur. Some arsenic compounds may cause an irritant dermatitis as well. Cancers that have been reported in association with arsenic exposure include lung cancer, leukemia, lymphoma, and angiosarcoma of the liver. Arsenic crosses the placenta and may cause fetotoxicity, decreased birth weight, or congenital malformations.

B. Laboratory Findings

Acute and chronic exposure to arsenic may cause anemia and leukopenia, and arsine-induced hemolysis results in anemia, hyperbilirubinemia, and hemoglobinuria. Hematuria and proteinuria indicate renal injury. Liver damage may result in elevation of serum enzymes and bilirubin. The electrocardiogram (ECG) may reveal rhythm or conduction disturbances. Delayed sensory conduction velocities in a distal symmetric distribution may be seen on nerve-conduction studies.

Total urine arsenic levels are useful in confirming recent exposure. The measurement of DMA and MMA eliminate confusion with dietary sources of organic arsenic compounds. Nonexposed persons will have levels of less than 10 μg/g of creatinine. Workers exposed to 0.01 mg/m^3 will have levels of 50 μg/g of creatinine. Acute poisoning usually causes levels exceeding 1000 μg/g of creatinine. Hair and nail arsenic levels may be useful in detecting systemic absorption of arsenic, primarily from ingestion. These are also subject to external contamination and are of little use for monitoring exposed workers.

Tissue biopsy will confirm the diagnosis of skin or respiratory cancer. Careful medical and occupational histories are necessary to determine the relationship of these common cancers to arsenic exposure.

Prevention

The use of engineering controls to contain sources of exposure to arsenic compounds will reduce exposure in smelting, metallurgy, and pesticide manufacturing operations. Personal protective equipment should be worn when performing maintenance work or during application of arsenic compounds. Medical surveillance should concentrate on skin and respiratory complaints, as well as liver, hematologic, renal, and nervous system function. Biologic monitoring of arsenic in urine will complement industrial hygiene efforts to control exposure.

Treatment

Treatment following acute ingestion is by induced emesis followed by administration of activated charcoal and a cathartic. Shock is treated with aggressive intravenous fluid resuscitation and pressor agents as indicated. If the diagnosis is confirmed, therapy with dimercaprol, 3–4 mg/kg every 4 hours for the first 2 days, is administered. This should be continued at 3 mg/kg every 12 hours until urine arsenic is below 50 μg/d. Sources of further exposure should be eliminated after treatment.

Arsine poisoning requires careful monitoring of the hematocrit and renal function. Alkaline diuresis will reduce the precipitation of hemoglobin in renal tubules and the resulting renal impairment. Elevation of plasma-free hemoglobin greater than 1.5 mg/dL or oliguria is an indication for exchange transfusion. Hemodialysis is indicated if acute renal failure develops. Dimercaprol is not effective in arsine poisoning.

Prognosis

In acute arsenic poisoning, survival for more than 1 week is usually followed by complete recovery. Complete recovery from chronic arsenic poisoning may require 6 months to 1 year.

REFERENCES

Agency for Toxic Substances and Disease Registry: Toxicological profile of arsenic, www.atsdr.cdc.gov/toxprofiles/tp2.html.

Chen CJ et al: Biomarkers of exposure, effect, and susceptibility of arsenic-induced health hazards in Taiwan. Toxicol Appl Pharmacol 2005;206:198 [PMID: 15967209].

Duker AA et al: Arsenic geochemistry and health. Environ Int 2005;31:631 [PMID: 15910959].

Lee L, Bebb G: A case of Bowen's disease and small-cell lung carcinoma: Long-term consequences of chronic arsenic exposure in Chinese traditional medicine. Environ Health Perspect 2005;113:207 [PMID: 15687059].

Marcus S: Toxicity, arsenic, www.emedicine.com/EMERG/topic42.htm.

Schoen A et al: Arsenic toxicity at low doses: Epidemiological and mode of action considerations. Toxicol Appl Pharmacol 2004;198:253 [PMID: 15276404].

Sun G: Arsenic contamination and arsenicosis in China. Toxicol Appl Pharmacol 2004;198:268 [PMID: 15276405].

Tchounwou PB et al: Carcinogenic and systemic health effects associated with arsenic exposure: A critical review. Toxicol Pathol 2003;31:575. [PMID: 14585726].

BERYLLIUM

Essentials of Diagnosis

- Tracheobronchitis, pneumonitis
- Granulomatous pulmonary disease
- Dermatitis (ulceration and granulomas)
- Eye, nose, and throat irritation
- Lung cancer

Exposure Limits

ACGIH TLV: 0.2 μg/m^3
OSHA PEL: 2.0 μg/m^3
NIOSH REL: Do not exceed 0.5 μg/m^3

General Considerations

Beryllium is a lightweight gray metal with high tensile strength. It is extracted from beryl ore after grinding and heating using electrolytic reduction. Bertrandite (4BeO·2SiO$_2$·H$_2$O), although lower in beryllium content (0.1–3%), provides a source of acid-soluble beryllium that is extracted more easily.

Use

The unique properties of beryllium are ideally suited for the production of hard, corrosion-resistant alloys for use in the aerospace industry. Beryllium alloys (primarily copper) are used in tools, bushings, bearings, and electronic components. Beryllium is used in nuclear reactors as a neutron moderator and a fuel source. Beryllium oxide combines high thermal conductivity with high electrical resistance for use in ceramics, microwave tubes, and semiconductors. Beryllium had been used historically in the manufacture of fluorescent and neon lamps, leading to numerous cases of beryllium disease.

Occupational & Environmental Exposure

The health risks from exposure to beryllium vary based on the purity of the material and the particle size. Mining of beryl ore appears to result in a relatively low risk of berylliosis. In contrast, the purification and use of refined beryllium compounds, particularly beryllium oxide, continues to result in a substantial risk of sensitization and disease. The aerospace, nuclear, electronics, and beryllium alloy industries continue to search for methods of providing adequate worker protection. Exposure to minute, ultrafine particles, rather than total mass, may be the key factor in exposure and sensitization. Assessment and control of beryllium exposure remain challenging.

Absorption, Metabolism, & Excretion

Beryllium compounds are poorly absorbed after inhalation, ingestion, or skin contact. Beryllium may be retained in the lung or deposited in bone, liver, and spleen. Renal excretion is slow but may used to confirm exposure because levels usually are not detectable in nonexposed individuals. The development of berylliosis does not have a clear dose-response, suggesting that particle size and individual sensitivity are the key factors. Pathologically, beryllium toxicity is a systemic disease evidenced by the presence of noncaseating granulomas in numerous tissues, including lung, liver, skin, and lymph nodes.

Clinical Findings

A. SYMPTOMS & SIGNS

1. Acute or subacute exposure—Acute or subacute exposure to beryllium dusts or fumes has irritant effects on the eyes, mucous membranes, and respiratory tract. Burning eyes, sinus congestion, epistaxis, and sore throat may be presenting complaints. Affected tissues may be swollen, hyperemic, and ulcerated. Tracheobronchitis is characterized by cough, chest pain, and dyspnea. In severe cases, a chemical pneumonitis may develop, manifested by tachypnea, hemoptysis, cyanosis, and rales. Death has occurred as a result of pulmonary edema and respiratory failure.

2. Chronic exposure—Chronic berylliosis may develop after months or years of exposure or following a single acute exposure. Exertional dyspnea is the usual presenting complaint, often accompanied by fatigue, weight loss, cough, and chest pain. On physical examination, there may be rales, hepatosplenomegaly, lymphadenopathy, and clubbing. In long-standing cases, there may be evidence of pulmonary hypertension such as jugular venous distension, a right ventricular heave, and an accentuated P_2 on cardiac auscultation. Exacerbations of symptoms may occur following trauma, systemic illness, or pregnancy.

After skin contact, beryllium may cause an irritant or allergic dermatitis characterized by erythema, papules, and vesiculation. After penetration of the skin through a cut or abrasion, a granuloma might develop that can ulcerate through the skin surface. Beryllium compounds are animal carcinogens, and numerous studies suggest that workers are at an excess risk for developing lung cancer.

B. LABORATORY FINDINGS

In cases of acute pneumonitis, there is arterial hypoxemia with diffuse pulmonary infiltrates. Chronic beryllium disease may present with hypergammaglobulinemia, anemia, elevated liver enzymes, hyperuricemia, and hypercalciuria. Pulmonary function studies show either an obstructive or restrictive pattern. The first sign may be a drop in diffusing capacity. In contrast to sarcoidosis, serum angiotensin-converting enzyme levels usually are normal. Biopsy of affected tissues reveals noncaseating granulomas.

While skin testing can confirm hypersensitivity to beryllium, this carries a risk of sensitization. Bronchoalveolar lavage (BAL) may demonstrate lymphocyte alveolitis with an increase in T cells. The beryllium lymphocyte proliferation test (BeLPT) confirms sensitization. Radiographic findings include diffuse bilateral nodular or linear infiltrates, often with bilateral hilar adenopathy. Nodular densities suggestive of possible lung cancer need to be assessed carefully.

Prevention

While standard exposure control measures appear to be effective in the processing of beryl ores, prevention of berylliosis in other industry sectors remains a challenge. Standard medical surveillance should include periodic pulmonary function testing, including the diffusing capacity. BeLPT testing also should be conducted. The frequency should be adjusted to the experience of the operation, recognizing that sensitization can occur shortly after first exposure.

Treatment

Persons with beryllium disease should be removed from exposure. Treatment of acute pneumonitis should include supplemental oxygen and corticosteroids. Chronic beryllium disease also may respond to steroids, starting with prednisone, 60 mg orally daily, and tapering slowly. Skin lesions should be cleansed thoroughly and treated with topical steroids. The management of asymptomatic workers with a positive BeLPT test remains controversial.

Prognosis

Berylliosis is a chronic disease that may persist and progress even after cessation of exposure. Prevention and early detection are critical.

REFERENCES

Henneberger PK et al: Industries in the United States with airborne beryllium exposure and estimates of the number of current workers potentially exposed. J Occup Environ Hyg 2004;1: 648 [PMID: 15631056].

Schuler CR et al: Process-related risk of beryllium sensitization and disease in a copper-beryllium alloy facility. Am J Indust Med 2005;47:195 [PMID: 15712254].

Schuler CR et al: Process-related risk of beryllium sensitization and disease in a copper-beryllium alloy facility. Am J Ind Med 2005;47:195 [PMID: 15712254].

Stange AW et al: The beryllium lymphocyte proliferation test: Relevant issues in beryllium health surveillance. Am J Indust Med 2004;46:453 [PMID: 15490468].

Stanton ML et al: Sensitization and chronic beryllium disease among workers in copper-beryllium distribution centers. J Occup Environ Med 2006;48:204 [PMID: 16474270].

Welch L et al: Screening for beryllium disease among construction trade workers at Department of Energy nuclear sites. Am J Indust Med 2004;46:207 [PMID: 15307119].

CADMIUM

Essentials of Diagnosis

A. Acute Effects

- Chemical pneumonitis
- Renal failure

B. Chronic Effects

- Proteinuria
- Osteomalacia
- Emphysema
- Anemia
- Anosmia
- Lung cancer

Exposure Limits

OSHA PEL: 5.0 $\mu g/m^3$ 8-hour TWA

ACGIH TLV: 2.0 $\mu g/m^3$ 8-hour TWA

NIOSH REL: Reduce exposure to lowest feasible concentration

ACGIH BEI: 5.0 $\mu g/g$ of creatinine

General Considerations

Cadmium is a soft, silver-white electropositive metal that provides unique properties to metal coating, glass, paints, and pigments. Pure cadmium sulfide (greenrockite) is rare; however, cadmium is commonly present in zinc, lead, and copper ores. Cadmium is produced as a by-product of the smelting and refining of these ores and is recovered by electrolysis and distillation. Cadmium is a nonessential biologic contaminant.

Use

Cadmium compounds are used extensively in electroplating. Cadmium imparts corrosion resistance to steel, iron, and a variety of other materials for use in automotive parts, aircraft, marine equipment, and industrial machinery. Cadmium alloys are used in high-speed bearings, solder, and jewelry. Cadmium sulfides and selenides are used as pigments in rubber, inks, plastics, paints, textiles, and ceramics, particularly where heat stability and alkali resistance are desirable. Nickel-cadmium batteries are used in motor vehicles and rechargeable household appliances. Cadmium is also used in photoelectric cells and in semiconductors.

Occupational & Environmental Exposure

The recovery and refining of cadmium compounds are associated with potential exposure to high levels of both dusts and fume. Workers also may have exposure to cadmium in the smelting of zinc, lead, and copper. Cadmium plating is used to impart a protective coating for aerospace and other applications. Workers may be exposed to cadmium mist from plating baths, as well as to fine cadmium dust when handling or machining plated parts. Cadmium compounds are used in the manufacture of batteries, paints, and plastics. Welders and brazers may be exposed to cadmium oxide fumes when working with cadmium-containing silver solders.

Nonoccupational exposure occurs primarily through dietary intake. Liver and meat by-products, shellfish, and vegetables are potential sources of intake. Air and water contamination may be significant in areas surrounding zinc smelters. Irrigation of rice paddies with contaminated water in Japan led to an epidemic of osteoporosis in postmenopausal women (*Itai-Itai disease*) in the 1940s, demonstrating that environmental contamination can lead to significant health impact. Food also may become contaminated when stored in ceramic containers that have been glazed with cadmium. The tobacco plant accumulates environmental cadmium, and cigarette smoke is an important source of chronic cadmium exposure in humans.

Absorption, Metabolism, & Excretion

Cadmium is absorbed primarily through inhalation or ingestion. Skin absorption is negligible under ordinary circumstances. After inhalation, 10–40% may be absorbed, depending on particle size and chemical composition. Gastrointestinal absorption is usually 5% but may be increased in the presence of iron, protein, calcium, or zinc deficiencies.

Absorbed cadmium is bound to plasma proteins. Cadmium accumulates in the liver and kidneys, where intracellular binding to metallothionein protects against cellular damage. Liver stores are released slowly and taken up by the kidney. There is a gradual increase in the body burden of cadmium, peaking at age 60 years.

Excretion is primarily renal, with a biologic half-life of 8–30 years. Transient peaks in urinary excretion also may occur after short-term, high-dose exposure. Renal excretion of cadmium increases after chronic exposure

Table 27–1. Biologic monitoring program for cadmium.

Actions	Biologic Monitoring Result
Annual biologic monitoring Medical examination every 2 years	Urine cadmium < 3 μg/g creatinine β_2-Microglobulin < 300 μg/g creatinine Cadmium in blood < 5 μg/L whole blood
Semiannual biologic monitoring Medical examination annually Exposure assessment Exposure control	Urine cadmium 3–7 μg/g creatinine β_2-Microglobulin 300–750 μg/g creatinine Cadmium in blood 5–10 μg/L whole blood
Mandatory removal Medical examination Exposure assessment	Urine cadmium > 7 μg/g creatinine β_2-Microglobulin > 750 μg/g creatinine Cadmium in blood > 10 μg/L whole blood

because of impaired proximal tubular reabsorption, a manifestation of cadmium-induced nephrotoxicity.

Clinical Findings

A. SYMPTOMS & SIGNS

1. Acute exposure—Acute inhalation of cadmium oxide fume has resulted in industrial fatalities. After a delay of several hours, victims complained of sore throat, headache, myalgias, nausea, and a metallic taste. Fever, cough, dyspnea, and chest tightness progress to a fulminant chemical pneumonitis and death from respiratory failure. Hepatic and renal injury also may occur following acute exposure. Ingestion of cadmium compounds results in nausea, vomiting, headache, abdominal pain, liver injury, and acute renal failure.

2. Chronic exposure—The most frequent manifestation of chronic exposure to cadmium is proteinuria. Initially, there is increased excretion of low-molecular-weight proteins, such as β_1- and β_2-microglobulins. With continued exposure, this can progress to Fanconi syndrome, with aminoaciduria, glycosuria, hypercalciuria, and phosphaturia. Cadmium-induced renal failure may be difficult to distinguish from diabetic nephropathy. Renal tubular dysfunction can result in nephrolithiasis and osteomalacia. Bone pain and pathologic fractures may occur owing to renal calcium and phosphorus loss and impaired synthesis of vitamin D. Chronic inhalation of cadmium dusts and fumes also may result in pulmonary fibrosis and emphysema. Other effects that have been reported include anosmia and anemia. Cadmium is potentially neurotoxic and also may cause testicular injury. Cadmium is a human carcinogen and is associated with an excess risk of lung cancer and prostate cancer.

B. LABORATORY FINDINGS

1. Acute inhalation—Evaluation of acute inhalations should include an arterial blood gas evaluation, a chest radiograph, spirometry, and assessment of renal and hepatic function. Hypoxemia, diffuse pulmonary infiltrates, and a reduction in forced expiratory volume in 1 second (FEV_1), forced vital capacity (FVC), and diffusing capacity for carbon monoxide indicate acute cadmium oxide exposure and impending respiratory failure. In subacute cases, bronchopneumonia may develop. Normal blood and urine cadmium levels are 1 μg/L and 1 μg/g of creatinine, respectively. After acute cadmium fume inhalation, these may rise as high as 3 and 0.36 mg/L.

2. Chronic exposure—Workers exposed to cadmium should participate in periodic biologic monitoring and medical examinations. The biologic monitoring should include urine and blood cadmium levels, as well as measurement of urinary β_2-microglobulin levels. Tables 27–1 and 27–2 summarize the requirements of the programs for cadmium-exposed workers in the United States.

Table 27–2. Medical examination for cadmium workers.

Medical and occupational history
Focusing on cadmium exposure; smoking; renal, cardiovascular, musculoskeletal, and respiratory conditions; reproductive concerns; use of nephrotoxic medications, recent physical exercise, recent febrile illnesses
Physical examination
Blood pressure, respiratory system, genitourinary system, prostate examination (men older than age 40 years), respirator medical clearance
Diagnostic testing
Pulmonary function testing
Chest radiograph
Complete blood count
Blood urea nitrogen, creatinine
Urinalysis, urinary protein measurement

β_1- and β_2-microglobulin levels are a sensitive indicator of cadmium nephrotoxicity, although exercise, febrile illness, nephrotoxic medications, and other kidney disorders also may affect these tests. A loss of sense of smell, mild anemia, and airway obstruction also may be observed in workers with chronic exposure.

Prevention

Processes that result in the production of cadmium oxide fumes should be enclosed. Local exhaust ventilation and personal protective measures should be used to minimize exposure to cadmium dusts. Strict attention to workplace and personal hygiene are critical to prevent chronic exposure. Smoking must be prohibited in work areas that use cadmium. Welding on cadmium-treated metal or brazing with cadmium solders should be performed only in areas that are properly ventilated. Air-supplied respirators must be used in enclosed spaces.

Biologic monitoring should focus on the minimizing cadmium exposure to prevent proteinuria. Urine cadmium levels should be kept below 3 μg/g of creatinine to prevent chronic renal damage. Because of the long half-life of cadmium, the ongoing protection of workers who have heavy past exposure is difficult using biologic monitoring.

Treatment

Persons who have suffered acute inhalation of cadmium oxide fumes should be thoroughly evaluated for evidence of acute lung injury. Admission to the hospital for observation is indicated because respiratory support may be required. In severe acute poisoning, chelation with calcium disodium edetate (CaNa$_2$ EDTA) may enhance cadmium excretion. Renal function should be monitored closely. Dimercaprol should not be used. Individuals with evidence of chronic cadmium toxicity should be removed from further exposure.

REFERENCES

Il'yasova D, Schwartz GG: Cadmium and renal cancer. Toxicol Appl Pharmacol 2005;207:179 [PMID: 16102569].

Jarup L, Alfven T: Low level cadmium exposure, renal and bone effects: The OSCAR study. Biometals 2004;17:505 [PMID: 15688854].

Kazantzis G: Cadmium, osteoporosis and calcium metabolism. Biometals 2004;17:493 [PMID: 15688852].

Sahmoun AE et al: Cadmium and prostate cancer: A critical epidemiologic analysis. Cancer Invest 2005;23:256 [PMID: 15945511].

Trzcinka-Ochocka M et al: The effects of environmental cadmium exposure on kidney function: The possible influence of age. Environ Res 2004;95:143 [PMID: 15147919].

Wu X et al: Lack of reversal effect of EDTA treatment on cadmium induced renal dysfunction: A fourteen-year follow-up. Biometals 2004;17:435 [PMID: 15259364].

CHROMIUM

Essentials of Diagnosis

- Sinusitis, nasal septum perforation
- Allergic and irritant dermatitis, skin ulcers
- Respiratory irritation, bronchitis, asthma
- Lung cancer

Exposure Limits

Chromium metal
  ACGIH TLV: 0.5 mg/m^3 TWA
Chromium(III) compounds
  ACGIH TLV: 0.5 mg/m^3 TWA
Chromium(VI) compounds
  OSHA PEL: 5.0 μg/m^3 TWA
  ACGIH TLV: 0.05 mg/m^3 TWA (soluble)
  ACGIH TLV: 0.01 mg/m^3 (insoluble)
  NIOSH REL: 1 μg/m^3 TWA
  ACGIH BEI: 30 μg/g of creatinine (end of week/end of shift)

General Considerations

Chromium is a hard, brittle gray metal that is widely distributed as chromite (FeOCr$_2$O$_3$) or ferrochromium. Chromite is extracted through both underground and open-cast mining. Chromium metal is produced through reduction of chromic oxide with aluminum. Chromates are produced by high temperature roasting of chromite in an oxidizing atmosphere. The valence state is a critical factor in determining the toxicity of chromium compounds. Hexavalent chromium [Cr(VI)] is the most toxic and is carcinogenic. In contrast, trivalent chromium [Cr(III)] is an essential element for normal glucose metabolism in humans.

Use

Chrome plating is used on automotive parts, household appliances, tools, and machinery, where the coating imparts corrosion resistance and a shiny, decorative finish. Chromium-iron alloys alone or with the addition of nickel or manganese produce a variety of durable, high-strength stainless steels. Chromium compounds also provide heat resistance in refractory materials. Chromate pigments and preservatives are added to paints, dyes, textiles, rubber, plastics, and inks. Chrome-based implantable orthopedic devices are used for joint replacement. The radioisotope ^{56}Cr is used in nuclear medicine to label erythrocytes.

Occupational & Environmental Exposure

Mining and crushing operations result in exposure primarily to chromic oxide. The greatest occupational hazards historically have been in chromate production, where exposure to Cr(VI) resulted in a high incidence of lung cancer. Exposure to chromium fumes occurs in the production of stainless steel. Arc welding of stainless steel also results in exposure to chromium compounds. Electroplaters are exposed to chromic acid mists. Erosion of the nasal septum was a common finding in chrome platers before the implementation of proper ventilation. Workers also may be exposed to chromates through their use in the paint, textile, leather, glass, and rubber industries and in lithography, printing, and photography. Certain cements have a high chromium content. Chromium is found in low concentrations in water, urban air, and a variety of foods. Chromium in jewelry is a common cause of skin allergies.

Absorption, Metabolism, & Excretion

Chromium compounds may be absorbed after ingestion, inhalation, or skin contact. The soluble Cr(VI) forms are absorbed much more readily than the insoluble trivalent forms. Cr(VI) readily enters cells, where it is converted to Cr(III). Intracellular Cr(III) binds to proteins and nucleic acids. Ingested Cr(III) is absorbed less readily and crosses into cells much more slowly. Chromium generally does not accumulate in tissues, although inhaled insoluble forms may remain in the lung. Excretion is primarily renal.

Clinical Findings

A. SYMPTOMS & SIGNS

Acute exposure to high concentrations of chromic acid or chromates will cause immediate irritation of the eye, nose, throat, and respiratory tract. Chronic exposure may cause ulceration, bleeding, and erosion of the nasal septum. Cough, chest pain, and dyspnea may indicate exposure to irritant levels of soluble chromium compounds or the development of chromium-induced asthma.

Dermatologic manifestations are common in chromium workers. Penetration of the skin will cause painless erosive ulceration (*chrome holes*) with delayed healing. These occur commonly on the fingers, knuckles, and forearms. Localized erythematous or vesicular lesions at points of contact or generalized eczematous dermatitis should suggest sensitization.

Ingestion of chromium compounds has caused nausea, vomiting, abdominal pain, and prostration. Death is a result of uremia.

Chromium is a proven human carcinogen. Workers involved in chromate production, chrome plating, and chrome alloy work all have been found to have an increased incidence of lung cancer. The carcinogenicity of chromium compounds is attributed to Cr(VI).

B. LABORATORY FINDINGS

With massive exposure, there will be evidence of renal and hepatic damage. Proteinuria and hematuria precede anuria and uremia. A reduction in the FEV_1:FVC ratio on spirometry may be seen after acute irritant exposure or in workers with chromium-induced asthma. Skin allergy can be confirmed by patch testing. Persistent cough, hemoptysis, or a mass lesion on chest radiograph in a chromium worker should prompt a thorough evaluation for possible lung cancer.

Prevention

Reduction of exposure to Cr(VI) will reduce the respiratory and nasal complications. Surveillance for nasal irritation or septal perforation will identify high-risk jobs to direct exposure-control efforts. Avoidance of skin contact—particularly contact with damaged or inflamed skin—will reduce the risk of developing chrome ulcers or skin sensitization. Prompt evaluation for skin sensitization will prevent the development of severe or chronic dermatitis.

Exposure to Cr(VI) should be reduced to the lowest feasible levels to reduce the risk of lung cancer. Chromium workers also should be encouraged to stop smoking. Biologic monitoring of urine chromium levels may be useful as an assessment of recent exposure. Exposure to 0.05 mg/m^3 of Cr(VI) in air will result in levels of 30–50 µg/g of creatinine at the end of the workweek.

Treatment

Persons who have suffered acute inhalation injury should be admitted to the hospital for observation. Supplemental oxygen and bronchodilators may be required. Careful attention to fluid and electrolyte balance is indicated in the setting of acute renal injury. Chromium-induced nasal and skin ulcerations should be treated with a 10% ointment of CaNa$_2$ EDTA and an impervious dressing with frequent application to prevent formation of persistent, insoluble Cr(III). Persons who develop chromium respiratory or skin allergy should be removed from further exposure if they cannot be protected adequately.

REFERENCES

Birk T et al: Lung cancer mortality in the German chromate industry, 1958 to 1998. J Occup Environ Med 2006;48:426 [PMID: 16607199]

Goon AT, Goh CL: Metal allergy in Singapore. Contact Dermatitis 2005;52:130 [PMID: 15811025].

Halasova E et al: Lung cancer in relation to occupational and environmental chromium exposure and smoking. Neoplasma 2005;52:287 [PMID: 16059643].

Luippold RS et al: Low-level hexavalent chromium exposure and rate of mortality among US chromate production employees. J Occup Environ Med 2005;47:381 [PMID: 15824629].

Nurminen M: On the carcinogenicity risk assessment of chromium compounds. Am J Indust Med 2004;45:308 [PMID: 14991859].

Park RM et al: Hexavalent chromium and lung cancer in the chromate industry: A quantitative risk assessment. Risk Anal 2004;24:1099 [PMID: 15563281].

LEAD

Essentials of Diagnosis

A. INORGANIC: ACUTE EFFECTS

- Abdominal pain (colic)
- Encephalopathy
- Hemolysis
- Acute renal failure

B. INORGANIC: CHRONIC EFFECTS

- Fatigue and asthenia
- Arthralgias and myalgias
- Hypertension
- Anemia
- Peripheral neuropathy (motor)
- Neurobehavioral disturbances and chronic encephalopathy
- Impaired fertility
- Gout and gouty nephropathy
- Chronic renal failure

C. ALKYL LEAD COMPOUNDS

- Fatigue and lassitude
- Headache
- Nausea and vomiting
- Neuropsychiatric complaints (memory loss, difficulty in concentrating)
- Delirium, seizures, coma

Exposure Limits

Lead, inorganic, dusts, and fumes
  ACGIH TLV: 0.05 mg/m^3 TWA
  OSHA PEL: 0.05 mg/m^3 TWA
  ACGIH BEI: 30 µg/dL whole blood
Tetraethyl lead
  ACGIH TLV: 0.1 mg/m^3 TWA (skin)

General Considerations

Lead is a soft, malleable, blue-gray metal characterized by high density and corrosion resistance. The ores of commercial interest include the sulfide (galena), the carbonate (cerussite), and the sulfate (anglesite). Lead is concentrated through flotation and smelted in a three-step process: blending, sintering, and furnace reduction. Raw lead is further refined to remove copper, arsenic, antimony, zinc, tin, bismuth, and other contaminants. Much of the lead produced today is recovered from secondary sources of lead scrap.

Lead serves no useful biologic function in humans. The release of lead into the environment from automobile emissions, lead-based paint, incineration of waste containing lead additives, and the burning of coal—and its subsequent bioaccumulation—has had profound public health implications. There continues to be new evidence for physiologic alterations and potential health effects with low levels of lead exposure and a "normal" body burden of lead. The "safe" level of lead exposure is constantly being reassessed to protect the health of workers and the general public, particularly children.

Use

The primary use of lead is in storage batteries. Lead is also used widely in plastics and rubber materials in pipes and cable sheathing. Electrical solder and yellow traffic paint contain lead. Lead glazes impart brilliance and hardness to ceramics. Lead compounds still may be found in crayons and art supplies, and it is a frequent contaminant of herbal remedies. Lead is used in cosmetics, munitions, glassware, and jewelry. Lead is used in construction for attenuation of sound and vibration and for radioactive shielding. Tetraethyl lead and tetramethyl lead are used primarily as antiknock agents in gasoline, a practice that is still common in many areas in the world.

Occupational & Environmental Exposure

Inhalation of lead fume during burning or sintering operations is the most common source of acute occupational poisoning. Burning of lead-based paints during home remodeling can result in similar intense exposures. Chronic lead exposure is usually a combination of inhalation and ingestion of lead dust. Exposure is a constant hazard in lead reclaiming operations and in the manufacture of lead batteries. Paint and plastic manufacturers also may handle lead compounds, added as stabilizers and pigments. Welders and brazers may be exposed to lead alloys, fluxes, and coatings. Workers in munitions plants and police and military personnel may have exposure to lead dust, particularly in poorly ventilated indoor firing ranges. Glassmakers, artists, and pottery workers unknowingly may be exposed to high levels of lead in pigments and glazes.

Environmental exposure may occur near lead smelters or incinerators as a result of air, soil, and water contamination. Urban residents have exposure to lead from automobile exhausts. Ingestion of moonshine whiskey and the drinking of acidic beverages in improperly fired ceramics glasses are other sources of ingestion.

Herbal remedies, lead-based cosmetics, gasoline sniffing, and retained bullets are less conventional sources of lead poisoning. Lead contamination of tap water from lead pipes is an important source of lead exposure in many older homes.

The primary source of lead exposure for children is house dust. Lead contamination may arise from slow decay of lead-based paint, particulate from automobile emissions, or contaminated soil tracked into the home. Standard vacuuming only serves to distribute fine lead particles throughout the residence. Children, particularly crawling toddlers, are exposed by placing contaminated fingers or objects into their mouths. Home remodeling, including sanding and burning of lead paint, causes significant internal contamination and is an important cause of acute poisoning in children.

Absorption, Metabolism, & Excretion

Inhalation and ingestion are the primary routes of absorption. Approximately 40% of inhaled lead oxide fume is absorbed through the respiratory tract. Respiratory absorption of particulate lead dust is enhanced with fine particle size and solubility. Roughly 5–10% of ingested lead compounds are absorbed from the gastrointestinal tract. Iron and calcium deficiencies and high-fat diets may increase the gastrointestinal absorption of lead. Gastrointestinal absorption is greater in infants and children than in adults.

In the bloodstream, the majority of the absorbed lead is bound to erythrocytes. The free diffusible plasma fraction is distributed to brain, kidney, liver, skin, and skeletal muscle, where it is readily exchangeable. The concentrations in these tissues are highest with acute, high-dose exposure. Lead crosses the placenta, and fetal levels correlate with maternal levels. Bone constitutes the major site of deposition of absorbed lead, where it is incorporated into the bony matrix similar to calcium. The lead in dense bone is only slowly mobilized and gradually increases with time.

Intracellularly, lead binds to sulfhydryl groups and interferes with numerous cellular enzymes, including those involved in heme synthesis. This binding accounts for the presence of lead in hair and nails. Lead also binds to mitochondrial membranes and interferes with protein and nucleic acid synthesis.

Excretion is slow over time, primarily through the kidney. Fecal excretion, sweat, and epidermal exfoliation are other routes of excretion. Blood lead levels decline with a half-life of 60 days, although the biologic half-life of stored lead is much longer, estimated to be 5–10 years. This varies with the intensity and duration of exposure and the total-body burden. Aging, bone diseases (osteoporosis, fractures), pregnancy, and hyperthyroidism all

lead to mobilization of bone lead, increasing blood lead levels and potentially causing toxicity.

Water-insoluble alkyl lead compounds are absorbed readily through skin contact, inhalation, and ingestion. Tetraethyl and tetramethyl lead are converted to the trialkyl metabolites that are responsible for toxicity. The fat solubility of these compounds accounts for their accumulation in the central nervous system. Alkyl lead compounds ultimately are converted to inorganic lead and excreted in the urine.

Clinical Findings

A. Symptoms & Signs

1. Inorganic lead—

a. Acute exposure—After acute or subacute exposure to lead through either ingestion or inhalation, the presenting symptoms usually are gastrointestinal. Cramping, colicky abdominal pain, and constipation often are present early. Abdominal pain may be severe, suggesting biliary colic or appendicitis. Nausea, vomiting, and black, tarry stools also may accompany the acute presentation.

Headache and fatigue are common complaints. The more severe neurologic manifestations of lead encephalopathy, confusion, coma, and seizures are more common in children. Funduscopic examination may reveal papilledema or optic neuritis. In severe cases, oliguria and acute renal failure may develop rapidly.

b. Chronic exposure—In the occupational setting, chronic lead intoxication is a slow, insidious disease with protean manifestations. Fatigue, apathy, irritability, and vague gastrointestinal symptoms are early signs of chronic lead intoxication. Arthralgias and myalgias may involve the extremities of axial structures. As exposure continues, central nervous system symptoms progress, with insomnia, confusion, impaired concentration, and memory problems. Long-term exposure can lead to a distal motor neuropathy presenting with wrist drop. Progression to frank lead encephalopathy with seizures and coma is rare in adults but may occur.

Other presenting symptoms include loss of libido and infertility in men and menstrual disturbances and spontaneous abortion in women. Hypertension and elevated blood pressure readings have been associated with increased blood lead levels. Gouty arthritis and nephropathy also have associated with chronic lead exposure.

Physical examination may reveal pallor owing to anemia. Jaundice may be present in the setting of acute hemolysis. A blue-gray pigmentation (*lead line*) may be present on the gums. Neurologic examination may reveal weakness, particularly of the distal extensor muscles.

In men, lead also may affect spermatogenesis. Lead crosses the placenta, and both maternal exposure and release of bone lead stores can result in fetal exposure and neurotoxicity.

2. Alkyl lead—The presenting symptoms of alkyl lead intoxication are neurologic. Anorexia, insomnia, fatigue, weakness, headache, depression, and irritability are early symptoms. These progress to confusion, memory impairment, excitability, dysesthesias (e.g., insects crawling on the body), mania, and toxic psychosis. In severe cases, delirium, seizures, coma, and death may occur in several days.

B. LABORATORY FINDINGS

Blood lead levels are an indication of recent exposure (days or weeks). Whole blood lead levels in nonexposed individuals range from 1–5 μg/dL. The correlation of blood lead levels with symptoms depends on the duration and intensity of exposure. A new worker with high-level exposure may have symptoms with lead levels of 30–60 μg/dL, whereas long-term workers may be asymptomatic with levels greater than 80 μg/dL. In adults, subtle effects of lead on the central and peripheral nervous systems may occur with levels between 30 and 50 μg/dL. In the United States, the OSHA standard requires that lead levels be maintained below 40 μg/dL. The Centers for Disease Control and Prevention (CDC) recommends that the lead levels of children be below 10 μg/dL; however, ongoing research suggests that this may not be protective for the developing nervous system.

Anemia is a frequent manifestation of lead intoxication in children but is unusual in adults. The anemia is usually normochromic. Increased red cell turnover and frank hemolysis may be present, with basophilic stippling of the red blood cells and reticulocytosis. Altered heme synthesis, evidenced by an increase in protoporphyrin—measured as either free erythrocyte protoporphyrin (FEP) or zinc protoporphyrin (ZPP)—begins when blood lead levels exceed 40 μg/dL.

Proximal renal injury may result in Fanconi syndrome, with aminoaciduria, glycosuria, and phosphaturia. Impaired uric acid excretion results in hyperuricemia. Elevations of blood urea nitrogen (BUN) and serum creatinine indicate impaired renal function. Liver involvement may be suggested by mild elevations of serum aminotransferases. Nerve-conduction studies may reveal delayed motor-conduction velocities even without overt peripheral neuropathy. Neuropsychiatric evaluation may reveal evidence of intellectual impairment and behavioral alterations.

In the past, a CaNa$_2$ EDTA lead mobilization test was used to assess lead in individuals with normal blood lead levels. The test will confirm past lead exposure (postchallenge levels > 350 μg/L) but is still only indirect evidence of lead toxicity. Chronic exposure to lead is perhaps best assessed by K-band x-ray fluorescence of bone.

Prevention

Workplace hygiene is critical in the prevention of excessive lead exposure. Clean areas for eating should be provided. Showering and cleaning of work garments are mandatory and should be provided at the plant to prevent exposure of children in the home. For processes that have the potential for generation of airborne dusts and fumes, respiratory protection must be provided.

Medical surveillance (required under the OSHA Lead Standard for workers exposed to air levels greater than 30 μg/m^3) includes the following:

Whole blood lead levels:

1. Every 6 months if less than 40 μg/dL
2. Every 2 months if greater than 40 μg/dL until two consecutive determinations are less than 40 μg/dL
3. Monthly during medical removal from exposure

Medical examinations (Table 27–3):

1. Yearly, if any blood lead level exceeded 40 μg/dL
2. Prior to assignment
3. Whenever a worker develops signs or symptoms or lead toxicity

Removal from exposure to lead:

1. Workers whose lead levels exceed 60 μg/dL
2. Workers whose average lead levels exceed 50 μg/dL
3. Workers at risk of health impairment

Workers may be returned to exposure if two consecutive blood lead levels are less than 40 μg/dL.

Table 27–3. Medical examination of lead-exposed workers.

Medical and occupational history
Focusing on lead exposure history; personal and workplace hygiene; gastrointestinal, hematologic, renal, reproductive, and neurologic problems
Physical examination
Focusing on the gums and on the gastrointestinal, hematologic, renal, reproductive, and neurologic systems
Pulmonary status should be evaluated in workers required to wear respiratory protective devices
Blood pressure measurement
Blood testing
Blood lead level
Zinc protoporphyrin or free erythrocyte protoporphyrin
Hemoglobin, hematocrit, and peripheral smear
Serum creatinine
Urinalysis, with microscopic examination
Other tests
As clinically indicated

Removal based on the risk of health impairment is a medical decision and should not be based solely on blood lead levels. Workers must not be returned until the final medical determination is that they are no longer at risk.

Eliminating lead from gasoline and abatement of lead-based paint remain the primary measures to eliminated exposure to children. The CDC recommends that all children with lead levels greater than 10 μg/dL receive follow-up evaluations. Parental lead education is important in preventing childhood lead poisoning. Children with levels between 20 and 45 μg/dL should have an environmental investigation and remediation of sources of exposure. Children with levels greater than 45 μg/dL must be referred for medical evaluation and possible treatment.

Treatment

In all cases of suspected lead intoxication, identification and elimination of the sources of exposure are critical. This may mean removal from the workplace (or the home) if hygienic conditions are such that secondary exposure is significant. The decision to use chelation therapy depends on the intensity and duration of exposure and the clinical picture. Adults with a rapid rise in blood lead levels and acute symptoms should be provided chelation therapy. The combined measurement of blood lead and ZPP may help in management: An elevated blood lead level (>60 μg/dL) with a normal ZPP (<100 mg/dL) suggests a recent increase in exposure.

The management of adults and workers with vague complaints is more difficult. In a young worker with short-term exposure and an elevated blood lead level (>40–60 μg/dL), treatment should be considered both to ameliorate symptoms and to reduce lead body burden. In long-term lead workers, removal from exposure remains the treatment of choice, chelation being reserved for those with cardiovascular, renal, or neurologic impairment. Children with elevated blood levels should be treated by experienced professionals. The critical factor in the management of children remains elimination of the sources of exposure.

A. Acute Poisoning

After poisoning by ingestion, emesis and then catharsis should be induced. Hydration will reduce acute renal injury. The patient should be hospitalized and treatment overseen by a physician who has experience with chelation therapy. Urinalysis, BUN, and serum creatinine should be monitored daily; if proteinuria, hematuria, or renal dysfunction is observed, $CaNa_2$ EDTA treatment should be discontinued.

For subacute cases of lead toxicity, chelation with an oral agent, 2,3-dimercaptosuccinic acid (succimer, Chemet), is appropriate. This also is approved in the United States for the treatment of children with lead levels in excess of 45 μg/dL. The dose is 10 mg/kg every 8 hours for 5 days. Higher doses (up to 30 mg/kg) have been used in adults. Treatment must be supervised carefully to monitor for side effects (e.g., neutropenia, gastrointestinal complaints, and skin rashes). Rebound elevation of lead levels also may occur after treatment.

B. Chronic Overexposure

For workers with mild symptoms, removal from exposure is the treatment of choice. Chelation may not be effective for workers with long-term exposure (and an excessive body burden of lead), and treatment with $CaNa_2$ EDTA actually may cause acute tubular necrosis. Prophylactic chelation should not be used and is prohibited by the OSHA Lead Standard. Oral chelation may be considered for persons with elevated body burdens of lead, although there is only limited evidence that this will affect clinical outcome on an individual basis.

C. Organic Lead

In acute alkyl lead intoxication, chelation therapy is of no benefit. Treatment should be directed at the presenting symptoms as indicated.

Prognosis

Early diagnosis and treatment of lead toxicity generally will result in complete recovery. Once renal or neurologic impairment has occurred, only partial recovery may be expected. The relationship of long-term health effects, such as hypertension, to lead exposure remains difficult to assess on an individual basis but is important in driving occupational and environmental health standards.

REFERENCES

American Academy of Pediatrics Committee on Environmental Health: Lead exposure in children: Prevention, detection, and management. Pediatrics 2005;116:1036 [PMID: 16199720].

Bellinger DC: Lead. Pediatrics 2004;113:1016 [PMID: 15060194].

Brewster UC, Perazella MA: A review of chronic lead intoxication: An unrecognized cause of chronic kidney disease. Am J Med Sci 2004;327:341 [PMID: 15201648].

Chuang HY et al: Reversible neurobehavioral performance with reductions in blood lead levels: A prospective study on lead workers. Neurotoxicol Teratol 2005;27:497 [PMID: 15939209].

Krieg EF et al: The relationship between blood lead levels and neurobehavioral test performance in NHANES III and related occupational studies. Public Health Rep 2005;120:240 [PMID: 16134563].

Lanphear BP et al: Low-level environmental lead exposure and children's intellectual function: An international pooled analysis. Environ Health Perspect 2005;113:894 [PMID: 16002379].

Marcus SM: Toxicity, lead, www.emedicine.com/EMERG/topic293.htm.

Muntner P et al: Continued decline in blood lead levels among adults in the United States: The National Health and Nutrition Examination Surveys. Arch Intern Med 2005;165:2155 [PMID: 16217007].

Needleman H: Lead poisoning. Annu Rev Med 2004;55:209 [PMID: 14746518].

MANGANESE

Essentials of Diagnosis

- Manganese-induced parkinsonism
- Behavioral changes, psychosis
- Respiratory symptoms and disease

Exposure Limits

Manganese elemental and inorganic compounds
ACGIH TLV: 0.02 mg/m^3 TWA
Manganese cyclopentadienyl tricarbonyl
ACGIH TLV: 0.1 mg/m^3 TWA

General Considerations

Manganese is a brittle gray metal that is abundant in soils and sediments. The most important source of manganese for commercial use is manganese dioxide, occurring as pyrolusite. Manganese is an essential trace element in humans with an average daily requirement of 2–5 mg for adults.

Use

Ferromanganese, an iron alloy containing more than 80% manganese metal, is used in steel production. Manganese serves as a depolarizer in dry-cell batteries and an oxidizing agent for chemical syntheses. Manganese is used in the manufacture of matches, paints, and pesticides (Maneb). The manganese carbonyls, particularly methylcyclopentadienyl manganese tricarbonyl (MMT), have been used as antiknock agents in fuel and as sources of manganese in the electronics industry.

Occupational & Environmental Exposure

Exposure to manganese dioxide occurs in the mining, smelting, and refining of manganese ores. Manganese exposure also occurs near crushing operations and reduction furnaces engaged in the production of alloys and steel. These operations historically had the highest levels of exposure and the greatest risk for manganese toxicity.

Exposures may occur in battery production, chemicals plants, and the electronics industry. Workers engaged in the manufacture of fuels containing MMT may have respiratory or skin contact with this highly toxic liquid. Combustion of manganese-containing fuels results in environmental release of manganese oxides. Welding rods and steel alloys are other sources of occupational manganese exposure.

Absorption, Metabolism, & Excretion

Manganese fume is readily absorbed after inhalation. There also may be uptake via the olfactory nerve. Larger particles are ingested after mucociliary clearance from the lungs. Gastrointestinal absorption generally is low (10%) but may be increased in persons who are iron deficient. MMT may be absorbed after ingestion, inhalation, or skin contact.

Manganese is excreted primarily in the bile. The biologic half-life of manganese is approximately 30 hours. Blood, urine, and hair levels are elevated in exposed workers, but individual results do not correlate with symptoms or toxicity. Variations in manganese or iron homeostasis may account for variable individual susceptibility to toxicity.

Clinical Findings

A. Symptoms and Signs

1. Acute exposure—Dermal and respiratory exposure to MMT results in slight burning of the skin followed by headache, a metallic taste, nausea, diarrhea, dyspnea, and chest pain. Acute overexposure to MMT can cause chemical pneumonitis and hepatic and renal toxicity.

2. Chronic exposure—Industrial exposure to manganese can result in chronic nervous system damage. The earliest manifestations are fatigue, headache, apathy, and behavioral changes. Episodes of excitability, garrulousness, and sexual arousal have been termed *manganese psychosis.* With continued exposure, there is development of a syndrome that is similar to idiopathic parkinsonism, with slow speech, masked facies, bradykinesia, gait dysfunction, and micrographia. Tremor is less common in manganism. Salivation, sweating, and vasomotor disturbances also may occur.

Inhalation of manganese dust has been associated with increased respiratory symptoms and susceptibility to respiratory infections.

B. Laboratory Findings

Laboratory findings usually are normal. Minor decreases in leukocyte and red blood cell counts may be seen. Liver enzyme elevations also have been reported. T_1-weighted images on magnetic resonance imaging (MRI) demonstrate high signal changes in the globus pallidus indicating manganese accumulation. Measurement of elevated urine or blood manganese levels confirms exposure. These measurements can discriminate exposed from nonexposed groups but do not correlate well with individual exposure or the degree of toxicity.

Prevention

Manganese exposure should be reduced by the use of closed systems, local exhaust ventilation, and respiratory protection. Dermal and respiratory exposure to MMT should be prevented through the use of proper personal protective equipment. Medical surveillance should focus on the nervous system and the respiratory system. Careful neurologic examinations and pulmonary function testing should be performed routinely on all exposed workers. Workers with exposure to MMT also should have periodic assessment of respiratory, liver, and kidney function.

Treatment

Workers suspected of having manganese-induced parkinsonism should be removed from exposure. Manganese-induced symptoms are resistant to treatment with levodopa, a factor that distinguishes this from idiopathic Parkinson's disease. Pneumonia, bronchitis, and asthma should be treated with appropriate therapy while the worker is removed from exposure.

After skin contact with MMT, the affected areas should be cleansed immediately to reduce skin absorption. Workers who develop respiratory symptoms after inhalation of MMT should be admitted to the hospital for observation. Liver and kidney function should be monitored.

REFERENCES

Cersosimo MG, Koller WC: The diagnosis of manganese-induced parkinsonism. Neurotoxicology 2006;27:340 [PMID: 16325915].

Dobson AW et al: Manganese neurotoxicity. Ann NY Acad Sci 2004;1012:115 [PMID: 15105259].

Finley JW: Does environmental exposure to manganese pose a health risk to healthy adults? Nutr Rev 2004;62:148 [PMID: 15141430].

Jankovic J: Searching for a relationship between manganese and welding and Parkinson's disease. Neurology 2005;64:2021 [PMID: 15985567].

Olanow CW: Manganese-induced parkinsonism and Parkinson's disease. Ann NY Acad Sci 2004;1012:209 [PMID: 15105268].

MERCURY

Essentials of Diagnosis

A. INORGANIC MERCURY

- Acute respiratory distress
- Tremor
- Erethism (shyness, emotional lability)
- Proteinuria, renal failure

B. ORGANIC MERCURY (ALKYL MERCURY COMPOUNDS)

- Mental disturbances
- Ataxia, spasticity
- Paresthesias
- Visual and auditory disturbances

Exposure Limits

Alkyl compounds
ACGIH TLV: 0.01 mg/m^3 TWA, 0.03 mg/m^3 short-term exposure limit (STEL)

Vapor (all forms except alkyl)
ACGIH TLV: 0.025 mg/m^3 TWA

Aryl and inorganic compounds
ACGIH TLV: 0.1 mg/m^3
ACGIH BEI: urine: 35 µg/g of creatinine; blood: 15 µg/L (end of week/end of shift)

General Considerations

Mercury is a heavy silvery-white metal that is a liquid at room temperature. The high vapor pressure of mercury results in continuous release into the atmosphere, a major factor contributing to occupational exposure and environmental contamination. Mercury is recovered primarily from cinnabar ore (HgS). The release of mercury into the atmosphere from both natural sources, such as volcanoes, and industrial emissions has led to global distribution of this element. Rainwater captures oxidized mercury and returns the element to bodies of water, where it is taken up and biomethylated by marine organisms. From there it enters the food chain, resulting in accumulation in animals and humans. Mercury is not considered an essential element in humans, and the environmental exposure is an international concern.

Use

Elemental mercury is used in control instruments, tubes, rectifiers, thermometers, barometers, batteries, and electrical devices. Mercury in brine cells catalyzes the electrolytic production of chlorine. Historical use of alkyl mercury compounds (methyl mercury and ethyl mercury) as grain fumigants caused serious human poisoning. Mercury is used in plating, jewelry, tanning, and taxidermy. Use in the felt industry in the nineteenth century led to extensive poisoning ("mad as a hatter"). Mercury dental amalgams remain an important source of low-level exposure, along with vaccines containing the mercury preservative thiomersal. While both clearly contribute to background population exposures, the health impact of these uses remains uncertain.

Occupational & Environmental Exposure

Workers involved in the extraction and recovery of mercury are at high risk for exposure to mercury vapor. Maintenance work on furnaces and flues is another source of exposure. Chloralkali workers can have significant exposure from contamination if workplace hygiene is not maintained.

Mercury is being phased out of medical equipment, although health care workers still may be exposed from damaged or broken equipment or past workplace contamination. Dentists and dental technicians may have short-term peak exposures during certain dental procedures. Workers may be exposed to alkyl mercury compounds during the production and application of organic mercury fungicides or the use of these agents in paints and plastics.

Two serious epidemics of organic mercury poisoning occurred owing to environmental contamination of food sources. Release of mercury wastes from a chemical plant into Minamata Bay in Japan led to accumulation of methyl mercury in seafood. *Minamata disease* resulted in neurologic impairment and birth defects in thousands of the affected area residents. Distribution of grain contaminated with organic mercury fungicides similarly poisoned over 50,000 persons in Iraq. These clear demonstrations of the toxicity of organic mercury continue to drive regulations to reduce mercury emissions and lower the acceptable levels of mercury in fish and seafood.

Absorption, Metabolism, & Excretion

Elemental mercury is efficiently absorbed after the inhalation but not ingestion. Soluble mercurial salts (Hg^{2+}) and aryl mercury compounds have similar uptake. Alkyl mercury compounds are absorbed readily through all routes, including skin contact.

Inorganic and aryl mercury compounds are distributed to many tissues, primarily the brain and kidney. There they bind to sulfhydryl groups and may interfere with numerous cellular enzyme systems. Metallothionein, a protein rich in sulfhydryl groups, binds mercury and exerts a protective effect in the kidney. Alkyl mercury in the bloodstream is taken up rapidly by red blood cells and also accumulates in brain tissue.

Both organic and elemental mercury compounds readily cross the placenta and are secreted in breast milk. Peak exposures to both organic and inorganic mercury compounds are more hazardous because of the intense effects on the central nervous system. Mercury compounds are eliminated slowly in the urine, feces, saliva, and sweat. The average half-life is 60 days for inorganic mercury and 70 days for alkyl mercury compounds. Mercury also may be measured in the hair and nails.

Clinical Findings

A. SYMPTOMS & SIGNS

1. Inorganic mercury—Inhalation of high concentrations of mercury vapor or salts causes cough and dyspnea. Inflammation of the oral cavity and gastrointestinal complaints occur shortly after exposure, followed by a chemical pneumonitis. Renal injury is a particular concern after exposure to mercuric chloride and presents as an initial diuresis followed by proteinuria and oliguric renal failure. After recovery from the acute illness, neurologic symptoms similar to those seen with chronic overexposure may develop. Chronic exposure to inorganic mercury compounds primarily affects the nervous system. Neuropsychiatric manifestations include changes in personality, shyness, anxiety, memory loss, and emotional lability. Tremor is an early sign of neurotoxicity. Initially, the tremor is fine and occurs at rest, progressing with further exposure to an intention tremor interrupted by coarse jerking movements. A head tremor and skeletal ataxia also may occur. A sensory peripheral neuropathy usually is present with distal paresthesias. Hallucinations and dementia are serious late manifestations.

Other reported findings after include salivation, gingivitis, and dental erosions. A bluish linear pigmentation may be present on the teeth or gums. Reddish brown pigmentation of the lens may be apparent on slit-lamp examination. Excessive sweating and an eczematous skin eruption also may be present.

2. Organic mercury—Exposure to alkyl mercury compounds results in the delayed, insidious onset of progressive nervous system damage that may be fatal. The earliest symptoms are of numbness and tingling of the extremities and lips. Loss of motor coordination follows, with gait ataxia, tremor, and loss of fine movement. Constriction of the visual fields, central hearing loss, muscular rigidity, and spasticity occur with exaggerated deep tendon reflexes. Behavioral changes and intellectual impairment may be prominent. Erythroderma, desquamation, and other skin rashes may be present. Renal disease is rare. Neurotoxicity in infants exposed in utero in the Minamata Bay epidemic resembled cerebral palsy.

B. LABORATORY FINDINGS

After acute inhalation, there may be hypoxemia and diffuse infiltrates on chest x-ray. Proteinuria indicates renal injury. The earliest manifestations of renal effects are increased excretion of low-molecular-weight proteins, including N-acetyl-β-glucosaminidase, β_2-microglobulin, and retinol-binding protein.

Measurement of mercury in blood and urine will confirm the diagnosis. Gross renal or neurologic manifestations are unusual unless urine mercury levels exceed 500 μg/g of creatinine. Subtle nervous system effects have been detected in workers with levels of 50–150 μg/g of

Table 27–4. Biologic monitoring program for mercury.[1]

Air Exposure	Urine Hg Level	Action
$> 50\,\mu g/m^3$	$> 100\,\mu g/g$ creatinine	Remove from exposure until < 50 Medical examination if over 150 or if two consecutive levels exceed 100 Repeat measurement weekly
$50\,\mu g/m^3$	$75–100\,\mu g/g$ creatinine	Monitor weekly Perform hygiene assessment to limit exposure
$25–50\,\mu g/m^3$	$50–75\,\mu g/g$ creatinine	Monitor monthly
$25\,mg/m^3$	$35–50\,\mu g/g$ creatinine	Monitor quarterly
$< 25\,\mu g/m^3$	$< 35\,\mu g/g$ creatinine	Monitor semiannually

[1]Approximate equivalents if adjusted to a specific gravity of 1.024: $100\,\mu g/g$ creatinine = $150\,\mu g/L$; $75\,\mu g/g$ creatinine = $100\,\mu g/L$; $50\,\mu g/g$ creatinine = $75\,\mu g/L$; $35\,\mu g/g$ creatinine = $50\,\mu g/L$.

creatinine, and early renal effects (low-molecular-weight proteinuria with normal renal function) have been detected when urine mercury levels chronically exceed 50 µg/g of creatinine. Normal concentrations in nonexposed individuals are less than 0.01 mg/L in whole blood and less than 10 µg/g of creatinine in urine. Substantial seafood consumption may result in high blood levels with low urine levels. A high ratio of whole blood mercury to plasma mercury suggests alkyl mercury intoxication. Hair and nail levels may be used to document exposure but do not correlate well with toxicity.

Prevention

Awareness of the constant hazard of mercury vapor exposure along with proper handling of materials and meticulous attention to workplace hygiene will reduce potential exposures. Use of proper ventilation and respiratory protection is required in all operations that use mercury compounds. Special attention should focus on maintenance workers. Care in the handling and disposal of mercury compounds will prevent inadvertent contamination of the workplace. Control of industrial emissions will prevent contamination of waterways and seafood.

Medical surveillance of mercury-exposed workers should include a careful history and neurologic examination as well as periodic urinalyses. Table 27–4 provides a sample biologic monitoring program. Urine levels fluctuate, and periodic monitoring or group monitoring is more representative of ongoing exposure. Greater accuracy may be obtained by adjusting to urine creatinine.

Treatment

After acute exposure to mercury, prompt treatment with dimercaprol (5 mg/kg intramuscularly) should be instituted. Respiratory distress and renal failure should be treated appropriately. Succimer and dimercaptosuccinic acid are also effective and are indicated for organic mercury intoxication. Individuals manifesting symptoms of chronic mercury toxicity should be removed from further exposure. The decision to give treatment in such cases depends on the severity of the symptoms and whether evidence of neurologic or renal toxicity is present. Chronic mercury poisoning also may respond to chelation therapy. The chronic neurologic sequelae of alkyl mercury poisoning are irreversible.

REFERENCES

Bast-Pettersen R et al: A neurobehavioral study of chloralkali workers after the cessation of exposure to mercury vapor. Neurotoxicology 2005;26:427 [PMID: 15935213].

Bhan A, Sarkar NN: Mercury in the environment: Effect on health and reproduction. Rev Environ Health 2005;20:39 [PMID: 15835497].

Horsted-Bindslev P: Amalgam toxicity: Environmental and occupational hazards. J Dent 2004;32:359 [PMID: 15193783].

Rohling ML, Demakis GJ: A meta-analysis of the neuropsychological effects of occupational exposure to mercury. Clin Neuropsychol 2006;20:108 [PMID: 16393923].

THALLIUM

Essentials of Diagnosis

A. ACUTE EFFECTS

- Alopecia
- Gastrointestinal distress
- Ascending paralysis, coma

B. CHRONIC EFFECTS

- Alopecia

- Weakness, fatigue
- Peripheral neuropathy

Exposure Limits

ACGIH TLV: 0.1 mg/m^3 TWA
OSHA PEL: 0.1 mg/m^3 TWA

General Considerations

Thallium is a heavy metal that occurs in the earth's crust as a minor constituent in iron, copper, sulfide, and selenide ores. Thallium can be recovered from flue dusts either from pyrite (FeS$_2$) roasting or from lead and zinc smelting. Thallium can be prepared as both water-soluble (sulfate, acetate) and water-insoluble (halide) salts.

Use

Thallium sulfate was used as a medicinal in the treatment of syphilis, gonorrhea, gout, and tuberculosis in the nineteenth century. Abandoned because of its toxicity, it enjoyed a brief resurgence as a depilatory in the 1920s. [^{201}Tl]Cl is currently used in myocardial imaging for the diagnosis of cardiac ischemia.

Thallium salts have been used extensively as rodenticides in the form of impregnated grain (Thalgrain) and pastes (Zelio). Numerous accidental and suicidal poisonings led to the banning of these compounds in the United States in 1972. Currently, thallium is finding increasing uses in the manufacture of electronic components, optical lenses, imitation jewelry, dyes, and pigments.

Occupational & Environmental Exposure

At highest risk for exposure are those engaged in the production of thallium salt derivatives. In addition, workers in the electronics and optical industries have potential exposure to thallium compounds. Thallium exposure can occur at smelters, particularly in the maintenance and cleaning of ducts and flues. Environmental exposure can occur in the vicinity of smelting operations through air and water contamination. Consumption of contaminated grain remains an important cause of accidental poisoning. Thallium chloride has been found in potassium chloride salt substitutes.

Metabolism & Mechanism of Action

Thallium—and especially its soluble salts—is absorbed readily through the gastrointestinal tract, skin, and respiratory system. Ingestion of 0.5–1 g may be lethal. Elimination is slow and occurs through intestinal and renal secretion in a ratio of 2:1. Thallium behaves much like potassium and binds avidly to several enzyme systems, including Na$^+$,K$^+$-ATPase. Thallium binds to

sulfhydryl groups and interferes with cellular respiration and protein synthesis. Binding to riboflavin may contribute to its neurotoxicity.

Clinical Findings

A. SYMPTOMS & SIGNS

1. Acute exposure—Gastrointestinal symptoms predominate early and include pain, nausea, vomiting, hemorrhage, and diarrhea. Cardiac abnormalities include tachycardia and hypertension. Neurologic manifestations usually begin with pain, hyperesthesia, and hyperreflexia in the lower extremities. This may progress rapidly to areflexia, hypesthesia, and paralysis depending on the amount ingested. Ataxia, agitation, hallucinations, and coma may occur in severe cases. Alopecia, primarily of scalp and body hair, occurs at the end of the first week; however, black pigmentation of the hair root may be seen earlier. Mees lines of nails and gingival pigmentation occur. Proximal erosion of the nail beds also has been reported. Anhidrosis occurs early owing to destruction of sweat glands.

2. Chronic exposure—In chronic intoxication, the onset of symptoms is insidious. Alopecia and dry skin may be the only complaint. Fatigue and asthenia are frequent. Insomnia and behavioral dysfunction, cranial nerve involvement, and dementia may be presenting symptoms.

B. LABORATORY FINDINGS

Findings generally are nonspecific. Hypokalemia and alkalosis may be present. Elevated liver enzyme levels in severe cases reflect centrilobular necrosis. Proteinuria and renal tubular necrosis can occur. The ECG may show signs of hypokalemia. The electroencephalograph (EEG) reveals nonspecific slow-wave activity in severe cases. Nerve-conduction studies are consistent with axonal degeneration. The diagnosis is confirmed by demonstrating elevated thallium levels in the urine. Normal levels range from 0–10 μg/L. Hair and nail levels may be elevated in chronic exposure. Levels in workers should be maintained below 50 μg/L.

Differential Diagnosis

Thallium intoxication should be considered in cases of peripheral neuropathy of unknown cause. The absence of urobilinogen in the urine distinguishes thallium poisoning from acute intermittent porphyria. In chronic intoxication from industrial exposure, the presentation may suggest depression, hypothyroidism, or organic brain syndrome.

Prevention

Proper skin and respiratory protection are essential. Eating and smoking should not be permitted in areas where thallium compounds are handled. Thallium is a cumulative toxin, and biologic monitoring of urine levels should be considered where there is chronic exposure to thallium compounds. The banning of thallium-containing pesticides has reduced the frequency of thallium poisoning in the United States, but these compounds still may be encountered and are still available in other countries.

Treatment

In acute cases, emesis should be induced. Treatment with Prussian blue (potassium ferric cyanoferrate II) in a dose of 1 g three times daily will bind secreted thallium in the gut. This should be administered with a cathartic to avoid constipation. Activated charcoal should be used as an alternative. Potassium chloride will exchange with thallium in cells and increase renal excretion. This should be administered cautiously because the rise in serum thallium levels may transiently worsen symptoms. Chelating agents have not been shown to be effective. In chronic intoxication, removal from exposure is the treatment of choice. Recovery generally is complete, although permanent blindness and hair loss have been reported.

REFERENCES

Ibrahim D et al: Heavy metal poisoning: Clinical presentations and pathophysiology. Clin Lab Med 2006;26:67 [PMID: 16567226].

Peter AL, Viraraghavan T: Thallium: A review of public health and environmental concerns. Environ Int 2005;31:493 [PMID: 15788190].

Saha A et al: Erosion of nails following thallium poisoning: A case report. Occup Environ Med 2004;61:640 [PMID: 15208382].

OTHER METALS

1. Aluminum

General Considerations

Aluminum is a lightweight metal and is easy to form and process, leading to widespread application in automobiles, aircraft, tanks, and military equipment. Aluminum metal is produced through refining of ore and electrolytic reduction. Recycling of aluminum cans and containers is now a primary source of industrial aluminum. This is a nonessential element in humans.

A significant portion of aluminum is used for containers and wrapping. Aluminum siding is used in construction. Aluminum chloride is used in antiperspirants. Medically, aluminum hydroxide is used as an antacid and to reduce phosphate accumulation in uremia.

Occupational & Environmental Exposure

Exposure to aluminum occurs from exposure to fume during welding and dust from handling of aluminum oxide powders. In the aluminum reduction industry, workers may be exposed to aluminum fume, as well as to fluorides and polynuclear aromatic hydrocarbons.

Aluminum may be absorbed after inhalation of dust and fume. Gastrointestinal absorption is minimal, although accumulation and toxicity have been observed after intake of high doses of aluminum hydroxide in persons with chronic renal failure. Urinary excretion is the primary route of elimination. The biologic half-life is variable (days to months) and depends on the source and duration of exposure.

Clinical Findings

Aluminum oxide and other aluminum dusts can cause drying and irritation of the eyes, nose, and throat. Nosebleeds may occur if exposures are excessive. Chronic inhalation of dusts and powders reportedly causes pulmonary fibrosis. Increased respiratory symptoms, airway obstruction, and asthma also may occur in more heavily exposed workers and welders. Excessive intake of aluminum compounds in uremia has been a cause of encephalopathy (*dialysis dementia*) in patients with uremia. The association between aluminum accumulation in the brain and the development of Alzheimer disease and other neurologic disorders remains controversial. Laboratory testing may reveal either obstructive or restrictive deficits in pulmonary function. Chest radiographs and high-resolution computed tomographic (CT) scans may show nodules or granulomas or merely a diffuse increase in interstitial markings. Biologic monitoring of either blood or urine levels may correlate with exposure.

Treatment & Prevention

Removal from exposure is the primary treatment when potential health effects related to aluminum occur in the workplace. Deferoxamine has been used to treat dialysis dementia but is associated with side effects such as hypotension and skin rash. Workers exposed to aluminum powders should use proper respiratory protection. Irritant symptoms are prevented through ventilation and dust-control measures. Medical surveillance should include periodic assessment of respiratory symptoms, spirometry, and chest radiographs.

2. Antimony

General Considerations

Antimony is a soft metal that is found as oxides and sulfides in a variety of ores. Antimony ores often contain significant quantities of arsenic and lead. Pure antimony metal is used in the manufacture of semiconductor devices both as a dopant compound for silicon and as a substrate material in the manufacture of intermediate crystals. Antimony alloys are used in the production of battery grids, type castings, bearings, and cable sheaths. Antimony compounds are also used in munitions, glass and pottery, fire retardants, paints and lacquers, rubber compounds, chemical catalysts, and solder. Antimonials have been used medicinally in the treatment of leishmaniasis, schistosomiasis, and filariasis.

Occupational & Environmental Exposure

Mining and smelting operations have resulted in significant worker exposure to antimony dusts and fumes. Health effects attributed to exposure to antimony during refining include respiratory tract irritation and pneumoconiosis. Exposure to antimony trisulfide has been associated with electrocardiographic abnormalities and sudden death. Antimony trioxide and antimony trichloride used in the microelectronics industry are strong irritants.

Stibine gas (SbH_3), a hemolytic toxin similar to arsine, may be formed when antimony alloys are processed with certain reducing acids. Stibine is also used as a grain fumigant. Parenteral administration of antimonial compounds for medicinal purposes is associated with electrocardiographic changes, alterations in liver function, and hemolysis. Soluble forms of antimony are readily absorbed after inhalation. Antimony is excreted largely in the urine. Insoluble forms are excreted slowly in the urine and may be detectable years after exposure has ceased.

Clinical Findings

Acute exposure to antimony dusts and fumes causes intense irritation of the eyes, throat, and respiratory tract. Nausea, vomiting, abdominal pain, and bloody diarrhea also may be present. Inhalation of stibine causes headache, fatigue, abdominal pain, jaundice, and anuria as a consequence of massive hemolysis. Chronic inhalation may result in dryness of the throat, dysosmia, and bronchitis. Chronic skin exposure to antimony compounds may cause pustular dermatitis. Antimony is suspected of being a human carcinogen.

Hemoglobinuria and red blood cell casts are a sign of stibine-induced hemolysis and suggest acute renal and hepatic failure. Electrocardiographic changes after therapeutic use or industrial exposure include T-wave changes and rhythm disturbances.

Acute inhalation of antimony trichloride can cause pulmonary edema. Rounded opacities in the middle lung fields on chest radiograph or CT scan are consistent with pneumoconiosis. The presence of antimony in urine is diagnostic of past exposure but does not necessarily correlate with severity of exposure or health effects.

Prevention

Chelation with dimercaprol or penicillamine is indicated when significant cardiovascular, pulmonary, or hepatic impairment occurs after acute exposure. Stibine-induced hemolysis requires exchange transfusion.

Personal protective devices should be worn where there is potential exposure to antimony dusts or fumes. Biologic monitoring of urinary antimony levels confirms exposure and may be useful for diagnosis if markedly elevated in acute overexposure.

3. Nickel

General Considerations

Nickel is a hard, silver-white, malleable, magnetic metal that has wide industrial application. Nickel is refined by electrolysis or the Mond process, in which treatment with carbon monoxide leads to the formation of nickel carbonyl [$Ni(CO)_4$]. Nickel occurs naturally in a variety of vegetables and grains.

The major use of nickel is in the production of stainless steel. Nickel alloys provide durability for use in food and dairy processing equipment. Coins, tableware and utensils, springs, magnets, batteries (nickel-cadmium), and spark plugs use nickel alloys. Nickel salts are used in electroplating to impart lustrous, polishable, corrosion-resistant surfaces to parts and equipment. Nickel compounds are also used as catalysts and pigments.

Occupational & Environmental Exposure

Exposure to nickel compounds may occur during mining, milling, and refining operations. In the Mond process, workers also may be exposed to highly toxic nickel carbonyl gas. In electroplating shops, workers may have respiratory and skin exposure to soluble nickel salts. Workers using nickel as a catalyst may be exposed to nickel powders.

Nickel is poorly absorbed from the gastrointestinal tract. Soluble nickel compounds and nickel carbonyl are readily absorbed after inhalation. Absorbed nickel does not accumulate in tissues and is excreted in the urine with a half-life of approximately 1 week. Insoluble nickel compounds may accumulate in the respiratory tract—a factor that may contribute to carcinogenicity.

Clinical Findings

The most common manifestations of exposure to soluble nickel compounds are dermatologic. Nickel is a common cause of allergic contact dermatitis. Exposure to high levels of soluble nickel aerosols also may cause rhinitis, sinusitis, and anosmia. Cough and wheezing should suggest the possibility of nickel-induced asthma. Exposure to nickel carbonyl causes headache, fatigue, nausea, and vomiting. In severe cases, there is a delay of 12–36 hours before development of a diffuse interstitial pneumonitis, with fever, chills, cough, chest pain, and dyspnea. Delirium, seizures, and coma may occur prior to death. Nickel is considered a human respiratory tract carcinogen.

The diagnosis of nickel skin allergy can be confirmed by patch testing or lymphocyte transformation testing. After exposure to nickel carbonyl, there is a moderate leukocytosis, hypoxemia, and a reduction in lung volumes and carbon monoxide diffusing capacity consistent with acute pneumonitis.

Treatment & Prevention

Nickel dermatitis should be treated with topical steroids and removal from further exposure. Individuals who have been exposed to nickel carbonyl should be monitored for the development of pulmonary complications and systemic toxicity. If exposure is found to be excessive (urine nickel = 100 µg/L), treatment should be instituted with sodium diethyldithiocarbamate (ditiocarb sodium) or disulfiram.

Skin and respiratory protection should be used where there is potential exposure to nickel dusts, fumes, or soluble nickel aerosols and liquids. Extreme caution should be used in handling gaseous nickel carbonyl. Medical surveillance should concentrate on the skin and respiratory system, with prompt removal of those who develop dermal or respiratory allergy. A biologic threshold level of 10 µg/L in plasma is recommended for workers exposed to nickel compounds. A maximum level of 10 µg/L in the urine is recommended for workers exposed to nickel carbonyl.

4. Selenium & Tellurium

General Considerations

Selenium and tellurium are metalloid elements that are distributed widely in mineral ores, particularly in sulfur and copper deposits. Selenium is an essential trace element in humans, serving as a cofactor for glutathione peroxidase in the prevention of oxidative damage in erythrocytes. Although present in various concentrations in human tissues, tellurium is not considered an essential trace element for humans.

Selenium is used in the manufacture of glass and plastics to impart a red tint or to neutralize green discoloration. The photoconducting properties of selenium are useful in rectifiers and photoelectric cells. Selenium is used medicinally in dandruff shampoos and topical antifungal lotions. Selenium is used in paint pigments, animal feeds, and veterinary medicines. Tellurium is used in the vulcanization of rubber to increase durability. Like selenium, tellurium is finding increasing use in electronics, primarily in the manufacture of rectifiers and semiconductors.

Occupational & Environmental Exposure

Workers engaged in the refining of copper and silver may be exposed to airborne selenium and tellurium fumes and dust. Selenium and tellurium are encountered in the electronics, glass, ceramics, plastics, and rubber industries. Formulators may be exposed to selenium in the production of pharmaceuticals and animal feed. Agricultural use of sodium selenite as a pesticide and selenium contamination of phosphate fertilizers has led to soil and groundwater contamination.

Selenium and tellurium compounds may be absorbed through the lungs, gastrointestinal tract, or damaged skin. Selenium is metabolized to organic forms in the liver. Dimethyl selenium and dimethyl telluride are excreted through the lungs and impart a garlic odor to the breath. Tellurium accumulates in liver and bone, and excretion may be prolonged after exposure.

Clinical Findings

Acute inhalation of selenium or tellurium fumes, oxide dusts, halide vapors, hydrogen selenide, or telluride may cause severe respiratory irritation, resulting in cough, chest pain, and dyspnea. Neurologic, hepatic, and renal damage may occur. Selenium oxide may cause severe skin burns. Both can cause a garlicky odor of the breath, and tellurium exposure often causes a blue-black discoloration of the skin.

Chronic exposure to selenium and tellurium compounds may result in nonspecific complaints of fatigue and lassitude. There is often a strong garlic odor to the breath and sweat. Chronic airborne selenium exposure may cause conjunctivitis, termed *rose eye*. Dermatologic manifestations include irritant or allergic dermatitis, painful paronychia, and loss of hair and nails. Reddish skin and hair discoloration also may be present.

Laboratory evaluation usually is nondiagnostic. Liver enzyme elevations and anemia may be seen. Measurement of selenium in the urine will confirm overexposure, normal concentrations being less than 150 µg/L.

Treatment & Prevention

Prompt evacuation and resuscitation should be undertaken in cases of acute inhalation. Burns of the skin should be irrigated with a solution of 10% aqueous sodium thiosulfate followed by use of a 10% sodium thiosulfate cream. Administration of ascorbic acid may lessen the offensive garlic odor of exposed individuals. Chelation is contraindicated and may cause renal damage.

Respiratory and skin protection should be used where exposure to high levels of airborne selenium and tellurium compounds cannot be controlled through other means. Medical surveillance should focus on gastrointestinal and dermatologic complaints. Urine selenium should remain below 100 μg/L in individuals exposed to air levels of 0.1 mg/m³. Urinary tellurium levels should be kept below 0.05 mg/L. Pregnant women should not work directly with tellurium compounds.

5. Tin

General Considerations

Tin is a soft, pliable, silvery metal that is used extensively for its corrosion-resistant properties. The primary use of tin is for plating, where it imparts corrosion resistance. Tin-plated iron and steel are used for canning, household utensils, and decorative purposes. Tin-lead solder is used to join electronic components. Tin alloys (bronze, babbitt metal, and pewter) are used in printing, bearings, and jewelry. Stannous fluoride is used in toothpastes. Organotin compounds are used as stabilizers in plastics and oils, as catalysts in curing silicone rubber, as preservatives in textiles and leather, and as biocides in marine paints.

Occupational & Environmental Exposure

The primary risk for tin miners is exposure to silica. Both smelting and plating operations may expose workers to tin oxide fumes and dust. Workers engaged in the manufacture of tin solder and other alloys also use tin oxide as a raw material. Exposure to the highly toxic organotin compounds may occur in paint and plastics production and biocides. Organotin paint on boat hulls is a source of marine contamination in harbors.

Inorganic tin is poorly absorbed from the gastrointestinal tract. Most of the ingested dose is excreted in the feces. Renal excretion is minor. Inhaled compounds remain in the lung. Organic compounds may be absorbed by inhalation, ingestion, or through the skin. Excretion depends on chemical composition and is through both the biliary tract and the kidney.

Clinical Findings

Workers exposed to tin dusts in high concentrations may complain of eye, throat, and respiratory irritation. Long-term exposure may result in interstitial opacities on chest radiographs, termed *stannosis*. Changes in pulmonary function are not associated with exposure to tin compounds.

Acute exposure to trimethyl and triethyl tin may cause severe skin irritation followed by headache, lassitude, and visual disturbances. In severe cases, this may progress to seizures and coma. Chronic exposure to organotin compounds may cause an erythematous skin rash and folliculitis, particularly over the lower abdomen and thighs.

Chest radiographic findings consist of large nodular densities throughout the lung fields. Abnormal spirometry should prompt evaluation for concomitant exposure to silica or other fibrogenic agents. Acute organotin toxicity results in renal, hepatic, and central nervous system injury.

Treatment & Prevention

After dermal exposure to organotin compounds, the skin should be cleansed extensively with a strong detergent and water to prevent delayed absorption. Neurologic, hepatic, and renal toxicity should be treated as indicated clinically.

Process enclosure, ventilation, and respiratory protection will reduce exposure to tin oxide dusts and fumes. Organotin compounds must be handled with extreme care to avoid inhalation and skin contact. Medical surveillance should focus on the respiratory system of inorganic tin workers and the skin and nervous system in workers exposed to organic tin compounds.

6. Vanadium

General Considerations

Vanadium is a soft gray metal that is derived commercially from vanadium sulfide ores. Vanadium is found in fossil fuels, contributing to environmental contamination. Vanadium imparts strength and elasticity to steel. Vanadium alloys supply hardness and durability for high-speed cutting and drilling tools. Vanadium is also used as a catalyst for high-temperature polymerization, as a mordant in dyeing, and as a colorant in ceramics and glass. Organic vanadium compounds are used as catalysts and coatings.

Occupational & Environmental Exposure

Exposure to vanadium pentoxide dusts and fumes may occur during milling and roasting. A particular inhalation hazard exists in cleaning fuel dusts from oil and coal furnaces where high levels of vanadium pentoxide may accumulate. Fossil-fuel-burning power stations may emit vanadium compounds, resulting in environmental contamination and air pollution. Vanadium compounds may be absorbed after inhalation or ingestion. Excretion is primarily renal, with little bioaccumulation.

Clinical Findings

Acute exposure to high levels of vanadium pentoxide dusts or fume results in eye irritation, epistaxis, cough, and bronchitis. Pneumonia may follow acute exposures. Sensitivity to vanadium may result in occupational asthma or allergic dermatitis. An unusual presentation of chronic exposure is a green discoloration of the tongue. Patch testing may be used to confirm dermal sensitization to vanadium compounds.

Treatment & Prevention

Persons who develop respiratory or dermatologic allergy should be permanently removed from exposure. Proper respiratory protection is critical when handling vanadium compounds and during the cleaning of oil and coal furnace flues. Medical surveillance focuses on respiratory and dermatologic complaints, looking for respiratory or skin sensitization. Biologic monitoring of vanadium in urine (end of shift/end of workweek) may be useful in controlling exposure.

7. Zinc

General Considerations

Zinc is a silver-white metal that is widely distributed with cadmium, iron, lead, and arsenic. Zinc is an essential element for humans, found in all tissues. Many enzyme systems require zinc, and daily intake is between 10 and 15 mg.

A major application of zinc is in the protective galvanizing of steel and other metals. Purified zinc metal is die cast for use in automotive parts, electrical equipment, tools, machinery, and toys. Zinc oxide is used as a pigment and in the vulcanizing of rubber. Zinc chloride is used in welding and soldering fluxes, wood preservatives, dry-cell batteries, oil refining, smoke bombs, dental cement, and deodorants. Zinc copper alloys form brass for fixtures and fittings.

Occupational & Environmental Exposure

Zinc roasting operations expose workers to zinc oxide dusts and fumes. Welding of galvanized metal also results in exposure to zinc oxide fumes. Zinc chloride exposure occurs in welding, soldering, and manufacturing.

Only 20–30% of ingested zinc is absorbed from the gastrointestinal tract. Zinc also may be absorbed after inhalation of fumes. Circulating zinc is bound to plasma proteins and is found in erythrocytes. Zinc is distributed widely in tissues. Absorbed zinc is excreted in pancreatic fluid, bile, and sweat, with only 20% excreted in the urine.

Clinical Findings

The most common manifestation of occupational zinc exposure is the development of metal fume fever. Several hours after exposure to zinc oxide fume (usually from welding on galvanized metal), the worker develops headache, a sweet metallic taste, muscle and joint pains,

and fatigue. Fever, chills, profuse sweating, cough, and chest pain occur 8–12 hours after exposure. The symptoms resolve spontaneously and completely after 24–48 hours. Metal fume fever presents with leukocytosis and a transient fall in lung volumes and diffusing capacity. The chest radiograph usually is normal. Urine and plasma zinc levels also may be elevated.

Contact with zinc chloride may cause serious skin and eye burns even after brief contact. Chronic skin exposure may cause an eczematous dermatitis or skin sensitization. Inhalation of zinc chloride fumes causes sinus and throat irritation, cough, hemoptysis, and dyspnea. Pulmonary edema and pneumonia may develop following excessive exposure. Ingestion of soluble zinc compounds causes nausea, vomiting, and diarrhea caused by irritation of the gastrointestinal tract.

Treatment & Prevention

No specific treatment is indicated for metal fume fever. Zinc chloride skin and eye burns should be irrigated immediately with copious amounts of water. Eye irrigation with 1.7% $CaNa_2$ EDTA for 15 minutes should be instituted to prevent the development of corneal opacities. Persons with suspected zinc chloride inhalation should be observed closely. Persons who develop chronic dermatitis and zinc skin allergy should be removed from further exposure.

Proper ventilation of high-temperature processes involving zinc will reduce exposure to zinc oxide dusts and fumes. Eye and skin protection should be used when handling zinc chloride. Medical monitoring for zinc-exposed workers should concentrate on dermatologic and respiratory effects.

REFERENCES

Bogle RG et al: Aluminium phosphide poisoning. Emerg Med J 2006;23:3 [PMID: 16373788].

De Boeck M et al: Cobalt and antimony: Genotoxicity and carcinogenicity. Mutat Res 2003;533:135 [PMID: 14643417].

Grimsrud TK et al: Can lung cancer risk among nickel refinery workers be explained by occupational exposures other than nickel? Epidemiology 2005;16:146 [PMID: 15703528].

Hartikainen H: Biogeochemistry of selenium and its impact on food chain quality and human health. J Trace Elem Med Biol 2005;18:309 [PMID: 16028492].

Hassaballa HA et al: Metal fume fever presenting as aseptic meningitis with pericarditis, pleuritis and pneumonitis. Occup Med (Lond) 2005;55:638 [PMID: 16314334].

Liao YH et al: Biological monitoring of exposures to aluminium, gallium, indium, arsenic, and antimony in optoelectronic industry workers. J Occup Environ Med 2004;46:931 [PMID: 15354058].

McCallum RI: Occupational exposure to antimony compounds. J Environ Monit 2005;7:1245 [PMID: 16307078].

Seet RC et al: Inhalational nickel carbonyl poisoning in waste processing workers. Chest 2005;128:424 [PMID: 16002966].

Sivulka DJ: Assessment of respiratory carcinogenicity associated with exposure to metallic nickel. Regul Toxicol Pharmacol 2005;43:117 [PMID: 16129532].

Tinggi U: Essentiality and toxicity of selenium and its status in Australia. Toxicol Lett 2003;137:103 [PMID: 12505436].

Yarema MC, Curry SC: Acute tellurium toxicity from ingestion of metal-oxidizing solutions. Pediatrics 2005;116:319 [PMID: 15995006].

WELDING

Welding is a joining process with wide application in manufacturing and the building trades. Through the application of heat or pressure, welding joins metals with a lightweight bond, with strength and resistance approaching that of the parent metal. Welding is a labor-intensive activity. Even though automated welding methods are finding increasing applications, manual arc welding remains the principal welding process.

Health Hazards of Welding

Welders work with a wide variety of materials under varied conditions and are exposed to many health hazards, including air contaminants (metal fumes, particulates, gases); physical agents such as radiation (infrared, ultraviolet), noise, and electricity; and ergonomic stress. Tables 27–5 and 27–6 list the common air contaminants of different welding processes. Shielded metal arc (SMA) welding of mild steel, or "stick welding," is the most common use of welding. The main exposure is to iron oxide, and pulmonary deposition of this nonfibrogenic particulate has resulted in the development of a benign pneumoconiosis. Exposure to manganese and

Table 27–5. Air contaminants of selected welding processes.

Process	Base Metal	Contaminants
Shielded metal arc (stick welding)	Mild steel	Dust, iron oxide, manganese
Shielded metal arc (stick welding)	Stainless steel	Chromium, nickel, manganese, fluorides
Gas metal arc (MIG)	Stainless steel	Chromium, nickel, manganese, nitrogen oxides, ozone
Tungsten inert gas (TIG)	Aluminum	Ozone, aluminum oxide
Gas, brazing, cutting	Variable	Nitrogen oxides, cadmium oxide, metal fume

Table 27–6. Potential hazards of welding processes.

Air contaminants

Metals

Iron oxide	Benign pneumoconiosis
Manganese	Neurotoxicity, pneumonia
Cadmium oxide	Acute lung injury
Zinc oxide	Metal fume fever
Chromium	Lung cancer, allergy
Nickel	Lung cancer, allergy
Fluoride	Skin or respiratory irritation

Gases

Ozone	Respiratory irritation, asthma
Nitrogen oxides	Acute lung injury
Carbon monoxide	Systemic poisoning

Physical hazards

Radiation

Ultraviolet	Photokeratitis, skin erythema
Infrared	Burns, cataracts(?)
Electricity	Electric shock, electrocution
Noise	Hearing loss
Ergonomic stress	Muscle strain

fluoride fumes may be considerable when certain welding rods are used.

The corrosion-resistant properties of stainless steel are a result of a high concentration of chromium (18–30%). Nickel and manganese also may be present in different stainless steel alloys. Exposure to chromium (including Cr[VI]), nickel, and manganese may be considerable, particularly with gas metal arc processes. The stainless steel surface reflects ultraviolet radiation, with formation of oxides of nitrogen and ozone. Low-hydrogen welding of stainless steel generates high concentrations of fluoride fumes.

Most aluminum welding uses the tungsten inert gas method. As with stainless steel, the gas-shielded process results in formation of ozone as a consequence of the action of ultraviolet radiation on the nascent oxygen in the atmosphere. Total dust and aluminum oxide generation are also considerable.

Brazing and gas welding both generate metal fume. An acetylene torch is used to generate an intense flame. Exposure to cadmium oxide from cadmium-containing silver solder has caused acute lung injury and death after brazing in enclosed spaces. Similar consequences have occurred from generation of the oxides of nitrogen during gas welding. In all cases, improper ventilation was the critical factor in creating the hazard.

Radiation and heat result in the most common injuries to welders: photokeratitis (welder's flash) and thermal burns. These are often related to improper use of protective goggles, gloves, and screens. Flying sparks or

Table 27–7. Coatings and contaminants encountered in welding.

Galvanized metal	Zinc oxide
Paints	Lead, cadmium, isocyanates, aldehydes, epoxies
Biocides	Organic mercury, organic tin
Chlorinated solvents	Phosgene
Rustproofing	Phosphorus, phosphine
Alloys, sheet metal	Cadmium, nickel, manganese, beryllium
Solders	Rosin, colophony

debris may cause burns or eye injury as well. Noise exposure may exceed 80 dB in welding processes, particularly cutting or gouging operations; in plasma welding (where intense heat is generated), levels may approach 120 dB. Environmental conditions also will influence noise generation. Electrical shock is a constant hazard and requires careful grounding and shielding of cables and equipment. Most manual processes place isometric stress on the welder, particularly involving the shoulders and the upper extremities.

Coatings or contaminants may present additional hazards (Table 27–7), particularly when their presence and potential hazard are unknown or unsuspected. The formation of toxic gases, fumes, or vapors usually is due to the heating of a coated or treated metal, although phosgene exposure is related to the action of ultraviolet radiation or heat on chlorinated hydrocarbon vapors (similar to the formation of ozone from oxygen and oxides of nitrogen from nitrogen).

Soldering is not associated with significant exposure to metal fumes because the temperatures are low. Potential contamination of the workplace with lead dust requires careful attention to hygiene. Some fluxes, such as rosin, are skin sensitizers and may cause allergic dermatitis or asthma.

Clinical Findings

A. Acute Exposure

1. Photokeratitis—Photokeratitis is the result of exposure of the cornea to ultraviolet B radiation (UVB) in the range of 280–315 nm. The duration of exposure necessary to induce this effect varies with the distance from the arc and the light intensity. Following exposure of the unprotected eye to the welding arc for several seconds, the worker develops pain, burning, or a feeling of "sand or grit" in the eye. Physical examination shows conjunctival injection, and slit-lamp examination may reveal punctate depressions over the cornea. The condition is self-limited, resolving in several hours. Careful examination for foreign bodies or evidence of thermal ocular injury is mandatory.

2. Metal fume fever—(See "Zinc," above.) Metal fume fever is a benign, self-limited condition characterized by the delayed onset (8–12 hours) of fever, chills, cough, myalgias, and a metallic taste. A history of welding on galvanized metal suggests the diagnosis.

3. Upper respiratory irritation—Upper respiratory tract irritation may result from exposure to a variety of welding contaminants, including dusts, ozone, aluminum oxide, nitrogen oxides, cadmium oxide, and fluorides. Asthma also may be triggered as a result of nonspecific irritation or allergy (chromium, nickel).

4. Lung injury—While unusual, exposure to oxides of nitrogen and cadmium oxide may cause acute lung injury and delayed pulmonary edema. A history of gas welding or brazing in enclosed or poorly ventilated spaces or sheet metal work should raise this concern and serve as an indication for careful medical evaluation and observation.

5. Musculoskeletal trauma—Injuries resulting from isometric stress on the upper extremity during welding may present as symptomatic shoulder and neck pain following prolonged activity. Asymptomatic muscle damage may result in slight increases in creatine phosphokinase levels in serum.

6. Thermal burns and electrical injuries—See Chapter 11.

B. Chronic Exposure

1. Siderosis—Siderosis results from accumulation of nonfibrogenic iron oxide particles in the lung. While the radiographic appearance may be dramatic, with evidence of diffuse reticulonodular densities, reports of deficits of pulmonary function are inconsistent, suggesting a mild or minimal effect. In welders who also have been exposed to crystalline silica or asbestos, radiographic differentiation of hemosiderosis from pulmonary fibrosis is difficult. Pleural thickening or calcification has not been related to welding in the absence of asbestos exposure.

2. Other chronic effects—Welders report an excess of respiratory symptoms and have increased work absences from respiratory diseases. Demonstration of clear deficits in pulmonary function attributable to welding have been inconsistent. At present, there is limited evidence that welding results in chronic respiratory impairment. In the evaluation of a welder with chronic lung disease, a careful medical and occupational history is essential, focusing on both welding exposures and other confounding factors.

Studies of lung cancer in welders also have been inconsistent, sharing the limitations of many of the respiratory studies. The excess in lung cancer in welders may be related to exposure to chromium and nickel in welding of stainless steel. Studies involving welders who worked in shipyards during the first half of this century are confounded by significant secondary exposure to asbestos.

Other studies indicate that welders may have decreased sperm counts and be at risk for adverse reproductive outcomes. Whether welders are at risk for the development of neuropsychological symptoms or manganese toxicity is an area of active research and controversy.

Prevention

Most acute injuries or poisonings related to welding processes are preventable. Strict adherence to appropriate safety procedures will prevent burns, eye injuries, and electric shock. Awareness of the potential hazards, with attention to the provision of adequate ventilation, is the best safeguard against accidental overexposure to air contaminants. In enclosed spaces, air-supplied respirators are essential, particularly with processes that result in generation of nitrogen oxides.

Carefully designed and controlled studies in the future will better assess the potential impact of welding on respiratory function and on the development of lung cancer. These effects, if present, certainly will be minimized by measures to reduce welding exposures through engineering, ventilation, and proper use of personal protection.

Treatment

Photokeratitis and metal fume fever require no specific treatment, although other diagnoses should be excluded. Welders suspected of having acute overexposure to nitrogen oxides, phosgene, or cadmium oxide should be observed for possible development of pulmonary edema. Treatment of pulmonary edema and respiratory insufficiency related to these agents is supportive. Asthmatics bothered by nonspecific irritant effects related to welding may benefit from improved ventilation and respiratory protection, although cartridge respirators will not prevent exposure to irritant gases. Frank allergic asthma to specific agents may require removal from further exposure. Burns and radiation injuries are discussed in Chapter 11.

REFERENCES

El-Zein M et al: Is metal fume fever a determinant of welding related respiratory symptoms and/or increased bronchial responsiveness? A longitudinal study. Occup Environ Med 2005;62:688 [PMID: 16169914].

Findan F et al: Oxidant-antioxidant status and pulmonary function in welding workers. J Occup Health 2005;47:286 [PMID: 16096352].

Jankovic J: Searching for a relationship between manganese and welding and Parkinson's disease. Neurology 2005;64:2021 [PMID: 15985567].

Kim JY et al: Exposure to welding fumes is associated with acute systemic inflammatory responses. Occup Environ Med 2005; 62:157 [PMID: 15723880].

Lu L et al: Alteration of serum concentrations of manganese, iron, ferritin, and transferrin receptor following exposure to welding fumes among career welders. Neurotoxicology 2005;26: 257 [PMID: 15713346].

Maier R et al: Welder's maculopathy? Int Arch Occup Environ Health 2005;78:681 [PMID: 16021465].

Palmer KT et al: Inflammatory responses to the occupational inhalation of metal fume. Eur Respir J 2006;27:366 [PMID: 16452594].

Chemicals

Robert J. Harrison, MD, MPH

This chapter covers selected chemicals of particular importance to the occupational health practitioner. Solvents, pesticides, and gases are covered in subsequent chapters.

ACIDS & ALKALIS

Acids and alkalis are of great importance as industrial chemicals. When ranked by volume of production, the inorganic acids and alkalis (including chlorine and ammonia) are 8 of the 50 major chemicals produced yearly in the United States.

1. Acids

Essentials of Diagnosis

A. ACUTE EFFECTS

- Irritative dermatitis, skin burn
- Respiratory irritation, pulmonary edema

B. CHRONIC EFFECTS

- Hydrofluoric acid: osteosclerosis
- Nitric acid (oxides of nitrogen): bronchiolitis fibrosa obliterans
- Chromic acid: nasal ulceration, perforation, skin ulceration
- Sulfuric acid: laryngeal cancer

Exposure Limits

A. SULFURIC ACID

American Conference of Governmental Industrial Hygienists (ACGIH) threshold limit value (TLV): 1 mg/m^3, 3 mg/m^3 short-term exposure limit (STEL)

Occupational Safety and Health Administration (OSHA) permissible exposure level (PEL): 1 mg/m^3 time-weighted average (TWA)

National Institute for Occupational Safety and Health (NIOSH) recommended exposure limit (REL): 1 mg/m^3 TWA

B. PHOSPHORIC ACID

ACGIH TLV: 1 mg/m^3 TWA, 3 mg/m^3 STEL
OSHA PEL: 1 mg/m^3 TWA
NIOSH REL: 1 mg/m^3, 3 mg/m^3 STEL

C. HYDROCHLORIC ACID

ACGIH TLV: 5 ppm ceiling
OSHA PEL: 5 ppm ceiling
NIOSH REL: 5 ppm ceiling

D. CHROMIC ACID (CR[VI])

ACGIH TLV: 0.05 mg/m^3 TWA
OSHA PEL: 0.1 mg/m^3 ceiling
NIOSH REL: 0.001 mg/m^3

E. HYDROFLUORIC ACID

ACGIH TLV: 3 ppm TWA
OSHA PEL: 3 ppm TWA
NIOSH REL: 3 ppm TWA, 6 ppm ceiling

F. NITRIC ACID

ACGIH TLV: 2 ppm TWA, 4 ppm STEL
OSHA PEL: 2 ppm TWA
NIOSH REL: 2 ppm TWA, 4 ppm STEL

General Considerations

An inorganic acid is a compound of hydrogen and one or more other elements (with the exception of carbon) that dissociates to produce hydrogen ions when dissolved in water or other solvents. The resulting solution has the ability to neutralize bases and turn litmus paper red. Inorganic acids of greatest industrial use are chromic, hydrochloric, hydrofluoric, nitric, phosphoric, and sulfuric acids. Inorganic acids share certain fire, explosive, and health hazards.

Organic acids and their derivatives include a broad range of substances used in nearly every type of chemical manufacture. All have primary irritant effects depending on the degree of acid dissociation and water solubility.

Use, Production, & Occupational Exposure

A. INORGANIC ACIDS

1. Sulfuric acid—Sulfuric acid is the leading chemical in production volume. It is less costly than any other acid, can be handled easily, reacts with many organic compounds to produce useful products, and forms a slightly soluble salt with calcium oxide or calcium hydroxide. The majority of sulfuric acid is used in the manufacture of phosphate and other fertilizers, petroleum refining, production of ammonium sulfate, iron and steel pickling, manufacture of explosives and other nitrates, synthetic fiber manufacture, and as a chemical intermediate. Workers with potential exposure to sulfuric acid include electroplaters, jewelers, metal cleaners, picklers, and storage-battery makers. Occupational exposure can occur both by skin contact and by inhalation of sulfuric acid mist.

2. Phosphoric acid—Phosphoric acid is used predominantly in the manufacture of fertilizers and agricultural feeds, in water treatment, and as a component of detergents and cleansers. Other uses include the acid treatment (pickling) of sheet metal, chemical polishing of metals, as a tart flavoring agent for carbonated beverages, as a refractory bonding agent, and for boiler cleaning, textile dying, lithographic engraving, and rubber latex coagulation. Occupational exposure occurs primarily to the liquid acid by skin contact.

3. Chromic acid—Chromic acid is produced by roasting chromite ore with soda ash and treatment with sulfuric acid to form chromic acid anhydride, chromic acid (chromium trioxide), and dichromic acid. Chromic acid is used in chromium plating, process engraving, cement manufacturing, anodizing, metal cleaning, tanning, and the manufacture of ceramic glazes, colored glass, inks, and paints. Without local exhaust ventilation, occupational exposure to chromic acid mist during metal-plating operations can range up to several milligrams per cubic meter, but with a local exhaust system, this can be reduced markedly to nearly undetectable limits.

4. Nitric acid—Nitric acid is produced from the oxidation of ammonia in the presence of a catalyst to yield nitric oxide, which is then further oxidized and absorbed in water to form an aqueous solution of nitric acid. Nitric acid is used to produce ammonium and potassium nitrate, explosives, adipic acid, isocyanates, fertilizers, nitroparaffins, and nitrobenzenes. Occupational exposure can occur by topical contact with the liquid acid, as well as by inhalation of nitrogen oxides evolved when nitric acid reacts with reducing agents (e.g., metals or organic matter) or during the combustion of nitrogen-containing materials (e.g., welding, glass blowing, underground blasting, and decomposition of agri-

cultural silage). Reports of occupational exposure to nitric acid are limited to measurements of nitrogen oxides that evolved by these reactions.

5. Hydrochloric acid—Hydrochloric acid is an aqueous solution of hydrogen chloride and is used in steel pickling, chemical manufacturing, oil- and gas-well acidizing, and food processing. Hydrochloric acid gas also may evolve from thermal degradation of polyvinyl chloride, a hazard to firefighters.

6. Hydrofluoric acid—Hydrofluoric acid (hydrogen fluoride) is a colorless liquid manufactured by reaction of sulfuric acid with calcium fluoride in heated kilns. It evolves as a gas and then is condensed as liquid anhydrous hydrogen fluoride. Hydrofluoric acid is used as an intermediate in the production of fluorocarbons, aluminum fluoride, and cryolite; as a gasoline alkylation catalyst; and as an intermediate in the production of uranium hexafluoride. It is used in metal cleaning, glass etching, and polishing applications. Occupational exposure can occur both by direct skin contact and by inhalation of fumes.

7. Organic acids—Among the saturated monocarboxylic acids, formic acid is used mainly in the textile industry as a dye-exhausting agent, in the leather industry as a deliming agent and neutralizer, as a coagulant for rubber latex, and as a component of nickel plating baths. Propionic acid is used in organic synthesis, as a mold inhibitor, and as a food additive. The unsaturated monocarboxylic acid acrylic acid is used widely in the manufacture of resins, plasticizers, and drugs. The aliphatic dicarboxylics maleic, fumaric, and adipic acids find use in the manufacture of synthetic resins, dyes, surface coatings, inks, and plasticizers. The halogenated acetic acids are highly reactive chemical intermediates used in glycine, drug, dye, and herbicide manufacture. Glycolic acid and lactic acid are used widely in the leather, textile, adhesive, and plastics industries, and lactic acid is also used as a food acidulant.

Metabolism & Mechanism of Action

Both inorganic and organic acids, by virtue of their water solubility and acid dissociation, will cause direct destruction of body tissue, including mucous membranes and skin. The extent of direct skin damage depends on the concentration of acid and length of exposure, whereas the damage to the respiratory tract by inhalation of acid mists will depend in addition on particle size. Hydrofluoric acid, one of the most corrosive of the inorganic acids, readily penetrates the skin and travels to deep tissue layers, causing liquefaction necrosis of soft tissues and decalcification and corrosion of bone. The intense pain that may accompany hydrogen fluoride burns is attributed to the calcium-precipitating property of the fluoride ion, which produces immobilization of tissue calcium and an excess of potassium that stimulates nerve endings. The fluoride ion also may bind body calcium, causing life-threatening systemic hypocalcemia after acute skin exposure or osteosclerotic bone changes after chronic exposure to hydrogen fluoride mist.

Clinical Findings

A. Symptoms & Signs

1. Acute exposure—All acids act as primary irritants of the skin and mucous membranes.

a. Skin—All acids on contact with the skin cause dehydration and heat release to produce first-, second-, or third-degree burns with pain. Sensitization is rare. Hydrofluoric acid solutions of less than 50% may cause burns that may not become apparent for 1–24 hours; stronger solutions cause immediate pain and rapid tissue destruction, appearing reddened, pasty-white, blistered, macerated, or charred.

b. Respiratory effects—Inhalation of vapors or mists causes immediate rhinorrhea, throat burning, cough, burning eyes, and conjunctival irritation. High concentrations may cause shortness of breath, chest tightness, pulmonary edema, and death from respiratory failure. Inhalation of acid vapors or mists generally causes immediate symptoms because of high water solubility in mucous membranes, but respiratory effects may be delayed for several hours. Noncardiogenic pulmonary edema has been reported following acute inhalation exposure to sulfuric acid fumes, with almost complete recovery except for slightly decreased diffusion capacity on pulmonary function testing. For nitric acid exposure with oxides of nitrogen, overexposure tends to produce delayed symptoms 1–24 hours after inhalation, beginning with dyspnea followed by pulmonary edema and cyanosis. Rapidly progressive pulmonary edema of delayed onset may follow the inhalation of fumes from accidental nitric acid exposure. In these cases, postmortem electron microscopy of lung tissue suggests increased permeability as a result of microvascular injury.

Chlorine species are highly reactive, resulting in a variety of dose-related lung effects ranging from respiratory mucous membrane irritation to pulmonary edema. Obstructive or restrictive pulmonary defects can result immediately following exposure, with complete resolution over a few days to weeks in most individuals. A few patients have long-term, persistent obstructive or restrictive pulmonary deficits or increased nonspecific airway reactivity after high-level exposure to chlorine gas.

Exposure to lower levels of acid vapors or mists over months may increase the risk of developing irritant-associated asthma. Aluminum potroom workers with exposure to fluorides have an increased risk of respira-

tory symptoms, with a greater prevalence of airway responsiveness as measured by nonspecific airway challenge. Occupational asthma also has been reported following exposure to chloramines in indoor swimming pool air.

c. Systemic effects—Several deaths have been reported as a result of persistent hypocalcemia and hypomagnesemia following exposure to concentrated hydrofluoric acid, with the exposures involving as little as 2.5% of total body surface area. Systemic toxicity involving gastrointestinal hemorrhage, acute renal failure, and hepatic injury has been reported following chromic acid ingestion.

2. Chronic exposure—

a. Skin—Chromate compounds can be allergens and can cause pulmonary as well as skin sensitization, but chromic acid results only in direct irritant dermatitis. Ulceration of the skin and ulceration and perforation of the nasal septum have been reported following chronic exposure to chromic acid.

b. Dental erosion—Exposure to inorganic and organic acid fumes is reported to cause tooth surface loss. An increase in periodontal pockets but not oral mucous membrane lesions was found among acid-exposed workers.

c. Respiratory effects—Bronchiolitis fibrosa obliterans, a chronic interstitial lung disease, has been described after acute pneumonitis from nitric acid and oxides of nitrogen. No significant change in lung function has been found among workers exposed to phosphoric acid while refining phosphorus. Acids and a variety of other irritants have been recognized to cause vocal cord dysfunction, with chronic symptoms of hoarseness and loss of voice.

d. Systemic effects—Osteosclerosis has been found in workers exposed to hydrofluoric acid and fluoride-containing compounds. Farmers with formic acid exposure have increased renal ammoniagenesis and urinary calcium excretion, possibly as a result of interaction with the oxidative metabolism of renal tubular cells.

e. Cancer—Studies of workers exposed to sulfuric acid mists show an excess risk of laryngeal and nasopharyngeal cancer. The International Agency for Research on Cancer (IARC) concludes that there is sufficient evidence that occupational exposure to strong inorganic acid mists containing sulfuric acid is carcinogenic (group 1). Battery manufacturers and steel workers exposed to mineral acid mists have an increased risk of upper aerodigestive tract cancer. For chromic acid, IARC concludes that there is sufficient evidence of carcinogenicity in humans and animals (group 1). Airborne hexavalent chromium exposure results in an increased risk of lung cancer among chromium platers. NIOSH recommends that chromic acid be regulated as a carcinogen. An increase in the number of sister-chromatid exchanges has been found in lymphocytes of workers exposed to acid aerosols at a phosphate fertilizer factory. IARC finds that hydrochloric acid is not classifiable in terms of carcinogenicity to humans (group 3). The cancer risk was not increased among cohorts of chemical manufacturing workers exposed to hydrogen chloride and nitric acid.

B. LABORATORY FINDINGS

In cases where inhalation exposure may cause more extensive mucosal irritation, the chest radiograph may show interstitial or alveolar edema, and hypoxemia may be evident by arterial blood gas analysis. Nonspecific abnormalities in liver and kidney function have been reported following massive inhalation exposures to sulfuric acid and hydrofluoric acid. Urine fluoride levels can be used as biologic indices of exposure in hydrofluoric acid intoxication, with a normal mean value in urine of 0.5 mg/L (recommended occupational postshift urinary biologic standard of 7 mg/L).

Differential Diagnosis

There are many respiratory irritants, including gases such as ammonia, phosgene, halogens (chlorine, bromine), sulfur dioxide, and ozone; solvents such as glycol ethers; and dusts such as fibrous glass. The symptoms and clinical course of lung disorders caused by these substances and by the acids discussed in this chapter do not differ; thus the history is essential. Likewise, hundreds of industrial chemicals may cause direct irritant dermatitis.

Prevention

A. WORK PRACTICES

When possible, highly corrosive acids should be replaced by acids that present fewer hazards, and if use of corrosives is essential, only the minimum concentration should be used. Proper storage practices should include fire-resistant buildings with acid-resistant floors, retaining sills, and adequate drainage; containers should be adequately protected against impact, kept off the floor, and labeled clearly. Wherever possible, handling should be done through sealed systems or the substances transported in safety-bottle carriers. Decanting should be done with special siphons or pumps. The potential for violent or dangerous reactions (e.g., when water is poured into nitric acid) can be avoided by appropriate training.

Where processes produce acid mists (as in electroplating), local exhaust ventilation should be installed. Workers potentially exposed to splashes or spills must wear acid-resistant hand, arm, eye, and face protection, and respiratory protection should be available for emer-

gency use. Emergency showers and eyewash stations should be strategically located.

B. MEDICAL SURVEILLANCE

Preplacement and periodic examinations should include medical history of skin and respiratory disease and examination of the skin, teeth, and lungs. For potential hydrofluoric acid exposure near or above the permissible exposure limit, periodic postshift urinary fluoride in excess of 7 mg/L (adjusted for urine specific gravity of 1.024) may indicate poor work practices. Elemental analysis of hair for fluoride has been correlated with fluoride levels in serum and urine.

Treatment

Immediate on-site first aid treatment of acid burns to the eye or skin includes copious flushing with running water with removal of all contaminated clothing. First- or second-degree burns involving a small area generally can be treated at the on-site medical facility with debridement and application of suitable burn dressings. All other acid burns should be treated at a hospital emergency facility.

For hydrofluoric acid burns, the definitive treatment is aimed at deactivation of the fluoride ion in tissue with calcium, magnesium, or quaternary ammonium solution. If the hydrogen fluoride concentration is 20% or more, if the patient has been exposed to a long delay of a lower concentration, or if a large tissue area has been affected by a lower concentration, then calcium gluconate solution should be used. Calcium gluconate solution is prepared by mixing 10% calcium gluconate with an equal amount of saline to form a 5% solution and is infiltrated with a small needle in multiple injections (0.5 mL/cm^2 of tissue) into and 5 mm beyond the affected area. Dramatic pain relief should occur. Vesicles and bullae should be debrided carefully, with removal of necrotic tissue; if periungual or ungual tissues are involved, the nail should be split to the base. A burn dressing then is applied along with calcium gluconate 2.5% gel or magnesium sulfate paste. Hydrofluoric acid burns of the hand have been treated successfully with repeated application of an occlusive glove over topical calcium carbonate gel. Repeated intraarterial infusion over 4 hours with 10 mL of 10% calcium chloride diluted with 40 mL of normal saline also has been recommended for the treatment of hydrofluoric acid extremity burns. Careful monitoring of serum magnesium and calcium levels is required. If the hydrogen fluoride concentration is 20% or less and only a small surface area is involved, the burn can be flushed with water and then treated with 10% magnesium sulfate solution under a soft dressing. The eye burned with hydrogen fluoride should be irrigated copiously and then evaluated by an ophthalmologist. Calcium gluconate 1% in normal saline can be used as an irrigant.

Systemic effects from absorption should be anticipated from skin burns from hydrogen fluoride of greater than 50% concentration or from extensive burns at any concentration. Hypocalcemia can be life-threatening and should be monitored by repeated measurement of serum calcium and electrocardiography for QT-interval prolongation. Calcium gluconate 10% intravenously with adequate hydration should be used for calcium depletion.

For inhalation of acid vapors or mists, the victim should be removed immediately from the source of exposure and treated on-site with 100% oxygen. If there are symptoms of shortness of breath, chest tightness, or persistent cough, the patient should be evaluated at the hospital. Patients who are minimally symptomatic with normal peak expiratory flow rate and oxygen saturation values can be discharged from the emergency department after several hours of observation and instructed to return if dyspnea occurs. Upper body or facial burns are a clue that inhalation may have occurred with possible serious lower airway damage. Evaluation should include a chest radiograph and arterial blood gas analysis for oxygen. Hypoxemia should be treated with 100% oxygen by mask or by intubation in the event of severe hypoxemia, acidosis, or respiratory distress. Fluid balance should be monitored carefully and intracardiac pressure measured directly if necessary. Bronchospasm may be treated with inhaled bronchodilators or intravenous aminophylline and steroids if necessary. The benefits of steroids in the management of noncardiogenic pulmonary edema caused by acid inhalation are unknown, but the drugs may be used empirically to speed recovery and prevent the subsequent development of interstitial lung disease. Nebulized calcium gluconate 5% solution has been used successfully for treatment of inhalational exposure to hydrofluoric acid.

REFERENCES

Edlich RF et al: Modern concepts of treatment and prevention of chemical injuries. J Long-Term Effects Med Implants 2005;15: 303 [PMID: 16022641].

Franzblau A, Sahakian N: Asthma following household exposure to hydrofluoric acid. Am J Ind Med 2003;44:321 [PMID: 12929153].

Hulten P et al: Hexafluorine vs standard decontamination to reduce systemic toxicity after dermal exposure to hydrofluoric acid. J Toxicol Clin Toxicol 2004;42:355 [PMID: 15461243].

Medina-Ramon M et al: Asthma, chronic bronchitis, and exposure to irritant agents in occupational domestic cleaning. Occup Environ Med 2005;62:598 [PMID: 16109815].

Vianna MI et al: Occupational exposures to acid mists and gases and ulcerative lesions of the oral mucosa. Am J Indust Med 2004; 45:238 [PMID: 14991850].

2. Alkalis

Essentials of Diagnosis

A. ACUTE EFFECTS

- Skin and eye burns
- Respiratory irritation

B. CHRONIC EFFECTS

- Corneal opacities of the eye (untreated)
- Obstructive lung disease

Exposure Limits

A. SODIUM HYDROXIDE

ACGIH TLV: 2 mg/m^3 TWA
OSHA PEL: 2 mg/m^3 TWA ceiling
NIOSH REL: 2 mg/m^3 ceiling (15 minutes)

B. POTASSIUM HYDROXIDE

ACGIH TLV: 2 mg/m^3 ceiling (15 minutes)
OSHA PEL: None

C. CALCIUM OXIDE

ACGIH TLV: 2 mg/m^3 TWA
NIOSH REL: 2 mg/m^3 TWA
OSHA PEL: 5 mg/m^3 TWA

General Considerations

Alkalis are caustic substances that dissolve in water to form a solution with a pH higher than 7.0. These include ammonia, ammonium hydroxide, calcium hydroxide, calcium oxide, potassium hydroxide, potassium carbonate, sodium hydroxide, sodium carbonate, and trisodium phosphate. The alkalis, whether in solid form or concentrated liquid form, are more destructive to tissue than most acids. They tend to liquefy tissues and allow for deeper penetration, depending on concentration, duration of contact, and area of the body involved.

Use, Production, & Occupational Exposure

In the United States, all sodium hydroxide (caustic soda) is produced by the electrolysis of sodium or potassium chloride in mercury cells. In this process, pure saturated brine is decomposed by electric current to liberate chlorine gas at the anode and sodium metal at the cathode. The latter reacts with water to form sodium hydroxide. Most caustic soda is produced as a 50% aqueous solution. Sodium hydroxide is used in pulp and paper production, water treatment, and manufacture of a wide variety of organic and inorganic chemicals, soaps and detergents, textiles, and alumina. Annual U.S. production is more than 22 billion pounds.

Sodium carbonate (soda ash) is produced by the ammonium chloride process, by the reaction of sodium chloride and sulfuric acid, or by leaching out of rock deposits. Sodium carbonate is used in glass manufacturing, as a component of cleaning-product formulations, in pulp and paper processing and water treatment, and as a chemical intermediate.

Potassium carbonate (potash) is produced by carbonating potassium hydroxide solutions obtained by electrolysis. Potassium carbonate is used in the manufacture of soap, glass, pottery, and shampoo; in tanning and finishing leather; in photographic chemicals, fire-extinguishing compounds, and rubber antioxidant preparations; and as an alkalizer and drainpipe cleaner.

Potassium hydroxide (caustic potash) is produced by electrolysis of potassium chloride solution and is used as a chemical intermediate in the manufacture of potassium carbonate, potassium phosphate, soaps, tetrapotassium pyrophosphate, liquid fertilizers, dyestuffs, and herbicides.

Calcium oxide (quicklime) is made by calcining limestone. Calcium oxide is used in metallurgy as a flux in steel production, for ammonia recovery in the Solvay process for sodium carbonate, in construction applications and water purification and softening, in beet and sugar cane refining, in kraft paper pulp production, and in sewage treatment.

Metabolism & Mechanism of Action

Occupational exposure to the alkalis is primarily by direct contact with the eyes, skin, and mucous membranes. Inhalation of caustic mists generally is limited by the irritant properties of the compound. Contact of the eyes with alkalis causes disintegration and sloughing of corneal epithelium, corneal opacification, marked edema, and ulceration. Alkaline compounds will combine with skin tissue to form albuminates and with natural fats to form soaps. They gelatinize tissue and result in deep and painful destruction. Accidental or intentional ingestion of alkalis may cause severe esophageal necrosis with subsequent stenosis.

Clinical Findings

A. Symptoms & Signs

1. Acute exposure—In contrast to acids, skin contact with the alkalis may not elicit immediate pain but may start to cause immediate damage with erythema and tissue necrosis within minutes to hours. Splashes of alkali to the eyes, if not treated within minutes, may result in corneal necrosis, edema, and opacification.

Irreversible obstructive lung injury has developed after acute inhalation of sodium hydroxide in a poorly venti-

lated space. Workers have suffered severe skin and inhalational injuries following exposure to "black liquor" used in the pulp and paper industry. Fatal injury has occurred after a relatively brief inhalation and dermal contact with a hot concentrated caustic solution. Acute tracheobronchitis and respiratory failure as a result of high-dose ammonia inhalation may result in permanent, severe, and fixed airways obstruction. Bronchiolitis obliterans caused by occupational exposure to incinerator fly ash has been reported.

2. Chronic exposure—Chronic exposure to caustic dusts does not increase the mortality rate significantly. Long-term sodium hydroxide inhalation has been reported to cause severe obstructive airway disease with significant air trapping. Chronic exposure to ammonia of over 7.5 ppm is associated with pulmonary function decrements among swine production facility workers. An increased prevalence of coughing, wheezing, and ocular and nasal irritation was reported among community residents exposed to alkali dust. Corneal opacities have resulted from untreated corneal alkali burns. An increased risk of nasopharyngeal carcinoma has been observed among Chinese textile workers exposed to acid and caustics.

B. Laboratory Findings

No specific laboratory tests are of value in the diagnosis and management of problems resulting from alkali exposure.

Differential Diagnosis

Many other industrial chemicals, including acids, may cause eye and skin burns.

Prevention

A. Work Practices

Insofar as possible, solutions of caustics should be handled in closed systems that will prevent contact with or inhalation of the chemical. All persons with potential exposure to caustics should wear proper protective clothing and equipment, such as a full-face shield, safety goggles, apron or suit, rubber gloves, and boots. Emergency showers and eyewashes must be located where eye or skin contact may occur.

B. Medical Surveillance

Medical examination of the eyes, skin, and respiratory tract is recommended for all workers with caustic exposure.

Treatment

Sodium and potassium hydroxide may cause more extended and deeper damage as a result of rapid penetration through ocular tissues. Alkali burns of the eye and skin should be treated within minutes by copious irrigation with tap water and removal of all contaminated clothing. Irrigation with a weak acid such as 5% acetic acid also has been suggested. First aid treatment with prompt and continuous eye irrigation is essential to prevent permanent corneal damage and visual loss. Topical use of a synthetic metalloproteinase inhibitor has been shown to reverse or stop the progression of corneal ulceration following an experimental alkali burn. A relatively new hypertonic, polyvalent, amphoteric chelating compound (Diphoterine) also appears to be of benefit for emergent eye and skin decontamination. A physician or health practitioner should be consulted for eye burns and careful examination of the eye performed. If eye damage is suspected, follow-up with an ophthalmologist is recommended. Intensive topical steroids, antibiotics, and amniotic membrane transplantation may be required.

REFERENCES

Andrews K et al: The treatment of alkaline burns of the skin by neutralization. Plast Reconstr Surg 2003;111:1918 [PMID: 12711953].

Kompa S et al: Effect of different irrigating solutions on aqueous humour pH changes, intraocular pressure and histological findings after induced alkali burns. Acta Ophthalmol Scand 2005;83:467 [PMID: 16029272].

ACRYLAMIDE & ACRYLONITRILE

1. Acrylamide

Essentials of Diagnosis

A. ACUTE EFFECTS

- Dermatitis

B. CHRONIC EFFECTS

- Peripheral neuropathy

Exposure Limits

ACGIH TLV: 0.035 mg/m³ TWA
OSHA PEL: 0.3 mg/m³ TWA
NIOSH REL: 0.3 mg/m³ TWA

General Considerations

Pure acrylamide is a white crystalline solid at room temperature and is highly soluble in water. It is a vinyl monomer with high reactivity with thiols and with hydroxy and amino groups. Commercial acrylamide is shipped in 50% aqueous form in stainless steel drums, tank trucks, and cars. Acrylamide manufacture is from the catalytic hydration of acrylonitrile.

Use

The major use of acrylamide monomer is in the production of polymers, which are useful as flocculators. Polyacrylamides are used for waste and water treatment flocculents, in products for sewage dewatering, and in a variety of products for the water treatment industry. Other uses include strengtheners for papermaking and retention aids, drilling-mud additives, textile treatment, and surface coatings. One of the more important uses is as a grouting agent, particularly in mining and tunnel construction.

Occupational & Environmental Exposure

Monomer manufacturing workers are potentially exposed to acrylamide, as are papermaking workers, soil-stabilization workers, textile workers, tunnel workers, and well drillers. Biomedical laboratory workers can be exposed to arcylamide used to make polyacrylamide gels. Intoxication has been reported in the manufacture of acrylamide monomer, in the handling of a 10% aqueous solution in a mine, in the production of flocculators, in the use of a resin mixture containing residual monomer, and in the production of polymers while manufacturing paper coating materials. One nonoccupational incident occurred in Japan, where a family ingested well water containing 400 ppm acrylamide.

Acrylamide may be formed at elevated temperatures in cooking, particularly of carbohydrate-rich foods such as potatoes (e.g., crisps, chips, and fries). Residual levels of acrylamide also can be found in cosmetic products.

Metabolism & Mechanism of Action

Acrylamide is absorbed easily in animals following all routes of administration. The peripheral nerve terminal is a primary site of acrylamide action, with possible inhibition of membrane-fusion processes impairing neurotransmitter release. Quantitative data on absorption or excretion in humans are not available. Following intravenous administration in rats, acrylamide is distributed throughout total-body water within minutes and then excreted largely in the urine with a half-life of less than 2 hours. Protein-bound acrylamide or acrylamide metabolites have a half-life in blood and possibly in the central nervous system of about 10 days. The primary metabolite of acrylamide is *N*-acetyl-*S*-(3-amino-3-oxypropyl) cysteine, and it is excreted predominantly in the urine.

Clinical Findings

A. SYMPTOMS & SIGNS

Acrylamide polymer may cause dermatitis but does not cause neurotoxicity. The monomer can produce numbness and tingling of hands and weakness of the hands and legs. Acrylamide is neurotoxic in many experimental animals, causing distal axonopathy and central neuronal degeneration.

More than 60 cases of acrylamide-associated neurotoxicity have been reported in humans. Subclinical peripheral neuropathy has been found in tunnel workers exposed to acrylamide during grouting work. Similar to the neuropathy associated with the hexacarbons n-hexane and methyl-n-butyl ketone, acrylamide neuropathy is considered a typical example of a dying-back disorder, where degeneration begins at the distal ends of the longest and largest fibers and spreads proximally. In most cases, toxicity results from skin contact and dermal absorption, although acrylamide may be absorbed by inhalation as well. The cellular and molecular site of acrylamide neurotoxicity may involve alterations in fast anterograde transport or sulfhydryl groups on presynaptic proteins. The neurologic features of acrylamide intoxication vary depending on the speed of intoxication. In the Japanese family that ingested contaminated well water, encephalopathy with confusion, disorientation, memory disturbances, hallucinations, ataxia, and peripheral neuropathy developed in approximately 1 month. Reported time to onset of symptoms in occupational cases has varied from 4 weeks to approximately 24 months. Clinically, acrylamide peripheral neuropathy affects both motor and sensory nerve fibers predominantly in the distal limbs. Difficulty in walking and clumsiness of the hands are usually the first symptoms, followed by numbness of the feet and fingers. Distal weakness is found on examination, with loss of tendon reflexes and vibration sensation. Evidence of excessive sweating affecting predominantly the extremities has been reported commonly, along with redness and exfoliation of the skin. In acute cases, central nervous system involvement may result in truncal ataxia, lethargy, and dysarthria. Major histologic findings are swelling of axons and/or a decrease in large-diameter axons. The axonopathy is reversible slowly over time, but complete recovery depends on the severity of intoxication.

Acrylamide has been found to increase the tumor yield in mice and is genotoxic in animal studies. Acrylamide reacts with hemoglobin to form DNA adducts and heritable translocations in animal studies. Human studies have shown increased DNA adducts and chromosomal aberrations among workers exposed to acrylamide. Cohort mortality studies have shown no significant excess of cancer among acrylamide-exposed workers, and initial studies suggest that there is not an excess of cancer owing to consumption of acrylamide in food. There is some evidence to suggest that acrylamide results in adverse developmental or reproductive effects in animal studies.

The State of California has listed acrylamide as a carcinogen since 1990. The IARC has concluded that there is sufficient evidence in experimental animals for acrylamide to be classified as a carcinogen (group 2A).

B. LABORATORY FINDINGS

Electrophysiologic studies of workers with signs and symptoms of neurotoxicity have shown only a slight effect on maximal conduction velocity of either motor or sensory fibers. Sensory nerve action potentials usually are reduced and are the most sensitive electrophysiologic test.

Sural nerve biopsies performed on two patients during recovery from acrylamide neuropathy showed axonal degeneration affecting mainly large-diameter fibers. Recent studies have suggested the use of urinary S-carboxyethyl cysteine and mercapturic acid metabolites of acrylamide for biomonitoring use in the workplace and general populations, respectively.

Differential Diagnosis

The combination of truncal ataxia with peripheral neuropathy—predominantly motor—accompanied by excessive sweating and redness and peeling of the skin makes the diagnosis of acrylamide-associated neurotoxicity likely. Other occupational toxic agents associated with peripheral neuropathy must be considered (see Chapter 7), along with the presence of other underlying metabolic diseases, drug use, and endocrine disorders.

Prevention

A. WORK PRACTICES

Mechanized bag loading of polymerization reactors, closed-line transfer of liquid acrylamide, and other closed-system processes are important to minimize exposure. Where necessary, personal protective equipment designed to prevent dermal and inhalation exposure to acrylamide should be available. General population consumption of acrylamide in foods can be reduced by changes in food-manufacturing raw materials and preparation methods.

B. MEDICAL SURVEILLANCE

Preplacement and periodic examinations should exclude symptomatic peripheral neuropathies. Hemoglobin adducts have been used to monitor occupational exposure to both acrylamide and acrylonitrile. A neurotoxicity index involving electrophysiologic measures was correlated with urinary 24-hour mercapturic acid levels, hemoglobin adducts of acrylamide, employment duration, and vibration sensitivity. Vibration threshold may be a sensitive indicator of early neurotoxicity caused by acrylamide exposure.

Treatment

Skin contaminated with acrylamide should be washed immediately with soap and water, and contaminated clothing should be removed. There is no known treatment for acrylamide intoxication. Removal from exposure is the only effective measure that can be taken. Full recovery has been observed in most cases after 2 weeks to 2 years, although in severe cases some residual neurologic abnormalities have been noted.

REFERENCES

Kjuus H et al: Chromosome aberrations in tunnel workers exposed to acrylamide and N-methylolacrylamide. Scand J Work Environ Health 2005;31:300 [PMID: 16161713].

National Toxicology Program Report on Carcinogens: Acrylamide, http://ntp.niehs.nih.gov/ntp/roc/eleventh/profiles/s003acry.pdf.

Pelucchi C et al: Dietary acrylamide and human cancer. Int J Cancer 2006;118:467 [PMID: 16003724].

State of California Office of Environmental Health Hazard Assessment: www.oehha.ca.gov/prop65/acrylamide.html.

World Health Organization: Acrylamide, www.who.int/foodsafety/chem/chemicals/acrylamide/en/.

2. Acrylonitrile

Essentials of Diagnosis

A. ACUTE EFFECTS

- Respiratory irritation, nausea, dizziness, and irritability, followed by
- Convulsions, coma, and death

B. CHRONIC EFFECTS

- Nausea, dizziness, headache, apprehension, fatigue

Exposure Limits

ACGIH TLV: 2 ppm TWA

OSHA PEL: 2 ppm TWA, 10 ppm ceiling (15 minutes)

NIOSH REL: 1 ppm TWA, 10 ppm ceiling (15 minutes)

General Considerations

Acrylonitrile is a volatile colorless liquid with a characteristic odor resembling that of peach seeds, discernible at 20 ppm or less. It is a highly reactive compound. Pure acrylonitrile polymerizes readily in light, and storage requires the addition of polymerization inhibitors. Its vapors are explosive and flammable and may release hydrogen cyanide on burning.

Use

Acrylonitrile was not an important product until World War II, when it was used in the production of oil-resistant rubbers. Nearly all world production of acrylonitrile is now based on a process where propylene, ammonia, and air react in the vapor phase in the presence of a catalyst. Hydrogen cyanide and acrylonitrile are the chief by-products formed; the latter undergoes a series of distillations to produce acrylonitrile.

Much of acrylonitrile monomer is used for the manufacture of acrylic fibers for the apparel, carpeting, and home furnishings industries. Acrylonitrile-containing plastics, particularly the resins acrylonitrile-butadiene-styrene (ABS) and styrene-acrylonitrile (SAN), are used in pipe and pipe fittings, automotive parts, appliances, and building components. Nitrile elastomers are used for their oil- and hydrocarbon-resistant properties in the petrochemical and automobile industries. Acrylonitrile is also used to make acrylamide.

Occupational & Environmental Exposure

Potential exposure to acrylonitrile may occur in monomer-, fiber-, resin-, and rubber-producing plants. Potential exposure to acrylonitrile in acrylic fiber production is greatest when the solvent is removed from newly formed fibers and during decontamination of acrylonitrile processing equipment, loading, surveillance of the processing unit, and product sampling.

Metabolism & Mechanism of Action

Acrylonitrile is absorbed readily in animals following ingestion or inhalation. There is a biphasic half-life of 3.5 hours and 50–77 hours, with elimination predominantly in the urine. Acrylonitrile is metabolized to cyanide, and its metabolites are eliminated in the urine. In humans, absorption can occur through both inhalation and skin contact. The acute toxicity of acrylonitrile in humans is thought to be due to the action of cyanide, and thiocyanate is detected in blood and urine of workers. Acrylonitrile is an electrophilic compound and binds covalently to nucleophilic sites in macromolecules. Hemoglobin adducts have been used for exposure assessment in experimental animal studies and for follow-up of acute exposure to acrylonotrile in accidentally exposed workers. It has been postulated that the mutagenic effect of acrylonitrile is caused by glycidonitrile, a reactive intermediate able to alkylate macromolecules.

Clinical Findings

A. SYMPTOMS & SIGNS

A few deaths have been reported from acrylonitrile exposure, with respiratory distress, lethargy, convulsions, and coma at 7500 mg/m^3. Acrylonitrile was implicated in four cases of toxic epidermal necrosis that developed 11–21 days after the victims returned to houses fumigated with a 2:1 mixture of carbon tetrachloride and acrylonitrile. One patient had measurable blood cyanide levels at autopsy. Symptoms of acute poisoning are described as irritability, respiratory irritation, limb weakness, respiratory distress, dizziness, nausea, cyanosis, collapse, convulsions, and cardiac arrest; these resemble cyanide poisoning.

Chronic human toxicity has been reported in rubber workers exposed to 16–100 ppm of acrylonitrile for periods of 20–45 minutes, with complaints of nasal irritation, headache, nausea, apprehension, and fatigue. Acrylonitrile is carcinogenic in rats after 2 years of feeding and inhalation, inducing brain tumors and stomach papillomas. An excess risk of colon and lung cancers occurred among acrylonitrile polymerization workers from a textile fibers plant. Epidemiologic studies suggest that acrylonitrile is associated with an increased lung cancer risk with a latency period of 20 years and that it should be regarded as probably carcinogenic in humans. However, meta-analyses of mortality studies among acrylonitrile-exposed cohorts do not reveal consistent evidence for carcinogenicity. The IARC has concluded that there is sufficient evidence in experimental animals for acrylonitrile to be classified as a carcinogen (group 2A).

B. Laboratory Findings

The use of biomarkers such as chromosomal aberrations and hemoglobin adducts has shown some promise as a tool to understand susceptibility for health effects and to monitor acutely exposed workers. Elevated serum cyanide or urine thiocyanate levels may be found in cases of acute intoxication.

Differential Diagnosis

Acute poisoning with acrylonitrile may mimic cyanide intoxication.

Prevention

A. Work Practices

Controls have proved effective in reducing employee exposure to acrylonitrile. NIOSH has recommended that acrylonitrile be handled in the workplace as a potential human carcinogen and has published detailed recommendations for adequate work practices.

B. Medical Surveillance

Preplacement and annual medical examinations should include special attention to the skin, respiratory tract, and gastrointestinal tract, as well as to the nonspecific

symptoms of headache, nausea, dizziness, and weakness that may be associated with chronic exposure. Treatment kits for acute cyanide intoxication (see Chapter 30) should be immediately available to trained medical personnel at each area where there is a potential for release of or contact with acrylonitrile.

Biologic monitoring may be useful to reflect exposure to acrylonitrile. The relationship between the degree of exposure to acrylonitrile and the urinary excretion of thiocyanate and acrylonitrile was determined in Japanese workers from acrylic fiber factories. A mean postshift urine thiocyanate concentration of 11.4 mg/L (specific gravity 1.024) was found to correlate with an 8-hour average acrylonitrile exposure of 4.2 ppm. Normal urinary thiocyanate levels in nonsmokers do not exceed 2.5 mg/g of creatinine. Mean urinary acrylonitrile levels of 30 µg/L in Dutch plastics workers were found to correlate with a mean 8-hour TWA exposure level of 0.13 ppm and were used to monitor adequate work practices.

Treatment

Treatment of acute intoxication with acrylonitrile is similar to that of cyanide poisoning (see Chapter 30). A combination of N-acetylcysteine with sodium thiosulfate has been suggested as an appropriate measure for acrylonitrile intoxication.

REFERENCE

National Toxicology Program Report on Carcinogens. http://ntp. niehs.nih.gov/ntp/roc/eleventh/profiles/s004acry.pdf

AROMATIC AMINES

Essentials of Diagnosis

A. Acute Effects

- Dermatitis
- Asthma
- Cholestatic jaundice
- Methemoglobinemia

B. Chronic Effects

- Bladder cancer

Exposure Limits

A. Aniline

ACGIH TLV: 2 ppm TWA
OSHA PEL: 5 ppm TWA
NIOSH REL: Reduce exposure to lowest feasible concentrations

B. P,P′-METHYLENE DIANILINE

ACGIH TLV: 0.1 ppm TWA
OSHA PEL: 0.010 ppm TWA, 0.100 ppm STEL
NIOSH REL: Reduce exposure to lowest feasible concentration

C. NAPHTHYLAMINES

ACGIH TLV: Confirmed human carcinogen
OSHA PEL: Stringent workplace controls; occupational carcinogen
NIOSH REL: Reduce exposure to lowest feasible concentrations

D. BENZIDINE-BASED DYES

ACGIH TLV: 0.01 ppm TWA
OSHA PEL: Stringent workplace controls; occupational carcinogen
NIOSH REL: Reduce exposure to lowest feasible concentration

E. O-TOLUIDINE

ACGIH TLV: 2 ppm TWA
OSHA PEL: 5 ppm TWA
NIOSH REL: Reduce exposure to lowest feasible concentrations

General Considerations

The aromatic amines are a class of chemicals derived from aromatic hydrocarbons, such as benzene, toluene, naphthalene, anthracene and diphenyl, by the replacement of at least one hydrogen atom by an amino group. Some examples are shown below.

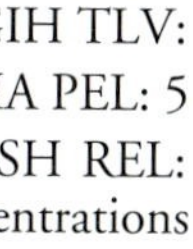

Aniline

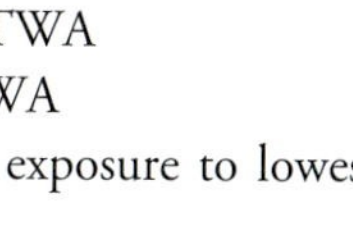

o-Toluidine

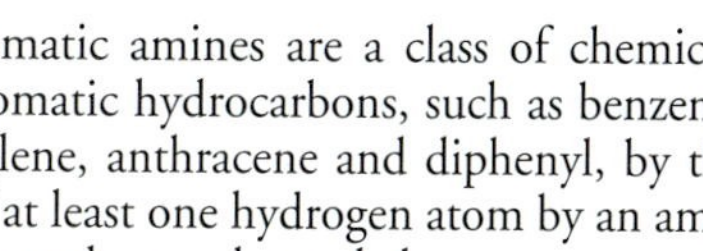

Benzidine

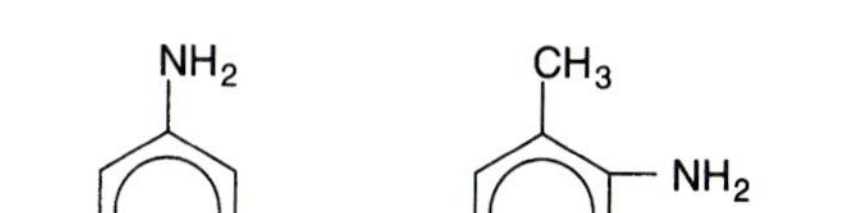

MBOCA

Use

Aromatic amines are used mainly in the synthesis of other chemicals. The principal commercial use of benzidine was as a chemical intermediate in dye manufacture, especially for azo dyes in the leather, textile, and paper industries. Benzidine once was used in clinical laboratories for the detection of blood, but this has been discontinued because of safety concerns. Benzidine is no longer produced for commercial sale in the United States. Any benzidine production must be captive consumption and maintained in closed systems.

Aniline is used as a chemical intermediate in the production of methylene diisocyanate, rubber products, dyes, pesticides, pigments, and hydroquinones. $p,p′$-Methylene dianiline is used as a chemical intermediate in the production of polyurethanes, dyes, and polyamide and polyimide resins and fibers and as a laboratory analytic reagent. o-Toluidine is used as a component of printing textiles, in the preparation of ion-exchange resin, as an antioxidant in rubber manufacture, and in the synthesis of dyestuffs. 1,4-Phenylenediamine may be found in some hair dyes. 4,4-Methylenebis(2-chloroaniline) (MBOCA) has been used as a curing agent in urethane and epoxy resins. It is no longer manufactured commercially in the United States.

Because of the demonstrated carcinogenicity of b-naphthylamine, its manufacture and use have been banned in many countries. Production of b-naphthylamine ceased in the United States in 1972.

Metabolism & Mechanism of Action

The aromatic amines are nearly all lipid-soluble and are absorbed through the skin. Metabolism is largely via the formation of hydroxylamine intermediates. These metabolites are transported to the bladder as N-glucuronide conjugates and hydrolyzed by the acid pH of urine to form reactive electrophiles that bind to bladder transitional epithelial DNA. The polymorphic enzyme N-acetyltransferase-2 is involved in the metabolism of the aromatic amines; slow acetylator status is a genetic risk factor for bladder cancer. Increased susceptibility for bladder cancer also may be related to glutathione S-transferase M1 gene deficiency. Urine pH (influenced by diet) may have a strong effect on the presence of free urinary aromatic compounds and on urothelial cell DNA adduct levels.

Clinical Findings

A. SYMPTOMS & SIGNS

1. Acute exposure—
   a. Dermatitis—Because of their alkaline nature, certain amines constitute a direct risk of dermatitis. Many

aromatic amines can cause allergic dermatitis, notably *p*-aminophenol and *p*-phenylenediamine. The latter was known as *fur dermatitis* and caused asthma among fur dyers and currently may cause contact dermatitis among hairdressers.

b. Respiratory effects—Asthma caused by *p*-phenylenediamine has been reported.

c. Hemorrhagic cystitis—Hemorrhagic cystitis can result from exposure to *o*- and *p*-toluidine and 5-chloro-*o*-toluidine. The hematuria is self-limited, and no increase in bladder tumors has been noted.

d. Hepatic injury—Cholestatic jaundice has resulted from industrial exposure to diaminodiphenyl methane, which also caused toxic jaundice as a consequence of contaminated baking flour (*Epping jaundice*). The hepatitis is reversible after cessation of exposure. Acute liver dysfunction has been reported among workers exposed to 5-nitro-*o*-toluidine.

e. Methemoglobinemia—Acute poisoning by aniline and its derivatives results in the formation of methemoglobin. A significant elevation of methemoglobin levels has been demonstrated in adult volunteers after ingestion of 25 mg aniline. The mean lethal dose is estimated to be between 15 and 30 g, although death has followed ingestion of as little as 1 g aniline. It has been postulated that a toxic metabolite, phenylhydroxylamine, is responsible for the methemoglobin. Peak levels of methemoglobin are observed within 1–2 hours of ingestion. Cyanosis becomes apparent at levels of methemoglobin of 10–15%, and headache, weakness, dyspnea, dizziness, and malaise occur at levels of 25–30%. Concentrations of methemoglobin greater than 60–70% may cause coma and death.

2. Chronic exposure—An excess of bladder tumors was recognized in 1895 among German workers who used aromatic amines in the production of synthetic dyes. British dyestuffs workers had a high risk for the development of bladder cancer. In the United States, bladder cancer has occurred in workers exposed to β-naphthylamine or benzidine in the manufacture of dyes and in chemical workers exposed to *o*-toludine.

Workers involved in the production of auramine and magenta from aniline and those working with 4-aminobiphenyl have an increased risk of bladder tumors. Workers exposed to 4-chloro-*o*-toluidine have a 73-fold excess of bladder cancer. Animal studies show an increased risk of bladder tumors after exposure to benzidine, *o*-toluidine, *o*-dianisidine-based dyes, MBOCA, and other aromatic amines. European studies of individual susceptibility to the development of aromatic amine–associated bladder cancer suggest some modulation by genetic polymorphisms.

The IARC considers benzidine carcinogenic to humans (group 1A) and MBOCA probably carcinogenic to humans (group 2A). The IARC has concluded that there is sufficient evidence in experimental animals for the carcinogenicity of *o*-toluidine and *p,p'*-methylene dianiline (group 2B) and finds limited evidence for the carcinogenicity of aniline in animals (group 3).

Results from cohort and case-control studies strongly support the association between occupational aromatic amine exposure (i.e., benzidine, naphthylamines, MBOCA, and *o*-toluidine) and bladder cancer. Since these compounds have been declining in use, the population-attributable risk for bladder cancer (approximately 25%) also may decline.

B. Laboratory Findings

Methemoglobin levels can help in the detection of excess absorption of the single-ring aromatic compounds. Normal individuals have methemoglobin concentrations of 1–2%. A biologic threshold limit value of 5% has been proposed.

Determination of the metabolites *p*-aminophenol and *p*-nitrophenol can be useful to monitor exposure to aniline and nitrobenzene. After 6 hours of exposure to 1 ppm nitrobenzene, the urinary concentration of *p*-aminophenol should not exceed 50 mg/L, and the recommended biologic threshold value is 10 mg/L. Levels of free MBOCA in the urine can be used to monitor exposure to this compound. Levels of free MBOCA in urine should be minimized to the limit of detection and used as an index of the adequacy of existing work practices and engineering controls. For workers exposed to the known or suspected carcinogenic aromatic amines, periodic screening of urine for red blood cells and evidence of dysplastic epithelium may detect early bladder cancer.

Differential Diagnosis

Aliphatic nitrates (e.g., ethylene glycol dinitrate), aliphatic nitrites, inorganic nitrites, and chlorates also may cause methemoglobinemia. Occupation-associated bladder cancer may account for 10–15% of all cases of bladder cancer. Exposure to arsenic in drinking water also causes an increased risk of bladder cancer. Cigarette smoking, with inhalation of carcinogenic arylamines (e.g., 2-aminonaphthalene), is also a significant risk factor.

Prevention

A. Work Practices

Every effort should be made to eliminate use of the carcinogenic aromatic amines by substitution of safer alternatives. Appropriate engineering controls for manufacturers of polyurethane products who use MBOCA—particularly the use of automated systems and local exhaust ventilation—can reduce the potential for exposures successfully. Because most cases of aniline exposure occur through skin and clothing contamination, emphasis should be placed on providing appropriate gloves and protective clothing.

For the benzidine-based dyes, worker exposure should be reduced to the lowest feasible levels through appropriate engineering controls, including the use of closed-process and liquid metering systems, walk-in hoods, and specific local exhaust ventilation. Dust levels can be minimized by the use of dyes in pellet, paste, or liquid form. Restricted access to areas with potential exposure and provision of suitable protective clothing and respirators should be instituted.

B. Medical Surveillance

Preemployment and periodic measurement of postshift urinary *p*-aminophenol is useful for biologic monitoring of aniline exposure. Similarly, periodic postshift urine samples for free MBOCA can be an important adjunct to industrial hygiene measures of exposure.

The ACGIH-recommended biologic exposure limit (BEL) for *o*-toluidine, MBOCA, and aniline is methemoglobin in blood in excess of 1.5% during or at the end of the work shift. Biologic monitoring by high-pressure liquid chromatographic (HPLC) methods for analysis of urinary *o*-toluidine, aniline, and MBOCA may be useful. Measurement of methylene dianaline (MDA) using the sensitive gas chromatography–mass spectrometry (GC-MS) assay in urine correlates with hemoglobin adducts of MDA in polyurethane production workers and may serve as a sensitive index of exposure (particularly for dermal exposure) at levels below air-monitoring-detection limits. Hemoglobin adducts also have been used for biologic monitoring of workers exposed to 3-chloro-4-fluoroaniline.

High-risk populations with past or current exposure to carcinogenic aromatic amines should be screened on a periodic basis with exfoliative bladder cytology. Positive findings are followed up with direct urologic examination. Biomolecular screening using voided urine samples for DNA ploidy, bladder tumor–associated antigen p300, and a cytoskeletal protein has been used in one cohort of workers exposed to benzidine.

Treatment

The definitive treatment of methemoglobinemia caused by aniline poisoning is administration of the reducing agent methylene blue. However, an excessive amount of methylene blue may itself provoke the formation of methemoglobin. Additionally, the ability of methylene blue to reduce methemoglobin can be impaired by hereditary glucose-6-phosphate dehydrogenase (G6PD) deficiency and can precipitate frank hemolysis. The recommended dose of methylene blue for the initial management of methemoglobinemia is 1–2 mg/kg of body weight intravenously, equivalent to 0.1–0.2 mL of a 1% solution. Maximal response to methylene blue usually occurs within 30–60 minutes. Repeated doses should be spaced about 1 hour apart and based on methemoglobin levels; most patients, unless they are anemic, can tolerate a level of 30% or less. Methylene blue administration should be discontinued if either a negligible response or an increase in methemoglobin levels results after two consecutive doses or if the total dose exceeds 7 mg/kg. It is advisable to continue to monitor methemoglobin levels even after an initial response to methylene blue because there is a potential for continued production of methemoglobin by aniline.

Treatment of bladder cancer associated with aromatic amine exposure is identical to that of nonoccupationally associated bladder tumors. Early detection through screening programs may improve prognosis.

REFERENCES

Chen HI et al: Bladder cancer screening and monitoring of 4,4′-methylenebis(2-chloroaniline) exposure among workers in Taiwan. Urology 2005;66:305 [PMID: 16098360].

Markowitz SB, Levin K: Continued epidemic of bladder cancer in workers exposed to *ortho*-toluidine in a chemical factory. J Occup Environ Med 2004;46:154 [PMID: 14767218].

Rosenman KD, Reilly MJ: Cancer mortality and incidence among a cohort of benzidine and dichlorobenzidine dye manufacturing workers. Am J Indust Med 2004;46:505 [PMID: 15490466].

CARBON DISULFIDE

Essentials of Diagnosis

A. Acute Effects

- Irritability, manic delirium, hallucinations, paranoia
- Respiratory irritation

B. Chronic Effects

- Coronary artery disease
- Neurobehavioral abnormalities
- Retinal microaneurysms
- Peripheral neuropathy with ascending symmetric paresthesias and weakness

Exposure Limits

ACGIH TLV: 10 ppm TWA

OSHA PEL: 20 ppm TWA, 30 ppm STEL (30 minutes), 100 ppm maximum peak

NIOSH REL: 1 ppm TWA, 10 ppm ceiling

General Considerations

Carbon disulfide is a colorless volatile solvent with a strong, sweetish aroma. The average odor threshold of 1 ppm is below the permissible exposure limit; therefore, carbon disulfide is a material with good warning properties. It evaporates at room temperature, and its vapor is 2.6 times heavier than air; it may form explosive mixtures in a range of 1–50% by volume in air.

Use

Carbon disulfide is used in the manufacture of rayon, cellophane, carbon tetrachloride, and rubber chemicals and as a grain fumigant.

Occupational & Environmental Exposure

In the production of viscose rayon, carbon disulfide is added to alkali cellulose to yield sodium cellulose xanthate. The latter is dissolved in caustic soda to yield viscose syrup, which can be spun to form textile yarn, tire yarn, or staple fiber or cast to form cellophane. Exposure to high concentrations of carbon disulfide can occur during the opening of sealed spinning machines and during cutting and drying.

Metabolism & Mechanism of Action

Inhalation is the major route of absorption in occupational exposure, and 40–50% of carbon disulfide in inhaled air is retained in the body. Excretion of carbon disulfide by the lung accounts for 10–30% of absorbed dose, and less than 1% is excreted unchanged by the kidney. The remainder is excreted in the form of various metabolites in the urine.

Carbon disulfide is metabolized by formation of dithiocarbamates and reduced glutathione conjugates, as well as by oxidative transformation. Thiourea, mercapturic acids, and the glutathione conjugate 2-thiothiazolidine-4-carboxylic acid (TTCA) can be detected in urine of exposed workers. Formation of dithiocarbamate may account in part for the nervous system toxicity of carbon disulfide, whereas oxidation yields carbonyl sulfide, a hepatotoxic metabolite. Carbon disulfide reacts with protein amino functions to form adducts of dithiocarbamate, which then undergo oxidation or decomposition to an electrophile, which reacts with protein nucleophiles to result in protein cross-linking. Cross-linked neurofilaments then may accumulate within axonal swellings.

Clinical Findings

A. SYMPTOMS & SIGNS

1. Acute exposure—Acute carbon disulfide intoxication was described in the 1920s among workers in the viscose rayon industry, involving exposure to concentrations of hundreds or thousands of parts per million. Signs and symptoms included extreme irritability, uncontrolled anger, rapid mood changes (including manic delirium and hallucinations), paranoid ideas, and suicidal tendencies.

Exposure to 4800 ppm of carbon disulfide for 30 minutes may cause rapid coma and death. High concentrations of vapor may cause irritation of the eyes, nose, and throat; liquid carbon disulfide may cause second- or third-degree burns.

2. Chronic exposure—Chronic effects of lower-level exposure to carbon disulfide include the following:

a. Eye—Viscose rayon workers have been reported to have a high incidence of eye irritation. A high incidence of retinal microaneurysms and delayed fundal peripapillary filling by fluorescein angiography has been reported in Japanese and Yugoslavian workers exposed to carbon disulfide. Color vision has been reported to be disturbed in Chinese workers below the current TLV.

b. Ear—Carbon disulfide exposure enhances noise-induced high-frequency hearing loss. Vestibular symptoms of vertigo and nystagmus also may occur.

c. Heart—Epidemiologic studies indicate that workers exposed to carbon disulfide are at increased risk for cardiovascular disease mortality. There is a correlation between blood pressure, elevated triglyceride, and decreased lipoprotein levels and exposure to carbon disulfide. The pathophysiologic mechanism is unclear but may include an effect on oxidative stress in plasma or alteration of arterial elastic properties. Carbon disulfide may cause increased heart rate variability with persistent effects after exposure has ended. A greater risk of ischemic electrocardiographic changes has been seen in a longitudinal study of viscose rayon workers.

d. Nervous system—Studies show persistent neurobehavioral changes in psychomotor speed, motor coordination, and personality in workers exposed to low concentrations (5–30 ppm) of carbon disulfide. There is a reduction in peripheral nerve conduction on exposure to less than 10 ppm, although clinical symptoms of polyneuropathy are not present. Distal latency, motor nerve-conduction velocity, and sensory amplitude were found to be sensitive indicators of polyneuropathy in viscose rayon workers exposed to carbon disulfide. Lower levels of exposure have been correlated with decreased slow-fiber-conduction velocity with prolongation of the refractory period of the peroneal nerve. Impaired motor and sensory nerve conduction has been demonstrated in prospective studies of workers exposed to carbon disulfide near the TLV. Cerebellar atrophy with extrapyramidal symptoms with atypical parkinsonism and cerebellar signs has been reported. Small-vessel disease with cerebral lesions in the basal ganglia, subcortical white matter, and brainstem has been reported. Peripheral nerve signs and symptoms may persist for as long as 3 years after exposure has ceased.

e. Reproductive effects—Carbon disulfide exposure was associated with a significant effect on libido and potency but not on fertility or semen quality. Women exposed to concentrations of less than 10 ppm may have an increased rate of menstrual abnormalities, spontaneous abortions, and premature births. No other effects on general endocrine function have been observed.

B. Laboratory Findings

Nonspecific elevations of liver enzymes and creatinine have been reported in acute intoxication. With chronic exposure, peripheral nerve-conduction velocity can be decreased, and neurobehavioral testing may show abnormalities in psychomotor skills and measures of personality function.

Urinary metabolites that catalyze the reaction of iodine with sodium azide can be used to detect exposure above 16 ppm (iodine-azide reaction). The concentration of end-of-shift urinary TTCA is related to exposure and can detect uptake as low as 10 ppm over the whole working shift. The ACGIH BEI is 5 mg TTCA per gram of creatinine in urine at the end of a shift. Heavy physical work and greater skin contact are correlated with higher TTCA levels. Biopsy of the sural nerve in cases of suspected peripheral nerve damage may be indicated and may show degeneration of both axon and myelin with a predominant loss of large myelinated fibers.

Differential Diagnosis

Cardiac disease from carbon disulfide intoxication must be differentiated from atherosclerotic heart disease from other causes. Peripheral polyneuropathy should be distinguished from that caused by alcohol, drugs, diabetes, and other toxic agents. Neuropsychiatric symptoms may be a result of depression, posttraumatic stress syndrome, or other toxic exposures such as organic solvents.

Prevention

A. Work Practices

Control of exposure must rely largely on engineering controls, with enclosure of processes and machines and proper use of ventilation systems. Operator rotation and respiratory protection during peak exposures should be implemented. Potential sources of ignition are prohibited in areas where carbon disulfide is stored or handled, and the substance must not be allowed to accumulate to concentrations higher than 0.1%. Impervious clothing, gloves, and face shields should be worn to prevent skin contact.

B. Medical Surveillance

Initial medical examination should include the central and peripheral nervous systems, eyes, and cardiovascular system. Visual acuity and color vision should be mea-

sured and a baseline electrocardiogram obtained. Periodic medical surveillance to detect early signs or symptoms of toxicity should include questions regarding cardiac, nervous system, and reproductive function, with evaluation of blood pressure, peripheral nerve function, and mental status. Neurobehavioral testing, exercise electrocardiography, and nerve-conduction velocity testing may be indicated. Reduced color discrimination may be a sensitive marker for carbon disulfide neurotoxicity. Measurement of finger tremor frequencies may provide an early indication of chronic carbon disulfide intoxication. Magnetic resonance imaging (MRI) may show periventricular hyperintensity and lacunar infarct, which may be of diagnostic use in selected patients with neurobehavioral effects from carbon disulfide exposure.

Measurement of TTCA in urine collected at the end of the work shift following the first workday is the test of choice for biologic monitoring. Skin disease and increased absorption of carbon disulfide may be important in exposure assessment. Five milligrams per gram of creatinine corresponds to an 8-hour exposure (TWA) to the current TLV. The widely used iodine-azide test is insensitive at carbon disulfide levels of less than 16.7 ppm. The presence of preexisting neurologic, psychiatric, or cardiac disease should be considered relative contraindications for individual exposure.

Treatment

Skin and eye contact with carbon disulfide should be treated immediately by washing with large amounts of water, and all contaminated clothing should be removed. No specific treatment is available for chronic carbon disulfide toxicity.

REFERENCES

ATSDR: Toxicological profile for carbon disulfide, www.atsdr.cdc.gov/toxprofiles/tp82.html.

Huang CC: Carbon disulfide neurotoxicity: Taiwan experience. Acta Neurol Taiwan 2004;13:3 [PMID: 15315294].

State of California Office of Environmental Health Hazard Assessment: Prioritization of Toxic Air Contaminants: www.oehha.ca.gov/air/toxic_contaminants/pdf_zip/carbondisulfide_final.pdf.

Takebayashi T et al: A six-year follow-up study of the subclinical effects of carbon disulphide exposure on the cardiovascular system. Occup Environ Med 2004;61:127 [PMID: 14739378].

CHLOROMETHYL ETHERS

Essentials of Diagnosis

A. Acute Effects

- Respiratory irritation
- Skin rash

B. CHRONIC EFFECTS

- Lung cancer

C. EXPOSURE LIMITS

ACGIH TLV: 0.001 ppm TWA
OSHA PEL: Stringent workplace controls
NIOSH REL: Reduce exposure to lowest feasible concentration

General Considerations

The haloethers bis(chloromethyl) ether (BCME) and chloromethylmethyl ether (CMME) are highly volatile, colorless liquids at room temperature, miscible with many organic solvents. The haloethers are alkylating agents that are highly reactive in vivo. Technical-grade CMME contains 1–8% BCME as an impurity.

Use

BCME is formed when formaldehyde reacts with chloride ions in an acidic medium. It has been used in the past primarily for chloromethylations (e.g., in the preparation of ion-exchange resins), where a polystyrene resin is chloromethylated and then treated with an amine.

Occupational & Environmental Exposure

Occupational exposure to the chloromethyl ethers occurs in anion-exchange resin production. Since 1948, approximately 2000 workers have been exposed to BCME in ion-exchange resin manufacture, where exposure levels ranged from 10–100 ppb. Small quantities are produced in the United States and only in closed systems to make other chemicals.

BCME also may be a potential hazard in the textile industry, where formaldehyde-containing reactants and resins are used in fabric finishing and as adhesives in laminating and flocking fabrics. Thermosetting emulsion polymers containing methylacrylamide as binders may liberate formaldehyde on drying and curing and then form BCME in the presence of available chloride. A NIOSH study of textile finishing plants found from 0.4–8 ppb BCME in the workroom air. This led to the use of low-formaldehyde resins and chloride-free catalysts.

Clinical Findings

A. SYMPTOMS & SIGNS

1. Acute exposure—The chloromethyl ethers are potent skin and respiratory irritants. There are no reported cases of acute overexposure to either BCME or CMME.

2. Chronic exposure—Both BCME and CMME are carcinogenic and mutagenic in animal and cellular test systems. When rats are exposed to 0.1 ppm BCME by inhalation for 6 hours a day, 5 days a week, a high incidence of esthesioneuroblastomas and squamous cell carcinoma of the respiratory tract is observed. Both BCME and CMME produce skin papillomas and squamous tumors on direct application or subcutaneous injection. In humans, an excess of lung cancer has been suspected. An industry-wide survey of plants using chloromethyl ethers has documented a strikingly increased risk of lung cancer in exposed workers. More than 60 cases of BCME-associated lung cancer have been identified, with oat cell the principal histologic type. The historical average time-weighted exposure in these cases is estimated to be between 10 and 100 ppm, and the latency period between exposure and lung cancer ranges from 5–25 years. An increasing incidence is observed with intensity and length of exposure. In addition, the risk of lung cancer is increased in smokers versus nonsmokers. The mortality rate from respiratory tract cancer is significantly (almost three times) higher among chloromethyl ether–exposed workers, with a latency of 10–19 years. The risk of cancer among exposed workers declines after 20 years from first exposure. NIOSH recommends that BCME be regulated as a potential human carcinogen. The IARC considers BCME carcinogenic to humans (group 1A).

B. LABORATORY FINDINGS

The lung carcinoma associated with BCME and CMME presents in similar fashion to nonoccupationally associated carcinoma. Chest radiography may show a mass that should lead to appropriate diagnostic testing. Alternatively, sputum cytology may be abnormal in the presence of a normal chest radiograph and thus may be useful as a screening technique in individual cases. Sputum cytology may be of limited value in the follow-up of workers exposed to known carcinogens who remain at risk for many years following exposure.

Differential Diagnosis

Known occupational lung carcinogens include asbestos, arsenic, chromium, and uranium; consequently, a careful occupational history should be obtained from an individual who presents with lung carcinoma.

Prevention

A. WORK PRACTICES

Enclosed chemical processes are essential to reduce exposure below 1 ppb, and continuous monitoring has been used successfully to warn of excessive exposures to BCME and CMME. Since the number of potentially exposed workers has markedly declined since the 1970s, medical follow-up of past exposed workers has assumed a greater role.

B. MEDICAL SURVEILLANCE

Preplacement and annual lung examination should be included in medical surveillance of exposed workers. Periodic sputum cytology may be of limited value in detecting early lung cancer.

Treatment

The treatment of lung carcinoma associated with BCME/CMME exposure does not differ from that of nonoccupational cases.

REFERENCES

US Department of Health and Human Services Public Health Service (USPHS) Agency for Toxic Substances and Disease Registry: Toxicological profile for bis (chloromethyl) ether, www.atsdr.cdc.gov/toxprofiles/tp128.html.

US Department of Health and Human Services Public Health Service (USPHS National Toxicology Program Substance Profile): http://ntp.niehs.nih.gov/ntp/roc/eleventh/profiles/s039bcme.pdf.

US Environmental Protection Agency Integrated Risk Information System (IRIS): Bis(chloromethyl)ether (BCME) (CASRN 542-88-1), www.epa.gov/iris/subst/0375.htm.

DIBROMOCHLOROPROPANE

Essentials of Diagnosis

A. ACUTE EFFECTS

- Oligospermia, azoospermia

Exposure Limits

OSHA PEL: 0.001 ppm TWA
NIOSH REL: Reduce exposure to lowest feasible concentration

General Considerations

Dibromochloropropane (DBCP) is a brominated organochlorine nematocide that was used extensively since the 1950s on citrus fruits, grapes, peaches, pineapples, soybeans, and tomatoes. Millions of pounds were produced in the United States. In 1977, employees at a California pesticide formulation plant were found to be infertile, and further investigation documented azoospermia and oligospermia among workers exposed to DBCP. In the United States, its use has been restricted since 1980 to a soil fumigant against plant-parasitic nematodes in pineapples. However, two American companies continued to export DBCP to less developed countries for use on bananas. This practice has largely stopped in recent years, but DBCP is one of many pesticides still in use in developing countries that lack regulation and enforcement.

DBCP may remain persistent in soil and continues to be detected as a groundwater contaminant in areas of high past use.

In DBCP-exposed men with both azoospermia and elevation of follicle-stimulating hormone (FSH) levels, follow-up evaluation generally has shown permanent destruction of germinal epithelium. A 17-year follow-up of DBCP-exposed workers found sperm count recovery at 36–45 months in three of nine azoospermic and three of six oligozoospermic men, with no improvement thereafter. A significant increase in plasma levels of FSH and luteinizing hormone was found in the most severely affected workers, with incomplete recovery of sperm count and motility.

In vitro, in vivo, and human genotoxicity studies indicate that DBCP can act as a mutagen and clastogen. No correlation has been found between DBCP contamination in drinking water and mortality rates from leukemia or gastric cancer. Birth outcomes (low birth weight and birth defects) did not differ among DBCP-exposed workers or community residents exposed to DBCP-contaminated drinking water.

NIOSH recommends that DBCP be regulated as a potential human carcinogen. The IARC finds that there is sufficient evidence of carcinogenicity in animals (group 2B).

REFERENCES

Clark HA, Snedeker SM: Critical evaluation of the cancer risk of dibromochloropropane (DBCP). J Environ Sci Health C Environ Carcinog Ecotoxicol Rev 2005;23:215 [PMID: 16291528].

Winker R, Rudiger HW: Reproductive toxicology in occupational settings: An update. Int Arch Occup Environ Health 2006; 79:1 [PMID: 16010576].

DIMETHYLAMINOPROPIONITRILE

Dimethylaminopropionitrile was a component of catalysts used in manufacture of flexible polyurethane foams. In 1978, NIOSH reported urinary dysfunction and neurologic symptoms among workers at facilities that used dimethylaminopropionitrile. Workers at polyurethane-manufacturing plants developed neurogenic bladder dysfunction after the introduction of a catalyst containing dimethylaminopropionitrile. Workers had urinary retention, hesitancy, and dribbling. Examination showed a pattern of decreased sensation confined to the lower sacral dermatomes, abnormal retention of contrast material on intravenous pyelogram, or abnormal cystometrograms. Nerve-conduction velocity studies were normal. Symptoms of persistent sexual dysfunction were found 2 years after the original epidemic, and one worker had residual sensorimotor neuropathy. Following these findings, production of catalysts containing dimethylaminopropionitrile was discontinued voluntarily.

Dimethylaminopropionitrile appears to be a unique example of a neurotoxin that produces localized autonomic dysfunction without peripheral nervous system damage. Urotoxic effects may be related to metabolism via a cytochrome P450–dependent mixed-function oxidase system, with formation of reactive intermediate metabolites that interfere with axoplasmic transport. The discovery of this toxicity by an alert clinician underscores the role of the community practitioner in the discovery of new occupational diseases.

ETHYLENE OXIDE

Essentials of Diagnosis

A. Acute Effects

- Respiratory tract irritation
- Skin rash
- Headache, drowsiness, weakness

B. Chronic Effects

- Increased sister chromatid exchanges in lymphocytes
- Possible increased risk of cancer

Exposure Limits

ACGIH TLV: 1 ppm TWA

OSHA PEL: 1 ppm TWA, 5 ppm excursion limit (15 minutes)

NIOSH REL: <0.1 ppm TWA, 5 ppm ceiling (10 min/d)

General Considerations

Ethylene oxide is a colorless flammable gas with a characteristic ether-like odor. At elevated pressures, it may be a volatile liquid. It is completely miscible with water and many organic solvents. The threshold of detection in humans is about 700 ppm but is quite variable, and smell cannot be relied on to warn of overexposure. To reduce the explosive hazard of ethylene oxide used as a fumigant or sterilant, it is often mixed with carbon dioxide or halocarbons (15% ethylene oxide and 85% dichlorofluoromethane).

Use

Ethylene oxide is used in the manufacture of ethylene glycol (used for antifreeze and as an intermediate for polyester fibers, films, and bottles), nonionic surface-active agents (used for home laundry detergents and dishwashing formulations), glycol ethers (used for surface coatings), and ethanolamines (for soaps, deter-gents, and textile chemicals). It is used as a pesticide fumigant and as a sterilant in hospitals, medical products manufacture, libraries, museums, beekeeping, spice and seasoning fumigation, animal and plant quarantine, transportation vehicle fumigation, and dairy packaging.

Occupational & Environmental Exposure

Most ethylene oxide is used as a chemical intermediate in plants where closed and automated processes generally maintain exposure levels below 1 ppm. The greatest potential for worker exposure occurs during loading or unloading of transport tanks, product sampling, and equipment maintenance and repair.

Although only approximately 0.02% of production is used for sterilization in hospitals, NIOSH estimates that 75,000 health care workers have potential exposure to ethylene oxide. Approximately 10,000 ethylene oxide sterilization units are in use in 8100 hospitals in the United States. Field surveys of hospital gas sterilizers generally have found that 8-hour TWA exposures to ethylene oxide are below 1 ppm. However, occupational exposure may be several hundred parts per million for brief periods during the opening of the sterilizer door, in the transfer of freshly sterilized items to the aeration cabinet or central supply area, during tank changes, and at the gas-discharge point.

Metabolism & Mechanism of Action

Ethylene oxide is absorbed through the skin and respiratory tract. It is an alkylating agent that binds to DNA and may cause cellular mutation.

Clinical Findings

A. Symptoms & Signs

1. Acute exposure—Ethylene oxide is irritating to the eyes, respiratory tract, and skin, and at high concentrations it can cause respiratory depression. Symptoms of upper respiratory tract irritation occur at between 200 and 400 ppm, and above 1000 ppm ethylene oxide may cause headache, nausea, dyspnea, vomiting, drowsiness, weakness, and incoordination. Direct contact of the skin or eyes with liquid ethylene oxide can result in severe irritation, burns, or contact dermatitis.

2. Chronic exposure—

a. Reproductive effects—Ethylene oxide is toxic to reproductive function in both male and female experimental animals. Retrospective studies of reproductive function show a higher rate of spontaneous abortions and preterm birth in women exposed to ethylene oxide.

b. Carcinogenic effects—Ethylene oxide is genotoxic in a variety of animal test systems. Chronic inhalation bioassays in rats have shown that ethylene oxide results in a dose-related increase in mononuclear cell leukemia, peritoneal mesothelioma, and cerebral glioma. Intragastric administration of ethylene oxide in rats produces a dose-dependent increase of squamous cell carcinomas of the forestomach. Studies show a dose-related increase in chromosomal aberrations, sister chromatid exchange in lymphocytes and micronuclei in bone marrow cells of exposed workers; and a dose-related increase in the level of hemoglobin adducts. The *GSTT1-null* genotype is associated with increased formation of hemoglobin adducts in relation to ethylene oxide exposure, suggesting that individuals with homozygous deletion of the *GSTT1* gene may be more susceptible to the genotoxic effects of ethylene oxide.

Retrospective cohort mortality studies have suggested an excess of lymphatic and hematopoietic cancers in ethylene oxide–exposed workers. The IARC considers ethylene oxide to be carcinogenic to humans (group 1). NIOSH recommends that ethylene oxide be treated as a potential human carcinogen.

c. Neurologic toxicity—Impairment of sensory and motor function has been observed in animals exposed to 357 ppm ethylene oxide over 48–85 days, and four cases of peripheral neuropathy were described among workers exposed to a leaking sterilizing chamber for 2–8 weeks. Central neurotoxicity has been reported following chronic ethylene oxide exposure, including neuropsychological abnormalities, lower P300 amplitude, and peripheral neuropathy.

d. Other—Occupational asthma also has been reported following acute exposure.

B. LABORATORY FINDINGS

No specific finding is characteristic of ethylene oxide exposure. Lymphocytosis has been noted after acute exposure. Where inhalation results in respiratory symptoms, the chest radiograph may show interstitial or frank alveolar edema. Where suspect, a complete blood count may be helpful in the diagnosis of leukemia. Cytogenetic analysis (i.e., sister chromatid exchange) of peripheral lymphocytes cannot be used in individual cases to quantitate exposure or estimate cancer risk.

Differential Diagnosis

The mixture of chlorofluorocarbons found in sterilant cylinders also may produce upper respiratory symptoms on inhalation exposure. Many other genotoxicants, including cigarette smoke and other alkylating agents, can cause an increase in sister chromatid exchanges and chromosomal aberrations.

Prevention

A. WORK PRACTICES

Proper engineering controls are essential for reducing short-term exposures to hospital sterilizer staff during procedures where ethylene oxide levels have been found to be greatest. A NIOSH survey found that engineering controls are extremely effective in hospitals in reducing ethylene oxide exposure during sterilization. These controls include effective sterilization chamber ethylene oxide purging, local exhaust ventilation at the sterilizer door, adequate ventilation of floor drains, efficient handling of product carts from sterilizer to aerator, and installation of ethylene oxide tanks in ventilated cabinets. Self-contained breathing apparatus or airline respirators are the only respirators acceptable for ethylene oxide and must be worn when concentrations of ethylene oxide are unknown, such as when entering walk-in chambers or for emergency response. With the implementation of effective engineering controls, work shift exposures to ethylene oxide may decrease, but intermittent peak excursions and accidental exposures still may occur.

B. MEDICAL SURVEILLANCE

Preplacement and periodic examinations should include attention to the pulmonary, hematologic, neurologic, and reproductive systems. Consistent changes in hematologic parameters have not been demonstrated among workers monitored for ethylene oxide exposure. The mean absolute numbers of eosinophils and red blood cells and percentage of hematocrit were significantly elevated among a group of workers with higher cumulative doses of ethylene oxide. Other studies have not demonstrated the utility of the complete blood count as a screening test for medical surveillance of ethylene oxide–exposed hospital workers. Biologic monitoring studies of ethylene oxide–exposed workers show an increase in chromosomal aberrations, sister chromatid exchanges, micronuclei, and hemoglobin adducts. Personnel trained in emergency response for use of self-contained breathing apparatus should be evaluated for cardiorespiratory fitness with pulmonary function or exercise testing.

Treatment

Removal from the work environment after inhalation of the gas should be immediate. If respiratory symptoms are evident, oxygen should be administered and the victim brought to the emergency room. Any contaminated clothing should be removed immediately and, where appropriate, the skin thoroughly washed with soap and water. A chest radiograph should be obtained if warranted by respiratory symptoms, and the patient should be observed for several hours for the onset of pulmonary edema. No other specific treatment is indicated.

REFERENCES

Coggon D et al: Mortality of workers exposed to ethylene oxide: Extended follow up of a British cohort. Occup Environ Med 2004;61:358 [PMID: 15031395].

LaMontagne AD et al: Long-term ethylene oxide exposure trends in US hospitals: Relationship with OSHA regulatory and enforcement actions. Am J Public Health 2004;94:1614 [PMID: 15333324].

Steenland K et al: Mortality analyses in a cohort of 18 235 ethylene oxide exposed workers: Follow-up extended from 1987 to 1998. Occup Environ Med 2004;61:2 [PMID: 14691266].

US Public Health Service Agency for Toxic Substance and Disease Registry: Medical management guidelines for ethylene oxide. www.atsdr.cdc.gov/MHMI/mmg137.html.

FORMALDEHYDE

Essentials of Diagnosis

A. ACUTE EFFECTS

- Eye irritation causing lacrimation, redness, and pain
- Cough, chest tightness, shortness of breath
- Skin irritation, contact dermatitis

B. CHRONIC EFFECTS

- Bronchitis, exacerbation of asthma

Exposure Limits

ACGIH TLV: 0.3 ppm ceiling
OSHA PEL: 0.75 ppm TWA, 2 ppm STEL
NIOSH REL: 0.016 ppm TWA, 0.1 ppm ceiling (15 minutes)

General Considerations

Formaldehyde is a colorless flammable gas with a pungent, irritating odor. Known to physicians as a tissue preservative and disinfectant, formaldehyde is a basic feedstock of the modern chemical industry. It also may be encountered as formalin (37–50% formaldehyde), methyl aldehyde, methanal (methanol-formaldehyde mixture), methylene glycol, paraform, or paraformaldehyde (a linear copolymer of formaldehyde).

Use

The largest use for formaldehyde is the manufacture of urea-formaldehyde and polyacetal and phenolic resins and as an intermediate in the manufacture of ethylenediaminetetraacetic acid, methylene dianiline, hexamethylenetetramine, and nitriloacetic acid. Other important uses include wood industry products, molding compounds, foundry resins, adhesives for insulation, slow-release fertilizers, manufacture of permanent-press finishes of cellulose fabrics, and formaldehyde-based textile finishes. Formaldehyde is used in relatively small quantities for preservation and disinfection. It is a by-product of the incomplete combustion of hydrocarbons and is found in small amounts in automobile exhaust and cigarette smoke.

Occupational & Environmental Exposure

Occupational exposure to formaldehyde above 1 ppm occurs in the production of formaldehyde resin and plastics and in the manufacture of apparel, plywood particle board and wood furniture, paper, and paperboard; workers at risk include urea-formaldehyde foam insulation dealers and installers, mushroom farmers, embalmers, and laboratory workers. NIOSH industrial hygiene surveys have found formaldehyde levels of up to 8 ppm in hospital autopsy rooms and up to 2.7 ppm in gross anatomy laboratories. Wildland firefighters may be exposed to formaldehyde as a result of vegetation combustion.

Residential exposure to formaldehyde up to several parts per million occurs from urea-formaldehyde foam insulation (UFFI) and particle board in mobile homes. Levels of formaldehyde are highest in new residences and decline with a half-life of 4–5 years for mobile homes and of less than 1 year for UFFI homes. Mean levels for mobile homes are about 0.5 ppm and for UFFI homes about 0.1 ppm. Diurnal and seasonal variations in exposure levels may occur.

Metabolism & Mechanism of Action

Formaldehyde is formed intracellularly as N_5,N_{20}-methylenetetrahydrofolic acid, an important metabolic intermediate. Exogenous formaldehyde can be absorbed by inhalation, ingestion, or dermal absorption. More than 95% of an inhaled dose is absorbed and metabolized rapidly to formic acid by formaldehyde dehydrogenase. Formaldehyde disappears from plasma with a half-life of 1–1.5 minutes, so an increase cannot be detected immediately following inhalation exposure to high concentrations. Most formaldehyde is converted to CO_2 via formate, and a small fraction is excreted in the urine as formate and other metabolites. Formaldehyde interacts with macromolecules such as DNA, RNA, and protein. This probably accounts for its carcinogenic effect.

Clinical Findings

A. SYMPTOMS & SIGNS

1. Acute exposure—Formaldehyde vapor exposure causes direct irritation of the skin and respiratory tract.

Both direct irritation (eczematous reaction) and allergic contact dermatitis (type IV delayed hypersensitivity) occur. After a few days of exposure to formaldehyde solutions or formaldehyde-containing resins, the individual may develop a sudden urticarial eczematous reaction of the skin of the eyelids, face, neck, and flexor surfaces of the arms. Allergic contact dermatitis may occur from exposure to phenol-formaldehyde resins, water-based paints, or photographic products. There appears to be no relationship between cutaneous disease from formaldehyde and personal or family history of atopy. Direct irritation of the eyes, nose, and throat occurs among most people exposed to 0.1–3 ppm of formaldehyde vapor.

The odor threshold is 0.05–1 ppm; some individuals may note irritation of the upper respiratory tract at or just above the odor threshold. Shortness of breath, cough, and chest tightness occur at 10–20 ppm. Exposure to 50–100 ppm and above can cause pulmonary edema, pneumonitis, or death. Irritant symptoms caused by formaldehyde exposure do not elicit a consistent immunologic response with elevated levels of immunoglobulin (Ig) E or IgG antibody to formaldehyde–human serum albumin.

Several studies show respiratory irritation from exposure to formaldehyde and wood dust. Embalmers report more frequent symptoms of respiratory irritation with exposures during embalming exceeding permissible limits. Formaldehyde exposures in gross anatomy dissection may exceed exposure limits, causing significantly increased upper respiratory symptoms and decrements in airflow during exposure. Respiratory irritant effects are significantly associated with formaldehyde exposure in mobile homes. Residents of homes insulated with urea-formaldehyde foam had a higher prevalence of respiratory symptoms than did residents of control homes but had no demonstrated changes in various hematologic or immunologic parameters.

2. Chronic exposure—

a. Cancer—Squamous cell carcinomas of the nasal epithelium were induced in rats and mice exposed for prolonged periods (up to 2 years). Biochemical and physiologic studies in rats have shown that inhaled formaldehyde can depress respiration, inhibit mucociliary clearance, stimulate cell proliferation, and cross-link DNA and protein in the nasal mucosa.

Epidemiologic studies have suggested that occupational exposure to formaldehyde increases the risk for lung and thyroid cancer and myeloid leukemia, whereas other studies have found no association between formaldehyde exposure and deaths from malignant respiratory disease. Generally consistent results have been found in studies of nasopharyngeal and hypopharyngeal cancer and exposure to formaldehyde, with several studies showing an increased risk of sinonasal cancer (particularly adenocarcinoma) with exposure to formaldehyde. Three cases of malignant melanoma of the nasal mucosa have been reported in persons occupationally exposed to formaldehyde. An increased risk of pancreatic cancer has been observed among embalmers exposed to formaldehyde. The IARC has found sufficient evidence to conclude that formaldehyde is carcinogenic in humans (nasopharyngeal cancer). NIOSH recommends that formaldehyde be regulated as a potential human carcinogen.

b. Respiratory—Occupational asthma has been reported as a result of exposure to formaldehyde resin dust, with studies reporting workers with asthma and positive specific bronchial challenge to formaldehyde. However, exposure-chamber studies have not demonstrated increased airway responsiveness among asthmatics following formaldehyde challenge. Tests of formaldehyde-specific IgE antibodies and cutaneous reactivity also generally have been negative, and formaldehyde sensitization does not correlate with symptoms. A study of students exposed to formaldehyde showed short-term decrements in peak expiratory flow rates. Workers exposed to formaldehyde have significantly greater cross-shift reduction in forced expiratory volume in 1 second (FEV_1) and significantly more lower respiratory symptoms than do unexposed controls. However, the rate of decline of lung function in formaldehyde-exposed workers is not greater than expected.

c. Other effects—Chronic formaldehyde exposure has been linked in case reports to a variety of neuropsychological problems, but cohort studies have not been performed to confirm these findings. Spontaneous abortions in cosmetologists and laboratory workers have been associated with the use of formaldehyde-based disinfectants and formalin, respectively. Wood workers exposed to formaldehyde had significantly delayed conception. However, a meta-analysis does not confirm these findings.

B. Laboratory Findings

1. Liver and kidney—Routine tests of hepatic and renal function generally are unremarkable. Measurement of formic acid in the urine generally is not helpful because of the short half-life of formaldehyde.

2. Skin—If contact dermatitis is suspected, patch testing should be performed with appropriate concentrations of formaldehyde.

3. Respiratory system—Cough, shortness of breath, or wheezing may be associated with decreased FEV_1 by pulmonary function testing. Peak-flow recordings while at work may show a decrease in maximal airflow during or after exposure to formaldehyde. After exposure to over 20–30 ppm of formaldehyde, chest radiographs may show interstitial or alveolar edema with a resulting reduction in arterial oxygen content on blood gas analysis.

Differential Diagnosis

Numerous workplace gases and vapors may produce symptoms of upper respiratory tract irritation. Symptoms of eye and throat irritation among office workers may be a result of inadequate ventilation, cigarette smoke, or glues and solvents emitted from newly installed synthetic materials. Asthmatics may be particularly sensitive to the effects of formaldehyde exposure to indoor environments.

Prevention

A. Work Practices

Ventilation engineering controls are effective at significantly reducing exposure to formaldehyde in anatomy laboratories and during embalming procedures. Safety goggles or a full-length plastic face mask should be worn where splashing is possible. At air concentrations above the permissible exposure limit, a full-facepiece respirator with organic vapor cartridge is required. Protective neoprene clothing and boots and gloves impervious to formaldehyde should be worn to prevent skin contact.

B. Medical Surveillance

A preplacement history of asthma or allergy should be obtained, along with a baseline FEV_1 and forced vital capacity (FVC). Biologic monitoring using urinary formate concentration is not useful with the possible exception of populations where ambient formaldehyde concentrations are greater than 1 ppm.

Low-level exposure to formaldehyde during embalming is associated with cytogenetic changes in epithelial cells of the mouth and in blood lymphocytes. These cytogenetic effects may be useful markers in biologic monitoring of formaldehyde-exposed workers. Various pathologic changes have been observed in the nasal mucosa of formaldehyde-exposed workers, including ciliary loss, goblet cell hyperplasia, squamous metaplasia, and mild dysplasia.

Treatment

In case of eye and skin contact, immediately flush the contaminated area with water for 15 minutes and remove any contaminated clothing. Immediate removal to fresh air is required for inhalation exposure, with administration of oxygen for shortness of breath or hypoxemia. For formaldehyde exposure exceeding 20–30 ppm, emergency department observation with periodic evaluation of respiratory status is necessary for 6–8 hours.

REFERENCES

Greenberg M: Extended follow-up of a cohort of British chemical workers exposed to formaldehyde. J Natl Cancer Inst 2004; 96:1037 [PMID: 15240788].

International Agency for Research on Cancer (IARC): Evaluation of carcinogenic risks to humans, http://monographs.iarc.fr/htdocs/monographs/vol88/formal.html.

Tarone RE, McLaughlin JK: Mortality from solid cancers among workers in formaldehyde industries. Am J Epidemiol 2005; 161:1089 [PMID: 15901630].

US Public Health Service Agency for Toxic Substance and Disease Registry: Medical management guidelines for formaldehyde, www.atsdr.cdc.gov/MHMI/mmg111.html.

Vandenplas O et al: Persistent asthma following accidental exposure to formaldehyde. Allergy 2004;59:115 [PMID: 14674947].

NITRATES: NITROGLYCERIN & ETHYLENE GLYCOL DINITRATE

Essentials of Diagnosis

A. Acute Effects

- Headache
- Angina
- Fall in blood pressure

B. Chronic Effects

- Sudden death
- Increased incidence of ischemic heart disease

Exposure Limits

A. Nitroglycerin

ACGIH TLV: 0.05 ppm TWA
OSHA PEL: 0.2 ppm ceiling
NIOSH REL: $0.1 \ mg/m^3$ ceiling (15 minutes)

B. Ethylene Glycol Dinitrate

ACGIH TLV: 0.05 ppm TWA
OSHA PEL: $1 \ mg/m^3$ ceiling
NIOSH REL: $0.1 \ mg/m^3$ ceiling (20 minutes)

General Considerations

Nitroglycerin (glyceryl trinitrate, trinitropropanetriol) and ethylene glycol dinitrate (dinitroethanediol) are liquid nitric acid esters of monohydric and polyhydric aliphatic alcohols. Those of the tetrahydric alcohols (erythritol tetranitrate, pentaerythritol tetranitrate) and the hexahydric alcohol (mannitol hexanitrate) are solids. They are less stable than aromatic nitro compounds.

Nitroglycerin is readily soluble in many organic solvents and acts as a solvent for many explosive ingredients, including ethylene glycol dinitrate. It is an oily liquid at room temperature with a slightly sweet odor. The sensitivity of nitroglycerin decreases with decreasing temperature, so ethylene glycol dinitrate may be added to nitroglycerin-bearing dynamites to depress the freezing point. Explosions of nitroglycerin may occur when the liquid is heated or when frozen nitroglycerin is thawed. Ethylene glycol dinitrate is an oily colorless liquid that is more stable and less likely than nitroglycerin to explode when it burns.

Use, Production, & Occupational Exposure

Alfred Nobel first used a mixture of nitroglycerin with diatomaceous earth and later a more stable mixture of nitroglycerin, sodium nitrate, and wood pulp to form dynamite. The major application of nitroglycerin is in explosives and blasting gels, as in low-freezing dynamite in mixture with ethylene glycol dinitrate. Other explosive uses are in cordite in mixture with nitrocellulose and petroleum and in blasting gelatin with 7% nitrocellulose. Nitroglycerin also has medical therapeutic applications for the treatment of angina.

Nitroglycerin may be manufactured by a process in which glycerin is added to a mixture of nitric and sulfuric acids. Dynamite is formed by adding "dope," or mixtures of sodium nitrate, sulfur, antacids, and nitrocellulose. Ethylene glycol dinitrate is made by nitration of ethylene glycol with mixed acid.

Occupational exposures to nitroglycerin and ethylene glycol dinitrate can occur during their manufacture and during the manufacture and handling of explosives, munitions, and pharmaceuticals. Skin absorption for both nitroglycerin and ethylene glycol dinitrate has not been quantified but is generally greater than respiratory absorption. Air sampling in dynamite plants where both nitroglycerin and ethylene glycol dinitrate are manufactured and used to produce explosives has shown that short-term higher exposures (in the range of 2 mg/m^3 of ethylene glycol dinitrate) occur among mixers, cartridge fillers, and cleanup or maintenance workers.

Metabolism & Mechanism of Action

Both nitroglycerin and ethylene glycol dinitrate pass readily through the skin. Although there is an excellent correlation between blood nitrate ester levels and airborne exposures, skin absorption is more significant. Both nitroglycerin and ethylene glycol dinitrate are hydrolyzed to inorganic nitrates. The biologic half-life of both nitroglycerin and ethylene glycol dinitrate is about 30 minutes. Both act directly on arteriolar and venous smooth muscle, causing vasodilation within minutes with a consequent drop in blood pressure and an increase in regional myocardial blood flow. The headache associated with nitrate esters is secondary to cerebral vessel distension.

The tolerance that develops after 2–4 days of continuous exposure appears to be the result of an increased sympathetic compensatory mechanism. The pathogenesis of sudden death caused by nitroglycerin and ethylene glycol dinitrate is postulated to be a rebound vasoconstriction resulting in acute hypertension or myocardial ischemia. NIOSH recommends that workplace exposure to nitroglycerin and ethylene glycol dinitrate be controlled so that workers are not exposed at concentrations that will cause vasodilation, as indicated by the development of throbbing headaches or decreases in blood pressure. At this exposure level, workers should be protected against work-related angina pectoris, other signs or symptoms of ischemia or cardiac damage, and sudden death.

Clinical Findings

A. Symptoms & Signs

1. Acute exposure—Symptoms of acute illness include loss of consciousness, severe headache, difficulty breathing, weak pulse, and pallor. Tolerance to these effects develops in dynamite production workers after 1 week of exposure, but symptoms recur on return to work after an absence of 2 days or more. The headache associated with nitroglycerin (*powder headache*) frequently begins in the forehead and moves to the occipital region, where it can remain for hours or days. Associated symptoms include depression, restlessness, and sleeplessness. Alcohol ingestion may worsen the headache.

An acute drop in mean blood pressure of 10 mmHg systolic and 6 mmHg diastolic occurs on return to work after 2–3 days off. Mean blood pressure measurements increase over the week as compensatory mechanisms develop.

Blood pressure reduction has been noted after exposure to 0.5 mg/m^3 for 25 minutes, and some workers develop headaches after inhalation exposure of more than 0.1 mg/m^3. Both irritant and allergic contact dermatitis as a consequence of nitroglycerin exposure have been reported.

2. Chronic exposure—Angina pectoris and sudden death have been described among dynamite workers handling nitroglycerin and ethylene glycol dinitrate. In affected workers, the angina usually occurs on the weekend or early in the work shift following periods away from work. The angina is relieved by reexposure to nitroglycerin or ethylene glycol dinitrate in contaminated clothes or by taking nitroglycerin sublingually. Sudden deaths without premonitory angina also have been recorded in dynamite workers. There is an excess risk of cardiac disease among nitroglycerin and ethylene glycol dinitrate workers.

Other reported chronic effects include symptoms of Raynaud phenomenon and peripheral neuropathy. At high concentrations, the aliphatic nitrates may give rise to methemoglobinemia. A retrospective cohort mortality study of munitions workers exposed to nitroglycerin and dinitrotoluene showed an increase in ischemic heart disease mortality for those younger than age 35 years.

B. Laboratory Findings

Coronary angiography has shown normal coronary arteries in workers with angina, and atheromatous coronary vessels generally have not been found on autopsy of workers who died suddenly. The incidence of ectopy is not increased in dynamite workers, and electrocardiograms may be normal. Abnormalities in digital plethysmography show changes in the digital wave pulse with inhalation exposures of 0.12–0.41 mg/m^3.

Differential Diagnosis

An increased incidence of cardiovascular disease has been found in carbon disulfide–exposed workers. Sudden cardiac death may occur after exposure to carbon monoxide or to hydrocarbon solvents.

Prevention

A. Work Practices

Avoidance of headaches, blood pressure reduction, angina, or sudden death is achieved by reduction of exposure through proper work practices. Control of exposure is best accomplished by closed systems, local ventilation, and the use of proper seals, joints, and access ports. The danger of detonation can be minimized by the use of nonsparking equipment, prevention of smoking and open flames, and other safety measures. Natural and synthetic rubber gloves accelerate absorption of nitrate esters, so only cotton or cotton-lined gloves should be worn. Dermal contact with nitrates should be minimized because this may be an important route of absorption.

B. Medical Surveillance

Preplacement and periodic examination should stress a history of cardiovascular disease and physical examination of cardiac abnormalities. Urinary glycerol dinitrates may have potential as a biologic monitoring tool. A small experimental study in humans has shown that urinary N-methylnicotinamide may have potential as a biomarker for nitrate exposure, but further studies are necessary to determine its importance in the occupational setting. Methemoglobin is not sensitive for routine monitoring of exposure.

Treatment

Treatment of cardiac symptoms caused by nitrate ester exposure does not differ from that of symptoms of coronary insufficiency caused by underlying coronary artery disease. Sublingual nitroglycerin should be used immediately for anginal symptoms. New-onset angina or a change in anginal patterns should be evaluated by noninvasive cardiac imaging or angiography if indicated.

REFERENCE

Price AE: Heart disease and work. Heart 2004;90:1077 [PMID: 15310715].

NITROSAMINES

Essentials of Diagnosis

A. Acute Effects

- Liver damage

B. Chronic Effects

- Probable human carcinogen (selected)

Exposure Limits

ACGIH TLV: Suspected human carcinogen
OSHA PEL: Stringent workplace controls
NIOSH REL: Reduce exposure to lowest feasible concentration

General Considerations

N-Nitrosamines have the general structure shown below:

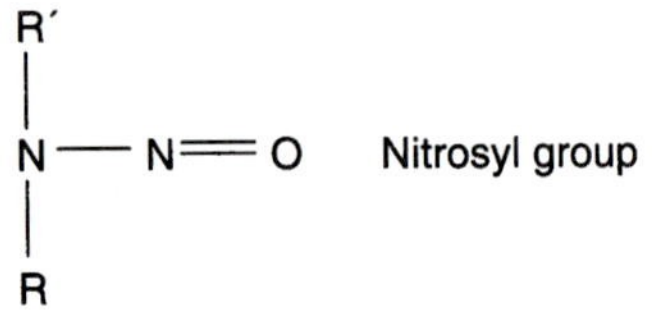

where R and R can be alkyl or aryl or aryl, for example, N-nitrosodimethylamine (NDMA), N-nitrosodiethylamine (NDEA), N-nitrosodiethanolamine (NDELA), and N-nitrosodiphenylamine (NDPhA). Derivatives of cyclic amines also occur, for example, N-nitrosomorpholine (NMOR) and N-nitrosopyrrolidine (NPyR). N-Nitrosamines are volatile solids or oils and are yellow because of their absorption of visible light by the NNO group.

Reactions of nitrosamines involve mainly the nitroso group and the CH bonds adjacent to the amine nitrogen. Enzymatic reactions leading to the formation of carcinogenic metabolites are thought to occur at the alpha carbon.

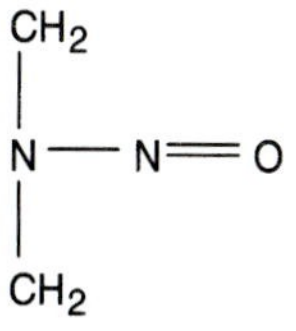
NDMA

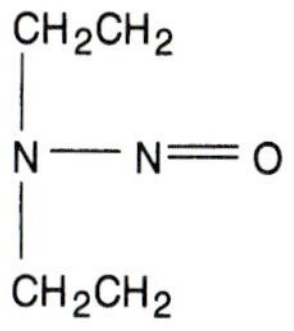
NDEA

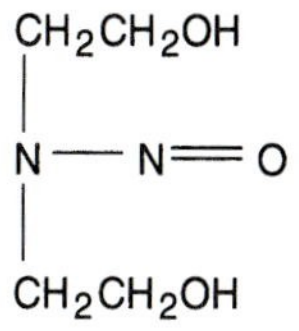
NDELA

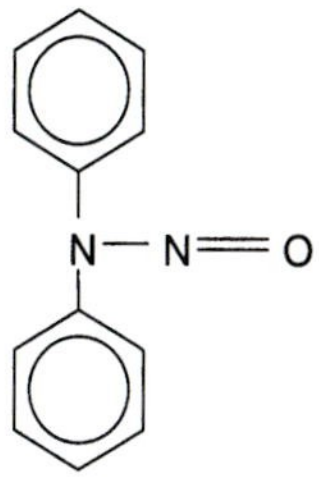
NDPhA

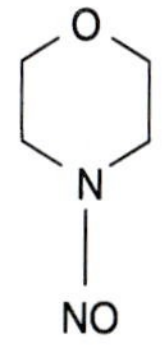
NMOR

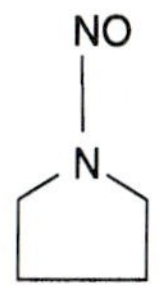
NPyR

Use, Production, & Exposure

Nitrosamines are formed by the reaction of a secondary or tertiary amine with nitrite ion in an acidic medium, according to the general equation shown below:

$$NH + NO_2^- \xrightarrow{H^+} N-N=O$$

Appreciation of the carcinogenicity of the nitrosamines has led to their characterization in many occupational and environmental circumstances. Humans may be exposed to nitrosamines in several ways: formation in the environment and subsequent absorption from food, water, air, or industrial and consumer products; formation in the body from precursors ingested separately in food, water, or air; from the consumption or smoking of tobacco; and from naturally occurring compounds. There is no commercial production in the United States of nitrosamines. Prior to 1976, NDMA was used in the production of dimethylhydrazine, a rocket propellant. NDMA now is used primarily as a research chemical. Other uses of NDMA include the control of nematodes, inhibition of nitrification in soil, as a plasticizer for rubber and acrylonitrile polymers, in the preparation of thiocarbonyl fluoride polymers, as a solvent in the plastics and fiber industry, and as an antioxidant. NDELA is a known contaminant of cosmetics, lotions, shampoos, certain pesticides, antifreeze, and tobacco. NDEA is used primarily as a research chemical, a gasoline and lubricant additive, an antioxidant, a stabilizer in plastics, a fiber industry solvent, a copolymer softener, and a starting material for synthesis of 1,1-diethylhydrazine. The major uses of NDPhA have been in the rubber industry as an antiscorching agent or vulcanization retarder. NDPhA reacts with other amines in the rubber to form *N*-nitrosamines.

The largest nonoccupational exposure to preformed nitrosamines is derived from tobacco products and tobacco smoke, which may contain NDMA, NDEA, NPyR, and others. Nitrosamine content is greater in sidestream smoke and from cigars. Low levels of nitrosamines occur in several types of food, including cheese, processed meats, beer, and cooked bacon. Many cosmetics, soaps, and shampoos are contaminated with NDELA as a result of the nitrosation of triethanolamine by bactericides.

Nitrate can be reduced to nitrite in vitro and in human saliva in vivo. The reaction of ingested nitrites with amines will yield in vivo nitrosamines in the acidic medium of the stomach. Main contributors to gastric nitrite load are vegetables, cured meats, baked goods, cereals, fruits, and fruit juices.

Occupational Exposure

NDMA has been detected in the workroom air of a rubber sealing factory, fish meal producer, manufacturer of surface-active agents, rubber footwear plant, and chrome and leather tanneries. Approximately 750,000 workers are employed by about 1000 cutting-fluid manufacturing firms, and an undetermined number of machine shop workers have the potential to be exposed to nitrosamines in cutting oils. Direct contact with cutting fluids and the presence of airborne mists provide the opportunity for ingestion or skin absorption.

The greatest exposure to the population as a whole occurs from cigarette smoking and the ingestion of nitrite-preserved meats. Certain classes of pesticides have been found to contain identifiable *N*-nitroso contaminants formed during synthesis or as a result of interaction with nitrate fertilizers applied simultaneously to crops. The Environmental Protection Agency (EPA) requires testing for nitrosamines of suspect formulation. NDMA has been found in drinking water, probably associated with the chloramine drinking water disinfection process when nitrogen species are added for chloramination.

Metabolism & Mechanism of Action

The nitrosamines are metabolized rapidly after skin or gastrointestinal absorption with a biologic half-life for NDMA of several hours. NDMA is enzymatically demethylated to form monomethylnitrosamine, which then yields an unstable diazohydroxide. The carcinogenic action of the nitrosamines is attributed to this electrophilic species, which can react covalently with DNA.

Clinical Findings

A. Symptoms & Signs

1. Acute exposure—Two cases of industrial poisoning caused by NDMA were reported in 1937 in chemists producing an anticorrosion agent. They developed headaches, backache, abdominal cramps, nausea, anorexia, weakness, drowsiness, and dizziness; both workers developed ascites and jaundice, and one died with diffuse hepatic necrosis. Five family members who ingested lemonade accidentally contaminated with NDMA developed nausea, vomiting, and abdominal pain within a few hours, and two died 4 and 5 days later with generalized bleeding. Postmortem examination showed hepatic necrosis.

2. Chronic exposure—Approximately 85% of more than 200 nitrosamines tested in animals are carcinogenic, inducing tumors of the respiratory tract, esophagus, kidney, stomach, liver, and brain. *N*-Nitrosodimethylamine, NDMA, NDEA, NDPhA, NDELA, NPyR, and NMOR are carcinogenic in many animal species and are transplacental carcinogens.

Analyses of lung tissue have found higher levels of 7-methyl-dGMP (a metabolic product of *N*-nitrosamines) in association with specific genotypes. Genetic polymorphisms may be predictive of carcinogen adduct levels and therefore may predict the risk of cancer following carcinogen exposure. DNA adducts derived from exposure to aromatic amines have been detected in pancreatic tissues in relation to cancer risk. Exposure to nitrosamines among rubber workers is associated with a significantly increased mortality from cancers of the esophagus, oral cavity, and pharynx. Studies of workers exposed to metalworking fluids indicate an association between metalworking fluid and stomach, pancreatic, laryngeal, liver, and rectal cancer. Although it remains to be determined which specific constituents of metalworking fluids are responsible for the increased risk of various cancers, *N*-nitrosamines are one of the suspect chemicals. The IARC considers that NDEA and NDMA are probably carcinogenic to humans (group 2A) and that NDELA, NMOR, and NPyR are possibly carcinogenic to humans (group 2B). NIOSH recommends that NDMA be regulated as a potential human carcinogen.

Nitrates may be found in drinking water and have been associated in epidemiologic studies with a greater risk of gastric cancer. Case-control studies of gastric cancer and occupational exposures have suggested a slight increase in risk associated with exposure to nitrosamine. Maternal dietary exposure to *N*-nitroso compounds (NOC) or to their precursors during pregnancy has been associated with risk of childhood brain tumors.

Liver cirrhosis has been reported following chronic exposure to NDMA.

B. LABORATORY FINDINGS

In the few fatalities reported, elevated liver enzymes consistent with hepatic necrosis were noted.

Prevention

A. WORK PRACTICES

Nitrosamines should be handled in well-ventilated fume hoods. To minimize the potential for formation of nitrosamines, nitrate-containing materials should not be added to metalworking fluids containing ethanolamines. Reduction of nitrosamine exposure in the rubber industry includes the avoidance of compounds that give rise to nitrosamines. Adequate engineering controls should be instituted for working with raw polymers, elastomers, and rubber parts containing dialkylamine compounds that may emit nitrosamine when heated.

B. MEDICAL SURVEILLANCE

Increased single-strand DNA breaks in peripheral mononuclear cells have been found in metalworkers exposed to NDELA in cutting fluids. Screening for mutagenicity of cutting fluids containing nitrite and NDELA has been suggested as a means to assess risk of hazardous exposure. Use of biologic samples for exposure to NDELA has been employed to monitor exposure of workers to metalworking fluids. No specific medical surveillance for nitrosamines is recommended.

Treatment

There is no treatment for nitrosamine exposure.

REFERENCES

California Department of Health Services: Studies on the Occurrence of NDMA in Drinking Water. California Department of Health Services, www.dhs.ca.gov/ps/ddwem/chemicals/ndma/ndmaindex.htm.

Dietrich M et al: A review: Dietary and endogenously formed *N*-nitroso compounds and risk of childhood brain tumors. Cancer Causes Control 2005;16:619 [PMID: 16049800].

Gordon T: Metalworking fluid: The toxicity of a complex mixture. J Toxicol Environ Health A 2004;67:209 [PMID: 14681076].

National Institute for Occupational Safety and Health: Topic page: Metalworking fluids, www.cdc.gov/niosh/topics/metalworking/.

National Toxicology Program Report on Carcinogens: http://ntp-server.niehs.nih.gov/index.cfm?objectid=32BA9724-F1F6-975E-7FCE50709CB4C932.

PENTACHLOROPHENOL

Essentials of Diagnosis

A. ACUTE EFFECTS

- Skin and respiratory tract irritation
- Systemic collapse

B. Chronic Effects

- Skin rash (chloracne secondary to chlorodibenzo-dioxin)

Exposure Limits

ACGIH TLV: 0.5 mg/m^3 TWA
OSHA PEL: 0.5 mg/m^3 TWA
NIOSH REL: 0.5 mg/m^3 TWA

General Considerations

Pentachlorophenol (PCP) is a crystalline solid with low water solubility and a characteristic pungent phenolic odor. Its commercial production proceeds by the direct chlorination of phenol in the presence of chlorine and a catalyst or by the alkaline hydrolysis of hexachloroben-zene; both processes result in 4–12% tetrachlorophe-nol and less than 0.1% trichlorophenol in the final product. In addition, the required elevated tempera-tures to produce PCP result in the formation of con-densation products, including the toxic dimers dibenzo-*p*-dioxin and dibenzofuran. Analyses of com-mercial PCP have reported ranges of chlorinated diox-ins and furans from 0.03–2510 ppm. Tetrachloro-dibenzodioxin has been found in a commercial sample of PCP, but it was not the most toxic 2,3,7,8-isomer. High serum dioxin levels have been reported among chlorophenol workers after occupational exposures. Thus evaluation of the health effects of PCP must be considered separately from those of its impurities.

Use

PCP is used as a wood preservative, herbicide, defoliant, fungicide, and chemical intermediate in the production of pentachlorophenate. A 0.1% solution in mineral spir-its, fuel oil, or kerosene is commonly applied as a wood preservative. PCP is used in pressure treatment of lumber at a 5% concentration. About 80% of PCP is used by the wood-preserving industry to treat products such as rail-way ties, poles, pilings, and fence posts. Treated wood products have a useful product life five times that of untreated wood, resulting in significant economic savings and conservation of timber resources. PCP is usually applied to wood products as a 5% solution in mineral spirits, fuel oil, or kerosene. In the United States, com-mercial and industrial use of PCP as a preservative is con-centrated in the South, Southeast, and Northwest. The remaining 20% is used in production of sodium PCP, in plywood and fiberboard waterproofing, in termite con-trol, and as an herbicide for use in rights of way and industrial sites. PCP is registered by the EPA as a termiti-cide, fungicide, herbicide, algicide, and disinfectant and as an ingredient in antifouling paint. It can be applied as a microbial deterrent in the preservation of wood pulp, leather, seeds, rope, glue, starch, and cooling-tower water. It may not be used for domestic purposes because it is a restricted-use pesticide by the EPA.

Because of the risk of teratogenicity and fetotoxicity, the EPA, since 1984, has required that PCP products in concentrations of 5% or less be used only by certified applicators and has restricted the use of PCP on prod-ucts that may come in contact with bare skin, food, water, or animals.

Occupational & Environmental Exposure

Occupational exposure to PCP occurs primarily in the gas, electric service, and wood preservative industries. Air sampling at 25 wood treatment plants using PCP showed an average exposure of 0.013 mg/m^3, and newer automated processes and closed systems at larger facili-ties are further reducing exposure. Acute exposure may occur with the opening of pressure-vessel doors or in tank cleaning, solution preparation, and the handling of wood after treatment. Hand application of PCP also may pose a risk of overexposure. Dermal exposure is the principal route, either through direct contact with PCP or through contact with treated wood.

Nonoccupational exposure to PCP can occur after the wood has been treated and shipped, where handling may result in dermal exposure. Six months after treat-ment, PCP will be present on the wood surface at a concentration of about 0.5 mg/ft^2. Elevated levels of PCP have been found in the blood and urine of resi-dents of log homes where the logs have been dipped in PCP prior to construction; air samples showed an indoor air concentration of up to 0.38 μg/m^3 five years after construction.

Metabolism & Mechanism of Action

Absorption of PCP in the occupational setting is largely through inhalation and skin absorption. The latter is increased when PCP is dissolved in organic solvents. Metabolic studies in rodents and human liver homoge-nates indicate that PCP undergoes oxidative dechlori-nation to form tetrachlorohydroquinone, which results in lipid peroxidation and cell death. PCP is excreted mainly in urine as free PCP and as a conjugate with glucuronic acid. Pharmacokinetics are characterized in a single-dose oral administration study by first-order absorption, enterohepatic circulation, and first-order elimination, with 74% of the oral dose of PCP excreted unchanged within 8 days. The half-life for elimination was approximately 30 hours. However, in chronically exposed workers during 2- to 4-week vacations, the ter-minal half-life of elimination ranges from 30–60 days.

Acute intoxication with PCP is caused by interfer-ence with cellular electron transport and the uncoupling of oxidative phosphorylation in mitochondria and endoplasmic reticulum. Interaction with energy-rich phosphate compounds results in hydrolysis and free-energy release, leading to a hypermetabolic state with peripheral tissue hyperthermia.

Clinical Findings

A. SYMPTOMS & SIGNS

1. Acute exposure—

a. Skin—Commercial PCP can cause skin irritation after single exposures to more than a 10% concentration of the material or after prolonged or repeated contact with a 1% solution. Skin sensitization has not been demonstrated. Chloracne may occur after exposure to PCP contaminated with dioxins and dibenzofurans, particularly associated with direct skin contact.

b. Eye, nose, and throat—Irritation can occur at levels above 0.3 mg/m^3.

c. Systemic intoxication—Systemic intoxication caused by PCP became evident in the 1950s after two workers died following cutaneous exposure in a wood-dipping operation. Since that time, fatalities from PCP have occurred among chemical production workers, herbicide sprayers, and wood manufacturers. A unique poisoning tragedy occurred in 20 babies wearing diapers inappropriately laundered in 23% sodium pentachlorophenate; two babies died.

Acute intoxication is characterized by the rapid onset of profuse diaphoresis, hyperpyrexia, tachycardia, tachypnea, weakness, nausea, vomiting, abdominal pain, intense thirst, and pain in the extremities. An intense form of muscle contraction is observed before death. Postmortem examination of one acutely intoxicated worker showed cerebral edema with fatty degeneration of the viscera. The minimum lethal dose of PCP in humans is estimated to be 29 mg/kg.

2. Chronic exposure—Long-term exposure to PCP is associated with conjunctivitis, sinusitis, and bronchitis. Chloracne may occur among PCP-exposed workers and may persist for years after exposure has ceased. Occupational exposure to PCP does not cause adverse effects on the peripheral nervous system, and consistent immunologic effects have not been demonstrated following prolonged exposure to PCP.

Paternal exposure to chlorophenate wood preservatives is associated with congenital anomalies in offspring of sawmill workers. Bone marrow aplasia has been reported after exposure to PCP. Cytogenetic studies of PCP-exposed workers have not demonstrated increased sister chromatid exchanges or chromosomal breakage.

An increased risk for non-Hodgkin lymphoma has been observed following exposure to PCP and phenoxy-acetic acids. The IARC finds that pentachlorophenol is possibly carcinogenic to humans (group 2B). The EPA concluded that the use of PCP poses a risk of oncogenicity because of the contaminants hexachlorodibenzo-dioxin and hexachlorobenzene. PCP and its contaminants cause teratogenic and fetotoxic effects in test animals, but little is known concerning adverse reproductive outcomes in humans.

B. LABORATORY FINDINGS

Acute intoxication with PCP can result in elevation of blood urea and creatinine, with metabolic acidosis and increased anion gap. Increased serum lactic acid dehydrogenase activity and reduced creatinine clearance have been measured in chronically PCP-exposed workers.

Blood levels of PCP in fatal cases have ranged from 40–170 mg/L. Urine levels have ranged from 29–500 mg/L in fatal cases and from 3–20 mg/L in nonfatal cases of intoxication. In PCP-exposed workers, mean urine PCP levels were 0.95–1.31 mg/L. In nonoccupationally exposed individuals in the United States, urine values of PCP average 6.3 μg/L, with a range from 1–193 μg/L and an average of 15 μg/L in hemodialysis patients.

Differential Diagnosis

Acute intoxication can be confused with hyperthermia from other causes, including heat stroke or sepsis. Symptoms of respiratory irritation may be due to the solvent carrier or other occupational irritants. Chloracne is associated with polychlorinated biphenyls, polychlorinated dibenzodioxins, or polychlorinated dibenzofurans.

Prevention

A. WORK PRACTICES

Appropriate respiratory protection must be worn where exposure to PCP may exceed permissible limits, particularly in higher-risk operations such as formulating plants and pressure-vessel and tank maintenance. Gloves of nitrile and polyvinyl chloride provide the best protection against both aqueous sodium pentachlorophenate and PCP in diesel oil. Clothing contaminated with PCP must be removed, left at the workplace, and laundered before reuse. Washing and showering facilities should be available to prevent contamination of food, drink, and family. Coating PCP-treated logs of home interiors with a sealant will reduce PCP exposure to the residents.

B. MEDICAL SURVEILLANCE

Preemployment urine analysis for PCP should be performed and repeated at intervals. Samples should be collected prior to the last shift of the work week and

PCP measured by methods that incorporate hydrolysis. The recommended ACGIH BEI is 2 mg of total PCP per milligram of creatinine in urine or 5 mg of free PCP per milligram of creatinine in plasma before the last shift of work. Discontinuation of PCP exposure will not result in persistent excretion of total PCPs in urine.

Routine medical surveillance should include attention to skin rash and mucous membrane irritation. Hot weather appears to be a predisposing factor for PCP intoxication, so exposure to PCP should be minimized during those times. Significant skin absorption of PCPs may occur and can be documented by urinary PCP monitoring.

Treatment

Solutions of PCP spilled on the skin are treated with prompt and thorough washing with soap and water. Eyes contaminated with PCP should be flushed for 15 minutes with water. All contaminated shoes and clothing should be removed immediately.

In the event of acute PCP intoxication, adequate intravenous hydration and efforts to maintain normal body temperature are essential to prevent cardiovascular collapse. Rapid onset of muscular spasms may prevent intubation and resuscitation, so careful monitoring of respiratory status is critical. Metabolic acidosis should be treated with sodium bicarbonate. Atropine sulfate is contraindicated.

REFERENCES

ATSDR: Toxicological profile for pentachlorophenol, www.atsdr.cdc.gov/toxprofiles/tp51.html.

Proudfoot AT: Pentachlorophenol poisoning. Toxicol Rev 2003; 22:3 [PMID: 14579543].

US Environmental Protection Agency Preliminary Risk Assessment for Pentachlorophenol, www.epa.gov/oppad001/.

POLYCHLORINATED BIPHENYLS

Essentials of Diagnosis

A. ACUTE EFFECTS

- Skin rash (chloracne)
- Eye irritation
- Nausea, vomiting

B. CHRONIC EFFECTS

- Weakness, weight loss, anorexia
- Skin rash (chloracne)
- Numbness and tingling of extremities
- Elevated serum triglycerides
- Elevated liver enzymes

Exposure Limits

ACGIH TLV: 0.5 mg/m³ TWA (54% chlorine)
OSHA PEL: 1 mg/m³ TWA (42% chlorine)
NIOSH REL: 0.001 mg/m³ TWA

General Considerations

Polychlorinated biphenyls (PCBs) are a large family of chlorinated aromatic hydrocarbons prepared by the chlorination of biphenyl. Commercial products are a mixture of PCBs with variable chlorine content and are named according to the percentage of chlorine. In addition, all PCBs are contaminated with small but highly toxic concentrations of polychlorinated dibenzofurans.

Use

Between 1930 and 1975, approximately 1.4 billion pounds of PCBs were produced in the United States. The fire-resistant nature of PCBs, combined with their outstanding thermal stability, made them excellent choices as hydraulic and heat-transfer fluids. They also were used to improve the waterproofing characteristics of surface coatings and were used in the manufacture of carbonless copy paper, printing inks, plasticizers, special adhesives, lubricating additives, and vacuum-pump fluids. In the United States, commercial PCBs were marketed under the name Aroclor. In 1977, Congress banned the manufacture, processing, distribution, and use of PCBs.

Occupational & Environmental Exposure

Leakage of PCBs from capacitors and transformers while in storage, shipment, or maintenance results in transient exposure risks for utility repair crews, railroad maintenance workers, building engineers, and custodians. Improper storage of used PCB electrical equipment may result in environmental contamination and community exposure. Electrical fires occurring in transformers containing PCBs may release polychlorinated dibenzofurans and polychlorinated dibenzodioxins formed through incomplete combustion of PCBs and chlorinated benzenes. Incidents of widespread building contamination caused by PCB transformer fires have occurred in many cities. The EPA maintains a database of PCB transformers that were in use or in storage for reuse that may pose a significant risk to the general public if leakage or fire should occur.

Metabolism & Mechanism of Action

Chlorinated biphenyl compounds are readily absorbed through the respiratory tract, gastrointestinal tract, and skin. Distribution is primarily into fat. Biphenyls are metabolized in the liver as the primary site of biotransformation. PCB mixtures cause induction of the hepatic microsomal monooxygenase systems. Induction is related to chlorination, and PCB mixtures containing higher percentages of chlorine are more potent than mixtures with lower levels of chlorination. More highly chlorinated isomers are also more resistant to metabolism and therefore are more persistent. Hydroxy metabolites can be detected in bile, feces, and breast milk, but urinary excretion is quite low. This leads to bioaccumulation in fat at low exposure levels and the persistence of PCBs in fatty tissue years after exposure. The formation of electrophilic arene oxide metabolites may cause DNA damage and the initiation of tumor growth.

Clinical Findings

A. SYMPTOMS & SIGNS

1. Acute—Acute exposure to PCBs results in mucous membrane irritation and nausea and vomiting. Transient skin irritation may result from direct handling of PCBs containing mixtures of solvents.

In the mass food poisoning incident, which was a result of rice oil contamination, in western Japan in 1968 (*yusho,* or *rice oil disease*), ingestion of PCBs resulted in chloracne. Chloracne probably results from interference with vitamin A metabolism in the skin, with disturbances of the epithelial tissues of the pilosebaceous duct. Typical chloracne presents with cystic or comedonal lesions over the face, ear lobes, retroauricular region, axillae, trunk, and external genitalia and may occur at any age. Yusho patients also showed dark pigmentation of the gingivae, oral mucosa, and nails, with conjunctival swelling. It is not clear whether all or some of these findings were a result of trace contamination of the PCBs with dibenzofurans; the latter compound may have increased during cooking.

2. Chronic—In addition to the acute symptoms of upper respiratory tract irritation, chronic workplace exposure to PCBs also has resulted in chloracne. The relationship between dose of exposure and the appearance of chloracne is inconsistent, although chloracne persists for years after exposure has ceased.

PCBs have an efficient transplacental transfer, and adverse reproductive effects of PCBs have been reported in many animal species; these include failure of implantation, increased number of spontaneous abortions, and low birth weight of litters. In *yu-cheng* (*oil disease*), mothers were exposed to PCBs and their heat-degradation products from the ingestion of contaminated rice oil in 1979. Children of these mothers were born growth retarded, with dysmorphic physical findings, delayed cognitive development, and increased activity levels. Rare cases of chloracne and, more commonly, nail abnormalities have been found in *yu-cheng* chil-

dren. Higher prenatal exposure to PCBs predicts poorer cognitive abilities, impaired development, and endocrine abnormalities in the offspring of women with exposure to PCBs in the environment or from eating PCB-contaminated fish; these effects appear long-lasting in follow-up studies.

Cytogenetic analysis of peripheral blood lymphocytes has shown increased chromosome aberrations and sister chromatid exchanges among PCB-exposed workers. PCBs fed to test animals produce hepatocellular carcinomas. Some cohort studies and case reports of workers exposed to PCBs show an increased risk of malignant melanoma and brain, liver, biliary, stomach, thyroid, and colorectal cancer. Other studies found no evidence of excess cancer risk associated with PCB exposure.

PCBs are known as environmental endocrine-disrupting chemicals, with a variety of end-organ hormonal effects. For example, low doses of PCBs potentially can interfere with thyroid hormone receptor–mediated transactivation and alter prenatal steroid hormones. Some PCBs exert dioxin-like activity mediated through receptors that can interfere with sexual hormone–mediated processes. To determine whether these exert an important clinical effect, several studies of environmental PCB exposure and breast cancer incidence have been performed over the past several years. A significant association between PCB levels and breast cancer risk has been demonstrated in some but not all studies. One recent study indicated that PCB-exposed women had an excess of amyotrophic lateral sclerosis and, among those most highly exposed, an excess of Parkinson disease and dementia.

B. LABORATORY FINDINGS

Mild elevations of serum triglyceride concentrations have been found in *yusho* patients and occupationally exposed individuals. PCB-exposed workers have been reported to have significant correlations between the serum PCB level and the gamma-glutamyl transpeptidase level.

If exposure to PCB is suspected, serum or fat levels of PCBs may be measured to document absorption. In a steady state, serum is as good a reflection of body burden as is fat. Results must be interpreted in light of established normal values for geographic area and laboratory technique. PCBs can be measured in human tissue by a variety of analytic methods and have been variously reported as total PCB content related to a commercial mixture, as quantification of chromatographic peaks, or by characterization of specific congeners. Analysis of coplanar mono-*ortho*-substituted and di-*ortho*-substituted PCB levels in human blood may be useful following acute or chronic exposure. These more toxic congeners contribute significantly to dioxin toxic equivalents in blood from U.S. adults. Normative PCB values among U.S. adults have been published recently by the Centers for Disease Control and Prevention (CDC).

Differential Diagnosis

Occupational exposure to PCBs may be accompanied by exposure to chlorinated dibenzodioxin and dibenzofuran contaminants and may be responsible for chronic toxicity. Concurrent exposure to solvents is important because these substances may cause chronic fatigue and elevated liver enzymes. Mild chloracne should not be confused with other papular rashes. A biopsy may be necessary to establish the diagnosis.

Prevention

A. Work Practices

Work practices to avoid exposure to PCBs include the use of special PCB-resistant gloves and protective clothing. Adequate ventilation should be maintained during spill cleanup or maintenance of vessels containing PCBs; if this is not possible, approved respirators should be provided. Provision should be made for proper decontamination or disposal of contaminated clothing or equipment. Locations where PCBs are stored should be clearly posted as required by law. Environmental sampling may be necessary to ensure adequate worker protection or safety for public reentry to contaminated areas. Reentry or cleanup levels have been established for dioxins and PCBs to protect workers who reoccupy buildings following a PCB fire.

B. Medical Surveillance

Workers intermittently exposed to PCBs should have a baseline skin examination and liver function tests. Follow-up examination can be limited to symptomatic individuals and those exposed as a consequence of accidental contamination. Routine serum measurements are not recommended.

Treatment

Acute exposure should be treated by immediate decontamination of the skin with soap and water to prevent skin absorption. No specific measures are available for respiratory tract or skin absorption. No treatment is available for chronic PCB toxicity. Chloracne is treated with topical therapy for symptomatic relief.

REFERENCES

ATSDR: Toxicological profile for polychlorinated biphenyls (PCBs), www.atsdr.cdc.gov/toxprofiles/tp17.html.

California Environmental Protection Agency Office of Environmental Health Hazard Assessment: Prioritization of Toxic Air Contaminants, www.oehha.ca.gov/air/toxic_contaminants/pdf_zip/dioxin_final.pdf.

Centers for Disease Control and Prevention, National Centers for Environmental Health: National Report on Human Exposure to Environmental Chemicals. www.cdc.gov/exposurereport/.

De Roos AJ et al: Persistent organochlorine chemicals in plasma and risk of non-Hodgkin's lymphoma. Cancer Res 2005;65: 11214 [PMID: 16322272].

POLYCYCLIC AROMATIC HYDROCARBONS

Essentials of Diagnosis

A. Acute Effects

- Dermatitis, conjunctivitis (coal tar pitch volatiles)

B. Chronic Effects

- Excess cancer rates in selected occupations

Exposure Limits

A. Coal Tar Products (Volatiles)

ACGIH TLV: Confirmed human carcinogen
OSHA PEL: 0.2 mg/m^3 TWA (benzene-soluble fraction)
NIOSH REL: 0.1 mg/m^3 TWA

B. Naphthalene

ACGIH TLV: 10 ppm TWA, 15 ppm STEL
OSHA PEL: 10 ppm TWA
NIOSH REL: 10 ppm TWA, 15 ppm STEL

C. Bitumens

NIOSH REL: 5 mg/m^3 ceiling (15 minutes)

D. Carbon Black

ACGIH TLV: 3.5 mg/m^3 TWA
OSHA PEL: 3.5 mg/m^3 TWA
NIOSH REL: 3.5 mg/m^3 TWA; in presence of polycyclic aromatic hydrocarbons, 0.1 mg/m^3 TWA

E. Anthracene

ACGIH TLV: 0.2 mg/m^3 TWA
OSHA PEL: 0.2 mg/m^3 TWA
NIOSH REL: 0.01 mg/m^3 TWA (cyclohexane extractable fraction)

F. Benzo(A)pyrene

ACGIH TLV: Suspected human carcinogen, no TWA

OSHA PEL: 0.2 mg/m³ TWA
NIOSH REL: 0.1 mg/m³ (cyclohexane extractable fraction)

General Considerations

Polycyclic aromatic hydrocarbons (PAHs) are organic compounds consisting of three or more aromatic rings that contain only carbon and hydrogen and share a pair of carbon atoms. They are formed by pyrolysis or incomplete combustion of such organic matter as coke, coal tar and pitch, asphalt, and oil. The composition of the products of pyrolysis depends on the fuel, the temperature, and the time in the hot area. PAHs are emitted as vapors from the zone of burning and condense immediately on soot particles or form very small particles themselves. Such processes always lead to a mixture of hundreds of PAHs. Compounds with three or four aromatic rings predominate. Carcinogenic PAHs are found among those with five or six rings. The simplest fused ring is naphthalene. Some important PAHs in the occupational environment are shown below:

Naphthalene   Anthracene

Benzo(a)pyrene

Use, Production, & Exposure

Pure PAHs have no direct use except for naphthalene and anthracene. Anthracene is used in the manufacture of dyes, synthetic fibers, plastics, and monocrystals; as a component of smoke screens; in scintillation counter crystals; and in semiconductor research. Benzo(*a*)pyrene is used as a research chemical and is not produced commercially in the United States. Bitumens are contained in road-paving, roofing, and asphalt products. The majority of carbon black is used as a pigment for rubber tires, with the remainder used in a variety of products such as paint, plastics, printing inks, pigment in eye cosmetics, carbon paper, and typewriter ribbons.

Creosote is used extensively as a wood preservative, usually by high-pressure impregnation of lumber, and as a constituent of fuel oil, lubricant for die molds, and pitch for roofing. Creosote contains over 300 different compounds, the major components of which are PAHs, phenols, cresols, xylenols, and pyridines.

Coal tar pitch is used as a raw material for plastics, solvents, dyes, and drugs; crude or refined coal tar products are used for waterproofing, paints, pipe coatings, roads, roofing, and insulation; as a sealant, binder, and filler in surface coatings; and a modifier in epoxy resin coatings.

Naphthalene is used as a chemical intermediate in the production of phthalic anhydride, carbamate insecticides, -naphthol, sulfonic acids, and surfactants and as a moth repellent and tanning agent. PAHs as contaminants can be found in air, water, food, and cigarette smoke, as well as in the industrial environment.

Occupational Exposure

A. Coal Tars & Products

Exposures to PAHs may occur among carbon black production workers, wildland firefighters, petroleum tanker deck crews, meat smokehouse workers, and printing press room operators. The most important source of PAHs in the air of the workplace is coal tar. Tars and pitches are black or brown liquid or semisolid products derived from coal, petroleum, wood, shale oil, or other organic materials. Coal tars are by-products of the carbonization of coal to produce coke or natural gas. The coke-oven plant is the principal source of coal tar. Coal tar pitch and creosote are derived from the distillation of coal tar. Numerous PAHs have been identified in coal tar, coal tar pitch, and creosote. Coal tar pitch volatiles are the volatile matter emitted into the air when coal tar, coal tar pitch, or their products are heated, and they may contain several PAHs.

The major use for coal tar pitch is as the binder for aluminum smelting electrodes; other uses include roofing material, surface coatings, pipe-coating enamels, and as a binder for briquettes and foundry cores. Creosote is used almost exclusively as a wood preservative.

Occupational exposure to PAHs in coal tar and pitches may occur in gas and coke works, aluminum reduction plants, iron and steel foundries, and coal gasification facilities and during roof and pavement tarring and the application of coal tar paints.

B. Carbon Black

Carbon black is derived from the partial combustion (pyrolysis) of natural gas or petroleum. It is used primarily in pigmenting and reinforcing rubber products and in inks, paints, and paper.

C. Bitumens

Bitumens are viscous solids or liquids derived from refining processes of petroleum. They are used principally for road construction when mixed with asphalt, in roofing felt manufacture, in pipe coatings, and as binders in briquettes. Occupational exposure may occur in these operations.

D. Soots

Soots are mixtures of particulate carbon, organic tars, resins, and inorganic material produced during incomplete combustion of carbon-containing material. Occupational exposure is primarily to chimney soot; potential exposure occurs to chimney sweeps, brick masons, and heating-unit service personnel.

E. Diesel Exhaust

Exposure to PAHs (methylated naphthalenes and phenanthrenes) has been documented among several occupational groups exposed to diesel exhaust, including truck drivers, underground miners, and railroad workers.

Environmental Exposure

PAHs occur in the air primarily as a result of coal burning and settle on soil, where they may leach into water. They are found in smoked fish and meats and form during the broiling and grilling of foods. They are inhaled in cigarette smoke from the burning of tobacco.

Metabolism & Mechanism of Action

PAHs are absorbed readily by the skin, lungs, and gastrointestinal tract of experimental animals and are metabolized rapidly and excreted in the feces. In humans, they are largely absorbed from carrier particles via the respiratory route. They are activated by aryl hydrocarbon hydroxylase to a reactive epoxide intermediate and then conjugated for excretion in urine or bile. The reactive epoxide may bind covalently with DNA and probably accounts for the carcinogenic activity.

Clinical Findings

A. Symptoms & Signs

1. Acute exposure—Acute inhalation exposure to naphthalene may cause headache, nausea, diaphoresis, and vomiting. Accidental ingestion has caused hemolytic anemia. Naphthalene also may cause erythema and dermatitis on repeated skin contact. Exposure to coal tar products may cause phototoxicity, with skin erythema, burning, and itching, and eye burning and lacrimation.

2. Chronic exposure—The PAHs are genotoxic, as demonstrated by increased DNA adducts, micronuclei, and chromosomal aberrations among exposed workers. Many PAHs are carcinogenic in animals. Often benzo(*a*)pyrene (BaP) is measured to indicate the presence of PAHs where exposure to carcinogens is suspected.

Evidence for human carcinogenicity was described initially by Percivall Pott in 1775, when he associated scrotal cancer in chimney sweeps with prolonged exposure to tar and soot. Subsequently, scrotal cancer has

been reported among mulespinners exposed to shale oil and among workers exposed to pitch.

Excess cancer mortality has been found among coke oven workers (lung and prostate), foundry workers (lung), aluminum smelter workers (lung and bladder), and roofers (lung and stomach). Workers exposed to diesel exhaust have an increased risk of lung and, possibly, prostate cancer. In one study, exposure to carbon black experienced by dockyard workers was associated with a twofold increased risk of bladder cancer. Road-paving workers may have a slightly higher rate of lung cancer and a moderately higher rate of stomach cancer than their nonexposed counterparts.

The IARC considers coal tar pitch volatiles to be carcinogenic to humans (group 1), BaP and creosote possibly carcinogenic to humans (group 2A), and carbon black possibly carcinogenic to humans (group 2B). NIOSH considers that coal tar products, carbon black, and anthracene are carcinogenic and recommends that exposures be limited to the lowest feasible level. There is evidence that extracts of refined bitumens are carcinogenic in animals. There are insufficient data to assess cancer risk among workers exposed to bitumens (such as highway maintenance workers and road pavers).

Exposure-related respiratory effects in carbon black–exposed workers have included reduction in airflow, symptoms of chronic bronchitis, and small opacities on chest radiograph. Elevated liver enzymes have been found in a group of coke oven workers heavily exposed to PAHs, and excess mortality from cirrhosis of the liver has been observed in a cohort of workers heavily exposed to chlorinated naphthalenes. Some studies have indicated that occupational PAH exposure causes fatal ischemic heart disease with a consistent exposure-response relationship. Occupational creosote exposure is a risk for squamous papilloma and carcinoma of the skin.

B. Laboratory Findings

Photopatch testing may demonstrate photodermatitis in workers with occupational exposure to coal tar pitch and fumes.

Differential Diagnosis

Exposure to other known or potential carcinogens in the work environment should be investigated.

Prevention

A. Work Practices

Reduction of emissions from coke ovens, aluminum works, foundries, and steel works is essential. Where gaseous emissions occur during loading or transferring of heated coal tar products, fume and vapor control systems will reduce personal exposure. Skin exposure to tars, pitches, and oils containing PAHs is avoided by wearing gloves and changing contaminated work clothes.

B. MEDICAL SURVEILLANCE

Periodic examination of workers exposed to coal tar pitch volatiles should include a history of skin or eye irritation and physical examination with attention to the skin, upper respiratory tract, and lungs. Urinary 1-hydroxypyrene (1-OHP) has been used for biologic monitoring of many worker populations, including coal liquefaction workers, coke oven workers, foundry workers, aluminum smelter potroom workers, underground miners, electrode paste plant workers, fireproof stone manufacturing workers, graphite electrode production workers, artificial shooting target factory workers, automotive repair workers, carbon black production workers, roofers, road pavers, asphalt workers, firefighters, and policemen. Good correlation has been found between airborne PAH exposure and urinary 1-OHP, with significant contribution from dermal exposure. Urinary 1-naphthol has been used as a biomarker of PAH exposure among naphthalene oil distillation workers, foundry workers, and creosote-impregnated wood assemblers. Urinary PAHs also may be useful biomarkers of occupational exposure. Enzyme radioimmunoassay techniques to measure PAH-DNA adducts in white blood cells also have been used as a biomarker of PAH exposure among several types of PAH-exposed workers, including foundry workers, coke oven workers, fireproof material workers, aluminum smelter potroom workers, roofers, and wildland firefighters. Dietary sources of PAHs (e.g., charbroiled food) and cigarette smoking contribute to PAH-DNA adduct or urinary 1-OHP levels and should be evaluated as confounding factors. Tetrahydrotetrol metabolites of BaP in urine also may prove to be useful for biomonitoring of PAH exposures.

Treatment

Photodermatitis should be treated with cortisone-containing preparations, barrier creams, or removal from exposure.

REFERENCES

Armstrong B et al: Lung cancer risk after exposure to polycyclic aromatic hydrocarbons. Environ Health Perspect 2004;112:970 [PMID: 15198916].

Burstyn I et al: Polycyclic aromatic hydrocarbons and fatal ischemic heart disease. Epidemiology 2005;16:744 [PMID: 16222163].

California Environmental Protection Agency Office of Environmental Health Hazard Assessment: Prioritization of Toxic Air Contaminants. http://cfpub.epa.gov/ncea/cfm/recordisplay.cfm?deid=29060.

National Institute for Occupational Safety and Health: Health Effects of Occupational Exposure to Asphalt. www.cdc.gov/niosh/01-110pd.html.

U.S. Environmental Protection Agency: Health Assessment Document for Diesel Engine Exhaust, http://cfpub.epa.gov/ncea/cfm/recordisplay.cfm?deid=29060.

STYRENE

Essentials of Diagnosis

A. ACUTE EFFECTS

- Eye, respiratory tract, and skin irritation

B. CHRONIC EFFECTS

- Weakness, headache, fatigue, dizziness
- Neuropsychological deficits, color vision loss, sensory nerve conduction slowing

Exposure Limits

ACGIH TLV: 20 ppm TWA, 40 ppm STEL
OSHA PEL: 100 ppm TWA, 200 ppm (15 minutes), 600 ppm (5 minutes in any 3-hour period)
NIOSH REL: 50 ppm TWA, 100 ppm ceiling (15 minutes)

General Considerations

Styrene, also known as vinyl benzene and phenylethylene, has the chemical formula $C_6H_5CH:CH_2$. It is a colorless volatile liquid at room temperature with a sweet odor at low concentrations. The odor threshold of 1 ppm is below the permissible exposure limit, and the material has adequate warning properties. Styrene monomer must be stabilized by an inhibitor to prevent exothermic polymerization, a process that may cause explosion of its container.

Use

Commercial styrene was first produced in the 1920s and 1930s. During World War II, styrene was important in the manufacture of synthetic rubber. More than 90% of styrene is produced by the dehydrogenation of ethylbenzene. Styrene is used as a monomer or copolymer for polystyrenes, acrylonitrile-butadiene-styrene (ABS) resins, styrene-butadiene rubber (SBR), styrene-butadiene copolymer latexes, and styrene-acrylonitrile (SAN) resins. Styrene is also used in glass-reinforced unsaturated polyester resins employed in construction materials and boats and in the manufacture of protective coatings.

Occupational & Environmental Exposure

In closed polymerization processes, worker exposure to styrene generally is low, but exposure peaks may occur during cleaning, filling, or maintenance of reaction vessels or during transport of liquid styrene. Styrene exposure during manual application of resins (hand lamination) or spraying in open molds may exceed exposure limits. The most significant exposure to styrene occurs when it is used as a solvent-reactant for unsaturated polyester products that are reinforced with fibrous glass. Reinforced plastics/composites are used in the manufacture of boats, storage tanks, wall panels, tub and shower units, and truck camper tops. In this process, alternating layers of chopped fibers or woven mats of fibrous glass are hand applied with catalyzed resin; up to 10% of the styrene may evaporate into the workplace air as the resin cures. Average styrene exposures in plants where the reinforced products are manufactured can range from 40–100 ppm, with short-term individual exposures of up to 150–300 ppm. In a NIOSH study of the reinforced-plastics industry, directly exposed workers engaged in the manufacture of truck parts and boats had the highest exposure to styrene, with a mean 8-hour TWA of 61 and 82 ppm, respectively.

Metabolism & Mechanism of Action

Occupational exposure occurs mainly via inhalation, with approximately 60% of inhaled styrene retained by the lungs. The odor threshold is 0.02–0.47 ppm. Percutaneous absorption is not significant. Styrene is metabolized by the microsomal enzyme system to styrene oxide, which is hydrated to phenylethylene glycol (styrene glycol). Styrene glycol then is metabolized to mandelic acid or to benzoic acid and then hippuric acid. Mandelic acid is further metabolized to phenylglyoxylic acid. Styrene oxide is also metabolized directly to hydroxyphenylethyl mercapturic acid. The styrene oxide intermediate is genotoxic and is probably the key factor in the carcinogenic effect of styrene. Genetic polymorphisms of xenobiotic-metabolizing enzymes (*EPHX1, GSTT1, GSTM1, GSTP1*) appear to play an important role in styrene biotransformation.

After short-term exposure, the venous half-life of styrene is approximately 40 minutes. The half-lives of mandelic acid and phenylglyoxylic acid are about 4 and 8 hours, respectively. In the chronically exposed worker, the half-life for mandelic acid excretion may range from 6–9 hours.

Clinical Findings

A. Symptoms & Signs

1. Acute exposure—Concentrations of styrene from 100–200 ppm may cause eye and upper respiratory tract irritation. Styrene is a defatting agent and a primary skin irritant, resulting in dermatitis. Experimental human exposure to several hundred parts per million causes typical organic solvent anesthetic symptoms, with listlessness, drowsiness, impaired balance, difficulty in concentrating, and decrease in reaction time. Styrene exposure acutely enhances serum pituitary hormone secretion. There are no reports of fatalities as a consequence of styrene exposure.

2. Chronic exposure—Weakness, headache, fatigue, poor memory, and dizziness can occur in workers chronically exposed to styrene in concentrations of less than 100 ppm. Mean reaction time and visuomotor performance may be decreased in exposed workers. The incidence of abnormal electroencephalographs (EEGs) is significantly greater as well.

Studies of styrene-exposed workers have shown detectable blood levels of styrene-7,8-oxide, with dose-related increases in lymphocyte DNA adduct levels, styrene-7,8-oxide hemoglobin adduct levels, single-strand DNA breaks, chromosomal aberrations, lymphocyte micronuclei, and sister chromatid exchanges. Higher hypoxanthine–guanine phosphoribosyl transferase (*HRPT*) gene mutant frequencies have been detected in styrene-exposed individuals, associated with years of employment and styrene in blood. Several studies of styrene-exposed workers have demonstrated an association between styrene exposure and degenerative disorders of the nervous system, pancreatic cancer, and lymphohematopoietic cancer. Significant associations have been observed in large European studies between the risk of leukemia and exposure to styrene. Other authors suggest that these findings may be confounded by concomitant exposures to other solvents (1,3-butadiene, benzene). The IARC considers styrene possibly carcinogenic to humans (group 2B).

A number of neurotoxic effects have been observed after styrene exposure, including electroencephalographic abnormalities, sensory nerve-conduction slowing, prolonged somatosensory evoked potentials, and neuropsychological deficits. Neuropsychological symptoms generally are reversible, but some deficits such as visuomotor performance and perceptual speed persist. Neuropsychological effects may correlate with microsomal epoxide hydrolase activity. Styrene exposure among glass-reinforced-plastic workers and plastic-boat manufacturing workers has been associated with early color and contrast vision dysfunction. The effects on contrast sensitivity increase with long-term cumulative exposure, probably reflecting chronic damage to the neurooptic pathways. An effect on hearing acuity has been observed, possibly owing to disorganization of the cochlear membranous structures.

Moderate exposure to styrene has been associated with an altered distribution of lymphocyte subsets in worker populations and may alter leukocyte adherence in experimental test systems. Results of these studies suggest that styrene may alter the cell-mediated immune response of T lymphocytes and result in leukocyte alterations in exposed workers. Styrene also has been found to increase the risk of acute ischemic heart disease mortality among the most highly exposed workers at a synthetic rubber plant.

Styrene may be embryotoxic or fetotoxic in animals. Human reproductive studies (spontaneous abortions, congenital malformations, low birth weight, or reduced fertility) have been inconsistent or limited by methodologic shortcomings.

B. Laboratory Findings

A dose-response relationship exists between styrene exposure and hepatic transaminase, direct bilirubin, and alkaline phosphatase concentrations. However, these tests are nonspecific and should be interpreted in light of other confounders.

The most reliable indicator of styrene exposure is mandelic acid in the urine. Postshift mandelic acid levels in urine show a good correlation with average TWA styrene exposure over the range of 5–150 ppm. Levels of 500 mg mandelic acid per liter of urine may indicate recent exposure to at least 10 ppm styrene. A concentration of 1000 mg mandelic acid per liter of urine corresponds to an average 8-hour TWA styrene exposure of 50 ppm.

Differential Diagnosis

Exposure to other solvents during the production of styrene and in the manufacture of reinforced-plastic products may cause similar symptoms of central nervous system toxicity such as headache, fatigue, and memory loss.

Prevention

A. Work Practices

Styrene poses a significant fire hazard, and proper handling and storage are essential to prevent ignition of the liquid and vapor and a potential explosive reaction. Exposures should be reduced through general and local ventilation systems or through the use of automated processes and closed molds. Intensive local exhaust ventilation is the best way to reduce styrene vapor concentrations during construction of large reinforced-plastic objects, although dilution ventilation is used widely to reduce styrene vapor exposure in the boat industry.

When worker exposure cannot be controlled adequately by engineering controls, protective clothing and respirators may be needed. Where workers may come into contact with liquid styrene, appropriate gloves, boots, overshoes, aprons, and face shields with goggles are recommended. Polyvinyl alcohol and polyethylene gloves and protective clothing give good protection against styrene. To prevent eye irritation at moderately low concentrations, full-facepiece respirators are recommended.

B. Medical Surveillance

Initial medical evaluation should include a history of nervous system disorders and an examination with particular attention to the nervous system, respiratory tract, and skin. Annual medical examinations should be performed on all workers with significant air exposure above the action level or with potential for significant skin exposure. The ACGIH recommended BEI is 240 mg phenylglyoxylic acid per gram of creatinine, 300 mg mandelic acid per gram of creatinine in urine, or 0.55 mg/L in venous blood at the end of the work shift. Styrene in exhaled air also has been used as an indicator of low-level styrene exposure. Measurement of monoamine oxidase type B activity in platelets and the glycophorin A assay also have been suggested as biomarkers of styrene exposure.

Treatment

Hands should be washed after skin exposure, and clothing saturated with styrene should be removed immediately. In the case of eye contact, flush the eye immediately with copious amounts of water for 15 minutes. No specific treatment is recommended for acute or chronic styrene exposure.

REFERENCES

Benignus VA et al: Human neurobehavioral effects of long-term exposure to styrene: A meta-analysis. Environ Health Perspect 2005;113:532 [PMID: 15866759].

California Environmental Protection Agency Office of Environmental Health Hazard Assessment: Chronic Toxicity Summary: Styrene, www.oehha.ca.gov/air/chronic_rels/pdf/100425.pdf.

Nestmann ER et al: Perspectives on the genotoxic risk of styrene. J Toxicol Environ Health B Crit Rev 2005;8:95 [PMID: 158047].

Paramei GV et al: Impairments of colour vision induced by organic solvents: A meta-analysis study. Neurotoxicology 2004;25:803 [PMID: 15288511].

2,3,7,8-TETRACHLORODIBENZO-*P*-DIOXIN

Essentials of Diagnosis

A. Acute Effects

- Eye and respiratory tract irritation
- Skin rash, chloracne
- Fatigue, nervousness, irritability

B. Chronic Effects

- Chloracne
- Soft-tissue sarcoma, non-Hodgkin lymphoma, Hodgkin disease

Exposure Limits

NIOSH REL: Lowest feasible concentration

General Considerations

Polychlorinated dibenzo-*p*-dioxins (PCDDs) and polychlorinated dibenzofurans (PCDFs) are two large series of tricyclic aromatic compounds that exhibit similar physical, chemical, and biologic properties.

PCDFs

PCDDs

However, there is a pronounced difference in potency among the different PCDD and PCDF isomers. The most extensively studied is the 2,3,7,8-tetrachlorodibenzo-*p*-dioxin isomer (2,3,7,8-TCDD). *Dioxin* is the name used for at least 75 chlorinated aromatic isomers, including 22 isomers of the tetrachlorinated dioxin. 2,3,7,8-TCDD is the specific dioxin identified as a contaminant in the production of 2,4,5-trichlorophenol (TCP), 2-(2,4,5-trichlorophenoxy)propionic acid (Silvex), and 2,4,5-trichlorophenoxyacetic acid (2,4,5-T). In its pure form, 2,3,7,8-TCDD is a colorless crystalline solid at room temperature, sparingly soluble in organic solvents, and insoluble in water. The degree of toxicity of the dioxin compounds is highly dependent on the number and position of the chlorine atoms; isomers with chlorination in the four lateral positions (2,3,7,8) have the highest acute toxicity in animals. Under laboratory conditions, 2,3,7,8-TCDD is one of the most toxic synthetic chemicals known. The chlorinated dibenzofurans are contaminants found in some PCBs used in transformers and capacitors, including the most toxic 2,3,7,8-tetrachlorinated dibenzofuran.

Use

2,3,7,8-TCDD is formed as a stable by-product during the production of TCP. Normally, 2,3,7,8-TCDD persists as a contaminant in TCP in amounts ranging from 0.07–6.2 mg/kg. Production of 2,4,5-T and Silvex ceased in the United States in 1979, although stockpiles are still being distributed and used. Agent Orange, used in Vietnam as a defoliant during the 1960s, was a 50:50 mixture of esters of the herbicides 2,4-D and 2,4,5-T. Between 10 and 12 million gallons was sprayed over 3–4 million acres in Vietnam; in Agent Orange, the 2,3,7,8-TCDD concentration was about 2 ppm.

The combustion of 2,4,5-T can result in its conversion to small amounts of 2,3,7,8-TCDD. Polychlorinated biphenyls can be converted to PCDFs. Soot from PCB transformer fires may be contaminated with more than 2000 µg/g PCDFs, including the most toxic 2,3,7,8 isomers. A complex mixture of PCDDs and PCDFs may occur in fly ash from municipal incinerators. 2,3,7,8-TCDD is not used commercially in the United States.

Occupational & Environmental Exposure

Occupational exposure to 2,3,7,8-TCDD can occur during the production and use of 2,4,5-T and its derivatives. Since 1949, there have been 24 accidents in chemical plants manufacturing chlorinated phenols in which workers were exposed to PCDDs. The explosion of a TCP chemical plant in 1976 in Seveso, Italy, exposed some 37,000 residents of surrounding communities to 2,3,7,8-TCDD.

Workers may be exposed to PCDDs during the production of TCP, 2,4,5-T, and pentachlorophenol. Herbicide sprayers using 2,4,5-T or Silvex have been exposed to 2,3,7,8-TCDD during application. Environmental contamination occurred from spraying waste oil that contained 2,3,7,8-TCDD for dust control on the ground in Missouri. Workers exposed to slag and fly ash from municipal waste incinerators may have increased blood concentrations of PCDDs and PCDFs. The EPA banned most uses of 2,4,5-T and Silvex in 1979, although their use was allowed on sugar cane and in orchards, and miscellaneous noncrop uses were permitted. In October 1983, the EPA published its intent to cancel the registration of all pesticide products containing 2,4,5-T or Silvex. It is not possible to accurately estimate the number of U.S. workers currently exposed to 2,3,7,8-TCDD during decontamination of work sites, from waste materials contaminated with 2,3,7,8-TCDD (such as metal recycling), or from cleanup after fires in transformers containing PCBs.

Metabolism & Mechanism of Action

2,3,7,8-TCDD is an extremely lipophilic substance that is absorbed readily following an oral dose in rats. It accumulates mainly in the liver and after a single dose is largely eliminated unmetabolized in the feces with a whole-body half-life of about 3 weeks. After repeated dosing in small laboratory animals, it is stored in adipose tissue. The half-life of 2,3,7,8-TCDD in humans is 9 years. Dermal absorption may be important in workers exposed to phenoxy acids and chlorophenols. Exposure to 2,3,7,8-TCDD as a vapor normally is negligible because of its low vapor pressure.

Dioxin-like compounds are characterized by high-affinity binding to the Ah receptor, and most biologic effects are thought to be mediated by the ligand-Ah receptor complex. A second protein is required for DNA-binding capability and transcriptional activation of target genes. Growth factors, free radicals, the interaction of 2,3,7,8-TCDD with the estrogen-transduction pathway or protein kinases also may play a role in signal-transduction mechanisms. Relative potency factors have been assigned to the dioxin-like compounds on the basis of a comparison of potency with that of 2,3,7,8-TCDD. Each chemical is assigned a toxic equivalency factor (TEF), some fraction of 2,3,7,8-TCDD, and the total toxic equivalency of the mixture (TEQ) is the sum of the weighted potencies. TEF values have been calculated for PCDDs, PCDFs, and dioxin-like PCBs.

Clinical Findings

A. SIGNS & SYMPTOMS

1. Acute exposure—In some animals, 2,3,7,8-TCDD is lethal in doses of less than 1 μg/kg. Acute toxicity results in profound wasting, thymic atrophy, bone marrow suppression, hepatotoxicity, and microsomal enzyme induction.

In humans, the acute toxicity of 2,3,7,8-TCDD is known from accidental release caused by runaway reactions or explosions. A process accident in Nitro, West Virginia, in 1949, was followed by acute skin, eye, and respiratory tract irritation, headache, dizziness, and nausea. These symptoms subsided within 1–2 weeks and were followed by an acneiform eruption; severe muscle pain in the extremities, thorax, and shoulders; fatigue, nervousness, and irritability; dyspnea; and complaints of decreased libido and intolerance to cold. Workers exhibited severe chloracne, hepatic enlargement, peripheral neuritis, delayed prothrombin time, and increased total serum lipid levels. Long-term follow-up studies of dioxin-exposed workers have found persistence of chloracne and some evidence of liver disease.

2. Chronic exposure—In animals, 2,3,7,8-TCDD is a teratogen and is toxic to the fetus. Two-year feeding studies in rats and mice have demonstrated an excess of liver tumors; the feeding level at which no observable effects in rats occurred was 0.001 μg/kg per day.

Chloracne can result within several weeks after exposure to 2,3,7,8-TCDD and can persist for decades.

Among production workers, the severity of chloracne is related to the degree of exposure. In some workplaces, exposed persons had chloracne but no systemic illnesses; in others, workers experienced fatigue, weight loss, myalgias, insomnia, irritability, and decreased libido. The liver becomes tender and enlarged, and sensory changes, particularly in the lower extremities, have been reported. In exposed production workers, systemic symptoms—except for chloracne—have not persisted after exposures ceased.

Immunotoxic, reproductive, and endocrine effects appear to be among the most sensitive indicators of dioxin toxicity. Research indicates that 2,3,7,8-TCDD inhibits multiple estrogen-induced responses in rodent uterus and mammary tissue and in human breast cancer cells. Antiestrogenic effects are thought to be mediated via the aryl hydrocarbon receptor. Laboratory studies in animals suggest that dioxin-like compounds cause altered development (low birth weight, spontaneous abortions, congenital malformations) and adverse changes in reproductive health (fertility, sex organ development, reproductive behavior). 2,3,7,8-TCDD may be transferred transplacentally and via breast milk, and elevated levels of 2,3,7,8-TCDD have been detected in adult children of female chemical production workers exposed to dioxins. A correlation has been found between serum dioxin levels and menstrual cycle characteristics, particularly among premenarcheal women. Minimal effects were observed on the incidence of endometrioses in this cohort. Epidemiologic studies suggest an association between paternal herbicide exposure and an increased risk of spina bifida in offspring. No effect on the risk of spontaneous abortion or sex ratio of the offspring has been observed.

A number of immunologic effects also have been seen in animal studies. Human studies show alteration in delayed-type hypersensitivity after exposure to dioxins. A relation between serum 2,3,7,8-TCDD concentration and a decrease in circulating CD26 cells and decreased spontaneous background proliferation has been observed. Evidence for an effect of dioxin on the humoral immune system is sparse, and no consistent cytogenetic effects have been seen from 2,3,7,8-TCDD exposure.

2,3,7,8-TCDD may inhibit uroporphyrinogen decarboxylation, and cases of porphyria cutanea tarda among exposed workers have been reported. However, recent studies have failed to find an association between 2,3,7,8-TCDD and porphyrin levels. No association has been observed among former chlorophenol production workers between 2,3,7,8-TCDD exposure and serum transaminase levels, induction of cytochrome P450 activity, peripheral neuropathy, chronic bronchitis or chronic obstructive pulmonary disease, and porphyria cutanea tarda. Serum dioxin levels have been positively associated with levels of luteinizing and follicle-stimulating hormones and inversely related to total testosterone levels. This finding is consistent with dioxin-related effects on the hypothalamic-pituitary-Leydig cell axis in animals.

An increased risk of peripheral neuropathy, heart disease and liver disorders has been seen in studies of Vietnam veterans exposed to dioxin (Operation Ranch Hand). No significant clinical effect on acne, hematologic parameters, immunologic function, or cognitive functioning has been observed in this population. Combined analyses of the Ranch Hand subjects and a NIOSH cohort of industrial workers show modest evidence that exposed workers are at higher risk than nonexposed workers of diabetes or abnormal fasting glucose levels. There is a slight influence of serum 2,3,7,8-TCDD on lipid concentrations in the NIOSH cohort.

Excess risk of soft-tissue sarcoma has been associated with exposure to 2,3,7,8-TCDD and phenoxy herbicides. In a recent reanalysis of U.S. chemical workers with 2,3,7,8-TCDD exposure, a positive trend was found between estimated log cumulative 2,3,7,8-TCDD serum level and overall cancer mortality. Long-term follow-up studies of the Seveso population and a large international cohort show an increase in all-cancer mortality, with increases in soft-tissue sarcoma and lymphohemopoietic neoplasms. Studies of the Operation Ranch Hand cohort suggest a modest increase in the risk of prostate cancer. Serum 2,3,7,8-TCDD levels were significantly related to breast cancer incidence in a long-term follow-up of women in the Seveso Womens' Health Study. However, another study indicates that breast cancer risk does not appear to be associated with adipose levels of PCDDs. The IARC finds that 2,3,7,8-TCDD to be carcinogenic to humans (group 1). NIOSH recommends that 2,3,7,8-TCDD be treated as a potential human carcinogen and that exposure be reduced to the lowest feasible concentration.

B. Laboratory Findings

Abnormalities reported most consistently are elevated liver enzymes, prolonged prothrombin time, and elevated cholesterol and triglyceride levels. Urinary porphyrins may be elevated. Following the Seveso accident, the incidence of abnormal nerve-conduction tests was significantly elevated in subjects with chloracne.

Very low levels of 2,3,7,8-TCDD (4–130 ppt) can be detected in adipose tissue of nonexposed populations. Concentration of polychlorinated compounds in plasma may be 1000-fold less than in adipose tissue. There is a high correlation between adipose and serum 2,3,7,8-TCDD levels; serum levels are a valid measure of body burden. The correlation between plasma and adipose tissue concentrations of 2,3,7,8-TCDD with signs and symptoms is uncertain. Normative PCDD and PCDF serum values among U.S. adults have been published recently by the CDC.

Differential Diagnosis

Known causes of an acneiform eruption in the workplace include petroleum cutting oils, coal tar, and the chlorinated aromatic compounds. With systemic complaints, such as weight loss, headache, myalgias, and irritability, other underlying medical illnesses should be ruled out before attributing the disorder to 2,3,7,8-TCDD.

Prevention

A. Work Practices

NIOSH recommends that 2,3,7,8-TCDD be considered a potential occupational carcinogen and that exposure in all occupational settings be controlled to the fullest extent possible. Specific guidelines for safe work practices must begin with environmental sampling to determine the presence of 2,3,7,8-TCDD contamination, including sampling of air, soil, and settled dust and wipe sampling of surfaces. For site cleanup, specific decontamination procedures should be adhered to for adequate worker protection. Protective clothing and equipment should consist of both outer and inner garments, with outer coveralls, gloves, and boots made of nonwoven polyethylene fabric. Appropriate respiratory protection must be worn, ranging from an air-purifying respirator to a self-contained breathing apparatus. Follow-up sampling should be conducted after decontamination of a site to ensure adequate cleanup.

B. Medical Surveillance

Production workers exposed to compounds contaminated with 2,3,7,8-TCDD, as well as site-decontamination personnel, should undergo baseline and periodic medical examinations with special attention to the skin and nervous system. Baseline laboratory testing should include liver enzymes, cholesterol, and triglycerides, with follow-up as required. Effective safety measures for dioxin cleanup workers will prevent clinical or biochemical disease (chloracne, liver disease, peripheral neuropathy, porphyria cutanea tarda). There has been considerable progress in the use of serum 2,3,7,8-TCDD levels, with the characterization of 2,3,7,8-TCDD body burdens in the Ranch Hand cohort, Seveso residents, herbicide production employees, and Vietnamese civilians. Serum dioxin levels may be useful for research purposes or to assess health-outcome risks for exposure reconstruction, but they are not recommended for routine medical monitoring.

Treatment

Skin contaminated with 2,3,7,8-TCDD should be washed immediately and any contaminated clothing removed and placed in marked containers and disposed of appropriately. Except for symptomatic treatment of chloracne, there is no treatment for acute or chronic health effects resulting from 2,3,7,8-TCDD exposure.

REFERENCES

California Environmental Protection Agency Office of Environmental Health Hazard Assessment: Draft Public Health Goal for TCDD in Drinking Water, www.oehha.ca.gov/water/phg/pdf/dioxin%20_draft.pdf.

US Environmental Protection Agency: Exposure and Human Health Reassessment of 2,3,7,8-Tetrachlorodibenzo-*p*-Dioxin (TCDD) and Related Compounds. www.epa.gov/ncea/pdfs/dioxin/nas-review/.

VINYL CHLORIDE MONOMER

Essentials of Diagnosis

A. ACUTE EFFECTS

- Respiratory tract irritation
- Lethargy, headache

B. CHRONIC EFFECTS

- Acroosteolysis, Raynaud phenomenon, skin thickening
- Hepatosplenomegaly
- Hepatic angiosarcoma

Exposure Limits

ACGIH TLV: 5 ppm TWA

OSHA PEL: 1 ppm TWA 5 ppm ceiling (15 minutes)

NIOSH REL: Reduce exposure to lowest feasible concentration

General Considerations

Vinyl chloride monomer (chloroethene) is a colorless, highly flammable gas at room temperature. It usually is handled as a liquid under pressure containing a polymerization inhibitor (phenol). It is soluble in ethanol and ether. The odor threshold is variable, so odor cannot be used to prevent excess exposure.

Use

The vast majority of vinyl chloride monomer is used for the production of polyvinyl chloride resins. Polyvinyl chloride is used primarily in the production of plastic piping and conduit, floor coverings, home furnishings, electrical applications, recreational products (records, toys), packaging (film, sheet, and bottles), and transportation materials (automobile tops, upholstery, and mats).

Occupational & Environmental Exposure

A 1977 NIOSH survey of three vinyl chloride monomer plants found that the 8-hour TWA ranged from 0.07–27 ppm. Following promulgation of the OSHA Standard in 1974, exposures were reduced to less than 5 ppm. The highest exposures occur in polymerization plants, particularly during reactor-vessel cleaning.

Metabolism & Mechanism of Action

The chief route of exposure to vinyl chloride monomer (VCM) is through inhalation of the gas, although dermal absorption may be significant during manual reactor-vessel cleaning. Vinyl chloride is absorbed readily through the respiratory tract. Its primary metabolite is chloroethylene oxide, which forms the reactive intermediate epoxide that can bind to RNA and DNA in vivo and may be responsible for the carcinogenicity observed in animal and human studies. There may be increased risk of hepatic angiosarcoma in association with *p53* gene mutations. Studies have suggested that polymorphisms of *CYP 2E1, GSTT1,* and *ADH2* may be a major reason for genetic susceptibility in VCM-induced hepatic damage.

The half-life of VCM in expired air is 20–30 minutes. Thiodiglycolic acid (TdGA) is the major urinary metabolite, but it is of limited value in biomonitoring because of metabolic saturation of vinyl chloride, variable metabolism rates, and nonspecificity. One study has suggested that TdGA can be used as an exposure marker for polyvinyl chloride workers when the air VCM level to which they are exposed is greater than 5 ppm.

Clinical Findings

A. SYMPTOMS & SIGNS

1. Acute exposure—VCM has relatively low acute toxicity, causing respiratory irritation and central nervous system depression at high concentrations (10,000–20,000 ppm).

2. Chronic exposure—Chronic toxicity from VCM exposure can result in liver disease, osteolysis, Raynaud phenomenon, vasculitic purpura, mixed connective-tissue disease, and scleroderma-like skin lesions.

   a. Acroosteolysis—Symptoms of Raynaud phenomenon, osteolysis in the terminal phalanges of some of the fingers, and thickening or raised nodules on the hands and forearms occurred in workers employed in production and polymerization, especially in workers assigned to clean the reactors. *Vinyl chloride disease* is a syndrome consisting of Raynaud phenomenon, acroosteolysis, joint and muscle pain, enhanced collagen deposition, stiffness of the hands, and scleroderma-like skin changes. An increase in circulating immune complex levels, cryoglobulinemia, B-cell proliferation, hyperimmunoglobulinemia, and complement activation has been found in these patients. Susceptibility to this disease has been associated with the HLA-DR5 allele. Vascular changes in the digital arteries of the hand associated with acroosteolysis have been demonstrated by arteriography, and circulating immune complexes have been identified.

b. Liver disease—Hepatic fibrosis, splenomegaly, and thrombocytopenia with portal hypertension have occurred. The characteristic pattern of changes consists of hypertrophy and hyperplasia of hepatocytes and sinusoidal cells, sinusoidal dilation associated with damage to the cells lining the sinusoids, focal areas of hepatocellular degeneration, and fibrosis of portal tracts, septa, and intralobular perisinusoidal regions.

In 1974, three cases of hepatic angiosarcoma among polyvinyl chloride polymerization workers were reported at a plant in Louisville, Kentucky. Since then, many cohort mortality studies have documented an increased risk of hepatic angiosarcoma, hepatocellular carcinoma, and liver cirrhosis. There have now been almost 200 cases of hepatic angiosarcoma reported worldwide, with an average latency of 22 years. Vinyl chloride is genotoxic, causing increased chromosomal aberrations, sister chromatid exchanges, and lymphocyte micronuclei among exposed workers. Specific gene mutations at the *p53* locus and mutant p21 proteins have been linked to vinyl chloride angiosarcoma. These findings suggest an effect of chloroethylene oxide, a carcinogenic metabolite of vinyl chloride. The risk of hepatic angiosarcoma is related to the time since the first exposure, duration of employment, and the extent of exposure. The IARC finds that vinyl chloride is carcinogenic to humans (group 1), and NIOSH recommends that vinyl chloride be regulated as a potential human carcinogen.

Only two cases of hepatic angiosarcoma have been documented in the polyvinyl chloride processing industry, suggesting a significantly lower vinyl chloride–related neoplastic risk among fabrication workers. Hemangioendothelioma also has been reported after both vinyl chloride and polyvinyl chloride exposure.

c. Pulmonary effects—Cases of pneumoconiosis have been reported in workers exposed to polyvinyl chloride dust. Some polyvinyl chloride production and fabrication workers with high (>10 mg/m^3) exposure to polyvinyl chloride dust have reduced pulmonary function and an increased incidence of chest radiograph abnormalities. Cumulative polyvinyl chloride dust exposure is associated with mild obstructive airway disease and a higher prevalence of small opacities on chest radiograph. One case of pneumoconiosis and systemic sclerosis following a 10-year exposure to polyvinyl chloride dust has been reported.

d. Reproductive effects—Decreased androgen levels and complaints of impotence and decreased libido and sexual function have been found among male vinyl chloride–exposed workers. Few studies have evaluated the effects of vinyl chloride exposure on the reproductive function of female workers. A significant increase in congenital abnormalities has been found in communities located near a vinyl chloride processing plant, although other studies have failed to report significant developmental toxicity in association with parental exposure to vinyl chloride or proximity to vinyl chloride facilities.

B. LABORATORY FINDINGS

There may be elevated levels of liver enzymes and alkaline phosphatase in workers with vinyl chloride exposure, although in some workers with hepatic angiosarcoma the liver enzymes remain normal until the final stages of disease. Fasting levels of serum bile acids and urinary coproporphyrins have been suggested as clinically useful indicators of early chemical injury in VCM-exposed worker populations with asymptomatic liver dysfunction.

Differential Diagnosis

Hepatic angiosarcoma has been associated with a history of arsenic exposure and thorium dioxide (Thorotrast) ingestion. The VCM-associated sclerotic changes in skin, with skin nodules, Raynaud phenomenon, and osteolysis, are clinically very similar to idiopathic scleroderma; however, sclerodactyly, calcinosis, and digital pitting scars are unusual in VCM disease.

Prevention

The risk of hepatic angiosarcoma should be greatly reduced if the 8-hour TWA is less than 1 ppm.

A. WORK PRACTICES

Worker isolation is achieved in most polyvinyl chloride plants through the use of isolated process control rooms. For operators, cleaners, and utility employees, extensive engineering controls in polyvinyl chloride polymerization plants are required to reduce 8-hour TWA worker exposures to less than 1 ppm. Preventing worker exposure during routine maintenance and cleanup operations by adequate degassing of autoclaves and reaction vessels is essential. Online gas chromatographic VCM-specific detectors can identify leaks before large emissions develop.

Employees should be required to wear half-face supplied-air respirators when the concentration of VCM exceeds 1 ppm. A full-face supplied-air respirator is required for reactor cleaning or other maintenance. Where skin contact is possible, protective uniforms, gloves, head coverings, and impervious boots are necessary.

B. MEDICAL SURVEILLANCE

Preplacement medical examination should evaluate the presence of liver disease. Concurrent viral hepatitis and alcohol consumption should be evaluated because these factors increase the risk of liver disease in vinyl chloride-exposed workers. Preplacement and periodic measurements of liver enzymes are recommended by NIOSH, although the specificity and sensitivity of these tests are poor. An increased γ-glutamyl transpeptidase level is associated with vinyl chloride exposure and may offer greater specificity for medical surveillance. However, a recent study concluded that liver function assessment only including liver function tests is not able to detect VCM-induced liver damage and only revealed alterations owing to nonoccupational factors, such as dietary and/or metabolic dysfunction. Fasting levels of serum bile acids or plasma clearance of technetium-labeled iminodiacetate have been suggested as a sensitive measure of liver dysfunction among vinyl chloride–exposed workers. Liver ultrasonography is a useful diagnostic test for medical surveillance of vinyl chloride workers, with an increased incidence of periportal fibrosis among more highly exposed workers. Surveillance using biomarkers such as *p53* gene mutations and DNA adducts are under investigation but have not yet been proven as useful screening tools.

Treatment

The mean survival after diagnosis of hepatic angiosarcoma is several months. Computed tomography with intravenous contrast dynamic scanning shows a characteristic isodense appearance on delayed postcontrast scans. Chemotherapy may slightly improve the duration and quality of survival. Acroosteolysis appears to be irreversible after cessation of exposure.

REFERENCES

ATSDR: Toxicological profile for vinyl chloride, www.atsdr.cdc.gov/toxprofiles/tp20.html.

Bolt HM: Vinyl chloride: A classical industrial toxicant of new interest. Crit Rev Toxicol 2005;35:307 [PMID: 15989139].

California Environmental Protection Agency Office of Environmental Health Hazard Assessment: Prioritization of Toxic Air Contaminants, www.oehha.ca.gov/air/toxic_contaminants/pdf_zip/VC-final%20doc.pdf.

Maroni M, Fanetti AC: Liver function assessment in workers exposed to vinyl chloride. Int Arch Occup Environ Health 2006;79:57 [PMID: 16091976].

Solvents

Jon Rosenberg, MD, & Elizabeth A. Katz, MPH, CIH

GENERAL PROPERTIES & HEALTH EFFECTS OF SOLVENTS

A solvent is any substance—usually a liquid at room temperature—that dissolves another substance, resulting in a solution (uniformly dispersed mixture). Solvents may be classified as aqueous (water-based) or organic (hydrocarbon-based). Most industrial solvents are organic chemicals because most of the industrial substances they are used to dissolve are organic. Solvents are used commonly for cleaning, degreasing, thinning, and extraction.

Many solvent chemicals are also used as chemical intermediates in the manufacture and formulation of chemical products. However, more workers are exposed to high levels of solvents during use of the substances as cleaners and thinners and in pesticide formulations.

Hundreds of individual chemicals are used to make more than 30,000 industrial solvents. There are physical, chemical, and toxicologic properties that help to classify this large group of chemicals into families with shared or distinguishing features. These features are discussed first, followed by a brief summary of the commonly used industrial solvents according to their chemical families.

PHYSICAL & CHEMICAL PROPERTIES OF SOLVENTS

Solubility

Lipid solubility is an important determinant of the efficiency of a substance as an industrial solvent and a major determinant of a number of health effects. The potency of solvents as general anesthetics and as defatting agents is directly proportionate to their lipid solubility.

Dermal absorption is related to both lipid solubility and water solubility (because the skin behaves like a lipid-water sandwich), so solvents such as dimethyl sulfoxide, dimethylformamide, and glycol ethers, which are highly soluble in both (amphipathic), are well absorbed through the skin. All organic solvents are lipid-soluble, but this solubility may differ to a significant degree.

Flammability & Explosiveness

Flammability and explosiveness are the properties of a substance that allow it to burn or ignite, respectively. Some organic solvents are flammable enough to be used as fuels, whereas others (e.g., halogenated hydrocarbons) are so nonflammable that they are used as fire-extinguishing agents. Flash point, ignition temperature, and flammable and explosive limits are measures of flammability and explosiveness. The National Fire Prevention Association (NFPA) rates flammability hazards by a numerical code from 0 (no hazard) to 4 (severe hazard). Table 29–1 lists flash points and NFPA codes. These properties are important to consider when selecting a solvent or substituting one solvent for another on the basis of undesirable health effects or efficacy.

Volatility

Volatility is the tendency of a liquid to evaporate (form a gas or vapor). Other conditions being equal, the greater the volatility of a substance, the greater is the concentration of its vapors in air. Because the most common route of exposure to solvents is inhalation, exposure to a solvent is highly dependent on its volatility. Solvents as a class are all relatively volatile over a wide range. Vapor pressure and evaporation rate are two measures of volatility listed in Table 29–1.

Chemical Structure

Solvents can be divided into families according to chemical structure and the attached functional groups. Toxicologic properties tend to be similar within a group, such as liver toxicity from chlorinated hydrocarbons and irritation from aldehydes. The basic structures are aliphatic, alicyclic, and aromatic. The functional groups include halogens, alcohols, ketones, glycols, esters, ethers, carboxylic acids, amines, and amides.

PHARMACOKINETICS OF SOLVENTS

Absorption (Route of Exposure)

A. PULMONARY

Because organic solvents are generally volatile liquids, and because the vapors are lipid-soluble and therefore

Table 29–1. Industrial solvents: Properties, odor thresholds, and exposure limits.

	Flash Point (°F)	NFPA Flamma-bility Code[1]	Vapor Pressure (mmHg 25 °C)	Evapo-ration Rate[2]	TLV[3] (ppm)	Odor Thresh-old[4] (ppm)	Biologic Monitor[5]	General Hazards of Chemical Family and Unique Hazards of Specific Compounds
Aliphatic								Anesthetic > irritant.
Pentane	–40	4	500	1	600	400		
n-Hexane	–10	3	150	1.9	50-S	130	+	Peripheral neuropathy.
Hexane (other)	–10	3	150	1.9	500	130		Hazard relative to concentra-tion of n-hexane.
Heptane	25	3	50	2.7	400	150		
Octane	55	3	15	5.9	300	50		
Nonane	90	0	5	2.9	200	50		
Alicyclic								Anesthetic > irritant.
Cyclohexane	10	3	95	2.6	100	25		
Aromatic								Anesthetic > irritant.
Benzene	10	3	75	2.8	0.5-S	10	+	Leukemia and aplastic anemia.
Toluene	40	3	30	4.5	50-S	5	+	Renal tubular acidosis, cere-bellar dysfunction.
Xylenes (all)	85	3	10	9.5	100	1	+	
Ethyl benzene	60	3	5	9.4	100	1	+	
Cumene	95	2	10	14	50	0.1	+	
Styrene	90	3	5	12.4	20	0.5	+	
Petroleum distillates								Hazard relative to aliphatic and aromatic components:
Petroleum ether	~ –50	3	~ 40	~ 1.1	...	...		100% aliphatic, extremely volatile, flammable.
Rubber solvent	~ –20	3	...	~ 2.3	400	...		Mostly aliphatic, extremely volatile, flammable.
VM & P naphtha[6]	~ 30	3	~ 20	~ 7.1	300	...		Mostly aliphatic.
Mineral spirits (Stoddard Solvent)	~ 100	3	~ 5	~ 4.4	100	...		
Aromatic petroleum naphtha	~ 110	3	~ 5	...	...	...		Mostly aromatic.
Kerosene/Jet fuels	~ 115	3	~ 5	200 mg/m³-S	...	...		
Alcohols								Irritant > anesthetic.
Methyl alcohol	50	3	90	5.2	200-S	100	+	Acidosis, optic neuropathy.
Ethyl alcohol	55	3	45	~7	1000	85		"Fetal alcohol syndrome" (ingestion).
1-Propyl alcohol	75	3	20	7.8	200	2		
Isopropyl alcohol	55	3	35	7.7	200	20		
n-Butyl alcohol	85	3	10	19.6	20	1		Auditory, vestibular nerve injury reported.
sec-Butyl alcohol	75	3	15	12.3	100	2		
tert-Butyl alcohol	50	3	15	...	100	50		
Iso-octyl alcohol	185	2	0.05	300	50-S	...		
Cyclohexanol	155	2	1	150	50-S	0.1		
Glycols								Extremely low volatility.
Ethylene glycol aerosol	230	1	0.05	...	...[8]			Acidosis, seizures, renal fail-ure (ingestion).

(continued)

Table 29–1. Industrial solvents: Properties, odor thresholds, and exposure limits. (continued)

	Flash Point (°F)	NFPA Flammability Code[1]	Vapor Pressure (mmHg 25 °C)	Evaporation Rate[2]	TLV[3] (ppm)	Odor Threshold[4] (ppm)	Biologic Monitor[5]	General Hazards of Chemical Family and Unique Hazards of Specific Compounds
Phenols								Irritant > anesthetic; cytotoxic, corrosive.
Phenol	175	2	0.5	...	5-S	0.05	+	Dermal absorption of vapors.
Cresol	180	2	0.2	> 400	5-S	...		
Ketones								Irritant, strong odor > anesthetic.
Acetone	−5	3	20	1.9	500	15	+	
Methyl ethyl ketone	15	3	70	2.7	200	5	+	
Methyl isobutyl ketone	70	3	5	5.6	50	1		
Diacetone alcohol	140	2	1	~60	50	0.1		
Mesityl oxide	90	3	10	8.4	15	0.5		
Cyclohexanone	110	2	3	22.2	20-S	1		
Esters								Irritant, strong odor > anesthetic.
Methyl formate	−2	3	475	1.6	100	600		Optic neuropathy from metabolism to formic acid.
Ethyl formate	−5	3	200	1.8	100	30		
Methyl acetate	15	3	175	2.2	200	5		Optic neuropathy from metabolism to methanol.
Ethyl acetate	25	3	75	2.7	400	5		
n-Propyl acetate	55	3	35	4.8	200	0.5		
n-Butyl acetate	75	3	10	5.2	150	0.5		
n-Amyl acetate	85	3	5	11.6	50	0.05		Odorant ("banana oil").
Ethers								
Ethyl ether	−50	4	450	1	400	10		Extremely volatile, flammable, explosive.
Dioxane	54	3	27	14	20-S	24		Carcinogenic in animals.
Methyl tert-butyl ether (MTBE)	14	3	245	...	50	...		Reproductive, renal
tert-Amyl methyl ether (TAME)	12	3	75	...	20	...		Neurologic, reproductive
Glycol ethers								Skin absorption without irritation.
2-Methoxyethanol	100	2	10	21.1	5-S	2	+	Reproductive toxicity in male and female animals.
2-Ethoxyethanol	110	2	5	28.1	5-S	3	+	Reproductive toxicity in male and female animals.
2-Butoxyethanol	340	2	1	85	20	0.1		Anemia.
Propylene glycol monomethyl ether	100	3	10	...	100	10		
Dipropylene glycol monomethyl ether	185	2	0.5	...	100-S	...		
Glycidyl ethers								Sensitizers, genetic and reproductive toxins.
Phenyl glycidyl ether	...	...	0.01	...	0.1-S	...		Carcinogenic in animals.
Diglycidyl ether	...	...	0.1	...	0.1	...		
Acids								Irritant > anesthetic.
Formic	...	...	...	45	5	0.1		
Acetic	105	2	15	11	10	0.5		
Propionic	...	...	...	5	10	0.2		

(continued)

484 / CHAPTER 29

Table 29–1. Industrial solvents: Properties, odor thresholds, and exposure limits. (continued)

	Flash Point (°F)	NFPA Flamma-bility Code[1]	Vapor Pressure (mmHg 25 °C)	Evapo-ration Rate[2]	TLV[3] (ppm)	Odor Thresh-old[4] (ppm)	Biologic Monitor[5]	General Hazards of Chemical Family and Unique Hazards of Specific Compounds
Amines								Irritant > anesthetic; corneal edema, visual halos.
Methylamine	...	...	gas	gas	5	3		
Dimethylamine	...	...	gas	gas	5	0.5		
Trimethylamine	...	...	gas	gas	5	0.0005		
Ethylamine	< 0	4	gas	gas	5-S	1		
Diethylamine	–9	3	240	2.2	5-S	0.2		
Triethylamine	20	3	70	2.7	1-S	0.5		
n-Butylamine	10	3	70	5.1	... -S[9]	2		
Cyclohexylamine	90	3	10	82.9	10	2.5		
Ethylenediamine	95	2	10	> 5000	10-S	1		Allergic contact dermatitis, asthma.
Dethylene triamine	215	1	0.5	> 400	1-S	...		
Ethanolamine	185	2	0.5	> 5000	3	2.5		
Diethanolamine	280	1	0.05	> 5000	0.46-S	0.5		
Chlorinated hydrocarbons								Cancer in animals; liver, kidney, cardiac effects.
Methyl chloroform (1,1,1,-trichloro-ethane)	NF	0	120	2.7	350	120	+	
Trichloroethylene	...	1	75	3.1	50	30	+	Alcohol intolerance, de-greaser's flush.
Perchloroethylene (tetrachloroethylene)	NF	0	20	6.6	25	25		Carcinogenic in animals.
Methylene chloride	NF	0	420	1.8	50	250	+	Metabolized to carbon mon-oxide, suspect human carcinogen.
Carbon tetrachloride	NF	0	110	2.6	5-S	100		Cirrhosis, liver cancer.
Chloroform	NF	0	190	2.2	10	85		Suspect human carcinogen.
1,1,2-Trichloroethane;	NF	0	20	12.6	10-S	...		
1,1,2,2-Tetrachloro-ethane	NF	0	10	19.1	1-S	1.5		
Chlorofluorocarbons								Weak anesthetic, irritant; cardiac effects.
Trichlorofluoro-methane (F-11)	NF	0	330	1.6	1000[7]	5		
Dichlorodifluoro-methane (F-12)	NF	0	...	...	1000	...		
Chlorodifluoromethane (F-22)	NF	0	...	...	1000	...		
1,1,2,2-Tetrachloro-2,2-difluoroethane (F-112)	NF	0	...	...	500	...		
1,1,2-Trichloro-1,2,2-tri-fluoroethane (F-113)	NF	0	325	2	1000	45		
1,2-Dichlorotetra-fluoroethane (F-114)	...	...	...	...	1000	...		
Chloropentafluoro-ethane (F-115)	...	...	...	...	1000	...		

Table 29–1. Industrial solvents: Properties, odor thresholds, and exposure limits. (continued)

	Flash Point (°F)	NFPA Flamma-bility Code[1]	Vapor Pressure (mmHg 25 °C)	Evapo-ration Rate[2]	TLV[3] (ppm)	Odor Thresh-old[4] (ppm)	Biologic Monitor[5]	General Hazards of Chemical Family and Unique Hazards of Specific Compounds
Miscellaneous								
Turpentine and selected monoterpenes	100	3	...	~ 375	20	...		Irritant> anesthetic; allergic contact dermatitis.
Dimethylsulfoxide	200	1	...	>300	...	...		Hepatotoxic > anesthetic; skin absorption.
Dimethylformamide	140	2	5	45	10-S	2		Smell in breath after exposure; skin absorption,
Tetrahydrofuran	5	3	175	2	50=S	2		Anesthetic, irritant.
1-Bromopropane	70	3	139	>1	10	...		Neurotoxicity, hepatotoxicity, reproductive, developmental

[1] See text for explanation.
[2] Ether = 1, see text for explanation.
[3] American Conference of Governmental Industrial Hygienists (ACGIH) threshold limit value, 8-hour time-weighted average, 2005. adopted. S = "skin" designation.
[4] Population odor threshold determined by testing.
[5] Information available on biological monitoring; see Chapter 38.
[6] Varnish makers' and painters' naphtha.
[7] No TWA; ceiling limit 1000 ppm.
[8] No TWA; ceiling limit 100 mg/m³ (aerosol only).
[9] No TWA; ceiling limit 5 ppm.

well absorbed across the alveolar-capillary membrane, inhalation is the primary route for occupational exposure. The pulmonary retention or uptake (percentage of inhaled dose that is retained and absorbed) for most organic solvents ranges from 40–80% at rest. Because physical labor increases pulmonary ventilation and blood flow, the amount of solvent delivered to the alveoli and the amount absorbed are likewise increased. Levels of physical exercise commonly encountered in the workplace will increase the pulmonary uptake of many solvents by a factor of two to three times that at rest.

B. PERCUTANEOUS

The lipid solubility of organic solvents results in most being absorbed through the skin to some degree following direct contact. However, percutaneous absorption is also determined by water solubility and volatility. Solvents that are soluble in both lipid and water are absorbed most readily through the skin. Highly volatile substances are less well absorbed because they tend to evaporate from the skin unless evaporation is prevented by occlusion by gloves or clothing. Skin absorption rates vary widely among individuals by at least a factor of 4. Factors that affect skin absorption include anatomic location, gender, age, condition (including hydration) of skin, personal hygiene, and environmental factors.

For a number of solvents, dermal absorption contributes to overall exposure sufficiently to result in a "skin" designation for the American Conference of Governmental Industrial Hygienists (ACGIH) threshold limit values (TLVs), as set forth in Table 29–1. For a few solvents, significant absorption of vapors through the skin also can occur. This is most likely to occur when solvents with a "skin" designation and low TLV are used in a situation that results in very high airborne concentrations, such as in an enclosed space with respiratory protection.

Distribution

Because organic solvents are lipophilic, they tend to be distributed to lipid-rich tissue. In addition to adipose tissue, this includes the nervous system and liver. Because distribution occurs via the blood, and because the blood–tissue membrane barriers are usually rich in lipids, solvents are also distributed to organs with large blood flows, such as cardiac and skeletal muscle. Persons with greater amounts of adipose tissue accumulate greater amounts of a solvent over time and, consequently, excrete larger amounts at a slower rate after cessation of exposure. Most solvents cross the placenta and also enter breast milk.

Metabolism

Some solvents are metabolized extensively, and some not at all. The metabolism of a number of solvents plays a key role in their toxicity and, in some cases, the treatment of intoxication. The role of toxic metabolites is discussed in their respective sections for *n*-hexane, methyl *n*-butyl ketone, methyl alcohol, ethylene glycol, diethylene glycol, methyl acetate, methyl formate, and glycol ethers. A number of solvents, including trichloroethylene, are metabolized in common with ethyl alcohol (ethanol) by alcohol and aldehyde dehydrogenase. Competition for these limited enzymes accounts for synergistic effects (*alcohol intolerance* and *degreaser's flush*) and may result in reactions in workers exposed to these solvents while taking disulfiram (Antabuse) for alcoholism. Chronic ethanol ingestion may induce solvent-metabolizing enzymes and lower blood solvent concentrations. Other solvents may have acute and chronic interactions similar to those of ethanol.

Excretion

Excretion of solvents occurs primarily through exhalation of unchanged compound, elimination of metabolites in urine, or a combination of each. Solvents such as perchloroethylene that are poorly metabolized are excreted primarily through exhalation. The biologic half-life of parent compounds varies from a few minutes to several days, so some solvents accumulate to some degree over the course of the work week, whereas others do not. However, bioaccumulation beyond a few days is not an important determinant of adverse health effects for most solvents.

Biologic Monitoring

Biologic monitoring can provide a more accurate measure of exposure than environmental monitoring for some solvents (see Table 29–1 and Chapter 38). This is particularly true for substances whose pulmonary absorption is affected to a large degree by physical work and for substances with significant dermal exposure and absorption (i.e., those with ACGIH "skin" designations; see Table 29–1). Unfortunately, solvents have properties that tend to make biologic monitoring less useful or practical. First, they tend to be absorbed and excreted rapidly, so biologic levels change rapidly over time. Second, exposure over very short intervals is often a more important determinant of adverse health effects than 8-hour or longer exposures. However, biologic monitoring has been investigated for a number of solvents. The ACGIH has recommended biologic exposure indices (BEIs) for the following solvents: acetone, benzene, carbon disulfide, chlorobenzene, cyclohexanol, cyclohexanone, dichloromethane (methylene chloride), dimethylformamide, 2-ethoxyethanol and 2-ethoxyethanol acetate, ethyl benzene, *n*-hexane, methanol, 2-methoxyethanol and 2-methoxyethanol acetate, methyl *n*-butyl ketone, methyl ethyl ketone, methyl isobutyl ketone, perchloroethylene (tetrachloroethylene), phenol, styrene, tetrahydrofuran, toluene, trichloroethane (methyl chloroform), trichloroethylene, and xylenes. For many solvents, significant levels may be present only in exhaled air. A number of laboratories offer whole-blood or plasma analysis of solvents. For solvents with relatively slow excretion, such as perchloroethylene and methyl chloroform, analysis of blood is a reasonable alternative to analysis of exhaled air. However, for those with relatively fast excretion (most of the rest), the timing of the sample is critical—even within minutes—and the results therefore are difficult to interpret. Most solvents distribute into several compartments in the body so that the decline in blood levels exhibits several consecutive half-times, with the first being very short, on the order of 2–10 minutes. A blood sample taken immediately after an exposure will reflect primarily peak exposure at that time. A sample taken 15–30 minutes after termination of exposure will reflect exposure over the preceding few hours, whereas a sample taken 16–20 hours after exposure (prior to the next shift) will reflect mean exposure over the preceding day. The distribution of exposure over an 8-hour shift also will affect the validity of the biologic sample.

■ HEALTH EFFECTS OF SOLVENTS

SKIN DISORDERS

Up to 20% of cases of occupational dermatitis are caused by solvents (see Chapter 18). Almost all organic solvents are primary skin irritants as a result of defatting, or the dissolution of lipids from the skin. The potency of solvents for defatting the skin is related directly to lipid solubility and inversely to percutaneous absorptivity and volatility. In addition to concentration and duration of exposure, a critical factor in the development of solvent dermatitis is occlusion of the exposed area of skin, such as by clothes and leaking protective clothing. A few industrial solvents also can cause allergic contact dermatitis. A form of contact dermatitis, contact urticaria, reportedly is caused by several specific solvents. Scleroderma has been found to be significantly associated with exposure to organic solvents in a number of case-reference studies.

The most common work practice leading to solvent dermatitis is washing the hands with solvents. The occupations most commonly associated with solvent dermatitis are painting, printing, mechanics, and dry cleaning, although workers are at risk wherever solvents are used.

Clinical Findings

A. SYMPTOMS & SIGNS

Diagnosis is based on the typical appearance of the skin and a history of direct contact with solvents. The typical appearance ranges from an acute irritant dermatitis manifested by erythema and edema to a chronic dry, cracked eczema. Areas of skin affected by solvent dermatitis are more permeable to chemicals than unaffected skin and are susceptible to secondary bacterial infection.

B. LABORATORY FINDINGS

Patch testing is rarely indicated because few solvents (principally turpentine, *d*-limonene, and formaldehyde) cause allergic contact dermatitis. Patch testing with actual material used in the workplace may be necessary on occasion.

Differential Diagnosis

Consideration sometimes must be given to the possibility of other sources of irritant or allergic contact dermatitis. Use of waterless hand cleansers that contain alcohols and emollients that contain sensitizers may exacerbate or cause irritant or allergic dermatitis.

Treatment & Prevention

Treatment of dermatitis caused by solvents is the same as for contact dermatitis from other causes: topical corticosteroids, emollients, and skin care. Prevention depends on education of workers about proper handling of solvents, use of engineering controls to minimize direct contact with solvents, provisions for alternatives to washing with solvents, and the use of solvent-resistant barrier creams or protective clothing where appropriate.

Prognosis

The resolution of solvent dermatitis depends on elimination of direct solvent contact with involved areas of skin.

REFERENCE

Rowse DH, Emmett EA: Solvents and the skin. Clin Occup Environ Med 2004;4:657 [PMID: 15465473].

CENTRAL NERVOUS SYSTEM EFFECTS

1. Acute Central Nervous System Effects

Almost all volatile lipid-soluble organic chemicals cause general, nonspecific depression of the central nervous system, or general anesthesia. Beginning with ethyl ether, a number of industrial solvents were used historically as surgical anesthetics. There is good correlation between lipid solubility, as measured by the air–olive oil partition coefficient, and anesthetic potency. However, the mechanism of action of general anesthesia by any agent is unknown. Excitable tissue is depressed at all levels of the central nervous system, both brain and spinal cord. Lipid solubility—and therefore anesthetic potency—increases with length of carbon chain, substitution with halogen or alcohol, and the presence of unsaturated (double) carbon bonds.

Clinical Findings

A. SYMPTOMS & SIGNS

The symptoms of central nervous system depression from acute intoxication by organic solvents are the same as those from drinking alcoholic beverages. Indeed, there is currently no evidence that ethyl alcohol has any acute effects on the central nervous system other than general anesthesia. Symptoms range from headache, nausea and vomiting, dizziness, light-headedness, vertigo, disequilibrium, slurred speech, euphoria, fatigue, sleepiness, weakness, irritability, nervousness, depression, disorientation, and confusion to loss of consciousness and death from respiratory depression. A secondary hazard from these effects is increased risk of accidents. Excitatory manifestations of early intoxication are the result of depression of inhibitory functions and correspond to stage I anesthesia.

The acute effects are related to the concentration of the chemical in the nervous system, so resolution of symptoms correlates with the biologic half-life, which ranges from a few minutes to less than 24 hours for most industrial solvents. However, it must be kept in mind that many solvent exposures are to mixtures of solvents and that the effects of each solvent are at least additive and may be synergistic.

Tolerance to the acute effects can occur, particularly for those compounds with longer half-lives, and generally is not metabolic in nature (i.e., not a result of increased rates of metabolism and excretion). The development of tolerance may be accompanied by morning "hangovers" and even frank withdrawal symptoms on weekends and during vacations, alleviated by ingestion of alcohol. Additive and synergistic effects both have been described for interactions between organic solvents and drinking alcohol.

B. LABORATORY FINDINGS

Biologic monitoring may provide an accurate assessment of exposure to some solvents, but there is little information on the correlation of biologic levels with degrees of intoxication.

Differential Diagnosis

Acute solvent intoxication must be distinguished from that resulting from the use of alcohol or psychoactive drugs on the basis of exposure.

Treatment

The sole treatment for acute solvent intoxication is removal from exposure to solvents or any other anesthetic or central nervous system depressant until the signs and symptoms have resolved completely. The use of alcohol or other central nervous system depressant medication should be avoided. Analgesics for headache may be necessary, but nonnarcotic medication usually is adequate.

Prognosis

Most symptoms resolve in a time course parallel to the elimination of the solvent and any active metabolites, although headaches may persist for up to a week or more following acute exposure. Persistence of central nervous system dysfunction following severe overexposure with coma suggests hypoxic brain damage. The occurrence of persistent neurobehavioral dysfunction following acute overexposure has been reported anecdotally and in a few case series, particularly impairment of memory.

2. Chronic Central Nervous System Effects

Alcohol is now well recognized as causing neurobehavioral dysfunction in chronic alcoholics. It is reasonable to assume that sufficient chronic exposure to organic solvents also could cause chronic adverse neurobehavioral effects. A number of terms have been applied to these effects when associated with solvent exposure: *chronic toxic encephalopathy, presenile dementia, chronic solvent intoxication, painter's syndrome, psychoaffective disorder,* and *neurasthenic syndrome.*

A number of epidemiologic studies of workers chronically exposed to organic solvents have demonstrated an increased incidence of adverse neurobehavioral effects. These effects have been best demonstrated in groups of workers with relatively high exposures, such as boat builders and spray painters, and with specific types of exposure, such as to carbon disulfide. Such effects include subjective symptoms, changes in personality or mood, and impaired intellectual function, as assessed by batteries of neurobehavioral tests. Decrements in short-term memory and psychomotor function are consistent findings. Chapter 24 discusses the nature of these tests and uncertainty about the significance of the results. Dose-response data and correlation of chronic with acute effects are becoming more available. Correlation of symptoms with test results is often lacking, so interpretation of neurobehavioral test results in an individual must be done by experienced observers. Solvent-exposed workers are at increased risk of requiring disability pension for neuropsychiatric disorders in a number of industrialized countries.

Chronic brain damage from chronic alcoholism or drug abuse is not well understood, but similar mechanisms may be present with chronic solvent exposure. Cortical atrophy may represent the underlying pathologic change. Recent studies have found conflicting results regarding the association between Alzheimer disease and history of solvent exposure.

In addition to neuropsychological dysfunction, there are other potential chronic central neurotoxic effects of solvents that can be considered briefly here. Acute and perhaps chronic intoxication with solvents can result in vestibulooculomotor disturbances, presumably because of effects on the cerebellum. A syndrome called *acquired intolerance to organic solvents,* in which there is dizziness, nausea, and weakness after exposure to minimal solvent vapor concentrations with normal vestibular test results, has been reported.

Clinical Findings

Symptoms commonly reported are headache, mood disturbance (depression, anxiety), fatigue, memory loss (primarily short-term memory), and difficulty in concentrating. Clinical examination may reveal signs of impairment in recent memory, attention span, and motor or sensory function. The Swedish Q16 questionnaire (Table 29–2) may be useful in the evaluation of workers with long-term solvent exposure.

Diagnosis

Test results associated with solvent exposure in group studies include alteration of a variety of neurobehavioral tests; electroencephalography, pneumoencephalography, computed tomographic (CT) scan, magnetic resonance imaging (MRI), positron-emission tomography, and cerebral blood flow studies showing evidence of diffuse cerebral cortical atrophy; and electroencephalographic abnormalities, particularly diffuse low wave patterns. These tests should not be used in the evaluation of individual patients without incorporating information from other sources.

The following criteria have been used for the diagnosis of chronic neurobehavioral toxicity from solvents:

A. Verified quantitative and qualitative exposure to organic chemicals that are known to be neurotoxic.

B. Clinical picture of organic central nervous system damage:

   1. Typical subjective symptoms

Table 29–2. Swedish Q16 questionnaire for long-term solvent-exposed workers.

This questionnaire is used to help determine whether long-term overexposure to solvents has affected the central nervous system (brain)—answer "yes" or "no" to each question.[1]
  1. Do you have a short memory?
  2. Have your relatives told you that you have a short memory?
  3. Do you often have to make notes about what you must remember?
  4. Do you often have to go back and check things you have done (turned off the stove, locked the door, etc.)?
  5. Do you generally find it hard to get the meaning from reading newspapers and books?
  6. Do you have problems with concentrating?
  7. Do you often feel irritated without any particular reason?
  8. Do you often feel depressed without any particular reason?
  9. Are you abnormally tired?
  10. Are you less interested in sex than what you think is normal?
  11. Do you have heart palpitations even when you don't exert yourself?
  12. Do you sometimes have a feeling of pressure in your chest?
  13. Do you perspire without any particular reason?
  14. Do you have a headache at least once a week?
  15. Do you often have a painful tingling in some part of your body?

---

[1]If a solvent-exposed worker answers "yes" to six or more of these questions, referral to more in-depth evaluation may be indicated.

  2. Pathologic findings in some of the following:
    a. Clinical neurologic status
    b. Electroencephalography
    c. Psychological tests
  C. Other organic diseases reasonably well excluded
  D. Primary psychiatric diseases reasonably well excluded.

Differential Diagnosis

Primary psychiatric disease may be excluded by the presence of signs of organic brain dysfunction, but these signs are not always entirely objective or clear-cut. Drug or alcohol abuse may result in a clinical state identical to chronic solvent toxicity, distinguished only by history and other evidence of exposure. Diffuse organic brain disease—particularly Alzheimer disease or, less commonly, Creutzfeldt-Jakob disease—also must be considered.

Treatment

Removal from exposure is recommended in all suspected cases. Alcohol and other central nervous system depressants should be avoided.

Depression may respond to antidepressants or other measures. Other neuropsychological symptoms may respond to psychological counseling. Treatment of chronic solvent-induced headaches involves empirical trials of medications, psychological counseling, and biofeedback therapy. Cognitive retraining is useful in some individuals with persistent memory loss documented on neuropsychological testing.

Prognosis

A number of follow-up studies of workers diagnosed as having solvent-associated neurobehavioral changes have been conducted. In general, those having symptoms but no impairment of psychometric test performance improved after removal from or reduction of solvent exposure. Severe impairment of initial test performance often was associated with persistent and sometimes worsening follow-up test performance, even if exposure was eliminated. Persistent impairment often was associated with persistent disabilities and considerable adverse social consequences.

REFERENCES

Jin CF et al: Industrial solvents and psychological effects. Clin Occup Environ Med 2004;4:597 [PMID: 15465471].

Lee CR et al: Neurobehavioral changes of shipyard painters exposed to mixed organic solvents. Ind Health 2005;43:320 [PMID: 15895847].

Rutchik JS, Wittman RI: Neurologic issues with solvents. Clin Occup Environ Med 2004;4:621 [PMID: 15465472].

EFFECTS ON PERIPHERAL NERVOUS SYSTEM & CRANIAL NERVES

All organic solvents may be capable of causing or contributing to peripheral neuropathies (see also Chapter 24). However, only a few are specifically toxic to the peripheral nervous system, including carbon disulfide and the hexacarbons n-hexane and methyl n-butyl ketone. These three cause a symmetric, ascending, mixed sensorimotor neuropathy of the distal axonopathy type that can be replicated in animals. This may be referred to as a *central peripheral distal axonopathy* because the nerves in the spinal canal are also affected. Of the three substances, only n-hexane is currently in general use as an industrial solvent. Most industrial hexane is a mixture of isomers with 20–80% of n-hexane content. Methyl ethyl ketone, a common solvent, potentiates the neurotoxicity of the hexacarbons (n-hexane and methyl n-butyl ketone). 1-Bromopropane, recently used as a chlorofluorocarbon substitute in spray adhesives, in cleaning metal and electronic components, and as a solvent for fats, waxes, or resins, has been found to cause a variety of central and peripheral nervous system effects.

Trichloroethylene is associated with isolated trigeminal nerve anesthesia. Other organic solvents such as methyl chloroform (1,1,1-trichloroethane) are associated with peripheral neurotoxicity in case reports of occupational exposure, following exposure to mixtures of solvents, or in persons exposed to extremely high levels from deliberate "sniffing" of solvents.

There is increasing evidence that solvent exposure can result in sensorineural hearing loss, particularly in combination with noise. Some aromatic solvents (e.g., toluene, p-xylene, styrene, and ethylbenzene) show, in the rat, ototoxicity characterized by an irreversible hearing loss. The loss was measured by behavioral or electrophysiologic methods and was associated with damage to outer hair cells in the cochlea of the exposed animals.

Acquired color vision disturbances have been found in association with occupational exposure to several solvents, including toluene, styrene, carbon disulfide, n-hexane, and mixed solvents. Disturbances of olfactory function (hyposmia and parosmia) have been reported in cases of solvent-exposed individuals and anecdotally in a high percentage of long-term painters. Effects on olfaction could be a result of local destruction of olfactory nerve endings in the nasal mucosa or action at a central site.

Studies of general solvent exposure have paid little attention to the peripheral nervous system. The few that have been performed suggest that at exposures more likely to result in central nervous system effects, symptoms of peripheral neurotoxicity are uncommon, but neurophysiologic function may be altered. Analogous to the effects of chronic alcoholism, solvents may be only weakly toxic to the peripheral nervous system but capable of acting additively or synergistically with dietary deficiencies or other neurotoxic agents.

Clinical Findings

Typical symptoms of solvent-induced neuropathy are slowly ascending numbness, paresthesias, and weakness. Pain and muscle cramps are present occasionally. Physical findings include diminished sensation and strength in a symmetric pattern and, in most cases, depressed distal reflexes. Trigeminal neuropathy from trichloroethylene is restricted to loss of sensory function in the distribution of the trigeminal nerve. Complaints of hearing or vision impairment in individual workers attributed to solvent exposure have not been reported.

Diagnosis

The diagnosis of solvent-induced neuropathy is based on a history of illness and exposure, clinical examination, and neurophysiologic testing, as described in Chapter 24. Nerve conduction velocities may be normal or slightly depressed. Sensory conduction velocities and sensory action potential amplitude are the most sensitive. Electromyography may indicate denervation

(fibrillations and positive sharp waves). The use of evoked potentials (visual and somatosensory) shows promise. Symptoms and other clinical findings often are found with absent or slight neurophysiologic abnormalities. A sural nerve biopsy may be helpful and in the case of hexacarbons show accumulation of neurofilaments in the terminal axon.

Neurophysiologic testing may be helpful in screening large numbers of workers but has not been shown to be more sensitive in early detection of clinical neuropathy than are clinical examinations, although periodic monitoring of n-hexane–exposed workers with nerve conduction velocity testing has been recommended.

Hearing may be assessed using standard techniques but has not been shown to be related to individual exposure. Color vision testing using various techniques has been shown to be useful in evaluating groups of workers but not in clinical evaluation of individual workers. Odor threshold testing and other tests of olfactory function should be performed in individuals with complaints of disturbances in either smell or taste.

Differential Diagnosis

The primary differential diagnosis for peripheral neuropathy includes diabetes, alcoholism, drugs, familial neuropathies, and renal failure. Approximately 25–50% of cases of peripheral neuropathy remain without etiologic diagnoses after initial evaluation excludes these causes. A chemical-related cause should be considered in all such cases.

Treatment

Treatment consists of removal of exposure to all substances toxic to the peripheral nervous system, including alcoholic beverages. Physical therapy should be encouraged for patients with weakness; this increases muscular strength to counteract loss of neuromuscular function, improves psychological outlook, and may even improve the ability of nerves to regenerate effectively. Careful clinical monitoring of workers exposed to substances toxic to the peripheral nervous system is important for early detection and prevention of permanent disability.

Prognosis

Symptoms may worsen initially and then improve for up to 1 year or more. The rate of recovery is related to the rate of axonal regeneration, which is approximately 1 mm/d. An axon from the tip of the toe that has died back to the cell body in the spinal cord may take 1 year to recover. The degree of residual disability, if any, is usually proportionate to the degree of injury at the time of diagnosis and cessation of exposure. However, permanent disability should not be judged until at least 1 year after diagnosis.

REFERENCES

Gagnaire F, Langlais C: Relative ototoxicity of 21 aromatic solvents. Arch Toxicol 2005;79:346 [PMID: 15660228].

Kim J et al: Combined effects of noise and mixed solvents exposure on the hearing function among workers in the aviation industry. Indust Health 2005;43:567 [PMID: 16100934].

RESPIRATORY SYSTEM

All organic solvents irritate the respiratory tract to some degree. Irritation is a consequence of the defatting action of solvents, and so the same structure-activity relationships hold true for the respiratory tract as for the skin. Addition of functional groups to the hydrocarbon molecule also may increase the potency of the solvent as an irritant, as in the case of organic amine bases and organic acids, which are corrosives, and alcohols, ketones, and aldehydes, which denature proteins at high concentrations.

Respiratory tract irritation from solvents usually is confined to the upper airways, including the nose and sinuses. Solvents that are both highly soluble and potent irritants, such as formaldehyde, cannot reach the lower respiratory tract without intolerable irritation of the upper tract. However, it is possible for less potent irritants to reach the alveoli in sufficient concentrations following extremely high overexposures, such as in spills and in confined spaces, to cause acute pulmonary edema. Severe central nervous system depression is usually also a result of such exposure. Pulmonary edema without effects on the nervous system can result from exposure to phosgene gas produced by the extreme heating (as in welding) of chlorinated hydrocarbon solvents. Exacerbation of asthma or, less commonly, induction of reactive airways dysfunction syndrome after acute exposure can occur, as with any other airway irritant.

There are few studies of chronic pulmonary effects from exposure to organic solvents; in general, solvents are less damaging than tobacco smoke in this regard. Chronic bronchitis may occur as a result of long-term exposure to the more potent irritant compounds, such as the aldehydes.

Clinical Findings

A. SYMPTOMS & SIGNS

Irritation of the upper respiratory tract is marked by sore nose and throat, cough, and possibly chest pain. If the eyes are not protected by vapor goggles, irritation of the eyes possibly accompanied by tearing also may occur. A few solvents are specific lacrimators and induce pronounced tearing such that exposure may be sufficient to preclude inhalation and irritation of the respiratory tract. A productive cough indicates chemical bronchitis or the imposition of an infectious bronchitis. Manifestations of pulmonary edema include a productive cough, dyspnea, cyanosis, and rales.

B. LABORATORY FINDINGS

Upper airway irritation should not be associated with any laboratory abnormalities. Pulmonary edema is marked by infiltrates on chest radiograph, hypoxia and perhaps hypocapnia on arterial blood gas analysis, and impaired diffusion, as shown by pulmonary function tests.

Differential Diagnosis

Infectious bronchitis may be distinguished from chemical bronchitis by sputum analysis and possibly sputum culture, although chemical bronchitis may be followed by a superimposed infection. Solvent-induced pulmonary edema must be distinguished from infectious or aspiration pneumonitis.

Treatment

Management of the acute pulmonary effects of solvents is the same as for any acute pulmonary irritant: administration of oxygen, bronchodilators, and other respiratory support as indicated.

Prognosis

Upper respiratory tract irritation should resolve quickly without sequelae in the absence of infection. Once treated appropriately, patients with acute pulmonary edema from solvent overexposure should recover completely if protected from the effects of hypoxic tissue damage. Rarely, induction of reactive airways dysfunction syndrome occurs (see Chapter 20).

EFFECTS ON THE HEART

The principal effect of organic solvents on the heart is *cardiac sensitization*, a state of increased myocardial sensitivity to the arrhythmogenic effects of epinephrine (see also Chapter 21). It can be demonstrated in animals—typically unanesthetized beagle dogs—by administration of epinephrine, either in fixed or multiple doses, before and after administration of a solvent and observation of the frequency of epinephrine-induced ventricular arrhythmias. Cases of sudden, otherwise unexplained death during abuse of solvents such as toluene in glue and trichloroethane in spot remover, usually associated with physical activity (*sudden sniffing deaths*), and occasional reports of sudden death in otherwise healthy workers overexposed to industrial solvents are probably a result of cardiac sensitization.

From animal studies it appears that high—near-anesthetic or anesthetic—levels are required for this effect on an otherwise healthy heart and that all organic solvents may be capable of causing it, although potencies vary. Halogenated hydrocarbons, particularly 1,1,1-trichloroethane, trichloroethylene, and trichlorotrifluoroethane, were of higher potency in the dog, with thresholds to a particular dose of epinephrine at 0.5% (5000 ppm) of solvent vapors for 5 minutes, as compared with approximately 5% (50,000 ppm) for heptane, hexane, toluene, and xylene; 10% (100,000 ppm) for propane; and 20% (20,000 ppm) for ethyl ether. Thresholds for these effects in humans, particularly with any condition predisposing to arrhythmias, are unknown.

A few solvents appear to have specific cardiovascular effects. Carbon disulfide exposure is associated with increased risk of coronary artery disease in a number of epidemiologic studies. Methylene chloride can affect cardiac function acutely, possibly on a long-term basis, through its metabolism to carbon monoxide.

Clinical Findings

A. SYMPTOMS & SIGNS

Cardiac sensitization should be considered when a worker exposed to high concentrations of a solvent reports dizziness, palpitations, faintness, or loss of consciousness in conjunction with or in the absence of symptoms of central nervous system depression (see above). If the victim is examined promptly, an irregular pulse or low blood pressure may be detected.

B. LABORATORY FINDINGS

A resting electrocardiogram (ECG) may be normal or abnormal and is rarely diagnostic. For workers with symptoms suggestive of cardiac sensitization, ambulatory cardiac monitoring during exposure may be helpful.

Differential Diagnosis

In the presence of high levels of exposure, the distinction between central nervous system depression alone and depression plus cardiac sensitization is difficult—and may not be important if all symptoms resolve with correction of overexposure. The need for evaluation for primary cardiac disease must be made on a case-by-case basis. The presence of cardiac disease does not preclude the possibility of solvent-related arrhythmias, which may occur at levels of solvent exposure lower than those usually associated with cardiac sensitization.

Treatment

Given the high levels of exposure usually associated with cardiac sensitization, evaluation and appropriate correction of exposure are essential. If arrhythmias appear to be related to exposure and the exposure is not excessive or cannot be controlled adequately, removal from exposure is preferable to treatment with antiarrhythmic medication and continued exposure.

Prognosis

Cases solely caused by excessive exposure should resolve with correction of the workplace situation.

EFFECT ON THE LIVER

Although it is possible that any organic solvent may cause hepatocellular damage in sufficient doses for a sufficient duration, some solvents, particularly those substituted with halogen or nitro groups, are particularly hepatotoxic. Others, such as the aliphatic hydrocarbons (e.g., cycloparaffins, ethers, esters, aldehydes, and ketones), are only weakly, if at all, hepatotoxic. The aromatic hydrocarbons (i.e., benzene, toluene, and xylene) appear to be weakly hepatotoxic, with only a few reports of possible liver toxicity in exposed workers. A few solvents, such as acetone, with little direct hepatotoxicity themselves are reported to potentiate the effects of alcohol on the liver.

Acute hepatic injury was reported frequently in the past from acute overexposure to carbon tetrachloride. More recently, acute hepatic necrosis and death from liver failure were reported from exposure to 2-nitropropane used as a solvent in specialty paint products.

Dimethylformamide, present in glues and fabric coatings, is reported to cause toxic hepatitis occasionally with persistent elevations of liver enzyme levels. Subacute liver disease is reported rarely in modern times, whereas chronic liver disease, including cirrhosis, is reported occasionally in workers exposed to carbon tetrachloride.

Clinical Findings

A. SYMPTOMS & SIGNS

Liver injury may be symptomless or associated with right upper quadrant pain, nausea, and vomiting. Hepatic tenderness, jaundice, dark urine, and light stool may be present.

B. LABORATORY FINDINGS

Diagnosis of acute hepatic injury is based on the presence of abnormal liver function tests in a pattern consistent with hepatocellular dysfunction and a history consistent with exposure to a hepatotoxic solvent in the absence of exposure to any other known hepatotoxin. A pattern of liver enzyme abnormality different from alcohol hepatitis has been reported anecdotally for a few solvents. Serum bilirubin may be elevated. Evaluation of liver injury caused by occupational exposure to solvents has been hampered by the lack of sensitivity and specificity of liver function tests and their often high incidence of abnormalities in working populations. The use of serum bile acid measurements and antipyrine metabolism rates has been proposed as a sensitive screening method for solvent-related liver dysfunction. Occasionally, liver biopsy is necessary to distinguish solvent-induced hepatitis from chronic active hepatitis.

Routine monitoring of liver function tests is not recommended unless there is potential exposure to a hepatotoxic dose of a solvent. Monitoring a patient after abstinence from alcohol may be necessary to evaluate the possible role of drinking. Removal of exposure with monitoring of liver function tests may be helpful in making a diagnosis.

Differential Diagnosis

The major entity that must be differentiated is alcohol-induced liver injury; if excessive use of alcohol cannot be ruled out, a diagnosis of solvent-induced liver injury often cannot be made with confidence. Viral and other infectious forms of hepatitis also must be considered.

Treatment

Treatment consists of removal from exposure and correction of any workplace situation that can be identified as having caused or contributed to the condition.

EFFECT ON THE KIDNEYS

Although many organic solvents, particularly halogenated aliphatic hydrocarbons, show evidence of nephrotoxicity to animals in relatively high doses, there are few reports of renal effects in exposed workers perhaps partly because of the lack of sensitivity and specificity of renal function tests. Acute renal failure from acute tubular necrosis has been observed in workers with acute intoxication from halogenated hydrocarbons such as carbon tetrachloride.

Animal studies indicate that halogenated aliphatic hydrocarbons damage primarily the proximal renal tubular cells. Renal tubular dysfunction, particularly renal tubular acidosis of the distal type, has been reported in solvent abusers using mainly toluene but is not associated with occupational exposure. Acute renal failure from intrarenal deposition of oxalic acid can result from ingestion of ethylene glycol but has not been reported from other routes of exposure.

There are few studies of chronic renal effects in solvent-exposed workers. Cross-sectional studies have suggested that chronic exposure to a number of solvents or solvent mixtures may result in mild tubular dysfunction evidenced by enzymuria (increased excretion of murami-

dase, β-glucuronidase, and N-acetyl-β-glucosaminidase) and either normal urinalyses or proteinuria. Case-control studies have suggested an association between solvent exposure and primary glomerulonephritis, particularly rapidly progressive glomerulonephritis associated with anti–glomerular basement membrane antibodies (the renal component of Goodpasture syndrome).

Clinical Findings

A. SYMPTOMS & SIGNS

Solvent abusers with renal tubular acidosis present with weakness and fatigue probably as a result of electrolyte abnormalities. Signs of acute intoxication (central nervous system depression) are often present. If it occurs, chronic renal tubular dysfunction as a result of chronic solvent exposure is usually subclinical.

B. LABORATORY FINDINGS

Renal tubular dysfunction from solvents may be manifested by polyuria, glycosuria, proteinuria, acidosis, and electrolyte disorders. Hypokalemia, hypophosphatemia, hyperchloremia, and hypocarbonatemia have been seen as manifestations of renal tubular acidosis in toluene abusers. Acute renal failure from halogenated solvents is similar to that from any other cause. Routine monitoring of renal function generally is not recommended for workers exposed to solvents. However, the measurement of urinary excretion of low-molecular-weight enzymes such as N-acetyl-β-glucosaminidase, β-glucuronidase, and muramidase appears to offer promise as a monitor for evidence of early tubular dysfunction.

Differential Diagnosis

Renal tubular dysfunction, including acidosis, can be a primary disease that first manifests in early adulthood or may occur secondary to a variety of metabolic and hyperglobulinemic states and exposure to toxic agents, including antibiotics and heavy metals.

Treatment

If renal tubular dysfunction is found in a worker with a high level of exposure to a solvent, observation of renal tubular function during cessation and then reinstitution of exposure may be helpful in both establishing a diagnosis and determining the effectiveness of removal from exposure.

REFERENCES

Brautbar N: Industrial solvents and kidney disease: A review. Int J Occup Environ Health 2004;10:79 [PMID: 15070029].

Phillips SD, Waksman JC: Hepatorenal solvent toxicology. Clin Occup Environ Med 2004;4:731 [PMID: 15465474].

EFFECTS ON BLOOD

Hematologic effects from solvents are uncommon. Benzene causes a dose-related aplastic anemia after months to years of exposure that may be a precursor to leukemia. Chlorinated hydrocarbons are associated with a number of reported cases of aplastic anemia that may be idiosyncratic or simply a spurious association. Some glycol ethers can cause either a hemolytic anemia because of increased osmotic fragility or a hypoplastic anemia because of bone marrow depression.

Clinical Findings

A. SYMPTOMS & SIGNS

Workers with anemia from solvents generally have presented with weakness and fatigue. Aplastic anemia can present with bleeding from thrombocytopenia or infections owing to neutropenia.

B. LABORATORY FINDINGS

Aplastic anemia from benzene may be manifested by reductions in any or all of the three cell lines, which may occur suddenly without preceding changes. The bone marrow may be hyperplastic or hypoplastic and does not always correlate with abnormalities in the peripheral blood. Hemolytic anemia from glycol ethers or other hemolytic agents is indicated by low red blood cell concentration and reticulocytosis. Monitoring of blood counts is recommended only for exposure to benzene and perhaps for the hematotoxic glycol ethers, but the results may not be predictive of anemia even for these agents.

Differential Diagnosis

The usual causes of anemia, particularly hypoplastic anemia, must be considered.

Treatment

The treatment of solvent-induced anemia is removal from exposure, transfusion if needed, and correction of the workplace situation if appropriate. Workers with aplastic anemia from benzene should not be reexposed to benzene.

Prognosis

A significant percentage of workers with aplastic anemia from benzene subsequently will develop leukemia, which is frequently fatal. Other solvent-induced hematologic effects should resolve with cessation of exposure.

CANCER POTENTIAL

Benzene is the only commonly used solvent for which there is sufficient evidence of carcinogenicity in humans. It is associated with all types of acute and chronic leukemia. It is possible that other solvents also increase the risk of leukemia.

Investigation of many of the halogenated hydrocarbons has produced limited to sufficient evidence of carcinogenicity in animals, particularly hepatocellular carcinomas in mice. Most have not been studied adequately in humans. Recent evidence suggests that trichloroethylene exposure may be associated with elevated risk for non-Hodgkin lymphoma and renal cancer. Mixed solvent exposures have been associated with increases in lymphatic and hematopoietic malignancies in some studies.

Solvents may increase skin absorption of carcinogens. An animal study indicated that absorption of carcinogenic polycyclic aromatic hydrocarbons (applied as a component of used gasoline-engine oil) increased when contaminated skin was washed with kerosene.

REFERENCES

Bird MG et al: International symposium: Recent advances in benzene toxicity. Chem Biol Interact 2005;153:1 [PMID: 15935795].

Harth V et al: Renal carcinogenicity of trichloroethylene. Rev Environ Health 2005;20:103 [PMID: 16121833].

Wernke MJ, Schell JD: Solvents and malignancy. Clin Occup Environ Med 2004;4:513 [PMID: 15325319].

EFFECTS ON REPRODUCTIVE SYSTEM

Most organic solvents easily cross the lipid barrier of the placenta and, to a lesser degree, the testes. There is concern for their potential to cause reproductive toxicity. A meta-analysis of retrospective case-control studies shows a significant increase in major malformations and a trend toward more spontaneous abortions. One prospective study supported this association and also found that symptoms of solvent overexposure only occurred in case mothers. Eye and upper airway irritation was the only type of symptom experienced by subjects. Several maternal exposure studies have suggested decreased fertility (increased time to pregnancy). A prospective study of solvent-exposed women showed an association between occupational exposure during pregnancy and visual deficiencies in offspring, including both color vision and visual acuity. Evidence for paternal effects is much more limited than for maternal effects.

With the exception of the glycol ethers, toluene, and ethyl alcohol, available animal studies generally have not revealed evidence of significant teratogenicity. Ethyl alcohol causes both structural and behavioral teratogenic effects [i.e., fetal alcohol syndrome (FAS)] in both animals and women drinking more than three or four glasses of alcoholic beverages per day. Controversy exists over whether pregnant women should be advised not to drink alcoholic beverages at all during pregnancy. Because all organic solvents readily cross the placenta and reach the fetal nervous system and affect the nervous system in ways similar to alcohol, the possibility of a "fetal solvent syndrome" has been discussed. If a fetal solvent syndrome exists, important questions about dose-response relationships need to be addressed. For instance, would effects occur in offspring only at levels that produced acute intoxication in the mother, such as the FAS-like syndrome reported in offspring of women overtly intoxicated during dermal exposure (involving both 2-methoxyethanol and ethylene glycol)? Decisions regarding exposure of pregnant workers to solvents currently must be made in the absence of definitive toxicologic data (see Chapter 25). Many solvents show evidence of fetotoxicity in animals at or near maternally toxic levels. Exposure that produces acute reversible effects on the mature maternal nervous system may produce developmental effects on the fetal nervous system. Therefore, it is prudent to ensure that women who may be pregnant not be overexposed to any organic solvent. In addition, because of distribution to a possibly vulnerable fetal nervous system and the possibility of behavioral teratogenicity, exposure to organic solvents should be kept as low as possible throughout pregnancy.

One study of printers suggested that low occupational exposure to toluene was associated with subfecundity (increased time to pregnancy) in women but not in men. Solvent exposure of males may affect reproduction directly by affecting male reproductive capacity or indirectly via damaged sperm. This is best studied in male workers chronically exposed to glycol ethers (2-methoxyethanol or 2-ethoxyethanol) who had an increased prevalence of oligospermia and azoospermia and an increased likelihood of low sperm counts compared with unexposed workers (see Chapter 26). Recent studies have found that 1-bromopropane, which is used as a chlorofluorocarbon substitute in spray adhesives and in cleaning metal and electronic components; as a solvent for fats, waxes, or resins; and as an intermediate in the synthesis of pharmaceuticals, insecticides, quaternary ammonium compounds, flavors, or fragrances, causes adverse effects on reproduction and development in animals at levels well below occupational exposure. There is limited evidence of similar effects in exposed workers. 2-Bromopropane appears to have similar properties.

REFERENCES

Ichihara G: Neuro-reproductive toxicities of 1-bromopropane and 2-bromopropane. Int Arch Occup Environ Health 2005;78:79 [PMID: 15812677].

Ichihara G et al: Neurologic abnormalities in workers of a 1-bromopropane factory. Environ Health Perspect 2004;112:1319 [PMID: 15345346].

PREVENTION OF SOLVENT TOXICITY

SELECTION & SUBSTITUTION OF SOLVENT

Selection of an initial solvent—or substitution of a less hazardous for a more hazardous solvent—must take into account both the desirable and undesirable properties of the solvents. This involves comparing not only health hazard (i.e., toxicity, dermal absorptivity, and volatility) but also flammability, explosiveness, reactivity, compatibility, stability, odor properties, and environmental fates. For example, carbon tetrachloride, perchloroethylene, trichlorotrifluoroethane, and mineral spirits all are used to some extent at the present time as dry-cleaning agents, although to different degrees than in the past. Carbon tetrachloride is by far the most toxic and, for that reason, is used chiefly as a spot-removal agent. Perchloroethylene is less toxic than carbon tetrachloride and has replaced it for that reason. Perchloroethylene replaced mineral spirits because of the flammability of the latter; perchloroethylene and carbon tetrachloride are virtually nonflammable. Solvent substitution increasingly has been driven by the need to replace smog-forming and ozone-depleting chemicals.

However, perchloroethylene is now considered a probable human carcinogen. Trichlorotrifluoroethane is the least toxic, but it is expensive and may contribute to depletion of the ozone layer. It is used in closed systems to decrease cost and environmental pollution by recycling, but this requires an initial capital outlay for equipment. Obviously, the choice of solvent is complicated when advantages and disadvantages exist in different categories.

ENGINEERING CONTROLS

The volatility of organic solvents makes engineering ingenuity to control vapors of paramount importance in many situations. Process enclosure, such as the closed-system use of trichlorotrifluoroethane for dry cleaning, is common in chemical manufacturing but not in other circumstances. Spray painting and other spray operations create large quantities of aerosols and vapors, so engineering controls such as paint spray booths are particularly critical. Effective functioning of ventilation systems depends on proper design and regular mechanical maintenance, but these are commonly lacking. The substitution of water-based for solvent-based paints has been the most effective means of reducing solvent exposure from painting. Aqueous cleaning for metal parts shows promise for reducing solvent use in vehicle repair and parts manufacturing.

PERSONAL PROTECTION

Respiratory protection should be used only when engineering controls are not feasible, such as in construction, confined space, and emergency-response situations. The employer must conduct a comprehensive respiratory protection program. Frequently, there is improper fitting, selection, and maintenance of respirators for solvent work, resulting in poor or inconsistent protection. Knowledge of the odor threshold of a substance (see Table 29–1) is useful before using a respirator for levels above the TLV for that substance. If the average odor threshold is well below the TLV (e.g., at least 10-fold), the odor will serve as an adequate warning to signal breakthrough or other failure of the respirator to provide adequate protection. A decrease in the ability to detect odors (hyposmia) has been reported from chronic exposure to solvents, and a history of hyposmia should be sought as part of the initial medical evaluation for ability to use a respirator. Use of a respirator with an approved end-of-service life indicator may improve respirator effectiveness in these cases. Some solvents, such as methanol, methyl chloride, and formaldehyde, are not removed by standard organic vapor filters.

Protective clothing made of the proper material should be selected on the basis of studies that show the rate of penetration of materials by the solvent used. *Guidelines for the Selection of Chemical Protective Clothing*, published by the ACGIH, is a good source of this information. Inappropriate glove material may be porous to solvents while retaining an intact appearance, leading to occlusion and increased hand exposure. Plasticizers used in polyvinyl chloride gloves are vulnerable to solvents. Glove selection for mixed solvents is difficult; multilayer materials or costly specialty products may be required. Some workers, such as mechanics, may be unable to use gloves and adequately perform their work. Barrier creams are not recommended as substitutes for gloves. Protective (barrier) creams can correct or prevent loss of oils from the skin and may provide very limited protection against percutaneous absorption of solvents.

■ SPECIFIC SOLVENTS & THEIR EFFECTS

ALIPHATIC HYDROCARBONS

Essentials of Diagnosis

A. ACUTE EFFECTS

- Anesthesia: dizziness, headache, nausea, vomiting, sleepiness, fatigue, "drunkenness," slurred speech, disequilibrium, disorientation, depression, and loss of consciousness
- Respiratory tract irritation: cough and sore nose and throat

B. CHRONIC EFFECTS

- Dermatitis: dry, cracked, and erythematous skin
- Neurobehavioral dysfunction: headache, mood lability, fatigue, short-term memory loss, difficulty concentrating, decreased attention span, neurobehavioral test abnormalities, computed tomographic (CT) scan (cerebral atrophy), electroencephalography (EEG) (diffuse slow waves)
- Peripheral neuropathy (*n*-hexane): slowly ascending numbness, paresthesias, and weakness; normal or slightly depressed nerve conduction velocity and electromyography (denervation)

General Considerations

Aliphatic hydrocarbons consist of carbon and hydrogen molecules in straight or branched chains. They are further divided into alkanes, alkenes, and alkynes.

1. Alkanes (Paraffins)

Alkanes are aliphatic hydrocarbons with single-bonded (saturated) carbons:

with the empirical formula C_nH_{2n+2}

The physical state of an alkane depends on its number of carbons:

Carbons	State	Name
1–4	Gas	Methane, ethane, propane, butane
5–16	Liquid	Pentane, hexane, heptane, octane, nonane
>16	Solid	Paraffin wax

The gases are essentially odorless, whereas the vapors of the liquids have a slight "hydrocarbon" odor.

Use

A number of liquid alkanes are used in relatively pure form as solvents and also are the major constituents of a number of petroleum distillate solvents (see below). The liquid alkanes are important ingredients in gasoline, which accounts for most of the pentane and hexane used in the United States. Hexane (generally a mixture of isomers including *n*-hexane) is an inexpensive general-use solvent in solvent glues, quick-drying rubber cements, varnishes, inks, and extraction of oils from seeds. The alkane gases are used as fuels, whereas paraffin wax is used for candles and other wax products.

Occupational & Environmental Exposure

The National Institute for Occupational Safety and Health (NIOSH) estimates that approximately 10,000 U.S. workers are potentially exposed to pentane and heptane, 300,000 to octane, and 2.5 million to hexane annually. Many more individuals may be exposed to these and other alkanes in gasoline, naphthas, and other petroleum products. They are common contaminants of ambient air, with levels of methane reported to be 1.2–1.5 ppm in rural areas and 2–3 ppm in urban air, whereas other alkanes generally are detected at more than 10-fold lower concentrations.

Pharmacokinetics

The alkanes are well absorbed by inhalation and, to a lesser but still significant extent, through the skin. Approximately 75% of most inhaled alkanes are absorbed at rest, decreasing to 50% with moderate physical labor. Unbranched hydrocarbons such as *n*-hexane and *n*-heptane are metabolized by microsomal cytochrome P450 enzymes to alcohols, diols, ketones, and diketones, which are further metabolized to carbon monoxide or conjugated with glucuronic acid and excreted in urine.

Health Effects

The alkanes generally are of low toxicity. The first three gases (methane, ethane, and propane) are simple inert asphyxiants whose toxicity is related only to the amount of available oxygen remaining in the environment and to their flammability and explosiveness. The vapors of the lighter, more volatile liquids (pentane through nonane) are irritants and anesthetics, whereas the heavier liquids (known as liquid paraffins) are primarily defatting agents. Hexane and heptane are used most commonly as general-purpose solvents. They cause anesthesia, respiratory tract irritation, and dermatitis and are associated with neurobehavioral dysfunction, and the associated clinical findings, differential diagnosis, treatment, and prognosis are not different from those of other solvents (see above). A meta-analysis concluded that hydrocarbon exposure may worsen renal function in glomerulonephritis.

One isomer of hexane, *n*-hexane, causes peripheral neuropathy. A number of outbreaks of peripheral neuropathy have been described, particularly in cottage industries such as shoe and sandal making, where glues

have been used containing *n*-hexane as a solvent. More recently, *n*-hexane in brake-cleaning aerosol products was associated with neuropathy in auto mechanics.

The proximate neurotoxin is the metabolite 2,5-hexanedione. Other diketones with the same spacing between ketone (carbonyl) groups, such as 3,6-hexanedione, also can cause peripheral neuropathy. A metabolite of *n*-heptane, 2,5-heptanedione, causes peripheral neuropathy in laboratory animal studies, but *n*-heptane has not been implicated in human peripheral neuropathy in the absence of concomitant exposure to *n*-hexane. The clinical and neurophysiologic findings of *n*-hexane-induced peripheral neuropathy are typical of distal axonopathies (see above and Chapter 24). Nerve biopsies are notable for swollen axons that contain increased numbers of neurofilaments. Methyl ethyl ketone and possibly methyl isobutyl ketone potentiate the neurotoxicity of *n*-hexane.

Exposure to *n*-hexane can be assessed by measuring 2,5-hexanedione in the urine or *n*-hexane in end-exhaled air. A concentration of 2,5-hexanedione in urine of 5 mg/L measured at the end of a work shift corresponds to exposure to a time-weighted average (TWA) of 50 ppm.

REFERENCE

Spencer PS et al: Aromatic as well as aliphatic hydrocarbon solvent axonopathy. Int J Hyg Environ Health 2002;205:131 [PMID: 12018006].

2. Alkenes (Olefins) & Alkynes

Alkenes are aliphatic hydrocarbons with double (unsaturated) carbon bonds:

with the empirical formula C_nH_{2n}

Dienes are alkenes with two double bonds. Alkynes are aliphatic hydrocarbons with triple carbon bonds. The physical state of alkenes and alkynes is determined by the number of carbons, as for alkanes.

Use

The liquid alkenes are not used widely as solvents but are common chemical intermediates. The alkenes are more reactive than alkanes, a property that leads to their use as monomers in the production of polymers such as polyethylenes from ethylene, polypropylene from propylene, and synthetic rubber and resin copolymers from 1,3-butadiene.

Occupational & Environmental Exposure

Occupational exposure estimates are not available for most alkenes and alkynes. Occupational exposure to ethylene, propylene, and 1,3-butadiene occurs primarily through inhalation during monomer and polymer production. Approximately 10,000 workers have significant exposure to 1,3-butadiene. Propylene is a common air pollutant as a result of engine exhaust emissions and industrial activity, with urban atmospheric concentrations ranging from 2.6–23.3 ppb in the United States and Europe. Butadiene has been detected in urban atmospheres in the United States at concentrations ranging from 1–5 ppb, whereas other alkenes and alkynes have been detected at comparable concentrations.

Pharmacokinetics

There is little information on absorption or metabolism of alkenes and alkynes. Absorption of these compounds should be similar to their corresponding alkanes.

Health Effects

The alkenes are similar in toxicity to the alkanes. The unsaturated carbon bonds increase lipid solubility to some extent and therefore irritant and anesthetic potencies as compared with corresponding alkanes. *n*-Hexene does not cause peripheral neuropathy, unlike *n*-hexane.

The presence of double bonds makes the alkenes more reactive than alkanes and dienes more reactive than alkenes. This reactivity is used in the production of polymers but in some cases also may result in additional health hazards. 1,3-Butadiene is carcinogenic in animals, whereas propylene and ethylene are not.

1,3-Butadiene is a human and animal carcinogen; elevated rates of leukemia and lymphosarcoma are associated with occupational exposure. Because of the carcinogenicity of 1,3-butadiene, the Occupational Safety and Health Administration (OSHA) has instituted a comprehensive standard with a permissible exposure level (PEL) of 1 ppm (TWA), medical surveillance, and other provisions. Both in utero embryo toxicity and male-mediated reproductive toxicity have been shown in animals. Biologic monitoring can be accomplished by urinary sampling for the product of epoxybutene hydrolysis followed by glutathione conjugation.

REFERENCES

Graff JJ et al: Chemical exposures in the synthetic rubber industry and lymphohematopoietic cancer mortality. J Occup Environ Med 2005;47:916 [PMID: 16155477].

Tsai SP et al: A hematology surveillance study of petrochemical workers exposed to 1,3 butadiene. J Occup Environ Hyg 2005;2:508 [PMID: 16147472].

ALICYCLIC HYDROCARBONS (CYCLIC HYDROCARBONS, CYCLOPARAFFINS, NAPHTHENES)

Essentials of Diagnosis

A. Acute Effects

- Anesthesia: dizziness, headache, nausea, vomiting, sleepiness, fatigue, "drunkenness," slurred speech, disequilibrium, disorientation, depression, and loss of consciousness
- Respiratory tract irritation: sore nose and throat and cough

B. Chronic Effects

- Dermatitis: dry, cracked, and erythematous skin
- Neurobehavioral dysfunction: headache, mood lability, fatigue, short-term memory loss, difficulty concentrating, decreased attention span, neurobehavioral test abnormalities, CT scan (cerebral atrophy), EEG (diffuse slow waves)

General Considerations

Alicyclic hydrocarbons consist of alkanes or alkenes arranged into cyclic or ring structures:

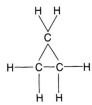

They have a slight "hydrocarbon" odor.

Use

Cyclohexane is the only alicyclic hydrocarbon that is used widely as an industrial solvent. Most of the U.S. production is used in the synthesis of nylon. Cyclopropane is used as a general anesthetic, but this is limited by its flammability and explosiveness.

Occupational & Environmental Exposure

The use of cyclohexane in nylon production results in only limited occupational exposure. The alicyclic hydrocarbons are not reported as common environmental contaminants.

Pharmacokinetics

Similar to their corresponding alkanes and alkenes, the alicyclic hydrocarbons are well absorbed by inhalation, whereas percutaneous absorption is less important. Approximately 70% of cyclohexane that is inhaled is absorbed and excreted unchanged in urine and exhaled air and as cyclohexanol in urine.

Health Effects

The alicyclic hydrocarbons are similar in toxicity to their alkane or alkene counterparts in causing irritation and central nervous system depression. They cause anesthesia, respiratory tract irritation, and dermatitis and are associated with neurobehavioral dysfunction. The associated clinical findings, differential diagnosis, treatment, and prognosis are not different from those of other solvents (see above). Cyclohexane does not cause peripheral neuropathy.

AROMATIC HYDROCARBONS

Essentials of Diagnosis

A. ACUTE EFFECTS

- Anesthesia: dizziness, headache, nausea, vomiting, sleepiness, fatigue, "drunkenness," slurred speech, disequilibrium, disorientation, depression, and loss of consciousness
- Respiratory tract irritation: cough and sore nose and throat

B. CHRONIC EFFECTS

- Dermatitis: dry, cracked, and erythematous skin
- Neurobehavioral dysfunction: headache, mood lability, fatigue, short-term memory loss, difficulty concentrating, decreased attention span, neurobehavioral test abnormalities, CT scan (cerebral atrophy), EEG (diffuse slow waves)

General Considerations

Aromatic hydrocarbons are compounds that contain one or more benzene rings:

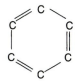

They are produced—directly or indirectly—chiefly from crude petroleum and to a lesser extent from coal tar. Aromatics used as solvents include benzene and the alkylbenzenes toluene (methyl benzene), xylenes (*o-*, *m-*, and *p-* isomers of dimethyl benzenes), ethyl benzene, cumene (isopropyl benzene), and styrene (vinyl benzene). They have a characteristic "aromatic" sweet odor.

Use

Although benzene currently has only limited use as a general industrial solvent, it is still used widely in manufacturing, for extraction in chemical analyses, and as a specialty solvent. Approximately half the benzene produced is used to synthesize ethyl benzene for the production of styrene. In the United States, gasoline contains approximately 2–3% benzene and 30–50% other aromatics. Aromatics constitute a significant percentage of a number of petroleum distillate solvents (see below). Toluene and xylenes are two of the most widely used industrial solvents—principally in paints, adhesives, and the formulation of pesticides—although about a third of the toluene used goes to produce benzene and only about one-sixth of the toluene produced is used as a solvent. The solvent uses of toluene and xylenes have been decreasing owing to environmental regulations because of their photochemical reactivity. Aqueous metal-cleaning methods are now available for cleaning metal parts as a substitute for xylene. Ethyl benzene is used chiefly as an intermediate in the manufacture of styrene and to a lesser extent as a solvent. Styrene is used chiefly as a monomer in the manufacture of plastics and rubber (see Chapters 28 and 31). Most of the cumene produced is used to manufacture phenol and acetone. Other aromatic compounds have a wide variety of uses but are not used commonly as solvents and so are not discussed here.

Occupational & Environmental Exposure

NIOSH estimates that 4.8 million workers are potentially exposed to toluene, the fourth largest number for an individual chemical. The NIOSH estimate for xylene exposure is 140,000 workers. Aromatic hydrocarbons are common environmental contaminants from engine exhaust and other industrial sources. Levels in urban air have been reported to be as high as 130 ppb toluene, 100 ppb xylenes, 60 ppm benzene, 20 ppb ethyl benzene, <1 ppb styrene, and 330 ppb total aromatics.

Pharmacokinetics

The pulmonary absorption values for aromatic hydrocarbons do not vary significantly as a group, ranging from approximately 50–70% at rest and decreasing to 40–60% with light to moderate work and to 30–50% with moderate to heavy work. Percutaneous absorption of aromatic hydrocarbons can be significant.

All the aromatic hydrocarbons are metabolized extensively, their metabolic profiles varying with the substituents on the benzene ring. Benzene is metabolized mainly to phenol and excreted in urine as conjugated phenol and dihydroxyphenols, with a slow elimination-phase half-time of about 28 hours. Approximately 10% of benzene is excreted unchanged in exhaled air. Toluene is metabolized primarily to benzoic acid and excreted in urine as the glycine conjugate hippuric acid with a half-time of about 1–2 hours. Approximately 15–20% of toluene is excreted unchanged in expired air. Xylene is metabolized almost entirely to the *o*-, *m*-, and *p*-methylbenzoic acids and excreted in urine as the glycine conjugates *o*-, *m*-, and *p*-methylhippuric acids with a slow elimination-phase half-time of about 30 hours. Approximately 64% of absorbed ethyl benzene is excreted in urine as mandelic acid and approximately 25% as phenylglyoxylic acid. The principal metabolites of the aromatic hydrocarbons are used for biologic monitoring, as indicated below.

Health Effects

The aromatic hydrocarbons generally are stronger irritants and anesthetics than the aliphatics. Substitution on benzene (toluene, xylene, ethyl benzene, and styrene) increases lipid solubility and these toxicities slightly. Aromatic hydrocarbons cause acute anesthetic effects, respiratory tract irritation, and dermatitis and are associated with neurobehavioral dysfunction. The associated clinical findings, differential diagnosis, treatment, and prognosis are not different from those of other solvents (see above).

Benzene is notable for its effects on the bone marrow: reversible pancytopenia, aplastic anemia that may itself be fatal or progress to leukemia, and all types of leukemia but predominantly acute nonlymphocytic leukemia. There is no evidence that the substituted benzenes have any of these myelotoxic effects. Earlier reports of effects of these substances on the bone marrow probably were due to their contamination with benzene.

There are a few anecdotal reports of liver function abnormalities in workers exposed to aromatic hydrocarbons. Renal tubular acidosis of the distal type, with serious but reversible electrolyte abnormalities, has been reported in solvent abusers exposed primarily to toluene. A syndrome of persistent cerebellar ataxia has been reported after exposure to toluene, chiefly in solvent abusers but also occasionally in workers. Toluene and xylenes have been reported to raise auditory thresholds in laboratory animals at relatively low levels of exposure.

Exposure to benzene, ethyl benzene, toluene, xylene, and styrene can be assessed by a variety of biologic monitoring techniques; Chapter 36 summarizes these techniques. Although extensive research has been conducted on the use of these techniques, given the short half-lives and acute effects of these compounds, the utility of biologic monitoring for the routine assessment of exposure is limited. Little information is available on the use of biologic levels in the diagnosis of acute intoxication from aromatic hydrocarbons.

REFERENCE

Bird MG et al: International symposium: Recent advances in benzene toxicity. Chem Biol Interact 2005;153:1 [PMID: 15935795].

PETROLEUM DISTILLATES (REFINED PETROLEUM SOLVENTS)

Essentials of Diagnosis

A. ACUTE EFFECTS

- Anesthesia: dizziness, headache, nausea, vomiting, sleepiness, fatigue, "drunkenness," slurred speech, disequilibrium, disorientation, depression, and loss of consciousness
- Respiratory tract irritation: cough and sore nose and throat

B. CHRONIC EFFECTS

- Dermatitis: dry, cracked, and erythematous skin
- Neurobehavioral dysfunction: headache, mood lability, fatigue, short-term memory loss, difficulty concentrating, decreased attention span, neurobehavioral test abnormalities, CT scan (cerebral atrophy), EEG (diffuse slow waves)

General Considerations

Petroleum distillate solvents are mixtures of petroleum derivatives distilled from crude petroleum at a particular range of boiling points. Each is a mixture of aliphatic (primarily alkane), alicyclic, and aromatic hydrocarbons, the relative concentration of each depending on the particular petroleum distillate fraction. They have a "hydrocarbon" or "aromatic" odor depending on the relative concentrations of aliphatic or aromatic hydrocarbons.

Table 29–3 lists the major petroleum distillate solvents, with the number of carbon atoms, typical percentages of components, and range of boiling points of each.

Use

Petroleum distillates are among the most common general-use solvents because they are available at low cost in large quantities. Petroleum ether (petroleum naphtha) represents an estimated 60% of the total industrial solvent usage. Approximately 1.4 billion gallons of petroleum solvents (see Table 29–3) were produced in the United States. Kerosene is used as a fuel, as well as a cleaning and thinning agent; about 2.3 billion gallons are produced in the United States each year.

Occupational & Environmental Exposure

NIOSH estimates that 600,000 workers are potentially exposed to the petroleum solvents (see Table 29–3) (naphtha solvents), 136,000 to the mineral spirits, and 310,000 to kerosene.

Table 29–3. Petroleum distillate solvents.

	Synonyms	Carbon Number	Class Components	Percentage (%)	Boiling Point (°C)
Petroleum ether	Petroleum, naphtha, ligroin, benzene	C_{5-6}	Alkanes (pentanes, hexanes)	100	30–60
Rubber solvent	Naphtha	C_{5-7}	Aliphatic Alicyclic Aromatic	60 35 5	45–125
Petroleum ether, high-boiling point	Light aliphatic solvent naphtha	C_{7-8}	...	...	80–130
V M & P naphtha[1]	...	C_{5-11}	Aliphatic Aromatic	> 80 < 20	95–100
Mineral spirits I	Stoddard solvent I, white spirits, petroleum distillate	C_{7-12}	Aliphatic Alicyclic Aromatic	30–50 30–40 10–20	150–200
Mineral spirits II	Stoddard solvent II, high-flash naphtha, 140-flash naphtha	C_{8-13}	Aliphatic Alicyclic Aromatic	40–60 30–40 5–15	175–200
Aromatic petroleum naphtha	Coal tar naphtha	C_{8-13}	Aliphatic Aromatic	< 10 > 90	95–315
Kerosene	Kerosine, stove oil	C_{10-16}	Aliphatic Alicyclic Aromatic	...	163–288

[1] Varnish makers' and painters' naphtha.

Pharmacokinetics

The pharmacokinetics of petroleum distillate solvents are those of the individual aliphatic, alicyclic, and aromatic constituents.

Health Effects

The hazard of a particular petroleum distillate fraction is related to concentrations of the various classes of hydrocarbons it contains (see Table 29–3). Petroleum distillate solvents cause anesthetic effects, respiratory tract irritation, and dermatitis and are associated with neurobehavioral dysfunction; the clinical findings, differential diagnosis, treatment, and prognosis are not different from those of other solvents (above).

Most of the aliphatic fractions are alkanes, including *n*-hexane. Therefore, the risk of peripheral neuropathy must be considered, particularly with exposure to petroleum ether, which may contain a significant percentage of *n*-hexane. The benzene content of petroleum distillates should be below 1%.

ALCOHOLS

Essentials of Diagnosis

A. ACUTE EFFECTS

- Respiratory tract irritation: cough and sore nose and throat
- Anesthesia: dizziness, headache, nausea, vomiting, sleepiness, fatigue, "drunkenness," slurred speech, disequilibrium, disorientation, depression, and loss of consciousness

B. CHRONIC EFFECTS

- Dermatitis: dry, cracked, and erythematous skin
- Optic neuropathy (methyl alcohol): blurred vision, blindness, hyperemic optic disk, and dilated pupil

General Considerations

Alcohols are hydrocarbons substituted with a single hydroxyl group:

$$—C — C — OH$$

They have a characteristic pungent odor. Examples of alcohols used as solvents are ethyl alcohol, methyl alcohol, and isopropyl alcohol (see Table 29–1).

Use

Alcohols are used widely as cleaning agents, thinners, and diluents; as vehicles for paints, pesticides, and pharmaceuticals; as extracting agents; and as chemical intermediates. Methyl alcohol is used widely as an industrial solvent—one-fourth of its production—and as an adulterant to denature ethanol to prevent its abuse when used as an industrial solvent. Approximately one-third of methyl alcohol used is in the production of formaldehyde. More than half the isopropyl alcohol produced is used to manufacture acetone and the rest in a variety of solvent and chemical formulation uses. Approximately 90% of cyclohexanol is used to produce adipic acid for nylon and the rest for esters for plasticizers. Alkyl alcohol is used solely as a chemical intermediate. The higher alcohols (>5 carbons) are divided into the plasticizer range (6–11 carbons) and the detergent range (≥12 carbons). About 500 kilotons of plasticizer-range alcohols are produced annually in the United States to make esters for plasticizers and lubricants, and about 260 kilotons of detergent-range alcohols are produced to make sulfate deionizers for detergents.

Occupational & Environmental Exposure

NIOSH estimates that approximately 175,000 workers are potentially exposed to methyl alcohol and 141,000 workers to isopropyl alcohol in the United States. Exposure to isopropyl alcohol in the home is common in the form of cleaners, cosmetics, and rubbing alcohol.

Pharmacokinetics

The pharmacokinetics of the simple (primary) alcohols are similar. Approximately 50% of inhaled alcohol is absorbed at rest, decreasing to 40% with light to moderate workloads. Some alcohols are sufficiently absorbed percutaneously to be given skin TLV designations.

The primary alcohols are metabolized by hepatic alcohol dehydrogenase to aldehydes and by aldehyde dehydrogenase to carboxylic acids. The metabolic acidosis and optic neuropathy caused by methyl alcohol have been attributed to its metabolism to formic acid. Metabolic interactions of ethanol with other organic solvents, such as *degreasers' flush* in workers exposed to trichloroethylene and other chlorinated hydrocarbons, frequently are due to competition for alcohol and aldehyde dehydrogenases, with subsequent accumulation of the alcohol and aldehyde and resulting reaction. Secondary alcohols are metabolized primarily to ketones.

Health Effects

The alcohols are more potent central nervous system depressants and irritants than the corresponding aliphatic hydrocarbons, but they are weaker skin and respiratory tract irritants than aldehydes or ketones. Respiratory tract and eye irritation usually occurs at lower concentrations than central nervous system depression and thus serves as a useful warning property. This may explain why occupational exposure to alcohols has not been implicated as causing chronic neurobehavioral effects. The TLVs for most alcohols are based on prevention of irritation.

Methyl alcohol is toxicologically distinct owing to its toxicity to the optic nerve, which can result in blindness. An extensive literature is available on this effect, which occurs primarily as a result of ingestion of methanol as an ethanol substitute or adulterant. A few poorly documented cases of blindness have been reported as a result of occupational inhalation exposure in confined spaces. The minimum oral dose causing blindness in an adult male has been estimated to be about 8–10 g; the minimum lethal dose is estimated to be 75–100 g. These amounts correspond to 8-hour exposure concentrations in air of approximately 1600–2000 and 15,000–20,000 ppm, respectively. Blurred vision and other visual disturbances have been reported occasionally as a result of exposures to levels slightly above the TLV of 200 ppm. Methanol in urine can be used for biologic monitoring, with 15 mg/L at the end of a work shift corresponding to an 8-hour exposure at 200 ppm.

Inhalation exposure to ethanol and propanols results in simple irritation and central nervous system depression, although propanols may be absorbed significantly through the skin. There are a few reports of auditory and vestibular nerve injury in workers exposed to *n*-butyl alcohol. Isooctyl alcohol is the most industrially important of the higher alcohols, but little toxicologic information about it is available.

GLYCOLS (DIOLS)

Essentials of Diagnosis

A. ACUTE EFFECTS

- Anesthesia (unusual because of low vapor pressure): dizziness, headache, nausea, vomiting, sleepiness, fatigue, "drunkenness," slurred speech, disequilibrium, disorientation, depression, and loss of consciousness

B. CHRONIC EFFECTS

- Dermatitis: dry, cracked, and erythematous skin

General Considerations

Glycols are hydrocarbons with two hydroxyl (alcohol) groups attached to separate carbon atoms in an aliphatic chain:

Examples include ethylene glycol, diethylene glycol, triethylene glycol, and propylene glycol (see Table 29–1). They have a slightly sweet odor.

Use

Glycols are used as antifreezing agents and as solvent carriers and vehicles in a variety of chemical formulations. Only ethylene glycol is in common general industrial use as a solvent, but large volumes of the others are used as vehicles and chemical intermediates. Approximately 40% of ethylene glycol is used as antifreeze, 35% to make polyesters, and 25% as solvent carriers. Glycols, for example, propylene glycol, are also used to generate artificial smoke or fog in entertainment and for emergency training.

Occupational & Environmental Exposure

NIOSH estimates that nearly 2 million workers potentially are exposed to ethylene glycol, 660,000 to diethylene glycol, and 226,000 to triethylene glycol, primarily as a result of their being directly handled, heated, or sprayed.

Pharmacokinetics

The glycols have such low vapor pressures that inhalation is only of moderate concern unless heated or aerosolized. Ethylene glycol does not have a skin TLV designation. Ethylene glycol and diethylene glycol are metabolized to glycol aldehyde, glycolic acid, glyoxylic acid, oxalic acid, formic acid, glycine, and carbon dioxide. Oxalic acid is the cause of the acute renal failure and metabolic acidosis that occur following ingestion of ethylene glycol. The first two steps in this metabolism use alcohol and aldehyde dehydrogenase and may be competitively blocked by administration of ethyl alcohol.

Health Effects

The low vapor pressures of the glycols result in little hazard in their customary industrial use. They are not significantly irritating to the skin or respiratory tract but can produce a chronic dermatitis from defatting of the skin. The systemic toxicity of ethylene glycol commonly seen after ingestion of commercial antifreeze compounds as an alcohol substitute—seizures, central nervous system depression, metabolic acidosis, and acute renal failure—have not been reported as a result of occupational exposure. When used to generate artificial smoke or fog, they may cause acute eye and upper airway irritation and decreased lung function from long-term exposure.

REFERENCE

Varughese S et al: Effects of theatrical smokes and fogs on respiratory health in the entertainment industry. Am J Indust Med 2005;47:411 [PMID: 15828073].

PHENOLS

Essentials of Diagnosis

A. Acute Effects

- Respiratory tract irritation: cough and sore nose and throat
- Tissue destruction (e.g., hepatic necrosis with abdominal pain, jaundice, abnormal liver function tests), kidney necrosis with acute renal failure, skin necrosis with blisters and burns
- Anesthesia: dizziness, headache, nausea, vomiting, sleepiness, fatigue, "drunkenness," slurred speech, disequilibrium, disorientation, depression, and loss of consciousness

B. Chronic Effects

- Dermatitis: dry, cracked, and erythematous skin

General Considerations

Phenols are aromatic alcohols:

Examples include phenol, cresol (methyl phenol), catechol (1,2,-benzenediol, 1,2-dihydroxybenzene), resorcinol (1,3-benzenediol, 1,3-dihydroxybenzene), and hydroquinone (1,4-benzenediol, 1,4-hydroxybenzene).

Use

The industrial use of phenols as solvents is limited by their acute toxicity. Phenol is used as a cleaning agent, paint stripper, and disinfectant, but its chief use is as a chemical intermediate for phenolic resins, bisphenol A for epoxy resins, and other chemicals and drugs. Cresol is used as a disinfectant and chemical intermediate. Catechol is used in photography, fur dyeing, and leather tanning and as a chemical intermediate. Resorcinol is used as a chemical intermediate for adhesives, dyes, and pharmaceuticals. Hydroquinone is used in photography, as a polymerization inhibitor, and as an antioxidant.

Occupational & Environmental Exposure

NIOSH estimates that more than 10,000 workers potentially are exposed to phenol.

Pharmacokinetics

Phenol is well absorbed both by inhalation of vapors and by dermal penetration of vapors and liquids. Phenol and cresols have skin TLV designations. Phenol is eliminated rapidly within 16 hours, almost entirely as conjugated phenol in urine.

Health Effects

Phenol and related compounds are potent irritants that can be corrosive at high concentrations. As a result of their ability to complex with, denature, and precipitate proteins, they can be cytotoxic to all cells at sufficient concentrations. Direct contact with concentrated phenol can result in burns, local tissue necrosis, systemic absorption, and tissue necrosis in the liver, kidneys, urinary tract, and heart. Central nervous system depression occurs, as it does with all volatile organic solvents. A concentration of total phenol in urine of 250 mg/g of creatinine at the end of a work shift corresponds to an 8-hour exposure to the TLV of 5 ppm.

KETONES

Essentials of Diagnosis

A. ACUTE EFFECTS

- Respiratory tract irritation: cough and sore nose and throat
- Anesthesia: dizziness, headache, nausea, vomiting, sleepiness, fatigue, "drunkenness," slurred speech, disequilibrium, disorientation, depression, and loss of consciousness

B. CHRONIC EFFECTS

- Dermatitis: dry, cracked, and erythematous skin

General Considerations

Ketones are hydrocarbons with a carbonyl group that is attached to two hydrocarbon groups (the carbonyl is nonterminal):

They are produced by the dehydroxylation or oxidation of alcohols. A great many ketones are in use; Table 29–1 lists some of the ketones that are used as industrial solvents. Acetone and methyl ethyl ketone (2-butanone) are in most common use. The ketones have a characteristic minty odor that some people find pleasant and others offensive.

Use

Ketones are used widely as solvents for surface coatings with natural and synthetic resins; in the formulation of inks, adhesives, and dyes; in chemical extraction and manufacture; and to a lesser extent, as cleaning agents. About one-fourth of the acetone produced is used in the manufacture of methacrylates and one-third as solvent. Almost all cyclohexanone is used to make caprolactam for nylon, but small amounts are used as solvents.

Occupational & Environmental Exposure

The wide use of ketones is reflected in the large numbers of potentially exposed workers estimated by NIOSH: acetone, 2,816,000; methyl ethyl ketone, 3,031,000; methyl isobutyl ketone, 1,853,000; cyclohexanone, 1,190,000; isophorone, 1,507,000; and diacetone alcohol, 1,350,000. The use of many ketones has decreased owing to their regulation as photochemical reactants. Consumer exposure to acetone is common in the form of nail polish remover and general-use solvent.

Pharmacokinetics

Ketones are well absorbed by inhalation of vapors and to a lesser extent after skin contact with liquid. Only cyclohexanone has a skin TLV designation. The pulmonary retention of acetone at rest has been estimated to be approximately 45%. Most ketones are eliminated rapidly unchanged in urine and exhaled air and by reduction to their respective alcohols, which are conjugated and excreted or further metabolized to a variety of compounds, including carbon monoxide. Acetone is excreted in the expired air of normal, healthy individuals at approximately 120 ng/L.

Health Effects

Ketones have good warning properties in that irritation or a strong odor usually occurs at levels below those that cause central nervous system depression. Headaches and nausea as a result of the odor have been mistaken for central nervous system depression. The TLVs for most ketones are set to prevent irritation. Methyl *n*-butyl ketone causes the same type of peripheral neuropathy as *n*-hexane. It is metabolized to the neurotoxic diketone 2,5-hexanedione to an even greater extent than *n*-hexane and therefore poses an even greater hazard. The neurotoxic potential of methyl *n*-butyl ketone was discovered following the occurrence of a large number of cases of peripheral neuropathy in a plastics manufacturing plant in Ohio in 1974. A large volume of research has been published since, from animal neurotoxicity and metabolism studies to cell culture and mechanistic studies. However, human exposure to this substance no longer occurs because the sole manufacturer ceased production a number of years ago. Other ketones used as solvents have not been shown to cause peripheral neuropathy, but methyl ethyl ketone potentiates the neurotoxicity of *n*-hexane and methyl *n*-butyl ketone probably through a metabolic interaction. Concentrations of methyl ethyl ketone and methyl isobutyl ketone of 2 mg/L at the end of a work shift correspond to 8-hour exposures to the TLVs of 200 and 50 ppm, respectively.

ESTERS

Essentials of Diagnosis

A. ACUTE EFFECTS

- Anesthesia: dizziness, headache, nausea, vomiting, sleepiness, fatigue, "drunkenness," slurred speech, disequilibrium, disorientation, depression, and loss of consciousness
- Respiratory tract irritation: cough and sore nose and throat

B. CHRONIC EFFECTS

- Dermatitis: dry, cracked, and erythematous skin

General Considerations

Esters are hydrocarbons that are derivatives of an organic acid and an alcohol:

$$\begin{array}{c} -C\!=\!O \\ \quad\backslash \\ \quad\; O\!-\!C- \end{array}$$

They are named after their parent alcohols and acids, respectively (e.g., methyl acetate for the ester of methyl alcohol and acetic acid). Table 29–1 lists examples of some of the many esters used as solvents. They have characteristic odors that range from sweet to pungent.

Use

Esters—particularly the lower esters—are used commonly as solvents for surface coatings. Vinyl acetate is used primarily in the production of polyvinyl acetate

and polyvinyl alcohol. Other lower esters are used to make polymeric acrylates and methacrylates. Higher esters are used as plasticizers.

Occupational & Environmental Exposure

NIOSH estimates that 70,000 workers potentially are exposed to vinyl acetate in polymer production in the United States. Large numbers of workers potentially are exposed to other esters used as industrial solvents, particularly in surface coatings.

Pharmacokinetics

Esters are metabolized very rapidly by plasma esterases to their parent organic acids and alcohols.

Health Effects

Many esters have extremely low odor thresholds, their distinctive sweet smells serving as good warning properties. Because of this property, *n*-amyl acetate (banana oil) is used as an odorant for qualitative fit testing of respirators. Esters are more potent anesthetics than corresponding alcohols, aldehydes, or ketones but are also strong irritants. Odor and irritation usually occur at levels below central nervous system depression. Their systemic toxicity is determined to a large extent by the toxicity of the corresponding alcohol. There is one report of optic nerve damage from exposure to methyl acetate as a result of metabolism to methanol and hence to formic acid (see "Alcohols" above). Similarly, methyl formate may cause optic neuropathy following metabolism directly to formic acid.

ETHERS

Essentials of Diagnosis

A. ACUTE EFFECTS

- Anesthesia: dizziness, headache, nausea, vomiting, sleepiness, fatigue, "drunkenness," slurred speech, disequilibrium, disorientation, depression, and loss of consciousness
- Respiratory tract irritation: cough and sore nose and throat

B. CHRONIC EFFECTS

- Dermatitis: dry, cracked, and erythematous skin

General Considerations

Ethers consist of two hydrocarbon groups joined by an oxygen linkage:

$$-C\!-\!O\!-\!C-$$

Examples include ethyl ether and dioxane (see Table 29–1). They have a characteristic sweet odor often described as "ethereal."

Use

Ethyl ether was used extensively in the past as an anesthetic but has been replaced by agents less flammable and explosive. It is too volatile for most solvent uses except analytic extraction. It is used as a solvent for waxes, fats, oils, and gums. Dioxane (1,4-diethylene dioxide) is used as a solvent for a wide range of organic products, including cellulose esters, rubber, and coatings; in the preparation of histologic slides; and as a stabilizer in chlorinated solvents. Methyl *tert*-butyl ether (MTBE) has been used widely as an oxygenated fuel additive to reduce carbon monoxide emissions.

Occupational & Environmental Exposure

Occupational exposure to ethyl ether is largely confined to analytic laboratories. NIOSH estimates that 2500 workers are exposed to dioxane in its use as a solvent, and many more may be exposed through its use as a stabilizer in chlorinated solvents. Inhalation exposure to MTBE is widespread because of its use in gasoline.

Pharmacokinetics

Ethyl ether is well absorbed by inhalation of vapors; its volatility limits percutaneous absorption. More than 90% of absorbed ethyl ether is excreted unchanged in exhaled air; the rest may be metabolized by enzymatic cleavage of the ether link to acetaldehyde and acetic acid. Dioxane is well absorbed by inhalation of vapors and through skin contact with liquid and has a skin TLV designation. It is metabolized almost entirely to β-hydroxyethoxyacetic acid and excreted in urine with a half-life of about 1 hour.

Health Effects

Ethyl ether is a potent anesthetic and a less-potent irritant. Higher ethers are relatively more potent irritants. Dioxane is also an anesthetic and irritant but also has caused acute kidney and liver necrosis in workers exposed to uncertain amounts. Animal cancer studies have indicated an increased incidence of tumors at about 10,000 ppm in the diet but not at about 100 ppm by inhalation. Studies in exposed workers have been inadequate. The issue of carcinogenic risk from exposure to dioxane is controversial. Exposure to gasoline containing MTBE is associated with headache, nausea, eye irritation, dizziness, vomiting, sedation, and nosebleeds. MTBE causes liver tumors in mice and other hematologic malignancies in rats. This has raised concern about possible synergistic effects with benzene, which is also present in gasoline.

REFERENCES

Ahmed FE: Toxicology and human health effects following exposure to oxygenated or reformulated gasoline. Toxicol Lett 2001;123:89 [PMID: 11641038].

Stickney JA et al: An updated evaluation of the carcinogenic potential of 1,4-dioxane. Regul Toxicol Pharmacol 2003;38:183 [PMID: 14550759].

GLYCOL ETHERS

Essentials of Diagnosis

A. ACUTE EFFECTS

- Anesthesia: dizziness, headache, nausea, vomiting, sleepiness, fatigue, "drunkenness," slurred speech, disequilibrium, disorientation, depression, and loss of consciousness

B. CHRONIC EFFECTS

- Dermatitis: dry, cracked, and erythematous skin
- Anemia: low erythrocyte count or pancytopenia and evidence of hemolysis or bone marrow suppression
- Encephalopathy: confusion and disorientation
- Reproductive toxicity: major malformations and fetal death with maternal exposure; low sperm count, testicular atrophy, and infertility with male exposure; there is evidence of human reproductive effects

General Considerations

The glycol ethers are alkyl ether derivatives of ethylene, diethylene, triethylene, and propylene glycol (an alkyl group linked to the glycol by substitution). The acetate derivatives of glycol ethers are included in and are considered toxicologically identical to their precursors. They are known by formal chemical names [e.g., ethylene glycol methyl ether (EGME)], common chemical names [2-methoxyethanol (2-ME)] as used here, and trade names (e.g., Methyl Cellosolve).

Use

The glycol ethers are widely used solvents because of their solubility or miscibility in water and most organic liquids. They are used as diluents in paints, lacquers, enamels, inks, and dyes; as cleaning agents in liquid soaps, dry-cleaning fluids, and glass cleaners; as surfactants, fixatives, desiccants, antifreeze compounds, and deicers; and in extraction and chemical synthesis. They are used extensively in the semiconductor industry. Because 2-methoxyethanol and 2-ethoxyethanol were found to be potent reproductive toxins in laboratory animals (and their TLVs were lowered on this basis), there has been a shift in use to 2-butoxyethanol and other longer-chained ethylene glycol ethers and to diethylene and propylene glycol ethers.

Occupational & Environmental Exposure

The most important exposures may occur as a result of skin contact with liquids, inhalation of vapors in enclosed spaces, and spraying or heating of the liquids to generate aerosols or vapors. Surprisingly, skin absorption of vapors also can be a significant route of exposure. Although glycol ethers have relatively low vapor pressures, some of their saturation vapor concentrations at room temperatures can greatly exceed TLVs. Exposures easily can exceed the doses of 2-methoxyethanol and 2-ethoxyethanol that cause reproductive toxicity in laboratory animals. Consumer and worker exposure to 2-butoxyethanol in glass cleaners is widespread; this glycol ether is apparently of lower toxicity.

Pharmacokinetics

The glycol ethers are well absorbed by all routes of exposure owing to their universal solubility. They have relatively low vapor pressures, so dermal exposure is often of primary importance. The acetate derivatives are hydrolyzed rapidly by plasma esterases to their corresponding monoalkyl ethers. The ethylene glycol monoalkyl ethers maintain their ether linkages and are metabolized by hepatic alcohol and aldehyde dehydrogenases to their respective aldehyde and acid metabolites. The acid metabolites 2-methoxyacetic acid and 2-ethoxyacetic acid are responsible for the reproductive toxicities of 2-methoxyethanol and 2-ethoxyethanol. These metabolites are excreted in urine unchanged or conjugated to glycine and can be used as biologic indicators of exposure; this is important because skin exposure easily can constitute the bulk of exposure.

Health Effects

Acute central nervous system depression has not been reported as an effect of occupational exposure. However, a number of cases of encephalopathy have been reported in workers exposed to 2-methoxyethanol over periods of weeks to months. Manifestations include personality changes, memory loss, difficulty in concentrating, lethargy, fatigue, loss of appetite, weight loss, tremor, gait disturbances, and slurred speech.

Bone marrow toxicity usually manifested as pancytopenia has been reported in workers and laboratory animals exposed to 2-methoxyethanol and 2-ethoxyethanol. The longer-chain ethylene glycol monoalkyl ethers cause hemolysis by increasing osmotic fragility in laboratory animals, an effect that has not been reported to date in humans.

Male reproductive toxicity has been demonstrated in experimental animals for 2-methoxyethanol, 2-ethoxyethanol, and their acetate derivatives. Acute or chronic exposure of mice, rats, and rabbits to low levels of these compounds by inhalation or dermal or oral routes resulted in reductions in sperm count, impaired sperm motility, increased numbers of abnormal forms, and infertility. These effects began about 4 weeks after the onset of exposure and—in the absence of testicular atrophy—were reversible following cessation of exposure.

The testicular toxicity of the glycol ethers decreases sharply with lengthening of the alkyl group such that beginning with and proceeding through n-propyl, isopropyl, and butyl, they are nearly or completely inactive. The acetic acid derivatives (alkoxy acids) appear to be the active testicular toxins. In limited testing, the dimethyl ethers of ethylene glycol and diethylene glycol—but not the monomethyl ether of diethylene glycol—show some evidence of causing testicular toxicity. Ethylene glycol hexyl ether, ethylene glycol phenyl ether, and the propylene glycol ethers do not appear to be toxic to either the male or female reproductive system.

The same glycol ethers that are testicular toxins have been shown to be teratogenic in the same and additional species of laboratory animals at comparable doses. The structure-activity relationships also appear to be similar; the alkoxy acid metabolites are apparently the proximate teratogens. Major defects of the skeleton, kidneys, and cardiovascular system have been observed, with some variation in their nature and severity with species, dose, and route of administration. The ethylene glycol monoalkyl ethers with longer alkyl chains and other glycol (propylene and dipropylene) ethers have not been shown to be teratogenic with the exception of the diethylene glycol ethers, which produced typical malformations.

Several studies of occupationally exposed men and women provide evidence that the effects in humans are the same as those in animals. A comprehensive study documented 44 cases of a birth-defect syndrome in children of mothers employed at a capacitor factory in Matamoros, Mexico. The case-control study component found that all case mothers, but none of the control mothers, had heavy or continuous hand immersion in both 2-methoxyethanol and ethylene glycol during their pregnancies. Frank maternal toxicity was reported in many workers. The syndrome resembled fetal alcohol syndrome but was distinct from it.

Maternal exposure to glycol ethers was associated with various major structural birth defects in a large European case-control study incorporating all occupations. Female workers exposed to ethylene glycol ethers (EGEs) in the semiconductor industry have been reported to have higher risks of spontaneous abortion, subfertility, and menstrual disturbances and prolonged waiting time to pregnancy.

Studies of male workers exposed to 2-methoxyethanol or 2-ethoxyethanol found evidence of spermatotoxicity.

Because reproductive effects have been produced consistently in all species tested and their metabolism and other health effects appear to be similar in humans and laboratory animals, those compounds with reproductive effects in animals should be assumed to be testicular toxins and teratogens in humans. Substitution of one glycol ether for another should be approached cautiously. Not all the compounds have been tested thoroughly, and not all propylene derivatives are safe (e.g., the beta isomer of propylene glycol methyl ether is a teratogen).

REFERENCES

Hsieh GY et al: Prolonged menstrual cycles in female workers exposed to ethylene glycol ethers in the semiconductor manufacturing industry. Occup Environ Med 2005;62:510 [PMID: 16046602].

LaDou J: Printed circuit board industry. Int J Hyg Environ Health 2006;209:211 [PMID: 16580876].

GLYCIDYL ETHERS

Essentials of Diagnosis

A. ACUTE EFFECTS

• Dermatitis (primary irritant): irritation, erythema, and first- and second-degree burns of skin

B. CHRONIC EFFECTS

• Dermatitis (allergic contact): itching, erythema, and vesicles

General Considerations

The glycidyl ethers consist of a 2,3-epoxypropyl group with an ether linkage to another hydrocarbon group:

They are synthesized from epichlorohydrin and an alcohol. Only the monoglycidyl ethers are in common use and discussed here.

Use

The epoxide or oxirane ring of glycidyl ethers makes these compounds very reactive, so their use is confined to processes that use this property, such as reactive diluents in epoxy resin systems. Epoxy resins have a wide range of applications in industry and consumer use.

Occupational & Environmental Exposure

The primary exposure of workers and consumers is in the application of uncured epoxy resins. The epoxide groups of the ethers react to form cross-linkages within epoxy resins so that glycidyl ethers no longer exist in a completely cured resin. However, workers may be exposed to the ethers in their manufacture and in the formulation and application of the resin system. NIOSH estimates that 118,000 workers in the United States potentially are exposed to glycidyl ethers and an additional 1 million to epoxy resins.

Pharmacokinetics

The glycidyl ethers have low vapor pressures, so inhalation at normal air temperatures usually is not a concern. However, the curing of epoxy resins often generates heat, which may vaporize some glycidyl ether. A number of uses such as epoxy paint require spraying and the generation of an aerosol. Although quantitative data are lacking, the glycidyl ethers should be well absorbed by all routes. They have a short biologic half-life owing to their reactivity. Three metabolic reactions have been proposed: reduction to diols by epoxide hydrase, conjugation with glutathione, and covalent bonding with proteins, RNA, and DNA.

Health Effects

Reported effects of glycidyl ethers from occupational exposure have been confined to dermatitis of both the primary irritant and allergic contact types. Dermatitis can be severe and may result in second-degree burns. Asthma in workers exposed to epoxy resins may be a result of exposure to glycidyl ethers.

Glycidyl ethers are positive in a number of short-term tests of genotoxicity, including mutagenicity, but none has been tested adequately for carcinogenicity. They are testicular toxins in laboratory animals, but few have been tested for teratogenicity.

ORGANIC ACIDS

Essentials of Diagnosis

A. ACUTE EFFECTS

• Respiratory tract irritation: sore nose and throat and cough

B. CHRONIC EFFECTS

• Dermatitis: dry, cracked, and erythematous skin

General Considerations

Organic acids are derivatives of carboxylic acid:

$$-C\!\!=\!\!O$$
$$\quad \searrow OH$$

Acetic acid (vinegar) is used in a variety of industrial settings, including photographic development. Other organic acids are used to a lesser extent. Most organic acids are such strong irritants that they can be considered as primary irritants and not anesthetics.

ALIPHATIC AMINES

Essentials of Diagnosis

A. ACUTE EFFECTS

- Eye irritation, corneal edema, and visual halos
- Respiratory tract irritation: sore nose and throat and cough
- Dermatitis (irritant): erythema and irritation of skin

B. CHRONIC EFFECTS

- Dermatitis (allergic contact): erythema, vesicles, and itching of skin
- Asthma (ethyleneamines): cough, wheezing, shortness of breath, dyspnea on exertion, and decreased FVC on pulmonary function testing with response to bronchodilators

General Considerations

Aliphatic amines are derivatives of ammonia in which one or more hydrogen atoms are replaced by an alkyl or alkanol group:

$$C-C-NH_2 \qquad\qquad -C-\overset{\displaystyle OH}{\underset{\displaystyle |}{C}}-NH_2$$

(primary amine)   (alkanolamine)

They can be classified as primary, secondary, and tertiary monoamines according to the number of substitutions on the nitrogen atom; as polyamines, if more than one amine group is present; and as alkanolamines, if a hydroxyl group is present on the alkyl group (an alcohol). They have a characteristic odor like that of fish and are strongly alkaline.

Use

There are a large number of aliphatic amines that have a number of uses. They are used to some extent as solvents but to a greater degree as chemical intermediates. They are also used as catalysts for polymerization reactions, preservatives (bactericides), corrosion inhibitors, drugs, and herbicides.

Occupational & Environmental Exposure

Given the diversity of their uses, accurate estimates of the number of workers exposed to aliphatic amines are not possible. They are not common environmental pollutants.

Pharmacokinetics

Little is known of the pharmacokinetics of the aliphatic amines in industrial use. They are well absorbed by inhalation, and some have skin designations as a result of their percutaneous absorption (see Table 29–1). Metabolism probably is primarily deamination to ammonia by monoamine oxidase and diamine oxidase.

Health Effects

The vapors of the volatile amines cause eye irritation and a characteristic corneal edema, with visual changes of halos around lights, that is reversible. Irritation will occur wherever contact with the vapors occurs, including the respiratory tract and skin. Direct contact with the liquid can produce serious eye or skin burns. Allergic contact dermatitis has been reported primarily from ethyleneamines, as has asthma.

CHLORINATED HYDROCARBONS

Essentials of Diagnosis

A. ACUTE EFFECTS

- Anesthesia: dizziness, headache, nausea, vomiting, sleepiness, fatigue, "drunkenness," slurred speech, disequilibrium, disorientation, depression, and loss of consciousness
- Respiratory tract irritation: cough and sore nose and throat

B. CHRONIC EFFECTS

- Dermatitis: dry, cracked, and erythematous skin
- Neurobehavioral dysfunction: headache, mood lability, fatigue, short-term memory loss, difficulty in concentrating, decreased attention span, neurobehavioral test abnormalities, CT scan (cerebral atrophy), EEG (diffuse slow waves)
- Hepatocellular injury: abdominal pain, nausea, jaundice, and abnormal liver function tests
- Renal tubular dysfunction: weakness, fatigue, polyuria, glycosuria, electrolyte abnormalities (acidosis, hypokalemia, hypophosphatemia, hypochloremia, and hypocarbonatemia), glycosuria, and proteinuria

General Considerations

The addition of chlorine to carbon and hydrogen

$$\begin{array}{c} \text{H} \\ | \\ -\text{C}-\text{Cl} \\ | \\ \text{H} \end{array}$$

increases the stability and decreases the flammability of the resulting compounds. They have characteristic slightly pungent odors. Six chlorinated aliphatic hydrocarbons are used commonly as solvents: trichloroethylene, perchloroethylene (tetrachloroethylene), 1,1,1-trichloroethane (methyl chloroform), methylene chloride (dichloromethane), carbon tetrachloride, and chloroform. Other chlorinated aliphatic hydrocarbons, such as ethylene dichloride and chlorinated aromatics such as chlorobenzenes, are used rarely as general industrial solvents and are not discussed here. Abbreviations such as TCE and TCA will not be used because they are not standardized and can lead to errors in identification.

Use

The chlorinated hydrocarbons are used extensively as cleaning, degreasing, and thinning agents and less so as chemical intermediates. Historically, trichloroethylene was the principal solvent used in vapor degreasers, but it has been largely replaced. Perchloroethylene has replaced mineral spirits and carbon tetrachloride as the primary dry-cleaning solvent in two-thirds of facilities because of the flammability of the former and the toxicity of the latter. In turn, efforts are in progress to replace solvent cleaning of fabrics with liquid carbon dioxide.

Methylene chloride is used as a paint stripper and extraction agent. Chloroform is used for extraction and spot cleaning. Carbon tetrachloride is used primarily as a chemical intermediate and in small quantities as a spot cleaning agent. 1,1,1-Trichloroethane is used as a general cleaning and thinning agent.

Occupational & Environmental Exposure

Current information on occupational exposure to chlorinated hydrocarbons is lacking. However, exposure to agents used in dry cleaning and metal degreasing, such as perchloroethylene and trichloroethylene, has been decreasing over the past 50 years. Chloroform is present in drinking water as one of the trihalogenated methanes produced as a result of chlorination. To avoid formation of trihalomethanes, some water suppliers now use chloramines instead of elemental chlorine for disinfection.

Pharmacokinetics

The chlorinated hydrocarbon solvents are all relatively volatile and moderately well absorbed by inhalation. Pulmonary uptake ranges from 60–80% at rest and decreases to 40–50% during activity. Percutaneous absorption of vapors is usually insignificant, but dermal absorption following prolonged or extensive contact of the skin with liquid can be significant.

Biologic monitoring of the chlorinated hydrocarbons is based on their pattern of metabolism and excretion, which varies with their structure. 1,1,1-Trichloroethane and perchloroethylene are excreted mainly unchanged in exhaled air and metabolized and excreted only slightly as trichloroethanol and trichloroacetic acid. Consequently, biologic monitoring is conducted chiefly with exhaled air and, to a lesser extent, with the parent compound in blood and metabolites in urine. Accumulation of both compounds occurs to some degree with daily exposure.

In contrast, less than 10% of trichloroethylene is excreted unchanged in exhaled air. The remainder is metabolized rapidly by alcohol and aldehyde dehydrogenases via chloral hydrate to trichloroethanol and trichloroacetic acid or to unidentified metabolites. Although the biologic half-life of the parent compound is very short, trichloroethanol is an active anesthetic and, with a half-life of 10–15 hours, accumulates to some extent over the course of a work week. Trichloroacetic acid, though inactive, has a much longer half-life of 50–100 hours and has been recommended for use in biologic monitoring. A value of 100 mg/L in urine voided at the end of the work week corresponds to exposure to a TWA of 50 ppm trichloroethylene. However, because of large individual variability, this value can be used only to assess groups of workers and not individuals.

Methylene chloride is both excreted unchanged in exhaled air and metabolized to carbon monoxide in a dose-dependent fashion. An 8-hour exposure to methylene chloride at its prior TLV of 100 ppm results in a carboxyhemoglobin level of approximately 3–5% in a nonsmoker, whereas with exposure at its current TLV, carboxyhemoglobin levels are indistinguishable from background (1–2%). Methylene chloride in blood and exhaled air also can be used as a biologic indicator of exposure.

Chloroform and carbon tetrachloride are each approximately 50% excreted unchanged in exhaled air and 50% metabolized. Both can be measured in blood and exhaled air, but little information is available on biologic monitoring for either.

Health Effects

As a class, the chlorinated hydrocarbons are more potent anesthetics, hepatotoxins, and nephrotoxins than other organic solvents. Most have been found to cause hepatocarcinomas in laboratory mice following oral administration. Evidence for carcinogenicity following inhalation was demonstrated for methylene chloride and perchloroethylene, whereas adequate inhalation bioassays of the remainder have not been completed. Because of their common industrial use, the issue of carcinogenic risk to humans from exposure to these compounds is one of the most controversial topics in regulatory toxicology. There are surprisingly few animal studies examining their potential for reproductive toxicity and almost none in male animals. Pertinent aspects of the toxicity of each compound are briefly discussed.

1. Trichloroethylene

The TLV of 50 ppm is based on prevention of central nervous system depression, which occurs at levels below those causing evidence of hepatic dysfunction. A National Toxicology Program (NTP) cancer bioassay in multiple rat strains conducted in an attempt to address the uncertainty over results in mice, unfortunately, inadequate owing to insufficient survival in dosed animals, so the carcinogenicity of trichloroethylene remains unresolved. Reproductive effects have been little studied. One study showed that trichloroethylene causes developmental effects and full-litter resorption in the presence of maternal toxicity (altered weight gain). It was associated with malformation suggestive of teratogenicity (microphthalmia).

2. Perchloroethylene

Perchloroethylene is approximately equipotent to trichloroethylene as an anesthetic and more potent as an irritant. Its TLV of 25 ppm is set to prevent both effects. Perchloroethylene is a probable human carcinogen (IARC group 2A), with the strongest epidemiologic evidence pointing toward esophageal and bladder cancers. Limited studies of the effects of perchloroethylene on reproduction in animals suggest that it may be spermatotoxic as well as fetotoxic. Semen quality was subtly affected in a group of dry-cleaning workers exposed to perchloroethylene, but clinical effects have not been reported. In several studies of female dry-cleaning workers, periconceptual exposure to perchloroethylene was associated with spontaneous abortion. Although these studies are weakened by the lack of quantitative exposure data, exposure to perchloroethylene during pregnancy should be minimized. One case has been reported of obstructive jaundice in a newborn that was nursed in a dry-cleaning shop where perchloroethylene was used and was found in the mother's breast milk. Dry-cleaning workers have shown subclinical decrements in color vision, visual reproduction, pattern memory, pattern recognition, immunologic parameters, and hepatic parenchymal indicators.

3. Trichloroethane

1,1,1-Trichloroethane is only weakly hepatotoxic, with minor injury reported following massive overexposure. It is the weakest anesthetic of this group; its TLV of 350 ppm is established to prevent this effect. Sudden deaths in situations indicative of acute overexposure have been attributed to cardiac arrhythmias as a result of cardiac sensitization. The compound is weakly positive for mutagenicity in *Salmonella*, but it has not been tested adequately for carcinogenicity or reproductive toxicity. Several case reports suggest the possibility of peripheral neuropathy associated with 1,1,1-trichloroethane.

4. Carbon Tetrachloride

Carbon tetrachloride is a potent anesthetic. Both acute and chronic effects on the liver and kidneys have been reported at levels not much higher than those causing central nervous system depression. The TLV of 5 ppm (skin) was established to prevent fatty infiltration of the liver demonstrated in animals. A case series showed that acute effects are potentiated by heavy alcohol ingestion. Deaths have occurred from both hepatic and renal necrosis, and liver cancer has been reported in workers following acute liver damage from acute overexposure. The TLV has a group A2 (suspected human carcinogen) designation. There is evidence that carbon tetrachloride is fetotoxic but not teratogenic, and it causes testicular and ovarian damage in animals at toxic doses—but there is no evidence about effects at nontoxic doses.

5. Chloroform

Chloroform is only slightly less potent than carbon tetrachloride as an anesthetic and liver toxin. Its TLV was lowered to 5 ppm by the ACGIH, and it is considered a suspected human carcinogen (group A2).

6. Methylene Chloride

Methylene chloride is similar to perchloroethylene and trichloroethylene in potency as an anesthetic and liver toxin. It is unique in that it is metabolized to carbon monoxide, with formation of carboxyhemoglobin. At methylene chloride exposure levels of 100 ppm and above, carboxyhemoglobin levels can exceed 10%, so the presence of anoxia in addition to anesthesia must be considered. The OSHA PEL was lowered from 500 to 25 ppm in 1997 as part of a new comprehensive standard that acknowledges methylene chloride as a potential occupational carcinogen. The standard includes an action limit of 12.5 ppm, exposure monitoring, medical surveillance, respiratory protection, and other requirements. Methylene chloride was not teratogenic to rats and mice exposed to 1225 ppm, although it was fetotoxic, causing delayed skeletal development typically seen with exposures that stress the maternal animal.

REFERENCES

Harth V et al: Renal carcinogenicity of trichloroethylene. Rev Environ Health 2005;20:103 [PMID: 16121833].

Hellweg S et al: Confronting workplace exposure to trichloroethylene and perchloroethylene in metal degreasing and dry cleaning. Environ Sci Technol 2005;39:7741 [PMID: 16245853].

CHLOROFLUOROCARBONS

Essentials of Diagnosis

A. ACUTE EFFECTS

- Respiratory tract irritation: cough and sore nose and throat
- Anesthesia: dizziness, headache, nausea, vomiting, sleepiness, fatigue, "drunkenness," slurred speech, disequilibrium, disorientation, depression, and loss of consciousness
- Cardiac sensitization: dizziness, palpitations, faintness, loss of consciousness, and arrhythmia on ambulatory cardiac monitoring

B. CHRONIC EFFECTS

- Dermatitis: dry, cracked, and erythematous skin

General Considerations

Chlorofluorocarbon (CFC) solvents are aliphatic hydrocarbons (methane or ethane) that contain one or more atoms each of chlorine and fluorine. Table 29–1 lists the commonly used CFC solvents.[1]

CFCs are often referred to as *Freons,* which is the trade name of CFCs manufactured by Dupont. A CFC may be formulated with another organic solvent, such as methanol or methylene chloride, in a proprietary solvent mixture.

Use

CFC production now has been largely phased out because of the depletion of stratospheric ozone. The completely

halogenated CFCs are those implicated in this effect; note that hydrochlorofluorocarbons are still permitted (see next category below). Reservoirs of CFCs persist in refrigeration and air-conditioning machinery; thus there is still occupational exposure potential. This machinery requires maintenance, and at the end of its service life, the CFC is removed and may be reused. CFCs eventually will be phased out of "essential" medical uses such as metered-dose inhalers, but many are still in use.

Occupational & Environmental Exposures

The widespread use of CFCs in industry and in consumer products in the past has resulted in exposure of large numbers of workers and consumers and in global contamination of the environment. Workers who service or dispose of refrigeration equipment, vehicle air conditioners, or building air-conditioning systems are still exposed. These workers are also exposed to numerous substitutes for CFCs, such as hydrochlorofluorocarbons (HCFCs).

Pharmacokinetics

Very little information is available on the pharmacokinetics of CFCs. Most probably are resistant to metabolism and are excreted rapidly unchanged in exhaled air. Correlations undoubtedly exist between exposure and concentrations in exhaled air, but information is too limited to recommend biologic monitoring.

Health Effects

The CFCs are of relatively low toxicity. All are anesthetics but require exposure to concentrations above 500–1000 ppm before this effect is manifested. Such levels most commonly are encountered in enclosed spaces (e.g., cleaning out a degreasing tank) or when the CFC is heated (e.g., using a heated-vapor degreaser) or sprayed (e.g., when used as a propellant). They are not associated with chronic neurobehavioral effects, nor are they strong irritants.

Prolonged or frequent skin contact can cause a typical solvent dermatitis. Cardiac sensitization was first demonstrated for CFCs after a number of cases of sudden death of persons abusing CFC-11 and CFC-12 beginning in the late 1960s. A National Cancer Institute bioassay of CFC-11 was negative for mice and inconclusive for rats, whereas CFC-22 may have caused a slight increase in salivary gland tumors in male rats. Two rarely used chlorofluorocarbons, CFC-31 and CFC-133a, were carcinogenic in a limited gavage assay in rats. CFC-22, CFC-31, CFC-142b, CFC-143, and CFC-143a are positive in one or more short-term genotoxicity tests. CFC-22, the only one of the genotoxic CFCs in common use, is a weak bacterial mutagen. A number of CFCs have been tested for teratogenicity,

---

[1]The numbering system for chlorofluorocarbons offers a convenient method of determining their chemical formulas. The "units" digit is the number of fluorine atoms (with CFC-113, this would be 3); the "tens" digit is the number of hydrogen atoms plus 1; and the "hundreds" digit is the number of carbon atoms minus 1. (Thus CFC-113 would contain 3 fluorine atoms, no hydrogen atoms, and 2 carbon atoms, thereby requiring 3 chlorine atoms to make trichlorotrifluoroethane.)

including CFC-11, CFC-12, CFC-21, CFC-22, CFC-31, CFC-114, CFC-123b, and CFC-142b, but because of either inadequate design or inadequate reporting, no conclusions about effects can be reached. Unpublished studies report that CFC-22 is teratogenic in rats but not rabbits, producing microphthalmia and anophthalmia at inhalation levels of 50,000 ppm.

HYDROCHLOROFLUOROCARBONS AND HYDROFLUOROCARBONS

HCFCs and hydrofluorocarbons (HFCs) share useful properties with CFCs but generally have much less environmental impact. Development of these alternatives has been rapid as CFCs are removed from use, so their toxicity is relatively untested. Most are sold as refrigerants, blowing agents for plastic foams, and fire-suppression agents. A few have been used as cleaning solvents (HCFC 141b, HCFC 225ca, and HCFC 225cb) or medical aerosol propellants (HCFC-134a and HFC 227ea).

The HCFCs and HFCs vary widely in toxicity, with some apparently quite benign, whereas others are toxic to the liver or heart. Some are suspect carcinogens or teratogens. It is advisable to monitor exposed workers to detect early signs of toxic effects.

HCFC-123 (2,2-dichloro-1,1,1-trifluorethane) has evidenced significant human liver toxicity. A group of 17 workers suffered liver damage in a 1997 outbreak. They were involved in containerizing this liquid. HCFC-123 is chemically similar to halothane and has the same toxic metabolite. HCFC-123 exposure also was implicated as the cause of liver disease in nine industrial workers who had repeated exposure because of a leaking air-conditioning system in 1996; the refrigerant also contained HCFC-124. HCFC-124 and HCFC-125 are also structurally similar to halothane.

ALDEHYDES

Essentials of Diagnosis

A. Acute Effects

- Respiratory tract irritation: cough and sore nose and throat

B. Chronic Effects

- Dermatitis: dry, cracked, and erythematous skin
- Asthma: cough, wheezing, shortness of breath, dyspnea on exertion, and decreased FVC on pulmonary function testing reversible with bronchodilators

General Considerations

The aldehydes are used primarily as preservatives, disinfectants, and chemical intermediates rather than as solvents. Glutaraldehyde is used commonly in hospitals as a disinfectant. The prototype aldehyde, formaldehyde, is discussed in Chapter 28. Most aldehydes are such strong irritants that at levels that would produce anesthetic effects, irritation would be intolerable. Asthma has been associated with exposure to formaldehyde and glutaraldehyde.

MISCELLANEOUS SOLVENTS

N-Methyl-2-Pyrrolidone

N-methyl-2-pyrrolidone (NMP) is a colorless liquid with a mild odor and low volatility. It is used increasingly as a substitute for methylene chloride and other solvents in microelectronics manufacture, degreasing, graffiti removal, furniture stripping, and industrial maintenance of painted surfaces. Headaches and eye irritation are reported. It is absorbed easily through skin and therefore is used in topical pharmaceuticals. Reproductive toxicity has become a concern based on animal test results and a stillbirth case report.

1-Bromopropane (n-Propyl Bromide) & 2-Bromopropane (Isopropyl Bromide)

These two isomers are attracting recent interest for use as substitutes for ozone-depleting solvents. 1-Bromopropane has been used in spray glue and as a degreaser in the United States. 1-Bromopropane is an experimental reprotoxicant in both males and females and shows dose-dependent neurotoxicity; there is limited evidence of these effects in exposed workers. The other isomer, 2-bromopropane, apparently caused ovarian failure, azoospermia, oligospermia, and anemia in a group of Korean workers. Experimental studies confirm specific reproductive effects in females and males. Hematopoietic effects and peripheral neuropathy also have been reported in animal studies. There is limited evidence of adverse effects in exposed workers similar to those seen in animals.

REFERENCE

Ichihara G: Neuro-reproductive toxicities of 1-bromopropane and 2-bromopropane. Int Arch Occup Environ Health 2005;78:79 [PMID: 15812677].

Turpentine and d-Limonene

Turpentine is a mixture of substances called *terpenes*, primarily pinene. Gum turpentine is extracted from pine pitch; wood turpentine, from wood chips. It has had greater home than industrial use as a solvent. It is irritating and anesthetic and is one of the few solvents that causes allergic contact dermatitis. The incidence of sensitization varies with the type of pine, being generally higher with European than American pines. Owing to the frequency of allergic dermatitis, the availability of turpentine is now extremely limited. One recent study suggested that occupational paternal exposure to turpentine was associated with neuroblastoma in offspring.

d-Limonene is a terpene used as a solvent for printing, art paints, and janitorial cleaning; it is usually derived from citrus peel oils. Air exposure transforms it into an oxide that causes allergic contact dermatitis. Containers should be kept tightly closed; skin protection is advised.

Dimethylformamide

Dimethylformamide is a useful solvent because of its solubility in both aqueous and lipid media. However, these properties also result in its being well absorbed by all routes of exposure. It is a potent hepatotoxin and has been associated with both hepatitis and pancreatitis following occupational exposure. This hazard precludes most general industrial solvent uses. Dimethylformamide exposure has been associated with alterations of sperm function and testicular cancer. Exposure can be monitored biologically by measuring monomethylformamide and related metabolites in urine. Alcohol intolerance, in the form of flushing of the face and upper body, develops in some exposed workers.

REFERENCES

Chang HY et al: Sperm function in workers exposed to *N,N*-dimethylformamide in the synthetic leather industry. Fertil Steril 2004;81:1589 [PMID: 15193482].

Kafferlein HU et al: The use of biomarkers of exposure of *N,N*-dimethylformamide in health risk assessment and occupational hygiene in the polyacrylic fibre industry. Occup Environ Med 2005;62:330 [PMID: 15837855].

Dimethyl Sulfoxide

Like dimethylformamide, dimethyl sulfoxide is soluble in a variety of media and is well absorbed by all routes of exposure. It appears to potentiate the absorption of other substances through the skin. Its use has not been associated with significant toxicity, but it has been subjected to little scientific study. It has a characteristic garlic-like or oyster-like odor that is present in the exhaled air of exposed persons. Its use as a dermally applied anti-inflammatory agent is not approved by the Federal Drug Administration, although it is used in that way in veterinary medicine.

Gases & Other Airborne Toxicants   30

Ware G. Kuschner, MD, & Paul D. Blanc, MD, MSPH

The airborne toxicants addressed in this chapter include gaseous and other substances dispersed in the air. These substances can exist in one or more of several physicochemical states, including gases, fumes, mists, aerosols, vapors, and smoke. Table 30–1 lists definitions of these terms. The physicochemical distinctions among categories of airborne toxicants may be of limited clinical relevance but can be important for industrial hygiene monitoring and in interpreting workplace exposure limits.

There are an estimated 85,000 chemicals commonly used in modern industrial and nonindustrial applications, many of which can be encountered as airborne toxicants. Web-based resources provide a wealth of information about specific airborne toxicants, most of which are encountered rarely by clinicians, and the overwhelming majority of which are not reviewed in this chapter (Table 30–2). The National Institute for Occupational Safety and Health (NIOSH) *Pocket Guide to Chemical Hazards* is a useful source of information on industrial hygiene recommendations and the most important health effects of 677 chemicals of occupational relevance, many of which are potentially respirable. This resource is available in a print version and on the Web at: www.cdc.gov/niosh/npg/npg.html. Additional information may be obtained by calling NIOSH at 1-800-35-NIOSH (outside the United States: 513-533-8328). The 800 number combines an automated voice-mail system with direct access to NIOSH technical information staff and the NIOSH Publications Office. The American Association of Poison Control Centers Web page provides contact information for regional poison control centers throughout the United States (see Table 30–2).

The airborne toxicants reviewed in this chapter include agents that cause local injury (respiratory tract and mucous membrane effects) and/or systemic injury through a variety of mechanisms. They are classified as asphyxiants, respiratory irritants, and systemic toxicants.

Victims of airborne toxicant exposure may be managed by a variety of health care providers. Victims of high-intensity exposures are more likely to be managed initially by first responders (e.g., paramedics and firefighters) or industry-based health care providers (e.g., employee health staff) and only subsequently by emergency department physicians and nurses. Patients presenting with symptoms attributable to low-intensity chronic exposure may be diagnosed and managed by consulting occupational physicians and other office-based community health care providers.

REFERENCES

Centers for Disease Control and Prevention (CDC): Public health consequences from hazardous substances acutely released during rail transit—South Carolina, 2005; selected states, 1999–2004. MMWR Morb Mortal Wkly Rep 2005;54:64 [PMID: 15674184].

Kaye WE et al: Surveillance of hazardous substance emergency events: Identifying areas for public health prevention. Int J Hyg Environ Health 2005;208:37 [PMID: 15881977].

Parrish JS: Toxic inhalational injury: Gas, vapor, and vesicant exposure. Respir Care Clin North Am 2004;10:43 [PMID: 15062226].

Ruckart PZ: Hazardous-chemical releases in the home. J Environ Health 2004;67:14 [PMID: 15628191].

Ruckart PZ et al: Risk factors for acute chemical releases with public health consequences: Hazardous Substances Emergency Events Surveillance in the U.S., 1996–2001. Environ Health 2004;3:10 [PMID: 15496226].

ROUTE OF EXPOSURE & TARGET ORGAN TOXICITY

The respiratory tract may be the route of exposure for a toxicant, the target organ of a toxicant, or both. All the toxicants discussed in this chapter enter the body principally, if not exclusively, through inhalation. In addition to being the primary route of exposure, the respiratory tract is also the target organ for many of these airborne toxicants. For example, irritant toxicants cause the abrupt onset of respiratory symptoms, including cough, wheeze, and breathlessness. In contrast, some nonirritant airborne toxicants exert their primary toxic effects on organs other than the lung. Carbon monoxide is a nonirritating chemical asphyxiant that exerts its most prominent toxic effects on the central nervous system and may be acutely lethal while causing no respira-

Table 30–1. Definition of terms.

Aerosol	A dispersion of solid or liquid particles in a gaseous medium, most commonly air.
Gas	A fluid at room temperature and pressure that occupies the space of enclosure; capable of being changed into the solid or liquid phase by both an increase in pressure and a decrease in temperature.
Vapor	The gaseous phase of a substance normally in the solid or liquid state; capable of being changed to liquid or solid either by increasing pressure or decreasing temperature.
Mist	An aerosol of liquid particles that may be visible and is generated by condensation from the gaseous to liquid state or by mechanical dispersion of a liquid.
Fume	An aerosol of solid particles generated by the condensation of vaporized materials, especially molten metals, often accompanied by oxidation.
Dust	Solid particles generated by disintegration of organic or inorganic materials such as rocks and minerals, wood and grain; capable of temporary suspension in a gaseous medium such as air.
Smoke	Aerosols of solids resulting from incomplete combustion.

tory symptoms. Finally, beyond the purview of this chapter are those toxicants that may cause lung toxicity but have a *non*respiratory route of exposure (e.g., paraquat, which may cause pulmonary fibrosis after gaining entry into the body by ingestion).

DOSE-RESPONSE & TIME COURSE OF EFFECT

The focus of occupational and environmental toxicology is frequently on low-intensity toxicant exposures that lead to chronic health effects (e.g., asbestos and lead exposure). In clinical practice, it is often challenging to establish a link between chronic toxicant exposure and a disease in an individual patient, especially in cases that are not "classic." This is not the typical scenario with the substances of concern in this chapter. High-intensity exposure to toxic gases and other airborne toxicants may result in clinical findings within seconds, minutes, or hours. These exposures are at an intensity that is at the far end of the dose-response curve, where most, if not all, exposed individuals will manifest some adverse effect. Under these exposure conditions, issues of susceptible subpopulations usually are not germane.

Some short-term, high-intensity exposures cause both acute adverse effects and long-term sequelae. Examples of long-term health effects resulting from single-exposure events include anoxic brain injury (e.g., owing to carbon monoxide), reactive airways dysfunc-

Table 30–2. Useful Web sites.

National Institute for Occupational Safety and Health (NIOSH)
www.cdc.gov/niosh/homepage.html
  NIOSH is the federal agency responsible for conducting research and making recommendations for the prevention of work-related disease and injury. The Institute is part of the Centers for Disease Control and Prevention (www.cdc.gov)

NIOSH Pocket Guide to Chemical Hazards
www.cdc.gov/niosh/npg/npg.html
  This very useful resource provides general industrial hygiene information on several hundred chemicals, most of which are inhalants, in a concise tabular form.

Agency for Toxic Substances and Disease Registry (ATSDR)
www.atsdr.cdc.gov
  The ATSDR is an agency of the U.S. Department of Health and Human Services (www.hhs.gov), charged with providing health information to prevent harmful exposures and disease related to toxic substances.

Agency for Toxic Substances and Disease Registry (ATSDR) About ToxFAQs
www.atsdr.cdc.govltoxfaq.html
  The ATSDR ToxFAQs is a very useful repository of summaries about important toxicants. Information for this series is excerpted from the ATSDR Toxicological Profiles and Public Health Statements. Each fact sheet serves as a quick and easy to understand guide. Answers are provided to frequently asked questions about hazardous exposures and the effects of exposure on human health.

Cornell University Department of Environmental Health and Safety Data Sheets
http://msds.ehs.cornell.edu
  A database containing 250,000 material safety data sheet files.

National Inhalant Prevention Coalition Web Site
www.inhalants.org
  This coalition, funded in part by the Robert Wood Johnson Foundation, is dedicated to promoting awareness and recognition of the problem of inhalant abuse ("recreational" inhalant use), especially among minors.

American Association of Poison Control Centers (AAPCC)
www.aapcc.org
  "Find your poison center" Web page: www.aapcc.org/findyour.htm
  The AAPCC is a nationwide organization of poison centers.

tion syndrome (RADS, e.g., owing to chlorine gas), and bronchiolitis obliterans with associated obstructive lung disease (e.g., owing to nitrogen dioxide).

Chronic health effects caused by repeated subclinical exposures to airborne toxicants are being recognized increasingly. Severe bronchiolitis obliterans was described recently in a cohort of microwave popcorn plant workers. The disease was attributed to long-term repeated exposures to airborne diacetyl, the predominant ketone flavorant in artificial butter. An earlier outbreak of severe lung disease marked by organizing pneumonia was reported among workers in Europe and North Africa exposed to a textile coating agent (Ardystil). Additionally, repeated *intentional* (i.e., recreational) exposure to volatile solvents, nitrites, and other inhalants can cause a spectrum of chronic health effects that includes liver disease, cognitive disorders, and bone marrow toxicities.

REFERENCES

Blanc PD: Exposure to vapors, gas, dust, or fumes: Assessment by a single survey item compared to a detailed exposure battery and a job exposure matrix. Am J Indust Med 2005;48:110 [PMID: 16032739].

Kanwal R et al: Evaluation of flavorings-related lung disease risk at six microwave popcorn plants. J Occup Environ Med 2006;48:149 [PMID: 16474263].

HISTORICAL CONSIDERATIONS

While the hazards of ingested poisons have been appreciated for thousands of years, it was not until the eighteenth century that scientists began to elucidate the elemental components of the atmosphere and a parallel perception evolved of "poisons that kill from a distance." Toxic gases were first recognized in three circumstances: naturally occurring events such as geothermal emissions, the combustion and decomposition of organic matter, and in mining operations. The toxic gases recognized earliest were asphyxiants. They were commonly given names that reflected their source. Only later were their chemical structures determined. For example, sewer gas is a generic descriptor of hydrogen sulfide. Marsh gas is methane. Methane also was known as "fire damp" in collieries, whereas "choke damp" referred to accumulated carbon dioxide in coal mines and "after damp" to carbon monoxide following a mine explosion or fire.

Nineteenth-century synthetic chemistry introduced a number of newly produced gases into commerce, especially as industrial intermediates. These included chlorine and anhydrous ammonia. In general, limitations in storage and transportation of these predominantly irritant gases dictated that synthesis on the one hand and end use on the other were carried out in close proximity to one another. Industrial point-source releases of these gases were a well-recognized hazard of the nineteenth century and led to some of the first zoning restrictions on the locations of workshops and factories.

The introduction of poison gas as a weapon of mass destruction in World War I fundamentally changed both scientific and public understanding of the importance of inhalational toxicology. This was followed by air pollution crises in both Europe and North America that illuminated the link between the workplace and the environment beyond the factory door. The disastrous release of the lethal irritant gas methyl isocyanate in Bhopal, India, in 1984, and the use of toxic gases against civilians by the government of Iraq during the Iran-Iraq war have shown the potential widespread importance of airborne toxicants for public health and safety.

Intentional respiratory exposure to inhalants such as glues, paint thinners, and other volatile compounds is an inexpensive and prevalent form of substance abuse. Recreational inhalants are especially prevalent among children and adolescents. Inhalant abuse among minors is receiving increased attention as a significant public health problem in the United States and other industrialized nations.

Finally, exposure to combustion by-products used for home cooking and heating remains a major public issue worldwide. Exposures range from high concentrations of particulates with biomass fuel consumption to predominantly gaseous by-products from combustion of fossil fuels.

REFERENCES

Broughton E: The Bhopal disaster and its aftermath. Environ Health 2005;4:6 [PMID: 15882472].

National Institute on Drug Abuse Research Report Series: Inhalant Abuse, www.nida.nih.gov/ResearchReports/Inhalants/ Inhalants.html.

SIMPLE ASPHYXIANTS: METHANE, CARBON DIOXIDE, NITROGEN, NITROUS OXIDE, ETHANE, PROPANE, ACETYLENE, NOBLE GASES

Essentials of Diagnosis

A. ACUTE EFFECTS

- Headache
- Nausea
- Confusion
- Loss of consciousness
- Coma
- Anoxic brain injury
- Cardiac arrest

B. CHRONIC EFFECTS

- Residual anoxic injury

Exposure Limits

Atmospheric oxygen should be greater than 19.5% at sea level [normal barometric pressure (partial pressure O_2 = 135 mmHg)].

Table 30–3. Common asphyxiant gases.

Simple asphyxiant	
Acetylene	Methane
Argon	Neon
Carbon dioxide	Nitrogen
Ethane	Nitrous oxide
Ethylene	Propane
Helium	Propylene
Hydrogen	

Chemical asphyxiants
Carbon monoxide
Hydrogen cyanide
Hydrogen sulfide

General Considerations

Physical asphyxiant gases displace oxygen and are toxicants insofar as they reduce the fractional inspiratory concentration of oxygen (Table 30–3). These otherwise "inert" gases contrast with toxic asphyxiants (see below) that exert toxicity by interfering with the delivery of oxygen to tissues or by disrupting the utilization of delivered oxygen at the cellular level.

Occupational & Environmental Exposure

Simple asphyxiants are health hazards most commonly in confined spaces (e.g., inside storage tanks or mines). Asphyxiant gases that are heavier than air also may be hazardous in low-lying semienclosed areas with little air movement allowing dispersion. Morbidity and death may occur if the exposure is overwhelming and rapid, insidious and occult, or if the victim is unable to flee the space. Although any inert gas could act as a simple asphyxiant, only a short list of substances is of practical importance.

Methane gas is encountered in coal mining, where, because it is lighter than air, it may accumulate in poorly ventilated upper pockets. Of historical interest, canaries once were used in mines to provide early warning of the presence of significant concentrations of methane and other simple asphyxiants. The high metabolic rate of canaries makes them especially vulnerable to low ambient oxygen concentration and, therefore, useful as biologic sentinels. A bird's death would provide warning of hazardous conditions.

Carbon dioxide is a clear and odorless gas used in food preservation. It also may be encountered in beer and wine fermentation; in settings where it is used as a refrigerant, including frozen carbon dioxide (dry ice),

especially if a large amount is allowed to sublimate within an enclosed space; and in mines, including off-gassing from abandoned mine sites. Natural release of carbon dioxide from a volcanic lake at Lake Nyos, Cameroon, Africa, in 1989, resulted in numerous deaths in surrounding population centers. This natural environmental calamity was an exception to the general rule that simple asphyxiants are only hazardous in small, confined spaces.

Nitrogen may be encountered in hazardous concentrations in a variety of work settings, including underwater work, mining, metallurgic operations, and pressurization of oil wells. In hyperbaric settings such as tunnels or in deep-sea diving occupations, nitrogen may cause narcosis, leading to behavioral changes and impaired judgment.

Propane, argon, and other agents may be associated with exposure in high concentrations while filling tanks or when there is a leak from a tank or fuel-delivery system. Whether the substance is heavier or lighter than air may drive exposure risk in the microenvironment.

Metabolism & Mechanism of Action

By definition, the simple asphyxiants act nonspecifically by displacing oxygen from inspired air. The reduction in the fractional inspired concentration of oxygen results in hypoxia and ultimately frank anoxia. The central nervous system and cardiovascular system are the organ systems most severely affected by hypoxia.

Although carbon dioxide is considered a simple asphyxiant, at high concentrations it also acts as a potent central nervous system depressant, which may account for some of its effects as well. Tachypnea and dyspnea may be noted with carbon dioxide concentrations greater than 2–3%. Exposure to carbon dioxide in concentrations greater than 10% may be lethal within minutes.

Clinical Findings

A. Symptoms & Signs

Responses to decreased concentrations of inspired oxygen are variable. Important predictors of clinical response include the concentration of the simple asphyxiant (i.e., the magnitude of the reduction in fractional inspired concentration of oxygen), the level of physical activity (i.e., metabolic activity) and the underlying health status of the exposed individual. Normal ambient air oxygen concentration is 21%. Moderate oxygen deprivation (oxygen concentrations of 10–16%) may cause tachycardia, tachypnea, and exercise intolerance. As the concentration of oxygen decreases to 6–10%, the victim may experience nausea, prostration, and coma. At oxygen concentrations of less than 6%, rapid loss of consciousness and death are typical.

B. LABORATORY FINDINGS

There are no specific findings other than the reduction of blood oxygen and associated metabolic derangements (e.g., lactic acidosis).

Differential Diagnosis

A brief occupational history may quickly identify a simple asphyxiant as the likely cause of anoxic injury, especially in the context of a confined-space injury. On clinical grounds alone it may be difficult to differentiate between physical and toxic asphyxia. Specific laboratory findings may suggest exposure to a chemical (toxic) asphyxiant. Other causes of collapse, such as primary cardiac and central nervous system events, may need to be excluded depending on the clinical context.

Prevention

Confined-space work should have engineering controls to ensure an adequate air supply. It is important to confirm that the air supply intake does not itself entrain other toxins (e.g., carbon monoxide from a compressor). Confined-space injury often occurs in the setting of inadequate safety training and lack of appropriate supervision.

Treatment

Immediate removal from the exposure can be lifesaving; however, rescuers themselves often are in equal danger without adequate air supply. Postexposure treatment is supportive and nonspecific but should include the administration of supplemental oxygen.

Prognosis

Although anoxic brain injury can occur, many survivors of simple asphyxiant gas inhalation make a complete and rapid recovery.

REFERENCES

Halpern P: Exposure to extremely high concentrations of carbon dioxide: A clinical description of a mass casualty incident. Ann Emerg Med 2004;43:196 [PMID: 14747808].

Hsieh CC et al: Carbon dioxide asphyxiation caused by dry ice. Am J Emerg Med 2005;23:567 [PMID: 16032635].

NIOSH: Worker deaths in confined spaces—A summary of NIOSH surveillance and investigative findings, www.cdc.gov/niosh/94-103.html.

■ TOXIC ASPHYXIANTS

CARBON MONOXIDE

Essentials of Diagnosis

A. ACUTE & SUBACUTE EFFECTS

- Headache
- Nausea
- Confusion
- Cardiac ischemia
- Coma
- Anoxic brain injury

B. CHRONIC EFFECTS

- Residual anoxic injury

Exposure Limits

Occupational Safety and Health Administration (OSHA) permissible exposure level (PEL): time-weighted average (TWA) 50 ppm (55 mg/m^3)

NIOSH recommended exposure limit (REL): TWA 35 ppm (40 mg/m^3), ceiling (C) 200 ppm (229 mg/m^3)

General Considerations

Carbon monoxide intoxication is the leading cause of death by gas inhalation. Most fatalities are a result of environmental rather than occupational exposures. In addition to unintentional exposures, carbon monoxide inhalation remains a common method of intentional self-poisoning.

Occupational & Environmental Exposure

Carbon monoxide is a product of the incomplete combustion of carbon-based fuels. The internal combustion engine is an important occupational and environmental source of carbon monoxide. Nonelectric fork lifts and other vehicles and gas-powered compressors and generators, especially when used indoors, represent important exposure sources. Carbon monoxide exposures also may be relevant among firefighters, petroleum refinery workers, traffic garage workers, and furnace operators. Home heating unit malfunction or misuse, structural fires, automobile exhaust, gas-powered recreation equipment, and cigarette smoke are the most common sources of significant nonoccupational environmental carbon monoxide exposure. Exposure also can occur after exposure to methylene chloride (see Chapter 29) because metabolism of this solvent releases carbon monoxide.

Metabolism & Mechanism of Action

Carbon monoxide acts by avidly binding to hemoglobin to form carboxyhemoglobin (COHb). This has two important effects. First, carbon monoxide competes with oxygen for binding sites on hemoglobin, thereby reducing the oxygen-carrying capacity of the blood. Second, the COHb unit interferes with heme-heme interactions such that the oxygen-hemoglobin dissociation curve is shifted to the left, resulting in decreased release of oxygen from hemoglobin carrier sites to the tissues. Carbon monoxide also may bind to other heme-containing moieties besides hemoglobin and also may affect the mitochondrial cytochrome oxidase system, thus compromising cellular respiration.

Clinical Findings

A. SYMPTOMS & SIGNS

The brain and heart are the organs most vulnerable to hypoxia. At high exposures, rapid loss of consciousness, coma, and death occur as with other asphyxiants. In subacute carbon monoxide exposure, symptoms are less marked and can be quite nonspecific, including headache, malaise, nausea, and vomiting. Cardiac ischemia may result from carbon monoxide exposure, particularly in individuals with underlying coronary artery disease.

B. LABORATORY FINDINGS

Elevated COHb is confirmed through co-oximeter blood gas analysis. COHb is increased in active cigarette smoking but should not exceed 10% on this account and usually is less than that (typically 4–7% in a two-pack-per-day cigarette smoker). COHb levels above 30% are associated with moderate to severe symptoms; levels of 50% and above can be associated with lethal carbon monoxide effects. There is a great deal of symptomatic heterogeneity, however, in relation to the absolute COHb level associated with specific findings. In pregnancy, a higher fetal level may be reached than that reflected by the maternal COHb level. A routine blood gas analysis (not done by co-oximetry) reports a calculated rather than measured oxygen saturation that will be falsely preserved in the setting of carbon monoxide intoxication. Similarly, pulse oximetry is unreliable in the presence of significant COHb. Electrocardiographic and biochemical monitoring (e.g., serial troponin assays) can be useful because myocardial infarction can occur in severe carbon monoxide intoxication, even in the absence of typical chest pain symptoms.

Differential Diagnosis

With severe exposure, the differential diagnosis is that of any anoxic injury. For fire victims, it is often difficult to rule out concomitant cyanide intoxication. The differential diagnosis of subacute carbon monoxide intoxication leading to nonspecific symptoms is quite wide, and it is likely that many cases go undiagnosed. A high index of suspicion is needed, particularly in winter months when space-heater malfunction is common. Group exposures can be misdiagnosed as food poisoning, for example.

Prevention

Carbon monoxide is odorless and has no warning properties. Internal combustion engines should not be used in indoor environments or near the intake of air supplies unless special precautions are taken. Heating units should be well maintained to ensure proper venting and to avoid partial combustion. Household carbon monoxide alarms are now employed widely. Properly used, these may serve to reduce home heating mishaps.

Treatment

Immediate removal from exposure together with supplemental oxygen (100% by non-rebreathing face mask or, in the comatose patient, by endotracheal tube) are the mainstays of initial treatment for carbon monoxide intoxication. On 100% oxygen, the half-life of COHb is reduced to approximately 60–90 minutes from 5–6 hours on room air alone. The role of hyperbaric treatment remains controversial in low-level poisoning. It is generally recommended in high-level intoxication, presuming that technical access to a hyperbaric chamber is logistically feasible. In one controlled study, such treatment was found to reduce the risk of selected long-term cognitive deficits following acute carbon monoxide poisoning.

Prognosis

Anoxic brain injury can occur after severe carbon monoxide exposure (i.e., intoxication to the point of loss of consciousness). Injury can be nonfocal and subtle, including neurobehavioral abnormalities. Parkinsonian deficits have been documented as a sequela of carbon monoxide poisoning.

HYDROGEN CYANIDE

Essentials of Diagnosis

A. ACUTE & SUBACUTE EFFECTS

- Dyspnea
- Headache

- Gastrointestinal distress
- Dizziness
- Loss of consciousness
- Anoxic brain injury

B. CHRONIC EFFECTS

- Residual anoxic injury

Exposure Limits

OSHA PEL: TWA 10 ppm (11 mg/m^3) (skin)
NIOSH REL: Short-term exposure limit (STEL) 4.7 ppm (5 mg/m^3) (skin)

General Considerations

Hydrogen cyanide is a colorless gas under standard atmospheric conditions. It can be encountered in a wide array of industrial applications. In addition to gas inhalation, exposures occur through ingestion and skin absorption of cyanide salts. The classic "bitter almond" odor of cyanide cannot be appreciated by a significant proportion of the population, apparently on a genetic basis. Because of its potency and rapidity of action, cyanide has long been important to forensic as well as occupational toxicology.

Occupational & Environmental Exposure

The major current industrial use of cyanide is in metal plating operations and in the extraction of silver and gold salts from ores. As with carbon monoxide, cyanide release is a potential hazard in structural fires, primarily as a thermolysis by-product of both natural and synthetic polymers. Toxicity also can occur after exposure to acrylonitrile (see Chapter 28) because metabolism of this solvent releases hydrogen cyanide. Cyanogenic glycosides are an environmental dietary exposure source in much of the developing world, principally from cassava.

Metabolism & Mechanism of Action

Cyanide is quickly absorbed through inhalation and skin exposures. Cyanide exerts its toxicity by binding to ferrous iron in cytochrome oxidase in the mitochondrial respiratory chain, blocking oxygen utilization. As aerobic metabolism is compromised, anaerobic metabolism develops, resulting in lactic acidosis.

Clinical Findings

A. SYMPTOMS & SIGNS

Low-level exposure leads to dyspnea, dizziness, headache, confusion, and gastrointestinal distress. Higher exposures cause rapid loss of consciousness, seizures, and death.

B. LABORATORY FINDINGS

Tests of blood cyanide levels are used in forensic examinations but generally are not available in a timely enough fashion to guide acute medical management. Thiocyanate levels do not accurately reflect the intensity of cyanide intoxication and should not be used as a proxy.

Differential Diagnosis

The differential diagnosis includes other asphyxiants, especially hydrogen sulfide and, in fire victims, carbon monoxide. Cyanide exposure should be suspected when collapse is very sudden after an inhalation or ingestion.

Prevention

Cyanide gas is released from cyanide salt solutions if the pH falls, such as may occur, for example, from inadvertent mixing of solutions with an acid. However, absorption following skin contact with salt solutions also occurs, leading to the same toxicity.

Treatment

The current standard of treatment for cyanide intoxication in the United States is induction of methemoglobin with nitrites (to compete for cyanide binding, sparing the cytochrome oxidase) and administration of thiosulfate to promote detoxification of cyanide to thiocyanate. Other treatment protocols are used outside the United States, some of which include hydroxycobalamin and other antidotes. Management details including specific antidote regimens are available at www.emedicine.com/emerg/topic118.htm and www.atsdr.cdc.gov/MHMI/mmg8.html.

Prognosis

As with other asphyxiants, anoxic brain injury can occur in survivors of severe acute exposure.

HYDROGEN SULFIDE

Essentials of Diagnosis

A. ACUTE EFFECTS

- Mucous membrane and respiratory irritation
- Loss of consciousness
- Anoxic brain injury

B. CHRONIC EFFECTS

- Residual anoxic injury

Exposure Limits

OSHA PEL: C 20 ppm, 50 ppm (10-minute maximum peak)

NIOSH REL: C 10 ppm (15 mg/m^3) (10 minutes)

General Considerations

Hydrogen sulfide is a naturally occurring toxicant generated from the breakdown of organic materials. It is associated with a pungent odor of rotten eggs and is detectable by smell in concentrations as low as 0.02 ppm, although this warning property may be lost through olfactory fatigue.

Occupational & Environmental Exposure

Geothermal and fossil-fuel energy extraction are the two major occupational sources of industrial hydrogen sulfide exposure, but other occupational risk groups include farmers (manure processing), sewage workers, fish processors, and roofers or surfacers who work with heated tar and asphalt. Hydrogen sulfide is a particular hazard in confined spaces such as fishing-ship holds, manure pits, and sewers. It is heavier than air and therefore accumulates in low-lying areas.

Metabolism & Mechanism of Action

Like cyanide, hydrogen sulfide exerts its toxicity by blocking oxygen utilization through the cytochrome oxidase pathway. Hydrogen sulfide also has irritant properties and can cause mucous membrane and respiratory tract irritation.

Clinical Findings

A. SYMPTOMS & SIGNS

High exposure leads to rapid loss of consciousness and death. At lower levels, irritant effects may predominate, including airway irritation and burning eyes. Other findings may include dermatitis, pneumonitis, and pulmonary edema, as well as headache, dizziness, nausea, and vomiting.

B. LABORATORY FINDINGS

Blood sulfide level measurements generally are not available in clinical laboratories.

Differential Diagnosis

The differential diagnosis includes other asphyxiants, most important of which is cyanide. Signs or symptoms of mucous membrane or respiratory tract irritation would support the diagnosis because the other toxic asphyxiants are not potent irritants.

Prevention

Confined-space precautions are particularly relevant to the prevention of hydrogen sulfide injury. The odor warning properties of hydrogen sulfide are not reliable as a protective factor.

Treatment

Sodium nitrite and amyl nitrite can be as antidotes, as is the case with cyanide poisoning (although thiosulfate is not administered). Additional details may be accessed at www.emedicine.com/EMERG/topic258.htm.

Prognosis

Anoxic brain injury may result from severe intoxication. In addition, the sequelae of acute irritant inhalant injury represent a potential adverse outcome (see "Irritant Inhalants" below).

REFERENCES

Domachevsky L: Hyperbaric oxygen in the treatment of carbon monoxide poisoning. Clin Toxicol (Phila) 2005;43:181 [PMID: 15902792].

Gracia R, Shepherd G: Cyanide poisoning and its treatment. Pharmacotherapy 2004;24:1358 [PMID: 15628833].

Hampson NB, Zmaeff JL: Carbon monoxide poisoning from portable electric generators. Am J Prev Med 2005;28:123 [PMID: 15626568].

Hendrickson RG: Coworker fatalities from hydrogen sulfide. Am J Indust Med 2004;45:346 [PMID: 15029566].

Kao LW: Carbon monoxide poisoning. Emerg Med Clin North Am 2004;22:985 [PMID: 15474779].

Nam B: Neurologic sequela of hydrogen sulfide poisoning. Indust Health 2004;42:83 [PMID:14964623].

Thorn J: Work-related symptoms and inflammation among sewage plant operatives. Int J Occup Environ Health 2004;10:84 [PMID: 15070030].

Walsh DW: Hydrogen cyanide in fire smoke: An underappreciated threat. Emerg Med Serv 2004;33:160 [PMID: 15553543].

Woodall GM: Proceedings of the hydrogen sulfide health research and risk assessment symposium, October 31–November 2, 2000. Inhal Toxicol 2005;17:593 [PMID: 16033755].

IRRITANT AIRBORNE TOXICANTS

Essentials of Diagnosis

A. ACUTE EFFECTS

- Mucous membrane irritation
- Cough
- Stridor
- Dyspnea
- Noncardiogenic pulmonary edema

Table 30–4. Major irritant airborne toxicants.

Substance	Selected Exposure Industries or Occupations	Exposure Limits (ppm)	
		OSHA PEL	**NIOSH REL**
Ammonia	Plastics and fertilizer manufacturing	TWA 50	TWA 25; STEL 35
Bromine	Specialty chemical manufacturing	TWA 0.1	TWA 0.1; STEL 0.3
Chlorine	Plastics industry; water treatment	C 1	C 0.5 (15 min)
Chlorine dioxide	Paper manufacturing; food preparation	TWA 0.1	TWA 0.1; STEL 0.3
Dibroane	Microelectronics industry	TWA 0.1	TWA 0.1
Ethylene oxide	Gas sterilizing systems	TWA 1	TWA < 0.1
		C 5 (15 min)	C 5 10 min/d
Formaldehyde	Embalmers, hospital workers, home furnishings textile industry, building materials	TWA 0.75 STEL 2	TWA 0.016 C 0.1 (15 min)
Hydrogen chloride	Chemicals industry; firefighters	C 5	C 5
Hydrogen fluoride	Plastics industry; microelectronics	TWA 3	TWA 3; C 6
Methyl isocyanate	Pesticide manufacturing, agricultural applications, cigarette smoke	TWA 0.02 (skin)	TWA 0.02 (skin)
Nitrogen dioxide	Gas shielded welding; agricultural workers	C 5	STEL 1
Ozone	Arc welding, textile and printing industries, photochemical smog (air pollution)	TWA 0.1	C 0.1
Phosgene	Isocyanate and pesticide manufacturing; welding	TWA 0.1	TWA 0.1; C 0.2 (15 min)
Sulfur dioxide	Petroleum refining; smelting; paper manufacturing; refrigerant exposure	TWA 5	TWA 2; STEL 5

Abbreviations: C = ceiling; min = minute exposure; PEL = permissible exposure limit; ppm = parts per million; REL = recommended exposure limit; STEL = short-term exposure limit; TWA = time-weighted average.

B. Chronic Effects

- Reactive airways dysfunction syndrome
- Bronchiolitis obliterans
- Chronic respiratory insufficiency

Exposure Limits

See Table 30–4.

General Considerations

Irritant airborne toxicants are a heterogeneous group of substances linked by common target-organ effects. The majority of these compounds (but not all) are moderately to highly *water soluble* and cause the abrupt onset of irritation of all mucous membranes with which they come in contact, including the eyes, nose, mouth, and throat. Exposure to water-soluble irritants such as chlorine, ammonia, sulfur dioxide, and the acid aerosols leads to tearing, rhinorrhea, and burning of the mouth and throat. Higher-dose exposures that may occur in confined-space mishaps or in large ambient releases can lead to lower respiratory tract injury. Water-*insoluble* irritants do not produce marked mucous membrane symptomatology but nonetheless do cause lower respiratory tract injury, including non-cardiogenic pulmonary edema and bronchiolitis oblit-

erans (an obstructive airways disease characterized by scarring of the small airways). The most important of these water-insoluble toxicants are nitrogen dioxide, phosgene, and ozone.

Occupational & Environmental Exposure

A. Water-Soluble Airborne Toxicants

Chlorine gas exposures occur through industrial leaks, especially in textile and pulp bleaching (where a related irritant, chlorine dioxide, is also common) and in the production of plastics and resins. Environmental releases occur primarily in transportation accidents, water-purification mishaps, swimming pool disinfectant accidents, and household cleaning product misadventures (when chlorine is released from hypochlorite up-mixing with an acid). Chlorine gas was used as a chemical weapon in World War I.

Acid aerosol exposure is widespread in a variety of industrial processes, including those involving plastics, microelectronics, and petroleum. Important compounds include hydrochloric, sulfuric, chromic, and hydrofluoric acids. The anhydrous acid analogues (e.g., hydrogen chloride) quickly form acid aerosols in normal atmospheric conditions where humidity is present.

Ammonia exposures result from refrigeration gas leaks, in the manufacture of plastics, and in petroleum refining. High-level exposures also occur when anhydrous ammonia is handled in fertilizer applications.

Other important but less widely encountered water-soluble irritant gases include diborane (microelectronics manufacture), bromine (chemical synthesis, including flame retardants), methyl isocyanate (pesticide manufacture; this is also a breakdown product of the pesticide metam sodium), and ethylene oxide (medical equipment sterilizing). Formaldehyde, a gas in pure form that also vaporizes easily from solutions (formalin) or off-gasses residual monomer from polymers (urea-formaldehyde resins), is an irritant that may be encountered in plastics, textiles, and paper industries, as well as in smoke and photochemical smog. Acrolein, structurally related to formaldehyde, is one of the most important combustion by-product irritants in fire smoke. As noted previously, chronic diacetyl exposure (which is not acutely irritating at low levels) is now recognized as causing a spectrum of chronic airways disorders, including bronchiolitis obliterans, informally termed "popcorn worker's lung."

B. Water-Insoluble Airborne Toxicants

Nitrogen dioxide exposure occurs in gas-shielded electric arc welding, in combustion engine exhaust, in the manufacture and use of explosives, and in the manufacture of fertilizers and dyes. Illness resulting from exposure to silage decomposition is the cause of silo filler's disease.

Phosgene, like chlorine, was important historically as a weapon in World War I. It is still encountered when certain volatile chlorinated hydrocarbons are exposed to heat or ultraviolet light, as in arc welding. It is used in the production of dyes and pharmaceuticals.

Ozone has becoming increasingly important as an alternative to chlorine in pulp paper bleaching and water disinfection. Ozone exposure in the paper industry in Sweden has been shown to be a risk factor for asthma.

Metabolism & Mechanism of Action

The irritants cause tissue injury through heterogeneous mechanisms that may include free-radical or oxidant pathways. In general, these are not substances that require metabolic activation in order to exert their toxic effect.

Clinical Findings

A. Symptoms & Signs

Low to moderate exposure to *water-soluble airborne toxicants* causes mucous membrane irritation marked by lacrimation, rhinorrhea, and burning of the mouth and face. These toxicants have good warning properties, prompting the victim to flee if possible. Higher exposure is associated with cough and respiratory irritation and also can lead to laryngospasm and lower respiratory tract injury. Lower respiratory tract injury

may range from mild pulmonary edema to severe injury that manifests clinically as acute respiratory distress syndrome (ARDS). Lower respiratory tract injury becomes evident in the hours immediately following exposure.

The *water-insoluble airborne toxicants* typically spare the mucous membranes and upper respiratory tract. These toxicants have poor warning properties, permitting significant exposure to occur before symptoms are manifest. In contrast with the immediate onset of symptoms following exposure to water-soluble toxicants, symptoms may be delayed for hours following inhalation of water-insoluble toxicants.

B. Laboratory Findings

After significant symptomatic exposure, laboratory evaluation should include pulmonary function testing, chest radiograph, and assessment of oxygenation.

Differential Diagnosis

The exposure history usually is sufficient to identify irritant inhalation as the cause of respiratory compromise. However, nitrogen dioxide or phosgene exposure sometimes may present as occult causes of ARDS, for which pneumonia and sepsis typically would be the leading alternative etiology. Lower respiratory tract injury without antecedent mucous membrane irritant symptoms is *inconsistent* with exposure to a water-soluble irritant such as ammonia or chlorine.

Prevention

Precautions in the storage and transport of irritant gases are critical to prevention. Household cleaning product misadventures can be prevented by avoiding hypochlorite mixing with other products, especially acid- or ammonia-containing cleaners. Nitrogen dioxide injury in agriculture can be prevented by proper silo ventilation. Precautions are particularly important during continuous-feed (high-volume) gas-shielded welding operations [e.g., tungsten inert gas (TIG) welding], especially in confined or poorly ventilated spaces. Ethylene oxide use in sterilizing systems should be accompanied by adequate venting, as well as by other engineering controls and specific overexposure monitoring.

Treatment

The treatment of irritant injury is supportive and non-specific and includes supplemental oxygen and bronchodilator therapy. Although corticosteroids are used frequently in the treatment of irritant injury in clinical practice, this has not been studied in a controlled manner. There is no proven role for prophylactic antibiotic use following such exposures.

Prognosis

In severe exposures leading to ARDS, mortality can be high, but injury of lesser severity resolves without sequelae in most cases. However, irritant-induced asthma (including reactive airways dysfunction syndrome) or, more rarely, bronchiolitis obliterans or bronchiectasis may result from acute irritant inhalation.

SMOKE & COMBUSTION BY-PRODUCTS

Essentials of Diagnosis

A. ACUTE EFFECTS

- Mucous membrane irritation and cough
- Stridor and dyspnea
- Noncardiogenic pulmonary edema
- Loss of consciousness

Exposure Limits

See Table 30–5.

General Considerations

Smoke is a complex mixture of gases and particulates (Table 30–5). The components of smoke depend on the material consumed, the temperature of combustion, and the amount of oxygen present. The principal relevant components of smoke include carbon monoxide, hydrogen cyanide, irritant gases and aerosols (particularly hydrogen chloride, formaldehyde, nitric oxide, and acrolein), and carbonaceous particulates (i.e., soot).

Occupational & Environmental Exposure

Firefighters are the largest occupational risk group for smoke inhalation. Home cooking and heating with biomass materials are ubiquitous sources of environmental smoke exposure in the developing world. Residential wood fireplaces are also used widely in industrialized nations for heating and ambiance. Passive cigarette smoke exposure has received a great deal of public health attention and is reviewed in Chapter 40. Incense is used worldwide for ceremonial purposes and as a source of aromatic aerosols. Incense is made of wood and other plant matter and is impregnated with fragrances. It represents a source of intentional smoke exposure and is used commonly in confined indoor spaces.

Metabolism & Mechanism of Action

Smoke can exert its toxicity through asphyxia (see "Carbon Monoxide" and "Cyanide" above) or irritant effects. In addition, combustion-related oxidants can cause methemoglobinemia (see Chapter 15). Direct thermal injury typically is not a major sequela of smoke inhalation, in contrast with steam inhalation, where this is an important cause of respiratory tract injury.

Clinical Findings

A. SYMPTOMS & SIGNS

Clinical findings in smoke inhalation injury can include features of both asphyxiant and irritant injury. Carbonaceous sputum represents a specific finding.

B. LABORATORY FINDINGS

Blood co-oximetry should establish the COHb level and document oxygenation status. After significant symptomatic exposure, laboratory evaluation also should include pulmonary function testing and chest roentgenogram.

Differential Diagnosis

The differential diagnostic questions following smoke exposure often center on identifying the potential toxicants of greatest concern, especially following chemical fires. Very acrid smoke suggests the presence of hydrochloric acid or other acid aerosols. These are frequently released when polyvinyl chloride and other halogenated polymers are burned.

Table 30–5. Common components of smoke from structural fires.

Substance	Exposure Limits (ppm, except where noted)	
	OSHA PEL	NIOSH REL
Carbon monoxide	TWA 50	TWA 35; C 200
Acrolein	TWA 0.1	TWA 0.1, STEL 0.3
Formaldehyde	TWA 0.75; STEL 2	TWA 0.016; C 0.1 (15 min)
Hydrogen chloride	C 5	C 5
Hydrogen cyanide	TWA 10	STEL 4.7
Nitric oxide	TWA 25	TWA 25
Nitrogen dioxide	C 5	STEL 1
Particulates (respirable)	TWA 15 mg/m^3 (total) TWA 5 mg/m^3 (respirable range)	Not specified

Abbreviations: C = ceiling; min = minute exposure; PEL = permissible exposure limit; ppm = parts per million; REL = recommended exposure limit; STEL = short-term exposure limit; TWA = time-weighted average.

Prevention

Appropriate use of a self-contained breathing apparatus is the principal preventive measure used for firefighters combating structural fires. The use of a breathing apparatus appears to be effective in preventing the development of pulmonary symptoms and in reducing both the deterioration in forced expiratory volume in 1 second and the increase in airway responsiveness caused by smoke inhalation. Limiting exercise in the afternoon is one way to prevent exposure to ambient-air smoke.

Treatment

The treatment of smoke inhalation includes supplemental oxygen, empirical bronchodilator therapy, and supportive care. As with other irritant exposures, corticosteroids sometimes are used but have not been studied in a controlled manner. Tracheal intubation and mechanical ventilation may be necessary.

Prognosis

Temporary deterioration in pulmonary function and increases in nonspecific airway reactivity have been well documented in persons exposed to smoke, including firefighters. In many states, firefighters can receive workers' compensation on a presumptive basis for lung cancer because of chronic fire smoke exposure. This compensation is based on social policy but does not reflect an established epidemiologic association. Community environmental exposures following conflagrations can lead to widespread concern over possible chronic effects. Acute respiratory symptoms, including aggravation of preexisting asthma and chronic obstructive pulmonary disease, can be anticipated. However, long-term sequelae in the absence of clear-cut acute effects would not be anticipated.

REFERENCES

Ernst KP: Releases from improper chemical mixing: Hazardous Substances Emergency Events Surveillance System, 1996–2001. J Occup Environ Med 2005;47:287 [PMID: 15761325].

Fedoruk MJ: Ammonia exposure and hazard assessment for selected household cleaning product uses. J Exp Anal Environ Epidemiol 2005;15:534. [PMID: 16030526].

Gorguner M: Reactive airways dysfunction syndrome in housewives due to a bleach–hydrochloric acid mixture. Inhal Toxicol 2004;16:87 [PMID: 15204781].

Koenig JO et al: Pulmonary effects of indoor- and outdoor-generated particles in children with asthma. Environ Health Perspect 2005;113:499 [PMID: 15811822].

Medina-Ramon M: Asthma, chronic bronchitis, and exposure to irritant agents in occupational domestic cleaning: A nested case-control study. Occup Environ Med 2005;62:598 [PMID: 16109815].

Ruckart PZ et al: Risk factors for acute chemical releases with public health consequences: Hazardous Substances Emergency Events Surveillance in the U.S., 1996–2001. Environ Health 2004;3:10 [PMID: 15496226].

Stefanidou M: Toxicological aspects of fire. Vet Hum Toxicol 2004;46:196 [PMID: 15303394].

Sundblad BM: Acute respiratory effects of exposure to ammonia on healthy persons. Scand J Work Environ Health 2004;30:313 [PMID: 15458015].

■ OTHER AIRBORNE RESPIRATORY TOXICANTS

ARSINE

Essentials of Diagnosis

A. ACUTE EFFECTS

- Malaise and weakness
- Gastrointestinal distress and dyspnea
- Hemolysis
- Hemoglobinuria and hematuria

B. CHRONIC EFFECTS

- Renal damage

Exposure Limits

OSHA PEL: TWA 0.05 ppm (0.2 mg/m^3)
NIOSH REL: C 0.002 mg/m^3 (15 minutes)

General Considerations

Hemolytic anemia is the most consistent clinical finding in humans. Other findings may include multi-organ-system dysfunction.

Occupational & Environmental Exposure

Arsine gas can be produced de novo in metal refining and other metal-working processes when arsenic reacts with an acid in the appropriate environment. Preformed arsine gas, often stored under pressure in large quantities, is used widely as a dopant in the microelectronics industry. In addition to a potential occupational hazard, this also presents an environmental risk to surrounding communities.

Metabolism & Mechanism of Action

Arsine is toxic to red blood cells, leading to hemolysis. Damage to other tissues may result from secondary damage from hemolysis (e.g., kidney deposition of hemoglobin) or from direct toxic effects.

Clinical Findings

A. SYMPTOMS & SIGNS

The signs and symptoms of arsine toxicity reflect both hemolysis with its sequelae and other systemic toxic manifestations. A triad of abdominal pain, hematuria, and jaundice is characteristic. Clinical findings also may include malaise, headache, renal failure, cerebral edema, intracerebral hemorrhage, dyspnea, cardiovascular collapse, and death. Delayed peripheral neuropathy may occur.

B. LABORATORY FINDINGS

The laboratory findings are those of intravascular hemolysis. The blood arsenic level may be elevated, although this is unlikely to be available rapidly enough to aid in early diagnosis. The free hemoglobin level may help to guide management; exchange transfusion has been advocated for free hemoglobin levels greater than 1.2–1.5 g/dL.

Differential Diagnosis

The principal differential diagnosis includes hemolysis as a consequence of other causes. Although chemical oxidant exposures also can cause hemolysis, this would occur in the context of significant methemoglobinemia, which is not present in arsine poisoning. Stibine (antimony hydride) exposure also can cause massive hemolysis, although it is rarely encountered industrially.

Prevention

Meticulous control measures and backup procedures should be in place whenever arsine gas is used. This should include hazardous materials (HAZMAT) incident planning relevant to community protection.

Treatment

There is no specific antidote for arsine poisoning. Treatment consists of measures to support vascular, renal, hematologic, and respiratory function. Treatment of massive arsine-caused hemolysis has required exchange transfusion. Alkalinization may reduce hemoglobin precipitation in the kidneys. Interim dialysis may be required if renal failure develops.

Prognosis

Severe arsine exposure is life-threatening. If adequate acute supportive care and transfusion are available, fatalities should be avoidable.

PHOSPHINE

Essentials of Diagnosis

A. ACUTE EFFECTS

- Respiratory distress
- Headache and dizziness
- Gastrointestinal distress
- Coma

Exposure Limits

OSHA PEL: TWA 0.3 ppm (0.4 mg/m^3)
NIOSH REL: TWA 0.3 ppm (0.4 mg/m^3), STEL 1 ppm (1 mg/m^3)

General Considerations

Phosphine is a systemic toxicant of high potency. It has a strong odor that is described either as "fishy" or "garlicky."

Occupational & Environmental Exposure

Like arsine, phosphine gas is used in the microelectronics industry. Phosphine is also generated from the hydrolysis of aluminum phosphide and zinc phosphide (which occurs spontaneously from contact with air moisture), both of which are employed as rodenticides and insecticides, especially in agricultural settings.

Metabolism & Mechanism of Action

When phosphine is inhaled, it can react with moisture to form phosphoric acid, which is an irritant. The systemic toxic mechanisms of phosphine are incompletely understood. A number of end organs are affected, including the central nervous, cardiac, respiratory, hepatic, and renal systems.

Clinical Findings

A. SYMPTOMS & SIGNS

Multi-organ-system dysfunction can be anticipated following phosphine exposure, with pulmonary, cardiovascular, and central nervous system morbidity most prominent. With lower-level exposure, pulmonary toxicity may be the primary manifestation, marked by dyspnea and delayed-onset pulmonary edema in the hours following exposure.

B. LABORATORY FINDINGS

There are no specific laboratory findings in phosphine poisoning. Phosphorus levels are not followed in routine practice in the management of phosphine intoxication.

Differential Diagnosis

Without a history of exposure, it may be difficult to identify phosphine as the cause of the acute multisystem injury this toxicant can induce. Exposure to silos or railroad cars that may have been fumigated should raise the index of suspicion for phosphine exposure.

Prevention

Adequate postuse ventilation and other appropriate reentry restrictions should prevent overexposure in agricultural settings. In industry, strict engineering controls must be enforced.

Treatment

There is no specific treatment for phosphine toxicity other than general supportive care. The potential for delayed onset of pulmonary edema should be recognized. Hemodialysis is recommended only if renal failure develops. The effectiveness of exchange transfusions is questionable. The value of steroids for phosphine-exposed patients who develop acute pulmonary edema has not been established.

Prognosis

Potential sequelae related to acute lung injury are a possible problem. There are no data on other chronic effects of phosphine poisoning.

METHYL BROMIDE
Essentials of Diagnosis
A. ACUTE EFFECTS

- Dyspnea and respiratory distress
- Seizures
- Coma

B. CHRONIC EFFECTS

- Genotoxicity

Exposure Limits

OSHA PEL: C 20 ppm (80 mg/m^3) (skin)
NIOSH REL: Lowest feasible concentration

General Considerations

Methyl bromide is a fumigant used to control insects and weeds in more than 100 crops. The United States has used about 60 million pounds each year (75% of which was to fumigate soil before crops are planted); however, its use is becoming increasingly restricted.

In the past, it has been used frequently in structural pest control in the urban environment. Methyl bromide, which is heavier than air, is a gas at room temperature but does condense at colder temperatures [<3.3°C (38°F)].

Occupational & Environmental Exposure

Pesticide applicators are the principal occupational risk group. Inadvertent environmental exposure occurs following misapplication or inappropriate reentry to areas treated with methyl bromide.

Metabolism & Mechanism of Action

Methyl bromide has multiple toxic actions, including alkylation and enzyme inhibition. It has two principal target-organ effects in humans: acute lung injury and central nervous system toxicity.

Clinical Findings
A. SYMPTOMS & SIGNS

Dyspnea and pulmonary edema may coincide with neurologic compromise marked by visual disturbance, tremor, and seizure. In severe cases, status epilepticus ensues.

B. LABORATORY FINDINGS

Serum bromide may be elevated, but the actual level correlates poorly with symptoms. In some assays, the serum chloride may be falsely elevated because of bromine.

Differential Diagnosis

The exposure history is critical. The combination of neurotoxicity and pulmonary injury represents an unusual constellation of symptoms that should suggest methyl bromide inhalation.

Prevention

Methyl bromide has few warning properties. For this reason, chloropicrin, which is a mucous membrane irritant even at low concentrations, frequently is added to the fumigant.

Treatment

Treatment is nonspecific. Control of status epilepticus is usually the primary focus of care. Dimercaprol and acetylcysteine have been suggested as antidotes based on the postulated mechanism of methyl bromide toxicity. However, no adequate studies have tested the efficacy of these therapies. Accordingly, they cannot be recommended for routine use.

Prognosis

Neurologic compromise that resolves very slowly or that may be persistent has been well documented following methyl bromide intoxication.

MILITARY & CROWD-CONTROL AGENTS & SELECTED AIRBORNE TOXICANTS WITH TERRORISM USE POTENTIAL

Essentials of Diagnosis

A. ACUTE EFFECTS OF IRRITANT AGENTS

- Lacrimation
- Mucous membrane irritation
- Dyspnea

B. ACUTE EFFECTS OF SELECTED INCAPACITANTS

Opioids, benzodiazepines, general anesthetics
  - Stupor
  - Sedation
  - Respiratory depression

Anticholinergics
  - Altered consciousness
  - Seizures
  - Dry mouth
  - Constipation

Exposure Limits of Selected Agents

A. ZINC CHLORIDE

OSHA PEL: TWA 1 mg/m^3
NIOSH REL: TWA 1 mg/m^3, STEL 2 mg/m^3

B. CHLOROACETOPHENONE (MACE)

OSHA PEL: TWA 0.3 mg/m^3 (0.05 ppm)
NIOSH REL: TWA 0.3 mg/m^3 (0.05 ppm)

General Considerations

Tear gases are well-dispersed aerosols. Another military agent, the "smoke bomb," releases zinc chloride aerosol. In October 2002, the Russian military used an incapacitating agent or mixture of incapacitating agents prior to a siege of a theater in Moscow where Chechen terrorists held 800 hostages. Carfentanil, a derivative of the opioid fentanyl, and halothane, a general anesthetic gas, are believed to have been the incapacitants used in that operation. 3-Quinuclidinyl benzylate (BZ) is an anticholinergic agent that has been weaponized and has a spectrum of effects including paranoid hallucinations and other responses typical for anticholinergic toxicity. More information about some of these agents may be found at www.sis.nlm.nih.gov/enviro/chemicalwarfare.html#a1 and other references listed below.

Occupational & Environmental Exposure

Occupationally, both military and police personnel can be exposed through accidental releases, in training exercises, and in the field. In the latter context, "environmental" exposure may be widespread.

Clinical Findings

A. SYMPTOMS & SIGNS

The tear gases, principally chloroacetophenone (CN, Mace) and *ortho*-chlorobenzylidenemalononitrile (CS), are designed to be lacrimators and mucous membrane irritants. Rarely, with severe exposure, lower respiratory injury also can occur. In contrast, zinc chloride, the principal component of smoke bombs, is a severe respiratory irritant. Nonirritant incapacitants cause a spectrum of effects, of which the most important is alterations in mental status.

B. LABORATORY FINDINGS

There are no specific laboratory findings.

Differential Diagnosis

All the lacrimators would be anticipated to have similar effects. Involvement of other organs or systemic toxicity suggests other chemical exposures. Other chemical warfare agents, especially the modern "nerve gases," cause an entirely different presentation, with systemic illness marked by severe cholinesterase inhibition. Another warfare agent, sulfur mustard, although commonly referred to as "mustard gas," is a vesicant aerosol that leads to skin blistering and bone marrow depression in addition to respiratory injury. Opioid incapacitants may induce respiratory failure, whereas anticholinergic incapacitants may cause systemic symptoms that include hypertension, dry mouth, constipation, and seizures.

Prevention

Confined-space exposures to any of these agents can be associated with adverse outcomes and should be avoided.

Treatment

Physostigmine may be used as an antidote for the anticholinergic incapacitants. Flumazenil and naloxone are antidotes for benzodiazepines and opioids, respectively. There are no specific treatments for irritant gases or other lacrimators. After removal from exposure, treatment is supportive.

Prognosis

There are no commonly observed chronic residual health effects of the lacrimators, although case reports of irritant-induced asthma have been documented. Smoke bomb inhalation may lead to the sequelae of acute lung injury.

REFERENCES

Arnold JL: CBRNE: Chemical warfare agents, www.emedicine.com/emerg/topic852.htm.

Centers for Disease Control and Prevention (CDC): Chemical agents, www.bt.cdc.gov/agent/agentlistchem.asp.

Hafazi M: Late respiratory complications of mustard gas poisoning in Iranian veterans. Inhal Toxicol 2005;17:587 [PMID: 16033754].

Hendrickson RG: Introduction: What critical care practitioners should know about terrorism agents. Crit Care Clin 2005;21:641 [PMID: 16168306].

Houston M: Decontamination. Crit Care Clin 2005;21:653 [PMID: 16168307].

Institute of Medicine of the National Academies: Long-term follow-up of army personnel potentially exposed to chemical warfare agents, www.iom.edu/project.asp?id=4911.

Kaye WE: Surveillance of hazardous substance emergency events: Identifying areas for public health prevention. Int J Hyg Environ Health 2005;208:37 [PMID: 15881977].

McManus J: Vesicants. Crit Care Clin 2005;21;707 [PMID: 16168310].

National Institutes of Health National Library of Medicine: Chemical warfare agents, www.sis.nlm.nih.gov/enviro/chemical-warfare.html.

Warden CR: Respiratory agents: Irritant gases, riot control agents, incapacitants, and caustics. Crit Care Clin. 2005;21:719 [PMID: 16168311].

INHALANT ABUSE ("RECREATIONAL" INHALANTS)

Essentials of Diagnosis

A. ACUTE EFFECTS

- Alcohol intoxication-like effects
- Excitation
- Euphoria
- Drowsiness
- Light-headedness
- Agitation
- Slurred speech
- Unconsciousness

B. CHRONIC EFFECTS

- Weight loss
- Inattentiveness
- Depression
- Impaired cognition
- Motor abnormalities
- Liver toxicity

Exposure Limits of Selected Agents

A. NITROUS OXIDE ("LAUGHING GAS")

> OSHA PEL: None
> NIOSH REL: 25 ppm

B. BUTANE

> OSHA PEL: None
> NIOSH REL: TWA 800 ppm

C. TOLUENE

> OSHA PEL: TWA 200 ppm, C 300 ppm, 500 ppm (10-minute maximum peak)
> NIOSH REL: TWA 100 ppm, STEL 150 ppm

General Consideration

Common household products that contain volatile solvents, propellants, gases, nitrites, and aerosols are widely abused to induce psychoactive effects. Products include glues, nail polish remover, lighter fluids, spray paints, deodorants, hair sprays, canned whipped cream, and cleaning fluids. The specific inhalants include amyl nitrite ("poppers"), butyl nitrite (found in video head cleaners), butane (found in lighter fluid), methylene chloride (found in paint thinners), nitrous oxide ("laughing gas"), n-hexane (found in glue), and toluene (found in correction fluid and glue). Inhalants may be sniffed from containers, sprayed into the mouth as aerosols, introduced into a bag as a vapor or aerosol and then inhaled, or inhaled from a soaked rag.

Occupational & Environmental Exposure

Recreational inhalant use refers to intentional inhalational exposure to chemicals in order to produce desired psychoactive and physical effects that may, in turn, have important acute and chronic adverse health consequences. Abuse of common consumer products may be viewed as a form of environmental toxicant exposure, particularly among young adults, adolescents, and children. It also may be viewed as a substance-abuse disorder. It is estimated that 12.5 million Americans have abused inhalants at least once in their lives. According to the National Institute on Drug Abuse, 20% of eighth-grade students have engaged in recreational inhalant use. Hair stylists, wood refinishers, and anesthesiologists are occupations that may be at increased risk of experiencing *unintentional* exposure to some of the same inhalants that have abuse potential.

Metabolism & Mechanism of Action

Inhaled chemicals are absorbed rapidly from the respiratory tract into the bloodstream and delivered quickly to the brain and other organ systems. Alcohol intoxication–like effects may be produced within seconds to minutes. Intoxication may only last a few minutes, which may result in repeated intentional exposures.

Clinical Findings

A. SYMPTOMS & SIGNS

Recreational inhalants produce a spectrum of acute effects, including euphoria, dizziness, slurred speech, hallucinations, headache, delusions, and loss of consciousness. A single session of inhalant abuse may cause a lethal cardiac dysrhythmia, a sequela termed *sudden sniffing death*. This can be related to the primary substance inhaled or to carrier propellants, especially if they are halogenated hydrocarbons that can sensitize the myocardium to catecholamine-related dysrhythmia. Long-term health effects from compulsive use include neurotoxicities such as cognitive abnormalities and movement disorders, as well as injury to the heart, liver, bone marrow, and kidneys.

B. LABORATORY FINDINGS

There are few specific laboratory findings. Macrocytic anemia has been described in chronic nitrous oxide abuse. Nitrates and oxidants induce methemoglobinemia. Forensic analysis may detect solvents in cases of acute mortality and very high-level exposure. Pathologic findings in chronic solvent exposure include brain atrophy (i.e., toluene), nerve demyelination (i.e., *n*-hexane), and cirrhosis (i.e., hepatotoxic chlorinated solvents).

Differential Diagnosis

An exposure history typically is sufficient to make a diagnosis of acute recreational inhalant use. A spectrum of recreational drugs with psychoactive effects may produce euphoria and other neurologic effects similar to those produced by abused inhalants. The clinical presentation of sudden sniffing death is indistinguishable from sudden cardiac death as a result of congenital or acquired heart disease unless a necropsy is performed. Chronic recreational inhalant use (especially solvents) may produce clinical and pathologic-neurologic syndromes difficult to distinguishable from multiple sclerosis and cirrhosis caused by alcohol.

Prevention & Treatment

The general strategies used to prevent and treat substance abuse are relevant to the public health problem of recreational inhalant abuse.

Prognosis

Intensity, duration, and frequency of exposure and, presumably, host factors are important determinants of prognosis. Chronic neurologic, cardiac, and liver disease may result from long-term abuse.

REFERENCES

Anderson CE: Recognition and prevention of inhalant abuse. Am Fam Phys 2003;68:869 [PMID: 13678134].

National Inhalant Prevention Coalition web site: www.inhalants.org.

National Institute on Drug Abuse research report series: Inhalant abuse, www.nida.nih.gov/ResearchReports/Inhalants/Inhalants.html.

Romanelli F: Poppers: Epidemiology and clinical management of inhaled nitrite abuse. Pharmacotherapy 2004;24:69 [PMID: 14740789].

Pesticides

31

Michael O'Malley, MD

In the currently registered pesticides in the United States, there are 1012 active ingredients formulated into 6981 separate products, including antimicrobial compounds. Both state and federal regulatory agencies classify antimicrobial compounds as pesticides, although many clinicians do not naturally think of them as such. Most of these can be divided into groups according to target pest or use categories and further subdivided by chemical structure (Table 31–1).

USE AND REGULATION OF PESTICIDES

The United States uses approximately 4.9 billion pounds of pesticides each year. Chlorine, hypochlorite, and other antimicrobial compounds account for 59.8%, wood preservatives for an additional 16%, sulfur and petroleum products for 6.3%, and "conventional pesticides" for 21%. Agricultural use accounts for the majority of use only in the "conventional pesticides" category. Approximately 1.7 billion pounds of pesticide were exported from the United States between the years 2001–2003. Included in this total were nearly 81 million pounds of Class 1* pesticides. Nearly 28 million pounds of pesticides whose use is forbidden in the United States were exported during this period. The vast majority of these hazardous exports were shipped to developing countries.

Pesticides are regulated differently from other chemicals in the United States and in most other countries that have chemical regulatory systems. Prior to enactment of the Federal Insecticide, Fungicide, and Rodenticide Act (FIFRA) in 1970, there was little regulation and testing of pesticides in the United States. Since then, the U.S. Environmental Protection Agency (EPA) has applied an increasingly strict testing scheme to registration for sale and use of pesticides in the United States. Since the discovery of irregularities and even fraud by certain commercial laboratories performing these tests under contract to manufacturers, greater attention has been paid to good laboratory practice and laboratory audits.

The data required by the EPA for registration of a pesticide include product chemistry, environmental fate,

acute and chronic toxicology, and studies of hazards to nontarget organisms and are set forth in Table 31–2. Access to the data on file with the EPA is limited by laws regarding confidential business information.

Despite testing requirements, gaps in the data have proved troublesome historically. In 1984, the National Academy of Sciences (NAS)–National Research Council (NRC) published the results of a survey on toxicity testing for chemicals, highlighting 104 pesticides and inert ingredients. Acute toxicity data were present for 49%, subchronic data for 41%, chronic data for 15%, reproductive data for 25%, and mutagenicity data for 20% of chemicals.

Because of the data call-in program initiated by the EPA in 1981 and legislation passed in California during the mid-1980s (California Senate Bill 950) that mandated filling of data gaps for all registered pesticides, a large number of new chronic studies were submitted for review by both the California and federal EPAs. By the year 2000, of 200 California-designated priority active ingredients, 55 were either withdrawn by their registrants or suspended by the state; adequate data were received on 142 of the remaining 145. For 703 compounds not on the priority list, 538 were suspended by the California Department of Pesticide Regulation (DPR), were withdrawn by their registrants, or were adjuvant compounds not subject to data requirements. Of the remaining 165 active ingredients, complete data were received for 127, 9 had submitted requests for waivers or exemptions, and 5 remained subject to suspension. Because of the complexities of the hazard and risk assessment process, regulatory review of these data is still ongoing.

Labeling Requirements

In the United States, the EPA regulates the registration, sale, and conditions of use of all pesticides and is responsible for the protection of agricultural workers exposed to pesticides. When a specific pesticide is approved for use, its use is specified as either general or restricted (to be applied only through permit to a licensed pest control operator), and it is registered and assigned an EPA registration number. The EPA also specifies use instructions, hazard information, and first aid information that must be listed on the product label. The hazard information

---

*In the classification system outlined in the U.S. Code of Federal Regulations, the most acutely toxic pesticides—those with an oral LD_{50} up to and including 50 mg/kg—are designated "Class 1."

Table 31–1. Occupational and environmental pesticide exposure situations.

Occupational exposures
  Research and development
  Manufacturing: technical grade material produced in en-
    closed and semi-enclosed operations; exposures during
    leaks/spill and process repairs—packaging operations
    vary in degree of enclosure
  Formulation: technical grade material mixed with "inert" in-
    gredients such as solvents, and adjuvants
  Transportation
  Pest control
  Mixing: commercial material diluted with water or other
    material
  Loading: into tanks in planes, ground rigs, backpacks, or hand-
    held sprayers. Closed versus open mix/loading systems
  Application: variable requirements in protective clothing
  Flagging: standing at the end of fields to mark the rows to
    be sprayed by crop-dusting aircraft. Flagging is currently
    being replaced by Global Positioning System flagging in
    some operations
  Farm work: field workers, pickers, sorters, packers, and oth-
    ers who come into contact with pesticide residues on
    leaves and fruit. High contact work tasks include hand
    labor in grapes; picking row crops, such as lettuce or
    strawberries, results in markedly less contact—as de-
    scribed in results of residue transfer studies
  Emergency and medical work: personnel exposed to con-
    taminated persons and equipment in the process of re-
    sponding to spills, accidents, and poisonings
Environmental and consumer exposures
  Accidents and spills, especially ingestion by children (floor
    level materials—ant traps, etc.)
  Suicide and homicide
  Home use: house and garden
  Structural use: residents and occupants of buildings
  Bystanders
  Contamination: food, water, air
  Agriculture-urban interface

Table 31–2. Environmental Protection Agency (EPA) requirements for pesticide registration.[1]

Product chemistry
  Production composition
  Physical and chemical characteristics
  Residue chemistry
Environmental fate
  Degradation studies (hydrolysis/photolysis studies); *metabolism studies; mobility studies* (leaching, adsorption/desorp-
  tion, and volatility of pesticides); *dissipation studies* (used to
  assess potential environmental hazards related to reentry,
  conditionally required foliar residue dissipation studies;
  hazards from residues in rotational crop and other food
  sources, the loss of land as well as surface and ground
  water resources); *accumulation studies* (to evaluate tendency for bioaccumulation in ecosystems)
Hazards to humans and domestic animals
  Acute studies
    Oral LD_{50}: rat
    Dermal LD_{50}: usually rabbit; inhalation LC_{50}: rat
    Primary eye irritation: rabbit
    Primary dermal irritation: rabbit
    Dermal sensitization
  Acute delayed neurotoxicity: organophosphates
  Subchronic studies: required depending on nature of
    exposure
    90-day feeding: rodent, nonrodent 21-day dermal,
      90-day dermal
    90-day inhalation: rat
    90-rat neurotoxicity: if acute studies positive
  Chronic studies: required for pesticides with allowable food
    residues (tolerances), or "significant" worker exposure
    Chronic feeding: two-species, rodent and nonrodent
    Carcinogenicity: two-species, rat and mouse preferred
    Teratogenicity: two species
    Reproduction: two generations
  Mutagenicity studies: a battery to include:
    Gene mutations
    Structural chromosomal aberrations
    Other genotoxic effects as appropriate
  Metabolism studies (pharmacokinetics)
Hazard to nontarget organisms
  Short-term studies
  Long-term and field studies
  Avian and mammalian testing
  Aquatic organism testing
  Plant protection
  Nontarget insect

[1]From US Environmental Protection Agency, 2006.
Abbreviations: LC_{50} = lethal concentration affecting 50% of test population; LD_{50} = lethal dose affecting 50% of test population.

depends on the assigned acute toxicity category (Table 31–3). Additional safety measures, such as postapplication field reentry, also may appear on the product labels.

Worker Protection Standard

Although labeling provides the chief means of regulating the use of pesticides by the EPA, some additional safety measures are imposed by regulations. For example, the Worker Protection Standard (WPS), promulgated in 1992, contains several detailed requirements: (1) prohibition against applications that may expose workers at the application site or allow off-site exposure to unprotected individuals, (2) restricted postapplication field reentry intervals, (3) personal protective equipment, (4) notifica-

Table 31–3. Environmental Protection Agency toxicity labeling categories.[1]

Hazard Indicator	Toxicity Category			
	I	II	III	IV
Oral LD$_{50}$	50 mg/kg	50–500 mg/kg	500–5000 mg/kg	> 5000
Inhalation LD$_{50}$	0.2 mg/L	0.2–2 mg/L	2–20 mg/L	> 20 mg/L
Dermal LD$_{50}$	200 mg/kg	200–2000 mg/kg	2000–20,000 mg/kg	> 20,000 mg/kg
Eye effects	Corrosive; corneal opacity not reversible within 7 days	Corneal opacity reversible; within 7 days; irritation for 7 days	No corneal opacity; irritation reversible within 7 days	No irritation
Skin effects in Draize dermal irritation (rabbits)	Corrosive	Severe irritation	Moderate irritation at 72 hours	Mild or slight irritation at 72 hours
Signal word	"Danger"	"Warning"	"Caution"	"Caution"
Precautionary statements regarding systemic toxicity	Fatal (poisonous) if swallowed, inhaled, absorbed through skin. Do not breathe vapor, dust, or spray mist. Do not get in eyes or on skin or clothing.	May be fatal if swallowed, inhaled, absorbed through skin. Do not breathe vapor, dust, or spray mist. Do not get in eyes or on skin or clothing.	Harmful if swallowed, inhaled or absorbed through skin. Avoid breathing vapor, dust, or spray mist. Avoid contact with skin, eyes or clothing.	No precautionary statements required.
Precautionary statements regarding topical effects on eye and skin	Corrosive, causes eye and skin damage or skin irritation.	Do not get in eyes, on skin, or on clothing. Wear goggles or face shield and rubber gloves when handling. Harmful or fatal if swallowed. (Appropriate first aid statement required.)	Causes eye (and skin) irritation. Do not get in eyes, on skin, or on clothing. In case of contact, wash eyes with plenty of water. Get medical attention if irritation persists.	No precautionary statements required.

[1]From: US Environmental Protection 40 CFR Part 156.

tion of workers regarding treated areas, (5) requirement for adequate supplies of water, soap, and towels for routine washing and emergency decontamination, (6) provisions for emergency assistance, (7) pesticide safety training for applicators and other handlers, and (8) access to pesticide labeling and application records. Responsibility for enforcement of the WPS requirements lies with the pesticide regulatory agency within each state, most often the state department of agriculture.

Other Federal and State Regulatory Bodies

The Occupational Safety and Health Administration (OSHA) is responsible for the protection of manufacturing and formulation workers; it also periodically investigates unusual hazardous conditions in industry. OSHA also has responsibility for enforcing regulations regarding field sanitation and hazard communication for agricultural workers.

Work by the National Institute for Occupational Safety and Health (NIOSH) relevant to pesticides has included criteria documents for engineering measures to control exposures in manufacturing and formulating operations and occupational exposure to parathion, methyl parathion, and ethylene dibromide. More recent activities at NIOSH have included a hazard alert regarding safety issues of phosphine-generating fumigants, mortality studies on phenoxy herbicide manufacturing workers, neurobehavioral studies of organophosphate (OP)–poisoned workers, and efforts to promote U.S. surveillance of pesticide-related illnesses.

State agriculture and health departments, along with county agriculture and health departments and other state and local agencies, as well as OSHA, may have a variety of regulatory or advisory functions with regard to the use of pesticides. Structural pest control—the application of pesticides to commercial and residential buildings—may fall under one or another of these jurisdictions or is regulated by separate state regulatory agencies.

PESTICIDES & ADDITIVES IN FOOD

There are more than 300 pesticides (active ingredients) used on food in the United States. The EPA [in conjunction with the Food and Drug Administration (FDA)] regulates the residues of pesticides and their breakdown products in foods by establishing tolerance levels, or the legal limits for residues in foods. Tolerances for raw agricultural commodities and processed foods are established through field trials to determine the highest residues likely to occur in the course of normal agricultural procedures and practices. Tolerances for processed foods are established by determining the degree to which the residues might become concentrated during processing, such as milling or juicing.

The Delaney Clause (see below) prohibiting tolerance for any additive found to cause cancer in humans or animals applied to processed foods but not to raw foods. New tolerances usually are denied for pesticides known to be carcinogenic, but many older pesticides were found to be carcinogenic only after food tolerances were established. This is the case with daminozide (Alar), an animal carcinogen used as a growth regulator in apples and the subject of a prolonged public controversy.

In 1996, the Delaney Clause was superseded by the Food Quality Protection Act (FQPA). The prohibition against tolerances for animal carcinogens was changed to "reasonable certainty of no harm" from exposure to residues. A requirement to screen for possible endocrine effects of pesticides also was added. The new law also required aggregate assessment of all nonoccupational sources of exposure, including drinking water, residential, and dietary exposure, and assessment of cumulative exposure to a pesticide and other substances with common mechanisms of toxicity. The implementation of the FQPA has in practice focused on the latter provision, leading particularly to changes in regulation of the use of organophosphates. Under another FQPA mandate, multiple new active ingredients with lower toxicity (e.g., the spinosad compounds and other biologicals) also have been registered.

Monitoring for pesticide residues in food is performed by the U.S. Department of Agriculture (USDA) in meat and poultry, by the FDA in domestic and imported raw and processed food, and by a number of individual states and private groups. Based on improved analytic methods, the percentage of the samples with detectable levels has increased from approximately 20% in 1987 to 37% in 2003. The fraction of samples within 50% or more of tolerance has remained constant at about 1%; another 1–2% of samples have illegal tolerances (samples over tolerance or detectable levels of compounds with no established tolerance).

OCCUPATIONAL & ENVIRONMENTAL PESTICIDE EXPOSURES

Table 31–1 lists typical occupational and nonoccupational pesticide exposure situations. The nature, extent, and route of exposure may vary among these different circumstances and the physical properties—particularly the vapor pressure—of individual pesticides (Table 31–4).

Table 31–4. Vapor pressures of common pesticides.

Pesticide	Vapor Material Pressure (mmHG)
Fumigants/nematocides	
Phosphine	23,369
Sulfuryl fluoride	760
Methyl bromide	1725
Chloropicrin	17
Metam-sodium	Not measurable
Metam-sodium by-products	
Methyl isothiocyanate	16.0
Methyl isocyanate	384
Carbon disulfide	334.3
Hydrogen sulfide	15,981
Methylamine	2324.3
Common solvents	
Water	24
Toluene	30
1,1-Dichloroethane	234
Organophosphate contaminants	
Methyl mercaptan	1261
Ethyl mercaptan	467
N-Butyl mercaptan	83
Organophosphates	
Dichlorvos (DDVP)	1×10^{-2}
Mevinphos	2×10^{-3}
Malathion	1.2×10^{-4}
Chlorpyrifos	2.02×10^{-5}
Dimethoate	8×10^{-6}
Phosalone	$< 10^{-9}$
Carbamates	
Methomyl	5.0×10^{-5}
Organochlorines	
Chlordane	1×10^{-5}
Herbicides	
2,4-Dichlorophenoxyacetic acid	1.4×10^{-7}
Cyanazine	1.6×10^{-9}
Alachlor	2.2×10^{-5}
Glyphosate	7.5×10^{-8}
Fungicides	
Hexachlorobenzene	1.09×10^{-5}
Zinc bisdithiocarbamate (ziram)	$< 7.5 \times 10^{-8}$
Benomyl	$< 3.75 \times 10^{-10}$
Chlorothalonil	5.72×10^{-7}
Triadimefon	1.5×10^{-7}

The nature of exposure depends on whether exposure is to the commercial formulation of a pesticide, as applied in a field or structure, or to the active ingredient, as occurs in a manufacturing facility. A pesticide, as applied, consists of the technical-grade chemical ("active" ingredient), diluents (often organic solvents), additives ("adjuvants"), and other "inert" ingredients. The pesticide then is applied mixed or unmixed as sprays, dusts, aerosols, granular, impregnated preparations, fumigants, baits, or systemics. Inert ingredients are not necessarily nontoxic; many are organic solvents. Most typical solvents used are petroleum distillates, but other organic solvents such as methylene chloride and propylene glycol have been used. Systemic pesticides are water-soluble chemicals that are taken up by a plant and translocated to a part of the plant where a pest, usually an insect, feeds on plant juices and ingests the pesticide. This term is also used for animal systemics, or feed-through pesticides, which are fed to an animal so that pests that feed on feces also ingest the pesticide. The use of systemic, granular, bait, and impregnated pesticide formulations can result in significantly reduced exposure during application.

Pesticides used by consumers for home and garden often are nearly identical in formulation to those used by commercial applicators or differ only in reduced concentration of active ingredient. The most serious exposures occur from accidental or deliberate ingestions. Although pesticides account for a relatively small percentage of the total childhood ingestions, childhood ingestions of organophosphates, carbamates, and dipyridyl herbicides (diquat and paraquat) may result in serious illness or death. Children also frequently attempt to ingest pesticides used at floor or ground level, such as anticoagulant rodenticides, snail baits, and ant traps, but these less often cause serious poisonings.

HIGH-RISK GROUPS

The highest exposures and incidences of poisonings occur in individuals involved in agricultural pest control operations: mixing, loading, applying, and flagging. Mixers and loaders are exposed to concentrated pesticides and large volumes, respectively. The use of closed systems for mixing and loading, required in California but not in other jurisdictions, has reduced these exposures and poisonings considerably. The exposure of applicators varies with the type of application, from backpack sprayers to enclosed-cab vehicles with filtered, cooled air. Leaking or poorly maintained equipment may fail and produce large overexposures with any type of application device, including closed mixing/loading systems. Exposures in most manufacturing facilities are low owing to the use of automated closed systems, but exposures that require unscheduled maintenance occur during development of new processes and process breakdowns or leaks. Exposures in formulating facilities may be much higher, particularly if dusty formulations (i.e., dusts, powders, and granules) are produced in open systems.

Communities with minimal zoning and mixed agricultural and urban or suburban land use may be at highest risk for environmental exposure to pesticides. In recent years, most problems have derived from high-volume applications of volatile soil fumigation products with low environmental effect levels. Additional details are discussed below in the section on fumigants and nematocides.

ROUTES OF EXPOSURE

Most pesticide inhalation exposures derive from aerosols generated at the time of application or from pesticide adsorbed to household or environmental dust. With fumigants and a few insecticidal compounds, exposures to vapors are also a significant issue (see Table 31–4).

The most important route for most occupational exposures is dermal. A high percentage of pesticides are absorbed across intact human skin because of a combination of relatively low molecular weight and high lipid solubility. This correlates with the requirement of many compounds to be absorbed through the protective coverings of insects or plants.

The ratio of dermal median lethal dose (LD_{50}) to oral LD_{50} values that are available for most pesticide provides a rough indication of degree of dermal absorption. A low ratio of dermal LD_{50} to oral LD_{50} indicates a probable high degree of dermal absorption (e.g., the organophosphate insecticide mevinphos has reported oral LD_{50}s ranging from 3.7–6.8 mg/kg and reported dermal LD_{50}s ranging from 4.2–7.0 mg/kg). For the carbamate insecticides, however, this general rule can be misleading. Because of rapid metabolic deactivation, dermal toxicity is best reflected by the dermal dose that causes 50% cholinesterase inhibition rather than the dermal LD_{50}. Other pharmacokinetic considerations vary considerably among pesticide families and so are discussed below, according to family.

REFERENCES

Grey CN et al: The use and disposal of household pesticides. Environ Res 2005;97:109 [PMID: 15476740].

Jaga K, Dharmani C: The epidemiology of pesticide exposure and cancer. Rev Environ Health 2005;20:15 [PMID: 15835496].

NIOSH: Pesticide illness and injury surveillance, www.cdc.gov/niosh/pestsurv/default.html.

OEHHA. California's Office of Environmental Health Hazard Assessment, http://www.oehha.ca.gov/pesticides.html.

EFFECTS, PREVENTION, & TREATMENT OF PESTICIDE TOXICITY

This section outlines general principles of diagnosis, treatment, and prevention for acute poisoning, skin effects of pesticides, and cancer and other chronic health effects.

Clinical Findings

A. SYMPTOMS & SIGNS

1. Acute exposure—The manifestations of acute toxicity vary among pesticide families, but diagnosis generally relies on the following features: (1) signs and symptoms consistent with exposure to one or more chemical families of pesticides [in which a relatively specific clinical constellation (toxidrome) is present], (2) a temporal relationship to known exposure to pesticides or field work, even in the absence of known recent pesticide application (temporal relationships vary depending on the type of pesticide, the route and duration of exposure, and the nature of the toxic effect), and (3) evidence of poisoning in other workers or family members.

Severe acute poisoning usually does not present a diagnostic challenge because a history of high-level acute exposure usually is available, and a full spectrum of clinical manifestations is normally present. Mild acute or subacute poisoning may not be readily apparent because the signs and symptoms are likely to be nonspecific and similar to influenza or other common illness. The history of exposure may not be particularly remarkable or even known to the patient.

B. LABORATORY FINDINGS

For acute pesticide poisoning, clinical laboratories are able to assess cholinesterase inhibition by organophosphate and possibly carbamate pesticides. Measurement of the pesticide or its metabolites in body fluids done at the time of initial presentation may not be helpful until the follow-up evaluation. The use of biologic levels is not helpful in the diagnosis of chronic toxicity because adequate dose-response data are unavailable for most pesticides, and biologic levels at the time of diagnosis, if present at all, may not reflect those present during exposure.

Prevention

A. WORK PRACTICES

Manufacturing and formulation workers, mixers, loaders, applicators, and flaggers all are exposed directly to the concentrated or dilute product and so can only be protected by engineering controls and personal protective clothing and devices. Field workers are exposed primarily to residues on plants and in soil. They are protected primarily by reentry intervals—the minimum time allowed between application of a pesticide on a field and entry into that field. The rate of degradation and the toxicity of the degradation products are important determinants of the extent and effect of exposure in this group. Pesticide degradation rates often vary among geographic regions, so reentry intervals may need to be specific to an area or climate. A common cause of acute pesticide intoxication in agriculture is the early entry of a group of field workers into a field where an acutely toxic pesticide was applied recently.

Because skin contamination is the most important route of most occupational exposures, the focus of prevention is on reducing dermal exposure though the use of respirators by manufacturing or formulation workers or pesticide applicators. Contamination of clothing, irritated skin, heat, and sweat are all factors common in agricultural work that promote absorption through the skin. The use of protective clothing in agriculture usually is impeded by the fact that most agricultural work takes place in hot and frequently humid environments. Therefore, the need for skin protection, which is difficult to quantify, must be balanced against the risk of heat-related disorders. The use of personal protective equipment for structural pest control sometimes is hampered by the need to work in tight areas, such as crawl spaces, but the confined nature of these spaces often makes their use necessary.

C. MEDICAL SURVEILLANCE

Specific medical and biologic monitoring is available for cholinesterase-inhibiting organophosphate pesticides, as discussed below. For most other pesticides, surveillance is limited to general and occupational histories and physical examinations, with available tests discussed under laboratory findings for each family.

Treatment

Treatment of pesticide poisoning in general proceeds in three steps, as described below.

A. DECONTAMINATION

Decontamination is the first priority, unless lifesaving measures are required. In the case of acute dermal overexposure, the skin and clothing are reservoirs for continued exposure, as is the gastrointestinal tract in the case of ingestion. All clothing should be removed and placed in double plastic bags for later analysis, decontamination, or disposal. The skin and, if necessary, the hair should be washed with soap. Contamination should be checked for under the fingernails. If the eyes have been contaminated, they should be irrigated. The need for gastrointestinal lavage or activated charcoal instillation should be determined on a case-by-case basis (i.e., depending on the pesticide, whether vomiting or diarrhea has occurred, and the level of consciousness). All procedures should be done in such a way as to minimize the contamination of medical personnel and equipment without compromising patient care.

B. SPECIFIC ANTIDOTES

Specific antidotes are available only in the form of atropine and pralidoxime for cholinesterase-inhibiting pesticides, as discussed in detail below, and chelating agents for heavy metal pesticides such as arsenic and mercury, which rarely result in the need for treatment, except in cases of ingestion.

C. SUPPORTIVE CARE

Supportive care may be the only treatment indicated and may be lifesaving. Assessment of respiratory status and provision of appropriate ventilatory support are critical because most fatal or serious acute pesticide poisonings are indicated, at least in part, through respiratory embarrassment or arrest. Certain medications that otherwise might be given based on clinical diagnosis may be contraindicated once the diagnosis of a specific pesticide intoxication is known. An example is the use of morphine, which can precipitate cardiac arrhythmia, for pulmonary edema in the presence of organophosphate poisoning.

REFERENCES

Kamanyire R, Karalliede L: Organophosphate toxicity and occupational exposure. Occup Med (Lond) 2004;54:69 [PMID: 15020723].

Rusyniak DE, Nanagas KA: Organophosphate poisoning. Semin Neurol 2004;24:197 [PMID: 15257517].

1. Dermatologic effects—Approximately one-third of all reported pesticide-related diseases are dermatologic—about the same percentage as estimated for other chemicals. Most skin reactions occur secondary to allergic or irritant contact dermatitis. A few pesticides have been reported to cause other reactions such as contact urticaria, erythema multiforme, chloracne, vitiligo, and porphyria cutanea tarda. Key structural factors related to irritation and sensitivity include protein reactivity and physicochemical properties related to increased absorption, binding, and transport. Important reactive elements (identified by structural acronyms) include reactive aliphatic/aromatic halides (IX), strong nucleophiles/reactive electrophiles (IUNIQ), simple aliphatic esters (ICOOR), conjugated olefins activated by SH/NH_2 groups or by Michael addition (ICONJ), easily metabolized phenols of quinone (IarOH), easily metabolized anilines (IarNH), and oxidizable primary alcohols (IOH). Factors that influence absorption include polarizable molecular volume (MR)

and lipophilic contribution of log P [octanol/water partition coefficient (PL)]. Hydrogen-bond acceptor (electron pairs on N and O, abbreviated HBA) and donor (protons on N—H and O—H moieties, abbreviated HBD) groups influence binding and transport. The effects of these factors are discussed below where relevant in the sections describing individual classes of compounds.

Diagnosis of contact reactions depends on careful evaluation of the pattern of exposure and its relation to the distribution and character of subsequent skin lesions. This task may be especially difficult in cases of dermatitis in field workers who may not know what pesticide residues are present on the plants they are in contact with. They also may be exposed to plants known to cause primary irritant or allergic contact dermatitis. (For a discussion of plant-related dermatitis, see Chapter 18.) Definitive diagnosis of irritant dermatitis depends on noting the above-described correspondence between pattern of exposure and pattern of skin reaction in addition to recognizing the irritant properties of the suspected material(s).

Allergic dermatitis can be confirmed only by diagnostic patch testing (type IV allergy), open patch applications, or prick testing (type I allergy). Patch tests are available for a number of pesticides and plants known to be sensitizers and may be made for others, provided preliminary testing of control subjects is conducted to identify the maximum nonirritating concentration of the new test material. The distinction between pesticide and plant allergy and allergic dermatitis is important from an exposure/management standpoint because irritant dermatitis often can be prevented by reducing exposure through use of personal protective equipment or administrative measures such as reentry intervals. Prevention of allergic contact dermatitis requires complete removal from exposure. Individual pesticides or weeds generally are simple to avoid, given a cooperative employer, but allergy to crop plants presents a greater problem. This is an infrequent problem with most food crops but may be relatively frequent among nursery workers handling *Alstromeria* (Peruvian lily), carnations, primrose, chrysanthemums, and other allergenic ornamental crops. The distinction is particularly important for field workers because a pesticide-related cause may mean transfer from the field for several days at one time during a season, whereas a plant-related cause may mean permanent avoidance of a particular crop for at least part of its growing cycle.

Medical treatment consists of alleviation of symptoms with corticosteroids and moisturizers. Prevention of further exposure sufficient to cause recurrence usually is possible with protective clothing. Additional details regarding the skin effects of pesticides are given in the sections on individual classes of pesticides below. Several reviews also cover the topic in detail.

REFERENCE

Penagos H et al: Pesticide patch test series for the assessment of allergic contact dermatitis among banana plantation workers in panama. Dermatitis 2004;15:137 [PMID: 15724348].

2. Chronic health effects—Chronic health effects can be divided into persistent aftereffects of acute poisoning and those that derive from cumulative exposure without prior acute effects. The former include teratogenicity and reactive airways following exposure to irritants, as well as persistent neurologic effects related to direct neurotoxicity or to hypoxia associated with respiratory depression.

ANIMAL TERATOGENS, REPRODUCTIVE TOXINS, ENDOCRINE DISRUPTORS, & RELATED EPIDEMIOLOGIC STUDIES

Animal studies of teratogenicity frequently employ albino rabbits but may use a variety of other species. Evaluation of study results depends on comparison of developmental abnormalities with controls and comparing doses producing fetal effects with doses producing maternal toxicity. Compounds with teratogenic effects at doses that do not cause maternal poisoning provoke special concern.

Individual compounds identified as teratogens or reproductive toxins in multigenerational studies in animals are identified in separate tables for each major pesticide use category (see below). No currently registered pesticides are recognized human teratogens or female reproductive toxins. However, case reports and a few epidemiologic studies have described either teratogenicity or fetotoxicity at doses that also cause maternal toxicity. For example, 35 workers developed acute organophosphate poisoning after entering a cauliflower field contaminated with residues of oxydemeton-methyl, mevinphos, and methomyl. A crew member who was 4 weeks pregnant at the time of the poisoning subsequently gave birth to a child with multiple cardiac defects, bilateral optic nerve colobomas, microphthalmia of the left eye, cerebral and cerebellar atrophy, and facial anomalies. Similarly, the massive amounts of methyl isocyanate (MIC) released from a plant producing the insecticide carbaryl at Bhopal, India, was associated with a fourfold increased incidence of spontaneous abortion in women who survived the acute pulmonary syndrome that it also provoked. In both examples, the adverse reproductive effects resulted from single short-term rather than cumulative exposures.

Endocrine Disruption

Since passage of the FQPA, the possible interference of pesticides with endocrine function has been an intensely studied topic. Environmental endocrine effects have been studied with epidemiologic studies, field observations of animal populations, and laboratory models. Epidemiologic studies of endocrine effects have included more or less direct measurement of hormonal function, and others have been studies of hormonally influenced endpoints, especially cancers of the male or female reproductive tract. Many studies have evaluated interactions between pesticides and reproductive hormones, especially estrogen, estrogen agonists, and estrogen receptors. However, potential effects may involve many other targets in the neuroendocrine axis. These include neurotransmitters and receptors in the hypothalamus and pituitary peptides that stimulate end-organ targets.

A study evaluated thyroid function, sister chromatid exchange (SCE), and chromosome translocations in 49 workers spraying the ethylenebis (dithiocarbamate) (EBDC) fungicides Maneb and Mancozeb on small tomato farms near Cuernavaca, Mexico. The mean urinary level of the EBDC metabolite ethylene thiourea (ETU) was 58 ppb in applicators compared with less than the 5 ppb limit of detection in 31 nonexposed controls. The mean age-adjusted thyroid-stimulating hormone (TSH) level was 2.13 mIU/L in applicators compared with 1.61 mIU/L in the controls. The difference was of borderline statistical significance ($p = 0.05$); both controls and applicators were well within the laboratory reference range (0.32–5.00 mIU/L). T_4 levels were comparable between exposed workers (7.68 µg/dL) and controls (7.59 µg/dL) and also within the reference range (4.5–11.5 µg/dL). Although the genotoxicity of ETU and the EBDC fungicides is equivocal, the authors reported a significant increase in SCE (8.52/cell), adjusted for age and smoking, for EBDC applicators compared with nonexposed controls (7.90/cell; $p = 0.03$). Translocations showed an age-adjusted increase (6.07/500 cell equivalents versus 4.59/500 cell equivalents) that was of borderline statistical significance ($p = 0.05$). A 2004 study from the Phillipines evaluated another population of EBDC applicators. The authors reported that there was a slight but nonsignificant increase in TSH (1.79 mIU/mL in 57 applicators and 1.77 mIU/mL in 31 indirectly exposed workers versus 1.52 mIU/mL in 43 unexposed controls). Nine of the 91 exposed workers had demonstrated thyroid abnormalities on ultrasound compared with 3 of 43 controls (relative risk = 1.7, $p = 0.34$).

Environmental and laboratory studies have evaluated the effect of pesticides on aquatic organisms, especially amphibian species. In a 2002 study, *Xenopus* (the

African clawed frog) larvae were exposed to 0.01–200 ppb of the triazine herbicide atrazine. Concentrations at or above 0.1 ppb induced hermaphroditism and demasculinized the larynges of male frogs. A 2005 Chinese field study following up these observations demonstrated no correlation between atrazine concentration and the environmental incidence of hermaphroditism. However, the presence of environmental atrazine did correlate with the occurrence of ectopic oocytes in the testes of male frogs.

REFERENCES

Colborn T: A case for revisiting the safety of pesticides: A closer look at neurodevelopment. Environ Health Perspect 2006;114:10 [PMID: 16393651].

Fenster L et al: Association of in utero organochlorine pesticide exposure and fetal growth and length of gestation in an agricultural population. Environ Health Perspect 2006;114:597 [PMID: 16581552].

Ropstad E et al: Endocrine disruption induced by organochlorines. J Toxicol Environ Health A 2006;69:53 [PMID: 16291562].

A. CHRONIC HEALTH EFFECTS WITHOUT RECOGNIZED ACUTE EFFECTS

Compounds and exposure situations that may cause no acute effects include male reproductive toxicity, as well as occupational cancer. Individual examples are described in the sections below.

MALE REPRODUCTIVE TOXICITY

In 1977, a number of male workers were discovered to have reduced or absent sperm, infertility or sterility, and testicular atrophy as a result of exposure to dibromochloropropane (DBCP) (see below). Similar effects were observed in animals. A short time later, workers exposed to chlordecone (Kepone) in a manufacturing facility were found to have similar testicular changes; subsequent animal tests were confirmatory. These episodes prompted an increase in the screening of pesticides for male reproductive toxicity.

Cancer

No pesticides currently in use are recognized human carcinogens, with the exception of inorganic arsenic. Arguable cases may be made for the wood preservatives creosote and chromic acid and for the fumigant ethylene oxide. Most occupational carcinogens have been identified in worker populations employed in chemical manufacturing. Because the current chemical industry is not labor-intensive, the number of workers required to produce chemical pesticides is relatively small, and the epidemiologic studies of these workers with unique exposures to individual pesticides

are necessarily limited by small numbers. For pesticides, these types of classic occupational cohort studies therefore are only capable of identifying very potent human carcinogens. Recently, 4-chloro-ortho-toluidine (4-COT), the principal metabolite of the insecticide chlordimeform, was found to be a carcinogen in a study of 120 manufacturing workers in Germany, provoking an incidence of bladder cancer 72 times higher than expected. Chlordimeform was taken off the market in 1986 when this information became known. Animal studies previously identified chlordimeform and 4-COT as carcinogens.

A. STUDIES OF FARMERS AND OTHER OCCUPATIONS WITH PESTICIDE EXPOSURE

Epidemiologic studies of cancer in farmers show a relatively consistent increase in certain cancers, notably leukemia, lymphoma, and multiple myeloma. Although these findings are suggestive of an increase in cancer caused by pesticides, specific pesticides could not be incriminated, and other causes related to farm work (e.g., viral exposures associated with animal handling) could not be ruled out. Studies of meat packing workers potentially exposed to biologic agents but not to pesticides provide inconsistent support for the viral hypothesis. Some case-control studies of lymphomas in this population have identified significant associations with phenoxy herbicides, atrazine, and organophosphate insecticides.

A few studies have examined cancer incidence in professional pesticide applicators. Two of these studies indicate elevated risks for lung cancer and one indicates an elevated risk for bladder cancer without being able to associate the effect with any specific pesticide.

B. PESTICIDES RECOGNIZED AS ANIMAL CARCINOGENS

As discussed earlier, epidemiologic information on carcinogenicity is constrained by the small populations with unique exposures to specific pesticides. Consequently, animal test data represent the only means for evaluating the effect of most compounds.

The EPA's scientific advisory panel devised a system for summarizing the large volume of cancer bioassay data in 1986. The system differentiates among the small number of compounds recognized to definitely cause cancer in humans, those likely to cause cancer in sufficiently exposed populations, possible carcinogens, and those unlikely to cause cancer. The panel revised the system again in 1996 and in 1999. The final result resembles both the 1986 EPA classification system and that used by the International Agency for Research on Cancer (IARC) (Table 31–5). The current list of carcinogens available from the EPA principally employs the 1986 system because the agency has reviewed relatively few individual compounds since the 1999 classifi-

Table 31–5. EPA versus IARC schemes for classification of carcinogens.[1]

	1986 Classification	1999 Classification	IARC Classification
Group A	Human carcinogen	Carcinogenic to humans	Group 1: The agent (mixture) is carcinogenic to humans
Group B	Probable human carcinogen	Likely to be carcinogenic to humans	Group 2A: The agent (mixture) is probably carcinogenic to humans
Group B1	Agents for which there is limited evidence of carcinogenicity from epidemiologic studies		
Group B2	Agents for which there is sufficient evidence from animal studies and for which there is inadequate evidence or no data from epidemiologic studies		
Group C	Possible human carcinogen	Likely to be carcinogenic to humans	Group 2B: The agent (mixture) is possibly carcinogenic to humans
Group D	Not classifiable as to human carcinogenicity	Data are inadequate for an assessment of human carcinogenic potential	Group 3: The agent (mixture, exposure circumstance) is not classifiable as to its carcinogenicity
Group E	Evidence of noncarcinogenicity for humans	Not likely to be carcinogenic to humans	Group 4: The agent (mixture, exposure circumstance) is probably not carcinogenic to humans

[1]List of Chemicals Evaluated for Carcinogenic Potential, 2006, available online at: http://www.epa.gov/pesticides/carlist/, and http://monographs.iarc.fr/.

cation changes. The sections below contain data on individual compounds and classes of compounds.

Data on the fungicide captan illustrate the principles of classification for probable carcinogens. Male and female rats fed ad libitum on a diet containing 8000 ppm captan [presumably a maximum tolerated dose (MTD)] for 21 weeks and containing 4000 ppm for an additional 59 weeks showed increased levels of benign and malignant endocrine tumors. Female mice also had increased numbers of neoplasms in the mammary glands, ovaries, and livers. Male rats also demonstrated testicular atrophy. Similar findings occurred in animals treated at 50% MTD dose. Mice fed on diets containing either 8000 or 16,000 ppm captan showed increased levels of duodenal neoplasms. In a separate study, male rats (70 per treatment group) fed captan at doses of 0, 25, 100, or 250 mg/kg per day for 2 years showed a slight but apparently dose-related increase in duodenal neoplasms with a tumor incidence of 1/70, 1/70, 3/70, and 4/70 in increasing dosage groups. Based on the demonstration of cancer effect in two rodent species at both the MTD and 50% of the MTD, captan is classified as a probable human carcinogen.

Compounds producing tumors only at the MTD in a single species are classified as class C or class D depending on the quality of the study demonstrating the effect. For example, the fungicide fosetyl-Al (Aliette or aluminum tris-[-O-ethyl-phosphonate]) received a group C classification because of benign and malignant urinary bladder tumors in a study involving male Charles River rats feeding ad libitum on food containing between 30,000 and 40,000 ppm. No tumors were seen in female rats in this study, nor in mice tested in another study (2500, 10,000, or 20,000/30,000 ppm). Because fosetyl-Al is a relatively simple compound, structurally unrelated to known classes of bladder carcinogens (aniline dyes or polynuclear aromatic hydrocarbons), the observed tumors probably represent no significance for human health.

C. STRUCTURAL ELEMENTS RELATED TO THE OCCURRENCE OF CANCER

Because of the complexity of carcinogenesis, its mechanisms remain incompletely understood. Nevertheless, evaluations of structural elements associated with positive animal bioassays have been studied for some time. Many animal carcinogens are potent electrophiles or have electrophilic metabolic activation products.

Data on the carcinogenicity of aromatic amines illustrate the current approach to modeling structure-activity relationships. Important parameters include fat solubility [as characterized by the octanol/water partition coefficient (log p)], the energy of the highest occupied and lowest unoccupied molecular orbitals, and the polarizability of substituent amino (NH_2) groups. These factors to some degree correspond with the elements in the scheme described earlier for predicting dermal irritation and allergenicity. As illustrated by data on fungicides such as chlorothalonil, many animal carcinogens also cause skin irritation, allergy, or both.

Male Reproductive Toxins

Identification of sterility related to the soil nematocide DBCP remains a landmark in the study of male reproductive toxicology. DBCP has moderate toxicity by oral administration (oral LD_{50} 100 mg/kg) and low dermal toxicity (dermal LD_{50} 1400 mg/kg). Although not producing other acute or subacute effects, rabbits inhaling 1.0 ppm DBCP for 14 weeks (estimated 490 mg/kg cumulative dose) showed reversible testicular effects. Rats also showed infertility after repeated exposures by gavage or injection (cumulative doses of 60 mg/kg or higher). Biochemical effects of the DBCP treatments include increases in leuteinizing hormone (LH) and follicle-stimulating hormone (FSH).

The clinical findings in the DBCP animal studies exactly mirror the effect of DBCP on humans. The dermal exposures most commonly occurring in the formulation of DBCP did not produce acute effects, but the effect on sperm production was proportional to the duration of exposure. Specific metabolic changes associated with DBCP include decreased metabolism of glucose by sperm cells and unscheduled DNA synthesis. Nevertheless, the mechanism of the toxic effect of DBCP on germinal epithelium remains incompletely understood. Crucial endpoints in the animal studies on DBCP include sperm count, sperm morphology, and histology of testicular seminiferous tubules and epididymis. Data on male reproductive compounds of other pesticides are discussed in sections on use categories and individual classes of compounds.

Studies of the cumulative effect of environmental as opposed to occupational exposure to pesticides have been reported recently. A 2004 study of men evaluated at a Massachusetts fertility clinic looked at sperm quality in relationship to presence of urinary metabolites of two cholinesterase-inhibiting insecticides: carbaryl and chlorpyrifos. The authors reported increased odds of below-normal sperm count associated increased levels of the carbaryl urinary metabolite 1-naphthol. [For low, medium, and high levels of 1-naphthol, the odds ratios (ORs) for decreased sperm count in the low, medium, and high groups were equal to 1.0, 4.2, and 4.2, respectively; p value for trend = 0.01.] These results were considered consistent with a 1981 study of workers formulating carbaryl, a group that presumably had markedly higher exposure than the participants in the 2004 study. The study showed a significantly higher level of abnormal sperm morphology in 50 carbaryl workers compared with 34 control subjects employed at the same plant.

A 2003 case-control study nested within a larger population fertility study (Study for Future Families)

evaluated urinary pesticide metabolites in relationship to subjects in Missouri and Minnesota with high (control) and low (case) mean sperm concentrations. No association with urinary 1-naphthol was found in either state. However, the case subjects from Missouri had high levels of metabolites for three herbicides (alachlor, metolachlor, and atrazine), as well as for the insecticide diazinon. Levels for all metabolites were comparable for Missouri control subjects and for both case and control subjects in Minnesota. The authors were not able to identify the source of exposure to the pesticide in question or rule out a multicomparison effect as the explanation for the study findings. They also acknowledged that the short biologic half-life of the pesticides evaluated relative to the approximately 2-month process of spermatogenesis strongly suggests that the metabolites measured were surrogate measures of some other exposure.

REFERENCES

Alavanja MC, Bonner MR: Pesticides and human cancers. Cancer Invest 2005;23:700 [PMID: 16377589].

Bhatia R et al: Organochlorine pesticides and male genital anomalies in the child health and development studies. Environ Health Perspect 2005;113:220 [PMID: 15687061].

Burns CJ: Cancer among pesticide manufacturers and applicators. Scand J Work Environ Health 2005;31:9 [PMID: 16190144].

John D et al: The relationship of urinary metabolites of carbaryl/naphthalene and chlorpyrifos with human semen quality. Environ Health Perspect 2004;112:1665 [PMID: 15579410].

Nelson NJ: Studies examine whether persistent organic agents may be responsible for rise in lymphoma rates. J Natl Cancer Inst 2005;97:1490 [PMID: 16234557].

ORGANOPHOSPHATE & CARBAMATE CHOLINESTERASE-INHIBITING INSECTICIDES

Essentials of Diagnosis

A. Acute Effects

- Acetylcholinesterase inhibition, acetylcholine excess
- Parasympathetic nervous system hyperactivity, neuromuscular paralysis, central nervous system dysfunction, and depression of red cell and plasma cholinesterase activity
- Irritant dermatitis from organophosphate compounds with irritant substructures in their nonphosphate portion (leaving groups, e.g., vinyl halogen compounds)

B. Chronic Effects

- Persistent central nervous system (CNS) dysfunction (organophosphates): irritability, anxiety, mood labil-

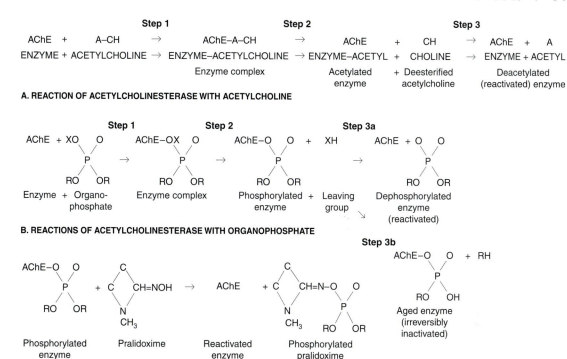

Figure 31–1. A. Reaction of acetylcholinesterase with acetylcholine. **B.** Reactions of acetylcholinesterase with orga-nophosphate. **C.** Reactivation of acetylcholinesterase by pralidoxime.

ity, fatigue, impaired short-term memory, and im-paired concentration for weeks or months after acute pesticide exposure; subclinical neurobehavioral ef-fects in multiple studies

- Organophosphate-induced delayed neuropathy: rapid onset of distal symmetric sensorimotor neuropathy

General Considerations

Organophosphates are esters of phosphoric acid that exist in two forms: -thion and -oxon. The latter is shown in Figure 31–1B. Potency depends on the three-dimensional shape of individual compounds and their ability to bind with the cholinesterase molecule. Irre-versible binding occurs with a serine molecule in the heart of the enzyme's active site and the nonphosphate portion of the molecule (leaving group) cleaved by hydrolysis. Under most circumstances, the inhibition becomes irreversible after 24–48 hours.

Carbamates are esters of carbamic acid. The organo-phosphates and *n*-methyl carbamates are considered here as a single class because they share a common mechanism of acute toxicity cholinesterase inhibition, with similar signs and symptoms of acute poisoning.

Carbamates differ in causing reversible rather than irre-versible cholinesterase inhibition and typically have a short clinical course. The thiocarbamates and dithiocar-bamates do not inhibit cholinesterase, but many have activity against plants and fungi.

Together the carbamates and organophosphates rep-resent one of the largest and most important classes of insecticides. Table 31–6 lists commonly used com-pounds according to acute toxicity. They vary widely in their cholinesterase-inhibiting potency, as reflected in their LD_{50} values.

As a result of their widespread use and acute toxicity, the organophosphates and carbamates are common causes of acute insecticide intoxication. Cholinesterase inhibi-tors produce a relatively stereotypical clinical presentation that in conjunction with determination of cholinesterase levels makes diagnosis more accurate than with other pes-ticides. Specific and nonspecific antidotes are available for treatment. A percentage of patients acutely poisoned by organophosphates display persistent CNS dysfunction for weeks or months after acute poisoning. A small number of organophosphate pesticides also cause a delayed neu-ropathy that is correlated with inhibition of the enzyme neurotoxic esterase (Table 31–7).

Table 31–6. Organophosphate and carbamate insecticides.

Common Name	Trade Name	Oral LD$_{50}$ (mg/kg)	Dermal LD$_{50}$ (mg/kg)

Organophosphates:
  Category I
  Parathion
		1–5	1–10

Mevinphos	Phosdrin	1–5	1–10
Methyl parathion		5–10	50–100
Carbophenothion	Trithion	5–10	20
EPN		5–10	20
Methamidophos	Monitor	10–20	100
Azinphos-methyl	Guthion	10–20	200
Methidathion	Supracide	20–30	400
Dichlorvos (DDVP)	Vapona	20–30	50–100

Organophosphates:
  Category II
  Chlorpyrifos
	Dursban
	Lorsban
		50–150	2000

Diazinon	Spectracide	50–150	400
Phosmet	Imidan	50–150	3000
Dimethoate	Cygon	150–500	150
Fenthion	Baytex	150–500	
Naled	Dibrom	150–500	1000
Trichlorion	Dipterex	150–500	2000
Organophosphates: Categories III and IV Acephate	Orthene	500–1000	2000
Malathion		500–1000	4000
Stirofos Gardona (tetrachlorvinphos)	Rabon	1000–5000	5000
Carbamates			
Aldicarb	Temik	1–5	1–10
Carbofuran	Furadan	5–10	>1000
Methomyl	Lannate	15–25	1000
Propoxur	Baygon	100	1000
Bandiocarb	Ficam	100–200	566
Carbaryl	Sevin	300–600	2000

Use

Organophosphate pesticides were developed following World War II as a consequence of the synthesis of the organophosphate nerve gases sarin, soman, and tabun. During the 1950s and 1960s, they began replacing inorganic pesticides and organochlorines as the principal insecticides used in agriculture. Mevinphos and ethyl parathion, two of the most toxic organophosphates, were prohibited from use in the United States during the 1990s. Subsequent to passage of the FQPA (see above), organophosphates have been replaced by pyrethroids for termiticide applications and for crops destined to be used in processed foods. California agricultural use statistics demonstrate reported use of cholinesterase-inhibiting insecticides decreased from 16,045,617 pounds in 1994 to 7,891,332 pounds in 2003. Over the same time interval, illnesses related to cholinesterase inhibitors reported to the California illness registry decreased from 363 cases (in 1994) to 62 cases (reported in 2003).

Table 31–7. Commonly used organophosphate pesticides with evidence for delayed neuropathy in humans and animals.

Compound	In Humans	In Animals
Trichlorphon	+	+
Merphos (Folex)	+	+
O-Ethyl-O-p-nitrophenyl-benzene-thiophosphonate (EPN)	?	+
Methamidophos	?	+
Fenthion	?	?
Trichloronate	NR	+
S,S,S-Tributyl phosphorotri-thioate (DEF)	NR	+
Diisopropylfluorophosphate (DFP)	NR	+
Dichlorvos	NR	?

NR = not reported; ? = uncertain; + = reliably reported.

A number of organophosphates are systemic insecticides, a property that correlates to some extent with the water solubility (sol) of individual compounds. Examples include demeton [sol 3.3 g/L at 20°C (68°F)], dimethoate [sol 25 g/L at 21°C (69.8°F)], disulfoton [sol 25 mg/L at 23°C (73.4°F)], phosphamidon, and trichlorphon [sol 120,000 mg/L at 20°C (68°F)].

Many are highly toxic and therefore restricted but still used extensively in agriculture (e.g., methyl parathion). However, even the low toxicity compounds such as diazanon and malathion are no longer sold for household use. Chlorpyrifos was perhaps the insecticide used most frequently by structural pest control operators against cockroaches and other structural pests, but its household use has also been curtailed under FQPA regulations.

A. CARBAMATES

The cholinesterase-inhibiting *n*-methyl carbamates have insecticidal properties. Carbaryl is used extensively because of its slow mammalian toxicity and relatively wide spectrum of activity. Aldicarb (sol 6000 mg/L), carbofuran (sol 320 mg/L), and methomyl (sol 57.9 g/L) are highly water-soluble, systemic insecticides with use limited to agriculture. Illegal applications of these compounds do occur occasionally in urban settings. Propoxur is used by structural pest control operators and in ready-to-use home formulations.

Occupational & Environmental Exposure

Organophosphates and carbamates are applied by a variety of techniques from aerial spraying to hand application. Granular and bait formulations significantly reduce exposure so that even hypertoxic compounds such as aldicarb (0.5 mg/kg) can be used safely given ordinary precautions.

Organophosphate compounds show variable dissipation times. Compounds with high vapor pressures, including dichlorvos, naled, and mevinphos, have environmental half-lives measured in hours and may dissipate completely in less than 24 hours. Residues of dimethoate (LD_{50} 180–330 mg/kg) have an environmental half-life ranging from 24–48 hours. Phosalone (LD_{50} 82–205 mg/kg) residues, by contrast, have half-lives of 30 days or longer. Many organophosphates degrade rapidly in wet coastal environments but may persistent for prolonged periods in hot, dry climates. Consequently, long reentry intervals (e.g., 90 days or more for ethyl parathion on San Joaquin Valley citrus crops) have proved necessary to prevent acute poisoning of field workers.

The risk posed by a given level of residue depends on the crop and work activity. Residues of 7 μg/cm² of phosalone, for example, cause no cholinesterase inhibition in workers picking citrus and peaches. Levels less than 1 μg/cm² are associated with poisoning of workers

harvesting wine and raisin grapes. A dermal residue transfer coefficient (in units of cm²/h) is used to summarize the relative levels of exposure associated with various agricultural tasks. Among various hand-harvested crops, transfer factors ranged from 5000–9000 cm²/h for row crops to 10,000 cm²/h for orchard crops and up 130,000 cm²/h for hand-labor tasks (cane turning) in production of table grapes.

The available literature contains comparatively few studies on dissipation of carbamate compounds. Environmental fate data required by EPA include basic physical and chemical properties such as the Henry law constant, vapor pressure, water solubility, ultraviolet spectra, and residue data at time of harvest but not residue dissipation studies. However, summary values exist for carbaryl, aldicarb, propoxur, and carbofuran. For propoxur, residual systemic activity has been reported for up to 1 month. Data on carbaryl do not give a half-life but indicate that residues generally dissipate in less than 2 weeks. The half-life of carbofuran leaf residue is reported as longer than 4 days. Aldicarb presents a complicated picture because of its tendency to leach into groundwater. Plants convert aldicarb to systemic sulfoxide and sulfone transformation products, previously associated with episodes of consumer poisoning from watermelons and cucumbers. Variability in dissipation observed in extensive studies on methomyl suggests the need for caution in generalizing from limited data. A study in California established a 0.1 μg/cm² safe-level for hand labor in methomyl treated vineyards. Residue monitoring later revealed much longer dissipation times. It was therefore necessary to adjust the hand labor re-entry interval from 7 days to 21 days.

Mechanism of Action & Clinical Findings

Organophosphates and carbamates are absorbed easily by inhalation, skin contact, and ingestion; the primary route of occupational exposure is dermal. They differ from one another in lipid solubility and therefore distribution in the body, particularly to the CNS.

Many commercial organophosphates are applied in the -thion (sulfur-containing) form but readily undergo conversion to the -oxon (oxygen-containing) form (see Figure 31–1B). Most of the -oxon forms have much greater toxicity than their corresponding -thion analogues. The conversion occurs in the environment, so the residues that crop field workers are exposed to may be more toxic than the pesticide that was applied. Some of the sulfur is released in the form of mercaptans, which produce the typical odor of the -thion form of organophosphates. The mercaptans have very low odor thresholds, and the reactions to their noxious odor, including headache, nausea, and vomiting, often are mistaken for acute organophosphate poisoning.

Table 31–8. Signs and symptoms of acute organophosphate poisoning by site of acetylcholine neurotransmitter activity.

System	Receptor Type	Organ	Action	Sign or Symptom
Parasympathetic	Muscarinic	Eye, iris muscle, ciliary muscle	Contraction	Miosis
Sympathetic			Contraction	Blurred vision
		Glands: lacrimal, salivary	Secretion	Tearing, salivation, bronchorrhea, pulmonary edema, nausea, vomiting
		Heart: sinus node	Slowing, refractory	Bradycardia, arrhythmias, heart block
		Smooth muscle: bronchial, gastrointestinal	Contraction	Bronchoconstriction
		Wall, sphincter	Contraction, relaxation	Vomiting, cramps, diarrhea
		Bladder, fundus, sphincter	Contraction, relaxation	Urination, incontinence
Neuromuscular	Nicotinic	Skeletal	Excitation	Fasciculations, cramps, followed by weakness, loss of reflexes, paralysis
Central nervous		Brain	Excitation (early)	Headache, dizziness, malaise, apprehension, confusion, hallucinations, manic or bizarre behavior, convulsions
			Depression (late)	Depression of, then loss of, consciousness; respiratory depression

The conversion from -thion to -oxon also occurs in vivo as a result of hepatic microsomal metabolism, so the -oxon becomes the active form of the pesticide in both animal pests and humans. Hepatic esterases rapidly hydrolyze organophosphate esters, yielding alkyl phosphates and phenols, which have little, if any, toxicologic activity and are excreted rapidly. Carbamates also are metabolized by the liver and excreted as metabolites in urine without evidence of significant accumulation.

Organophosphates and carbamates exert effects on insects and mammals, including humans, by inhibiting acetylcholinesterase at nerve endings. The normal function of acetylcholinesterase is the hydrolysis and inactivation of acetylcholine (see Figure 31–1A). Figure 31–1B shows the reactions of organophosphates and acetylcholinesterase. The enzyme then can be dephosphorylated spontaneously and reactivated (step 3a) or aged through the hydrolysis of an alkyl (—R) group, resulting in irreversible inactivation.

Carbamates initially react with acetylcholinesterase in the same fashion as organophosphates, resulting in accumulation of acetylcholine in the same distribution as organophosphates. The carbamyl enzyme product does not progress to an aging reaction but instead dissociates relatively rapidly. As a family, the carbamates have no known health effects other than those resulting from this acute, reversible inhibition of cholinesterase and resulting overactivity of acetylcholine.

The clinical manifestations of acute organophosphate or carbamate poisoning reflect the organs where acetylcholine is the transmitter of nerve impulses, (see Table 31–8). Rapid rates of cholinesterase inhibition are associated with clinical illness at levels of inhibition that may not be associated with symptoms following slower rates of inhibition. Asymptomatic subacute inhibition of acetylcholinesterase results in a state in which exposure to a dose of an organophosphate that previously would have had no effect now may lower acetylcholinesterase levels below a critical threshold and result in clinical illness. This type of cumulative inhibition of acetylcholinesterase is unlikely to occur from carbamates owing to the rapidly reversible nature of the enzyme inhibition.

For a large proportion of patients with acute intoxication, the clinician will not know the identity of the particular pesticide or pesticides at the time of initial presentation, and decisions regarding diagnosis and management will need to be made on the basis of clinical signs, symptoms, and laboratory data.

The only known systemic health effect of organophosphate pesticides that is entirely unrelated to cholinesterase inhibition is organophosphate-induced delayed neuropathy. Inhibition of an enzyme known as *neuro-*

toxic esterase (NTE), found in the central and peripheral nervous systems of various species, is an indicator of neurotoxic potential and a potential tool for biologic monitoring. Animal studies indicate that irreversible inhibition of NTE to 75% of initial activity will be followed 10–14 days later by a rapidly progressive ascending peripheral neuropathy. Currently used organophosphate pesticides with evidence of neurotoxicity (see Table 31–7) include such weak cholinesterase inhibitors as merphos (*S,S,S*-tri-*n*-butyl phosphorotrithioite) and DEF (*S,S,S*-tri-*n*-butyl phosphorotrithioate), which are used as cotton defoliants rather than as insecticides.

A. SYMPTOMS & SIGNS

Despite the popularity of mnemonics such as MUDDLES (miosis, urination, diarrhea, defecation, diaphoresis, lacrimation, excitation, and salivation), the signs and symptoms of acute intoxication with organophosphates and carbamates are best learned on a neurophysiologic basis by grouping them according to the affected class of cholinergic receptor (see Table 31–8). There is some variability in parasympathetic nervous system manifestations because they are opposed by the sympathetic nervous system, which has preganglionic cholinergic innervation. Thus the heart rate may be slow, normal, or fast and the pupils may be small, normal, or large depending on which system predominates. In one large series of organophosphate-poisoned patients, 90% had at least muscarinic manifestations, 40% both muscarinic and nicotinic manifestations, 30% had muscarinic and CNS manifestations, and 10% had all three. The number of systems involved increases with the severity of intoxication. Mild poisoning usually is manifested by mild muscarinic signs and symptoms only.

The cause of death in acute organophosphate poisoning usually is respiratory failure. Bronchorrhea or pulmonary edema, bronchoconstriction, and respiratory muscular paralysis all contribute to respiratory failure. Cardiac arrhythmias, such as heart block and cardiac arrest, are less common causes of death. Ventricular arrhythmias have been observed in some of these cases. Seizures are not uncommon in cases of severe poisoning but rarely persist long enough to require treatment. Severe poisoning from occupational exposure to carbamates is uncommon. Owing to the rapid spontaneous reactivation of acetyl cholinesterase, workers who become ill on the job are often better by the time they are seen at a medical facility.

B. LABORATORY FINDINGS

1. Cholinesterase—A number of nonspecific laboratory findings may be present in an individual with acute poisoning, including leukocytosis, proteinuria, glucosuria, and hemoconcentration. However, changes in cholines-

terase activity, along with the typical signs and symptoms, provide sufficient information for the diagnosis and management of most cases. Red cell cholinesterase is called "true" cholinesterase because it is the same enzyme present in nerve endings and because its activity more closely parallels that in the nervous system than does plasma cholinesterase, particularly in the time course of recovery, after inhibition. However, red cell cholinesterase is more difficult to measure and therefore more susceptible to analytic error than plasma cholinesterase. Organophosphates and carbamates may differentially inhibit one enzyme relative to the other, so if one and not the other appears depressed, it is conservative to assume that neuronal cholinesterase more closely corresponds to the lower of the two. For example, the commonly used organophosphate chlorpyrifos (Dursban, Lorsban) preferentially depresses plasma cholinesterase, causing illness without significant depression of red cell cholinesterase.

A number of analytic methods are used to measure both red cell and plasma cholinesterase. Results obtained by one method usually cannot be compared with results from another, even if the units expressed by each are the same. There is considerable variability in cholinesterase activity in unexposed persons, so reports of results relative to "normal" may not reflect the true level of inhibition present.

Individuals with a genetic trait for atypical plasma cholinesterase have lowered plasma but not red cell cholinesterase. They have prolonged muscular paralysis after administration of succinyl choline and other neuromuscular blocking agents that are normally metabolized by plasma cholinesterase, but they are not more susceptible to cholinesterase-inhibiting pesticides. Unlike red cell cholinesterase, plasma cholinesterase is not a reliable indicator of exposure or poisoning in these individuals.

Plasma cholinesterase production may be lowered as a result of liver disease extensive enough to impair the production of proteins such as albumin. Albumin-losing conditions, such as nephrotic syndrome, may be accompanied by elevated levels of plasma cholinesterase as a result of increased hepatic protein synthesis. The only medical conditions known to influence red cell cholinesterase activity are those associated with reticulocytosis, such as recovery from hemorrhage, pernicious anemia, and some other anemias.

Two circumstances in which cholinesterase determinations may be useful are (1) routine biologic monitoring of exposure to organophosphates and (2) diagnosis of acute poisoning. In assessing exposure to carbamates, cholinesterase depression may prove difficult to document unless treatment facilities can run cholinesterase assays on-site shortly after phlebotomy.

Severe poisoning usually is accompanied by cholinesterase levels well below normal for the laboratory. However, patients with mild to moderate poisoning often have cholinesterase levels reported as equivocal, normal, and even above normal. The diagnosis can be confirmed retrospectively by periodic (i.e., weekly or biweekly) determinations of cholinesterase until levels fluctuate by no more than 30%. If the average level at this time—the *retrospective baseline*—is more than 30% higher than the level at the time of illness, exposure to cholinesterase-inhibiting pesticides almost certainly was present, and the illness may have been due to that exposure. The rate of recovery of red cell cholinesterase, in the absence of treatment with pralidoxime and of further exposure, depends on the rate of formation of new red cells, which is approximately 1% per day. Red blood cell cholinesterase levels will reach a plateau in about 60–70 days and plasma cholinesterase in 30–50 days.

2. Intact pesticides and metabolites—Measurement of the parent organophosphate or carbamate, or their metabolites, in blood or urine has been investigated to a limited extent. No such measurements are currently likely to be helpful in the diagnosis of acute intoxication. Measurement of alkyl phosphate metabolites in urine has not been of use in biologic monitoring of exposure because of its lack of specificity and instability. Measurement of *p*-nitrophenol in urine can be useful for monitoring exposure to parathion; 0.5 mg/L in a sample collected at the end of an exposure interval corresponds to exposure to parathion at the current threshold limit value (TLV). Measurement of 1-naphthol in urine is used to monitor exposure to carbaryl.

Differential Diagnosis

Mild acute poisoning from organophosphates or carbamates most closely resembles acute viral influenza, respiratory infections, gastroenteritis, asthma, or psychological dysfunction. The most significant differential diagnosis is between severe organophosphate poisoning and acute cerebrovascular accident; unequal pupils caused by the local effect of a direct-inhibiting (oxon) organophosphate or *n*-methyl carbamate in one eye of a comatose patient is a potential source of misdiagnosis. Other conditions to be distinguished from acute organophosphate poisoning include heat stroke, heat exhaustion, and infections.

As noted earlier, the major disorder to be distinguished from organophosphate-induced delayed neuropathy is idiopathic acute symmetric polyneuropathy. Other toxic and disease-related neuropathies generally are insidious in onset and slowly progressive in course.

Treatment

Treatment that is otherwise indicated should never be delayed pending determination of cholinesterase levels. The initial diagnosis can be made on clinical grounds alone, samples sent to the laboratory, and a test dose of atropine delivered. Atropine blocks the effects of acetylcholine at muscarinic receptors. A dose of atropine sulfate (0.5 mg intravenously) produces signs of mild atropinization (i.e., dry mouth, dry eyes, increased heart rate, and large pupils) in a normal adult; it has no effect in an individual with organophosphate poisoning. A dose of 1–2 mg intravenously will produce marked signs of atropinization in a nonpoisoned adult and may reverse the signs of cholinergic excess in a case of poisoning.

Samples must be sent for cholinesterase measurement before administration of pralidoxime, which will regenerate cholinesterase in red cells and plasma as well as nerves. Atropine has no effect on cholinesterase levels.

Treatment of acute intoxication must be predicated on assessment of the severity of poisoning, which largely depends on clinical judgment and experience. For some occupational poisonings, removal from further exposure to cholinesterase-inhibiting insecticides may prove to be the only treatment necessary. Treatment with specific antidotes should be reserved for patients observed in the hospital setting.

Assessment of severity should focus primarily on the respiratory system because it is affected by all three types of cholinergic sites and is the critical one for survival and serious morbidity. The most commonly used severity rating defines mild toxicity as involving only muscarinic signs and symptoms, moderate toxicity as involving more than one system but not requiring assisted breathing, and severe toxicity as requiring ventilatory assistance.

Treatment modalities include the following:

1. Decontamination, including bathing of skin, shampooing of hair, or emptying of stomach, as dictated by route of exposure.

2. Atropine sulfate in a dosage of 1–2 mg intravenously for mild to moderate poisoning, 2–4 mg intravenously for severe poisoning, as often as every 15 minutes, as needed. There is no maximum dosage. Atropine blocks muscarinic activity but not the nicotinic (muscle paralysis) or CNS effects. Patients without evidence of muscle weakness or respiratory depression may be treated with atropine alone until one or more signs of mild atropinization appear (i.e., tachycardia, flushing, dry mucous membranes, or dilated pupils). Multiple doses may need to be administered over a prolonged time.

3. For organophosphate poisoning only, give pralidoxime chloride (2-PAM, Protopam) slowly, 1 g intravenously (no more than 0.5 g/min), repeated once in 1–2 hours and then at 10- to 12-hour intervals, if needed. Pralidoxime acts by breaking the bond between acetylcholinesterase and organophosphate, reactivating the enzyme and restoring

acetylcholine activity to normal (see Figure 31–1C). Its advantages over atropine include acting at the neuromuscular junction to reverse muscular paralysis and possibly crossing the blood-brain barrier to reverse CNS depression. Overdosage is not a problem if the drug is administered slowly to avoid inducing hypotension. The decision to use pralidoxime must be made reasonably soon after diagnosis because it is ineffective once aging has occurred. A high incidence of atropine toxicity may result from the often-recommended regimen of first using atropine until primary signs of atropine toxicity appear and then using pralidoxime if necessary. This may be avoided by making the decision to use pralidoxime early.

4. Artificial ventilation, ventilatory assistance, oxygen, and clearance of secretions.

The use of pralidoxime for carbamate poisoning is controversial. Fortunately, it is rarely indicated. There is experimental evidence that pralidoxime may be helpful in the management of poisoning by some rarely used carbamates, but for most of the commonly used carbamates, this drug has not been studied. One animal study indicated that pralidoxime may be harmful in the treatment of carbaryl poisoning.

Morphine, aminophylline, and phenothiazines are contraindicated because of the increased risk of cardiac arrhythmias. Diuretics for pulmonary edema and fluids for hypotension are also contraindicated. It is recommended that atropine be withheld until adequate ventilation has reversed hypoxia because atropine may generate arrhythmias in the presence of hypoxia.

By the time the diagnosis of organophosphate-induced delayed peripheral neuropathy is made, the initial manifestations of cholinesterase inhibition, if present, have resolved. Administration of atropine or pralidoxime, initially or later, does not influence the course of neuropathy. Treatment of delayed neuropathy is supportive; in a few cases, mechanical ventilation has been required because of respiratory failure caused by muscular paralysis.

Prognosis

If treatment for organophosphate or carbamate poisoning is initiated before hypoxia results in tissue damage, antidotal therapy and respiratory support should ensure complete recovery, even in the most severe cases. Persistence of manifestations beyond 24 hours indicates the possibility of continued absorption of pesticide and the need to carefully consider and examine the skin, fingernails, eyes, and gastrointestinal tract as possible reservoirs.

Sudden death occurs in a small percentage of organophosphate-poisoned patients (2% in one series) 24–

48 hours after apparent complete recovery from the acute phase of poisoning and is caused by, in at least some cases, ventricular arrhythmia. Sudden relapse of acute signs and symptoms within a few days of apparent recovery has been reported occasionally, perhaps as a result of release of pesticide from fat following mobilization of the patient from bed.

Deaths have been reported as a result of accidental or deliberate ingestion of carbamates, as a result of large doses and prolonged gastrointestinal absorption, and perhaps as a complication of delayed or inadequate treatment. Intoxication from occupational exposure may be serious but is rarely fatal and usually is of brief duration. Poisoning from contaminated fruits and vegetables with high water content also may be serious but not persistent.

A number of reports describe persistent CNS symptoms in a small percentage of patients following well-documented incidents of acute poisoning from organophosphates but not carbamates. Typical symptoms include irritability, depression, mood lability, anxiety, fatigue, lethargy, difficulty in concentrating, and short-term memory loss. Limited studies suggest that neurobehavioral test results and electroencephalograms may be different for such patients when compared with controls. Symptoms may persist for weeks or months after the initial intoxication and are difficult to distinguish from psychological reactions likely to occur after such an event. Sympathetic counseling and judicious use of antianxiety agents, when appropriate, generally will be more effective than intensive psychotherapy and antipsychotic medicine.

Skin Effects

Organophosphates generally have high octanol/water partition coefficients and high dermal absorption rates, but most cause minimal skin irritation. Skin effects derive from the reactivity of the nonphosphate portion (termed the *leaving group*) of individual compounds. For example, the irritant compounds dichlorvos and naled both have reactive halogen atoms (reactive element IX described earlier) in their leaving groups. Dichlorvos also has an unconjugated carbon-carbon bond–reactive element (ICONJ). Some organophosphate formulations produce transient irritation in the Draize assay, including acephate, diazinon, dimethoate, malathion, methamidophos, methidathion, oxydemeton-methyl, phosmet, and sulfotep; many cause mild primary irritation in the challenge (epicutaneous) phase of the guinea pig maximization test. Clinically, acute irritation with these compounds occurs most frequently with accidental direct exposure to pesticide handlers (mixer/loader/applicators). These types of exposures also may provoke systemic effects; in 202 cases of organophosphate-associated dermatitis reported from Japan, approximately 25% had at least mild coincident symptoms of systemic poisoning. Systemic poisoning also was reported in a case of irritant dermatitis caused by dichlorvos.

Buehler (epicutaneous) sensitization assays show negative findings for acephate, chlorpyrifos, dimethoate, malathion, methamidophos, methidathion, and phosmet. Nevertheless, several are sensitizers in the guinea pig maximization test (induction of allergy by subcutaneous injection), including diazinon, fenitrothion, and methidathion. Cases of possible contact sensitivity to organophosphates have been reported for omethoate and dimethoate. A case-control study of dermatitis in farmers identified allergic reactions to malathion and oxydemeton-methyl, as well as the carbamate compounds carbofuran and carbaryl. Further studies identified allergic contact dermatitis caused by malathion and naled, but the patch testing conducted did not meet current standards, especially with regard to identifying nonirritant concentrations to conduct of the patch procedure.

A case report from Australia identified an isomer and contaminant of diazinon called *isodiazinon* (2-isopropyl-6-methyl-4-*S*-pyrimidinyl diethylthiophosphate) as a possible cause of porphyria cutanea tarda in a sheep rancher. Investigation in a rat study showed that isodiazinon affected porphyrin synthesis by inhibiting the liver enzyme ferrochelatase. Other noncontact reactions include a case of erythema multiforme associated with indoor use of methyl parathion, an unusual contact reaction to ethyl parathion resembling erysipeloid, and a case of systemic organophosphate poisoning.

Chronic Health Effects

A. NEUROBEHAVIORAL EFFECTS

Conjectured persistent sequelae of organophosphate poisoning remains a subject of controversy. Numerous studies document subclinical neurobehavioral deficits relative to control subjects in previously poisoned workers and to a lesser extent in workers with applicators with long-term exposures who never experienced acute poisoning. The recorded deficits include vibrotactile sensitivity, decreased sustained attention, and decreased speed of information processing, memory and abstraction, and cognitive tests.

Poisoning by the organophosphate nerve agent sarin produced persistent neurobehavioral deficits, including significant amnesia in some victims of the 1995 terrorist attack on the Tokyo subway. The most severe deficits were seen in patients who experienced prolonged hypoxia. Cases of posttraumatic stress also occurred. Findings in less severely poisoned cases more closely resembled those seen in studies of applicators poisoned by organophosphate insecticides.

Studies of workers who handled organosphosphates without a history of overt poisoning show less consistent findings of subclinical neurobehavioral impairment. A British study of sheep dippers handling organophosphates showed findings similar to the studies of overtly poisoned workers. Other studies of nonpoisoned organophosphate handlers demonstrated equivocal or negative findings.

Although none of the studies of poisoned workers shows significant clinical impairment, all involve cross-sectional measurement of neurobehavioral function, most less than 10 years after poisoning. From currently available information, it cannot be ascertained if the subclinical deficits observed eventually might progress to clinically significant impairments. The Maastricht study of aging did show an association between pesticide exposure recorded at the outset of the study and mild cognitive defects recorded 3 years subsequently but did not identify exposures to particular pesticides or classes of pesticides.

B. REACTIVE AIRWAYS

Possible reactive airways cases, an asthma-like respiratory condition that occurs in some individuals exposed to environmental irritants, are commonly diagnosed by means of a specialized pulmonary function test called a *methacholine challenge*. Occasionally, cases of reactive airways disease or new-onset asthma are associated with organophosphate exposure or organophosphate contaminants. A cross-sectional study of applicators working in the Canadian grain industry showed an association between asthma and exposure to carbofuran, although confounding from grain dust exposure could not be completely eliminated as an explanation. A separate report on the same study identified an association between asthma and carbamate insecticides as a class.

C. CARCINOGENICITY, TERATOGENICITY, AND MALE REPRODUCTIVE TOXICITY

1. Carcinogenicity—Most of the carbamates and organophosphates show no evidence of carcinogenicity in animal tests (Table 31–9). Exceptions include probable (cancer classification B2) animal carcinogens propoxur (bladder cancer and liver cancer) and dichlorvos (gastric tumors in female mice, leukemia in male rats). Possible (cancer classification C) carcinogens include acetamide, a metabolite of methomyl and thidiocarb (liver cancer in male and female rats), acephate, dimethoate, parathion, methidathion, phosphamidon, tetrachlorvinphos, and tribufos.

Some cancer case-control studies conducted in the 1990s showed associations between handling organophosphates and occurrence of non-Hodgkin lymphoma and leukemia. Effects of the reported expo-

Table 31-9. Animal studies evaluating chronic effects of organophosphate and carbamate compounds.

Chemical, Use Category, or Structural Class	Cancer or Reproductive Effect	EPA Potency Factor –Q* $(mg/kg/d)^{-1}$	Cancer Classification
Organophosphate compounds			
Acephate	Mouse liver		C
Chlorpyriphos			E
Dichlorvos	Rat: 0, 4, 8 mg/kg/d, 5 d/wk; pancreatic adenomas, leukemias in males; 0, 10, or 20 mg/kg/d (M). Mice: 0, 20, 40 mg/kg/d (F), 5 d/wk, corn oil gavage; forestomach papillomas at high doses in males/females	2.0 E-1	B2
Dimethoate	Rats were treated twice weekly by gavage with 5, 15, or 30 mg/kg, or intramuscularly with 15 mg/kg. Doses of 30 mg/kg oral and 15 mg/kg intramuscularly resulted in statistically significant increases in the combined incidence of malignant tumors. Malignant tumors were found in 4 of 20 rats that had received 30 mg/kg orally. Several negative studies also reported		C
Ebufos			E
Ethion			E
Fenamiphos			E
Fenitrothion			E
Fonofos			E
Guthion			E
Imidan/Phosmet			E
Malathion	Combined oncogenicity/chronic feeding study rat: 100, 6000, 12,000 ppm; increase in female liver adenomas, male nasal adenomas at ≥ 6000 ppm		D
Methidathion	Male mouse liver		C
Parathion	Combined oncogenicity/chronic feeding study rat: 2, 8, 32 ppm pancreatic exocrine tumors at high dose; cholinesterase inhibition at low dose; oncogenicity study in rats: 0, 23, 45 ppm males, 32, 62 females; adrenal adenomas at mid/high dose Mouse oncogenicity study: 0, 60, 100,140 ppm; malignant lymphoma at 2 highest doses		C
Phorate			D
Phosphamidon			C
Phostebupirim (corn insecticide)			E
Tetrachlorovinphos	Female mouse liver	3.13 E-3	C
Tribufos (DEF) (cotton defoliant)			C
Carbamate compounds			
Acetamide	Metabolite of methomyl and thidiocarb: male and female rat liver	3.07 E-3	C
Carbaryl	Combined oncogenicity and chronic rat study: 250, 1500, 7500 ppm in diet; papilloma and carcinoma in the urinary bladder; single transitional cell carcinoma in males, liver adenoma, and thyroid (adenoma and a single carcinoma) at the high-dose level. Male reproductive: spermatotoxin in rodents; study in manufacturing and formulating workers indicating no effect at relatively low levels of exposure Teratogenicity: 3.1 to 50 mg/kg were fed to beagle dogs during pregnancy. At levels of 6.25 and above the defect rate was increased in the offspring. Midline abdominal wall defects skeletal defects were the most common type. Negative studies reported for rodent species	2.27 E-2	None
Methiocarb			D
Baygon/Propoxur	Male and female rat bladder, hepatocellular adenomas mice	3.70 E-3	B2

sures on the immune system were hypothesized as a possible mechanism. An effect of a specific compound, for example, dichlorvos, which is recognized as an animal carcinogen, also could explain the findings. A case-control study investigating causes of aplastic anemia in Thailand also revealed a strong association with dichlorvos and with the carbamate insecticide propoxur. In common with the studies of lymphoma, the study employed questionnaire information to assess exposure, and the findings could have been attributed to recall bias.

2. Teratogenicity—The organophosphate compounds generally are not teratogenic below maternally toxic doses. As discussed earlier, the carbamate compound carbaryl is a spermatotoxin in rodents; a study in manufacturing and formulating workers demonstrated, as discussed earlier, an effect on sperm morphology. Sperm effects related to environmental exposures to carbaryl also have been reported (see above). Carbaryl is also teratogenic to beagle dogs but not to rodent species.

The FQPA has inspired considerable work on animal models for developmental neurotoxicity. A recent study on chlorpyrifos included several endpoints, in addition to general measures of fetal and maternal toxicity, evaluating treatments given at time of neural tube formation (gestation days 9–12) and treatments given during peak neurogenesis (days 17–20). There were effects on cell packing density (DNA/g of tissue) in fetal brain at doses as low as 1 mg/kg, well below the level producing decreased maternal weight gain (5 mg/kg per day). Decreased development of cholinergic synapses also was observed at doses producing greater than 20% cholinesterase inhibition.

3. Male reproductive effects—The carbamate compound carbaryl, still used in agriculture and as a garden insecticide, showed clear-cut effects on sperm production in the rat at doses of 50 and 100 mg/kg in a 60-day feeding study. Effects on workers producing carbaryl and effects of environmental exposures also have been evaluated, as discussed earlier.

REFERENCES

Balali-Mood M et al: Effect of high doses of sodium bicarbonate in acute organophosphorous pesticide poisoning. Clin Toxicol 2005;43:571 [PMID: 16255339].

Barlow SM: Agricultural chemicals and endocrine-mediated chronic toxicity or carcinogenicity. Scand J Work Environ Health 2005;31:141[PMID: 16190161].

Eddleston M et al: Speed of initial atropinisation in significant organophosphorus pesticide poisoning. J Toxicol Clin Toxicol 2004;42:865 [PMID: 15533026].

Gordon RK et al: Oral administration of pyridostigmine bromide and huperzine A protects human whole blood cholinesterases from ex vivo exposure to soman. Chem Biol Interact 2005;157:239 [PMID: 16256090].

ORGANOCHLORINE INSECTICIDES

Essentials of Diagnosis

A. ACUTE EFFECTS

- CNS excitation: irritability, excitability, dizziness, disorientation, paresthesias, tremors, and convulsions

B. CHRONIC EFFECTS

- Cancer in animals
- Case reports of aplastic anemia

General Considerations

The organochlorine insecticides are chlorinated hydrocarbon compounds of cyclic structure and high molecular weight. In contrast to chlorinated hydrocarbon solvents and fumigants, they are of low volatility and are CNS stimulants rather than general anesthetics. The prototype organochlorine, dichlorodiphenyltrichloroethane (DDT), was discovered in 1939. Until it was banned from most uses in the United States in 1973, more than 4 billion pounds were applied in agriculture and in control programs aimed at mosquitoes and other insects that transmit human disease, such as yellow fever and malaria. From 1940 through the 1970s, a number of other organochlorine compounds were used widely as insecticides, but following recognition of their persistence in the environment, bioaccumulation in animals and humans, adverse effects on some wildlife, and carcinogenicity in laboratory animals, most were deregistered or severely restricted in use. Those compounds still in use in the United States include dicofol, endosulfan, and lindane (Table 31–10). These compounds have shorter environmental and biologic half-lives than the canceled organochlorines although longer than typical organophosphates or typical pyrethroids. For example, lindane has a half-life of 3–4 days in plants with a high water content, such as lettuce. In carrots, with a higher comparative lipid content, the half-life is 10 weeks. Soil half-life is approximately 15 months. By comparison, the half-life of DDT in the soil ranges from 2–15 years.

Table 31–10. Organochlorine pesticides still in use in the United States.

Compound	Oral LD$_{50}$ (mg/kg)	Dermal LD$_{50}$ (mg/kg)
Dicofol	575–960	1000–5000 mg/kg
Endosulfan	20–40	75–150
Benzene hexachloride (BHC), γ-BHC lindane	100–200	500–1000

In addition to agricultural use, the use of lindane as a scabicide remains legal in most of the United States. In California, use as a scabicide was canceled by legislation in 2000, with the ban in effect beginning in 2002.

Occupational & Environmental Exposure

There is little information on current occupational exposure to organochlorines. Owing to their persistence and bioaccumulation, environmental exposure to organochlorines will continue for years, even to compounds no longer in use, although there is evidence that levels are decreasing. Most of the world's population has measurable levels of DDT and its metabolites in fat and blood. Elimination times for dicofol are approximately 192 hours, for endosulfan days to weeks. Metabolism of lindane (γ-isomer of hexachlorocyclohexane) is rapid.

Mechanism of Action and Clinical Findings

The organochlorines are well absorbed by inhalation or ingestion but are absorbed more slowly through the skin. Most are highly fat soluble and are distributed to adipose tissue, the liver, and the nervous system. Most are metabolized by the liver and excreted in urine as metabolites. For some, this is a slow process, so accumulation in adipose tissue occurs during chronic exposure. DDT is metabolized and excreted slowly and is found in the fat of most persons; average DDT levels in the fat of Americans have been decreasing since cessation of its use in the United States.

Although the clinical picture of acute intoxication is similar for members of this family of compounds, their precise mechanism of action is unknown, and whether they share a common mechanism is, for that reason, uncertain. These chemicals cause CNS excitation and dysfunction with little pathologic change, presumably as a result of changes in the transmission of nerve impulses. They cause hepatocellular necrosis in high doses, hepatocellular hypertrophy, and carcinomas—particularly in mice—at lower doses, and are inducers of hepatic microsomal enzymes.

A. SYMPTOMS & SIGNS

Acute or subacute intoxication from organochlorines produces a picture of generalized CNS excitability and dysfunction: apprehension, excitability, dizziness, headache, disorientation, confusion, disequilibrium, weakness, paresthesias, muscle twitching, tremor, convulsions, and coma. Nausea and vomiting are common after ingestion but not after dermal exposure, which is the primary route in the workplace. Most organochlorines are formulated with organic solvents, which may account for CNS depression, particularly after ingestion. Fever commonly occurs after seizures but may be a result of seizure activity rather than an effect of the pesticide. Chlordecone, no longer in use, caused a unique chronic intoxication.

There are a number of case reports and case series suggesting an association between aplastic anemia and exposure to organochlorine insecticides. These reports cannot exclude the possibility of coincidental occurrence of this rare condition with relatively common exposures.

B. LABORATORY FINDINGS

With the exception of measurement of parent compounds or metabolites in biologic samples, laboratory findings are nonspecific. Electroencephalography may show generalized seizure activity. For some compounds, a correlation between biologic levels and degree of poisoning is known, but such levels are rarely available in time to assist in management of acute poisonings.

Differential Diagnosis

Severe organochlorine poisoning usually occurs following obvious overexposure and, as a result, does not present a problem in diagnosis. Other causes of CNS overactivity or seizures must be considered, particularly drug intoxications. Infections of the nervous system must be considered in the presence of seizures. Pneumonitis may be present as a result of aspiration of organic solvent.

Treatment

There are no antidotes, so treatment is supportive, directed primarily at maintenance of respiratory function and prompt management of seizures with anticonvulsant medication. Decontamination of the skin, hair, and gut (as appropriate) is important, as in all cases of acute intoxication. Cholestyramine has been shown to accelerate the elimination of chlordecone (from an average half-life of 165 days to a half-life of 80 days) but has not been studied for use in management of poisoning with any other organochlorine.

Prognosis

Uncontrolled seizures may result in anoxic brain or other organ damage. If hypoxia is prevented, recovery should be complete.

Chronic Effects

Chlordecone caused a constellation of nervousness, tremor, weight loss, opsoclonus, pleuritic and joint pain, and a syndrome resembling pseudotumor cerebri in overexposed production workers. These chronic effects were mitigated by treatment with cholestyramine to enhance elimination of chlordecone.

The other noteworthy concern regarding organochlorines is the risk of cancer. As shown in Table 31–11,

Table 31–11. Animal studies evaluating chronic effects of organochlorines.

Chemical, Use Category, or Structural Class	Cancer or Reproductive Effect	EPA Potency Factor –Q* $(mg/kg/d)^{-1}$	Cancer Classification
Chlordane	Mouse liver	1.3	B2
Chlordecone (canceled)	NTP summary: hepatocellular carcinomas in rats/mice of both sexes		None given
	Reproductive: fetotoxicity and malformations ranging from reduced ossification, edema, undescended testes, enlarged renal pelves, and enlarged cerebral ventricles		
	Male reproductive: testicular toxin in a number of species; infertility in manufacturing and formulating workers; no longer manufactured		
Chlorobenzilate (canceled)	Cancer: published studies show hepatocellular carcinomas in two strains of mice		
	Male reproductive: testicular toxin in rodents; inadequate human studies		
DDT, DDE, DDD	Female mouse stomach; male rat leukemia	0.24–0.34	B2
Dicofol/Kelthane	Mouse oncogenicity study: 471, 942 ppm males, 122, 243—lung and liver tumors, marginal effect at low dose		C
Dieldrin		16	B2
Endosulfan			E
Heptachlor	Mice: hepatomas at 10 ppm dose; rats: 40, 80, 160 ppm—thyroid adenomas at low/high dose	4.5	B2
Lindane	Liver tumors in mice and rats (NTP summary)	1.3	B2/C
Methoxychlor	Published studies show testicular tumors in some mouse strains 100 ppm in diet; carcinomas both sexes of rats 2000 ppm in diet		B2
Mirex	Hepatomas in mouse and rat at maximum tolerated dose and 50% MTD	1.8	B2
Toxaphene	Rat liver/thyroid	1.1	B2

most of the organochlorines cause liver cancer in one or more rodent species. Evidence for excess liver and biliary tract cancer in humans is equivocal. A 1992 NIOSH study of manufacturing workers showed excess biliary tract cancer in a facility producing aldrin, dieldrin, endrin, and DBCP and a nonsignificant increase in a plant producing DDT. Facilities producing other organochlorines (principally heptachlor and chlordane) did not show excess cancer. A principal limitation of the study was incomplete exposure information.

Serum levels of the DDT metabolite dichlorodiphenyl dichloroethylene (DDE) is a risk factor for breast cancer, with a fourfold increase in the relative risk of breast cancer for an elevation of serum DDE concentrations from 2.0 (10th percentile) to 19.1 ng/mL (90th percentile). This finding prompted widespread concern about organochlorines and breast cancer, and attempts were made to correlate secular trends in organochlorine exposures with trends in breast cancer incidence. A subsequent study of women in the San Francisco Bay Area found no relationship between serum DDE levels and breast cancer. Other follow-up case-control studies also

have shown negative or inconsistent results, but a positive study was reported recently from Belgium. A study from India found positive association for lindane or PCBs but a negative association for DDE and DDT.

Male Reproductive Effects

The organochlorine compound chlordecone (Kepone) produced demonstrable effects on spermatogenesis in both animal studies and workers. Adult male rats fed 15 or 30 ppm chlordecone for 90 days showed reversible changes in mobility and viability of spermatozoa.

Workers affected by neurologic symptoms also experienced oligospermia and decreased sperm motility and had abnormal testicular biopsies. Because organochlorines have recognized estrogenic properties, it appears possible that the decreased sperm production associated with chlordecone toxicity derives from an endocrine mechanism rather than a direct effect on germinal epithelium. However, this supposition has not been supported by the findings in animal studies investigating the compound's estrogenic properties.

REFERENCES

Beard J et al: DDT and human health. Sci Total Environ 2005;355:78 [PMID: 15894351].

McCready D et al: Breast tissue organochlorine levels and metabolic genotypes in relation to breast cancer risk. Cancer Causes Control 2004;15:399 [PMID: 15141140].

Toft G et al: Semen quality and exposure to persistent organochlorine pollutants. Epidemiology 2006;17:450 [PMID: 16755259].

PYRETHRUM & SYNTHETIC PYRETHROID INSECTICIDES

Essentials of Diagnosis

A. ACUTE EFFECTS

- Topical paresthesias and irritation of the skin, ocular and respiratory irritation, systemic poisoning on ingestion
- Allergic contact dermatitis: erythema, vesicles, papules, and itching
- Allergic rhinitis: nasal congestion and sore throat
- Asthma: wheezing, cough, chest lightness, and dyspnea

General Considerations

Pyrethrum is a partially refined extract of the chrysanthemum flower and has been used as an insecticide for more than 60 years. There are six known active compounds in pyrethrums, including two esters known as *pyrethrins* (pyrethrin I and pyrethrin II). Chrysanthemum and pyrethrum have long been recognized to cause allergies. In rodent acute toxicity tests, pyrethrin mixtures demonstrate remarkable variability in effect (Table 31–12), but most mixtures have oral LD_{50}s greater than 1000 mg/kg. Pyrethrum and pyrethrin mixtures do not cause systemic toxicity on dermal application.

Table 31–12. Pyrethrin and pyrethroid acute toxicity.

Compound	Oral LD_{50} (mg/kg)	Dermal LD_{50} (mg/kg)
Natural pyrethrins	200 > 26,000	Very low
Type I pyrethroid		
Permethrin	430–4000	> 4000
Resmethrin	1244–2500	> 3000
Cypermethrin	250	< 2000
Type II (cyano-halogen) pyrethroid		
Esfenvalerate	458	2500
Cyfluthrin	869–1271	> 5000
Deltamethrin	128	> 2000

Synthetic pyrethroids structurally resemble pyrethrins, with modifications that increase both toxicity and stability. Between two subtypes of synthetic pyrethroids, designated as type I and type II (cyanohalogen) compounds, the latter generally demonstrate greater toxicity. Animal studies also demonstrate some differential age-related toxicity of type II pyrethroids. Deltamethrin, for example, has an LD_{50} of 5.1 for 11-day-old male rats versus 81 mg/kg for 72-day-old male rats. Because of this possible increased susceptibility, illegally imported pyrethroid chalk products (containing deltamethrin), resembling a form of hard candy, pose a risk of systemic poisoning to children. A published case report describes poisoning of a 4-year-old child with a deltamethrin chalk at an estimated dose of 2 mg/kg.

Use

There are several hundred commercial products containing pyrethrum (active ingredients pyrethrin I and pyrethrin II) and pyrethroids. Most contain piperonyl butoxide as a synergist (see below) and often with an additional insecticide, such as a carbamate or organophosphate to delay pyrethroid metabolism in the target insects. Many are available for home use against flies, mosquitoes, and fleas. The usual household formulation contains about 0.5% active ingredient. The greater stability of the synthetic pyrethrins has made them useful in agricultural applications. The petroleum solvents contained in most ready-to-use mixtures and "bug bombs" as "inert ingredients" have their own toxicity. A number of spectacular fires and explosions have occurred with overapplication of the indoor "bug bomb" products presumably because the petroleum distillates and propellants achieve such high concentrations.

Occupational & Environmental Exposures

The low toxicity of pyrethrins has resulted in little interest in quantifying exposure levels apart from concern about hazards to small children from residues on interior surfaces from mixtures that contain organophosphates and carbamates. Occupational pyrethroid exposures in the United States principally result in topical symptoms, but systemic poisoning caused by pyrethroid compounds has been reported in applicators from China.

Indoor exposures to residue of pyrethroids also may produce irritant upper respiratory and ocular symptoms. Similar symptoms also have been reproduced in limited experimental studies in humans and in California orange harvesters working in orchards recently treated with cyfluthrin. These symptoms resemble acute allergy but probably represent an effect of the pyrethroids on nerve endings in the eye and the respiratory tract.

Residue dissipation for cyfluthrin has been characterized to only a limited extent, with available data showing marked variability. In some orchards in California's central valley, rapid dissipation occurred. In others, there was biphasic decay with an initial half-life of 11 days, followed by a half-life of 32 days. At 65 days postapplication, 10–20% of the initial residue still remained.

Pyrethroids generally have not been thought to accumulate in the environment. Nevertheless, a recent study demonstrated permethrin and bifenthrin accumulating in runoff sediment in southern California. Under both aerobic and anaerobic conditions, the half-life for bifenthrin ranged from 8–17 months. Concentrations in sediment may be high enough to affect growth of some crustaceans in soil sediment, such as the amphipod *Hyalella azteca.*

Indoor dissipation of pyrethroids also may be unpredictable. A German study, for example, demonstrated multiphasic dissipation of permethrin following indoor application, with a final slow-phase half-life of up to 2 years. The levels have been reported to be high enough to cause irritant symptoms in sensitive individuals.

Mechanism of Action & Clinical Findings

The pyrethrins and pyrethroids are absorbed from the gastrointestinal tract and hydrolyzed in the gut and tissues, and excreted rapidly. They are very slowly absorbed from the skin. They function principally by excitation of the sodium channels in the nervous system. Data on acute toxicity in animals shows moderate oral toxicity and very low systemic toxicity following skin contact (see Table 31–12).

Possible interactions between pyrethroids and other insecticides have received little notice. There may be a possible metabolic interaction with organophosphates and with the insect repellant diethyltoluamide (DEET). Workers exposed to the type II pyrethroid deltamethrin excreted principally metabolic transformation products. Workers also exposed to the organophosphate compound methamidophos excreted unchanged active pyrethroids (fenvalerate or deltamethrin) in the urine, implying an inhibition of pyrethroid metabolism by methamidophos. The effect has been documented clearly in fish exposed simultaneously to esfenvalerate and diazinon. In that experimental system, the esfenvalerate toxicity was enhanced by diazinon inhibition of the enzyme carboxylesterase, usually responsible for pyrethroid metabolism.

A. SIGNS AND SYMPTOMS

The most common effect of pyrethrum exposure is allergic contact dermatitis, which is manifested by itching and an erythematous vesicular rash. Bullae, edema, and photosensitivity also may occur. Allergic rhinitis is not uncommon, with nasal congestion, sneezing, and sore throat. Asthma and hypersensitivity pneumonitis have been reported but are uncommon. Dyspnea, cough, and wheezing indicate asthma, although these manifestations plus fever, malaise, and pulmonary infiltrates are indicative of hypersensitivity pneumonitis. Anaphylaxis with bronchospasm, laryngeal edema, and shock has been reported occasionally after inhalation of pyrethrum. A case report published in 2000 reported an apparent fatal allergic reaction in an 11-year-old using a pet shampoo containing 0.2% pyrethrins.

These allergic manifestations have been reported only infrequently from exposure to synthetic pyrethroids, but cases of related allergic contact dermatitis have been documented. The most common effect of the pyrethroids appears to be topical paresthesias and ocular or respiratory irritation (see examples cited earlier).

B. LABORATORY FINDINGS

Skin testing can aid in the diagnosis of sensitivity to pyrethrum. There are no biologic monitoring methods for exposure to pyrethrum or pyrethroids.

Differential Diagnosis

Allergy to other pesticides, plants or flowers, insect stings, and household products must be considered in the evaluation of one of the allergic manifestations of pyrethrum.

Treatment

The key to treatment of any allergy is removal from exposure to the allergen. Allergic contact dermatitis may be treated with application of topical steroid preparations. Allergic rhinitis may be treated with antihistamines, decongestants, and a steroid nasal spray, if needed. Asthma is treated with bronchodilators and steroids as appropriate. Anaphylaxis may require epinephrine, aminophylline, or a parenteral corticosteroid. Topical application of creams containing vitamin E may alleviate pyrethroid-related paresthesias if applied shortly after skin contact. Acute respiratory irritation is short lived and does not require medical treatment unless lower respiratory symptoms are also present.

Prognosis

If the diagnosis is correct, treatment is prompt, and removal from exposure is effective, recovery should be rapid and complete. In a pediatric ingestion case involving deltamethrin, transient CNS symptoms occurred, but recovery was rapid following gastric decontamination. The overall time course is comparable with an acute carbamate intoxication.

SYNERGISTS (PIPERONYL BUTOXIDE)

Although there are a few other examples, by far the most common synergistic insecticide combination is that of piperonyl butoxide with pyrethrins.

Use

Piperonyl butoxide is used as an insecticide synergist with pyrethrins in ratios of 5:1 or 20:1 in a variety of formula-

Table 31–13. Animal data evaluating chronic effects of pyrethroids.

Chemical, Use Category, or Structural Class	Cancer or Reproductive Effect	EPA Potency Factor –Q* $(mg/kg/d)^{-1}$	Cancer Classification
Bifenthrin	Male mouse bladder		C
Cyhalothrin (Karate)	Inadequate dose		D
Cypermethrin	Mouse lung	1.9 E-2	C
Fenpropathrin (Danitol)			E
Permethrin	Mouse lung and liver	1.84 E-02	C
Tetramethrin			C

tions, many of which are available for home use. They are used primarily for flies, mosquitoes, and fleas, often in combination with a carbamate or organophosphate.

Occupational & Environmental Exposure

Most exposure occurs with use of household ready-to-use formulations.

Mechanism of Action & Clinical Findings

Piperonyl butoxide is poorly absorbed from the gastrointestinal tract and probably poorly absorbed dermally. It is metabolized but also retained unchanged to an uncertain degree in rodents. Its mechanism of action is inhibition of hepatic mixed-function oxidase enzymes.

A. SYMPTOMS & SIGNS

There are no reports of clinical illness occurring as a result of isolated exposure to piperonyl butoxide.

B. LABORATORY FINDINGS

There is no evidence of enzyme inhibition from piperonyl butoxide in humans. A single oral dose of 50 mg did not change the metabolism of antipyrine in eight volunteers.

Differential Diagnosis

Any illness occurring in an individual exposed to a formulation containing piperonyl butoxide probably is caused by another ingredient, such as allergy to pyrethrum, an effect of a carbamate or organophosphate, or something other than the pesticide.

Treatment

Treatment, if required, would be symptomatic.

Prognosis

The outcome depends on the actual diagnosis.

Chronic Effects

Several of the synthetic pyrethroids cause cancer at maximum tolerated doses in animals, including bifenthrin, cypermethrin, permethrin, and tetramethrin (Table 31–13). However, none are classified as probable human carcinogens. The pyrethroid compounds do not cause teratogenic effects in animal studies. For example, in a study of cyfluthrin, offspring of animals dosed at 0, 3, 10, or 40 mg/kg per day on gestation days 6–15 showed no signs of malformations. Treatment-related maternal toxicity occurred at doses of 10 and 40 mg/kg per day, including decreased weight gain, hypoactivity, locomotor incoordination, increased salivation, and a 15% mortality rate. Piperonly butoxide has complex, often biphasic effects on mixed function oxidases (cytochrome p450 system) in laboratory animals. Following oral administration, initial enzyme inhibition occurs, followed by induction. This may increase the metabolism of other xenobiotic compounds. In experimental studies this has been associated with relative tolerance to the organophosphate compounds methyl parathion, dimethoate, azinphos methyl and the neurotoxic esterase inhibitor tri-ortho cresyl phosphate.

REFERENCES

Bradberry SM et al: Poisoning due to pyrethroids. Toxicol Rev 2005;24:93 [PMID: 16180929].

Proudfoot AT: Poisoning due to pyrethrins. Toxicol Rev 2005;24:107 [PMID: 16180930].

BIOLOGIC INSECTICIDES

A number of insect growth-regulator chemical substances that disrupt the action of insect hormones, controlling molting and other stages of development, were developed recently. Many of these are biorational pesticides, either naturally occurring organisms (such as *Bacillus thuringiensis*) or chemical analogues of naturally occurring biochemical substances (such as the sex-attractant pheromones). Epidemiologic studies have demonstrated a high prevalence of IgE reactivity to *B. thuringiensis* in European nursery workers and in vegetable harvesters in northern Ohio.

FUMIGANTS & NEMATOCIDES

Essentials of Diagnosis

A. ACUTE EFFECTS

- Respiratory tract irritation: burning eyes, nose, throat, cough, shortness of breath, and pulmonary edema
- CNS depression: headache, nausea, vomiting, dizziness, drowsiness, fatigue, slurred speech, loss of balance, disorientation, loss of consciousness, and respiratory depression
- Encephalopathy (methyl bromide): tremors, seizures, elevated serum bromide level, late personality changes, and cognitive dysfunction

B. CHRONIC EFFECTS

- Liver damage (halogenated hydrocarbons): anorexia, abdominal pain, jaundice, and abnormal liver function tests
- Peripheral neuropathy (methyl bromide): progressive distal symmetric sensorimotor neuropathy, ascending paresthesias, numbness, and weakness
- Asthma and reactive airways secondary to metam-sodium by-products and to chloropicrin
- Immune effects of metam-sodium and MITC in animal studies

General Considerations

Many fumigants are halogenated hydrocarbons and as such are lipid-soluble anesthetics and often alkylating agents. Most of the nematocides are soil fumigants. Ethylene oxide and propylene oxide are registered pesticides used to fumigate spices. Ethylene oxide is also used for the sterilization of medical instruments, a nonagricultural use that is regulated by OSHA (see Chapter 28).

Use

Fumigants are used to kill insects, insect eggs, and microorganisms. Cultivated crops, herbs and spices, and packaged products such as dried fruits, beans, and medical materials usually are treated in fumigation chambers. Structures such as houses, warehouses, grain elevators, and greenhouses may be sealed, fumigated, and then aerated before being reoccupied. Fumigants are highly penetrating and will pass through many types of material. For methyl bromide, soil usually is treated by application under a tarpaulin that provides a relatively tight seal. The nematocide vapors spread through soil and reach microscopic roundworms in the water that surrounds soil particles. Metam-sodium soil applications employ shank or sprinkler equipment.

The latter poses problems because the compound decomposes readily in water, and off-site movement of metam by-products may occur during the course of sprinkler treatment.

Occupational & Environmental Exposure

The fumigants are either gases at ambient temperatures or form vapors on heating (see Table 31–4). Because vapors can penetrate biologic tissue and protective clothing and can pass through absorbent filters, opportunities for direct exposure must be minimized. Workers applying fumigants may be exposed when leaks occur in equipment, when buildings are not sealed adequately, and when checking for leaks and entering chambers or buildings before complete aeration without appropriate protective equipment.

Exposure of applicators, field workers, and bystanders to soil fumigant nematocides most commonly occurs when tarpaulins are disturbed, usually by wind. Phosphine is applied in solid formulations of aluminum or zinc phosphide, which liberate phosphine gas when in contact with water in the environment or after ingestion by pests such as rodents.

The high volatility and rapid environmental degradation of fumigants and nematocides suggest little potential for leaving residues in food or contaminating water. Nevertheless, residues of ethylene dibromide have been found in raw and prepared foods.

The planned phaseout of methyl bromide has had a drastic effect on fumigant use patterns. To replace methyl bromide as a soil fumigant, increased levels of metam-sodium are being used, and concentrations of chloropicrin are being increased to replace a portion of methyl bromide used during soil fumigations. Because the metam-sodium degradation product methyl isothiocyanate (MITC) causes irritant symptoms over a period of 1 hour at concentrations near 800 ppb, the increased use of metam has coincided with a series of environmental exposures to businesses and communities near metam-treated fields. Similar problems may occur with chloropicrin because it causes mild ocular symptoms (or *chemesthesis*) after a 30-minute exposure to 75 ppb.

The search for alternative structural fumigants also has led to unexpected adverse consequences. A fumigator in southern California died of asphyxiation during an application of a novel pest control system that employed liquid nitrogen to freeze termites. Another approach, eradicating termites by application of heated propane, has been associated with drastic safety problems, including fires and explosions. Failure to disconnect household gas service properly during sulfuryl fluoride treatments also has been associated with safety hazards. Unspent residues of the phosphide fumigants are also associated with fires, explosions, and accidental injuries.

Table 31–14. Selected fumigants and nematocides historically used in the United States.

Fumigant or Nematocide	LC$_{50}$ ppm	Duration, Hours	LD$_{50}$ mg/kg
Halogenated hydrocarbon			
Ethylene dibromide	391	2	108
Methyl bromide	1158	1	214
Ethylene dichloride	3000	2.4	870–950
Carbon tetrachloride	7228	6	2920
Dibromochloropropane	153	1	100
Chlorpicrin	14.4	4	Not given
p-Dichlorobenzene	845	4	3863
Sulfur, phosphorus and other compounds			
Sulfuryl fluoride	1000	4	Not given
Phosphine	11	4	Not given
Sulfur dioxide	1000	4	Not given
Cyano compounds			
Hydrogen cyanide	142	0.5	Not given
Oxides			
Ethylene oxide	1462	4	Not given
Propylene oxide	1729–4007	4	690
Formaldehyde	3345–7751	4	800
Glutaraldehyde	23	4	134
Acrolein	8.3	4	46
MITC	180	4	175

LC$_{50}$ = lethal concentration for 50% of test animals, with durations as shown.

Mechanism of Action & Clinical Findings

A. HALOGENATED HYDROCARBONS

Most halogenated fumigants and nematocides are well absorbed by all routes of exposure and are excreted rapidly without significant bioaccumulation. Inhalation of vapors is the most common route of exposure, although dermal absorption of vapors or liquid also can occur. The vapors and liquids usually are primary irritants and in some cases are quite potent. Most are general anesthetics (CNS depressants), whereas some, such as methyl bromide, have specific neurotoxic effects. The halogenated hydrocarbon fumigants share most of the effects of the halogenated hydrocarbon solvents, including cardiac sensitization, direct cellular toxicity to the liver and kidneys, and carcinogenicity in laboratory animals. The potency, as measured by the lethal concentration required to kill 50% of test animals (LC$_{50}$), varies considerably among the individual compounds (Table 31–14).

1. Symptoms & signs—Halogenated hydrocarbon exposure is marked initially by general anesthetic effects: headache, nausea, vomiting, and dizziness, followed by drowsiness, fatigue, slurred speech, loss of balance, disorientation, and in severe poisoning, loss of consciousness, respiratory depression, and death. Tremors, myoclonus, and generalized seizures may occur, particularly

from methyl bromide poisoning. Acute and chronic poisoning from methyl bromide may be followed by prolonged and, in some cases, permanent organic brain damage marked by personality changes and cognitive dysfunction. Workers have been diagnosed as suffering from severe psychological disorders until a source of methyl bromide exposure was recognized. Direct contact with liquid halogenated hydrocarbons may result in erythema and blisters. Damage to the skin can be severe if liquid is spilled on clothing and shoes, which retard evaporation.

Chronic exposure to halogenated hydrocarbons may cause liver damage, manifested by anorexia, abdominal pain, nausea, vomiting, jaundice, dark urine, and light stools. Chronic exposure to methyl bromide can result in progressive peripheral neuropathy with ascending paresthesias, numbness, and weakness and with or without depressed deep tendon reflexes.

2. Laboratory findings—For the most part, laboratory findings in cases of fumigant poisoning and overexposure are nonspecific and related to the organ affected (e.g., abnormal liver function tests). Halogenated hydrocarbons can be measured in blood and exhaled air, but this is rarely helpful except in forensic cases. Methyl bromide is degraded rapidly to inorganic bromide, and measurement of serum bromide may be helpful in the diagnosis of methyl bromide toxicity. Background levels of serum bromide, in the absence of an external source of inorganic bromide, are usually less than 5 mg/L. Most reported acute poisoning cases have levels exceeding 50 mg/L and most fatalities have serum bromide levels exceeding 100 mg/L. Interpretation of the measurements is complicated by the 10–15 day half-life for serum bromide. Applicators with cumulative exposures to methyl bromide may have serum bromide measurements in the 50–100 mg/L range without having any apparent symptoms. To complicate matters, the reference range on laboratory reports frequently identify levels >500 mg/L as causing poisoning. This number actually refers to toxic levels of inorganic bromide, poisoning commonly associated with an over-the-counter bromide sedative popular in the 1950s and 1960s.

3. Chronic effects—Most of the halogenated hydrocarbons are carcinogenic in animals (Table 31–15). Ethylene dibromide, dibromochloropropane, and methyl bromide are alkylating agents that were positive in a number of short-term tests of genotoxicity, including mutagenicity. Ethylene dibromide and dibromochloropropane are rodent carcinogens and spermatotoxins and have been eliminated from use.

Methyl bromide has been tested for carcinogenicity, but the compound is so neurotoxic that this effect causes death of the animals prior to the occurrence of cancer (see Table 31–15). Carbon tetrachloride is an animal carcinogen. Liver cancer has been reported in workers following hepatic necrosis and cirrhosis from acute and chronic exposure.

Table 31–15. Animal studies evaluating chronic effects of fumigants and nematocides.

Chemical, Use Category, or Structural Class	Cancer or Reproductive Effect	EPA Potency Factor –Q* $(mg/kg/d)^{-1}$	Cancer Classification
Carbon tetrachloride	Liver carcinogen in mice/rats; multiple positive studies 47–2000 mg/kg/d		B2
Dibromochloropropane (DBCP)	Cancer: liver, kidney, stomach, nasal in the rat	1.4 oral; 8.3 inhalation	B2
	Reproductive: nematocide: testicular toxin in a number of species; alkylating agent, mutagen, carcinogen; number of reports and studies indicating infertility in formulating workers and applicators; almost all uses suspended		
Dichloropropene (Telone II)	Forestomach/liver tumors in male rats; forestomach tumors female rats; forestomach, lung, urinary bladder in female mice	Oral 1.8 E-1; inhalation 9.66 E-2	B2
Ethylene dibromide (EDB)	Cancer: stomach mouse; nasal rat; alkylating agent, mutagen	67 oral 1.4 inhalation	B2
	Reproductive: fumigant, nematocide, testicular toxin in a number of species; epidemiologic study indicating decreased sperm count		
Methyl bromide	Cancer: 1974 published rat study showed squamous cell cancer in stomach at doses of 50 mg/kg/d but this was reinterpreted as only inflammatory hyperplasia. Gliomas noted at 33% of MTD in male rats; effect not seen at MTD dose; mouse study limited by neurotoxicity		D
	Reproductive: omphalocele, arterial malformations, gallbladder agenesis in studies reported to California DPR		
Acrylonitrile	Cancer study by NTP: When administered orally (by gavage or in drinking water), acrylonitrile induced increased incidences of forestomach squamous cell papillomas, central nervous system microgliomas, mammary gland carcinomas, and Zymbal gland carcinomas in rats of both sexes. Inhalation of acrylonitrile induced Zymbal gland carcinomas, forestomach papillomas and acanthomas, and central nervous system neoplasms in rats of both sexes	5.4 E-1	B2

(continued)

Table 31–15. Animal studies evaluating chronic effects of fumigants and nematocides. (continued)

Chemical, Use Category, or Structural Class	Cancer or Reproductive Effect	EPA Potency Factor –Q* $(mg/kg/d)^{-1}$	Cancer Classification
Ethylene oxide	Cancer: Leukemia in rats and monkeys; mice show lung cancers, and lymphomas; human cancer in case reports; NIOSH study showed increased risk of leukemia in US cohort. IARC classification: limited evidence for human carcinogenicity Reproductive: Dominant lethal mutations produced when male mice injected with single 150 mg/kg dose of ethylene oxide. Similar effect produced by inhalation of 1000 ppm. Aberrations in cervical vertebrae in mice treated intravenously with 75–150 mg/kg; Male: Decreased sperm count and motility in monkeys inhaling 50–100 ppm		Refer to IARC classification
Propylene oxide	Sprague-Dawley rats receiving propylene oxide by stomach tube in doses of 15 or 60 mg/kg of body weight twice weekly for 109.5 weeks exhibited a dose-dependent increase in forestomach tumors. Additional rat study showed pheochromocytomas and mesotheliomas. Mouse inhalation study showed hemangiomas and hemangiosarcomas		B2
Carbon disulfide	Fetotoxicity at doses of 25, 75, 250 mg/kg/d; malformations in a multigeneration study: hydrocephalus, microcephalus, clubfoot, tail deformations Male reproductive: Interferes with sperm transport in rats exposed to 600 ppm CS2. Testes grossly and histologically normal		
Dazomet	Cancer: California DPR negative mouse and rat oncogenicity study; Male reproductive: 150 ppm in California DPR dog chronic study-testicular tubular atrophy		D
Metam-sodium	California DPR cancer: mouse liver masses at 240 ppm (high dose) in females Cancer: California DPR angiosarcomas in combined rat study at concentrations ≥0.056/mL Fetotoxicity in feeding studies; principal by-product methyl isothiocyanate negative in similar studies; other by-products include carbon disulfide and hydrogen sulfide. CS2 is noted to produce malformations in feeding studies	1.98 E-1	B2

B. PHOSPHIDE FUMIGANTS

The mechanism of multiorgan toxicity of phosphine and phosphides is unknown, but the compound probably poisons one or more enzymes involved in cellular metabolism, with a resulting toxic effect similar to cyanide.

1. Signs & symptoms—Cases of acute aluminum phosphide ingestion result in death from pulmonary edema, seizures, and respiratory depression. Nonfatal cases have been marked by liver injury with abdominal pain, nausea, vomiting, jaundice, elevated hepatic enzymes, and coagulopathy with bleeding. Occupational cases infrequently cause fatal outcomes but may result in symptoms severe enough to require hospitalization. Severe poisoning and fatal outcomes have occurred during fumigation in transit by either ship or rail.

Documentation of phosphine levels that cause symptomatic human illness is minimal. The ACGIH TLV documentation cites a study of Australian grain silo workers that does not contain individual data on symptoms and exposure, but many workers were symptomatic, and measured phosphine concentrations ranged from none detected to as high as 35.0 ppm. A study of Indian grain fumigation workers suffered from similar limitations. Most workers were intermittently symptomatic; measured phosphine concentrations ranged from 0.17–2.11 ppm.

2. Laboratory findings—Following inhalation exposure to phosphine, no specific tests are available in most laboratories to aid in diagnosis. However, in cases of phosphide ingestion, aluminum may be elevated in serum and other tissues. Phosphine can be measured in expired air in either inhalation or ingestion. It may prove possible to use colorimetric tubes or direct-reading industrial hygiene instruments.

3. Chronic effects—An investigation of excess lymphoid cancers in members of a Midwestern grain millers union demonstrated g-banded chromosomal translocations in workers handling phosphine and corresponding lesions in lymphocyte cultures exposed to the gas. No specific measures of exposure were reported. A follow-up study from New South Wales of applicators did not show any indication of genotoxicity. Passive-diffusion badges and colorimetric tubes were used to measure exposures; none exceeded 2.4 ppm.

C. SULFURYL FLUORIDE

1. Signs and symptoms—Sulfuryl fluoride appears to cause respiratory depression similar to the halogenated hydrocarbons, including numbness, weakness, abdominal pain, slowed speech or movements, coughing, and accumulation of fluid in the lungs. Ocular, dermal, and respiratory irritant symptoms produced by sulfuryl fluoride overlap with those produced by chloropicrin and may accompany accidental exposures.

Deaths have occurred on illegal entry into treated structures during the fumigation process or when sulfuryl fluoride had not dissipated to appropriate levels prior to reentry. Eight such deaths were recorded in California between 1982 and 1999. An additional 109 possible, probable, or definitely related cases occurred in the same time period. These cases included transient, mild systemic symptoms and irritation of the eyes or skin. Several cases involved police or other emergency-response workers pulling transients from inside treated structures, but most had only short-term symptoms of dizziness, nausea, dyspnea, and eye irritation. Because the irritant compound chloropicrin (see below) is applied as a warning agent in conjunction with sulfuryl fluoride, it is possible that not all the symptoms reported in the emergency responders are related directly to inhalation of sulfuryl fluoride.

2. Laboratory measurements—Exposure to sulfuryl fluoride can be evaluated by measuring fluoride levels in serum. Reference values range from 0.01–0.2 μg fluoride per milliliter of serum (equivalent to 1–20 μg fluoride/dL, 10–200 μg fluoride/L, 10–200 ppb, or 0.5–10.5 μmol/L). Two fatal cases reported in California during the 1990s demonstrated serum fluoride levels of 3200 and 3800 μg/dL.[1]

There appears to be a fairly limited awareness of the availability of fluoride monitoring. No monitoring data were available for 9 additional sulfuryl fluoride fatalities, 23 cases involving brief exposures to emergency-response personnel and application crews, and 9 brief nonoccupational exposures to sulfuryl fluoride–treated buildings reported to the California illness registry between 1982 and 2002.

3. Chronic effects—In one controversial compensation case, permanent neurologic injury related to sulfuryl fluoride was disputed between an applicator and his employer. However, cases of residual neurotoxicity similar to those caused by methyl bromide usually do not occur following exposure to sulfuryl fluoride. In a NIOSH study of sulfuryl fluoride applicators, repeated exposure in the year preceding examination was associated with subclinical effects on memory (in a test called the Pattern Memory Test) and also on the sense of smell.

D. METAM-SODIUM

The degradation products of metam-sodium include a complex mixture of irritant compounds: the primary pesticidal agent MITC, MIC (approximately 4% of the level of MITC), carbon disulfide, hydrogen sulfide, and methyl amine. The toxicologic effects of the mixture have not been characterized.

1. Signs and symptoms—Exposure to airborne MITC for 1 hour produces burning eyes and other irritant symptoms at concentrations of 800 ppb. Exposure for 4 minutes may produce similar symptoms at concentrations of 1900 ppb. Those with asthma or smoking-related pulmonary disease may experience respiratory problems at concentrations that only produce eye symptoms in others. In community exposures, nonspecific systemic symptoms such as nausea, headache, and diarrhea accompany the irritant symptoms in a portion of those exposed. The symptoms produced by hydrogen sulfide, carbon disulfide, and methyl amine have a high degree of overlap with those produced by MIC and MITC, but quantitative experimental data on dose-response for these compounds do not exist.

Irritant dermatitis was associated initially with direct skin contact in metam-sodium applicators in Germany. Mulitple cases also occurred in workers cleaning the upper Sacramento River in a large-volume spill of liquid metam-sodium. However, dermatitis has not been a frequent problem in community exposure to airborne metam-sodium by-products.

2. Laboratory findings—No specific clinical tool exists for monitoring exposure to MITC metam-sodium by-products. Measurement of environmental levels of MITC in excess of the 0.8-ppm irritation threshold clearly would suggest the cause of concurrent ocular or upper respiratory symptoms. However, permit conditions and the metam-sodium applicators trade

---

[1]Assuming a volume of distribution similar to that of bromide (approximately one-third of body weight), this represents 2504 mg sulfuryl fluoride. At a breathing rate equivalent to sedentary activity and an initial concentration of 1440–3580 ppm (5760–15,400 mg/m³) of sulfuryl fluoride, this represents approximately 1 hour of exposure prior to death.

association encourage the use of odor monitoring in the place of industrial hygiene techniques. Odor monitoring is a poor means of detecting MITC because the average odor threshold (1700 ppb) is approximately twice the 800-ppb 1-hour ocular irritation threshold.

Pulmonary function studies and methacholine challenge tests may prove of value in cases of residual airway reactivity. Following the spill of metam-sodium into the Sacramento River, pulmonary evaluation documented 20 cases of persistent irritant-induced asthma and 10 cases of persistent exacerbation of asthma.

3. Chronic effects—As indicated earlier, the irritant effects of MITC and other metam-sodium by-products on the lower airways may produce persistent respiratory problems in some cases.

Recent animal studies have demonstrated that exposure to metam-sodium administered by gavage decreased production of interleukins IL-1a, IL-1b, IL-18, IL-12, IL-12p35, and IL-12p40 and increased IL-10 production (induced by lipopolysaccharide in mice). Other cytokines affected included interferon-γ (IFN-γ), and macrophage migration inhibitory factor (MIF).

MITC by gavage caused effects on cytokine production at doses as low as 17 mg/kg. Working at a moderate rate outdoors (equivalent to walking 2.5 mi/h) for 1 hour would result in approximately 3 mg MITC for an adult female and 5 mg for an adult male. It is unknown if an MITC dose in this range could result in a significant human immune suppression. If suppression of interleukins did occur, it would result in increased vulnerability to some occupational infectious exposures. Recent work, for example, has demonstrated that the interleukin depressed by metam-sodium and MITC, IL-12, is essential for immunity to coccioidomycosis, the cause of San Joaquin Valley fever.

Differential Diagnosis

Anesthesia from halogenated hydrocarbons must be distinguished from exposure to other CNS depressants, including drugs and alcohol. The acute irritation produced by chloropicrin, formaldehyde, acrolein, and sulfur dioxide will be marked by the presence of their distinctive odors. Phosphine has a garlic-like odor that often can be detected on a victim's breath, especially in cases of ingestion. The encephalopathy and peripheral neuropathy from methyl bromide are similar to those from other organic causes of central or peripheral disease, such as alcohol, drugs, and other neurotoxins (see Chapter 24). Toxicity can occur from exposure to levels without a detectable odor, making diagnosis difficult without a history of exposure.

Treatment

Treatment of all fumigant poisonings except cyanide is symptomatic: Respiratory support and anticonvulsants

should be provided as indicated. Dimercaprol [British anti-Lewisite (BAL)] has been used in early methyl bromide poisoning but without evidence of benefit; given its toxicity, it cannot be recommended. Treatment to increase the excretion of inorganic bromide has no rational basis.

Prognosis

Toxicity from the irritants chloropicrin, formaldehyde, acrolein, and sulfur dioxide is limited to their acute reversible effects. On the other hand, deaths have been reported from the use of most of the other fumigant and nematocides. Recovery from nonfatal poisoning usually is complete, except for methyl bromide, which has caused permanent organic brain damage and a prolonged, if not permanent, peripheral neuropathy. Acute liver necrosis followed by cirrhosis and liver cancer has been reported from industrial solvent use of carbon tetrachloride, but not from use as an agriculture fumigant.

REFERENCES

O'Malley M et al: Modeling of methyl isothiocyanate air concentrations associated with community illnesses following a metam-sodium sprinkler application. Am J Indust Med 2004;46:1 [PMID: 15202120].

Pruett SB et al: Sodium methyldithiocarbamate inhibits MAP kinase activation through Toll-like receptor 4. Toxicol Sci 2005;87:75 [PMID: 15933225].

Sudakin DL: Occupational exposure to aluminium phosphide and phosphine gas. Hum Exp Toxicol 2005;24:27 [PMID: 15727053].

RODENTICIDES

Rats are the most prevalent pest in many developing countries and consume up to 20% of stored grain. They represent a significant threat to the food supply in developed countries as well. Other rodents and small mammals such as squirrels, gophers, and rabbits compete for food and act as reservoirs for diseases that affect humans and are considered pests for that reason.

Poisoning with rodenticides is the most widely used method of control of small mammals. To be effective, rodenticides must be attractive to a rat as food, which is difficult because they are fastidious eaters. Rodenticides also must be delayed in action if used as bait because rats will avoid returning to feed where another rat has died after eating. Unfortunately, what is attractive, edible, and ultimately lethal to a rat is also appealing to pets and other animals and small children. Because application of baits results in negligible exposure to applicators, the primary human health hazard from most rodenticides is childhood poisoning from ingestion, although serious poisoning from single ingestions of warfarin is rare.

Table 31–16. Rodenticides historically used in the United States.

Rodenticide	Oral LD$_{50}$ (mg/kg)
Alpha-naphthylenethiourea (ANTU)	6
Coumafuryl	25
Dicumarol	550
Diphacinone	3
Pindone	280
Strychnine	1–30
Warfarin	180
Zinc phosphide	50

Table 31–16 lists the rodenticides in current use. Yellow phosphorus and Vacor are no longer used because of their extreme human health hazard. Sodium fluoroacetate is similarly hazardous but may have some utility against coyotes and wolves. Strychnine may be useful against rats when anticoagulants are no longer effective, but it is toxic to all warm-blooded animals, is not always an effective rodenticide, and its use is controversial. No alpha-naphthylthiourea (ANTU) products are currently registered either with the EPA or with the state of California. The usefulness of rodenticides is limited primarily by the development of resistance in the target species.

Because anticoagulants are the principal chemical class used against rodents, the rest of this discussion is confined to members of this class. The phosphide fumigants, used for outdoor rodent control, were discussed earlier.

Use

The anticoagulants include short- and intermediate-acting compounds, represented by warfarin and diphacinone, and the long-acting compounds ("super-warfarins"), represented by 4-hydroxycoumarin, brodifacoum, bromodialone, difenacoum; and the indione derivative chlorphacinone.

Warfarin is formulated as a dust (10 g/kg of active ingredient, or 1%) for use in holes and runs and as a powder (1 and 5 g/kg, or 0.1% and 0.5%) for mixing with bait for a final concentration of 50–250 mg/kg (0.000050–0.00025%). Warfarin has been used extensively as an oral anticoagulant medication. Diphacinone is formulated as prepared baits in concentrations of 50–125 mg/kg (0.00005–0.000125%).

Occupational & Environmental Exposure

There are no reports of harmful exposure from the manufacture, formulation, or application of dry anticoagulant rodenticides. There is one report of bleeding in a farmer following extensive and prolonged skin contact with a liquid warfarin solution. Childhood ingestion of these compounds is common, although bleeding as a result is uncommon unless the compounds are ingested repeatedly. The long-acting anticoagulants require fewer doses to cause bleeding. From a human case report, the elimination half-life of brodifacoum appears to be approximately 20–25 days.

Mechanism of Action and Clinical Findings

Warfarin is well absorbed from the gastrointestinal tract. Diphacinone is absorbed following ingestion, but there is no information regarding its dermal absorption. All the anticoagulants act through inhibition of hepatic synthesis of prothrombin (factor II) and factors VII, IX, and X. In humans and rats, the half-lives of these factors are longer than the half-life of the anticoagulants, so repeated doses are necessary before significant depression and bleeding occur.

Resistance to warfarin in humans and rats appears to be genetic and may be a result of rapid metabolism.

The anticoagulants also produce capillary damage through an uncertain mechanism, although this, too, is reversed by administration of vitamin K. Skin necrosis and dermatitis have been reported as rare complications of therapeutic use of warfarin but have not been reported as a result of exposure to rodenticides. The indanediones cause neurologic and cardiovascular toxicity in some animal species, but these effects have not been reported in humans.

A. SYMPTOMS & SIGNS

Most cases of accidental ingestion do not result in evidence of toxicity even without treatment because doses usually are single and relatively small. Repeated doses could be followed by bleeding, primarily from the mucous membranes such as the gums and nasal passages and into the skin, joints, and gastrointestinal tract. Abdominal, flank, back, and joint pain reflect bleeding into those areas.

B. LABORATORY FINDINGS

Prolonged prothrombin time may appear 24–48 hours after ingestion of an anticoagulant and often is the only evidence of toxicity following a single exposure. Coagulation time will be increased in cases of significant poisoning, but bleeding time may be normal. Specific factors other than prothrombin may be depressed. Warfarin can be measured in plasma and its metabolites in urine, but these measurements have limited clinical value.

Long-acting warfarins—Prolonged follow-up may be necessary to monitor clotting status following ingestion of the newer long-acting synthetic anticoagulants or "super-warfarins." For example, a 2000 case report described ingestion of eight 43-g boxes of 0.005% brodifacoum. The initial measured level of brodifacoum was 170 ng/mL of serum 6 days after the ingestion. The level was 80 ng/mL 25 days later, 40 ng/mL 32 days, and 20 ng/mL at 40 days after the initial evaluation. Brodifacoum was estimated to reach a safe range (4–10 ng/mL) at 46 days. The disappearance of brodifacoum followed linear (zero-order) kinetics during the period from 6–40 days postingestion (90 ng/25 days, or 3.6 ng/day), although it is likely that the initial clearance was more rapid. Other reported "superwarfarin" cases have required treatment with vitamin K and even fresh-frozen plasma for as long as 1–2 years after initial medical evaluation. Compared with the case reported in 2000, the necessity for such prolonged treatment implies initial ingestion of a higher dose or multiple episodes of ingestion.

Differential Diagnosis

Most cases of rodenticide ingestion are observed or reported episodes and do not result in significant toxicity. In 1998, for example, only 301 of 16,109 ingestions of long-acting anticoagulants reported to U.S. poison centers resulted in overt symptoms or coagulopathy. Epistaxis, bleeding gums, bruising, hematomas, petechiae, hemoptysis, or gastrointestinal bleeding may be presenting symptoms. Symptomatic cases also may present with hematuria that may provoke concern about urinary tract stones or urinary malignancies.

Treatment

Treatment of single acute ingestions usually is unnecessary, but patients should be observed (at home) for 4–5 days following ingestion. Vitamin K may be administered orally in a dosage of 15–25 mg for adults and 5–10 mg for children with a history of ingestion or intramuscularly in a dosage of 5–10 mg for adults and 1–5 mg (up to 0.6 mg/kg) for children with prolonged prothrombin time or bleeding. Following treatment, prothrombin times should be determined every 6–12 hours and used as the basis for further treatment. If bleeding is severe, slow intravenous infusion may be considered but carries a risk of adverse reactions, including flushing, dizziness, hypotension, dyspnea, cyanosis, and death. Transfusion and iron to replace blood loss should be considered.

Treatment in cases of ingestion of brodifacoum or other long-acting warfarin compounds may be prolonged. In the case described earlier (see "Laboratory Findings"), 46 days of oral vitamin K was required.

Prognosis

Treatment is usually effective within 3–6 hours. The prognosis is determined by the extent and location of bleeding and is usually good.

REFERENCES

Painter JA et al: *Salmonella*-based rodenticides and public health. Emerg Infect Dis 2004;10:985 [PMID: 15207046].

Sarin S et al: Prolonged coagulopathy related to superwarfarin overdose. Ann Intern Med 2005;142:156 [PMID: 15657170].

FUNGICIDES (PHTHALIMIDES, DITHIOCARBAMATES, SUBSTITUTED AROMATICS, TRIAZOLES, COPPER FUNGICIDES, & MISCELLANEOUS COMPOUNDS)

Pesticides classified as fungicides overlap with compounds classed as algaecides and antibacterial agents. Most fungicides are distinct from other pesticides owing to the unique plant characteristics of fungi and the fact that the chemical must kill or inhibit the fungi without adversely affecting the host plant. Quantitative structure-activity relationship (QSAR) models of fungicide activity highlight the importance of hydrophobicity (measured by log P) and three-dimensional steric configuration, important in inhibiting fungal enzymes such as 14α-demethylase, involved in sterol synthesis.

Approximately 150 fungicides are available, mostly synthetic organic chemicals of relatively recent development. This discussion is confined to the most commonly used classes of compounds, the phthalimido compounds, dithiocarbamates, substituted aromatics, and miscellaneous compounds with important adverse effects (Table 31–17).

Most crops are susceptible to fungi and related diseases. Frequent application of fungicides often is necessary owing to the rapid replication of many fungi. With the exception of a few systemics, fungicides are only active where they have been left as a residue on a plant, making uniform application necessary. They are applied as sprays or dusts so that a film of residue is left on the plants. Many seeds are treated with fungicides. A limited number of general-purpose lawn and garden fungicides are available for home use.

Occupational & Environmental Exposure

Field workers and employees in greenhouses and nurseries are more apt to be exposed to fungicides than to other pesticides on a routine basis because fungicides are only effective as long as a residue is present on plant surfaces, and application is often necessary at the same time plants must be handled by these workers. Seed-treatment facilities are an important site of exposure to fungicide.

Homeowners are exposed to lawn and garden treatments. Most fruits and vegetables have allowable residues (tolerances) for one or more fungicides. Water contamination has not been a significant problem to date.

Table 31–17. Fungicides used in the United States.

Chemical Class	Oral LD$_{50}$ (mg/kg)
Phthalimido compounds	
Captan	9000
Folpet	10,000
Captafol	6000
Dithiocarbamates (ethylene-bis-dithiocarbamates [EBDCs])	
Ferbam	1000
Vapam	1700
Maneb	7000
Zineb	5000
Thiram	800
Ziram	1500
Substituted aromatics	
Chlorothalonil	10,000
Chloroneb	11,000
Pentachloronitrobenzene (PCNB)	12,000
Hexachlorobenzene	10,000
Pentachlorophenol (PCP)	200
Triazole compounds	
Bayleton (triadimefon)	300–600
Baytan (triadimenol)	90
Fenbuconazole (thiazopyr)	> 5000
Imazalil	227–343
Terrazole	4000
Miscellaneous compounds	
Inorganic Sulfur	None
Metalaxyl-Alanine derivative (Ridomil)	669
Aliette/Fosetyl-A1-Aluminum phosphonate	3700–5800
Triphenyltin (Organotin)	125
Fenarimol (Pyrimidine)	2500
Iprodione-Imidazolidine	3500–4400
Mercury compounds	1–200

Safety issues arise for few fungicides. Nevertheless, products are formulated with elemental sulfur because of its flammability. Hot-weather aerial applications present a particular risk, and several fires and crop-duster accidents associated with burning sulfur have occurred.

Clinical Findings

A. Thiocarbamate Compounds

Disulfiram (Antabuse), used to treat alcoholism because of its ability to produce an adverse reaction in the presence of alcohol, is a dithiocarbamate and shares a number of properties with other compounds in the class. Several dithiocarbamates, including the ethylene-bis-dithiocarbamates (EBDCs), are used as accelerators in the vulcanization of rubber. These compounds are not acutely toxic;

the primary recognized health effect is dermatitis, both irritant and allergic. An alcohol-dithiocarbamate reaction is marked by headache, nausea, vomiting, flushing, dizziness, confusion, and disorientation.

1. Chronic effects—Thiocarbamate compounds also contain varying levels of the contaminant ethylenethiourea (ETU), a material classified as a probable human carcinogen. ETU has affinity for the thyroid similar to the antithyroid drug propylthiouracil. Mancozeb and zineb both cause thyroid adenocarcinoma in animal tests. The IARC concluded that the mechanism of ETU-related thyroid cancer was not genetic and unlikely to cause cancer following low-dose exposure to humans. The EPA nevertheless classified the compound as a probable human carcinogen (Table 31–18).

Sprayers in Mexico heavily exposed to maneb and mancozeb showed increased levels of thyroid-stimulating hormone (TSH) compared with controls but normal levels of thyroxine (T$_4$). Sprayers also showed increased levels of sister chromatid exchange and chromosome translocations. In reproductive studies, ETU produces neural tube and brain malformations in rats. Other test species do not appear susceptible to this adverse effect.

B. Phthalimido Compounds

Captan and captafol have low systemic toxicity but can cause both immediate and delayed allergic reactions. Skin irritation also may occur given sufficient exposure. In QSAR terms, the phthalimido compounds act as reactive electrophiles (structural element IUNIQ). This property also accounts for the carcinogenicity of the compounds in rodent bioassays. Both captan and folpet cause intestinal tumors in rodent species. Captafol causes lymphosarcoma in feeding studies with mice. The EPA ranking system designates all three compounds as probable human carcinogens (see Table 31–18).

Structural analogies with the drug thalidomide have raised concerns that the phthalimido compounds could cause teratogenicity in agricultural workers. Studies of teratogenic effects of captan show positive effects in chick embryos but negative in Syrian hamsters, rabbits, and nonhuman primates.

C. Substituted Aromatics

The substituted aromatics include several compounds with a marked tendency to cause immediate and delayed allergy, including chlorothalonil and pentachloronitrobenzene (PCNB). Hexachlorobenzene (HCB) was used formerly as an antifungal seed treatment, but several episodes of accidental food contamination have curtailed its use. During the 1950s, HCB caused a widespread outbreak of acquired porphyria and adverse reproductive outcomes; serum levels of HCB showed a strong correlation with risk for spontaneous abortion.

Table 31–18. Animal studies evaluating chronic effects of fungicides.

Chemical, Use Category, or Structural Class	Cancer or Reproductive Effect	EPA Potency Factor –Q* $(mg/kg/d)^{-1}$	Cancer Classification
Thiocarbamates & ETU			
Mancozeb; maneb	Thyroid follicular cell adenomas and carcinomas, combined thyroid follicular cell adenomas and/or carcinomas in male and female rats		B2
Zineb	Cancer: 3500 mg/kg/wk for 6 weeks caused one of two mice strains tested to develop benign lung tumors after 3 weeks Reproductive: See ethylenethiourea below		3-IARC
Ethylenethiourea	Cancer: rat thyroid; mouse liver Reproductive: ETU produces neural tube and brain malformations in rats; other species not affected except at high-dose levels	1.1 E-1	B2
Phthalimido compounds			
Captafol (canceled)	Cancer: mouse lymphosarcoma	5.1 E-2	B2
Captan	Intestinal tumors occurred in multiple strains of male and female mice; renal and cortical/tubular cell neoplasms occurred in rats Female rats developed uterine sarcomas Reproductive: Positive studies in chick embryos reported in public literature; incomplete ossification observed in rabbit study reported to California EPA at 30 and 100 mg/kg/d; study in hamsters negative; literature report on teratogenicity on nonhuman primates negative	3.6 E-3	B2
Folpet (canceled)	Carcinoma and adenoma of the duodenum in male and female CD-1 and B6C3F1 mice	3.49 E-3	B2
Triazoles			
Bayleton (triadimefon)	Cancer: hyperplastic liver nodules at high dose; also thyroid follicular tumor		C
Baytan (triadimenol)	Male and female mouse liver		C
Cyproconazole	Male mouse liver	3.02 E-01	C
Fenbuconazole	Female mouse liver male rat thyroid	1.65 E-2	C
Hexaconazole	Rat testis	2.3 E-2	C
Propiconazole	Male mouse liver		C
Tebuconazole	Male and female mouse liver		C
Terrazole (etridazole-fungicide)	Cancer: male and female rats dose-related lung adenomas Male reproductive: chronic rat study showed testicular atrophy at mid and high dose	7.2 E-2 male 5.4 E-3 female rare tumor	B2
Triflumizole			E
Uniconazole	Male mouse liver		C
Substituted aromatics			
Chlorothalonil	Cancer: kidney and forestomach tumors in male/female rats at and below MTD	1.1 E-2	B2
Hexachlorobenzene	Thyroid adenomas, hepatomas (hamsters); mice hepatomas	1.7	B2
Pentachlorophenol (PCP)	Increases in hepatocellular adenomas and carcinomas, adrenal medulla pheochromocytomas, and malignant pheochromocytomas, and/or hemangiomas in mice. Some workers in NIOSH dioxin cohort with increased risk of all tumor types combined had extensive exposure to PCP		B2
Miscellaneous fungicides			
Benomyl and MBC (Benomyl and thiophanate methyl breakdown product)	Cancer: California CPR study: mouse liver adenomas at 500–1500 ppm in feed Reproductive: Encephalocele, hydrocephalus, microphthalmia, and anophthalmia in animal model systems over doses ranging from 15.6 mg/kg to 125 mg/kg Male reproductive: Dose-dependent decreases in mean testis weight and mean seminiferous tubular diameter and occlusions in efferent ductules in rodents dosed with 400 mg/kg of benomyl metabolite carbendazim (MBC)	4.20 E-03	C

(continued)

Table 31–18. Animal studies evaluating chronic effects of fungicides. (continued)

Chemical, Use Category, or Structural Class	Cancer or Reproductive Effect	EPA Potency Factor –Q* $(mg/kg/d)^{-1}$	Cancer Classification
Miscellaneous fungicides			
Methyl mercury, mercury, and mercury compounds (inactive or canceled registrations as seed treatment and paint preservative)	Reproductive: Pregnant mice treated with a single doses of 4–8 mg/kg methyl mercury had offspring with no structural birth defects, but showed cerebellar deficits in behavioral tests and pathologic changes in cerebellar Purkinje cells		
Furmecyclox-Furancarboxamide	Female rat liver	2.98 E-2	B2
Prochloraz-Imidazole	Male and female mouse liver	1.50 E-01	C
Iprodione-Imidazolidine	Male and female mouse liver at 4000 ppm in diet; rat testes—testicular adenomas at 1600 ppm in diet (California DPR)	4.39 E-2	Likely
Vinclozolin (Ronilan)-Oxazolidinedione			E
Coal tar creosote	Human/animal skin carcinogen		A
Tycor (Ethiozin)-Triazine	Male and female rat thyroid		C
Metalaxyl-Alanine derivative			E
Fosetyl-A1-(Aluminum phosphonate)	Male rat bladder at 30,000–40,000 ppm in diet		C

The EPA rankings designate both chlorothalonil and HCB as probable human carcinogens (see Table 31–18). Pentachlorophenol has complex dermal and systemic toxicity. Although no longer in use, it remains of concern because of residual contamination at some hazardous waste sites.

D. TRIAZOLE COMPOUNDS

This group structurally resembles ketoconazole and other antifungal compounds used in human medicine. Triadimefon, the prototypical compound in the group, has low to moderate toxicity but a maximum application rate of only 8 ounces/acre. As with most of the compounds in the group, triadimefon is a possible human carcinogen. Feeding studies show that it causes liver adenomas in mice. Terrazole is the only compound in the group classified as a probable human carcinogen. It also causes testicular atrophy in the rat (see Table 31–18).

E. MISCELLANEOUS COMPOUNDS

1. Benomyl—Benomyl and its breakdown product, carbendazim (MBC), also cause mouse liver adenomas. It produces developmental anomalies, including encephalocele, hydrocephalus, microphthalmia, and anophthalmia, in various animal model systems over doses ranging from 15.6–125 mg/kg. Clusters of anophthalmia have been reported in Britain and Wales, speculatively associated with benomyl exposure (by means of residence in a high-use area). Benomyl also causes dose-dependent male reproductive effects (see Table 31–18).

2. Mercury—Mercury fungicides are no longer used as either seed treatments or paint preservatives, but exposure to mercury remains a significant environmental issue. Because of its persistence in the nervous system, developmental toxicity for these compounds is significant (effect on cerebellar function in behavioral tests). Pregnant mice administered single doses of methyl mercury have anatomically normal offspring that demonstrate functional and histologic cerebellar abnormalities. Clinical cases of in utero mercury poisoning have resulted from episodes of grain contaminated with mercury in Iraq and from fish contaminated with mercury in Minamata, Japan. Currently, there are no mercury-containing seed-treatment fungicides with active U.S. registrations. Organic mercuries used as preservatives in latex paint were phased out following reported cases of acrodynia associated with their use in 1990.

3. Iprodione—The EPA also classifies iprodione as a likely carcinogen based on male and female rat liver adenomas. Testicular adenomas occurred in animals fed

1600-ppm iprodione diets. In these doses, the compound had a marked antiandrogenic effect.

4. Elemental sulfur—Between applications to grapes, tomatoes, and sugar beets, farmers use approximately 70 million pounds of inorganic sulfur annually. It has a low potency when compared with synthetic organic pesticides. Application rates for triadimefon, for example, range from 6–8 oz/acre compared with a range of 3–30 lb/acre for inorganic sulfur, often with multiple applications required to achieve control.

Animal data indicate that sulfur is basically nonreactive. It produces no irritation in the Draize dermal irritation assay and is negative in predictive allergy tests submitted for pesticide registration. Nevertheless, sulfur is among the most frequently reported sources of illness in agricultural workers, a discrepancy perhaps explained by transformation of elemental sulfur to various sulfur oxide compounds. Some, such as sulfur dioxide and sulfuric acid, are known to cause irritation, and others, notably the sulfite compounds, are recognized causes of allergic reactions.

In 155 California cases involving pesticide handlers directly exposed to sulfur, 68 (44%) involved ocular exposure, 70 (45%) involved dermatitis (typically in a contact pattern), and 34 (22%) involved either respiratory or systemic illness. Some cases had rhinitis or asthma symptoms that suggested a possible immediate allergy to sulfur, but no cases had documented provocation tests to demonstrate that the reactions were allergic rather than irritant in nature. Cases of allergic contact dermatitis, documented by patch testing, have been reported occasionally in sulfur applicators. In a cross-sectional study of California nursery workers, 6 of 39 subjects had positive patch test reactions to sulfur. Although none of the reactions was relevant to a specific episode of dermatitis, the positive reactions correlated with a history of doing pesticide application work in the nursery industry.

Safety issues also have arisen because of the tendency of sulfur to oxidize spontaneously. Cases reported in California included six cases of fires associated with loading or applying elemental sulfur. Several involved spontaneous combustion during summer months when temperatures routinely exceed 32.2°C (90°F). There were three additional fires that occurred when loads of sulfur ignited after a crop-duster crash.

5. Copper naphthenate, copper sulfate, and other copper compounds—Copper sulfate has been used as a fungicide for more than 200 years. Uses include control of downy mildew, blights, leaf spots, apple scab, and peach leaf curl. In vineyards, it is mixed with lime and applied as "Bordeaux mixture." It causes acute gastric irritation when ingested and also may cause irritation of the eyes and skin.

Systemic poisoning associated with ingestion of copper sulfate also may cause methemoglobinemia. This also has been reported in conjunction with ingestion of an organic copper fungicide, copper-8-hydroxyquinolate. A case reported to the California illness registry also demonstrated 16% methemoglobinemia and borderline elevated levels of serum copper in an adult with indoor exposure to copper naphthenate. Two children from the same residence had definite elevation of serum copper but did not demonstrate methemoglobinemia. Methemoglobinemia may be more likely in patients with partial or complete deficiency of glucose-6-phosphate dehydrogenase (G6PD). The majority of cases of indoor exposure to the compound have exhibited only upper respiratory irritation, eye irritation, and mild, nonspecific systemic symptoms. The tendency to cause irritant symptoms and the apparently long environmental half-life have led to prohibition of indoor applications of copper naphthenate. The compound is still legal to apply as an outdoor wood preservative.

A published case report documented elevation of serum copper following a residential application of copper naphthenate in Tennessee. The significance of the increased serum copper following such exposures is uncertain. However, elevated serum copper related to chronically contaminated water sources has been associated with childhood hepatic cirrhosis. Animal studies evaluating chronic inhalation exposure to copper naphthenate are lacking.

Laboratory Findings

Confirmation of a hypersensitivity response to a fungicide requires patch testing for allergic contact dermatitis and for asthma inhalation challenge or pre- and postshift spirometry. Diagnosis of an alcohol dithiocarbamate reaction is based on the history of concurrent exposures.

Serum copper levels and methemoglobin levels may be helpful in evaluating patients exposed to copper fungicides to ensure that only irritant symptoms are present. Normal levels of methemoglobin usually are less than 1%, and normal serum copper concentrations range between 65 and 145 µg/dL.

Differential Diagnosis

Fungicide-induced allergic contact dermatitis must be distinguished from contact dermatitis caused by irritants and allergic contact dermatitis caused by other pesticides or plants. Asthma in a phthalimide manufacturing worker may be due to an intermediate in the manufacturing process.

Elevated methemoglobin can derive from exposure to chromates, nitrobenzene, naphthalene, aniline dyes, and numerous nitrate- or sulfonamide-containing medications. Congenital enzyme deficiencies may contribute to the condition including NADH-dependent methemoglobin reductase deficiency and cytochrome-b$_5$ deficiency.

Serum copper may be elevated owing to increased levels of the copper-binding protein ceruloplasm. This is associated with smoking, inflammatory conditions, and high levels of endogenous or exogenous estrogens.

Treatment

Allergic contact dermatitis is treated by withdrawal of the offending agent and local steroids. Asthma is treated by removal from exposure and symptomatic treatment as needed.

Prognosis

Fungicide-related allergies should resolve following cessation of exposure. Irritant symptoms related to copper fungicides usually are short term unless sufficient inhalation exposure occurs to provoke persistent reactive airways.

REFERENCES

Gutierrez M et al: Occupational and environmental exposure to tribromophenol used for wood surface protection in sawmills. Int J Environ Health Res 2005;15:171 [PMID: 1613448].

Steenland K: Carcinogenicity of EBDCs. Environ Health Perspect 2003;111:266 [PMID: 12727609].

Yang CC et al: Prolonged hemolysis and methemoglobinemia following organic copper fungicide ingestion. Vet Hum Toxicol 2004;46:321 [PMID: 15587250].

■ HERBICIDES

MISCELLANEOUS HERBICIDES OF LOW TOXICITY

Herbicides are pesticides that are intended to prevent or control the growth of unwanted plants or kill them once they have appeared. They have largely replaced mechanical methods of weed control and are currently the largest category of pesticides used in agriculture, accounting for 58% of agricultural pesticide sales in the United States and 44% of sales worldwide in 2001. Included here are plant growth regulators that alter plant development, defoliants that cause leaves to drop prematurely, and desiccants that accelerate the drying of plant parts. Nonselective herbicides affect all plants, selective herbicides affect specific target weeds, contact herbicides affect plant parts that touch the chemical, and translocated herbicides are absorbed by the plant and act at distant sites.

Table 31–19. Some herbicides with little or no known acute toxicity to humans.

Herbicide	Oral LD$_{50}$ (mg/kg)
Alachlor	1000
Amitrole	1000
Ammonium sulfamate	4000
Atrazine	3000
Bifenox	6500
Dalapon	6500
Dicamba	1000
Ethafuralin	10,000
Glyphosphate	4300
Linuron	1500
Monuron	3500
Oryzalin	10,000
Oturon	3500
Oxadiazon	3500
Pictoram	8000
Prometon	3000
Pronamide	5500
Propanil	1500
Propham	9000
Simazine	5000
Terbutryn	2000
Trifluralin	3500

The herbicides that have serious recognized or suspected human health effects—the dipyridyls and the chlorophenoxyacetic acids—are considered separately in following sections. Substituted phenols used as herbicides were discussed earlier. The organophosphate defoliants differ from the organophosphate insecticides in causing relatively more inhibition of neurotoxic esterase (NTE) and relatively less inhibition of acetylcholinesterase (AChE). The rest of the synthetic organic herbicides have limited recognized acute effects on human health.

Several categories of herbicides demonstrate at least limited activity in animal cancer bioassays. Additional details are given in the section below entitled "Animal and Human Cancer Studies Implicating Herbicides."

The inorganic herbicides (e.g., arsenicals) are more hazardous and are being used with decreasing frequency. Table 31–19 lists examples of the organic herbicides.

Use

In addition to agriculture, herbicides are used to clear rights of way along roadsides, railroads, power lines, fence lines, and property lines; to reduce competition for seedlings in forests; and for fire prevention by reducing the amounts of combustible grasses and brush available as fuel. They are usually sprayed in bands or strips, broadcast over an entire area, or focused on one area or group of weeds (spot or directed treatment). The timing of application may be preplanting (before planting crop), preemergence (after planting but before emergence of weeds or crop), and postemergence (after weeds or crops emerge).

Occupational & Environmental Exposure

Occupational exposure to herbicides occurs as a result of dermal exposure to spray applicators and flaggers, whereas environmental exposure occurs in the form of residues on crops and food. Although a few studies suggest the possibility of health effects occurring in populations as a result of spray drift or other environmental contamination from herbicides, with the exception of cases of obvious spray drift with damage to nontarget plants, such exposure is difficult to document.

Pharmacokinetics & Mechanism of Action

Apart from the bipyridyl compounds paraquat and diquat, most herbicides have marked differential toxicity to plants. These compounds show little evidence of toxicity to mammals; consequently, there is little information on pharmacokinetics or mechanisms of action in humans.

Animal and Human Cancer Studies Implicating Herbicides

Classes of herbicides demonstrating some evidence of carcinogenicity (Table 31–20) in animals include acetanilides (i.e., acetochlor, alachlor, metolachlor, and butachlor), nitrobenzenes, phenol derivatives, and triazines. Human data for most of the compounds are lacking. However, a cohort study of 2045 workers manufacturing the triazine herbicide atrazine demonstrated a 75% excess of prostate cancer (11 cases versus 6.3 expected) with a significant excess among actively working employees (5 cases versus 1.3 expected). Nine of the 11 cases involved early-stage cancer. The finding occurred during the early 1990s coincident with the initial availability of the prostate-specific antigen (PSA) screening test for prostate cancer and may have been related to a screening program operated by the plant medical department. A follow-up case-control study with 12 cases and 130 controls did not show an association between case status and either the duration or intensity of exposure.

Clinical Findings

A. SYMPTOMS & SIGNS

Some formulations of herbicides contain organic solvents, surfactants, emulsifiers, or other vehicles and additives that may cause eye, nose, or throat irritation in applicators exposed to spray mists and dermatitis in mixers and loaders as a result of prolonged skin contact. Otherwise, these compounds have no known human health effects.

B. LABORATORY FINDINGS

There is little or no information regarding measurement of parent compounds or metabolites in biologic media.

Differential Diagnosis

It is always possible that these compounds have effects not yet appreciated in humans, particularly from accidental or deliberate ingestion. The toxicity of "inert" ingredients should be considered in evaluating persons with symptoms following exposure.

Treatment

Because these compounds have little or no known human health effects, treatment of any symptoms resulting from their use should be symptomatic only. For evaluation of symptomatic patients, the manufacturer should be consulted, particularly for identification of the inert ingredients.

Prognosis

Acute irritation and dermatitis from herbicide formulations should resolve shortly after cessation of exposure.

CHLOROPHENOXYACETIC ACIDS

Essentials of Diagnosis

A. ACUTE EFFECTS

- Topical irritation: redness of skin, burning, soreness in throat and chest, and cough
- Ingestion associated with CNS depression, myotonia, rhabdomyolysis, renal failure, nausea and vomiting, severe hypotension

B. CHRONIC EFFECTS

- Scattered cases of peripheral neuropathy following either ingestion of 2,4-D or occupational exposure

General Considerations

The principal herbicidal derivatives of phenoxy acetic acid include 2,4-dichlorophenoxyacetic acid (2,4-D), 2,4,5-trichlorophenoxyacetic acid (2,4,5-T), 2-methyl-4-chlorophenoxyacetic acid (MCPA), and their salts and ester derivatives. Silvex, kuron, and fenac are

Table 31–20. Animal studies evaluating chronic effects of growth regulators and herbicides.

Chemical, Use Category, or Structural Class	Cancer or Reproductive Effect	EPA Potency Factor –Q* $(mg/kg/d)^{-1}$	Cancer Classification
Growth regulator			
Daminozide	Rat: uterine sarcomas; unsymmetrical dimethylhydrazine contaminant—female liver tumors	8.70 E-03	B2
	Mouse: liver angiosarcomas at 10,000 ppm in diet; lung adenomas and adenomacarcinomas, angiosarcomas in mouse drinking water study 3000 mg/kg/d (California DPR)		
Calcium cyanamide	Mouse ovarian	6.74 E-2	C
Ethephon			E
Maleic hydrazide			D
Herbicide			
Acetanilides			
Acetochlor	Rat nasal; mouse multiple sites	1.69 E-02	B2
Alachlor	Rat nasal	8.0 E-2	B2
Metolachlor	Female rat liver	9.60 E-03	C
Butachlor			Known/likely
Aniline and nitroaniline derivatives			
Asulam	Male rat/adrenal pheochromocytomas—metabolite hydroquinone		C
Chloramben	Cancer: hepatocellular cancers in mice at 20,000 ppm in diet; other bioassays negative	1.60 E-04	
Ethalfuralin	Cancer: mouse study—hepatocellular hyperplasia without definite adenomas at 1500 ppm, less at 400 ppm in diet (California DPR)		
Pendimethalin	Male and female rat thyroid		C
Dipyridyls			
Diquat			E
Paraquat			E
Metallic			
Cacodylic acid	Female and male rat bladder		A
Chromate wood preservatives	Cancer: human lung carcinogen (NTP)		
	Reproductive: EPA lists as teratogen and fetotoxin		
Methanearsonic acid			B2
Nitrobenzene			
Acifluorfen	Mouse liver; male and female	1.1 E-1	B2
Dinocap	Reproductive: Torticollis and fetotoxicity in offspring at doses below those producing maternal toxicity		C
Dinoseb	Cancer: EPA evaluation incomplete; 1971 published mouse study negative at maximum tolerated dose		B2
	Reproductive: Abdominal distention, cleft palate, torticollis at MTD; torticollis at doses below MTD; fetotoxicity		B2
	Male: Diffuse tubular atrophy/reproductive failure in rats fed up to 200 ppm; decreased sperm motility at doses down to 125 ppm		
Nitrofen/TOK	Liver cancer male and female mice; pancreatic cancer female rats		B2
Phenoxy and phenol compounds and related contaminants			
Dichlorophenoxy-acetic acid (2,4-D)	Astrocytomas male rats at high dose only; several completely negative studies		C
Dicamba 2,3,7,8-Tetra-chlorodibenzo-para-dioxin (TCDD); contaminated by banned 2,4,5-trichlorophenol-related phenoxy compounds, not 2,4-D	Cancer: By gavage, TCDD increased thyroid follicular cell adenomas in male rats and neoplastic nodules of the liver in female rats, hepatocellular carcinomas in mice of both sexes and thyroid follicular cell adenomas in female mice. Also positive feeding and positive skin application studies. Other studies indicate that TCDD is most effective as a promoter, rather than an initiator of cancer		D
	Reproductive: Cleft palate, kidney anomalies mice/rats; fetotoxic to variety of experimental animals; mouse NOEL = 0.1 μg/kg/d; male toxin at doses above those producing above effects		B2

(continued)

Table 31–20. Animal studies evaluating chronic effects of growth regulators and herbicides. (continued)

Chemical, Use Category, or Structural Class	Cancer or Reproductive Effect	EPA Potency Factor –Q* (mg/kg/d)$^{-1}$	Cancer Classification
o-Phenyl-phenol and Na salt	Male rat bladder	2.20 E-03	B2
Pentachlorophenol; contamination by hexa- and higher chlorinated and dioxins	Cancer: Studies of two formulated PCP products (Dowcide and Penta) showed increases in cancers of the spleen, liver, and adrenal gland in test mice or rats at doses of about 17 to 18 mg/kg/d	1.29 E-01	B2
Thiocarbamates			
Butylate			E
Molinate (Ordram)	Reproductive: Decreased survival and growth of their young at 30 mg/kg/d; 50 mg/kg/d on 6–15, 8–11, 12–15 toxicity in the young in the form of resorptions, subcutaneous edema, dilated ureters, and skeletal anomalies. Only at maternally toxic doses		
Sulfallate	Positive in NCI mouse and rat bioassays		
Triallate	Mouse liver		C
Triazine			
Atrazine	Female rat mammary	2.22 E-1	C
Cyanazine	Cancer: female rat mammary	8.40 E-01	B2
	Teratogenicity, fetotoxicity—head anomalies 25 mg/kg 6–15 days; NOEL 10 mg/kg/d—no effect in Sprague Dawley rat; fetotoxicity NZ rabbits but no teratogenicity		
Hexazinone	Male and female mouse liver		C
Propazine	Rat mammary		C
Simazine	Female rat mammary	1.2 E-1	C
Terbutryn (herbicide)-(canceled)		8.9 E-3	C
Triazole			
Amitrole	Rat thyroid mouse liver	1.1	B2
Paclobutrazol			D
Trifluorobenzene			
Fluoridone			E
Fomesafen (herbicide)		1.90 E-01	C
Haloxyfop-Methyl Verdict (herbicide)	Male and female mouse liver	7.39	C
Lactofen	Mouse liver	1.70 E-01	B2
Oxyfluorfen	Mouse liver	1.28 E-01	C
Treflan/Trifluralin	Male rat thyroid	7.7 E-03	C
Prodiamine	Rat thyroid		C
Sulfosate			E
Urea herbicides			
Nicosulfuron			E
Primisulfuron-methyl			D
Bromacil	Male mouse liver		C
Bromoxynil	Cancer: male mouse liver		C
	Reproductive: Reported effects of bromoxynil are limited to skeletal abnormalities (a high incidence of supernumerary ribs as compared to controls) at doses that also produced some maternal toxicity		
Rimsulfuron			E
Tribenuron methyl	Female rat mammary		C
Linuron	Rat testicular		C
Halosulfuron Methyl			E
Tebuthiuron			D
Triasulfuron			C

(continued)

Table 31–20. Animal studies evaluating chronic effects of growth regulators and herbicides. (continued)

Chemical, Use Category, or Structural Class	Cancer or Reproductive Effect	EPA Potency Factor –Q* (mg/kg/d)$^{-1}$	Cancer Classification
Other herbicides			
Oxadixyl	Male and female rat liver	5.30 E-02	C
Desmedipham			E
Glyphosate	Cancer: equivocal effect—renal adenomas and a few carcinomas; not clearly dose related in mice oncogenicity studies; high dose tested was 30,000 ppm in diet		C
Dimethipin			C
Imazamethabenz-methyl			D
Pronamide	Mouse liver; rat thyroid and testes	1.54 E-02	C
Oryzalin	Female rat mammary	1.3 E-1	C
Dichlobenil	Male and female rat liver		C
Ethofumesate			D
Oxadiazon	Male and female mouse liver	1.4 E-1	C
Tridiphane		3.00 E-01	C
Nitrapyrin	Male rat kidney; mouse inadequate		D
Quizalofop-ethyl	Mouse liver equivoc		C
Diclofop-methyl	Female and male mouse liver	4.40 E-01	C
Norflurazon			C
Pyridaben			E
Dithiopyr			E
Thiazopyr	Rat thyroid		C
Flumetsulam			E
Quinclorac	Male rat pancreas		C
Dacthal			
Clofentezine	Rat thyroid		C
Bentazon			E
Picloram			D
Cinmethylin			D

homologues of 2,4,5-T, whereas 2,4-DB and MCPB, MCPCA, and MCPP are homologues of 2,4-D and MCPA, respectively. They are translocated herbicides relatively selective for broadleaf plants. 2,4,5-T and its homologues are no longer manufactured or used in the United States because of their combination contamination with 2,3,7,8-tetrachlorodibenzo-*p*-dioxin (TCDD) and the controversy over health effects in environmentally exposed populations and Vietnam veterans. While certain batches of 2,4-D have been found to be contaminated with low levels of other lesser chlorinated dioxins such as dichlorodibenzo-*p*-dioxin, none of its contaminants has been found to be of toxicologic importance. The toxicity of dioxins is discussed in Chapters 28 and 39.

Use

The chlorophenoxy herbicides have had a wide variety of uses, including control of undesirable perennial hardwood trees and plants for "release" of desirable evergreen softwood trees.

Occupational & Environmental Exposure

Occupational exposure occurs primarily as direct contact with liquid concentrate during mixing and loading and inhalation and contact with spray mist during application. Although concern has been expressed about environmental exposure of populations living near conifer forests where chlorophenoxy herbicides are applied, in the absence of obvious spray drift with nontarget crop damage, such exposure is difficult to document. 2,4-D is degraded rapidly in the environment, and water contamination has not been a major problem.

Pharmacokinetics & Mechanism of Action

The herbicidal mechanism of action of chlorophenoxy-acetic acids is uncertain but appears to involve a mimicking of plant auxins (growth hormones) and effects on plant metabolism. They are absorbed by inhalation, dermal contact, and ingestion and are excreted rapidly unchanged in urine. The mechanisms of any health effects on humans other than irritation are uncertain. They are weak uncouplers of oxidative phosphorylation and may produce hyperthermia at extremely high doses as a result of increased heat production. A study reported to the EPA indicated that 2,4-D caused an increase in brain tumors in rats given 40 mg/kg per day by mouth. A study of cancer deaths in farmers in Kansas was reported, in 1986, to show an association between lymphoma and the use of 2,4-D. A recent case-control study reported an association between Agent Orange exposure in Vietnam veterans and the occurrence of prostate cancer. However, exposure was assessed by a simple questionnaire, and the results could have been attributable to response bias.

Clinical Findings

A. SYMPTOMS & SIGNS

Some formulations produce skin irritation following contact with liquid; irritation of the eyes, nose, throat, and respiratory tract, with burning and cough from exposure to spray mist; and irritation of the gastrointestinal tract, with abdominal pain, nausea, and vomiting following ingestion. Ingestion of chlorophenoxyacetic acid herbicides has resulted in nausea, vomiting, abdominal pain, and diarrhea followed by muscle twitching, myotonia, metabolic acidosis, and a hypermetabolic state with fever, tachycardia, hypertension, sweating, convulsions, and coma.

Approximately six cases of peripheral neuropathy have been reported following relatively large dermal exposures to 2,4-D over the course of a few days. Clinically, these resembled idiopathic acute symmetric polyneuropathy (Guillain-Barré syndrome) and organophosphate-induced delayed neuropathy in their symptoms of an initial influenza-like illness associated with nausea, vomiting, diarrhea, and myalgias, followed by an asymptomatic interval and then, 7–10 days later, by rapidly ascending loss of both motor and sensory nerve function. Respiratory function was spared in most cases.

Chloracne has been reported as a result of exposure to TCDD in 2,4,5-T manufacturing plant workers. A number of epidemiologic studies have suggested an association between exposure to chlorophenoxyacetic acid herbicides and soft-tissue sarcomas. NIOSH has established a registry of cases of such tumors.

B. LABORATORY FINDINGS

Exposure to a chlorophenoxyacetic compound can be confirmed through analysis of blood or urine by gas-liquid chromatography. Urine samples should be collected as soon as possible after exposure because the chemical may be excreted completely within 24–72 hours. There is insufficient information to relate a spot urine level precisely to a level of exposure. However, because these compounds are excreted almost entirely unchanged in urine, a dose can be measured by collecting and analyzing all urine, provided collection is begun promptly after exposure. Other laboratory findings in cases of acute intoxication are entirely nonspecific. In the few cases of peripheral neuropathy associated with exposure to 2,4-D where testing was done, nerve conduction velocities were normal or slightly depressed, and spinal fluid analyses were unremarkable.

Differential Diagnosis

Acute irritation following direct exposure or acute intoxication following ingestion present with obvious diagnoses. The differential diagnosis for a patient with peripheral neuropathy following exposure to 2,4-D includes idiopathic acute symmetric polyneuropathy and exposure to other neurotoxic compounds, including organophosphates.

Treatment

Treatment of acute irritation and peripheral neuropathy is entirely symptomatic. Because chlorophenoxyacetic compounds are weak organic acids, they are preferentially excreted in alkaline urine. In severe poisoning from ingestion of large doses, alkalinization of the urine can hasten elimination of the chemical and may improve the course of intoxication. Administration of large fluid volumes to achieve "forced" diuresis should be avoided owing to the risk of precipitating pulmonary edema.

Prognosis

Although death from ingestion of a chlorophenoxyacetic acid has been reported, severe intoxications apparently have been infrequent, and most victims have survived. In cases of peripheral neuropathy following exposure to 2,4-D, maximum paralysis lasted approximately 1 week or less. Recovery of function usually was prolonged for up to 1 year following exposure, with some residual weakness in most cases.

Chronic Health Effects

A number of studies conducted in Sweden suggest an association between phenoxy herbicides and soft-tissue sarcoma, but these studies have not been consistently replicated in other populations. Nevertheless, manufacturing populations have shown dose-response relationships between exposure (characterized by high levels of serum dioxin) and total cancer mortality.

DIPYRIDYLS (PARAQUAT & DIQUAT)

Essentials of Diagnosis

A. ACUTE EFFECTS

- Contact with skin, eyes, and respiratory tract: irritation and fissuring of skin of hands, cracking and discoloration of fingernails, conjunctivitis, sore throat, and coughing
- Ingestion of paraquat: early (1–4 days), oral and abdominal pain, nausea, vomiting, and diarrhea; later (24–72 hours), liver injury, jaundice, elevated hepatocellular enzymes, and renal injury (proteinuria, hematuria, pyuria, elevated serum urea nitrogen and creatinine); late (3–4 days), pulmonary fibrosis (cough, dyspnea, tachypnea, cyanosis, and respiratory failure)
- Ingestion of diquat: same as paraquat without late pulmonary fibrosis

General Considerations

Paraquat is used extensively in the United States and worldwide, diquat to a lesser extent. They are nonselective contact herbicides.

Use

The dipyridyls are used extensively as general-purpose herbicides owing to their ability to kill most plants on contact. They are also used as defoliants and desiccants because the foliage of plants becomes dry and frostbitten in appearance, resulting in the premature dropping of leaves. Paraquat is used on cotton, potatoes, and soybeans, whereas diquat is used on alfalfa, clover, and soybeans.

Occupational & Environmental Exposures

The most important occupational exposures occur by direct contact of the skin with liquid concentrate during mixing and loading and inhalation and skin contact with spray mist during application. A case of acute paraquat intoxication was reported in a flagger who endured extensive dermal exposure to spray mist. Environmental exposure through field residues, food residues, and water contamination has not been a concern. The program of the U.S. Drug Enforcement Agency to spray marijuana fields with paraquat generated controversy over the possibility of inhalation of paraquat by marijuana smokers. Most of the paraquat probably undergoes thermal decomposition before it is inhaled, but the possibility of adverse effects from paraquat or its decomposition products has not been ruled out.

Pharmacokinetics & Mechanism of Action

The dipyridyls affect both plants and mammals by damaging tissue through the generation of oxygen free radicals. Their effect on plants requires the presence of sunlight. They are absorbed by inhalation, dermal contact, or ingestion. They damage epithelial tissues such as skin, nails, cornea, gastrointestinal tract, and respiratory tract, as well as the liver and kidneys.

Paraquat is more toxic to humans than diquat. A small sip of the liquid concentrate can kill an adult, which accounts for the hundreds of deaths reported worldwide from accidental and deliberate ingestion of this herbicide. An experimental trial that consisted of adding an emetic to formulations of paraquat was instituted recently in an attempt to reduce the frequency of fatal ingestions.

A relatively small number of cases of serious poisoning from paraquat have been reported as a result of large dermal exposures, whereas none has been reported from inhalation exposure in the absence of significant skin contact. Pulmonary injury from chronic dermal or inhalation exposure has not been reliably reported or found in the few epidemiologic studies performed with applicators. Neither paraquat nor diquat has been adequately tested for carcinogenicity.

Clinical Findings

A. SYMPTOMS & SIGNS

Direct contact with concentrated liquid dipyridyls results in skin irritation and fissuring and in cracking, discoloration, and sometimes loss of the fingernails. Liquid splashed in the eye can cause conjunctivitis and opacification of the cornea. Inhalation of spray mist can irritate the nose and throat, causing nosebleeds and sore throat.

Ingestion of either paraquat or diquat can result in an early phase (1–4 days) of inflammation of the mouth and gastrointestinal tract, with soreness, ulceration, burning pain, nausea, vomiting, diarrhea, and sometimes hematemesis and melena. These symptoms can range from mild to severe, and their intensity may not predict the severity of the following phases. The second phase begins 24–72 hours after exposure and is marked by evidence of hepatic and renal injury. Hepatocellular injury is indicated by abdominal pain, nausea, and jaundice. Renal injury usually is asymptomatic unless oliguria or anuria develops. Renal and hepatic injury from ingestion of paraquat is common and frequently severe, whereas that from ingestion of diquat is less common and often milder.

A late phase (72–96 hours) of pulmonary fibrosis occurs from paraquat, but not diquat, presumably because paraquat, but not diquat, becomes concentrated in pulmonary epithelial tissue. Pulmonary edema has occurred occasionally following ingestion of either paraquat or diquat. In cases of paraquat poisoning, pulmonary fibrosis is marked by cough, shortness of breath, and tachypnea. Advanced fibrosis is indicated by progressive cyanosis.

B. LABORATORY FINDINGS

In the early phase of acute poisoning, the findings are nonspecific and usually are related to dehydration from nausea and diarrhea. In the later phase, liver injury is indicated by elevated bilirubin and hepatocellular enzymes. Renal injury, primarily tubular, is indicated by proteinuria, hematuria, pyuria, and elevated serum urea nitrogen and creatinine. Oliguric renal failure typical of acute tubular necrosis may occur. Laboratory evidence of pulmonary fibrosis from paraquat in the form of a progressive decline in arterial oxygen tension and diffusion capacity for carbon monoxide commonly precedes the appearance of pulmonary symptoms. Later, pulmonary function findings are typical of restrictive lung disease. The diagnosis of acute intoxication from paraquat or diquat can be confirmed by analysis of either compound in blood and urine.

Differential Diagnosis

The early phase of acute intoxication from a dipyridyl may be mild and, in the absence of a history of ingestion, may be mistaken for gastroenteritis or ingestion of another irritant chemical. The combination of renal and hepatic injury could occur following exposure to a chlorinated hydrocarbon solvent such as carbon tetrachloride. In the absence of a history of paraquat exposure, the differential diagnosis of the pulmonary injury is the same as for acute pulmonary fibrosis (see Chapter 20).

Treatment

The primary treatment during any phase of intoxication from paraquat or diquat is supportive, particularly during periods of organ failure. Bentonite and Fuller's earth are more effective absorbents for dipyridyls in the gastrointestinal tract than activated charcoal. If available, they should be administered as a 7 g/dL suspension in normal saline in quantities of at least 2 L to any patient suspected of ingesting any quantity of a dipyridyl within the preceding several days. If neither bentonite nor Fuller's earth is available, a similar quantity of the usual concentration of activated charcoal should be administered.

Saline catharsis then is recommended, using sodium sulfate rather than magnesium salts because of the risk of magnesium retention in the presence of impaired renal function. This cycle may be repeated for several days. Given the high fatality rate following paraquat ingestion, this extreme degree of gut cleansing is probably worth the risk of fluid and electrolyte imbalance, which must be monitored closely.

The issue of enhanced excretion of dipyridyl is controversial. There is no basis for the recommendation that glucose and electrolyte infusions be given in large quantities to minimize toxicant concentrations in tissues and force diuresis of the compounds. Hemodialysis is clearly ineffective for removal of paraquat. Hemoperfusion with coated charcoal may be effective in removing paraquat from the blood if it is performed before the chemical has been distributed to tissues. However, few patients have a confirmed diagnosis and can be placed in a facility where the procedure can be performed early (24–48 hours after ingestion). The decision to perform hemoperfusion should be made by a physician with experience in the technique and familiarity with the issues and risks involved.

A number of therapies are available to attempt to retard pulmonary fibrosis from paraquat. Increased levels of alveolar oxygen increase the rate of production of oxygen free radicals and accelerate the process of pulmonary fibrosis. Animal studies show increased survival in low-oxygen atmospheres, but there are no comparable human studies. Early placement of a patient in an atmosphere of 15% oxygen has been recommended. Supplemental oxygen should be administered only as necessary to maintain minimally acceptable levels of oxygenation. Early experimental results with the free-radical scavenger superoxide dismutase have been disappointing. Corticosteroids and cytotoxic agents such as azathioprine have been tried with uncertain results.

Prognosis

Once pulmonary fibrosis occurs as a result of paraquat ingestion, death from respiratory failure can be expected. Survival with disability from restrictive lung disease also may occur. Occasionally, recovery of lung function may take place over a course of weeks to months. Although death from liver and kidney necrosis may occur following diquat ingestion, recovery is more common than following paraquat ingestion.

REFERENCES

Bradberry SM et al: Glyphosate poisoning. Toxicol Rev 2004;23:159 [PMID: 15862083].

Bradberry SM et al: Poisoning due to chlorophenoxy herbicides. Toxicol Rev 2004;23:65 [PMID: 15578861].

De Roos AJ et al: Cancer incidence among glyphosate-exposed pesticide applicators in the Agricultural Health Study. Environ Health Perspect 2005;113:49 [PMID: 1562664].

Gammon DW et al: A risk assessment of atrazine use in California: Human health and ecological aspects. Pest Manag Sci 2005;61:331 [PMID: 15655806].

Hou L et al: Pendimethalin exposure and cancer incidence among pesticide applicators. Epidemiology 2006;17:302 [PMID: 16452832].

Rusiecki JA et al: Cancer incidence among pesticide applicators exposed to metolachlor in the Agricultural Health Study. Int J Cancer 2006;118:3118 [PMID: 16425265].

DISINFECTANTS & ALGICIDES

If one includes the use of chlorine and chlorine compounds for water treatment, these are the most heavily used pesticides worldwide. They include the halogens (i.e., chlorine, hypochlorites, chloramine, and iodine), the phenols, the aldehydes (i.e., formaldehyde and glutaraldehyde), and the detergents.

The use of chlorine in water treatment generally is not a toxic concern, except for accidental releases. The use of hypochlorite in swimming pools is associated with thinning of dental enamel in people who swim regularly when the acidity produced from the generation of chlorine and hydrochloric acid is not buffered properly. The substitution of chloramine for chlorine has raised concern for dialysis patients and aquarium fish.

The hazards of phenol were discussed in Chapter 29 and those of formaldehyde in Chapter 28. Glutaraldehyde is chemically similar to formaldehyde but has not been tested for carcinogenicity. It is used commonly in hospitals as a disinfectant (Cidex) and causes eye, nose, and throat irritation when an aerosol is created. It has not been reported to cause asthma.

REPELLENTS

The best-known repellents are insect repellents for human application. The most common is DEET (diethyltoluamide), used primarily to repel mosquitoes. Its use generally has been without incident, with the exception of a single reported case of an acute neurologic reaction in a young child who underwent heavy aerosol exposure. Some concern has been expressed, however, regarding the heavy use of DEET by personnel working outdoors in mosquito-infested areas.

GROWTH REGULATORS & BIORATIONAL PESTICIDES

Growth regulators are substances that alter the behavior of the target organism, most often a plant, through a physiologic effect to hasten or retard growth or other biologic processes. They are generally without known or suspected adverse human health effects, but the discovery that the breakdown product of the plant growth regulator daminozide (Alar), or unsymmetric dimethylhydrazine (UDMH), causes cancer in animals has generated considerable controversy. Daminozide restricts growth of apples so that they remain on the trees longer and become firmer, making them resistant to insects.

UDMH is concentrated in processed or cooked-apple products, further increasing any cancer risk from daminozide residues. The registration of daminozide has been inactive in the United States since 1990.

There are six classes of plant growth regulators. The auxins are plant growth hormones that include indoleacetic acid and the phenoxy acetic acids; the latter was discussed earlier in the section on herbicides. The gibberellins are represented primarily by gibberellic acid, which has a variety of beneficial effects on fruit and no known adverse effects on humans. The cytokinins are naturally occurring compounds such as adenine, which are unlikely to affect humans in the amounts used as pesticides. Ethylene generators, including ethylene itself and ethephon, initiate degreening and ripening of many fruits without affecting humans. Inhibitors range from simple organic acids of low toxicity, such as benzoic, gallic, and cinnamic acids, to maleic hydrazide, for which preliminary evidence of carcinogenicity in animals has been reported. Finally, growth retardants include newly developed substances such as chlorflurenol that generally are without known human health effects.

INFORMATION SOURCES

Information on the identity, exposure, toxicity, and clinical management of specific pesticides is often difficult to obtain. It is therefore important to become familiar with the sources of such information that are available in any particular area of practice. This can include the county agricultural commissioner or extension agent, county health officer, regional poison control center, state departments of health and agriculture, union officials, and local growers. The annual editions of the *Farm Chemicals Handbook* are useful sources of information on the identity of brand-name products as well as individual active ingredients. A current online version includes a full-text copy of individual pesticide labels. For commonly used agricultural compounds, a consortium of university extension toxicologists also provides online information, often derived from data supplied by pesticide manufacturers, at Extoxnet. The EPA booklet, "Recognition and Management of Pesticide Poisonings," is a concise guide to diagnosis and treatment. The 1991 and 2001 editions of the misnamed *Handbook of Pesticide Toxicology* are a more definitive source of health-related information.

Although there have been regulatory requirements for toxicity testing of pesticides in the United States for a number of years, the regulatory and public health assessment of these data is still ongoing. The California Department of Pesticide Regulation makes available summaries of their current assessments of rodent chronic health studies, carcinogenicity bioassays, teratogenicity studies, and multigenerational reproductive studies.

SECTION V
Program Management

Occupational Stress

James P. Seward, MD, MPP, & Robert C. Larsen, MD, MPH

Stress is an increasingly important occupational health problem and a significant cause of economic loss. While *stress* remains a broad, somewhat elusive concept, research efforts have led to a clearer understanding of the problem, its causes, and its consequences. Occupational stress may produce both overt psychological and physiologic disability; however, it also may have more subtle manifestations that can affect personal well-being and outcomes of organizational importance such as productivity.

Although many of the factors in the workplace that may cause stress have been studied, the ability to predict a stress response in any given individual remains poor. The stress response should be seen as an interplay between exacerbating and modifying factors. When stress is deleterious, it may result in physical and/or mental disorders.

Most research on stress involves cross-sectional studies, although a growing number of longitudinal studies are being conducted with an increased ability to identify causal associations. The complexity of stress as a phenomenon requires different explanatory models than the biomedical and toxicologic approaches used elsewhere in occupational medicine. Considerations such as multicausality, intervening variables, time sequencing, and healthy-worker effects are important in stress research. Much of the occupational stress literature is found in social science and psychology publications that are not often read by occupational physicians. There are related concepts in the literature, such as *job burnout,* as well as the stress-related diagnosis of *posttraumatic stress disorder.* The study of stress is a broad field extending far beyond the disciplines usually associated with occupational medicine. However, this chapter focuses on stress and its relationship to work.

There is a growing body of evidence to indicate that the prevention of occupational stress may be accomplished by creating a healthy work environment based on recognized organizational principles. Organizational solutions for high-stress work units offer promise, although there is not much experimental information available to guide these interventions. It also may be possible to monitor and control stress in the workforce by recognizing problem situations as well as early clinical or behavioral signs. Not all employment stress is problematic. Work almost invariably is associated with some degree of struggle and conflict. Workplace and personal stressors can affect group and individual well-being and effectiveness. When individual dysfunction arises, then the stress response has crossed into an area in which clinical intervention may be necessary.

STRESS CONCEPTS & MODELS

Stress in general terms is a syndrome that involves a nonspecific response of the organism to a stimulus from the environment. In framing the concept to make it applicable to the occupational setting, *stress* might be defined as a perceived imbalance between occupational demands and the individual's ability to perform when the consequences of failure are important. The element of individual perception introduces subjectivity into the definition of stress, and this perceptual component has played an important role in the evaluation of stress in the workers' compensation system.

Models of stress attempt to integrate individual and environmental factors into a working scheme of how stress is generated. An ideal model for occupational stress would be useful both in ongoing theoretical research and in practical problem solving. Such a model would have to meet many criteria. It should offer a clear definition of how stress develops and allow for differentiation of stressful and nonstressful situations. The model should help to explain why certain events produce stress in some individuals but cause no detectable stress in others—and why stress may lead to different degrees of pathologic or even beneficial effects according to the circumstances.

All the major factors that determine the stress response should be considered in the model. In general terms, these factors would include occupational, social, familial, and individual characteristics. If such a conceptual framework were developed, it would help to integrate the results of past research and suggest new areas for inquiry. It also would allow accurate predictions. Unfortunately, none of the available models meets these stringent criteria.

Several good efforts have been made that reflect different viewpoints on the genesis of occupational stress, and three different approaches will be presented here. The models differ with respect to completeness and the principal explanatory variables. These models should be seen as complementary.

One of the earliest and most complete paradigms to explain the causation of stress is called the *person-environment fit model*. In this model, a distinction is made between the objective and subjective evaluations of the individual and the environment. Stress is produced by the subjective person-environment fit, which is mediated ultimately by the individual's perceptions of self and the environment. In this system, good mental health in the working situation depends on the outcome of four interactions: the objective environment–objective person, the objective environment–subjective environment, the objective person–subjective person, and the subjective environment–subjective person. A simple example will clarify these concepts.

A garment worker may be expected to produce 40 pieces per hour (objective environment), whereas she believes that she is required to produce 50 pieces (subjective environment). She actually may be capable of producing 45 pieces (objective individual), but she thinks that she can only produce 40 pieces (subjective individual).

In this case, there is a good match between the objective environmental demands (40 garments) and the objective person's ability (45 garments). However, the worker's perception that 50 garments are demanded (subjective environment) and underestimation of her own abilities (subjective person) lead to a stressful situation. Given this scenario, the worker might experience stress based on a poor subjective person–environment fit despite an adequate objective fit.

The person-environment fit model is relatively comprehensive and clearly places much emphasis on the individual's subjective interaction with the environment. Other models focus more on interactions with the work environment in an effort to understand the stress response.

The *demand-control model* concept holds that stress results from an imbalance between demands on a worker and the worker's ability to modify those demands. This model focuses on the adaptive response of the individual to a potentially stressful stimulus. When the worker can modify the response or alter the circumstances, less stress may result. Low decision-making control coupled with high job demands leads to high strain or to a stressful situation. In the demand-control model, high demands and low control work synergistically to have more impact than either factor alone. Proponents of the demand-control model tend to focus on work tasks, but other aspects of the work environment, such as organizational features or opportunities for creativity and independent thought, may be as important.

The demand-control model has received wide attention over the last two decades, and a number of research studies have attempted to validate its predictions. Higher decision latitude is associated with decreased cardiovascular morbidity. The model also has been used to show that workers who participated in company reorganizations and who had a resulting increase in job decision control experienced fewer health symptoms than did employees who moved into situations with less decision-making latitude.

Despite these successes, the demand-control model also has been criticized for its inconsistent ability to explain stress outcomes. There are concerns that the model does not apply equally across a range of occupations and social classes and that the relationships are more complex than the model allows. One study shows that social support is a more powerful predictor of stress outcome than job control.

A third model that figures prominently in the occupational stress literature is the *effort-reward imbalance model*. This approach places emphasis on the rewards of work (i.e., money, esteem, security, and career opportunities) rather than on job control. The model posits that stress results from an imbalance between the efforts expended and the rewards received at work. There are both extrinsic (situational) and intrinsic (personal) dimensions to this model. The model assumes that high efforts in combination with low rewards increase the risk for poor health and that a combination of extrinsic and intrinsic factors results in an even higher risk for poor health. The effort-reward imbalance model draws a somewhat wider boundary on the problem of stress at work than does the demand-control model because it considers the broader economic variables of job stability, pay, and the like. However, both models have had significant explanatory value in research efforts. Combining the two models achieves greater predictability of health status.

The research on stress has generated a number of other models that attempt to provide meaningful frameworks for understanding the phenomena. Some emphasize factors such as social support, that is, the amount of positive interpersonal contact and assistance a worker has on or off the job. Some research focuses on individual "hardiness" or the extent to which an individual feels challenged, committed, and in control of his or her work life.

No model is comprehensive or capable of explaining the stress experience with great accuracy. Despite this situation, a great deal still can be said regarding specific workplace and environmental conditions that produce stress, the effects of stress on the individual and the organization, and methods that may control or alleviate stress in the work setting. Subsequent sections consider these issues.

REFERENCES

Calnan M et al: Job strain, effort-reward imbalance and stress at work: Competing or complementary models. Scand J Public Health 2004;32:84 [PMID: 15255497].

Niedhammer I et al: Psychosocial work environment and mental health: A study of job strain and effort-reward imbalance model in a context of major organizational changes. Int J Occup Environ Health 2006;12:111 [PMID: 16722190].

van Vegchel N et al: Reviewing the effort-reward imbalance model: Drawing up the balance of 45 empirical studies. Soc Sci Med 2005;60:1117 [PMID: 15589679].

WORKPLACE STRESSORS

Various characteristics of working life may contribute to occupational stress (Table 32–1). These characteristics may be grouped with much overlap into five general categories: organization and organizational relationships, career development, role of the individual, job task or assignment, and working environment and conditions. The following sections discuss the contribution of each of these areas to the genesis of occupational stress.

Organization & Organizational Relationships

Most people in industrialized societies are now employed in some organizational context and are subject to fallout from factors that affect the organization as a whole. Issues inherent in organizational life, such as political conflict, communication difficulties, delegation of tasks, decision-making authority, and regulations, may be sources of conflict and stress. Relationships with supervisors are particularly important determinants of subjective well-being.

Stressful conditions often are produced when organizations undergo change. The situations encountered in producing new products or services, reorganizing institutional structure, and expanding or contracting

Table 32–1. Common workplace stressors.

Organizational
  Change
  Inadequate communication
  Interpersonal conflict
  Conflict with organizational goals
Career development
  Lack of promotional opportunity
  New responsibilities beyond level of training
  Unemployment
Role
  Role conflict
  Role ambiguity
  Inadequate resources to accomplish job
  Inadequate authority to accomplish job
Task
  Quantitative and qualitative overload
  Quantitative and qualitative underload
  Responsibility for the lives and well-being of others
  Low decision-making latitude
Work environment
  Poor aesthetics
  Physical exposures
  Ergonomic problems
  Noise
  Odors
  Safety hazards
Shift work

operations often challenge the individual's ability to adapt. Increased levels of anxiety and diminished job satisfaction and morale have been shown in companies during the process of introducing new product lines. Thus the process of change may disrupt an individual's equilibrium within an organization and place the individual at increased risk of a stress response.

Poor communication within organizations and a sense of not being either informed or heard by managers similarly can lead to stress as manifested by low job satisfaction. Conversely, good interpersonal support from colleagues—but especially from supervisors—may alleviate stress. Conflict with a supervisor or coworker is a powerful stressor. Moral or ideological conflict between the individual and the goals of the organization also can produce psychological strain. The salesperson required to promote what is perceived to be a second-rate or socially irrelevant product and the manager forced to fire a respected older employee both will experience substantial stress.

Career Development

Many transitions in working life are recognized as stressful situations. A change in jobs, getting a promotion or being passed over, and being laid off or fired are all high-risk events. Studies of workers undergoing periods of unemployment show increased rates of mental illness and alcohol and drug use. There is also a suggestion of increased rates of disease such as peptic ulcer and hypertension. Work stressors such as organizational disruption, layoff experience, and educational discordance are associated with ill health, whereas higher occupational status appears to be protective.

Promotion is a potential stressor. New job responsibilities, especially when calling for skills not previously exercised, can result in anxiety and psychological decompensation. Promotion to a position beyond one's abilities has the potential for inducing behavioral disorders. Frustrated career goals and underpromotion are associated with increased rates of mental hospitalization, as documented in a study of U.S. Navy enlisted men who achieved officer status. Thus symptomatic stress may result both from the frustration of thwarted ambition and from the inability to cope with new demands.

Role in the Organization

Role conflict exists when two or more competing expectations make simultaneous satisfaction of both difficult. Role ambiguity implies insufficient information or guidance on which to base decisions and behavior. In one survey, approximately half the workforce reported having role conflicts, and ambiguous expectations and duties were a concern for more than a third of the group.

Role conflict often occurs at interface positions. For example, a production supervisor occupies a position between management and staff, with an interest in keeping both sides happy without compromising production. Other examples of role conflict include differing opinions over what a given job should entail, contradictory job demands, and managing disputes between colleagues. Correlations have been observed between role conflict and increased heart rate as well as job dissatisfaction.

Role ambiguity may occur as a result of specific ill-defined responsibilities, unclear expectations of personal image, or hazy organizational objectives. The source of stress in these situations may be the lack of clarity itself or the inability to assess one's own performance.

Another type of role-related stress may result when individuals experience discrepancies between their supervisors' expectations and the resources available to meet them. Insufficient time, personnel, or funding puts a strain on the responsible individual who lacks the power to increase the availability of resources or to change expectations.

Task

Work overload and underload, decision-making ability, and level and type of responsibility are important task-related issues with relevance for occupational stress. Both quantitative overload and qualitative overload have been implicated in stress disorders. In quantitative overload, the individual is overwhelmed by the amount of work. In qualitative overload, the expected functional level is too high—that is, the work is too difficult. High quantitative overload is associated with coronary artery disease in several studies; there is also a relationship with alcohol and tobacco use, lost work time, poor motivation, and poor self-image.

Qualitative overload also has adverse physiologic effects. Blood cholesterol levels rise in medical students under conditions of qualitative overload during an evaluation process. Tax accountants have higher cholesterol levels at deadlines. University professors with personal expectations of very high quality work score poorly in terms of one stress indicator: self-esteem.

Qualitative and quantitative underload also may cause stress. One study of disease indicators in a large executive population shows higher rates of disease among individuals at the two extremes of the spectrum—the overworked and the underworked. Stress may be induced by understimulation and excessively routine activities; workers become bored and alienated and lose initiative.

Job responsibilities are significant sources of stress; work that involves responsibility for the lives of others is particularly stressful. Physicians, air traffic controllers, and first-line supervisors who make decisions affecting the lives of others may have higher rates of peptic ulcer; myocardial infarction and hypertension also may be related to work involving responsibility for others.

Several studies show a beneficial effect of higher job autonomy on stress indicators. Greater latitude to make basic decisions about the performance of one's work is associated with fewer myocardial infarctions and fewer job-related injuries. Conversely, low decision-making autonomy is related to higher levels of stress. Hospital employees with a higher perception of justice for decision making are at less risk for ill health than those perceiving low justice.

Work Environment

The physical environment of the workplace may present many potential stressors. Most environmental hazards are identified with specific health effects they may cause, such as hearing loss from noise exposure. However, these exposures also may contribute to stress in a variety of ways. Physical exposures, chemical exposures, crowding, and ergonomic problems may function independently or collectively as stressors.

Noise provides a good example of a multifaceted stressor. In addition to its cumulative effect on the cochlea, noise exposure may raise blood pressure acutely. In addition, high levels of sound isolate workers by preventing conversation and drowning out other auditory cues to events near the workers. In one experiment, many of the physiologic and psychological changes associated with excessive noise were eliminated by providing a button that could be used to control sound levels. The beneficial effect occurred whether or not the control option was used.

Other physical exposures, such as excessive heat or cold, extremes of lighting or glare, and vibration, may produce ill effects. While the magnitude of these effects may not itself be disabling, the associated discomfort can contribute to mental distress and to secondary physiologic changes characteristic of stress.

Physical comfort and pleasant surroundings correlate with mental health. Ergonomic factors in tool and workstation design also play a role in worker frustration, morale, and ultimately productivity.

Research on video-display terminal users indicates a complex relationship between workload, ergonomic factors, social factors in the workplace, and stress outcomes. Although the primary focus has been on the ergonomic design of computer workstations, work demands, as well as task structure, also have significant effects on symptoms.

Chemical exposures also may induce stress through a variety of mechanisms. There may be direct irritating or intoxicating effects. Anxiety may arise regarding personal welfare as a result of potentially hazardous exposures. Unpleasant chemical odors—regardless of toxicity—may be powerful stressors by themselves.

Safety hazards inherent in some workplaces, such as risks of explosion or falls, add the element of fear to other work concerns. Welding on a thousand-foot-high tower is clearly more stressful than welding at ground level. Thus psychological stress and physical environment characteristics can be additive and increase the risk for ill health.

The assumption should be made—even though good documentation is not available—that the effects produced by stressful conditions are additive. Combined environmental stressors even may operate synergistically in some situations. Any given job is likely to have a complex array of potential stressors acting in a variety of ways. More research is needed, specifically on the cumulative effects of environmental stressors.

Individual & Social Factors in Stress

Both personality traits and stressors from outside the workplace can influence the likelihood of work-induced stress. According to the person-environment fit model, individual response to a stressor is an important determinant of the outcome. Any comprehensive model of stress must help to explain why workers exposed to the same stressors will exhibit different responses. When attempting to reduce occupational stress, more empha-

sis should be placed on workplace stressors than on individual predisposition; however, the latter should not be ignored—especially as a precipitating factor.

Many variables may affect individual vulnerability to occupational stress. Personality structure, family life, stage in life, and social support systems are among the most important factors affecting the stress response. Many cases of occupational stress are precipitated by factors in the personal sphere. In addition to a thorough inquiry about stressors at work, physicians always should inquire about events in an individual's nonworking life when evaluating patients with stress symptoms.

Personality factors also may predispose certain individuals to a greater risk of stress-related disease. A case has been made for increased incidence of heart disease in individuals with aggressive, achievement-oriented personalities. Individuals with obsessive personality traits may depend on the structure of their jobs and undergo stress when changes occur. Preexisting psychiatric disorders as well as passive-aggressive, antisocial, and other maladaptive personality traits may affect the worker's ability to cooperate and be productive.

Changes in the workplace affect individuals differently according to their age and stage in life. According to the theory of life stages, adults undergo developmental changes that result in new needs and expectations from working life. Phases such as choosing a career, struggling for advancement, and reaching a high level of maturity and experience can be stressful depending on the individual's underlying personality organization and whether the phases are accompanied by appropriate recognition and reward. A transfer to very different job duties may be less taxing to a new employee who is just acquiring skills than to an established one who is trying to gain recognition for accomplishments in a specific area.

Social support by individuals outside the workplace can be an important mitigating factor in development of stress. The spouse is usually the most important person in this regard, but other family members and friends also can play an important role in supporting individuals in stressful occupations. An important concern here is that families often bear the burden of alleviating stress originating in the workplace. The deterioration of family or social support relationships may precede decompensation from stress at work.

With the growth in the number of employed women, more attention and research is needed on their status in relation to occupational stress. Women tend to occupy jobs different from those of men; these are often positions with lower status, fewer benefits, and less opportunity for growth. In addition, women often carry a double burden with substantial childrearing and homemaking responsibilities. It is relatively common for women to be single mothers. Women in managerial positions may face greater stressors than their male counterparts.

REFERENCES

Cohidon C et al: Exposure to job-stress factors in a national survey in France. Scand J Work Environ Health 2004;30:379 [PMID: 15529801].

Daniels K: Perceived risk from occupational stress: A survey of 15 European countries. Occup Environ Med 2004;61:467 [PMID: 15090671].

Jamison CS et al: Contemporary work characteristics, stress and ill health. Am J Hum Biol 2004;16:43 [PMID: 14689515].

Lallukka T et al: Working conditions and health behaviours among employed women and men: The Helsinki Health Study. Prev Med 2004;38:48 [PMID: 14672641].

Melchior M et al: Work factors and occupational class disparities in sickness absence. Am J Public Health 2005;95:1206 [PMID: 15933236].

SHIFT WORK

The rotating work shift is a common stressor that affects a growing proportion of the working population worldwide. Estimates are that between 20% and 25% of the U.S. workforce do some form of rotating schedule, evening, or night work. Rotating shifts usually involve regularly changing work hours. Employees' shifts change periodically (e.g., every 2–30 days) so that time spent working day, evening, and night shifts is shared by the workforce. These schedule changes have consequences for mental and physical well-being. Research has contributed to knowledge about the physiologic effects of shift rotation, leading to a number of practical applications (Tables 32–2 and 32–3). Many of the issues faced by rotating shift workers are shared by individuals who have permanent night-work schedules.

Despite numerous studies of the physiologic and health consequences of shift work and the relationship of shift work to accidents, social well-being, and productivity, there is uncertainty about both long-term health effects and the role of personal factors in adaptation to shift work. Some points of general agreement provide the basis for evaluating work schedules and advising shift workers.

Circadian Rhythms

Many physiologic systems in the human body display a regular circadian rhythm. Key examples include body

Table 32–2. Personal factors that may increase risk from shift work.

Advanced age
Cardiovascular disease
Chronic diseases (e.g., type I diabetes, epilepsy)
Gastrointestinal disorders
Psychological problems
Sleep disorders

Table 32–3. Factors requiring special consideration for shift workers.

Access to medical care
Availability of meals
Chemical exposures
Family and social circumstances
Medication schedules
Physical exposures
Safety factors, (e.g., lighting)
Sleeping conditions
Transportation to work
Type of shift schedule

temperature and glucocorticoid secretion. Diurnal variations have been found in cognitive function, gastric emptying, pulmonary function, metabolism of medications, and other physiologic and psychological processes. A key issue with nondiurnal and rotating schedules is the readjustment (entrainment) of these physiologic cycles.

With change from a day to a night schedule, the various physiologic circadian rhythms begin to readjust; however, each one adapts at its own rate, with resulting dyssynchrony. In theory, all the rhythms would reach a new homeostasis if the new schedule were maintained perfectly. In practice, there is seldom complete readjustment.

Most shift-work research has focused on diurnal temperature variations as a surrogate measure for adaptation to new schedules. In a normal daytime-adapted human, the body has a temperature trough in the early morning hours and a temperature peak in the late afternoon. In an individual who becomes adapted to a night-work schedule under isolated laboratory conditions, the temperature curve first flattens and then reverses completely.

Under real-life conditions, complete readjustment—or phase shifting—of the temperature curve fails to occur for several reasons. First, individuals usually revert to daytime schedules on their days off. This causes a partial reversal of any phase shifting that has occurred. Second, research shows the importance of light exposure as a synchronizing cue to the human organism; workers on night shift who have exposure to daylight during off-work hours have incomplete readjustment of the temperature curve. Experimental studies of exposure to bright light during the night hours combined with the wearing of dark goggles to avoid light exposure at other times has shown more effective adjustment. Third, the readjustment time required for a complete inversion of the temperature curve is usually several weeks, so workers on short rotation cycles of days or even a week do not have adequate time to adapt.

In addition to issues of circadian rhythm adjustment, another consideration in rotating shift work is the direction of the progression of the shift cycle [i.e., clockwise (day to evening to night) versus counterclockwise (day to night to evening)]. Humans adapt more easily to clockwise progression of their sleep cycles than to counterclockwise progression. It is generally more difficult to arise progressively earlier than to delay awakening by an hour (shifting the internal clock back). The same phenomenon may explain why adjustment to time-zone changes after air travel usually takes longer in the west-east direction; adapting to a more easterly time zone is essentially the same process as awakening earlier.

When this information is applied to rotating shift work, it becomes apparent that successful shift rotation should proceed from day to evening to night shifts rather than the reverse order. By following a clockwise progression to later shifts, the rotation order puts less strain on the adaptive ability of the internal clock. Application of the forward-rotation principle to a mining company in the United States resulted in increased productivity and subjective well-being, as well as less job turnover.

There are at least two schools of thought regarding the rate of rotation of a shift-work schedule. One approach is to assign shifts that rotate slowly so that workers have at least 5 days and often much longer on a given schedule. In theory, workers have a longer time to adapt to the schedule both physiologically and socially. The other viewpoint advocates a short rotation length of 1–3 days on a given schedule. Proponents of these fast rotations argue that workers never fully adapt to night shifts and that short night rotations cause less chaos with circadian rhythms. Physiology notwithstanding, the acceptability of a shift schedule will depend to a significant extent on environmental, social, and recreational factors.

Proponents of the long-cycle forward shift rotation suggest that humans are able to adapt at least partially to a new schedule, as evidenced by a flattening of the temperature curve, over a period of several weeks. The time recommended for a given shift schedule would be at least 21 days before a rotation forward. Advocates of this approach point out that numerous studies show that workers on prolonged or permanent night shifts get more hours of sleep (average 6.72 hours) than do workers on weekly rotation schedules (average 6.30 hours). The latter, in turn, get more sleep than those who rotate more rapidly (average 5.79 hours).

While there may be physiologic advantages to the long-cycle forward shift rotation, the short-cycle forward rotation (2–3 days per schedule) is much more acceptable to workers. The principal reason is personal convenience, because the more rapid progression allows more frequent intervals of normal social and family life. Days off between shift rotations appear to offer time for individuals to recoup their sleep. As yet, the evidence

regarding performance and accidents does not show a convincing difference between these two alternatives.

The physical and mental exertion involved in the work, the social and family support systems available, and the opportunities to eat well at the workplace are factors that should be considered in scheduling decisions.

Health Effects of Shift Work

There are few clearly established causal links between shift work and disease. Discussion of this subject draws on a balance of positive and negative findings in epidemiologic research and must be interpreted with some reserve. Based on the disruption of rotating and night work on circadian functions, the ability of these schedules to aggravate some preexisting chronic disorders is certain. Other physiologic functions, such as reproduction, also may be affected.

Sleep is affected in several ways, the major cause being alterations in circadian rhythms. Studies show that there is difficulty in maintaining sleep after a night shift and difficulty in initiating sleep (in the early evening) before a morning shift. Sleep may be interrupted by street noise, family activity, the telephone, or other causes. The quality of sleep also may be altered, with changes in the sleep cycles and less rapid-eye-movement sleep. Sleep disorders are common among night-shift and rotating-shift workers.

Gastrointestinal complaints are increased in rotating-shift workers. There are changes in appetite and increased constipation. Alimentation often is adversely affected by poor availability or poor quality of food for night-shift employees. Some studies show a high incidence of peptic ulcer among shift workers and an even higher incidence among workers who dropped out of shift work. Given the multifactorial causation of peptic ulcer disease, delayed gastric emptying, which can occur with circadian rhythm disruption, may be a contributing factor. Other factors related to the gastrointestinal problems may be the increased consumption of caffeine and tobacco among rotating-shift workers.

Shift work may complicate management of chronic diseases for which timing and adjustment of medications are important. Insulin-dependent diabetes mellitus may be more difficult to control in part because of the irregularity of meals. However, there is also evidence for a circadian variation in the effects of insulin. The alteration of the sleep cycle may cause increased seizure frequency in epileptics owing to sleep deprivation or medication regulation. Asthmatics also may experience difficulty with medication adjustments.

The risk of cardiovascular disease in shift workers is increased by 40%. Some studies have indicated increases in cholesterol and hypertension in shift workers. Other research has focused on behavioral factors such as diet, tobacco use, and lack of exercise as the likely cause. Some of these studies show an increased mortality among shift workers.

Research findings on reproductive outcomes among women shift workers include increased spontaneous abortions, preterm births, and intrauterine growth retardation. Although not definitive, these studies indicate a potential reproductive risk from shift work.

A few studies indicate a tendency toward depression in shift workers. In addition, workers with preexisting psychiatric disease, such as bipolar disorder, may undergo exacerbations in a shift-work setting. There are clearly social and familial stresses resulting from shift work. A shift worker often will have difficulty maintaining normal social contacts and community involvement. Altered sleep and leisure schedules can result in periods of low interaction with children and spouses. Shift workers tend to have higher scores on stress questionnaires than do nonshift workers.

Special considerations should be given to concerns of safety for night workers. Especially with boring and repetitive work, there is increased likelihood of reduced attention and increased errors. In situations where safety risk is high, alertness monitors, extra measures to protect against injury, and perhaps shorter shifts should be recommended.

Medical Advice on Shift Work

An important role for the occupational practitioner is to advise shift workers about possible health concerns and how best to adapt to them. Medical evaluation and advice for shift workers should include particular attention to a history of cardiovascular disease, gastrointestinal problems, sleep disorders, epilepsy, diabetes, asthma, difficulty with night vision, or other chronic disorders. In shift work, the timing of medication and the quality of nutrition for people with chronic diseases are concerns. While not conclusive, the potential reproductive concerns that are associated with shift work should be a consideration for women who are attempting to conceive.

Advice to shift workers also should cover social and familial concerns as well as sleeping habits, diet, and the use of caffeine and other stimulants (Table 32–4). While routine surveillance of all shift workers is not necessary, the clinician should consider periodic rechecks of individuals with conditions that put them at higher risk for maladaptation or for specific medical problems related to shift work. Occupational health professionals may advise clients that shift-work lifestyle training and involvement of employees in setting schedules may reduce fatigue, turnover, and absenteeism while increasing morale.

Some individuals adapt poorly to rotating shift work and night work. While the reasons are not fully understood, this intolerance may be based in the susceptibility of the individual's circadian rhythms to desynchro-

Table 32–4. Issues in medical evaluation of shift workers.

Accidents on and off the job
Cardiovascular disease
Gastrointestinal disease
Health and functioning at work
Other chronic diseases
Psychological problems
Sleep quality and quantity
Chronic fatigue, naps
Sleep environment, noise
Social and family problems
Use of alcohol, caffeine, tobacco, drugs
Use of medication

nization or their inability to readjust with the normal daylight cues. Shift-work-intolerant individuals may present with poor sleep quality, persistent fatigue, mood changes, and reliance on sleeping medications.

There is no practical predictive test to identify these individuals. However, older age and a history of sleep problems or rigid sleep requirements are associated with shift-work intolerance. Medical evaluation should assess and attempt to control exacerbating factors such as daytime noise, social and family interruptions of sleep, medication use, caffeine use, and adverse environmental sleep conditions. These individuals may require a daytime work schedule.

In summary, it is best to avoid scheduling shift work and night work when possible. When circumstances dictate, the shifts should rotate clockwise (day to evening to night). It is best to provide one or more rest days between shifts. Because many individuals have difficulty initiating sleep in the early evening, early-morning shift starts (e.g., 4–6 A.M.) should be avoided. Rapid rotations (2–3 days) are preferred by workers, even though there are some physiologic justifications for advocating longer rotation cycles. Night work carries a somewhat increased risk of attention lapses and accidents, as well as reduced productivity, when compared with the day shift.

REFERENCES

Folkard S et al: Shiftwork: Safety, sleepiness and sleep. Indust Health 2005;43:20 [PMID: 15732299].

Kerin A, Aguirre A: Improving health, safety and profits in extended hours operations (shiftwork). Indust Health 2005; 43:201 [PMID: 15732324].

Knutsson A: Health disorders of shift workers. Occup Med (Lond) 2003;53:103 [PMID: 12637594].

Lac G, Chamoux A: Biological and psychological responses to two rapid shiftwork schedules. Ergonomics 2004;47:1339 [PMID: 15370851].

Van Amelsvoort LG et al: Direction of shift rotation among three-shift workers in relation to psychological health and work-family conflict. Scand J Work Environ Health 2004;30:149 [PMID: 15143742].

STRESS & DISEASE

There have been significant research efforts attempting to clarify the links between stress and disease. While there is good epidemiologic evidence associating occupational stress with a number of disease states, the pathophysiologic mechanisms often remain obscure, and in most situations, a true causal relationship has not been demonstrated.

The question of how stress may produce disease has generated many models, as discussed earlier. In addition, there are ongoing research efforts to establish the physiologic pathways through which stress may produce disease. Neurologic, immunologic, and endocrine mediators of disease have been established. The hypothalamic-pituitary axis, the autonomic nervous system, and the catecholamine response are cited often as stress-sensitive systems. These and other neurologic, endocrine, and immunologic mediators may be important actors in the chain of events leading to cardiovascular, gastrointestinal, endocrine, and other potentially stress-related disorders.

Mental Illness

The mental health effects of stress exist on a continuum ranging from mild subjective symptoms to overt psychiatric disease with significant impairment of functioning (Table 32–5). Subjective reports regarding personal well-being constitute some of the earliest measures of stress. Frequently noted symptoms include anxiety, tension, anger, irritability, poor concentration, apathy, and depression. These manifestations of stress interfere with a sense of well-being and may be precursors of more severe illness.

Behavioral changes also may occur in response to occupational stress. Diminished participation in family activities, increased marital discord, and reduced participation in club activities have been attributed to stress. Rates of substance abuse often are increased. Studies show increased rates of alcohol abuse among individuals with high levels of stress and job dissatisfaction. Tobacco consumption is elevated among people with heavy workloads and tends to increase near deadlines. Other behavioral changes may include alterations in appetite and eating behavior, risk taking (e.g., when driving), and reduced interest in recreational activities.

Overt psychological dysfunction frequently is attributed to stress. Examples of such diagnoses include clinical depression, anxiety disorders, somatoform disorders (e.g., hypochondriasis and psychogenic pain), and exac-

Table 32–5. Examples of mental manifestations of stress.

Mild subjective
Anxiety
Tension
Anger
Depression
Decreased concentration
Irritability
Mild behavioral
Decreased participation in family
Marital discord
Reduced social activity
Risk taking
Clinical psychiatric disorders
Adjustment disorders
Affective disorders
Anxiety disorders including posttraumatic stress disorders
Somatoform disorders and psychophysiologic disorders
Exacerbation of existing psychiatric conditions
Substance abuse

erbation of existing physical conditions by psychological factors. The most frequent psychiatric diagnosis in the working population is that of an adjustment disorder or a time-limited emotional reaction to a specific psychosocial stressor. Stress may act as a nonspecific promoter of disease. Multiple studies show statistical associations between stressors and overt psychiatric disease. Unemployment and lack of opportunity for promotion both have been related to increased psychiatric hospitalizations and suicide rates.

There are increasing data on the specific types of psychiatric disorders that occur most frequently among stressed workers seeking medical attention. The annual prevalence of major depression is approximately 10% in the general population, whereas lifetime prevalence is estimated at 17%. According to a World Health Organization study, of the 10 leading causes of disability, 5 are psychiatric conditions. Major depression, alcoholism, bipolar disorder, schizophrenia, and obsessive-compulsive disorder are commonly associated with an inability to function at work or in the academic setting.

Life-threatening trauma at work may result in overwhelming fear or terror in an employee. Acute stress disorder and the more chronic condition of posttraumatic stress disorder (PTSD) are examples of psychiatric conditions that come forth as a result of a recognizably disturbing external stressor. Not uncommonly, the individual experiences dissociation at the time of the traumatic event. Persistent reexperiencing of the trauma takes place through recurrent intrusive recollections and disturbing dreams. Avoidant behavior is reported not uncommonly, along with sleep disturbance, hypervigilance, irritability, and startle reaction. PTSD has been studied in a variety of work groups, including flight attendants and security personnel. Cognitive functioning involving attention and memory can be adversely affected in individuals with chronic PTSD. Cognitive behavioral therapy and the use of selective serotonin reuptake inhibitor antidepressants have been found to be effective in addressing symptoms of the disorder, which include nightmares, sleep disturbance, intrusion, and hyperarousal. Furthermore, PTSD and clinical depression frequently occur as comorbid conditions in individuals exposed to trauma.

The psychiatric fitness-for-duty (FFD) examination is an assessment that the occupational physician at times may use in addressing troubled employees. This type of examination is governed by the same principles as other fitness-for-duty examinations. Situations that can trigger the psychiatric FFD exam include preplacement psychological screening as in law enforcement, the disruptive employee, the need for a psychiatric leave, failed attempts at return to work, and threat assessment. As in other types of FFD examinations, the report that is issued typically addresses functionality in essential and nonessential job functions relative to the worker's psychopathology. Violence, the threat of violence, and harassment are types of stressors that can have untoward effects on an individual employee and on a work group, resulting in liability for the employer. When there is concern for the potential of violence or aggression in the worksite, a skilled psychiatric consultant can provide important information allowing the employer to take appropriate action in safeguarding the worksite. Factors such as antisocial personality, paranoia, substance abuse, job loss, and a desire for retaliation have been associated with workplace violence.

Cardiovascular Disease

There is growing evidence for the designation of occupational stress as a risk factor for cardiovascular disease. Although causality is difficult to establish, a great number of retrospective and prospective studies have implicated workplace stressors in the etiology of coronary artery disease. Excessive workload has been associated with increased myocardial infarction rates; workers with more than one job or excessively long work hours had more heart disease than a control group with fewer work hours. Role conflict and coronary artery disease are associated for some white-collar workers.

An inverse relationship between job satisfaction and coronary artery disease has been well demonstrated. This factor seems most strongly predictive for white-collar workers. Self-esteem, which may be related to satisfaction, is also negatively correlated with coronary artery disease. These factors may, in turn, be related to another proposed predictor of coronary artery disease—job decision-making latitude. Many studies show that coronary artery disease mortality and morbidity are increased among individuals with demanding jobs that allow little decision-making latitude. Job strain is defined as high job demands with relatively low decision latitude. Increases in job strain are associated with an increased incidence of hypertension in young adults. Justice at work may have benefits for heart health among employees.

One of the most widespread concepts relating behavior to heart disease is the *type A personality hypothesis.* In this model, individuals with aggressive, competitive behaviors who also tend to show time urgency are thought to be more prone to coronary artery disease. The type A personality hypothesis has yielded gradually to more complex models of human behavior that move beyond personality predispositions to include other variables such as rewards and frustrations in the workplace, decision latitude, and social support.

Although there is a substantial epidemiologic foundation that strongly suggests an association between stress and cardiovascular disease, there is still considerable doubt regarding the mechanisms through which a causal chain might occur. One step in the causal process that has been proposed is a link between stress and cardiovascular reactivity. This step includes efforts to determine the relationships between stress and the physiologic processes that are believed to lead to heart disease.

Research has established links between stress and cardiovascular reactivity. In studies involving continuous blood pressure monitoring, short-term blood pressure has been shown to increase the stressful conditions on the job. In these studies, the pressures tended to return to normal when the subjects were at rest away from work. There is also evidence for increases in total cholesterol levels and declines in high-density lipoprotein cholesterol levels in workers under stress.

Cardiovascular reactivity appears to be mediated to a significant extent by the sympathetic nervous system and adrenal responsiveness. Catecholamine release is a frequent measure in research studies of the effect. Arterial constriction in response to stressful conditions has been demonstrated. In addition, cardiac arrhythmias, particularly premature ventricular contractions, have been noted in stressful situations.

Studies examining the relationship between stress-induced cardiovascular reactivity and hypertension are suggestive. One study showed a threefold increase in the risk of a sustained increase in diastolic blood pressure among workers with job strain. This study also demonstrated an increase in the left ventricular mass index, indicating a chronic effect. However, there is still insufficient evidence from long-term longitudinal studies to corroborate a causal relationship between work stress and sustained hypertension.

With respect to coronary artery disease, experiments with primate models show that the progression of atherosclerotic lesions correlate with experimentally induced psychological stresses over the long term. In one research effort, measures of cardiovascular reactivity to stressful psychological stimuli were better able to predict coronary artery disease than were the traditional cardiologic measures. Other research has suggested that stress may affect hematologic parameters, such as blood clotting and fibrinogen levels, that are involved in the etiology of myocardial infarction.

Occupational stress probably contributes to other behavioral and physiologic risk factors for coronary artery disease. Serum cholesterol levels have been shown to rise in tax accountants near deadlines, students taking exams, and shift workers. Statistically significant rises in blood pressure have been found with some stressful jobs such as telephone switchboard operators and air traffic controllers. Increased serum and urine catecholamine levels have been found in workers in competitive situations and those with high workloads. Tobacco use increases among some stressed workers. Some epidemiologic studies implicate sedentary work in increasing the risk of coronary artery disease.

Gastrointestinal Disease

Gastrointestinal disease, particularly peptic ulcer disease, historically has been associated with stress, although there is limited recent epidemiologic information in this area. The identification of *Helicobacter pylori* as a causative factor in peptic ulcer disease has not eliminated consideration of stress as a possible cofactor.

Epidemiologic evidence demonstrates an elevated prevalence of peptic ulcer disease among foremen whose stressors may include responsibility for the behavior and safety of others and an interface role between workers and management. Other occupations that involve responsibility for others—physicians and air traffic controllers—are also associated with high rates of peptic ulcer disease. Workers anticipating plant shutdowns also experience an increase in ulcer disease, as do rotating-shift workers. The incidence of duodenal ulcer—but not gastric ulcer—is also related to workload as measured by energy expenditure. The incidence of ulcer disease may be modified by good social support networks both at home and at work.

There are several possible physiologic mechanisms responsible for the relationship of stress to ulcer disease, even given the etiologic role played by an infectious agent. Gastric acid secretion in response to catecholamine stimulation also may be a contributing factor, although there is conflicting evidence on its significance. Stress may have an impact on wound healing as well as immune function. The etiologic importance of these factors in ulcer disease should be explored further.

Other gastrointestinal problems such as eating disorders, ulcerative colitis, functional bowel disease, and constipation are related to stress. However, there is generally very little information about their association with occupational factors. One exception is rotating-shift work, in which appetite disturbances and constipation have been noted frequently.

Other Diseases

The general model of stress as a stimulus producing a wide variety of physiologic adaptations suggests the possibility that many human diseases are precipitated or aggravated by occupational stress. In most cases, there are plausible hypotheses linking stress to a physiologic response that may play an etiologic role in the causation or aggravation of disease.

Diseases such as diabetes, headaches, and asthma are recognized as having a psychophysiologic component in some individuals, and it is probable that occupational stress factors can complicate their control. For example, there is suggestive evidence that air traffic controllers have higher than normal rates of non-insulin-dependent diabetes.

The role of occupational stress in the causation of a wide range of diseases from cancer to eczema is not confirmed or defined adequately. Such associations are the source of legitimate speculation, but few scientific studies have defined these relationships adequately.

Injury & Accidents

There is a multifactorial relationship between occupational stress and injury in the workplace. Although there is little consistent evidence to demonstrate either the magnitude of stress-related injury or to confirm the mechanisms of the problem, this remains a promising area of stress research. A study of bus drivers demonstrated that psychological job demands, frequency of job problems, and job dissatisfaction all were related to back injuries. An increased risk of low-back pain is found in employees who report insufficient support from supervisors. In addition to high job demands, interpersonal conflict at work also may represent a separate risk factor for occupational injury. Job stress and non-work-related stress reactions are consistently related with upper extremity pain disorders.

The stress of high workload demands may lead to compromise of safety measures to attain higher productivity. Workers paid on a piecework basis have increased numbers of injuries. Attention span may be altered by low levels of stimulation and long periods without breaks; inattention can lead to accidents. Changes of shift are associated with higher rates of injury on the first days of new shifts. There is mounting evidence to relate shift changes and sleeplessness to airplane pilot and air traffic controller errors. There also may be a relationship between job decision latitude and frequency of injury. The contribution of stress to substance abuse also leads to accidents; a large proportion of motor vehicle accidents on the job involve alcohol.

Some authors note a relationship between stressful events in an employee's life and subsequent occupational accidents. The possibility exists that stress from work or personal factors may contribute to the likelihood of an accident. Stressors should be assessed in evaluating injured employees; treatment of the physical impairment alone may not result in successful return to work.

Sickness, Absence, & Productivity

A clear relationship exists between sickness, absence from work, and lost productivity. Stress may be an independent variable influencing each of these three factors. The case for stress as a contributor to sickness already has been discussed. However, absence from work is a complex phenomenon involving not just organic disease but also mental health, motivation, satisfaction with employment, and other personal and work-related factors. Some research has demonstrated a relationship between organizational stressors, such as high-demand/low-control work, and subsequent absenteeism. However, research studies on stress and absenteeism are mixed. Some studies indicate that stressors appear to predict absences associated with a physician visit but not other absences.

Productivity on the job is a stress-sensitive function. Reduced output, production delays, and poor performance may be manifestations of stress. Declining productivity of an organization or individual should prompt a search for occupational stressors. A stress management program may promote increases in attendance and productivity. This has been demonstrated by experiments that increase employee decision-making participation, as well as by revisions of workers' rotating shifts, according to psychological principles.

REFERENCES

Belkic KL et al: Is job strain a major source of cardiovascular disease risk? Scand J Work Environ Health 2004;30:85 [PMID: 15127782].

Collins SM et al: Job strain and autonomic indices of cardiovascular disease risk. Am J Indust Med 2005;48:182 [PMID: 16094616].

Eriksen W et al: Work factors as predictors of intense or disabling low back pain: A prospective study of nurses' aides. Occup Environ Med 2004;61:398 [PMID: 15090659].

Karlsson B et al: Total mortality and cause-specific mortality of Swedish shift- and dayworkers in the pulp and paper industry in 1952–2001. Scand J Work Environ Health 2005;31:30 [PMID: 15751616].

Kivimäki M et al: Justice at work and reduced risk of coronary heart disease among employees. Arch Intern Med 2005; 165:2245 [PMID: 16246990].

Langlieb AM, Kahn JP: How much does quality mental health care profit employers? J Occup Environ Med 2005;47:1099 [PMID: 16282870].

MacDonald HA et al: Posttraumatic stress disorder (PTSD) in the workplace. J Occup Rehabil. 2003;13:63. [PMID: 12708101].

Swaen GM et al: Psychosocial work characteristics as risk factors for being injured in an occupational accident. J Occup Environ Med 2004;46:521 [PMID: 15213513.]

Yehuda R: Risk and resilience in posttraumatic stress disorder. J Clin Psychiatry 2004;65:29 [PMID: 14728094].

Stress & Workers' Compensation

While representing only a small portion of the costs of stress, workers' compensation claims for mental injuries have increased substantially in recent years. Most states in the United States recognize mental stress as a compensable disorder. In an attempt to restrict "stress claims," some jurisdictions have placed restrictions on claims during the probationary period of employment, eliminated claims resulting from appropriate personnel actions, and increased the causation threshold to substantial or predominant cause.

Stress-related workers' compensation claims may be divided into three categories: physical-mental, mental-physical, and mental-mental. Physical-mental claims usually result from well-defined work-related injuries such as crush injuries, amputations, or other sudden, significant, well-defined occurrences, although they also may result from illnesses. The claim is made for mental health effects such as posttraumatic stress, neuroses, or depression resulting from the physical event. Such claims are recognized in all U.S. jurisdictions, although some claim types pose a challenge to the system. For example, mental health effects that an individual claims as a result of a gradually developing occupational disease, such as asbestosis, expand the scope of the physical-mental claim and raise new issues.

The mental-physical category includes instances in which claimants contend that emotional stresses at work have caused physical ailments, including a wide variety of disorders such as myocardial infarction and neurologic, dermatologic, and gastrointestinal diseases. The epidemiologic evidence linking emotional stress to the initiation or aggravation of these disorders is variable and often weak. In the United States, most states limit these claims by requiring the presence of an unusual stressor or a close coupling of the events in time.

In recent years, mental-mental claims have drawn the most attention, and the number of claims has grown rapidly. Claimants file for compensation on the basis of mental health effects of conditions at work. There are fundamentally three kinds of situations that

Table 32–6. Psychiatric injury claims: Preventive measures.

Employee education
Supervisor training
Employee assistance programs
Early intervention
Mediation services
Outpatient mental health benefits
Comprehensive psychiatric exam
Claims review
Standardized personnel policy
Executive consultation

may precipitate these claims: stress resulting from involvement in sudden, emotionally disturbing events, such as witnessing a coworker's death; stress resulting from a continuing situation that is unusual in its demands on the worker (e.g., air traffic controllers and some types of police work); and stress arising out of the conditions of everyday work. These claims, particularly the last group, often are difficult to resolve. Many of these cases involve interpersonal conflict, predominantly conflict with supervisors. Both the extent of impairment and the causal factors are difficult to assess objectively. Legal precedent has allowed the claimant's subjective perception of events to be a factor in determining compensibility in many jurisdictions. As a result of concerns over rising claims, California has legislated that mental stress must be more than 50% occupational in origin to qualify for compensation.

Alternative schema for categorizing psychiatric claims include those that involve a reaction to an admitted or acknowledged physical injury, an obviously psychologically traumatic event, and cumulative stress associated with the nature of the job position. Psychiatric claims are contentious because of the subjective nature of the evidence presented. In jurisdictions that allow for cumulative stress injuries, those claims tend to be heavily litigated. Prevention and early intervention of psychiatric injuries involve employee education, employee assistance programs, reasonable mental health benefits, and appropriate personnel policies (Table 32–6).

REFERENCES

Cutler RB et al: Relationships between functional capacity measures and baseline psychological measures in chronic pain patients. J Occup Rehabil 2003;13:249 [PMID: 14671989].

Haines J et al: Workers' compensation for psychological injury: Personal and environmental correlates. Work 2004;22:183 [PMID: 15156084].

Haines J et al: Workers' compensation for psychological injury: Demographic and work-related correlates. Work 2006;26:57 [PMID: 16373980].

PREVENTION & MANAGEMENT OF STRESS

The prevention and management of occupational stress are a great challenge. There has been solid progress in understanding many of the organizational and personal factors that contribute to occupational stress. Evidence is accumulating that the models of stress introduced in this chapter have predictive value in the organizational setting. However, efforts to intervene to control stress at the individual, group, or organizational level have met with mixed success.

Stress management programs tend to focus on solutions at the individual level. One approach is to intervene through individual counseling with individuals who are experiencing adverse psychological impacts from stress. Another approach is to provide individuals or work groups with training and education on coping and adaptive techniques. These training and education interventions may be done either preventively or reactively with stressed individuals or groups.

Growing evidence and experience point to the need for solutions that focus on organizational factors, as described earlier, that appear to have a causal role in occupational stress. These interventions usually involve organizational changes directed at one of a number of factors—task control, role definition, workload, reward structure, job challenge and meaningfulness, and social support in the workplace. A growing number of well-designed applied research studies have begun to fill the void of knowledge about these organizational interventions. The results are not yet encouraging in terms of objective evidence for improved outcomes.

Role of the Health Professional

Occupational health physicians and other occupational health professionals should monitor their patients and, when possible, entire work groups for signs of stress. Many possible indicators should be considered. Individuals or clusters of patients may present with symptoms including mild mental distress, frequent absences from work, substance abuse, or severe mental impairment. Productivity may fall. Rates of injury may increase. Physical symptoms may be out of proportion to the type of injury.

Once alerted to the problem, the clinician may take steps to counsel individuals and offer assistance in stress reduction. The availability of programs designed for this purpose is a great asset; however, the clinician should take primary responsibility for helping the patient gain insight into the problem and for providing concrete advice and referrals to assist in its management (see "Individual-Level Approaches to Stress Management" below).

The role of health professionals in managing an organization-wide stress intervention often is more challenging. Managers often will seek help for the individual employee with stress-related problems. They usually expect the clinician to deal with the situation on an individual level and may not expect or welcome interventions that involve an entire work group or organization. The challenge for occupational health professionals is to bridge the gap between the traditional medical model and a population-based model of stress control.

It is important for the occupational health professional to recognize that organizational stress is not the domain solely of the medical department and that other professionals have a significant contribution to make. Human resources specialists, organizational development consultants, employee assistance professionals, and others have expertise that should be employed in shaping an organization's stress prevention or management program. The issues related to stress interventions are complex, and there has been limited demonstrated effectiveness with the interventions. It is best to proceed with care based on well-designed interventions and a thorough situation analysis. Efforts to achieve consensus of all the stakeholders in these situations will contribute to the likelihood of success.

Individual-Level Approaches to Stress Management

Most stress management approaches focus on the individual and attempt to teach coping skills for the management or reduction of stress. These programs may be offered to all employees of an organization, to targeted groups, or to individuals.

A great number of approaches have been developed. Information may be transmitted through methods ranging from simple self-study brochures to intensive individual counseling. Many programs rely on group training sessions. Educational efforts may involve the distribution of written materials, lectures, seminars, poster campaigns, and a variety of other methods.

The objectives of work-site stress programs usually are to educate employees about stress and its effects, to increase awareness of stress in their lives and jobs, and to teach coping skills for managing or reducing the problem. These programs aim to identify people in the early stages of stress before it has become a significant health problem.

In recent years, a number of standardized surveys have been developed to assess stress in individuals. Self-assessment questionnaires may help to educate employees about stressors and give feedback about personal levels of stress compared with norms.

In addition to the self-assessment questionnaires, an important advance in the ability to assess an individual's stress and coping style has been the development of validated surveys that are interpreted by researchers or health professionals. These instruments can be used

Table 32–7. Stress management techniques.

Biofeedback
Deep-breathing exercises
Exercise/physical activity
Meditation
Progressive relaxation exercise
Stress-inoculation training
Yoga

either in individual counseling or in organizational research and development. One such survey, the Occupational Stress Inventory (OSI), has been the subject of several validation studies. Its most appropriate use is to assist in the evaluation of individuals experiencing significant levels of occupational stress. The Finnish Institute of Occupational Health has developed another survey, the Occupational Stress Questionnaire, for research use. These and other similar stress-assessment questionnaires, some of which are available commercially, may assist clinicians to determine the prevalence of stress within a working population.

It is insufficient to increase awareness of occupational stress without teaching specific skills to improve the individual's ability to handle the stressful situation. Many stress management techniques involve teaching relaxation or meditation exercises (Table 32–7), some emphasize physical activity, and others teach the individual to be aware of and to manage the emotions related to stressful situations. The role of social support from spouses, friends, and coworkers is emphasized in some programs.

Another type of stress-coping program educates the individual to make adaptations to be able to better control the work environment and stress responses (Table 32–8). Some of these stress-coping methods involve strategies for dealing with stressful situations; others include time management, priority setting, improved planning abilities, and decision-making skills. These techniques all may be helpful to the individual whose job allows their implementation. Interpersonal skills such as assertiveness training, conflict resolution, and relationship building also may be useful. Another method of stress reduction involves teaching cognitive

Table 32–8. Examples of stress-coping skills.

Assertiveness training
Conflict resolution
Decision-making and problem-solving skills
Goal and priority setting
Interpersonal skills training
Time management

skills to help individuals to recognize what personal beliefs, perceptions, and expectations lead to stress.

The concept of acceptance on the part of the employee is a controversial approach to stress reduction. Acceptance involves a willingness to experience thoughts, feelings, and sensations without the need to control them. Acceptance on the part of customer service employees is predictive of mental health and positive job performance. Evaluation of stress-coping efforts in occupational settings is difficult; studies of these programs tend to show improvements in perceived stress, stress-related symptoms, and a variety of other endpoints, such as muscle tension, use of health services, and interference with job performance. However, the benefits of stress management programs tend to fade with time, and few long-term (1 year or more) follow-up evaluations have been done. There is relatively little information comparing the effectiveness of the various stress-coping techniques, and the effectiveness of specific programs varies according to the outcome measure used. The use of combinations of techniques appears to be more effective than single techniques. Refresher courses and periodic reinforcing of stress management skills help to ensure continuing effectiveness.

A consensus panel of experts evaluated the effectiveness and practicality of six stress management techniques, including relaxation, physical fitness, cognitive restructuring, meditation, assertiveness training, and "stress inoculation." The panel concluded that relaxation and physical fitness were the most effective approaches. Experts rated relaxation as the more practical option, given the acceptability and logistics associated with exercise. Meditation and assertiveness training were rated least effective.

Individual psychotherapy usually is reserved for individuals with significant stress-related problems. These individuals may self-refer, be identified by supervisors, or come to the attention of instructors who are teaching stress management programs. Referral of these individuals to employee assistance program professionals or to other health care providers with expertise in stress management counseling is appropriate. Personal counseling in these situations can involve a number of stress management and reduction techniques. One common technique is *stress scripting,* in which an individual is taught to recognize and reframe his or her internal dialog regarding stressful situations. Short-term therapy involving a few sessions may be sufficient to ameliorate the individual's condition; however, periodic follow-up is advised. For some workers, group psychotherapy may be more appropriate and acceptable. Others may experience symptoms of depression or anxiety amenable to a course of antidepressant or antianxiety medication in addition to measures to address the underlying circumstances. There is evidence indicating the effectiveness of individual counseling in stress reduction.

Organizational-Level Approaches to Stress Management

The development of organizational approaches to stress prevention and control is at the leading edge of occupational stress research. Although a great number of employers have introduced stress management programs directed at individuals, relatively few efforts have been made to focus on the "organization as the patient." However, there is growing theoretical knowledge and practical experience with interventions to protect the workforce against stress through appropriate design of the environment and relationships at work. Similarly, there are increasing efforts to resolve problems of high stress through institution-wide restructuring or other organizational-level interventions.

The field of organizational-level interventions is relatively new. There have been useful developments both at identifying the sources of stress within an organization and at designing solutions to the problem. The number of published experimental and "action research" studies has increased, much of it in the organizational development, administrative sciences, or psychology literature.

In the organizational-level approach, the objective is to reduce the stressors arising from within the organization itself. For example, interventions may be directed at altering hierarchical organizational structures, enhancing communication style, involving employees in decision making, or clarifying work roles.

Other approaches have included variation of work tasks, improving the physical tasks, improving the physical environment (including ergonomic design), and improving employee training. Increasing attention also has gone into social support systems in the workplace; efforts in this area usually have focused on team-building concepts.

Research done largely in Scandinavian countries has emphasized the development of criteria for a workplace that protects individual physical and psychological well-being and allows individual mastery of work skills. The emphasis has been on creating a good work environment, not merely one free of adverse stressors. The nature of the industry involved will have a major influence of the relative importance of various aspects of optimal job design and requires careful consideration. For example, the key factors to avoid in production work are quantitative and qualitative overload. In the hospital industry, the main tension is created by the conflicting demands of high workload and a need to maintain high standards in the face of qualitatively complex situations.

Apart from a balance of workload and content, other elements of the optimal work environment include a reasonable degree of control over the job task or process, an environment that favors the development of supportive social networks among coworkers, clarity in job roles, and training or other opportunities to learn fully about the job process and how to cope with its variations.

The ability to assess and measure stress in organizations has developed as a result of the application of survey instruments in these settings, as discussed earlier. While many different surveys exist, there is growing experience with aggregating individual responses to develop an organizational stress profile. The various scales on the survey give an indication of the sources of stress in the organization. This approach has been used successfully to direct the types of interventions needed. For example, an organizational intervention in a hospital as a result, in part, of survey data has led to reduced overall workers' compensation claims.

The survey approach has been applied more commonly in the assessment of the stressors for individuals in a given occupational category. Stress surveys have been done for police officers, schoolteachers, physicians, social workers, and bus operators. With a valid survey instrument, these studies can be revealing in terms of the underlying dynamics of stress in that profession.

Many organizational-level stress interventions have been attempted, although efforts with managerial or professional employees predominate. Reduced absenteeism and declines in role conflict and ambiguity have been demonstrated in a study of insurance company workers. The intervention consisted of enhanced goal setting and goal clarification. Several studies show positive effects from increased levels of employee involvement in decision making and increased job decision latitude. Increasing perceived time autonomy is also effective in reducing absenteeism and improving work performance.

Blue-collar interventions have included efforts to improve the work environment, reduce job overload, increase job autonomy, and increase social support. Improved teamwork has been a common theme. Workers have been given more self-determination in the organization of work through quality circles and work teams with shared production responsibility. Teamwork also has been seen to increase social support. Job rotation has been a technique to relieve boredom and to increase workers' understanding of the overall production process.

Organizational stress-reduction interventions often have had inadequate evaluations, and there are notably few controlled studies in this area.

NIOSH offers some general guidelines on organizational change to prevent occupational stress:

- Adjust workload to workers' abilities
- Define roles and responsibilities clearly
- Design jobs that are meaningful, stimulating, and allow workers to use their abilities
- Promote interaction among workers
- Facilitate worker participation in decisions regarding their tasks and how their job is accomplished
- Establish good communication about workplace issues

While this type of intervention offers much promise for the prevention of stress effects on the workforce, much remains to be studied and documented before standard approaches can be recommended. A recent review of organizational change interventions did not find convincing overall evidence for their effectiveness in improving employee well-being or organizational outcomes. Nonetheless, some intervention efforts have had demonstrated success. This area remains open for future research and efforts to evaluate approaches that may be more consistently successful.

REFERENCES

Bond FW, Bunce D: The role of acceptance and job control in mental health, job satisfaction, and work performance. J Appl Psychol 2003;88:12057 [PMID: 14640816].

Burton WN et al: The association of medical conditions and presenteeism. J Occup Environ Med 2006;48:252 [PMID: 16531829].

Chan AO, Huak CY: Influence of work environment on emotional health in a health care setting. Occup Med (Lond) 2004; 54:207 [PMID: 15133146].

Jones DL et al: Stress management and workplace disability in the US, Europe, and Japan. J Occup Health 2003;45:1 [PMID: 14605422].

Pransky G et al: Disability prevention and communication among workers, physicians, employers and insurers—current models and opportunities for improvement. Disabil Rehabil 2004; 26:625 [PMID: 15204500].

Substance Abuse & Employee Assistance Programs

33

Stephen Heidel, MD, MBA

Substance abuse is a major problem throughout the United States, including the workplace. In 2002, there were 19.8 million adults in the United States with a substance abuse problem. Of these, 15.3 million (77.1%) were employed. Alcohol is the most widely abused substance, whereas marijuana is the most widely used illicit drug. The cost of substance abuse in the United States is staggering. It is estimated to be $328 billion. Most of these costs are due to lost productivity, including $134 billion of lost productivity due to alcohol and $100 billion due to illicit drugs.

Substance abuse causes absenteeism, safety problems, poor-quality workmanship, friction with coworkers, and liability to the organization. Behavioral problems, including unscheduled absences, unsafe actions, and irritability, create a strain between substance abusers and coworkers, supervisors, and customers. Erratic and unsafe work practices while under the influence may expose the organization to significant liability, such as the case of the *Exxon Valdez.*

Substance abuse disorders usually are accompanied by a decline in social and occupational functioning, making the workplace a good place to observe this decline in an individual's functioning and to direct him or her to appropriate treatment. The structure of the workplace allows for this because there are clearly defined expectations on attendance, work performance, and behavior. The workplace is also less influenced by the emotional ties that family and friends of the substance abuser must confront in dealing with a substance abuser's dysfunctional behavior. This combination of factors allows the workplace to detect drug and alcohol abuse problems and, in conjunction with its employee assistance program (EAP), refer employees for assessment, treatment, and follow-up.

Dealing with substance abuse in the workplace is a challenge for the occupational medicine physician requiring special knowledge of the diagnosis and treatment of substance use disorders, the clinical presentation of substance abuse syndromes as they appear in the workplace, the pharmacologic and legal aspects of urine testing, and the legal aspects of patient confidentiality and reporting requirements. Occupational physicians also must consult with and refer to psychiatrists and partner with EAPs to identify, diagnose, and effectively treat substance-abusing employees.

REFERENCES

Cunradi CB et al: Alcohol, stress-related factors, and short-term absenteeism among urban transit operators. J Urban Health 2005;82:43 [PMID: 15738336].

Goetzel RZ et al: Health, absence, disability, and presenteeism cost estimates of certain physical and mental health conditions affecting US employers. J Occup Environ Med 2004;46:398 [PMID: 15076658].

DIAGNOSTIC CRITERIA

The definitions of *addiction, substance abuse,* and *dependency* have suffered from a lack of formal nomenclature. In the past, these terms often were used interchangeably. Significant strides in nomenclature have been made over the last 10 years. The American Psychiatric Association's *Diagnostic and Statistical Manual of Mental Disorders,* 4th edition (DSM-IV), text revision, uses a cluster of behavioral, physiological, and cognitive variables to define substance abuse–related conditions such as dependence, abuse, toxicity, and withdrawal. All have specific diagnostic criteria. The basic criteria for substance dependence are a maladaptive pattern of substance use that includes tolerance, withdrawal, and other patterns of use that are maladaptive (Table 33–1). *Abuse* is a less severe pattern of substance use extending over 12 months that leads to a failure to fulfill major obligations at work, school, or home (Table 33–2). These criteria serve as a useful common reference point for the physician attempting to establish a diagnosis of abuse or dependence on a psychoactive substance. Using these standardized criteria can be helpful for establishing a diagnosis and for documenting the need for treatment.

Many managed-care organizations will not authorize treatment for patients unless they meet the DSM-IV-TR criteria for abuse and/or dependence. These criteria are applicable to the major classes of abusable substances, including alcohol, amphetamines, cannabis, cocaine, hallucinogens, inhalants, opioids, phencyclidine, and minor tranquilizers.

A practical approach to evaluate an individual for an addiction includes evaluating continued use of a substance despite negative consequences. Addicts continue to abuse

Table 33–1. Criteria for substance dependence.

A maladaptive pattern of substance use leading to clinically significant impairment or distress, as manifested by three (or more) of the following, occurring at any time in the same 12-month period:

- A. Tolerance, as defined by either of the following:
  1. A need for markedly increased amounts of the substance to achieve intoxication or desired effect
  2. Markedly diminished effect with continued use of the same amount of the substance
- B. Withdrawal, as manifested by either of the following:
  1. The characteristic withdrawal syndrome for the substance (refer to criteria A and B of the criteria sets for Withdrawal from the specific substances)
  2. The same (or a closely related) substance is taken to relieve or avoid withdrawal symptoms
- C. The substance is often taken in larger amounts or over a longer period than was intended
- D. There is a persistent desire or unsuccessful efforts to cut down or control substance use
- E. A great deal of time is spent in activities necessary to obtain the substance (e.g., visiting multiple doctors or driving long distances), to use the substance (e.g., chain-smoking), or to recover from its effects
- F. Important social, occupational, or recreational activities are given up or reduced because of substance use
- G. The substance use is continued despite knowledge of having a persistent or recurrent physical or psychological problem that is likely to have been caused or exacerbated by the substance (e.g., current cocaine use despite recognition of cocaine-induced depression, or continued drinking despite recognition that an ulcer was made worse by alcohol consumption)

Specify if:

With psychologic dependence: evidence of tolerance or withdrawal (i.e., either item 1 or 2 is present)
Without psychologic dependence: no evidence of tolerance or withdrawal (i.e., neither item 1 nor 2 is present)

Table 33–2. Criteria for substance abuse.

- A. A maladaptive pattern of substance use leading to clinically significant impairment or distress, as manifested by one (or more) of the following, occurring within a 12-month period:
  1. Recurrent substance use resulting in a failure to fulfill major role obligations at work, school, or home (e.g., repeated absences or poor work performance related to substance use; substance-related absences, suspensions, or expulsions from school; neglect of children or household)
  2. Recurrent substance use in situations in which it is physically hazardous (e.g., driving an automobile or operating a machine when impaired by substance use)
  3. Recurrent substance-related legal problems (e.g., arrests for substance-related disorderly conduct)
  4. Continued substance use despite having persistent or recurrent social or interpersonal problems caused or exacerbated by the effects of the substance (e.g., arguments with spouse about consequences of intoxication, physical fights)
- B. The symptoms have never met the criteria for substance dependence for this class of substance.

alcohol and/or drugs despite financial, legal, medical, or marital problems. Evaluating each of these areas often will reveal a pattern of continued use despite negative consequences. For example, a history may reveal several lost jobs owing to substance use or several divorces or failed relationships owing to the use of alcohol and/or drugs.

SUBSTANCE ABUSE SYNDROMES

Alcohol-Related Disorders

Alcoholism is by far the most serious chemical dependency problem encountered in the workplace. An estimated 6.2 percent of adults working full time are "heavy drinkers" and likely would meet the diagnostic criteria for alcohol dependence. The workplace offers an ideal setting for early intervention for alcohol dependence because many of the subtle behavioral manifestations of alcoholism become apparent in the workplace long before they are seen at home or in everyday social life. Decreasing work performance in a previously high-functioning employee, excessive absenteeism (particularly on Mondays), and excessive uses of sick leave are all signs of alcohol or other drug impairment. The occupational medicine specialist must be able to recognize the early signs of alcohol-induced impairment and direct employees to appropriate treatment to minimize the economic impact that the untreated alcoholic can have on themselves, coworkers, employers, and the public.

Early identification of the alcoholic patient in the occupational setting can be facilitated by focused history taking, a carefully focused physical examination, and use of selective laboratory studies. An effective method for obtaining an alcohol history is to use a structured interview and to obtain history from independent sources. Inquiring about the patient's relationship, legal, and financial history is important because problems in these areas often are associated with substance abuse. Questions about quantity of alcohol drunk, time period of drinking, and choice of beverage usually are not fruitful because alcoholics tend to minimize and/or deny their alcohol intake. The CAGE questionnaire (Table 33–3) is a highly effective tool in establishing a diagnosis of alcohol abuse or dependency. Patients who answer two of four CAGE questions positively have a score that correlates in excess of 90% with the diagnosis of alcohol dependence. The CAGE questionnaire is easy to administer in the context of a workplace medical evaluation. The importance of obtaining independent reports of an employee's alcohol use from

Table 33–3. The CAGE questionnaire.

1. Have you ever felt you should **c**ut down on your drinking?
2. Have people **a**nnoyed you by criticizing your drinking?
3. Have you ever felt bad or **g**uilty about drinking?
4. Have you ever taken a drink first thing in the morning (**e**ye opener) to steady your nerves or get rid of a hangover?

coworkers, supervisors, and family members should not be underestimated. Reports from supervisors and coworkers on changes in work performance, absenteeism, and observed use of alcohol and drugs can be obtained during a workplace evaluation. Contacting a patient's family or friends outside the workplace, however, needs to be done with the patient's permission.

The physical examination can yield subtle clues to alcohol abuse. In many cases, employees abruptly cease alcohol use when asked to present for a medical evaluation. Temporary cessation of alcohol use will precipitate signs of mild withdrawal, including diaphoresis, tachycardia, mild hypertension, and an upper extremity symmetric tremor. In addition, signs of trauma, particularly in the lower extremities, associated with falls while intoxicated can be helpful clues. Fractures, particularly of the ribs, have been associated with alcohol abuse. Signs of frank organ injury such as spider angiomas and organomegaly are also helpful when present, but these injuries represent end-organ damage, usually seen only in cases of advanced alcoholism.

The judicious use of laboratory studies can further support the diagnosis of alcohol abuse and dependence. Blood alcohol determinations usually are helpful only if acute intoxication is suspected. Most employees presenting for evaluation will have stopped drinking hours or days prior to the evaluation; subsequently, blood alcohol determinations often are completely negative. Therefore, the determination of a zero blood alcohol level should not be used to conclude that there is no alcohol problem. One exception to this rule is when patients show signs of intoxication in the workplace. In this case, a breathalyzer test or blood alcohol determination can be quite useful. Results from a breathalyzer correlate quite well with blood alcohol levels, and such devices can be more convenient to use in the workplace.

Alcohol also can cause direct injury to certain organ systems, such as the liver and bone marrow, which can be reflected in the peripheral blood. The most useful blood studies are the complete blood count, especially the mean corpuscle volume (MCV), and certain liver enzyme studies, particularly γ-glutamyl transpeptidase (GGT), which commonly is elevated with significant alcohol use. A number of studies have shown that elevation of the MCV, particularly when combined with an elevated GGT, can identify more than 90% of alcohol-abusing patients. These tests alone, while sensitive, are not very specific and cannot

be used as a diagnostic marker for alcohol dependence. In evaluating a patient for any chemical dependency, laboratory studies, including urine testing, never should be used alone but rather to support findings obtained by careful history taking and a thorough physical examination.

Cannabis

Cannabis is the substance most commonly detected in workplace urine testing. It is usually smoked and is absorbed readily from the respiratory and intestinal mucosa. Tetrahydrocannabinol (THC) is the active ingredient of marijuana and produces a state of emotional and muscular relaxation and euphoria. In susceptible individuals, however, it can produce depression and psychosis. Chronic use is associated with apathy and both impaired judgment and problem-solving ability. Chronic use can lead to respiratory complications, including bronchitis and permanent lung injury. THC is lipid-soluble and tends to remain in body tissues for days to weeks. It can appear in the urine for weeks after chronic use.

Stimulants: Cocaine & Amphetamines

The central nervous system (CNS) stimulants include cocaine in its various forms and amphetamines. Cocaine is produced as an extract from the coca leaf in the form of pure alkaloid, or "free base," and crystalline hydrochloride salt, which is water-soluble and absorbed rapidly by the respiratory and enteric mucosa. The crystalline version usually is insufflated into the nose or taken orally. Free base cocaine is volatile and usually is smoked with a pipe. This form of ingestion results in rapid absorption, leading to an intense euphoria that lasts about 30–45 minutes. This intense but short-lived effect makes cocaine popular for users who do not desire a prolonged "high." This feature has implications for the workplace, where impairment may be short-lived and intermittent but quite severe. Acute cocaine intoxication can result in acute mania, paranoid psychosis, and impulsive and sometimes severe, violent behavior. Chronic use can lead to intense depression, suicidal ideation, and paranoid psychosis. The physical symptoms of cocaine intoxication resolve within days of removal of the drug, but psychiatric complications of cocaine use can be so intense that it creates an acute psychiatric emergency. Cocaine also produces an intense adrenergic discharge, resulting in tachycardia, hypertension, and mydriasis. These syndromes, in turn, can produce acute cardiovascular complications, including myocardial infarction, seizures, cerebral vascular accidents, and cardiac arrhythmias.

Amphetamines often are used as appetite suppressants and to boost energy. Initially, they do have positive effects for many individuals (weight loss and increased energy); however, long-term use leads to personality changes and psychiatric symptoms, including insomnia, depression, paranoia, and psychosis. Amphetamines are absorbed rapidly via the respiratory and gastrointestinal (GI) tract and are usually taken orally or intranasally. Methamphetamine is smoked in the same way as "crack" cocaine and is relatively volatile. The amphetamines differ from cocaine in that their half-life is longer, and they produce a prolonged period of intoxication. In a workplace evaluation, amphetamine-abusing workers are more likely to show acute autonomic signs of intoxication such as tachycardia, hyperemia, and mydriasis. Acute amphetamine intoxication is associated with severe toxic psychosis characterized by motor agitation, intense paranoia, and violence.

Opioids

Opiate problems in the workplace take two forms. The first type is the worker who is prescribed opiates for a medical reason, including medication prescribed for an industrial injury. Such patients can develop opiate abuse or dependency in the course of their medical treatment and can present a special challenge to the occupational medicine specialist. The challenge is to first diagnose the pattern of abuse or dependence. The occupational medicine physician then must work with the treating physician to develop a shared understanding of the problem. These patients need simultaneous treatment both for their medical condition and for the opiate dependence. Often these patients need a multidisciplinary approach to detoxification, rehabilitation, and workplace reentry. The second type of opiate abuse is the worker with a primary opiate dependency not associated with a medical condition. These patients are more likely to engage in intravenous drug use and usually obtain their drugs from illegal sources. These two factors place these patients at high risk for a variety of serious medical complications, including hepatitis B and C, human immunodeficiency virus (HIV) infection, endocarditis, and infections at the injection site (phlebitis and cellulitis).

Naturally occurring narcotics (opiates) and synthetic agents (opioids) act as CNS depressants. Opiates and opioids produce intense euphoria and feelings of emotional tranquility and sedation. The duration of these effects varies by route of administration and type of opioid used. The opiates with low protein binding, such as heroin, move into the CNS quickly but are absorbed slowly from the GI tract. This is the reason why addicts, in an attempt to achieve rapid euphoria, tend to use these drugs intravenously. The drugs differ in their half-life and potency. All are excreted in the urine and are readily detectable with urine drug testing. It is important to note that both heroin and codeine are metabolized by the body to morphine. Therefore, patients using either of these agents will test positive only for morphine on urine drug testing. Opiates produce profound mental and psychomotor slowing that

will interfere with almost any work task. Depression of cardiopulmonary function is a particular risk for workers in special environments that require the use of respirators or breathing apparatus. The varying concentration (drug versus "filler") of street drugs poses the risk of accidental overdose on and off the work site. Detection of opiate abuse, particularly in the nonprescription addict, can be somewhat challenging. Addicts also can be quite covert in their drug use. Careful history taking, with particular attention to the presence of apathy, depression, and sedation, can be quite helpful. Needle tracks, miosis, signs of constipation, weight loss (opiates induce anorexia), and infectious complications of intravenous drug use seen on physical examination all can alert the physician to a covert opiate addiction problem. Urine drug testing can be helpful in supporting such a diagnosis.

Tranquilizers: Sedative, Hypnotic, & Antianxiety Drugs

Minor tranquilizers are prescribed very widely. Benzodiazepines are used to treat anxiety disorders, including panic disorder and insomnia. Benzodiazepines, by and large, are safe; however, they can cause cognitive impairment, even at therapeutic doses. If intoxicated by these drugs, an individual may become lethargic, very sedated, and have impaired coordination. Since these are legally prescribed and used widely, this poses a risk in the workplace if an employee has a safety-sensitive job. All this is made worse by the fact that many individuals using benzodiazepines combine them with alcohol, which may aggravate the negative effects. There is a certain profile that can place patients at risk for dependence. These factors include long-term use of benzodiazepines, previous history of alcohol or sedative-hypnotic abuse, and concomitant chronic medical problems or psychiatric problems such as dysthymia, anxiety, and certain personality disorders.

The occupational medicine specialist should screen employees taking benzodiazepines, even for appropriate conditions and in therapeutic dosages. These employees may need to be excluded from duties that require a high degree of concentration and motor skills. Patients with a dependence on these drugs may require detoxification and stabilization before workplace reentry. Consultation with the patient's prescribing physician is extremely helpful to determine benzodiazepine dependency and to formulate a return-to-work treatment plan.

REFERENCES

Conway KP et al: Lifetime comorbidity of DSM-IV mood and anxiety disorders and specific drug use disorders. J Clin Psychiatry. 2006;67:247 [PMID: 16566620].

Hasin D et al: Diagnosis of comorbid psychiatric disorders in substance users. Am J Psychiatry. 2006;163:689 [PMID: 16585445].

McDonald AJ 3rd et al: US emergency department visits for alcohol-related diseases and injuries between 1992 and 2000. Arch Intern Med 2004;164:531 [PMID: 15006830].

ORGANIZATIONAL RESPONSE TO SUBSTANCE ABUSE

By taking certain steps, organizations will be ready to address substance abuse problems when they occur. The components necessary to respond to drug and alcohol problems include a drug and alcohol policy, urine drug testing, an employee assistance program, access to psychiatric fitness-for-duty exams and referrals, access to treatment, and a return-to-work plan.

Drug & Alcohol Policy

A written policy is the starting point for a company when setting a strategy to respond to substance abuse in its workplace. The policy should be tailored to the particular workplace; thus no two policies will be exactly alike. Policies will have common elements, however, with statements that include drug and alcohol problems are serious but treatable illnesses, alcohol and drug abuse are unacceptable in the workplace, what constitute violations of the policy, a description of consequences for violations, employees are responsible for seeking treatment and complying with treatment recommendations, the circumstances for drug testing (preplacement, for cause, random), and the consequences for a positive drug test.

Urine Drug Testing

Few topics have created more controversy in the workplace than urine drug testing. Urine testing was first adopted by the U.S. military in the 1980s. It was used subsequently by increasing numbers of employers in certain industries, particularly transportation and nuclear industries, both of which are required by federal statute to test employees. It is estimated that more than 7 million Americans now must participate in mandatory urine drug testing as required by federal law. This requirement, in turn, has led to the accreditation of drug-testing laboratories by the National Institute on Drug Abuse (NIDA). To acquire certification, laboratories must test for at least five drugs: amphetamines, cannabinoids, cocaine, opioids, and phencyclidine (PCP). If companies are not mandated to drug test their employees, they must decide whether and under which circumstances to test.

Drug testing typically is conducted in the following instances: (1) preplacement testing of new employees, (2) random employee drug testing on an ongoing basis, and (3) "for cause" testing to evaluate an employee in the context of an unusual event such as an accident on the job or acute behavioral changes.

One large study of prospective postal employees showed that preemployment test results that were positive for marijuana and cocaine use were associated with adverse employment outcomes as measured by accidents, absences, and turnover rates. The true preventive value of preplacement urine drug testing needs to be further evaluated from a safety-enhancement and cost-benefit viewpoint.

The rise of drug testing has led to the emergence of a new role as medical review officer (MRO) for physicians. The MRO is charged with reviewing positive urine test results and is responsible for ensuring the integrity of the "chain of custody" of the sample from employee to laboratory. The MRO also evaluates the mitigating circumstances related to a positive urine test (e.g., an employee who was taking prescribed medication at the time of the urine test). The MRO needs to be very knowledgeable of the pharmacology of the drugs being screened for, the causes of false-positive and false-negative results, the specificity of various laboratory techniques used in drug testing, and the legal issues surrounding drug testing. These legal issues include federal drug testing regulations, due process, and employee confidentiality. Only time and further research will define the role of drug testing in the workplace. It is clearly an area in which occupational medicine specialists need to be knowledgeable.

Employee Assistance Programs

Employee assistance programs (EAPs) are work-based programs designed to (1) help organizations resolve productivity problems and (2) identify employees with personal problems and refer them to appropriate resources to resolve their problems. These personal problems include relationship, family, psychological, stress, alcohol, drug, and financial, among others.

EAPs had their beginning in the 1940s in industries preparing for World War II. The pressure to mobilize industrial production during wartime led to the establishment of workplace alcohol intervention programs. These programs also were influenced by the development of Alcoholics Anonymous (AA). Originally run out of the company's medical department, they usually would involve medical evaluation and referral to AA. The introduction of mental health professionals in the EAP field led to the expansion of an EAP's focus to include personal and family crises, mental disorders, and substance abuse problems. Standards for certification of EAP professionals led to creation of the Certified Employee Assistance Professional (CEAP). More than 4500 professionals have attained EAP certification since 1993, including many licensed mental health professionals.

The EAP core technology defines the essential components of the employee assistance field. The seven components include

1. Consultation, training, and assistance to leaders to manage troubled employees
2. Confidential assessment of troubled employees
3. Use of confrontation and short-term interventions to deal with employees with job-performance problems
4. Referral of troubled employees for diagnosis, treatment, and follow-up
5. Help to organizations to establish and maintain relations with treatment personnel and facilities
6. Consultation with organizations to encourage access to adequate benefits to cover mental disorders and substance use disorders
7. Evaluation of the effectiveness of employee assistance services on organizations and individuals

Access to an EAP professional usually is a function of company size. One study found that 87% of employees of large companies had access to EAP professionals, but only 4% of employees of small companies had the same access.

Companies provide EAPs as an employee benefit. There is no out-of-pocket expense to use the EAP; therefore, they are very attractive to employees. Most employees who use an EAP refer themselves to the EAP program. The EAP professional will complete a confidential assessment and then may provide brief counseling or refer the individual to an appropriate treatment resource. A supervisor who is dealing with a troubled employee may initiate contact with the EAP. When an employee is having performance problems and has not attempted to get professional help, a supervisor, working closely with an EAP professional, may make a formal referral to the EAP. Supervisors will talk to an employee about his or her job-performance problem and warn him or her that disciplinary action will be taken if the job performance does not improve. The supervisor both recommends that the employee contact the EAP and continues to apply progressive discipline to the employee. The goal is to motivate the employee to seek assistance with the EAP, resolve the problem, and return to acceptable job performance. Unresolved personal problems, including drug and alcohol problems, usually will lead to continued poor job performance and often to termination.

The keys to a successful EAP are (1) a clear mandate for EAP services from management, (2) a nonpunitive policy on employees seeking the services of an EAP professional, and (3) support of all the constituencies within the company, including management, union officials, supervisors, and employees. EAP professionals are a major resource for the occupational medicine physician. The EAP professional can help the company retain employees who otherwise would be lost as a consequence of substance abuse disorders. In addition, they can train and supervise employees in the recognition of substance abuse–related performance

impairment, relieving line staff of these training responsibilities. They also help with appropriate referrals for impaired employees. By functioning as a monitor of workplace impairment and injury, the EAP professional can contribute to lower medical costs by making appropriate referrals to treatment programs and monitoring services that facilitate employee reentry into the workplace. One study revealed that 40% of employers see EAPs as a health care cost-control tool and 30% believe that they are helpful in reducing litigation. The data on the effectiveness of EAPs generally has been good. Most studies confirm a trend toward decreased absenteeism and improved work performance.

Psychiatric Fitness-for-Duty Exam

When an employee's behavior becomes disruptive, dangerous, or threatening, a psychiatrist may be asked to perform a fitness-for-duty exam to determine if the employee is able to perform his or her essential job functions in an effective and safe manner. This may arise with an employee who is known to have or suspected of having a substance abuse problem because alcohol and other drug abuse often cause severe symptoms, including suicidal and homicidal thoughts, agitation, paranoia, hallucinations, and severe cognitive impairment. Employees with any of these symptoms probably are not able to perform their job functions; may be at risk of causing an accident or injury to themselves, a coworker, or the public; and may be at risk of suicide or homicide. When an employee is felt to have such an impairment, the company should put the employee on administrative or medical leave and directly request or ask either the EAP professional or the occupational physician to determine if a psychiatric fitness-for duty-exam is necessary. Removing an impaired employee from the workplace is clearly in a company's best interest. Such an employee generally is not allowed back to work until he or she has been seen for the fitness exam by a psychiatrist, completed appropriate treatment, and been reevaluated by a psychiatrist to ensure that he or she can perform his or her normal job functions in a safe manner.

Treatment for Substance Abuse

An EAP professional or occupational physician often makes the diagnosis and referral for treatment for a substance abuse problem. They may, however, ask a psychiatrist to evaluate an employee that either has or is suspected to have a substance abuse disorder both to make the correct diagnosis and to ensure proper treatment. Acute psychiatric syndromes, including severe depression, anxiety, and psychotic disorders, are commonly induced by a substance abuse disorder, and comorbid psychiatric syndromes often are associated with but are not directly caused by substance abuse. Comorbid depressive and anxiety disorders are very common among substance abusers, as are personality disorders. Failure to recognize these psychiatric problems and treat them along with the substance use disorder can lead to treatment failure and a relapse of the substance abuse disorder.

The treatment of choice for most patients with a substance abuse disorder is an outpatient substance abuse treatment program followed by a longer course of aftercare. Those patients with medical complications or requiring detoxification first may need a brief hospitalization. Treatment programs involve education about substance abuse, problem-solving skills, stress and relationship management, and self-help programs such as AA and Narcotics Anonymous (NA). Substance abuse and dependence are chronic medical problems with a high risk of relapse; therefore, these patients require ongoing treatment that continues long after they complete an outpatient treatment program. Elements of treatment include involvement in self-help groups, including AA and NA; psychiatric treatment for psychiatric illnesses such as depression and anxiety disorders; and psychological treatment for family and personal problems. Some patients embrace self-help groups, but many are reluctant initially to become involved and to stay involved in them. Active involvement in 12-step programs, including working with a sponsor and continuing involvement in AA or NA, will greatly strengthen the chances for sustained recovery.

Return-to-Work Plan

Employers may choose to take an active role in making sure that there is a well-communicated return-to-work plan for an employee who has completed a substance abuse treatment program successfully. This might include use of a "last chance" agreement specifying that a condition of continued employment will be for the employee to sign an agreement specifying that the employee will be subject to random drug testing for a certain period of time. Often an EAP counselor, the supervisor, and the returning employee will have a meeting to talk about the employee's return to work. This is an opportunity to discuss the expectations of the employer and to talk about any special needs the employee has, including needing time off for medical appointments. Having a meeting of this nature a day or two before the employee resumes work also serves as an ice breaker to decrease the stress that naturally exists on the part of both the employer and the employee.

REFERENCES

Becker DR et al: Supported employment for people with co-occurring disorders. Psychiatr Rehabil J 2005;28:332 [PMID: 15895916].

Bennett JB et al: Team awareness, problem drinking, and drinking climate: Workplace social health promotion in a policy context. Am J Health Promot 2004;19:103 [PMID: 1555971].

Bogenschutz MP et al: The role of twelve-step approaches in dual diagnosis treatment and recovery. Am J Addict 2006;15:50 [PMID: 16449093].

Chan KK et al: Treating addictive behaviors in the employee assistance program: Implications for brief interventions. Addict Behav 2004;29:1883 [PMID: 15530733].

Department of Labor resource information on substance abuse statistics, sample policies, drug-free workplace programs, and relevant federal laws, www.dol.gov/asp.

Information on drug use in America, drug testing, and drug-free workplace programs, www.samhsa.gov.

Wickizer TM et al: Do drug-free workplace programs prevent occupational injuries? Health Serv Res 2004;39:91 [PMID: 14965079].

www.ensuringsolutions.org (a nonprofit organization offering resources for the workplace to curb costs associated with alcohol abuse).

Ziedonis DM et al: Improving the care of individuals with schizophrenia and substance use disorders. J Psychiatr Pract 2005;11:315 [PMID: 16184072].

Occupational Safety

34

Franklyn G. Prieskop, MS, MA, CSP

Occupational safety is the professional specialization that is concerned with the prevention and control of work-related accidents, injuries, illnesses, and other similarly caused harmful events. These events also may result in property damage, business interruption, and environmental incidents that threaten public health and safety, as well as product-related injuries and illnesses.

Safety professionals are trained to recognize that all occupational "accidents" and harmful incidents (other than those that result from unpredictable acts of nature) can be anticipated from and attributed to substandard work conditions, substandard job practices, or both. These substandard work conditions and job practices are called *hazards* and are considered the last link in a chain of accident causation.

The safety professional is concerned primarily with empowering managers, supervisors, and employees with information to identify and control occupational hazards and their enabling factors. A hazard is the proximate cause of an injury or illness. Enabling factors are the underlying deficiencies within the organization's operations that produce or permit the existence of exposure to a hazard.

The occupational health physician—whether employed directly by a company, retained on a consulting basis, or working in an occupational medicine clinic serving the industrial community—will be called on to work with safety professionals. In very large organizations, the physician and the safety professional may be part of a loss-control team or even may work in the same department. In smaller organizations, the internal safety professional often will be the point of contact for the outside occupational physician.

The physician's interactions with the safety professional will occur in the following spheres, among others:

- Cooperating in the establishment of emergency medical facilities or services
- Performing individual medical monitoring of employees potentially exposed to occupational health hazards
- Designing and implementing medical screening programs for potential employees
- Participating in employee training programs on health hazards, chemical safety, and the use of personal protective equipment
- Evaluating the effectiveness of personal protective equipment

- Serving on management oversight committees reviewing the safety program's effectiveness
- Assisting in accident investigations or reviews
- Providing medical expertise in the areas of ergonomics and the appropriate design of workstations
- Providing consultant services to management to interpret the medical aspects of safety analyses or outside regulatory standards

Whatever the level of contact between the occupational health physician and the safety professional, it will be useful for the physician to understand the safety professional's background, role, and concerns.

PROFESSIONAL EVOLUTION

Professional safety practice evolved in industrialized countries from the passage of workers' compensation laws in the early decades of the twentieth century and the enactment of employee protection laws and regulations in the decades following World War II. The workers' compensation laws require employers to compensate injured workers for a portion of their lost wages and medical expenses regardless of fault. The certainty of having to indemnify injured employees led employers to place greater emphasis on accident prevention. Prevention measures mostly consisted of work-site safety inspections, employee hazard awareness training, and the installation of guards around hazardous machinery. Gradually, the responsibilities and duties of the "safety engineer" and "safety inspector" became job classifications within many organizations.

The employee protection laws and regulations that have been passed in every industrialized country since World War II have greatly accelerated the growth of the safety profession and expanded its range of activities. In the United States, the Occupational Safety and Health Act of 1970 (OSH Act) created the Occupational Safety and Health Administration (OSHA), an administrative agency within the Department of Labor, and made it responsible for the promulgation and enforcement of safety standards applicable to employers. An increasing number of OSHA standards have recognized certified safety professionals, as well as certified industrial hygienists and physicians, as "qualified" and "competent" to evaluate and control regulated hazards.

PROFESSIONAL QUALIFICATIONS

The modern safety professional usually has a Bachelor of Arts degree but is no longer necessarily an engineer (fewer than 40% have engineering degrees). More valuable today than engineering expertise are degrees in management, business administration, or systems analysis. Several universities offer baccalaureate, masters, and even doctoral degrees specifically in occupational safety and health or safety management, with a few state and community colleges now offering associate degrees or technical certification in the field.

The highest professional designation in the safety profession in the United States is that of certified safety professional (CSP). This certification is awarded by an independent Board of Certified Safety Professionals. The certifications are granted to practitioners who have passed both core subject and comprehensive practice examinations. To be eligible to take the examinations, safety practitioners must submit two professional references and have 96 units of education and/or professional experience. Originally, 1 month's work experience was equal to 1 unit, and 48 units were allotted for a college degree.

Beginning in 1998, CSP candidates were required to have an associate or baccalaureate degree in safety from an accredited college or university to be eligible to take the examination, regardless of their number of years of professional experience. Currently at least two states, California and Massachusetts, license professional safety engineers. Candidates for the professional engineer (PE) in safety registration must have a bachelor's degree in engineering from an accredited engineering program and 5 years of professional experience and must have passed the engineering fundamentals examination and a professional safety practice examination. Many safety practitioners who received their safety PE registration in California, however, did not obtain their title by meeting these qualifications but rather were granted registration based on professional experience supported by professional engineering and safety references. Most safety PEs do not practice solely in the field of safety engineering.

There are any numbers of other safety certifications awarded by a wide assortment of professional and academic organizations, but the CSP and state-registered PE designation remain the most credible credential for the safety professional.

FUNCTIONAL RESPONSIBILITIES OF SAFETY PRACTITIONERS

At present, there are more than 20,000 safety practitioners in the United States. Their functional responsibilities vary widely depending on the size and type of organization, the degree of inherent risks within the workplace, and the level of safety management expertise. In a small service organization, for example, the "safety person" is often a nonprofessional whose responsibilities are limited to ensuring that the organization complies with applicable OSHA regulations. In a medium-sized manufacturing company, the safety practitioner may be a trained professional with a wide range of safety and loss-control responsibilities. In large, complex organizations, a staff of certified professionals from among several different departments usually covers the full scope of safety and loss-control responsibilities. The staff may include safety professionals, industrial hygienists, occupational physicians and nurses, engineers, environmental specialists, risk managers, insurance personnel, security officers, and fire-protection professionals.

The responsibilities of safety professionals may be grouped into six broad functional categories: (1) safety engineering: the systematic analysis of equipment, tasks, and processes to identify inherent hazards and failure modes, as well as the development of hazard prevention and control measures based on their findings; (2) safety management: the application of management principles and methods to establish, facilitate, coordinate, and achieve safety goals and objectives; (3) loss control: the application of safety engineering and safety management methods for the prevention and mitigation of all types of loss-producing events; (4) safety inspection and auditing: observation and evaluation of work sites, job tasks, and policies and procedures to identify deficiencies or omissions that could contribute to an occupational injury or illness; (5) regulatory compliance: communication of applicable safety and health regulations to affected personnel and monitoring of response activities to ensure compliance with the regulatory requirements; and (6) education and training: the development, conducting, and/or coordinating of safety training for employees, supervisors, and managers.

Many safety practitioners specialize within one or two of the functional categories, and some even concentrate on a subspecialty within a category (e.g., traffic safety engineering, electrical safety inspection, or hazardous materials training); most, however, perform some duties that fall within each of the broad functions. Some functional specialists and generalists work their entire careers in the same industry and become industry safety specialists. These may include construction safety professionals, chemical safety engineers, and railroad safety inspectors.

SAFETY & HEALTH MANAGEMENT SYSTEM

A principal responsibility of a safety professional in any organization is to facilitate and coordinate the development and implementation of an effective safety and health management system. The elements of this system are the related policies, goals, plans, programs, procedures, and standards. Their collective purpose is to systematically guide the organization to (1) prevent

Table 34–1. Elements of a safety and health management system.

Administrative Elements	Hazard Control Elements
Safety and Health (S&H) Policy Statement	Code of Safe Practices[1]
Statement of S&H Responsibilities	Hazard Identification and Control Program
Procedure for Communicating S&H Information[1]	Job Safety Analysis Program
Process & Criteria for Setting S&H Performance Goals & Indicators	Hazardous Energy Control Procedure[1] (Lockout/Tagout)
S&H Program Audit, Feedback, and Correction Program	Hazardous Substance Control and Communication Program (Haz/Com)[1]
S&H Education and Training Procedure[1]	Confined Space Safety Program[1]
Procedure for Development of Annual S&H Plan and Budget	Trenching and Shoring Safety Program[1]
Procedure for Establishing and Operating S&H Committees	Vehicle Operation Safety Program
S&H Procedure and Standards for Engineering Designs	Laboratory Hygiene Program[1]
Contractor S&H Procedure	Ergonomic Hazard Control Program[2]
OSHA Compliance Procedure	Indoor Air Quality Program[2]
Program for Employee S&H Participation	Personal Protective Equipment Standards[1]
Medical Management Program[1]	Respiratory Protection Program[1]
S&H Performance Evaluation Criteria Accountability Process	Hearing Conservation Program[1]
	Housekeeping Standards
	Accident/Incident Investigation Procedure[1]

[1]OSHA required program, procedure, or activity.
[2]Pending OSHA requirement.

work-related injuries and illnesses, (2) comply with applicable health and safety regulations, and (3) minimize injury/illness and compliance costs.

Safety professionals seek to make the occupational safety and health management system a self-regulating process by incorporating performance monitoring, feedback, and correction capabilities. These capabilities can be established either as a separate administrative policy/procedure or as an administrative section in each of the organization's hazard-control programs and procedures.

The administrative policies and procedures of a safety and health management system are developed to ensure that the system functions properly and consistently. The hazard-control programs and procedures are intended to guide affected personnel in the recognition and control of specified hazards.

Some of the system's administrative and hazard-control elements may be required by government regulation. The safety professional usually is responsible for ensuring that the safety and health management system

includes these required elements. Table 34–1 lists the elements of an organization's safety and health management system.

ELEMENTS OF THE SAFETY SYSTEM[1]

Training

The safety professional is concerned primarily with the prevention of accidents. This can be accomplished to a large extent through proper training of employees. The primary cause of accidents in the workplace is not unsafe machinery or dangerous chemicals—it is the lack of understanding by employees about the nature or severity of the hazards surrounding them.

---

[1]The safety and health management system of an organization is the same as its safety and health program. The term *management system* was chosen over the word *program* because it is more descriptive and less apt to be confused with its subprogram elements.

A prudent employer will provide employees with adequate training to warn them of hazards peculiar to their jobs and instruct them in safe operating practices. The OSH Act requires that workers be warned about hazardous materials through the use of warning labels and similar devices and that workers also be made aware of the relevant symptoms of overexposure and of emergency treatment procedures. The most important feature of the law, however, is that which requires employers to make workers understand appropriate precautions.

Since the passage of the OSH Act, many other federal and state hazard communication standards have been promulgated. These require the employer to train workers to understand the labeling of hazardous materials and to use the material safety data sheets (MSDSs) that must be maintained for all chemicals and other hazardous substances to which the worker may be exposed. Various OSH Act standards also require specialized training for employees operating specific types of equipment (e.g., forklifts, cranes, powered punch presses, etc.). These laws require that numerous training programs be established for workers in various job categories or working conditions.

Communication

Safety committees draw together individuals from throughout the workforce so that they can pool their experience and efforts to achieve greater safety. Several types of safety committees may be formed to fulfill various needs within the organization. The company physician may be asked to serve on an executive committee functioning as an oversight committee for the safety department or on a general planning committee. Other safety committees might include supervisory committees, joint union-management committees, and shop workers' committees.

Safety suggestion boxes are a form of communication. To make them effective, however, management—often through its delegated representative, the safety professional—must demonstrate that it listens to all serious suggestions and responds in a timely and serious manner.

Safety posters, placards, and signs are also forms of communication. They are effective only insofar as they are kept relevant to the hazards and, in the case of posters, if they are changed frequently to stimulate safety awareness.

Emergency-Response Programs

The safety professional must recognize the need to prepare for a disaster or emergency situation.

A. Evacuation Planning

Federal, state, and local authorities now require that businesses establish emergency evacuation plans. Items to consider in an evacuation plan include the following:

1. What events might precipitate an evacuation?
2. What other notifications are necessary—medical, fire department, police, others?
3. What medical facilities are likely to be needed?
4. Will electrical and gas services also be shut down?
5. Are there manufacturing processes that should be shut down in emergencies?
6. Who can authorize evacuation?
7. How will the employees be instructed to evacuate?
8. Who will be responsible to see that evacuation is carried out?
9. Where should evacuated employees go?
10. How will it be determined that all employees, contractor personnel, and visitors have been evacuated?
11. Who will do the shutdowns? How? Are they appropriately trained?

B. Chemical Response Teams

Plants that use large quantities of toxic or dangerous chemicals often will form specialized teams of employees to contain or control exposures to the employees, the general public, or the environment resulting from accidental discharge. The occupational physician often will be asked to help in the planning and training stages when these teams are formed.

C. Fire Brigades

Industries or operations located at remote sites or with special fire hazards often require the formation of firefighting teams. These trained employees are responsible for ensuring swift reaction to the outbreak of fire and for containing the fire until professional help arrives.

D. Emergency Medical Facilities

State regulations now require almost all places of employment to provide a minimum level of emergency medical capability. Depending on the exposures involved, the safety professional, in concert with the occupational physician, might wish to improve on this minimum requirement significantly.

For an office building with no special hazards, the Red Cross multimedia training certifications for two or three employees, perhaps with cardiopulmonary resuscitation (CPR) training added, very well might be sufficient. However, a hazardous chemical processing plant would require at least several emergency medical technician (EMT) level 1 trained personnel and perhaps even an occupational health nurse or an on-site occupational physician for each shift.

Personal Protective Equipment

One method of providing for employee safety in hazardous conditions is the use of personal protective equipment. These devices are intended to protect employees in case an accident occurs or to insulate the employee from a hazardous condition (e.g., noise, dusts, fumes, etc.) that is part of the normal operation.

The basic problem with personal protective devices is that the individual must understand the need to wear the protection, must wear it properly, and must maintain the device in good working condition. In situations where engineering or administrative controls are not yet effective in eliminating the hazard, protective devices must be issued as a last line of defense to prevent injury to the employee. The occupational health physician may be called on by the safety professional to consult about the appropriateness of the device chosen or to assist in educating employees about the necessity for the device.

Any program that provides personal protective equipment to employees must follow the same basic procedures. First, the hazards must be evaluated to ensure that the equipment will be appropriate. Second, the equipment itself must be checked to see that it meets all applicable government standards of manufacture. Employees must be informed of the hazards involved and be trained in how to wear protective equipment and maintain it properly. Supervisors must be trained to ensure that the protection is worn at all times when it is needed. Warnings must be posted to inform everyone of the need for protection.

Inspections & Monitoring

The safety professional, especially in the industrial environment, is responsible for numerous inspections and periodic monitoring. The principal monitoring technique is measurement of airborne chemical contamination levels and physical exposure levels to noise, vibration, and ionizing and nonionizing radiation. While an industrial hygienist usually performs monitoring, the safety professional often is required to perform some routine monitoring. Individual medical monitoring also is required under certain conditions. Again, while monitoring and testing usually are done under the direction of the occupational health physician, the safety professional often is charged with the administrative and record-keeping details of the program.

Physical inspections are the direct responsibility of the safety professional. Federal and state regulations now require periodic inspections of the work environment designed to recognize hazard potentials. Often this type of inspection actually is performed as part of the safety committee's duties so that various points of view are brought to bear in the attempt to identify accident potentials. However, even when this is the case, the safety professional must review the results and recommendations. Various pieces of equipment also require periodic inspection to ensure that they are in place, fully functional, certified, and suitable for the intended purposes.

Chemical Safety

Specific hazards to employees must be recognized and detailed for each chemical or process. Where feasible, engineering controls such as containment, automated processing, or ventilation systems should be installed. Administrative controls such as job rotation or multistationed work processes may be used to control exposures in some circumstances. Where applicable, personal protective equipment must be issued. Periodic monitoring of environmental chemical exposures should be established. Chemical safety training specific to the processes involved must be given to all employees. With certain chemicals, employee health monitoring may be required. Safe chemical handling rules and process instructions must be initiated. Emergency containment or evacuation systems must be initiated. Emergency shutdown and protection equipment must be installed and employees trained in their use. Finally, all the preceding procedures and equipment must be reviewed periodically to ensure proper functioning of control measures and to see that controls are adequate. MSDSs must be obtained and reviewed on all chemicals used in the work setting.

OTHER SAFETY PROGRAM ELEMENTS

Fire Protection

Safety professionals usually are required to take charge of fire-protection activities of the organization as well as employee safety functions. In fact, only organizations with extraordinary casualty exposure will employ a fire-protection engineer.

The primary duty is, of course, to prevent fires. The fire safety program follows much the same pattern as has been outlined for the employee safety program, which was designed to keep injuries from occurring: (1) training, (2) communications, (3) emergency protective equipment, (4) chemical safety, and (5) accident investigation.

The safety professional should be involved in the construction and remodeling of facilities, as well as occupancy plans, in order to create a relatively fire-protected office or plant environment. Once the facility has been constructed, fire-prevention activities usually are limited to monitoring of hazardous areas, fire emergency planning, training, and monitoring of the adequacy of fire-suppression equipment.

Vehicle Fleet Safety

Management usually does not realize the severity of its losses to vehicular accidents unless the company happens to operate an unusually large number of vehicles or is in the transportation industry. The safety professional should gain control of this area of responsibility because it frequently represents one of the major sources of injury within an organization.

The safety professional would begin with documentation to obtain clear-cut authority for a control program through the company's safety policy and directives. Employee or applicant screening probably is the major loss-control option available to the employer. This is one of the few areas where there is sufficient legal precedent to allow medical and driver-history screening of drivers. Therefore, the safety professional will rely on the occupational health physician to devise an adequate and responsible medical screening program to meet the employer's needs.

The second element of the fleet vehicle safety program must be a preventive-maintenance program on all vehicles. This program must be documented meticulously in order to be of any value in dealing with insurers or the government agencies that monitor them. The remaining fleet vehicle safety program elements again are training, communications, emergency planning, accident investigation, and inspections or monitoring.

Product Safety & Product Liability

Manufacturers—especially those whose products end up in the hands of the private consumer or in high-technology systems (e.g., nuclear reactors, commercial aircraft, or aerospace modules)—are vitally concerned with the safety of their products. It is not uncommon for the organization's safety professional to become involved in product safety or product liability reviews.

A product safety review must consider first the intended uses and foreseeable misuses of the product. The aim of the review is to provide the most painstaking analysis—often using the techniques known as *systems safety analysis* (see below)—to ensure the product's correct and safe functioning under the most adverse foreseeable use.

The product liability review is performed to determine how to assess or limit (to the extent possible) the legal liability of any unsafe operation of the product that might occur. From this review, the manufacturer—or its product liability insurance carrier—can determine the probable extent to which the manufacturer may be held liable in litigation for product operations or failures that cause personal injury or property damage.

MANAGEMENT APPROACHES TO ACCIDENT PREVENTION

Systems Safety

Systems safety analysis is not a single technique or process but rather a group of analytic techniques wherein operations (such as manufacturing a printed circuit board) or machines (such as punch presses) are viewed as if they were a single system. That system, in turn, should have each of its discrete parts, steps, or functions analyzed for potential hazards. All of this must be limited by practical considerations of operational effectiveness, time availability, and cost-effectiveness.

The traditional approach to safety is called the *fly-fix-fly method*, wherein an operation is initiated or a machine is designed and put into use. Then, if the operation or machine breaks down, causes an accident, or generally does not perform as expected, it is redesigned, reengineered, or otherwise changed. The operation or machine then is put back into use again until another problem is found with it. However, there are certain systems for which we cannot afford the first accident, such as the core meltdown of a nuclear reactor, an accidental nuclear weapons explosion, the crash of a commercial airliner, the loss of a manned space shuttle, or the release of a toxic gas cloud in an urban area.

This is not to say that these catastrophes cannot happen but rather that the manufacturers and operators involved must approach these potentials as if they cannot be allowed to happen. To guard against such potential safety calamities, the following safety approaches may be used.

A. FAILURE MODES AND EFFECTS ANALYSIS

One of the earliest "systems safety" approaches was developed by reliability engineers to identify problems that could arise from machinery malfunctions. The technique analyzes each of the components, subassemblies, and subsystems to find out how each might fail and what effect its failure would have on the system as a whole.

B. FAULT HAZARD ANALYSIS

This refinement of the foregoing considers only those failure modes that could cause an accident, ignoring all other failures or failure modes. This allows analysis of larger systems while not requiring the reviewer to be bogged down in extraneous detail. Criticality ratings are used to see which components or subsystems need design changes, tighter production controls, more comprehensive testing, specialized safeguards, monitoring, shielding, and the like.

C. FAULT-TREE ANALYSIS

Unlike the first two techniques, which consider all possible individual failures in order to find out what they would do to the system as a whole, fault-tree analysis takes a single undesirable event (such as leakage of a toxic gas from a process) and works backward, trying to establish what could cause leakage to occur. Quantitative values are assigned to individual failure points to show the likelihood that failure will occur. The use of flowcharting clearly demonstrates the relationships between the various components and thus encourages the analyst to consider cumulative failure possibilities (i.e., two or more simultaneous component failures that cause the event).

D. HUMAN FACTORS ANALYSIS

This technique was developed to fit the human operator into the system with maximum safety. Most machinery is designed for the convenience of the workflow or operation, and the operator is required to adapt to the machine's requirements. Because the human being is the most adaptable component in the system, it is relatively easy to make the system fit the "average" physical form. This leads designers and engineers to ignore the human element. Recognition that the "average" human physique and operating limits did not meet all the needs of industry gave emphasis to this discipline.

The most common need is for adjustability of workstations to fit the operator. The occupational health physician can be useful in this systems safety technique by providing consultation and physical data on body mobility, environmental stresses, repetitive-motion effects, and sensory inputs.

More challenging still is the fitting of the operator's psychological and cultural differences into the work environment. The fact that blue instead of red may be the color associated with "stop" or "emergency" in some cultures has cost the lives of workers.

Employee Operations & Management Reviews

Systems safety analysis was concerned initially only with equipment failures because it grew out of the quality-control discipline. Later, it was realized that the operator is more than just a physical element in the system. The human decisions and actions were in fact a major risk factor and therefore had to be considered as part of the system. Finally, systems safety practitioners began applying the techniques of this discipline to human organizations.

A. JOB SAFETY ANALYSIS

This technique was developed during World War II when large numbers of inexperienced workers had to be integrated into the workforce quickly and safely. By systematic observation and detailed analysis, one uncovers the inherent hazards in the work environment. This task can be performed by supervisors, who, in turn, gain great understanding and appreciation of the areas under their control. The employees who participate develop a better recognition of the hazards they face. Finally, use of this technique develops an effective teaching tool and documentation on which personnel

departments effectively may base their physical hiring requirements for certain jobs.

B. TECHNIQUES FOR HUMAN ERROR RATE PREDICTION

These techniques are primarily methods for quantifying what has been called *pilot error* in the broad sense of that term to determine probabilities of occurrence. Because they are directed solely toward human errors, they are often used in conjunction with fault-tree analysis or failure modes and effects analysis.

In this approach, all human tasks are broken down into the smallest possible discrete actions. Each component task is referenced to a set of tables reflecting basic human tasks, with the probability of functioning correctly considered for each of nine potential error states. A *basic error rate* can be obtained, expressed as errors per million operations. These values have been obtained through detailed clinical research.

C. MANAGEMENT OVERSIGHT RISK TREE

This technique was developed to combine the systems safety analysis techniques with modern management techniques. The result was a large analytic diagram or flowchart. It portrays the operation of a safety management program in a logical and orderly manner, with the actual safety program compared with an idealized system. The evaluator thus can detect omissions, oversights, and ineffective programs. The defects might be as diverse as poor training or employee misconduct, and the effective diagnosis of these problems provides the evaluator with a tool for loss control.

D. TECHNIQUE OF OPERATION REVIEW

This is a system for analyzing the root causes of accidents or other undesired events. The examiner starts with an undesired event and cross-references it on a chart with a large number of organizational processes (e.g., training, supervision, management, etc.). The technique provides a simplistic but systematic method of examining potential causes within an organization in relation to any specific failure event.

Root-Cause Identification & Control

Permanent control of unsafe work conditions and unsafe job practices requires elimination of their underlying support system. Correcting hazards without eliminating their *root causes* treats only the symptoms of the problem; the hazards eventually will reappear.

Safety professionals identify the enabling or root causal factors of hazards by systematically analyzing the events, conditions, and values that logic, experience, and training lead them to believe could have contributed to the existence of the hazard. The findings then are evaluated to determine where, how, and why the organization's safety and health management system failed to prevent or control the enabling factors. Permanent control of these factors is achieved by correcting identified inconsistencies, contradictions, and omissions in the organization's safety and health or operating policies, programs, and procedures.

Accident & Incident Investigation

Accidents are defined as unintended events that result in injury, illness, and/or material loss. Unintended events that have the potential to cause human and/or material harm but which do not only because of chance are called *incidents*. Many safety professionals prefer to use the term *incident* to describe both types of events because there is a general misconception that accidents are "freak," random occurrences that cannot be anticipated. This view can retard an organization's prevention efforts and lead to the recurrence of loss-producing events. Safety professionals regard accidents/incidents as preventable events that indicate correctable deficiencies in the organization's safety and loss-control system.

An injury or illness incident occurs when a harmful amount of energy or toxicity is transferred via an unsafe work condition or unsafe job practice to an exposed employee. This transference may occur acutely, as in the case of unprotected contact with a rotating saw blade or with a corrosive chemical, or chronically, from such hazardous exposures as frequent repetitive body motions and long-term inhalation of small amounts of toxic vapors.

Safety professionals conduct and/or coordinate accident/incident investigations to uncover their proximate and enabling causal factors so that measures can be identified and implemented to prevent a recurrence. The investigation process involves the systematic collection, analysis, documentation, and communication of relevant information.

Accidents almost never have just one cause but are the result of chains of events and circumstances. Finding the causes of an accident calls for more than simply reviewing the injured employee's actions at the scene; the physical conditions and all equipment must be scrutinized to determine what could be done to prevent recurrences. Such items as workflow patterns, environmental conditions, and stress levels also must be considered. A primary purpose of accident investigation is to initiate changes or measures to prevent repetitions.

In most routine accidents, it is helpful if the supervisor or manager conducts the accident investigation in order to learn from the experience, although the safety professional will have to instruct the supervisors or managers in how to proceed and should review the results. Safety professionals often develop a written procedure to systematically guide the investigative process.

The procedure typically identifies the types of accidents and incidents that are to be investigated and who is to conduct the investigation, when the investigation is to be commenced and ended, where it is to take place, how it is to be conducted, who is to communicate the findings, and the form in which communications will be made. The accident/incident investigation procedure is an important element of any organization's safety and health management system.

Safety Performance Goals & Indicators

An important function of safety professionals is to help their organizations develop and administer safety performance goals and indicators. There are two types of goals and indicators: results directed and behavior directed. Results-directed safety goals and indicators focus on the consequences of desired safety behaviors, whereas behavior-directed safety goals and indicators are concerned with the safety behaviors themselves.

The total injury and illness case rate is the principal results-directed safety performance indicator of most organizations. It can be compared against last year's rate and the industry average to help determine whether current safety performance is acceptable. An annual goal to reduce this rate below the industry average or below last year's total case rate would be an example of a results-directed goal.

The frequency and quality of employee safety meetings are examples of a behavior-directed performance indicator. The greater the frequency and the better the quality of employee safety meeting, the less likely are job errors and unsafe work practices. A behavior-directed goal would be to have qualified trainers hold structured safety meetings every month.

Safety professionals regularly monitor and analyze the safety performance indicators to help identify any significant behavioral or loss trends. This information helps management to track the organization's progress toward achievement of its stated performance goals and to implement timely corrections of indicated deficiencies in the safety and loss-control system. Table 34–2 lists key results-directed and behavior-directed performance indicators.

OSHA COMPLIANCE

Overseeing the organization's efforts to comply with OSHA regulations is a major responsibility for all safety practitioners. This responsibility is fulfilled by analyzing and interpreting the regulations to determine their applicability to the organization and then communicating the requirements to the affected personnel. Safety practitioners also develop written programs and procedures that are required by the regulations and conduct or arrange mandated training for employees.

Table 34–2. Key results-directed and behavior-directed indicators.

Results-Directed Indicators	Behavior-Directed Indicators
Total Case Rate: number of injuries and illnesses × 200,000 hours[1] ÷ number of hours worked	Frequency and quality of workplace safety and loss-control inspections
Lost Time Case Rate: number of lost time cases × 200,000 hours ÷ number of hours worked	Frequency and quality of job safety observations
Lost & Restricted Case Rate: number of lost time and restricted work cases x 200,000 hours ÷ number of hours worked	Frequency and quality of employee safety training
Lost & Restricted Day Rate: number of days lost and restricted × 200,000 hours ÷ number of hours worked	Frequency and quality of safety program audits
Total Workers Compensation Reserves: the amount of money reserved by the insurance company to pay for current year's injuries/illnesses	Frequency and quality of employee safety meetings
Experience Modification Factor: the multiplier based on injury/illness experience used by insurance companies to determine workers' compensation premiums. An "ex-mod" factor greater than 1 is high	Frequency and quality of safety communications to employees
Property Damage and Business Interruption Costs: the direct and indirect costs resulting from accidents involving property damage and/or business interruption	Frequency and quality of safety performance appraisals
Vehicle Accident Incidence Rate: the number of vehicle accidents × 25,000, 100,000, or 1,000,000 miles ÷ number of miles driven in a year	Frequency and quality of employee safety suggestions
Total Vehicle Accident Costs: the direct and indirect costs to pay for accident and to restore vehicles	Timeliness of required responses to employee safety suggestions
Annual Number of OSHA Citations: the total number of citations received in a year	Timeliness and quality of accident/incident investigations
Cost of OSHA Penalties: annual cost of penalties for OSHA citations	Frequency of personal protection equipment inspections and observations
Number and Cost of Product Liability Claims: the annual number and cost of customer injury/illness claims from product defects	Quality and frequency of safety committee meetings
Number and Cost of Environmental Accidents/Incidents: the annual number and cost of mishaps that impair the environment, injure members of the public, or both	Frequency and quality of employee involvement in program development and implementation activities

[1]200,000 hours is the number of hours 100 employees work in 1 year.

If industrial hygiene or medical specialists are employed with the organization, they usually have the lead responsibility for analyzing and interpreting complex health-related regulations. If these specialists are not available in the organization, the safety professional often will consult with an external industrial hygienist or occupational physician.

There are many safety and health regulations that pertain directly to occupational physicians. In the United States, OSHA specifically references medical practitioners in regulations covering such subjects as blood-borne pathogens; physical examinations for asbestos, lead, cadmium, arsenic, and other specified toxic substances; biologic monitoring; audiometric and hearing examinations; respiratory protection; pulmonary function testing; laboratory hygiene; regulated carcinogens; sanitation; and hazard communications.

The occupational physician who is well informed about OSHA regulations will be better prepared to provide the diagnostic and treatment methods required by government regulations. The physician also will be able to work with other safety and health professionals to identify deficiencies in the organization's regulatory compliance efforts that could adversely affect employee health and safety.

LOSS-CONTROL MANAGEMENT

Safety practitioners, like other occupational and safety and health professionals, have the well-being of employees as their primary concern, but unlike the other specialists (at least until recently); some safety professionals have the closely related secondary responsibility of loss-control management. Loss-control management involves planning, organizing, and leading the organization's efforts to prevent all types of loss-producing events and to control the monetary cost when such an event occurs. A loss-producing event is an incident in which either the value of an organizational asset declines or the cost of preserving it increases.

Losses are measured in monetary terms. Accidents and harmful exposures that cause employee injury or illness, property damage, business disruption, environmental impairment, lost worker productivity, adverse public relations, and labor strife are all loss-producing events; they directly or indirectly cost the organization money.

Employees are the most valuable assets of an organization, so the loss-control responsibilities of safety practitioners are consistent with and supportive of their injury- and illness-prevention interests. Nevertheless, there is a potential for conflict whenever cost considerations may compete with health and safety concerns. This potential for conflict is based on the same kinds of issues that characterize the debate over managed health care: Physicians wish to deliver the best care to their patients without interference and monetary restrictions from the care payers (health insurance companies), whereas the care payers wish to keep the cost of medical care as low as possible.

In the United States, employers pay for the cost of injury care and workers' compensation through their insurance premiums. They expect, therefore, loss-control managers and health care providers to protect employee health and safety cost-effectively. To achieve this objective, both prevention and case-management efforts are required, with the prevention efforts being the most cost-effective.

CASE MANAGEMENT

Employers want their loss-control representative and the treating physician to ensure that injured employees receive the proper medical care necessary to return them to full health in the shortest period of time for the least amount of money. The following are ways in which safety professionals and occupational physicians can and should collaborate for better case management.

Safety professionals can provide relevant work-history and exposure information to treating physicians as soon as possible after an employee injury and illness is reported. If the safety practitioner fails to provide such information in a timely manner, the physician or an assistant should contact the safety practitioner for input prior to completion of the diagnosis.

Nothing can sour the relationship between an employer and a health care provider more quickly than a controversial medical diagnosis that is (or is perceived to be) based on inaccurate or biased information. Physicians can prevent both the reality and perception of an inaccurate or biased diagnosis by obtaining prior input relative to the injured employee's work history and exposure. Information obtained by the occupational physician through annual facility visits and discussions with managers will help to preclude misdiagnoses and misperceptions and can obviate the need for case input from safety professionals except in unusual cases.

Safety professionals should provide and medical care providers should seek information on the organization's modified-duty program and available modified-duty jobs in advance of determination of a treatment protocol for an injured or ill employee. Insurance data indicate that employees with nondisabling injuries who are placed in a job they are able to perform recover sooner than they would have if they were given time off from work. A lack of a monetary incentive to return to work, insufficient physical and mental exercise, and/or the performance of stressful home chores probably account for the slower home healing rates. Safety professionals and occupational physicians can work together on presentations and programs to educate employers about the health and cost benefits of providing modified-duty jobs.

TOTAL SAFETY MANAGEMENT SYSTEM

The total quality management (TQM) movement was launched by Edward Deming and Joseph Juran in Japan in the 1950s and since has spread to every advanced country in the world. TQM principles and methods now form the foundation of modern management theory and practice, providing for continuous organizational improvement through dedicated leadership, a commitment to customer satisfaction, employee empowerment, team management, systems analysis, application of statistical quality controls, extensive training and retraining, and the balancing of cost concerns with quality considerations.

Some safety and health managers have long advocated similar views for improving the quality of safety performance in their organizations, and many more have adopted the TQM approach in recent years. Their goal is to establish a management system that provides for constant improvement in the quality of all the organization's safety and loss-control efforts and for continual reduction in the number, frequency, and severity of harmful events.

The safety quality movement has evolved to the point that a technical committee of the International Standards Organization (ISO) was formed to develop safety and health assessment criteria. Many safety and health professionals wish to have ISO occupational safety and health standards similar to the ones established under ISO 9000 for quality assurance and under the ISO 14000 draft for environmental management. The ultimate goal is to have universally applicable guidance and assessment documents for quality assurance of the design and performance of an organization's occupational safety and health management system.

REFERENCES

American Society of Safety Engineers: www.asse.org/.

Board of Certified Safety Professionals: www.bcsp.org/.

Geldart S et al: Have companies improved their health and safety approaches over the last decade? A longitudinal study. Am J Ind Med 2005;47:227 [PMID: 15712256].

Hoonakker P et al: The effect of safety initiatives on safety performance: A longitudinal study. Appl Ergon 2005;36:461 [PMID: 15892940].

Milczarek M, Najmiec A: The relationship between workers' safety culture and accidents, near accidents and health problem. Int J Occup Saf Ergon 2004;10:25 [PMID: 1502819].

Palassis J et al: Enhancing occupational safety and health through use of the national skill standards. Int J Occup Environ Health 2004;10:90 [PMID: 15070031].

Rikardsson PM, Impgaard M: Corporate cost of occupational accidents: An activity based analysis. Accid Anal Prev 2004;36:173 [PMID: 14642872].

US Department of Labor, Occupational Safety and Health Administration: www.osha.gov/.

Zacharatos A et al: High-performance work systems and occupational safety. J Appl Psychol 2005;90:77 [PMID: 15641891].

Industrial (Occupational) Hygiene

35

Douglas P. Fowler, PhD, CIH

The four definitive elements of industrial hygiene (often called *occupational hygiene* outside the United States) are the anticipation, recognition, evaluation, and control of health hazards arising in or from the workplace. (Hazards arising from the workplace include the potential harm that may arise in the community by poorly controlled emissions and such issues as familial exposures from harmful debris taken home on workers' clothing.) The anticipation and recognition of health hazards have primacy because they must take place before proper evaluation or control (if needed) can take place. On anticipation or recognition of a health hazard, the industrial hygienist should be able to identify measures necessary for proper evaluation. On completion of the evaluation, the industrial hygienist then is in a position (in consultation with other members of the occupational health and safety team) to recommend and implement controls needed to reduce risks to within tolerable limits.

ANTICIPATION OF HEALTH HAZARDS IN THE WORKPLACE

The duty to anticipate health hazards in the workplace is a relatively new addition to the industrial hygienist's traditional responsibilities for recognition, evaluation, and control; it is a heavy but necessary burden. Anticipation of health hazards may range from a reasonable expectation to mere speculation, but it implies that the industrial hygienist will understand the nature of changes in the processes, products, environments, and workforces of the workplace and how those changes might affect human health or well-being. As an example, transplanting a successful chemical process from a unionized workplace in the United States or Canada to another country without understanding important cultural factors or the extent of the industrial experience in that country might cause significant risk of harm to the workers in that new country. As another example, changing weekly work schedules from five 8-hour days to three 12-hour days almost certainly will produce dislocation among the workforce because of the psychosocial and physical effects of shift work but also may lead to the danger of chemical intoxication if the chemical exposures are such as to lead to the buildup of excessive body burdens without the usual 16-hour "rest" period.

An important aspect of anticipation will be an understanding of past exposures and practices and how that past experience may act to cause injury to those exposed. Such retrospective exposure assessment is, of course, essential to the performance of epidemiologic studies in order to come to a sound understanding of risks associated with occupational experience. The industrial hygienist is the person most likely to be able to perform such a retrospective study.

RECOGNITION OF HEALTH HAZARDS IN THE WORKPLACE

In a workplace where the processes are well established, the recognition of health hazards is the first step in the process that leads to evaluation and control through the identification of materials and processes that have the potential for causing harm to workers. Sources of information about health hazards include clinical data about health problems in exposed populations; information in scientific journals, bulletins of trade associations, and reports of government agencies; conversations with peers; and direct reports from workers, union representatives, supervisors, or employers.

Inspection of the workplace is the best source of directly relevant information about potential health hazards. There is no substitute for observation by an experienced observer of work practices, the use of chemical and physical agents, and the apparent effectiveness of control measures. The physician should be able to recognize major and obvious health hazards and distinguish those that require formal evaluation by the industrial hygienist.

The Walk-Through Survey

The *walk-through survey,* in the company of the occupational physician, is the first and most important technique used to recognize occupational health hazards. The survey should begin with a proper introduction to plant management, a discussion of the purpose of the survey, and an inquiry about any relevant recent complaints. If appropriate, a simplified process flow diagram also should be prepared at this time.

Following the process flow through the plant usually is most productive. The survey thus might begin at the loading dock, where materials entering the plant can be examined. Warning labels, descriptive language about the chemical composition of materials, and the packaging of incoming materials should be noted. Questions then should be asked regarding the handling of unknown materials or materials about which insufficient information is available. The incoming materials then should be followed into the process flow stream, and each of the processes of interest in the plant should be observed in action. Of interest throughout the survey will be the methods used for materials handling and the labeling of materials, particularly at points where they are transferred from manufacturers' containers into other vessels for use within the plant.

Observations to Be Made

At each point in the process, the industrial hygienist and physician should observe all handling procedures as well as any protective measures that are employed. Use of respiratory protection and protective clothing should be recorded, as well as other commonsense observations, such as the apparent effectiveness of engineering controls, as indicated by absence of characteristic odors, visible dust accumulations, and loud noise. The survey should continue through to the final product produced by the plant and its packaging. The surveyors also should follow the pathway of any waste materials and determine their disposal sites.

The numbers of employees at each process step should be noted, as well as any relevant data on gender, ethnicity, or age that might affect employees' sensitivity to chemicals in the workplace. It is also important to look for obvious stigmata such as drying and roughening of the skin, as might be expected where exposure to solvents occurs. It is usually appropriate to discuss work practices with the personnel directly involved because the perception of those practices is often very different on the shop floor from what it is in the executive offices.

On completion of the walk-through survey, the industrial hygienist ordinarily will have a closing conference with the plant management, at which time obvious concerns can be discussed and follow-up measures agreed on. Where the industrial hygienist is a regulatory agency representative, follow-up surveys may require special notices and interaction with agency officials as well as plant officials. In any case, a report on the walk-through survey, together with conclusions and recommendations, should be completed for the record.

Data Review

An important part of the industrial hygienist's role in recognition of health hazards in the workplace is data review. Such data may include reports from physicians on clinical findings that may be related to exposures in the workplace as well as a review of company records on materials coming into the workplace that may represent significant health hazards. The current Occupational Safety and Health Administration (OSHA) Workers' Right-to-Know regulation makes explicit (and subject to governmental investigation) the commonsense duty of the employer to inform workers of the nature and hazards of materials to which they may be exposed. Where exposures are to materials purchased from a third party, data on materials and their hazards usually are derived from material safety data sheets (MSDSs).

Value & Limitations of MSDSs

The industrial hygiene review of MSDSs and other information from suppliers should include attention to identifiable health hazards as well as recommended control measures. While recently MSDSs are far more informative than in the past, there are still substantial differences between the information provided by different manufacturers for the same (generic) materials. In addition, the MSDSs provided by a manufacturer or distributor may be prepared by people without substantial health science backgrounds and sometimes represent merely a reprinting of data from conventional sources that often are outdated and sometimes inappropriate. The industrial hygienist therefore must compare and balance the recommendations made by various manufacturers in order to provide a unified program for control of materials of similar sorts, regardless of their commercial sources.

As chemical manufacturers have become more sophisticated, the available MSDSs have begun to stress protective measures more completely than in the past. This has come about both from manufacturers' concerns that their materials were in some cases being misused and from fear of litigation. In some cases, recommended personal protective measures are unnecessarily complex, particularly where the chemicals are used in very small quantities. The industrial hygienist may be able to recommend less restrictive protection if the combination of quantities used, inherent toxicity, process controls, and other engineering control measures combine to reduce exposures to acceptable levels.

Materials of Uncertain Toxicity

In some cases, the industrial hygienist must assess the potential for harm of chemicals for which no reliable human toxicologic data are available. This need arises most often in research and development settings but also wherever chemical intermediates are produced. An important consideration is that the worker must be protected at all cost. If uncertainty exists, it should be resolved in favor of a higher standard of concern.

EVALUATION OF HEALTH HAZARDS IN THE WORKPLACE

Evaluation of health hazards within the plant includes measurement of exposures (and potential exposures), comparison of those exposures with existing standards, and recommendation of controls, if needed.

Exposure Measurements

Exposure measurements are intended to be surrogates for determinations of doses delivered to the individual. The mere existence of chemicals in the workplace or even in the workplace atmosphere does not necessarily mean that the chemicals are being delivered to a sensitive organ system in quantity sufficient to cause harm. The effective dose depends on such things as particle sizes of dust in the air, the use of protective devices (i.e., respirators and protective clothing), and the existence of other contaminants in the workplace. The task of determining the dose delivered to the worker may be further complicated by the existence of multiple pathways of absorption and metabolism. Such contaminants as lead are absorbed through both inhalation and ingestion, and both routes of intake must be considered in evaluation of the potential for harm. Similarly, many solvents are absorbed readily through the skin, and mere determination of airborne levels is not sufficient to determine the complete range of potential exposures.

Sampling & Analysis of Airborne Contaminants

Inhalation of airborne contaminants is the major route of entry for systemic intoxicants in the workplace. Thus evaluation and control of airborne contaminants is an important part of any occupational health program.

Sampling and analysis of airborne contaminants is the definitive function of the industrial hygienist. While it is the joint responsibility of the hygienist and physician to interpret the results of such measurements, measurement alone makes a contribution to the awareness of hazards as well as to their evaluation. Recent developments in instrumentation have made it possible to measure very low concentrations, with the result that previously unsuspected contamination is now being discovered.

In some cases, these more sophisticated measurements, coupled with evaluations of the health status of those exposed, have led to discoveries of connections between relatively low levels of airborne contaminants and health effects. The field of indoor air quality is one such general case. The determination of exposures to occupants of buildings (office workers) has not received substantial attention in the past, but health effects are now being found at concentrations of contaminants well below established occupational standards.

Maximum acceptable exposure limits typically have been lowered in recent years as both our ability to discern clinical effects and our expectations of no risk of (detectable or undetectable) health effects have increased. A good example of this phenomenon is concern about asbestos in buildings. A hygienist should attempt to ensure that avoidable exposure to asbestos is eliminated. There is no definitive evidence that there is a threshold dose below which the asbestos-related disease mesothelioma will not occur. In addition, substantial liability may attach to the building owner who permits unnecessary exposure to building employees or tenants. Thus measurements of asbestos concentrations down to and including ambient levels have become commonplace.

General Approaches to Air Monitoring

There are two major approaches to air monitoring for determination of airborne contaminant levels. In the personal, or breathing zone, sampling, the hygienist places a collection device near the breathing zone of a worker. The collection device may be either active, requiring that air be drawn through it, or passive, requiring no pump or other suction source (a *dosimeter*). The second approach (area sampling) employs fixed or mobile sampling stations in the work area.

A. Personal Breathing Zone Monitoring

Personal breathing zone monitoring usually is preferred because exposures are measured at the point nearest to the actual entry of airborne contaminants, and the sampling system moves with the worker. Thus measurements are more likely to represent actual potential exposures. Figure 35–1 shows an example of a worker with a breathing zone (personal) sampler in place.

B. Area Monitoring

There are disadvantages to the personal breathing zone approach, however. First, the volume of air sampled is limited by the capacity of the battery-operated pumps used (or the diffusion coefficient of a passive collection device), so trace contaminants may be difficult to measure. Second, where complex evaluations are required, the number of collection devices may be too cumbersome for practical installation in the worker's breathing zone. In these circumstances, or when direct-reading instruments (usually larger and often requiring line power) are to be used, area monitoring by means of fixed monitoring stations may be employed. Fixed monitoring stations also may be used to measure emissions from sources, to measure background concentrations, or to measure concentrations in several areas simultaneously in order to evaluate the effectiveness of controls. Figure 35–2 shows the application of both area sampling and personal sampling inside a work area.

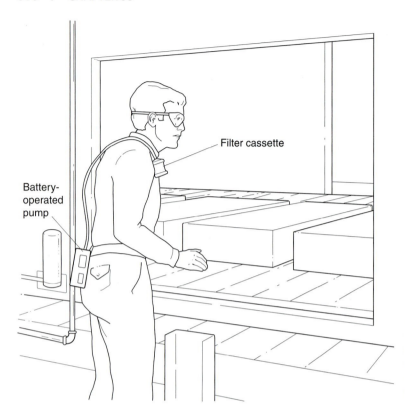

Filter cassette

Battery-operated pump

Figure 35–1. Worker wearing personal breathing zone monitor. The monitor samples air near enough to the nose and mouth to catch the same type of air that the worker is breathing.

DURATION AND TIMING OF MONITORING

Determination of Time-Weighted Average Exposures

The time course of exposure potential should be identified before beginning the sampling process so that all times during which exposure is possible will be appropriately sampled. Time-weighted average exposure determinations should be made for the entire period of work to be evaluated. In a continuous (assembly-line) process, the period of exposure usually will be the entire work shift. In other cases, exposures may occur only for a relatively short time within the work shift. The time-weighted average exposure throughout the workday usually is required for determination of compliance with relevant standards and also may be useful for comparison of exposures at various points within the plant.

Determination of the Time Course of Exposure

Although chronic diseases usually are the result of long-continued exposures, peak exposure levels can be important in causing acute effects and may be more directly rele-

vant even in long-term exposures than their relative contribution on a time-weighted average would indicate. In other words, peak exposures may overwhelm such defenses as the mucociliary pathway for removal of contaminants and may occur at times of maximal exertion and maximal intake of airborne contaminants. Peak exposures may be determined by taking an integrated sample for a relatively short period (for performance of a specific operation, or for 10–15 minutes at a time when maximum exposure is expected, or for such other period as may be required by a regulation or standard) or by using direct-reading instruments for real-time measurements.

SAMPLING FOR SPECIFIC CONTAMINANTS

The general approaches introduced earlier may be applied to determination of individual agents or groups of agents. In general, sampling and analytic methods are divided into those for gases and vapors and those for airborne particles.

1. Gas & Vapor Sampling

Gas and vapor sampling may be accomplished by any of five methods: (1) active collection, by drawing a

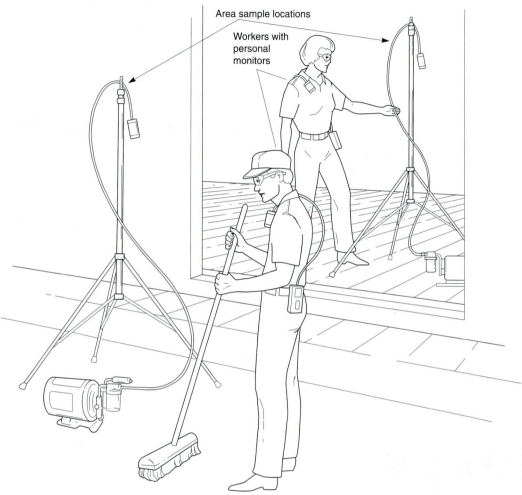

Figure 35–2. Worker wearing personal monitor. Industrial hygienist is gaining additional information by installing an area monitoring device.

measured volume of air through a collection system that is then analyzed, (2) passive collection, with a dosimeter that attracts gas or vapor molecules by diffusion from the atmosphere, (3) collection in a color-sensitive medium in a device in which color change is proportionate to concentration of the contaminant and which can be read directly, (4) collection in an evacuated container used to carry a sample of air to a convenient site for analysis, and (5) direct evaluation by direct-reading instruments sensitive to one or several atmospheric gases or vapors.

In general, the first and fourth methods—using active collection devices with subsequent laboratory analysis—are more sensitive and can be used to determine lower concentrations than can the other approaches listed. However, the direct-reading devices (both instrumental

and color-change) provide a more rapid (immediate) result and are useful when an immediate hazard must be assessed. Passive dosimeters offer the advantage of not requiring a suction source to draw air through the collection device and thus are more acceptable to workers because the need for carrying a pump is avoided.

Collection Media & Analysis

Collection media for gases and vapors may be either solid or liquid.

A. SOLID SORBENTS

The most commonly used solid sorbent is activated charcoal, which can be used for collection of many low-molecular-weight hydrocarbons, as well as for some inorganic gases and vapors. The most common analytic procedure employed in determining concentrations from the gases and vapors collected on the charcoal is gas-liquid chromatography (*gas chromatography*). The collected sample, with the molecules of gas or vapor adsorbed to the surface of the charcoal, usually is desorbed with a solvent (often carbon disulfide) compatible with those to be determined. Then either the solvent extract of the charcoal is injected directly into the gas chromatograph column, or the volume of the extract is reduced to provide greater sensitivity, followed by injection.

In some cases, particularly for oxygenated hydrocarbon species, silica gel is used in testing. Desorption often is accomplished with distilled water or oxygenated solvents, again followed by analysis by either gas chromatography or other analytic approaches. Another group of sorbents is used less commonly for routine industrial hygiene sampling but is finding increasing use in evaluation of indoor air quality and for collection of samples for analysis of higher-molecular-weight species. These are the solid sorbents that were developed initially as gas chromatographic column packings. Examples are Tenax and the variously numbered Chromosorb materials. Some of these sorbents can be characterized as *molecular sieves* and find particular use in collection of samples in environments where compounds that may bind irreversibly to charcoal are found. Desorption often is accomplished conveniently by heating the sample collection tube while injecting a carrier gas (nitrogen or another inert gas) through the sample tube during heating. This approach, coupled with analysis of the desorbed gas, by gas chromatography, mass spectrometry, or some other analytic method, often is useful where a complex environment with many trace components is suspected.

B. LIQUID MEDIA

Gases and vapors also may be collected effectively from the atmosphere using various liquids as the collection media. The air is drawn through the measured volume of the liquid into a device that may be called an *impinger* or *bubbler* or a *gas-washing bottle*. Sampling in liquid for gases and vapors has several disadvantages when personal breathing zone concentrations are to be determined. Some of the liquids that have been recommended are themselves toxic, and placing a glass vial on a worker's lapel may add to the risk in the workplace. There is a danger also of spillage from any liquid container, and the liquid may evaporate, either of which will complicate evaluation of the results.

C. EVACUATED CONTAINERS

Collection of samples of air in evacuated containers such as inert plastic bags, glass bottles, stainless steel cylinders, or other containers is appropriate only if it is certain that the samples will be analyzed before analytes of interest have had a chance to either degrade or react. In most cases, this limits the utility of the technique to relatively stable gases and vapors. The technique is particularly useful for inorganic and nonreactive gases such as carbon monoxide, although "passivated" stainless steel containers are used widely for collection of ambient air samples for trace hydrocarbon analysis. Reactions may include those with the walls of the container (or simple sorption to the walls), as well as reactions with other airborne contaminants held within the container. In addition, care must be taken to avoid exposure of the collected gas to sunlight or other sources of artificial light that may initiate photochemical reactions. This technique is very useful whenever such analytic procedures as gas-phase infrared spectrometry appear to be useful approaches and a laboratory-based instrument offers advantages in sensitivity or precision over field direct-reading instruments.

Direct-Reading Instruments

A variety of direct-reading battery-powered instruments is now available, so direct measurements of "real time" concentrations can be made conveniently in remote or isolated environments. Some of these units also measure oxygen concentrations, making them useful for evaluating the safety of entry into enclosed spaces. Others measure only one or two contaminants but are useful where the suspected contamination is relatively well known.

With the recent advent of small portable *data loggers* from which data may be downloaded to computer systems, it has become feasible to record the real-time output from very small direct-reading instruments. This has made it possible to construct some individual chemical exposure profiles over time because these units can be as small as a "pack of cigarettes" and are carried easily and are not intrusive. An important application of this approach has been in indoor air quality studies, where the relative contributions of various sources to overall exposures to carbon monoxide and other gases of interest have become much better understood.

Other available direct-reading instruments are less portable but may be more accurate and more easily and permanently calibrated. The detection principles employed are often the same as those in the small instruments, but the detection systems and associated electronics may be more reliable. Output may be directed to digital or analog meters, strip-chart recorders, or data loggers.

Several kinds of direct-reading instruments respond to a wide variety of airborne contaminants, although with differing sensitivities. Each of these must be calibrated for specific chemical mixtures because each of them may respond differently.

A. PORTABLE CHROMATOGRAPHS

A recent development in industrial hygiene instrumentation has been the adaptation of gas chromatographs to portable field use. With these instruments, a bolus of air may be drawn directly into the instrument through a gas sampling valve, or an evacuated container (often a syringe) may be used to collect a small sample of air that is then injected directly into the instrument. These instruments share the advantages (specificity and sensitivity) of laboratory gas chromatographs but have the disadvantage that a relatively extensive calibration effort may be required to obtain quantitative results. The detectors used may be selected to measure only the family of airborne contaminants of interest.

B. INFRARED SPECTROPHOTOMETERS

These instruments (an example of which is the family of MIRAN instruments manufactured by Foxboro-Wilks) can be used to measure concentrations of several hundred gases and vapors at or near the 1-ppm level. An advantage of the instrument is that corrections for background concentrations of water vapor and other gases and vapors than those of immediate interest can be performed on site.

C. DIRECT-READING INSTRUMENTS WITH SPECIALIZED DETECTORS

Some of these instruments may give a single-number response to the totality of the atmosphere they are measuring. Such a single number may be imputed to be "total hydrocarbons" or "volatile organic carbon" (VOC) based on the response of the detector. Each such detector has its own characteristic response to the mixture of hydrocarbons present in the air, and comparison of the results from one type of instrument (e.g., a photoionization detector) to another (e.g., a flame ionization detector) usually is inappropriate.

Other specialized instruments may measure one or several specific individual gases or vapors in the atmosphere, such as carbon monoxide, sulfur dioxide, hydrogen sulfide, or the like. Although these are less likely to be affected by other atmospheric components than those that purport to measure "total hydrocarbons," each may have idiosyncratic responses to other atmospheric components, and the nature of those responses must be known.

D. FIXED MONITORS

Any of the direct-reading instruments just described can be made substantially more reliable if installed permanently with line power. Such installations have been used for many years where potential for exposure to highly toxic gases exists.

E. COLORIMETRIC INDICATORS

These may be either passive or active. In the passive type, a "badge" that has a portion that changes color on exposure to specific gases or vapors at a given concentration for a sufficient period of time may be placed in an area or in the breathing zone of a worker. The system functions by diffusion of the molecules of interest from the atmosphere to the badge. Such devices can be useful to indicate the presence of potentially harmful concentrations of gases without having an industrial hygienist present in the workplace at all times. In the active type, a measured volume of air is drawn through a glass tube containing a reagent (usually adsorbed onto a solid support) that reacts with specified chemicals in the air. The degree of color change in the reagent—either the shade of coloration or the "length of stain" along the tube length—is proportionate to the concentration of contaminant and can be compared with standard charts. The major danger in their use is that they may not be reliable; they should not, generally speaking, be considered any more accurate than about plus or minus half of the indicated value. In addition, their reliable detection limit may be near to the level at which controls should be implemented.

2. Particulate Material Sampling

Measurement of airborne particulate contamination can be done either by collection of integrated samples with subsequent analysis or by use of direct-reading instruments. Integrated sample collection and analysis is by far the more common modality of evaluation both because of certain inherent difficulties associated with direct-reading measurements and because of the greater precision associated with laboratory analysis.

Filter Sampling

Modern airborne particle sampling ordinarily is done with filters. The filter selected for use must collect and retain the particles of interest, must not offer so much resistance to flow that pumps cannot draw air through it at a useful rate, and must be compatible with the analytic method of choice.

Size-Selective Sampling

Inhalation and retention of particulate material in the lung depend on the aerodynamic equivalent diameter (AED) of the particles. That is, only particles within a specific (small) size range (which also depends on the specific gravity and shape of the particles) will both penetrate to and be retained within the alveolar and lower bronchiolar (unciliated) airspaces. Somewhat larger particles may penetrate into the thoracic cavity, whereas those even larger will be collected in the upper respiratory system (nose and mouth). The very largest particles only rarely will be carried into the nose or mouth. Thus, sampling to evaluate hazards associated with agents such as crystalline silica is done with the aid of a size-selective sampling device preceding the filter on which the material is to be collected for analysis. When air is drawn through the sampling system at the proper rate, only particles small enough to both penetrate and be retained within the deep lung space will pass through the selective device and be captured on the filter for analysis. In recent years, general environmental sampling for particles also has used size-selective criteria to define the particles believed to be most likely to cause long-term harm to the respiratory system.

The size-selective criteria established and the devices used to collect the defined range(s) of particles differ from agency to agency, and it is important to verify the current status of regulations and scientific opinion in this rapidly changing field.

In addition to the cyclone, size-selective devices used in particulate material sampling include direct inertial collectors such as impingers and impactors. The former uses a wet collection system, wherein a jet of air is directed against a collecting surface within a liquid bath. While impingers are effective for the collection of large particles, they are not particularly suitable for collection of very small particles (<1 μm AED) owing to the limitations of the inertial forces employed for such collection. Impactors use a dry collection system, wherein particles are directed in a jet of air against a dry (or sometimes greased) collection surface. The final stage of the impactor is usually a filter, where the remaining (small) particles are collected. Size-selective sampling with greater detail than offered by the cyclone thus is provided.

Special versions of impactors are used widely for the evaluation of viable airborne particles (fungi and bacteria). The devices, having either one or several collection stages, are designed to accommodate Petri dishes of conventional microbiologic growth media as the collection surfaces. After air is drawn through the device, and the airborne particles are deposited on the surface of the selected medium, the dishes are taken to a laboratory, and the organisms are allowed to proliferate in the usual manner. The dishes are examined by a microbiologist, and the organisms are counted and identified by genus and species, if possible. The number of colony-forming units per cubic meter of air is reported.

Total Particulate Sampling

In circumstances where a biologically active material may be absorbed readily at many portals of entry, total particulate sampling may be the approach of choice. This is the case, for example, where such biologically active compounds as organophosphorus or carbamate pesticides require evaluation. For these and many other chemicals, it is important to collect all airborne particles if the full extent of the hazard is to be evaluated.

Analysis of Particulate Material Samples

Analysis of collected samples may be by any of a variety of techniques appropriate to the analyte of interest.

A. MICROSCOPY

In the case of materials such as asbestos, where the numerical concentration of particles in air is the most important dose factor, a sample is taken by drawing air through a filter, and the number of particles on the filter is counted by microscopic techniques.

The most common analytic procedure used for evaluation of asbestos is that involving optical phase-contrast microscopy as specified by the National Institute for Occupational Safety and Health (NIOSH) and by OSHA. The procedure is relatively simple but has the disadvantages that not all airborne asbestos fibers are visualized or counted and that other (nonasbestos) fibers are counted. However, because only the fibers most often considered to be harmful (those longer than 5 μm) are counted, the method gives an imperfect index of exposure to all asbestos fibers.

Where more detailed information on the total airborne fiber population is desired, transmission electron microscopy is used. This method, which is capable of visualizing all airborne asbestos fibers (and differentiating asbestos fibers from other fibers) is much more complex and costly. In the United States in 2003, the analytic cost of the phase-contrast method typically was in the range of $10–25 per sample, whereas transmission electron microscopy typically costs from $50–500 per sample depending on the level of detail required in the results (and the speed of analysis).

B. OTHER ANALYTIC APPROACHES

Other commonly used analytic approaches are atomic absorption or emission spectroscopy for analysis of elements in the particles, x-ray diffraction for identification of crystalline materials, and (where appropriate) any of the aforementioned organic analysis modalities where organic compounds exist in particulate form.

3. Combined Collection Devices

In some environments it may be appropriate to use combined particulate and gas or vapor collection devices. This may be the case where a substance exists in particulate form in the atmosphere but has an appreciable vapor pressure so that substantial amounts may evaporate following collection on a filter. In this case, a vapor-sorbing material would be used behind the filter to ensure complete collection. Such a combined sampling approach is used often for collection of pesticides and polynuclear aromatic hydrocarbons.

4. Surface Evaluation (Wipe Sampling)

Evaluation of surface contamination can be a useful supplementary technique to assist in the definition of exposure potential and particularly for evaluation of the effectiveness of control measures. Wipe sampling is useful also for identifying contaminated areas where a spill of a potentially hazardous material has occurred. As an example, wipe sampling is used routinely to evaluate the extent of contamination resulting from spills of such materials as polychlorinated biphenyls (PCBs), pesticides, and other materials for which absorption through the skin may be an important route of entry.

Wipe sampling also may be a useful adjunct to programs used to evaluate the effectiveness of housekeeping measures, particularly in manufacturing facilities where separation of manufacturing areas from cafeterias, offices, or dressing rooms is important. A typical program would call for the wipe sampling of identical areas monthly or quarterly.

Wipe sampling must be done according to a well-defined protocol if it is to have any significant utility for long-term evaluations. Most commonly, a template of a defined size (usually 10×10 cm) is prepared, and wiping is done within the exposed area of the template for the sake of uniformity. Any suitable substance may be used to perform the wiping, but filter papers (usually the low-ash, quantitative type papers) are used most commonly.

Other methods of surface evaluation also are sometimes useful. For example, the polynuclear aromatic hydrocarbons fluoresce readily when irradiated with ultraviolet light, and this characteristic can be used to make qualitative surveys of areas where contamination is feared.

PHYSICAL AGENT EVALUATION

Evaluation of physical agents requires specialized equipment that often is not available routinely (except for sound-level meters and noise dosimeters). Evaluation of ionizing or non-ionizing radiation requires specialized training, but many industrial hygienists have developed expertise in these evaluations.

Noise Exposure Evaluation

Evaluation of exposures to noise is a traditional industrial hygiene function. The equipment used is of two principal types.

A. SOUND-LEVEL METERS

Sound-level meters consist of a microphone and associated electronic circuitry, with a meter that gives a readout in decibels. The circuitry typically contains filtering circuits that permit evaluation of exposures to components of the noise spectrum weighted in accordance with their effects on hearing. The A-weighting network has been adopted as the standard for determination of occupational noise exposure. In this weighting scheme, the very low and very high frequencies are suppressed, and the middle frequencies (1000–6000 Hz) are slightly accentuated. This gives primacy to the speech frequencies.

Sound-level meters also may be fitted with filtering circuits for determination of noise levels within specified bandwidths. One octave or one-third octave (less commonly) bandwidth circuits are often employed. With such devices, it is possible to isolate and identify the specific frequencies of occurrence of the noise. This identification of sources is essential to control in complex noise environments.

Figure 35–3 shows a sound-level meter in use. Note that the instrument is used to measure noise intensity in an area and thus is analogous to area sampling for chemicals.

B. NOISE DOSIMETRY

Noise dosimeters employ a recording circuit consisting of a small microphone placed close to the ear of the worker to record noise exposure. The devices may either give an overall integrated average exposure for the course of the measurement period or a readout showing exposure as a function of time. Dosimetry is the preferred approach because the exposures measured are specific and unique to the individual, and dosimetry offers the same advantage over area sampling as indicated earlier for breathing zone sampling for airborne contaminants. Figure 35–4 shows the use of a dosimeter. Note that the microphone is located close to the worker's ear.

Evaluation of Other Physical Agents

Other physical agents ordinarily require specialized equipment for competent evaluation. However, many industrial hygienists are experienced in evaluations for such agents as electrical and magnetic fields, microwaves, and ultraviolet and infrared radiation. Similarly, the evaluation of a workplace to determine the extent of hazard because of heat or cold stress usually can be done by an experienced industrial hygienist.

OBSERVATIONS OF WORK PRACTICES & PROCESS VARIABLES

Exposures often vary substantially from time to time during a day, week, month, or year. The work practices employed by workers whose exposures are measured should be observed during the monitoring period. The description of the workplace must include personal protective devices so that an estimation of *true exposure* (actual intake of chemical into the worker's body) can be derived.

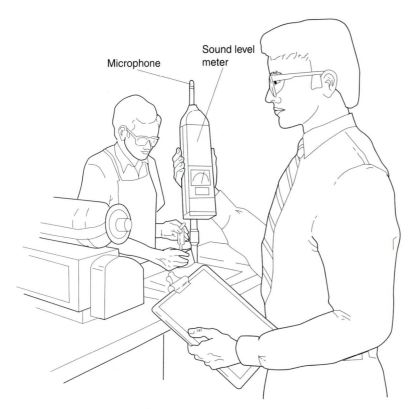

Microphone

Sound level meter

Figure 35–3. Industrial hygienist using a sound-level meter in a work area.

Ventilation equipment and other engineering controls also must be evaluated so that sampling results are placed in a sensible context. Workers and supervisors ordinarily will be able to estimate how closely conditions during the survey period approximate "usual" conditions. General conditions in the workplace, including such things as whether windows and doors are open or closed, also must be evaluated and recorded. The ideal industrial hygiene report will be detailed enough so that another industrial hygienist entering the workplace later will be able to determine whether conditions are the same as or different from those that existed during the survey period.

COMPARISON WITH STANDARDS

Statistical Considerations

The industrial hygienist must determine whether exposures measured are likely to cause harm to those exposed. If such harm seems likely, action must be taken to reduce exposures to tolerable levels (see "Control of Health Hazards" below). In most cases, the industrial hygienist will refer to a set of standards for various individual chemical contaminants or physical agents. Exposures usually are considered to be acceptable (1) if the measured concentrations are less than the allowable upper limit and (2) if

exposures are unlikely to rise above that allowable limit under reasonably foreseeable circumstances.

Certain precautions are needed in such comparisons. The monitoring process is, in the statistical sense, a sampling process. If the systematic biases and random error in the measurements made are within acceptable limits, it can be presumed that the measurements are accurate. That is, not only that the monitoring results are reflective of the true mean of the results that might be obtained if all possible subsets of samples were examined but also that the measurements reflect the "truth" about concentrations to which workers are exposed.

However, all industrial hygiene measurements are inaccurate to some degree owing to sampling and analytic errors and cannot be absolutely reflective of all possible workplace conditions because all possible workplace conditions cannot be evaluated owing to cost considerations. Therefore, it is prudent to construct confidence intervals about the sample means so that the range within which the true average concentration may be expected to fall is known. The upper 95% confidence limit should fall below the allowable exposure limit before it can be stated, with 95% certainty, that the true average concentration probably is below that standard, assuming that the samples taken can be presumed to be otherwise reflective of typical conditions in the workplace.

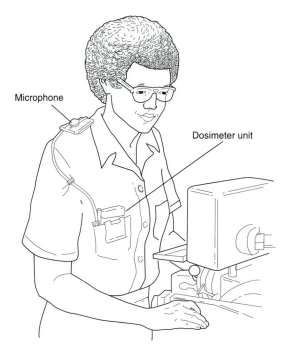

Figure 35–4. Worker wearing a noise dosimeter with a microphone located close to the ear.

A precautionary note is in order. Because of the inherently great dispersion of environmental data, it should be presumed that the data are log-normally distributed, and the logarithmic transformation of individual data points should be performed before the data are evaluated. The geometric mean (the inverse log of the average of the logarithms of the data points) is usually an appropriate measure of central tendency when evaluating environmental data, although the conventional arithmetic mean (the average) will more truly represent the exposures of the workforce.

Occupational Exposure Standards for Airborne Contaminants

Lists of occupational exposure standards for airborne contaminants have been available for more than 60 years. The first standards were for a few widely recognized health hazards such as lead, mercury, and benzene. Currently, hundreds of chemicals and physical agents are either regulated (e.g., by federal or state OSHA programs) or have recommended control limits (from NIOSH or voluntary organizations). In the United States, the most important standards are derived from the following sources:

1. The American Conference of Governmental Industrial Hygienists (ACGIH) threshold limit val-

ues (TLVs): *Threshold Limit Values and Biological Exposure Indices for 2006,* ACGIH Guidelines for Industrial Hygienists, www.acgih.org/TLV/.

2. The recommended exposure levels (RELs) of the National Institute for Occupational Safety and Health: *NIOSH Pocket Guide to Chemical Hazards* (*NPG*), www.cdc.gov/niosh/npg/npg.html.

3. The permissible exposure limits (PELs) of the Occupational Safety and Health Administration: *NIOSH Pocket Guide to Chemical Hazards* (*NPG*), www.cdc.gov/niosh/npg/npg.html.

These and similar lists prepared by some state OSHA programs are legally enforceable by regulatory agencies. The TLVs and RELs should be considered advisory.

All these standards typically are based on time-weighted average (TWA) exposures. That is, concentrations within each day are averaged, with weighting assigned depending on the time period of exposure to each of the concentrations measured. They each may have some upper limit of exposure for shorter periods as well, expressed as a ceiling or as a short-term exposure limit (STEL). A ceiling limit ordinarily will be assigned to those substances for which tolerance of overexposure is slight and where the consequences of even modestly exceeding the ceiling for short periods of time may be disastrous. (As an example, hydrogen cyanide is regulated most appropriately by a ceiling standard.) A STEL may be assigned to substances for which harmful effects (but not life-threatening or likely to cause permanent disability) may arise at short-term exposures to concentrations above the TWA exposure limit, even if there is sufficient time at lower concentrations to bring the TWA within the overall exposure limit. From a practical point of view, it must be recognized that short bursts of intense peak exposure to any substance may have harmful effects not anticipated in the usual workplace and that accumulating the entire exposure sufficient to reach the TWA in, say, an hour, would be unacceptable.

Threshold Limit Values

Of the sets of standards to which industrial hygienists have reference in this regard, the most important (in the United States) is the table of TLVs published annually by the Threshold Limit Values Committee of the American Conference of Governmental Industrial Hygienists (ACGIH). This listing has been published annually since the mid-1940s and is used in the United States and in other countries. In 1970, on enactment of OSHA, the 1968 TLVs were adopted and given the status of law. In their incarnation as OSHA regulations, they have been named PELs. ACGIH also publishes a loose-leaf binder (updated periodically) in which are set forth the data on which the TLVs are based.

The TLVs include values for chemical substances and physical agents (i.e., heat, ionizing radiation, lasers, noise and vibration, radiofrequency and microwave radiation, ultraviolet and infrared radiation, and visible light). A recently added section sets forth biologic exposure indices for about 50 chemicals for which well-established acceptable levels of the parent chemical or its metabolites in body fluids have been documented. The ACGIH biological exposure indices (BEIs) are discussed in Chapter 36.

Despite warnings to the contrary in the ACGIH booklet, many people improperly consider TLVs (and PELs) as "safe" levels, that is, that no harm may come to those exposed at concentrations less than the TLVs. However, TLVs always have been intended only as guidelines for control of workplace atmospheres by personnel with adequate training and experience in industrial hygiene. The following is quoted (emphasis in the original) from the ACGIH publication, *TLVs: Threshold Limit Values and Biological Exposure Indices for 2006*:

> These limits are intended for use in the practice of industrial hygiene as guidelines or recommendations in the control of potential health hazards and for no other use, e.g., in the evaluation or control of community air pollution nuisances, in estimating the toxic potential of continuous, uninterrupted exposures or other extended work periods, as proof or disproof of an existing disease or physical condition, or adoption by countries whose working conditions differ from those in the United States of America and where substances and processes differ. These limits *are not* fine lines between safe and dangerous concentrations nor are they a relative index of toxicity, and *should not* be used by anyone untrained in the discipline of industrial hygiene.

Too many personnel (both industrial hygienists and others) interpreting occupational exposure measurements have implied that exposures just beneath the TLVs are acceptable. In fact, it always has been considered good practice to hold exposures to the minimum practically possible; that is, no unnecessary exposure to any toxic material should be tolerated. In some cases it is necessary, because of economic or engineering factors, to expose workers to levels greater than zero (ambient) levels. In such cases, the TLVs should be used as a guide to the *maximum* tolerable exposure levels. (The equivalent German values are in fact entitled, in English translation, "Maximum Allowable Concentrations," which was the title of the TLVs for several years in the past.) It is emphasized again that the TLVs—or the OSHA PELs and the NIOSH RELs—represent *maximum allowable* time-weighted exposure levels. The industrial hygienist or physician should attempt to

hold exposures to the lowest level practically possible or to a level at which risk is acceptable, bearing in mind that there is no risk-free environment and that a "safe" environment is one in which the level of risk is acceptable.

Because some of those exposed may develop disease as a consequence of lifetime exposures even at the TLV level, many organizations have adopted a policy of setting standards at some fraction of the TLV. Thus 10%, 25%, or 50% of the TLV may be designated as the internal control level. Some companies have gone so far as to attempt to remove all contamination from workplace atmospheres. In such cases, any detectable odor or irritation is considered to be unacceptable, and control measures are instituted to reduce exposures when any process effluvia are detected.

The OSHA Permissible Exposure Limits

The OSHA PELs were first established in 1970, on implementation of the Occupational Safety and Health Act, by adopting in toto the 1968 ACGIH TLVs, as well as some other voluntary standards from the American National Standards Institute. It should be recognized that the OSHA PELs have not been modified significantly since 1970. Industrial experience, new developments in technology, and available scientific data clearly indicate that in many instances those adopted limits are now obsolete and inadequate. Furthermore, many new toxic materials commonly used in the workplace are not covered. These inadequacies are evidenced by the lower allowable exposure limits recommended by many technical, professional, industrial, and government organizations in the United States and elsewhere.

Only a few substances have been added to those regulated, and for a few more the allowable exposures were reduced. Substantial and significant changes were made in the TLVs in that period. Thus certain exposures that are generally agreed to be potentially harmful are officially acceptable to OSHA. In 1989, OSHA attempted a wholesale upgrade of their PELs, but the attempt was challenged in court by certain industrial interests, and the challengers prevailed. As a result, OSHA must now justify, in extreme detail, each change in each standard. Only a few such changes have been made since 1989.

Many of the individual states have established their own list of allowable exposures, often relying on the TLVs. These may be enforced in lieu of the federal PELs if they are at least as stringent as the PELs.

NIOSH-Recommended Exposure Limits

NIOSH has established recommendations for many workplace chemical and physical agents since its establishment in 1970, coincidentally with the establishment of OSHA. In fact, NIOSH was established in the same act with OSHA, with a legal mandate to provide research to support OSHA. A major function of NIOSH in the 1970s was the production of "criteria documents" for substances and agents, in which recommendations were made for relative exposure limits (RELs). In this set of documents, NIOSH has provided an evaluation of the literature, recommended control measures, and recommended upper limits for exposures. Since the early 1980s, fewer of these documents have been produced. Many of the allowable exposure recommendations of NIOSH are lower than the recommended TLVs or PELs for the same chemicals. In part, this is a result of NIOSH's practice of recommending exposure limits for 10-hour workdays rather than the 8-hour workdays assumed by ACGIH and OSHA.

Other Sources of Standards

Several other sources of recommended exposure limits are available to the industrial hygienist. Among these are the "Workplace Environmental Exposure Limits" promulgated by the American Industrial Hygiene Association for several chemicals not listed by the TLV Committee. Although many countries outside the United States have adopted the ACGIH TLVs without substantial modification, several have active committees evaluating allowable exposure limits. The ACGIH has published ("Guide to Occupational Exposure Values, 2006") a booklet giving the ACGIH TLVs, the OSHA PELs, the NIOSH RELs, the "Maximum Allowable Concentrations" from the German government, Chemical Abstracts Service (CAS) numbers, and carcinogenicity designations from ACGIH, OSHA, NIOSH, Germany, IARC, the U.S. National Toxicology Program, and the U.S. Environmental Protection Agency. Where no established standards are available for guidance, in-house research may be necessary to establish guidelines. Where a chemical not previously used is being widely adopted in a particular industry, a trade association study of the effects of that chemical may be an appropriate venue for such research. Because of the potential risks associated with subtle health effects not easily foreseen, such control limits should be established only with great caution.

Exposure Limits for Unusual or Extended Work Shifts

As noted earlier, the usual exposure limits have been established assuming regular work shifts of 8 (ACGIH and OSHA) or 10 (NIOSH) hours. Where the work shifts differ significantly from the usual day, consideration must be given to the effects of more protracted exposures on workers. A minimum adjustment can be made simply by cutting the allowable exposure limit in inverse proportion to the workday or workweek as a fraction of the usual 8-hour day or 40-hour week, depending on the effect of greatest concern and the biologic half-life of the chemical. A more conservative general approach is to take into account both the increased workday and the decreased period away from exposure, but this approach may yield unrealistically low allowable exposures. Finally, detailed physiologically based pharmacokinetic models may be established. These latter, although they may be the most accurate way to modify general exposure limits, require detailed knowledge of the metabolic pathways of each substance to be so regulated, including information on the biologic half-life of each of the substances.

CONTROL OF HEALTH HAZARDS

On completion of the evaluation, the industrial hygienist should be in a position to recommend appropriate controls, if needed. Recommendations should take into account not only the conditions found during the survey but also those that may be expected to prevail in the future. Planned process modifications should be taken into account, and recommendations should be adaptable to future needs. Controls should be adequate to prevent unnecessary exposure during accidents and emergencies, as well as during normal operating conditions. Consideration must be given to fail-safe operation of controls; that is, recommended controls always should operate to protect workers regardless of process fluctuations.

Substitution

All possibilities for substitution of a nontoxic for a toxic material or agent should be explored. If a toxic material can be dispensed with and a less-harmful material substituted, that should be done. Substitution, of course, can be done only if a useful substitute is available—one that is suitable for existing processes or for which the processes can be relatively easily adapted. This obvious approach must be undertaken with caution, however, because several instances are known where an apparently harmless substitute for an obvious hazard was later found to be harmful in and of itself.

Engineering Controls

Engineering controls on toxic exposures consist mainly of enclosure (building structures around the sources of emissions), isolation (placing hazardous process components in areas with limited human contact), and ventilation.

A. Ventilation

Ventilation for the control of health hazards may be either local exhaust ventilation or general ventilation. Local exhaust ventilation conforms to the principle that control should be implemented as near to the source as practically possible. Thus, for example, application of a local exhaust inlet on a specific tool, such as a grinder, is inherently more desirable than performing the grinding operation in a ventilated hood, which, in turn, is more desirable than installing general ventilation in the room where the grinding is performed. In a situation where a very toxic substance is being manipulated in such a way that exposure is possible, all three ventilation systems might be reasonable to use. Thus the operator would be protected by ventilation of the specific tool, nearby workers (as well as the operator) would be protected by the hood, and the remainder of the building would be protected by the general ventilation system. Figure 35–5 is a conceptual model of a typical operation showing the three zones of control required.

On the other hand, where sources are more diffuse or dispersed, or where many people must be protected from relatively low-level contaminants, such as in indoor air quality in an office building, general ventilation alone may be appropriate. Furthermore, for control of comfort and provision of heating or cooling, general ventilation may be essential. In any case, the general ventilation system must be considered and evaluated for its potential to distribute contaminants throughout a plant or other building.

Design of ventilation systems for contamination control ordinarily should not be left to engineers without specific background or experience. Similarly, an industrial hygienist without engineering training and experience in the processes to be controlled may produce an unsatisfactory design. ACGIH publishes a biennial document on industrial ventilation that provides guidance on the principles of ventilation control.

B. OTHER ENGINEERING CONTROLS

In addition to ventilation, enclosure, and isolation, some specific engineering controls may be appropriate in the specific process environment. It is, for example, often necessary to design process pipelines and valves to minimize splashes and ejection of toxic chemicals. Control systems that will permit safe and orderly shutdown of the process to avoid runaway reactions also may be of substantial benefit.

Controls on Human Behavior

These controls on human behavior can be subdivided into the general categories of administrative controls and work-practice controls.

A. ADMINISTRATIVE CONTROLS

Control of behavior patterns within the process environment includes such things as establishment of prohibited areas, where smoking and eating are either prohibited or allowed, and safe pathways through the work environment. Administrative controls also include scheduling of

work in such a way that dangerous operations are carried out when the fewest workers are present.

Less desirable is the practice of scheduling individual workers to perform tasks for short periods, where excessive exposures would be incurred over an extended period of time. This practice was at one time common in the nuclear power industry, where temporary employees were used to perform maintenance tasks in high-radiation environments. These "jumpers" were employed and paid by the day, although their actual work period may have been as short as 15 minutes. Such practices, where exposure to carcinogenic or genotoxic agents is spread across a larger population group, is entirely unacceptable, although individual exposures are lower. While the individual risk may be relatively low, the effect of distributing an exposure with potential genetic effects to many members of the population is inherently unsound.

On the other hand, administrative controls that include scheduling usually are essential to control of the work environment. An example is prohibiting personnel who do not have adequate training from entry into spaces where health or safety hazards exist.

B. WORK-PRACTICES CONTROL

Control of work practices implies control over the behavior of individual workers on the job. Such work-related details as handling of contaminated tools and appliances are included in this type of control. Education (on the hazards to be avoided) and training (on the desired practices) are, of course, required. Close supervision of workers is needed in order to enforce compliance with proper work practices. Controls on work practices are particularly important where engineering controls are either not adequate or not possible and where there is significant potential for generation of airborne contaminants outside of controlled spaces.

Personal Protection

Personal protective equipment use, though often essential, is less desirable than other approaches because of the difficulty in ensuring both that it is used and that it is also effective. For example, on construction sites, personal protective equipment may consist of hard hats and safety shoes, and in laboratory environments, it may consist of protective eyewear, gloves, and protective garments such as laboratory coats.

However, there are significant complexities in both design and function of the protective devices used to reduce exposures. A worker who is issued and is wearing a respirator, for example, may feel adequately protected from all potential hazards in the workplace and therefore may neglect the use of engineering controls, violate administrative control guidelines, and ignore required work practices. In fact, without substantial attention to selection, fitting,

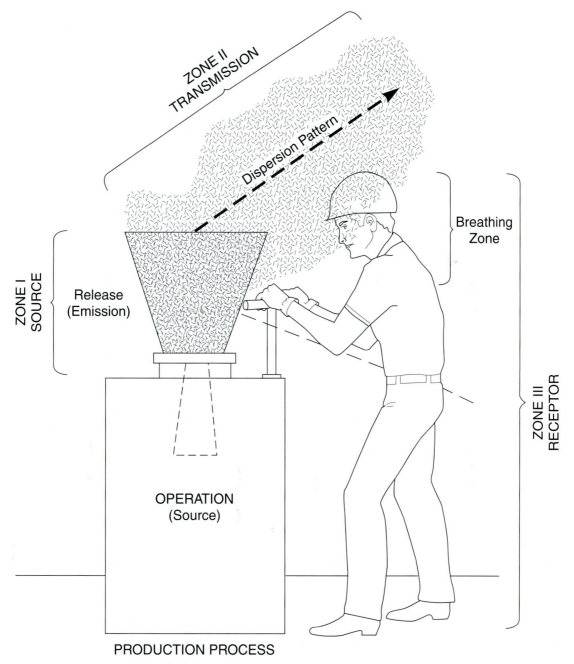

Figure 35–5. Conceptual model of the three zones of influence to control workplace hazards.

training, and maintenance of respirators, exposures during their use may be nearly as high as for those of unprotected workers.

Respirators often are handed out without adequate attention to any of these precautions. It is common, for example, to see workers with beards wearing negative-pressure air-purifying respirators in areas where contaminants are present in the air. The devices are, of course, useless unless they fit tightly, which is nearly impossible if the wearer has facial hair.

Similarly, gloves protect against exposure to solvents and other toxicants only if chosen with knowledge of what materials are suitable in each case. Ironically, prolonged wearing of gloves into which skin hazardous materials have either leached or leaked through holes may result in substantial exposure to the worker (sometimes higher than would occur without the gloves).

Integrated Control

A well-regulated control program in a company with diverse operations usually will employ all the modes just mentioned plus adequate housekeeping and disposal of waste materials. It is emphasized again that substitution should be the first consideration. Where substitution cannot be rationally adopted, isolation of workers from exposure and enclosure of sources should be considered next. If no substitute material is readily available, and if complete isolation and enclosure are not possible, local exhaust ventilation should be considered next. General exhaust ventilation is a useful supplement to local exhaust ventilation and should be part of the ventilation design. When none of these engineering controls can completely abate the hazard, administrative controls, work-practices controls, and personal protection may be necessary.

The controls process must be viewed as a continuing one in which existing controls are continually evaluated for their effectiveness. Equipment ages, personnel change, processes evolve, and the level of management attention to control varies with time. All these forces act to change the effectiveness of a given control. The evaluation of effectiveness is the province of the industrial hygienist, who must involve physicians, managers, engineers, and workers in the evaluation.

EMERGING ISSUES

Among the new workplace exposure issues is the emergence of nanotechnology, the use of extraordinarily small particles in industrial processes (see Chapter 13). It is not yet clear what the harmful effects of these small particles may be, and the prudent occupational physician and industrial hygienist will be cautious about both allowable exposures and clinical evaluation.

The European Parliament and the European Council are considering legislation, Regulation, Evaluation, and Authorization of Chemicals (REACH), that will require industry to prove that chemicals being sold and produced in the European Union are safe to use or handle. REACH policy will require registration of all substances that are produced or imported into the European Union. The amount of information required for registration will be proportional to the chemical's health risks and production volumes. Companies also will need to seek authorization to sell and produce problematic chemicals, such as carcinogens, mutagens, and teratogens. Toxic chemicals that persist in the environment or that bioaccumulate also will need authorization. The policy is slated for enactment in 2006.

In the United States and the European Union, the concept of *control banding* has arisen in the past few years. In this concept, the usual kinds of detailed evaluations performed by industrial hygienists are bypassed in favor of an overall process evaluation wherein the state (gas, liquid, vapor, or solid), vapor pressure, etc. and potential extent of disruption of the process materials are evaluated. Control schemes are established with due regard to allowable exposure limits. This new approach to control of workplace hazards has yet to be proven in practice, although it shows great promise.

REFERENCES

Brouwer DH et al: Personal exposure to ultrafine particles in the workplace: Exploring sampling techniques and strategies. Ann Occup Hyg 2004;48:439 [PMID: 15240340].

Castleman BI: Legacy of corporate influence on threshold limit values and European response. Am J Ind Med 2006;49:307 [PMID: 16526063].

Harper M: Assessing workplace chemical exposures: The role of exposure monitoring. J Environ Monit 2004;6:404 [PMID: 15152307].

Harper M, Pacolay B: A comparison of X-ray fluorescence and wet chemical analysis for lead on air filters from different personal samplers. J Environ Monit 2006;8:140 [PMID: 16395471].

Johnston KL et al: Evaluation of an artificial intelligence program for estimating occupational exposures. Ann Occup Hyg 2005;49:147 [PMID: 15734827].

NIOSH: Emergency response resources, www.cdc.gov/niosh/emres01.html.

NIOSH: *Manual of Analytical Methods,* www.cdc.gov/niosh/nmam/nmampub.html.

NIOSH: *Pocket Guide to Chemical Hazards,* www.cdc.gov/niosh/npg/pgdstart.html.

Oberdorster G et al: Nanotoxicology: An emerging discipline evolving from studies of ultrafine particles. Environ Health Perspect 2005;113:823 [PMID: 16002369].

Biologic Monitoring

Raymond K. Meister, MD, MPH, & Yuxin Zheng, MD, PhD

Biologic monitoring is the measurement of a chemical, its metabolite, or a biochemical effect in a biologic specimen for the purpose of assessing exposure. Biologic monitoring is an important tool to identify the nature and amount of chemical exposures in occupational and environmental situations. The term also may be used to denote drug abuse monitoring and other types of medical surveillance, but to avoid confusion it should be restricted to exposure monitoring.

Biologic monitoring uses *biologic markers* or *biomarkers.* Biomarkers are indicators of events in biologic systems or samples. There are three types of biomarkers: biomarkers of exposure, effect, and susceptibility. A biomarker of exposure is a chemical or its metabolite measured within a specimen. A biomarker of effect is a measure of molecular, biochemical, or physiologic change or other alteration within an organism that can be related to potential health effect. A biomarker of susceptibility is an indicator of an inherited or acquired limitation of an organism's ability to respond to the challenge of exposure to chemicals or other factors. The ideal biomarker should be sensitive, specific, biologically relevant, practical, inexpensive, and available. Seldom does a biomarker meet all these criteria; most represent a compromise.

Typically, specimens are blood, urine, or exhaled air. For example, exposure to organophosphorus insecticides can be confirmed by measuring the metabolite—alkyl phosphates—in the urine or by measuring a biochemical effect—the activity of the enzyme cholinesterase—in the blood. Most often, however, exposure is assessed by measuring the chemical or its metabolite in a body fluid.

Environmental monitoring is measurement of the ambient (external) exposure of a chemical in the workplace. Typically, samples are taken from the air or from surfaces at the workplace. Environmental monitoring provides information about potential exposure primarily from one route of exposure (e.g., air or workplace surfaces), whereas biologic monitoring provides a measure of the quantity of a chemical absorbed regardless of the route of absorption (e.g., inhalation, skin contact, and/or ingestion). Total exposure rather than only workplace exposure is measured.

The biologic level may not correlate well with environmental measurements (Figure 36–1). This variability occurs for several reasons: (1) Actual work practices vary among employees doing identical work. For example, one worker may have more skin contact or may inhale more of a chemical than another worker. (2) A high respiratory rate can increase pulmonary absorption of solvents by a factor of 3–4. (3) The rates of metabolism and excretion vary between individuals even when hepatic or renal function is normal. (4) Lipid-soluble chemicals may accumulate to a greater extent in a person with more adipose tissue. (5) There is variable effectiveness of personal protective equipment. And (6) other inheritable and acquired factors, such as disease status, diet, and pregnancy, may affect a person's biologic level.

Workplace exposure to more than 100 different chemicals can be estimated in an individual by measuring the chemical in the blood, urine, or exhaled air. Depending on the pharmacokinetics of the target substance, the body fluid sampled, and the time of sampling, the measured level will reflect the duration of exposure ranging from acute recent exposure or accumulated lifetime exposure (body burden).

New uses of biologic monitoring and advances in biomarkers continue. In some occupational environments it is well recognized that workers are exposed to multiple chemicals, and the contributions by the various chemicals to the expression of biomarkers needs to be considered. Recent research also has focused on the use of new biomarkers for susceptibility and genome-wide responses. In addition, there is a continued need to develop and apply biomarkers that can be used to provide real-time detection of excessive exposure to hazardous substances in the workplace. This chapter gives the clinician practical information on biologic monitoring.

Because some chemicals are cleared rapidly from the blood, interpretation of biologic levels depends on accurate timing of sample collection. Because significant errors can be introduced in the sampling process, following standard methods of sample collection will improve the clinician's ability to interpret a biologic level.

REFERENCES

Au WW et al: Biomarker research in occupational health. J Occup Environ Med 2005;47:145 [PMID: 15706174].

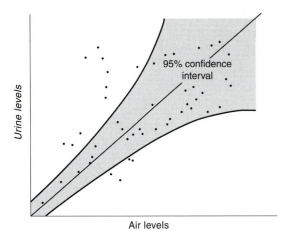

Figure 36–1. Relationship of levels of a substance measured in the breathing zone of workers to levels measured in urine.

Metcalf SW, Orloff KG: Biomarkers of exposure in community settings. J Toxicol Environ Health A 2004;28:715 [PMID: 15192864].

Watson WP, Mutti A: Role of biomarkers in monitoring exposures to chemicals: Present position, future prospects. Biomarkers 2004;9:211 [PMID: 15764289].

HOW TO USE BIOLOGIC MONITORING

Biologic monitoring of workers exposed to toxic agents is an accepted means of accurately determining exposure. It should be used to augment other sources of exposure assessment, such as occupational history and environmental monitoring. Biologic monitoring assesses the extent of exposure of workers and thus only indirectly the risk of health effects as a result of that exposure. Moreover, any action arising out of abnormal biologic monitoring levels should be based not on a single measurement but on multiple measurements.

It cannot be assumed that a biologic level necessarily represents a more accurate reflection of dose than an environmental level. All occurrences of elevated levels judged to be caused by excessive workplace exposure should be evaluated with the assistance of an industrial hygienist.

Before a biologic monitoring program is instituted, some scientific and practical issues must be considered. The program should be able to produce results that are meaningful, be implemented in a cost-effective fashion, and be used as indicated to reduce worker exposures to levels that avoid adverse effects. Tables 36–1 and 36–2 show, respectively, the necessary and sufficient conditions for the consideration of institution of biologic monitoring. Ethical and social aspects also should be considered: For example, confidentiality of results should be ensured; workers should be encouraged to maintain confidentiality (i.e., not share results); and participation should be voluntary. Communication of results and explanation of actions also must be considered.

Table 36–3 summarizes information for chemicals with data sufficient for consideration of biologic monitoring. It is useful in two situations. The first is the routine monitoring of a healthy employee who works with a toxic chemical. The clinician must determine whether the exposure is significant and potentially harmful. If the biologic level measured is below the "no adverse effect level," or if it is within the range "levels without occupational exposure," the exposure probably is not harmful. This situation is analogous to measuring airborne concentrations of a chemical and comparing them with recommended levels. For a few chemicals, biologic monitoring of exposed workers is mandated by law. In the case of an employee who works with lead, if the blood lead concentration is above a certain level,

Table 36–1. Necessary conditions to consider biologic monitoring (all must be present).

Item	Condition
A. Determinant (substance, metabolite, reaction product, nonadverse biochemical effect)	1. Present in media (blood, urine, exhaled air) 2. Suitable for sampling 3. Sampling method acceptable to population to be monitored
B. Method of analysis	1. Practical 2. Produces valid reproducible results over the range of concentrations present
C. Strategy of sample collection	Produces representative samples
D. Results	Can be interpreted in a meaningful fashion
E. Action for responding to aberrant results	Established prior to monitoring

Table 36–2. Sufficient conditions to consider biologic monitoring (one or more must be present).

Item	Condition
A. Environmental monitoring or other workplace exposure assessment	Conducted to complement biologic monitoring
B. Exposure routes to substance being monitored	Other than or in addition to workplace inhalation (skin, gastrointestinal, nonoccupational)
C. Environmental monitoring	1. Not adequate to assess exposure a. Respirators or other personal protection is used b. Absorption is uncertain because of particle size and/or solubility c. Individual variability in respiratory volume or work practices is extreme d. Exposure fluctuates rapidly over time 2. Not feasible a. Plants or sites are in multiple locations b. Physical constraints such as work in a closed space or protective clothing are present
D. Substances to be monitored	1. Cumulative toxicants a. Metals bound to tissues (Pb, Cd, Hg) b. Organics that are fat soluble and/or poorly metabolized (polychlorinated biphenyls, dioxin) 2. Multiple agents with shared biochemical effects a. Cholinesterase for organophosphate pesticides b. Methemoglobin for multiple inducers c. DNA adducts for antineoplastic drugs

that worker must be transferred to an area where he or she is not exposed to lead.

Table 36–3 also is useful in the clinical assessment of an ill employee who has been exposed to a toxic chemical. Is it possible that the employee's abnormal symptoms, signs, or laboratory tests are a result of exposure to that chemical? The *clinical-effect level* is one that is associated with illness typically caused by that chemical. If an employee has signs and symptoms consistent with those caused by the chemical, and if the measured level is at or above the clinical-effect level, there is a high probability that the chemical is causing the illness. However, samples from ill individuals usually are taken at variable and often unspecified times following exposure and therefore reflect an uncertain duration of exposure. A biologic level—no matter how high or low—still only reflects exposure and a given probability of illness and is never diagnostic of illness.

Between the "no adverse effect level" and the clinical-effect level there often lies a gray zone. Figure 36–2 illustrates these concepts. If the employee's level falls into this zone, the clinician may repeat the measurement, use other indices of exposure, or do further reading of the primary literature to refine the evaluation. The clinician also should carefully consider the chronicity of the exposure, the level of exposure, and timing of the sample collection in relation to exposure.

Individuals differ in their response to chemicals; one worker may develop peripheral neuropathy from *n*-hexane exposure, whereas another worker with the same exposure will not. This difference in sensitivity to a chemical may be a result of variable rates of metabolism or excretion, different sensitivity of end-organ receptors, different tolerance to discomfort, a preexisting illness, or simultaneous exposure to drugs or other toxins. Because of these differences between individuals, within a group of exposed workers, the biologic level associated with symptoms usually will follow a bell-shaped distribution.

In addition to individual differences in responses to chemicals, certain subgroups of workers also may need special consideration. For example, the level of concern regarding exposure to a reproductive toxicant may be lower in a woman of childbearing age.

The areas of application of biomonitoring of occupational exposure include determination of DNA and protein adducts; unchanged volatile organic compounds in urine; and monitoring of exposure to pesticides, heavy metals, and polycyclic aromatic hydrocarbons. Biomonitoring provides unequivocal evidence of exposure, but it could not identify the source of exposure. For many chemicals, testing must be conducted soon after exposure has occurred. Biomonitoring is finding wider application in many areas. Recent advances in analytic tech-

Table 36–3. Chemicals for which there are reliable data for determining reference biologic monitoring levels.

Chemical Determinant[1]	Media (units)	Levels without Occupational Exposure	No Adverse Effect Level	Clinical Effect Level	Timing of Sample[2]	Terminal Half-Time ($t_{1/2}$)	Comments
Inorganics: Metals							
Arsenic	Urine (μg/L)	< 15	35	> 300	EWW	1–2 d	No seafood for 2–3 days before collection.
Cadmium	Urine (μg/g Cr)	< 2	2–10	> 10	NC	10–30 y	Reflects chronic exposure (years) after 1 year of exposure.
	Blood (μg/L)	< 0.5	< 10	> 10	NC	10–15 y	Reflects recent exposure (months). Smokers may have blood levels of 1.4–4.5 μg/L.
Chromium	Urine (μg/g Cr)	< 1	25	...	EOS, EWW	15–40 h	Exposure from welding stainless steel.
Lead	Blood (μg/dL)	< 2	20	> 20	NC	...	Use lead-free needles and tubes, $t_{1/2}$ for soft tissue is 1 month; for skeleton, 20 years.
Zinc protoporphyrin (ZPP)	Blood (μg/dL)	16–35	< 35	...	NC	2–4 wk	Increase lags 2–6 weeks behind elevation of blood lead level. Free erythrocyte protoporphyrin (FEP) is interpreted similarly to ZPP.
Mercury (inorganic)	Urine (μg/L)	< 5	35–50	100	PNS	60 d	Reflects prior 2–4 months' exposure.
Nickel	Urine (μg/L)	< 5	70	...	EOS	17–39 h	Corrected to SG of 1018. Measures only soluble nickel.
	Plasma (μg/dL)	0.2–0.4	0.7	...	EOS	...	
Selenium	Plasma (μg/dL)	5–18	...	...	...	...	
	Urine (μg/g Cr)	7–79	25	...	...	100–150 d	
Vanadium	Urine (μg/g Cr)	< 1	50	...	EOS, EWW	20–40 h	
Inorganics: Other							
Carbon disulfide TTCA	Urine (mg/g Cr)	0	5	...	EOS	2–3 d	TTCA is 2-thiothiazolidine-4-carboxylic acid. Carbon disulfide is a metabolite of disulfiram (Antabuse) and dithiocarbamates.
Carbon monoxide COHb	Blood (%)	0.4–0.7	2	5	EOS	1–8 h	Blood COHb following: Cigarettes 1 ppd = 5–6%; 2–3 ppd = 7–9% Driving on urban highways = 5%

Table 36-3. Chemicals for which there are reliable data for determining reference biologic monitoring levels. (continued)

Chemical Determinant[1]	Media (units)	Levels without Occupational Exposure	No Adverse Effect Level	Clinical Effect Level	Timing of Sample[2]	Terminal Half-Time ($t_{1/2}$)	Comments
Cyanide *Thiocyanate*	Urine (mg/24 h)	0.11	6.5	...	...	...	Levels higher in smokers.
Fluorides	Urine (mg/L)	< 0.4	3	...	PNS	4–7 h	In unexposed persons, varies with drinking water fluoride, use of dental products.
		...	10	...	EWW	...	
Organics: Aliphatics and alicyclics Acetone	Urine (mg/g Cr)	< 2	20	46	DS	...	
	Blood (mg/dL)	< 0.2	2	...	DS	6 h	Elevated during diabetic or fasting ketoacidosis.
	Alveolar air (mg/m3)	...	53	...	DS	4 h	
Cyclohexane *Cyclohexanol*	Urine (mg/L)	...	3.2–5.5	...	L4H	...	
Cyclohexanol	Blood (μg/dL)	...	46–52	...	DS	...	
Cyclohexane	End-exhaled air (mg/m³)	...	780–880	...	DS	...	
Dioxane β-*Hydroxyeth-oxyacetic acid*	Urine (mg/L)	...	36.5	...	EOS	1 h	
Dioxane	Blood (mg/L)	...	12	...	DS	...	
Ethylene glycol *Oxalic acid*	Urine (mg/g Cr)	< 50	...	0.3–4.3 g/L	...	2–6 h	
Ethylene glycol monoethyl ether *Ethoxyacetic acid*	Urine (mg/L)	< 0.07	6	...	PNS	21–24 h	
			100	...	EOS, EWW		
n-Hexane *2,5-Hexanedione*	Urine (mg/L)	0.1–0.8	0.4	...	EOS	...	Large individual variability. Correlates best with air concentration.
n-Hexane	End-exhaled air (ppm)	...	40	...	DS	1–2 h	Large individual variability.
Methanol	Urine (mg/L)	0.3–2.6	15	...	EOS	1.5–2 h	
Formic acid	Urine (mg/g Cr)	5–50	80	...	PNS, EWW	...	

(continued)

Table 36–3. Chemicals for which there are reliable data for determining reference biologic monitoring levels. (continued)

Chemical Determinant[1]	Media (units)	Levels without Occupational Exposure	No Adverse Effect Level	Clinical Effect Level	Timing of Sample[2]	Terminal Half-Time ($t_{1/2}$)	Comments
Methyl ethyl ketone	Urine (mg/L)	< 0.5	2–5	...	EOS	0.5–1.5 h	Large individual variability.
2-Methyl pentane *2-Methyl-2-pentanol*	Urine (mg/L)	...	< 0.1–5.5	...	EOS	...	
3-Methylpentane *3-Methyl-3-pentanol*	Urine (mg/L)	0	< 0.1–1	...	EOS	...	
Propylene glycol monoethyl ether (PGME)	End-exhaled air (ppm)	0	4	...	EOS	...	
Organics: Aromatic							
Benzene							
Muconic acid	Urine (μg/g Cr)	< 500	500		EOS	5 h	
S-phenylmercapturic acid	Urine (μg/g Cr)	< 15	25		EOS	9 h	
Benzene	Blood (ng/dL)	< 50	...		PNS	8 h	Losses during sample storage or contamination are potential problems.
Ethyl benzene							
Mandelic acid	Urine (g/g Cr)	< 0.005	1.5	...	EOS	5 h	Large individual variability.
Ethyl benzene	End-exhaled air (ppm)	< 0.03	2	...	PNS, EWW	2 d	
Phenol	Urine (mg/g Cr)	0–20	250	...	EOS	3.5 h	Large individual variability.
Styrene							
Mandelic acid	Urine (g/g Cr)	< 0.005	0.3	...	EOS	20 h	Large individual variability.
Styrene	Blood (mg/L)	0 / 0	0.3 / 0.02	... / ...	EOS / PNS	5 h	Large individual variability.
Penylglyoxylic acid	Urine (mg/g Cr)	...	100	...	EOS	7–10 h	
Toluene							
Hippuric acid	Urine (g/g Cr)	< 1.6	1.6	...	EOS	< 5 h	Large individual variability.
Ortho-cresol	Urine (mg/g Cr)	< 0.3	0.5	...	EOS		
Toluene	Blood (mg/L)	< 0.005	0.05	> 1	EOS	< 5 h	

Table 36–3. Chemicals for which there are reliable data for determining reference biologic monitoring levels. (continued)

Chemical Determinant[1]	Media (units)	Levels without Occupational Exposure	No Adverse Effect Level	Clinical Effect Level	Timing of Sample[2]	Terminal Half-Time $(t_{1/2})$	Comments
Xylene							
Total methylhippuric acid	Urine (g/g Cr)	0	1.5	...	EOS	30 h	
Xylene	Blood (mg/L)	0	1.5	3–40	EOS	20–30 h	Fatalities reported at 3–40.
Organics: Halogenated							
Methyl bromide *Bromide*	Blood (mg/dL)	0.05–0.2	1.1	5	...	...	
Methylene chloride *Carboxyhemoglobin*	Blood (%)	0.4–0.7	2.5	> 10	EOS	10 h	Smoking and CO exposure additive in COHb levels. Longer $t_{1/2}$ than with CO exposure.
			1	...	PNS	...	
	End-exhaled air (ppm)	< 2	3–6	8–13	EOS	10–12 h	
Methylene chloride	Blood (mg/L)	0	0.5	3	EOS	< 1 h	
Perchloroethylene	End-exhaled air (ppm)	0	18	30	EOS	...	
			5	...	PNS, EWW	64 h	
	Blood (mg/L)	0	0.5	...	PNS, EWW	...	
Trichloroacetic acid	Urine (mg/g Cr)	0	3.5	...	EOS	80 h	
Polychlorinated biphenyl *Total chlorobiphenyl*	Blood (µg/L)	0–30	150	600	NC	3–7 y	Method of analysis critical. Results differ depending on specific polychlorinated biphenyl isomer.
1,1,1-Trichloroethane	End-exhaled air (ppm)	0	30	...	PNS, EWW	...	
	Blood (mg/dL)	0	0.5	...	EOS	...	
Trichloroethanol	Urine (mg/L)	0	30	...	EOS, EWW	10–15 h	
	Blood (mg/L)	0	1	...	EOS, EWW		
Trichloroacetic acid	1 Urine (mg/L)	< 5	10	...	EWW	70–100 h	

(continued)

Table 36–3. Chemicals for which there are reliable data for determining reference biologic monitoring levels. (continued)

Chemical Determinant[1]	Media (units)	Levels without Occupational Exposure	No Adverse Effect Level	Clinical Effect Level	Timing of Sample[2]	Terminal Half-Time ($t_{1/2}$)	Comments
Trichloroethylene							
Free trichloro-ethanol	Blood (mg/L)	0	4	...	EOS, EWW	12 h	
Trichloroethylene	End-exhaled air (ppm)	0	0.5	...	PNS, EWW	30 h	
Trichloroacetic acid	Urine (mg/L)	0	75	200	EWW	50–100 h	Large individual variability.
Trichloroacetic acid and tri-chloroethanol	Urine (mg/L)	0	300	...	EOS, EWW	...	
Organics: Nitrogen-containing							
Aniline							
p-Aminophenol	Urine (mg/g Cr)	0	50	...	EOS	...	Large individual variability.
Methemoglobin	Blood (%)	1–2	11.5	...	EOS	...	
Dimethylforma-mide							
N-Methylform-amide	Urine (mg/g Cr)	0	20–40	...	EOS	12 h	
Dinitrobenzene							
Methemoglobin	Blood (%)	1–2	5	...	EOS	...	
Ethylene glycol dinitrate	Blood (μg/L)	0	0.2	...	DS	30 min	
Nitrobenzene							
p-Nitrophenol and p-amino-phenol	Urine (mg/g Cr)	0	5	...	EOS, EWW	60 h	
Methemoglobin	Blood (%)	1–2	1.5	...	EOS	...	
Organics: Pesticides							
Organophosphates							
RBC cholinesterase	Blood (% depression)	< 20	< 30	> 40	NC	20–30 d	Levels are % depression from baseline. Symptoms depend on rate of decline in addition to absolute level.
Parathion							
RBC cholines-terase	Blood (% depression)	< 20	< 30	> 40	NC	20–30 d	Reflects chronic exposure.
p-Nitrophenol	Urine (mg/L)	0.01–0.03	0.5	2	EOS	4 h	Reflects recent exposure.
Carbamates							
RBC cholines-terase	Blood (% depression)	< 20	< 30	> 40	EOS	1–2 h	Cholinesterase is reacti-vated very quickly.

Table 36–3. Chemicals for which there are reliable data for determining reference biologic monitoring levels. (continued)

Chemical Determinant[1]	Media (units)	Levels without Occupational Exposure	No Adverse Effect Level	Clinical Effect Level	Timing of Sample[2]	Terminal Half-Time $(t_{1/2})$	Comments
Carbaryl							
RBC cholinesterase	Blood (% depression)	< 20	< 30	> 40	EOS	1–2 h	Cholinesterase is reactivated very quickly.
1-Naphthol	Urine (mg/g Cr)	1.5–4	10	...	EOS	...	
Chlordane	Blood (μg/L)	0	6	3000	...	...	
Dieldrin	Blood (μg/L)	...	150	200–1000	...	...	
Endrin	Blood (μg/L)	0	50		EOS	...	
Anti-12-hydroxy-endrin	Urine (mg/g Cr)	0	130	...	EOS	...	
Hexachlorobenzene	Blood (mg/L)	...	3	...	NC	2 y	
Lindane	Serum (mg/L)	0	20–30	500	...	20 h	

[1]If the laboratory determinant is other than the material itself, it is listed below it in italics.
[2]COHb = carboxyhemoglobin; DS = during shift; EOS = end of shift; EWW = end of work week; L2H = last 2 hours of shift; L4H = last 4 hours of shift; NC = not critical; PNS = prior to next shift; ppd = packs per day; ppm = parts per million; SG = specific gravity; ... = insufficient data.

niques are expanding the utility of biomarker testing in environmental health investigations.

REFERENCES

Harper M: Assessing workplace chemical exposures: The role of exposure monitoring. J Environ Monit 2004;6:404 [PMID: 15152307].

Jakubowski M, Trzcinka-Ochocka M: Biologic monitoring of exposure: Trends and key developments. J Occup Health 2005;47:22 [PMID: 15703450].

Metcalf SW, Orloff KG: Biomarkers of exposure in community settings. J Toxicol Environ Health A 2004;28:715 [PMID: 15192864].

METHODOLOGY

Ideally, the biologic level of a chemical is determined by its rate of absorption, elimination, and metabolism. Unfortunately, many other factors affect the measured level and are potential sources of error.

Timing of Collection

The timing of the sample collection relative to the exposure usually is the most critical methodologic fac-

tor and may be the greatest source of error. For chemicals with a short half-time, the difference between sampling 15 minutes versus 1 hour after the end of exposure may alter the results by as much as a factor of 10.

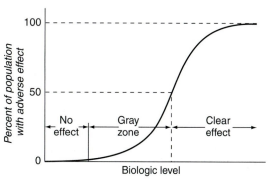

Figure 36–2. Percentage of population demonstrating adverse clinical effects from increasing biologic levels of the chemical.

Collection Methods

Before taking a specimen, it is advisable to consult the laboratory about proper collection methods. Errors in sampling will occur if standard collection methods are not followed. Once collected, chemicals may deteriorate if not analyzed rapidly. The specimens often must be centrifuged or frozen soon after collection. An improper container may bind (adsorb) the chemical of interest or contaminate the specimen (e.g., lead-free glass tubes should be used for measuring blood lead levels). A urine collection can be contaminated from unwashed hands or clothing.

Body Site Sampled

The most frequent sites sampled are blood, urine, and exhaled air. With very rare exceptions, hair analysis is unreliable and should not be used.

A. BLOOD

Blood usually is considered to provide the most accurate assessment of exposure. However, for volatile substances with short half-times, the variation in blood level can be considerable.

Unless otherwise indicated, blood sampling calls for whole venous blood. If the plasma-erythrocyte distribution ratio is not near unity, sampling may call for a serum specimen. The venous sample of a chemical that easily penetrates the skin—for example, nitroglycerin—may reflect skin absorption distal to the sampling site and not total-body exposure.

B. URINE

Urine is the easiest fluid to sample. A 24-hour urine collection provides the most accurate assessment of exposure, but for practical reasons in the workplace setting, the sample usually collected is the spot urine—a single sample collected at a specified time relative to exposure. Unfortunately, significant variation can occur in spot urine levels owing to fluctuation in urine concentrations. This variability may be reduced by adjusting levels to urine specific gravity (SG 1.014) or urine creatinine (1 g of creatinine). This type of standardization should be done on a case-by-case basis. For example, while correcting for urinary creatinine will decrease variability in the assessment of mercury exposure, it appears to have no effect on variability when one is assessing cadmium exposure. In Table 36–3, urine values refer to spot urine levels and, where appropriate, are corrected for specific gravity or creatinine. Highly concentrated (SG > 1.030 or Cr > 3 g/L) or highly dilute spot urine specimens (SG < 1.010 or Cr < 0.3–0.5 g/L) usually are not suitable for monitoring, and a new specimen should be collected. Urine monitoring may not be appropriate for workers with advanced renal disease.

C. EXHALED AIR

Measurements of chemicals in exhaled air are noted in the comments column of Table 36–3 to be either mid-exhaled or end-exhaled air. In general, the concentrations in end-exhaled air during exposure are smaller than in mid-exhaled air, and during postexposure the concentrations in mid-exhaled air are smaller than in end-exhaled air. Workers with emphysema should not be monitored by exhaled air sampling. Sampling must be performed in an area free of the chemical being measured. The process usually involves breathing into a Saran bag that is then exhausted through a charcoal-containing tube.

Selecting a Laboratory

Selection of a laboratory for analysis of specimens generally is the responsibility of the medical supervisor of a biologic monitoring program. Selection should be on the basis of analytic accuracy, convenience, turnaround time, and cost. Analytic accuracy is the most important factor but often is difficult, if not impossible, to assess. The only true assessment of accuracy is an independent intralaboratory and interlaboratory program of quality assurance. This is accomplished by submitting blind samples to laboratories and comparing the results with those of a reference laboratory, followed by certification of laboratories meeting minimum standards. Certification in this way has been implemented on a national basis in the United States only for blood lead determinations.

Determination of cholinesterase levels for state-mandated monitoring of pesticide handlers must be done by state-certified laboratories in California, the only state with such a program. The World Health Organization has conducted an international quality assurance program for blood lead and urine cadmium determinations.

Initial feedback from these testing and certification programs indicates that even the most experienced laboratories can fail to meet minimum standards and that without a regular quality assurance program, analytic quality cannot be ensured. The practitioner responsible for a monitoring program should request data on the laboratory's testing and certification status. It is more common, however, for the practitioner to rely on the use of "experienced" laboratories to produce reliable monitoring results. Analysis of a random sample of "split" specimens by another—preferably a reference—laboratory is an alternative to an internal quality assurance program.

For a number of compounds, the use of specific collection equipment is critical. Many laboratories provide such equipment as a service and may deliver and pick up samples on site. The laboratory should provide information on methods of sample collection, containers, and sources of contamination. Some laboratories have collected biologic specimens from unexposed populations and generated a range of "normal" or "background" levels. Careful attention must be paid to the interpretive information that is provided with the results of a biologic monitoring specimen. For example, some laboratories will reference regulatory levels that are not based on currently known adverse health effects. The amount of assistance and accuracy of information provided should help to indicate the level of experience and expertise of the laboratory in analyzing the compounds of interest.

REFERENCES

Cholinesterase Testing Program, Environmental Health Laboratory Branch (EHLB), California Department of Health Services (CDHS), www.dhs.ca.gov/ps/deodc/ehlb/BioChem/.

OSHA: Approved laboratories (lead), www.osha-slc.gov/SLTC/bloodlead/index.html.

HOW TO USE TABLE 36–3

Selection of Chemicals

Only agents for which there are adequate biologic monitoring studies are included in Table 36–3. Chemicals are arranged in the table first by major chemical group (i.e., metals, other inorganics, organics, etc.). Within each major group, the chemicals are arranged alphabetically.

Under each chemical name is listed the body media (i.e., blood, urine, or breath) in which the chemical or its metabolite can be measured and in what units. Only those media that have been studied adequately are included. The body fluids to be sampled are ranked so that the one with the greatest scientific validity is listed first. For practical reasons, the one ranked highest may not always be the measurement of choice.

Levels without Occupational Exposure

Biologic levels in populations without occupational exposure to that agent usually follow a Poisson distribution (skewed bell shape). The ranges listed in this column will include the majority, or 90%, of the unexposed population. The 5% of the population with the highest levels would be expected to be above this range.

The *National Report on Human Exposure to Environmental Chemicals* provides an assessment of the U.S. population's exposure to environmental chemicals using biomonitoring. This *Third Report* presents exposure information of the 148 chemicals. It provides the data including the concentrations of chemicals by measuring the chemicals or their metabolites in blood or urine. The report also provides general information on each chemical, geometric mean selected percentiles, and the values stratified by gender and age and ethnicity.

REFERENCES

Centers for Disease Control and Prevention (CDC), National Center for Environmental Health (NCEH): *Third National Report on Human Exposure to Environmental Chemicals, 2005,* NCEH publication no. 05-0570, www.cdc.gov/exposurereport.

Scherer G: Biomonitoring of inhaled complex mixtures—ambient air, diesel exhaust and cigarette smoke. Exp Toxicol Pathol 2005;57:75 [PMID: 16092718].

No Adverse Effect Level

This is the level at which almost all workers will be free of symptoms, signs, and adverse clinical laboratory test results. An adverse result is one that reflects end-organ damage. For example, an elevated serum aspartate transaminase (AST) level would be considered an adverse laboratory result, whereas an abnormal serum aminolevulinic acid (ALA) synthetase level would not. A very small number of people with biologic levels below the "no adverse effect" level may have clinical findings. Unless otherwise noted, reproductive or carcinogenic effects of chemicals are not considered in calculating this level.

Only a limited number of chemicals have been studied for the purpose of determining the biologic level associated with absence of adverse health effects. If such data do not exist, the "no adverse effect level" may be based on extrapolation from limit values of environmental monitoring recommended by the American Conference of Governmental Industrial Hygienists (ACGIH) or the National Institute for Occupational Safety and Health (NIOSH). For example, almost all workers exposed to perchloroethylene (a cleaning solvent) below ambient air levels of 100 ppm will fail to experience the irritant and central nervous system depressant properties of perchloroethylene. The corresponding perchloroethylene blood or exhaled air level would be the biologic "no adverse effect" level. This does not take into account the theoretical risk of cancer from animal cancer data. "No adverse effect" levels that have been arrived at by extrapolation from recommended environmental levels are identified with an asterisk.

Biologic exposure indices (BEIs) are reference biologic monitoring levels established by the ACGIH. A BEI is a level that corresponds to the level measured in a worker exposed to a substance at the threshold limit value time-weighted average (TLV-TWA) (see Chapter 35). Where a BEI has been established, it is in essential agreement with Table 36–3 unless otherwise noted in the comments to that table.

Clinical-Effect Level

This is the level that is commonly associated with symptoms, signs, or abnormal laboratory tests. This level is most useful for diagnostic purposes, that is, for evaluating a worker with an abnormal clinical presentation whose degree of exposure is uncertain. For example, the differential diagnosis of a worker exposed to pentachlorophenol includes salicylate poisoning, hyperthyroidism, and pentachlorophenol poisoning. The latter would be confirmed by a blood pentachlorophenol level near or above the clinical-effect level.

Timing of Sample Collection

The interpretation of a biologic level is critically dependent on the timing of sample collection. The following abbreviations are standard times for biologic sample collections and should be considered relative to standard workdays and workweeks. For example, PNS (prior to next shift) means sampling 16 hours after the last shift, and EOS (end of shift) means sampling 15–30 minutes after the last exposure. The time recommendations are most important for the number that appears in the "no adverse effect level" column.

DS	during shift
EOS	end of shift
EWW	end of workweek
L2H	last 2 hours of shift
L4H	last 4 hours of shift
NC	not critical
PNS	prior to next shift

Terminal Half-Time

The rate of elimination of an agent—its *terminal half-time*—is useful for interpreting measured levels relative to the timing of sample collection. If the half-time is short (minutes to hours), the timing of collection is critical. If the half-time is long (days to weeks), the timing of collection is not critical.

Most organic chemicals have two half-times—an initial short half-time and a terminal longer one. The short half-time usually is a measure of the rate at which the solvent equilibrates from the blood to other tissues (e.g., fat, muscle, or brain) and may be very rapid. The terminal half-time more accurately reflects the rate of elimination of the bulk of the chemical from the body.

Biologic levels of chemicals with short half-times should be interpreted with caution when they are evaluated by using an average elimination half-time. The rates of metabolism and elimination may vary significantly between individuals. For example, the average half-time of carboxyhemoglobin is about 5 hours, with a range of 1–8 hours. Consequently, a carboxyhemoglobin level obtained 1 hour after exposure represents somewhere between 50% and 95% of the end-of-shift level depending on the individual's elimination half-time.

ADDITIONAL RESOURCES

Agency for Toxic Substances and Disease Registry: www.atsdr.cdc.gov.

American Academy of Clinical Toxicology (AACT): www.clintox.org.

American College of Medical Toxicology (ACMT): www.acmt.net.

American Conference of Governmental Industrial Hygienists (ACGIH): www.acgih.org/home.htm.

American Industrial Hygiene Association: Biologic monitoring of exposure to organophosphate pesticides: www.aiha.org/aihce02/handouts/62 files/frame.htm.

Association of Public Health Laboratories (APHL): www.aphl.org.

California Department of Health Services (DHS), Occupational Health Branch: www.dhs.ca.gov/ohb.

Health & Safety Executive: www.hse.gov.uk/pubns/indg245.htm.

Massachusetts Division of Occupational Safety: www.state.ma.us/dos/Index.htm.

Clinical and Laboratory Standards Institute (CLSI): www.nccls.org

National Institute of Environmental Health Sciences (NIEHS): www.niehs.nih.gov.

National Institute for Occupational Safety and Health (NIOSH): www.cdc.gov/niosh/homepage.html.

New Jersey Environmental and Occupational Health: www.state.nj.us/health/eoh/survweb/.

OSHA: Cadmium biologic monitoring advisor: www.osha.gov/dts/osta/oshasoft/gocad2.html.

US Environmental Protection Agency (EPA): www.epa.gov/.

SECTION VI
Environmental Health

| Environmental Exposures & Controls | 37 |

Gina Solomon, MD, MPH, Joseph LaDou, MS, MD, & Catharina Wesseling, MD, PhD

As globalization has transformed developing countries into newly industrialized countries, environmental pollution has developed on a global scale never before encountered. The experience with the costs of environmental programs is that a very substantial financial burden is being shifted from developed countries to newly industrialized countries. The cost of future industrial accidents, mitigation of environmental damage, and effects on the public health, are not often discussed with candor. The greatest challenge of contemporary occupational and environmental medicine is in the international arena, and environmental health is a central issue.

Pollution of air and water, contamination of food, releases from nearby industrial facilities or waste sites, and environmental hazards in the home environment are all common causes for concern among patients, community members, and public health officials. Physicians today increasingly are called on to address questions or problems related to environmental health. All physicians must understand the effects of common environmental exposures and the similarities and differences between environmental health and occupational health.

THE MAGNITUDE OF ENVIRONMENTAL CONTAMINATION

All nations are faced with problems of environmental contamination, and the developing countries are beginning to realize the extent of these difficulties as their industrialization progresses. In the United States, more than 4 billion pounds of toxic chemicals were released by industry into the nation's environment in 2004, including nearly 72 million pounds of recognized carcinogens. At least two-thirds of the U.S. population live in areas where toxic chemicals pose an elevated cancer risk. About 11 million people in the United States, including 3–4 million children, live within 1 mile of a federal Superfund site.

The air in urban areas is heavily polluted by the annual release of hundreds of millions of pounds of hazardous air pollutants such as xylene, toluene, and benzene, as well as by criteria air pollutants such as ozone and particulate matter. At least 20 million Americans live in areas where their lifetime cancer risk simply from breathing ambient air exceeds 1 in 10,000. Mobile sources such as cars and trucks contribute more than three-quarters of the total risk. Approximately 170 million people live in counties where monitored air in 2003 was unhealthy at times because of high levels of at least one of the six criteria air pollutants.

In the United States, more than 4000 water systems used by more than 20 million people violate Environmental Protection Agency (EPA) drinking water standards for at least one contaminant. Drinking water may contain volatile organic compounds, pesticides, nitrates, arsenic, and pathogens. Traditional water treatment, designed primarily for purposes of infection control, often is ineffective against chemical contaminants.

The vast size of the exposed population and the proliferation of new materials with unknown effects introduced by advancing technology have made it critical that we find some means of controlling the possible deleterious health effects of environmental contaminants. Unfortunately, we know little about what these effects will be, particularly over the long term, and epidemiologic studies—our primary source of information—cannot answer many of our questions.

Pollution is particularly critical in developing countries, where unsafe water, poor sanitation and hygiene, indoor air pollution, urban air pollution, agricultural pesticides, and toxic waste constitute important environmental health threats. Poverty and short-term survival needs go hand in hand with the use of outdated hazardous technologies and poor legal enforcement, all this underscored by international double standards and dumping practices. The global disease burden owing to environmental pollution has been estimated at 8–9%, being considerably higher in developing countries. Environmental degradation in the developing world is also of special concern because the natural ecosystems are the basis for the economies of many developing countries, for example, through ecotourism, and many people depend on the diversity in these ecosystems for food, energy, and natural medicines. Their loss places these people at risk for hunger, the worst of all environmental health threats.

REFERENCES

Cohen AJ et al: The global burden of disease due to outdoor air pollution. J Toxicol Environ Health A 2005;68:1301 [PMID: 16024504].

Environmental Defense scorecard, www.scorecard.org/.

EPA: Drinking water and ground water statistics for 2006, www.epa.gov/safewater.

EPA: Hazardous waste facts, www.epa.gov/epaoswer/osw/basifact.htm.

Ezzati M et al: Environmental risks in the developing world. J Epidemiol Commun Health 2005;59:15 [PMID: 15598721].

MAJOR ISSUES IN ENVIRONMENTAL MEDICINE

Although workplace exposures to industrial chemicals often are far higher than environmental pollution levels, the latter still may be a significant concern. Lower-level exposures are an issue when the size of the exposed population is sufficient to suggest that even rare or subtle health effects may have public health importance. For example, a chemical that confers a cancer risk at environmental exposure levels of 1 extra case per 100,000 people is of considerable importance when the base population exposed includes millions of people.

While many workers in chemically exposed industries are healthy adult males, the general population includes pregnant women, young children, those with underlying disease, and the elderly. Each of these groups may face increased risk from lower environmental levels of exposure. Children, for example, may be more exposed to contaminants because they breathe more air, drink more water, and eat more food per kilogram of body weight than do adults. In addition, toddlers engage in frequent hand-to-mouth activity, meaning that they may be exposed to contaminants (such as lead or pesticides) in dust and dirt. Young children are more susceptible to long-term damage from neurotoxicants because of the critical phases of brain development in infancy. Finally, a child has a lifetime to manifest delayed health effects, and low-level exposures to carcinogens such as ionizing radiation have been shown to be more likely to cause cancer when the exposure occurs in childhood.

Environmental health often is difficult to assess because of difficulties in designing and carrying out studies to pinpoint subtle toxic effects from specific exposures in the general population. Frequently the only data available are from animal toxicology tests, and these results often are used in risk assessments in an attempt to quantify risk to sensitive members of the public. Risk assessment, although based on scientific principles, is subject to judgment and is criticized by both industry and environmental health advocates as being either overprotective or insufficiently protective of public health.

Environmental epidemiology is a challenge because of inevitable problems of study design, including selection of appropriate control groups, difficulties with exposure assessment, and issues related to confounding by multiple low-level exposures. Prospective cohort studies are rare, and many epidemiologic studies simply do not have the statistical power to reliably detect a small effect that may be of public health relevance.

Clinicians may encounter patients known to have been exposed to an environmental toxicant or who believe that they may have sustained such an exposure. In some cases, an entire community may become concerned because of a natural or human disaster or because of a new discovery such as contaminants in the water supply or an apparent disease cluster. These situations require a careful evaluation, including a thorough exposure history and quantification, where possible, of exposure levels. Principles of thoughtful risk communication are important in environmental exposure situations. Risk is perceived differently by scientists, industry experts, government regulators, and community groups. Often there is no fully objective way to evaluate risk, and the physician should listen seriously to the community viewpoint and be available as a fair and honest resource for information.

New issues in environmental health include a rapidly evolving ability to test for a wide range of contaminants in biologic samples. Although tests for a wide range of pesticides, phthalates, volatile organics, and other compounds are not yet widely available, ongoing research spearheaded by the Centers for Disease Control and Prevention (CDC) is developing normative data for a range of contaminants in blood and urine. These assays are revolutionizing research and soon may contribute to patient care. Environmental health also is refocusing from acute toxicity and cancer to a more careful consideration of delayed functional effects such as endocrine disruption, developmental toxicity, and neurotoxicity.

New technologies and methods of assessing human exposure to chemicals, dietary and lifestyle factors, infectious agents, and other stressors provide an opportunity to extend the range of human health investigations and advance our understanding of the relationship between environmental exposure and disease. The methods use environmental sensors, geographic information systems, biologic sensors, toxicogenomics, and body-burden (biologic) measurements. Improved methods for exposure assessment will result in better means of monitoring and targeting intervention and prevention programs. New techniques are evolving for evaluation of risks to susceptible subpopulations, including attention to gene-environment interactions. Opportunities exist for applying the tools of genomics to clinical and public health research, especially for conditions with known or suspected environmental causes. This research is likely to lead to population-wide health-promotion and disease-prevention efforts. Ethical, legal, and social issues are becoming increasingly more complex as genetic and molecular techniques are used to study environmental toxicants and their potential influence on human and ecologic health.

In addition, researchers are giving attention to the problem of mixtures and combined chemical exposures in environmental settings. The need for studies on chemical mixtures has been proposed as one of the six priority areas the CDC identified in its agenda for public health environmental research. The five other priority research areas the agency identified are exposure, susceptible populations, community and tribal involvement, evaluation and surveillance of health effects, and health promotion/prevention.

Precautionary Principle

The precautionary principle, proposed as a new guideline in environmental decision making, has four central components: taking preventive action in the face of uncertainty, shifting the burden of proof to the proponents of an activity, exploring a wide range of alternatives to possibly harmful actions, and increasing public participation in decision making. Scientists in many fields have recognized the need for innovative approaches and tools to address increasingly complex, uncertain risks on a global scale.

The precautionary principle recently has been formally introduced into national and international law. The key element is the justification for acting in the face of uncertainty. The precautionary principle is a tool for avoiding possible future harm associated with suspected, but not conclusive, environmental risks. Under the precautionary principle, the burden of proof is shifted from demonstrating the presence of risk to demonstrating the absence of risk, and it is the responsibility of the producer of a technology to demonstrate its safety rather than the responsibility of public authorities to show harm. Past experiences demonstrate the costly consequences of disregarding early warnings about environmental hazards. New research is needed to expand current insight into disease causation, to elucidate the full scope of potential adverse implications resulting from environmental pollutants, and to identify opportunities for prevention.

REFERENCES

ATSDR: Primer for health risk communication principles and practices, www.atsdr.cdc.gov/HEC/primer.html.

Brulle RJ, Pellow DN: Environmental justice: Human health and environmental inequalities. Annu Rev Public Health 2006;27:103 [PMID: 16533111].

CDC: Third national report on human exposure to environmental chemicals, July 2005, www.cdc.gov/exposurereport/3rd/.

Goldstein BD: Advances in risk assessment and communication. Annu Rev Public Health 2005;26:141 [PMID: 15760284].

Khoury MJ et al: Do we need genomic research for the prevention of common diseases with environmental causes? Am J Epidemiol 2005;161:799 [PMID: 15840611].

Pirkle JL et al: National exposure measurements for decisions to protect public health from environmental exposures. Int J Hyg Environ Health 2005;208:1 [PMID: 15881972].

Saunders P: A discussion of precautionary tools for reshaping environmental policy. Environ Health Perspect 2006;114:254 [PMID: 16581532].

Weis BK et al: Personalized exposure assessment: promising approaches for human environmental health research. Environ Health Perspect 2005;113:840 [PMID: 16002370].

PRIMARY SOURCES OF CONTAMINATION

The world's environmental challenge is evident from the growth in energy demand. Global energy demand—excluding the 1.6 billion people dependent on biomass in the developing world—is at present 9.2 billion tons of oil equivalent. It will increase to 15.3 billion by 2030. Oil, gas, and coal account for around 85 percent of the total and are projected to account for at least as much in 2030.

Population growth and rising standards of living invariably are accompanied by increases in energy generation. The burning of coal, oil, and wood adds to the global burden of pollution and provides an explanation for the greenhouse effect now recognized as an ecologic disaster in the making. China and India, as they expand their industrial production and increase the standard of living of their citizens, will add significantly to world energy demands. Total energy demand in Asian developing economies will double by 2030 and represent half the world consumption.

The environmental impact of fossil fuel use on the climate is proven beyond doubt to the vast majority of environmental scientists. Climate change is having a profound impact on the global environment. The effects will include major shifts in agriculture, sea-level rise, changes in the distribution of diseases, and extreme weather conditions with droughts in some areas and hurricanes causing floods and landslides in others. These phenomena have profound political and humanitarian implications, particularly for the poorer countries. The response to global warming by the governments of countries that consume the most energy has been inadequate. Global warming may have been beyond reversal long before Kyoto, but the recalcitrance of many governments has ensured that the effects are likely to be greater than if early action had been taken.

Environmental contamination arises from a combination of heavy industry, small industry, agriculture, and mobile sources. Chemical manufacturing, power plants, incinerators, pulp and paper milling, petroleum production, textile manufacturing, mining, and metal smelting are major point sources of pollution. Small sources such as dry cleaners, gas stations, and electroplating shops can create significant pollution problems in local areas. Mobile sources, including gasoline and diesel engines, are a growing part of the overall pollution problem, and for some pollutants such as particulate matter, ozone, and aromatic organics, mobile sources eclipse all others. Biomass accounts for about one-third of all energy, and nearly 90% in some of the least-developed countries. Wood burning is highly inefficient with high CO_2 emissions, contributing to both climate change and the depletion of natural resources. The indoor environment also deserves special consideration because many contaminants have been shown to concentrate inside buildings and vehicles. Consumer product use also can result in direct or airborne exposures or can create residues that sometimes linger for a significant time in carpets, where they may result in exposures to toddlers. Carpet dust has been shown to be a dominant exposure pathway for children in the case of lead, pesticides, and polycyclic aromatic hydrocarbons (PAHs).

Modern agriculture is a major contributor to environmental contamination through the extensive use of pesticides and fertilizers, spray drift into nearby communities, irrigation and damming projects, and conversion of the remaining natural reserves of the earth into pasture and agricultural lands. Unsustainable agriculture leads to groundwater and surface water pollution, eutrophication of water resources, acidification and salinization of soils or waters, bioaccumulation of toxins in the food chain, pesticide resistance, biodiversity losses, and directly and indirectly to human health degradation.

REFERENCES

Intergovernmental Panel on Climate Change, www.ipcc.ch.

Morgan MG et al: Learning from the US national assessment of climate change impacts. Environ Sci Technol 2005;39:9023 [PMID: 16382921].

UNDP Energy and Environment, www.undp.org/energyandenvironment and www.undp.org/biodiversity/pdfs/CCF_Report_2005_final.pdf.

US Department of Energy, Office of Scientific & Technical Information, www.osti.gov/energyfiles.

MAJOR ENVIRONMENTAL CONTAMINANTS

Asbestos

Asbestos is a general term applied to certain fibrous minerals long popular for their thermal resistance, tensile strength, and acoustic insulation properties. Asbestos minerals are divided into two groups: serpentine and amphibole. There is only one type of asbestos derived from serpentine minerals, chrysotile, also known as *white asbestos.*

More than 30 million tons of asbestos in its various forms have been mined in the past century. More than 2 million tons of chrysotile are mined and shipped around the world each year. Asbestos industry advocates allege that amphibole groups are the fibers with the greater risk for lung cancer and that chrysotile can be handled safely. Actually, on a per-fiber basis, the highest risks of lung cancer have been shown for chrysotile.

Asbestos is one of the most pervasive environmental hazards in the world, present in more than 3000 manufactured products. All forms of asbestos can result in asbestosis, lung cancer, and mesothelioma.

Asbestos exposure affects not only asbestos workers but also their families, users of asbestos products, and the public exposed to building materials and asbestos in heating and ventilating systems. In developing countries, where protection of workers and communities is scanty or nonexistent, the asbestos cancer epidemic may be even more devastating than it has been in the developed countries. Worldwide, about 20–40% of adult men report some past jobs that may have entailed asbestos exposures. In the most affected age groups, mesothelioma may account for 1% of all deaths. In addition to mesotheliomas, 5–7% of all lung cancers can be attributable to occupational exposures to asbestos. The asbestos cancer epidemic may take as many as 10 million lives before asbestos is banned worldwide and exposures are brought to an end.

Today, the largest asbestos producers are Russia, China, Canada, Kazakhstan, Brazil, and Zimbabwe. Canada dominates world trade sales with an annual export of about 300,000 tons of chrysotile asbestos. Over 70% of the world production is used in Eastern Europe, Latin America, and Asia, in countries desperate for industry and naive to the health effects of occupational and environmental exposures to asbestos. Brazil, China, India, Japan, Russia, and Thailand account for more than 80% of the world's apparent consumption of asbestos.

The only way to ensure an end to the asbestos cancer epidemic is to ban asbestos mining and to ban all asbestos manufacture. This approach, which has been taken in many developed countries, is even more necessary in developing countries, where enforcement of health and safety regulations is not a viable alternative to a ban. There is no indication at this time that a global ban on asbestos is likely to be accepted by all countries, and international enforcement of a ban on asbestos is unlikely to occur. In developing countries, where little or no protection of workers and communities is taking place, the asbestos cancer epidemic may be even more devastating and continue indefinitely.

REFERENCES

ATSDR: Asbestos exposure and your health, www.atsdr.cdc.gov/asbestos/index.html.

LaDou J: The asbestos cancer epidemic. Environ Health Perspect 2004;112:285 [PMID: 14998741].

Landrigan PJ, Soffritti M: Collegium Ramazzini call for an international ban on asbestos. Am J Indust Med 2005;47:471 [PMID: 1589809].

Lemen RA: Chrysotile asbestos as a cause of mesothelioma: Application of the Hill causation model. Int J Occup Environ Health 2004;10:233 [PMID: 15281385].

Tossavainen A: Global use of asbestos and the incidence of mesothelioma. Int J Occup Environ Health 2004;10:22 [PMID: 15070022].

Lead

Toxic lead exposure accounts for the most significant and prevalent disease of environmental origin in the world today. Despite all that is known regarding the hazards of lead exposure for young children, it has taken more than a century for primary prevention to be adopted in the most highly developed countries. The rest of the world is woefully behind in the development of programs to protect children from lead poisoning. The phasing out of lead in gasoline in the United States has resulted in an approximately eightfold reduction in median blood lead levels in children. The demonstrable success and social benefits of preventing lead exposure are inarguable.

Lead is a heavy metal that is not biodegradable. It is indestructible and cannot be transformed into a nontoxic form. Worldwide mining each year produces nearly 3 million tons of lead. Well over half the 300 million tons of lead ever removed from the earth has been released as contamination and is available to human exposure.

The ever-increasing global use of lead is occurring at a time when lead uses in gasoline, canning, and paints are restricted or banned in most developed countries. Lead is used increasingly in storage batteries and other electronic equipment, major areas of international economic growth. The greatest global demand for lead has occurred in Asia over the past 20 years.

Lead is absorbed and largely deposited in bone. Although lead serves no useful physiologic purpose, lead stays in the body for many years. Young children and fetuses are especially vulnerable to the toxic effects of lead. Lead impairs brain development in children, retarding mental and physical development and causing behavioral and learning disabilities. Lead exposure demonstrably lowers intelligence quotients (IQs) in school-age children. A 10 µg/dL increase in blood lead is associated with a 2.5-point decrease in the IQ of exposed children. Although a slight decrease in IQ may not seem like much on an individual basis, across a population, such a decrement results in a substantial increase in the number of children falling into categories that require special education. More recent research links elevated lead levels in childhood to behavior disorders in older children and teens, including delinquency and criminal behavior.

The U.S. Centers for Disease Control and Prevention (CDC) designates a blood lead level of 10 µg/dL as a threshold of concern in children and 20 µg/dL as a level requiring medical intervention. Despite these guidance numbers, however, there is no blood lead level above zero that has not been shown to cause adverse neurologic effects in children.

The CDC estimates that 310,000 children aged 1–5 in the United States have blood lead levels at or above 10 µg/dL. Blood lead levels of urban populations, especially children, often reach alarmingly high levels. It is estimated that among urban children in developing countries, 100% of those younger than 2 years of age and more than 80% of those between the ages of 3 and 5 years have blood lead levels greater than 10 µg/dL. Preliminary studies show that blood lead levels of virtually all children in Africa and Latin America exceed 10 µg/dL.

Lead is also toxic to adults in concentrations once thought to be safe. Several studies relate increased blood pressure and hypertension in adults to elevated blood lead levels. This, in turn, increases the risk of cardiovascular disease. The impact of lead on blood pressure, a major risk factor for coronary artery disease and stroke, is seen at levels quite prevalent in the general population. A review of available studies indicates that a 1-μg increase in ambient lead concentrations may cause substantial increases in hypertension, nonfatal heart attacks, and premature deaths. Other health effects in adults associated with environmental lead exposure include accelerated cognitive decline in the elderly, cataracts, and dental caries.

The use of lead in gasoline, uncontrolled point sources such as smelters, lead in plumbing, and lead solder in food canning are major sources of lead exposure in many countries. Lead is used around the world for bullets and other ammunition. There is no reliable estimate of the amount of lead introduced into the environment by military training, wars, hunting, and target practice. Ceramic containers and cooking vessels with lead paint or glazes are important sources of lead poisoning. Old lead-based paint and lead in soil from historical use of leaded gasoline are the most important sources of lead exposure for children in the United States. Lead is found in a number of consumer products, children's toys, jewelry, cosmetics, candy, and folk remedies.

Lead is far from necessary for many of its current industrial applications. Substitution has reduced the use of lead in building construction, electrical cable covering, cans, and containers. Aluminum, tin, iron, and plastics compete with lead in other packaging and protective coatings, and tin has replaced lead in solder for new or replacement potable water systems in the United States.

Exposure to lead causes an economic loss to society. The reduction of intellectual performance results in reduced productivity and diminished lifetime earnings. Children with learning disabilities may require special assistance. Adults with cardiovascular problems lose work days, require medical care, and may die prematurely. In the United States, for example, the benefits of phasing out lead are estimated to outweigh the costs by more than 10 times.

In the European Union, since July 1, 2003, electronics products have not been allowed to deliberately contain lead, mercury, cadmium, or hexavalent chromium. Lead was classified as category 1, toxic to reproduction (embryotoxic), and as a precaution, the EU classified lead chromate pigments as category 3 carcinogens.

REFERENCES

American Academy of Pediatrics Committee on Environmental Health: Lead exposure in children: Prevention, detection, and management. Pediatrics 2005;116:1036 [PMID: 16199720].

ATSDR: Public health statement for lead, www.atsdr.cdc.gov/toxprofiles/phs13.html.

CDC Childhood Lead Poisoning Prevention Program, www.cdc.gov/nceh/lead/lead.htm.

Global Lead Network, www.globalleadnet.org/.

Ozkaynak H et al: Exposure assessment implications for the design and implementation of the National Children's Study. Environ Health Perspect 2005;113:1108 [PMID: 16079086].

Pirkle JL et al: National exposure measurements for decisions to protect public health from environmental exposures. Int J Hyg Environ Health 2005;208:1 [PMID: 15881972].

Schwartz BS et al: Occupational lead exposure and longitudinal decline in neurobehavioral test scores. Epidemiology 2005;16:106 [PMID: 15613953].

Tsaih SW et al: Lead, diabetes, hypertension, and renal function: The normative aging study. Environ Health Perspect 2004;112:1178 [PMID: 15289163].

Organic Mercury

Mercury is a heavy metal that persists in the environment. It is mined and used widely or emitted by industry in the metallic or inorganic forms. Once discharged into the environment, mercury may travel long distances on air currents but eventually will wash into water bodies. Bacteria in the sediments absorb the mercury and methylate the metal. Methyl mercury then can concentrate by thousands of fold as it makes its way up the food chain into fish that then are consumed by people. Methyl mercury was the toxic agent responsible for the mass poisoning in the 1950s in Minamata, Japan, where an industrial facility released mercury into the bay in its wastewater. The mercury accumulated in the fish, the main source of protein in this community.

Mercury is a potent neurotoxin, and exposure to methyl mercury can cause symptoms such as paresthesia, blurred vision, malaise, speech difficulties, and constriction of the visual fields. More recent research has shown associations between mercury at lower environmental exposure levels and increased risk of cardiovascular disease and myocardial infarction. When women are exposed to methyl mercury during pregnancy, even low-dose exposures can cause developmental toxicity. Infants born in Minamata during the epidemic had mental retardation, ataxia, blindness, and cerebral palsy, even when their mothers showed minimal symptoms. Very low-level exposures can cause subtle delays in attention span, learning, memory, language acquisition, and visuospatial and motor skills in infants and children. Recent studies in a cohort of children followed since birth found associations between prenatal mercury exposure and abnormalities in brain stem auditory evoked potentials, as well as abnormal cardiac autonomic activity, in these children at age 14.

The EPA currently defines a safe upper limit (reference dose) for dietary methyl mercury exposure at 0.1 μg/kg per day. Because of the relatively high levels of mercury in fish such as tuna and swordfish, a pregnant woman would exceed the EPA reference dose after eating more than about 1.5 ounces of swordfish or 7 ounces of canned albacore tuna per week. Data from the CDC suggest that about 6% of women of reproductive age in the United States may exceed recommended exposure limits.

There are alternatives for many current uses of mercury. For example, chloralkali facilities can use membrane diffusion processes that do not require mercury as a catalyst. Thermometers, sphygmomanometers, switches, and thermostats increasingly are manufactured without mercury. Mercury generation from incinerators and coal-fired power plants can be reduced through source elimination or after-treatment devices.

Mercury is an enormous problem in the Amazon basin and in Africa as a result of gold-mining activities. Mercury is used widely in mining because of its ability to amalgamate with gold. This use can result in direct discharges to water and rapid bioaccumulation in fish. In addition, slash and burn agricultural practices in the Amazon have resulted in deforestation and erosion with leaching of mercury into the water sources. The dramatic increase in mercury pollution in the Amazon is creating an environmental health disaster that likely will dwarf that of Minamata Bay.

REFERENCES

Booth S, Zeller D: Mercury, food webs, and marine mammals: Implications of diet and climate change for human health. Environ Health Perspect 2005;113:521 [PMID: 15866757].

Canuel R et al: New evidence on variations of human body burden of methylmercury from fish consumption. Environ Health Perspect 2006;114:302 [PMID: 16451872].

Davidson PW et al: Mercury exposure and child development outcomes. Pediatrics 2004;113:1023 [PMID: 15060195].

EPA: Home page for mercury-related issues, www.epa.gov/mercury/.

Needham LL et al: Concentrations of environmental chemicals associated with neurodevelopmental effects in US population. Neurotoxicology 2005;26:531 [PMID: 16112319].

Stern AH: A revised probabilistic estimate of the maternal methyl mercury intake dose corresponding to a measured cord blood mercury concentration. Environ Health Perspect 2005;113:155 [PMID: 15687052].

Inorganic Arsenic

Inorganic arsenic is a common environmental contaminant of major worldwide concern. Although industrial and mining activities have caused widespread contamination, naturally occurring arsenic is also a problem in drinking-water sources throughout the world. Wells in countries such as Bangladesh, parts of India, Chile, and Taiwan have caused epidemics of illness among local inhabitants. Taiwanese blackfoot disease is caused by arsenic contamination in wells, resulting in peripheral vascular disease. Nearly 150 million people in Bangladesh and West Bengal, India, have been exposed to very high levels of arsenic in water because of contaminated wells that were drilled by an international relief effort to provide a safe water supply for villages. The deep aquifer tapped by the wells is not contaminated with pathogens, but unfortunately, it runs through arsenic-bearing rock. Thousands of villagers in these regions, including children, exhibit the characteristic skin changes of arsenic poisoning, neuropathy, and early-onset cancers. Even at levels more than an order of magnitude lower than those found in Bangladesh and other highly contaminated areas, arsenic poses a significant cancer risk. In the United States, an estimated 12 million people consume water containing more than 10 ppb arsenic. The National Academy of Sciences estimates that such a level could confer a cancer risk as high as 1 in 500.

Arsenic has been used for more than a century as a pesticide, sometimes in the form of lead arsenate, although this use is banned in many countries. Chromium copper arsenate (CCA) is still used in the United States as a wood preservative, and CCA-treated wood has been used to build decks, playground equipment, picnic tables, and fences. CCA-treated wood has been withdrawn from consumer use recently but still will be available for use by professionals. Arsenic is also a key ingredient in the manufacture of silicon wafers in the semiconductor industry. Although this use is generally considered to be an occupational risk, there is the potential for accidental emissions of arsine gas from these facilities, as well as potential discharges into water.

Arsenic is a known human carcinogen. Inorganic arsenic is known to cause bladder, lung, and skin cancer and also may cause kidney and liver cancers. Arsenic also can cause neurotoxicity, cardiovascular disease, and hyperkeratosis and scaling of the skin—particularly of the palms and soles. Some research indicates that environmental arsenic exposure also may be associated with an increased risk of diabetes mellitus. In several studies, arsenic also has been linked to birth defects, lower birth weight, and male reproductive toxicity. Children apparently are less able to detoxify and eliminate arsenic efficiently compared with adults.

In the United States, the drinking-water standard for arsenic was set at 50 ppb in 1942, before arsenic was known to cause cancer. An effort to update the health standard began in 1962. In 2001, after decades of regulatory development, public comment, research, and at least three missed statutory deadlines, the EPA finally issued a new 10-ppb standard.

REFERENCES

ATSDR: Toxicological profile for arsenic, www.atsdr.cdc.gov/toxprofiles/tp2.html.

Kalia K, Flora SJ: Strategies for safe and effective therapeutic measures for chronic arsenic and lead poisoning. J Occup Health 2005;47:1 [PMID: 15703449].

Katz SA, Salem H: Chemistry and toxicology of building timbers pressure-treated with chromated copper arsenate: A review. J Appl Toxicol 2005;25:1 [PMID: 15669035].

Smith AH, Smith MM: Arsenic drinking water regulations in developing countries with extensive exposure. Toxicology 2004; 198:39 [PMID: 15138028].

Endocrine-Disrupting Chemicals

In the mid-1990s, scientists from various fields of research began to realize that they were all seeing toxic effects on the endocrine system from environmental exposures. Some common chemicals were found to bind to the estrogen receptor and cause transcriptional activation in a manner that mimics estrogen itself. Some of these chemicals also cause breast cancer cells to proliferate in vitro, thereby confirming an estrogenic effect. Many of these same chemicals also were found to cause hormonally related developmental disorders in laboratory animals or in wildlife living in contaminated areas.

Although there was initial skepticism about the theory that environmental chemicals could cause endocrine disruption in animals and humans, the existence of this problem is now a matter of general consensus. A rapidly increasing number of chemicals or their degradation products are being recognized as weakly estrogenic or as possessing other hormonal activities. Hormonally active agents can occur naturally in the diet, such as the phytoestrogens coumestrol and genistein, or from industrial processes (Table 37–1). Exogenous industrial chemicals or pesticides have been found to mimic or block estrogen, androgens, thyroid hormone, and hypothalamic and pituitary hormones. Thyroid disruptors have received special attention because subclinical hypothyroidism during brain development is known to cause neurologic deficits. Irreversible damage can occur during prenatal and early postnatal development in organs that respond to endocrine signals. In addition, endocrine-disrupting chemicals that accumulate in body fat can be mobilized during pregnancy or lactation, giving rise to transgenerational effects. Chemicals that are known endocrine disruptors include some pharmaceuticals, some pesticides, and some chemicals in detergents and plastics. Two important endocrine-disrupting chemical groups are the dioxins and polychlorinated biphenyls (PCBs). These are addressed in more detail below.

There is considerable controversy over the public health importance of endocrine-disrupting agents. While some observers assert that the exposure levels are low and that there are few documented human health effects, others point out that hormones can be active at very low doses and are particularly sensitive to perturbation during fetal development. Some public health experts point to documented increases in potentially hormone-related disorders in the general population such as hypospadias, cryptorchidism, and various cancers of the reproductive organs. These increases remain unexplained, and parallel health effects are observed from some endocrine disruptors in laboratory animals and wildlife.

REFERENCES

Colborn T: Neurodevelopment and endocrine disruption. Environ Health Perspect 2004;112:944 [PMID: 15198913].

Environmental Estrogens and Other Hormones Web site, www.tmc.tulane.edu/ECME/eehome/.

Trubo R: Endocrine-disrupting chemicals probed as potential pathways to illness. JAMA. 2005;294:291 [PMID: 16030264].

Vidaeff AC: In utero exposure to environmental estrogens and male reproductive health: A systematic review of biological and epidemiologic evidence. Reprod Toxicol 2005;20:5 [PMID: 15808781].

Dioxins and Furans

Dioxins and furans are a group of environmentally persistent chlorinated organic chemicals. Dioxin congeners differ in toxicity according to the number and placement of chlorine atoms on the two six-carbon rings. Furans are closely related to dioxins in structure and toxicity. Dioxins and furans with chlorine substitutions in the 2, 3, 7, and 8 positions are the most toxic. By international agreement, the dioxins, furans, and even the dioxin-like PCBs are grouped together, and their relative toxicity is summed into 2,3,7,8-tetrachlorodibenzodioxin (TCDD) toxic equivalents (TEQs). When the singular word *dioxin* is used, it refers to these 2,3,7,8-TCDD TEQs.

Dioxin is one of the most toxic substances known. It has adverse biologic effects at doses measured in picograms. Moreover, it is highly stable in the environment, is lipophilic, and bioaccumulates by thousands of fold as it moves up the food chain. It was distributed widely in herbicides throughout the United States and was a contaminant of the defoliant Agent Orange [a mixture of equal parts of 2,4-D (2,4-dichlorophenoxyacetic acid) and 2,4,5-T (2,4,5-trichlorophenoxyacetic acid)], used during the Vietnam War. Dioxins also are released from many industrial sources, including incinerators, power plants, cement kilns, pulp and paper mills, refineries, and diesel engines. Dioxins are also trace contaminants in other chemicals, including the wood preservative pentachlorophenol and potentially in the common topical disinfectant triclosan. Dioxins may be formed in the incineration of municipal solid waste, sewage sludge, and hospital and household waste. Some dioxins are released in forest fires and, possibly, volcanic eruptions. Furans share many of these sources, and human exposures also can result from pyrolysis of polychlorinated biphenyls (PCBs) and explosions of electrical transformers. Except in the case of industrial acci-

Table 37–1. Chemicals in the environment reported to have reproductive and/or endocrine-disrupting effects.

Herbicides
2,4-D (2,4-dichlorophenoxyacetic acid)
2,4,5,-T (2,4,5-trichlorophenoxyacetic acid)
Acetochlor
Alachlor
Amitrole
Atrazine
Bromacil
Bromoxynil
Cyanazine
DCPA (Dacthal)
Ethiozin
Glufosinate-ammonium
Ioxynil
Linuron
Metribuzin
Methyl bromide
Molinate
Nitrofen
Oryzalin
Oxyacetamide/fluthamide (FOE 5043)
Paraquat
Pendimethalin
Picloram
Prodiamine
Pronamide
Simazine
Terbutryn
Thiazopyr
Trichlorobenzene
Trifluralin

Fungicides
Benomyl
Carbendazim
Etridiazole
Fenarimol
Fenbuconazole
Hexachlorobenzene
Mancozeb
Maneb
Metiram
Nabam
Pentachloronitrobenzene
Triadimefon
Tributyltin
Vinclozolin
Zineb
Ziram

Insecticides
Aldrin
Bifenthrin

Carbaryl
Carbofuran
Chlordane
Chlordecone
Chlorfentezine
γ-Cyhalothrin
DDT (dichlorodiphenyltrichloroethane) and metabo-
    lites (DDE [dichlorodiphenylichloroethylene], DDD
    [dichlorodiphenyldichloroethane])
Deltamethrin
Diazinon
Dibromoethane
Dicofol
Dieldrin
Dimethoate
Dinitrophenol
Endosulfan (α and β)
Endrin
Ethofenprox
Fenchlorfos (Ronnel)
Fenitrothion
Fenvalerate
Fipronil
β-HCH (hexachlorocyclohexane)
Heptachlor and H-epoxide
Lindane (γ-HCH)
Malathion
Methomyl
Methoxychlor
Mirex
Oxychlordane
Parathion (methylparathion)
Photomirex
Pyrethrins
Synthetic pyrethroids
Toxaphene
Transnonachlor

Nematocides
Aldicarb
DBCP

Rodenticides
n-2-Fluorenylacetamide

Pesticide By-products and Additives
Ethylene thiourea (ETU)
Pentachlorobenzene
Piperonyl butoxide

Industrial Chemicals
4-OH-alkylphenol
Aluminum

(continued)

Table 37–1. Chemicals in the environment reported to have reproductive and/or endocrine-disrupting effects. (continued)

Industrial Chemicals, Cont.	2,2′,4,4′-tetrachlorobiphenyl (PCB 47)
Arsenic	2,2′,4,5′-tetrachlorobiphenyl (PCB 48)
Benzopyrene	2,2′,5,5′-tetrachlorobiphenyl (PCB 52)
Bisphenol-A	2,3,4,5-tetrachlorobiphenyl (PCB 61)
4-hydroxybiphenyl	2,4,4′,6-tetrachlorobiphenyl (PCB 75)
t-butylhydroxyanisole (BHA)	3,3′,4,4′-tetrachlorobiphenyl (PCB 77)
Cadmium	PCB Aroclor 1242
Carbon disulfide	PCB Aroclor 1248
Dioxins	PCB Aroclor 1254
1,2,3,7,8-pentachlorodibenzodioxin	PCB Aroclor 1260
2,3,7,8-tetrachlorodibenzo-*p*-dioxin (TCDD)	2 to 4-OH 2′,5′ dichlorobiphenyl
Epichlorohydrin	2,3,4 trichlorobiphenyl
Furans	4-OH trichlorobiphenyls (2,2′,5,2′,4,′6′)
1,2,3,7,8-pentabromodibenzofuran	Polybromodiphenyl ether (PBDE)
1,2,3,7,8-pentachlorodibenzofuran	Pentachloropherol
1,2,3,7,9-pentachlorodibenzofuran	Penta- to nonylphenols
1,2,7,8-tetrachlorodibenzofuran	Perchlorate
1,3,6,8-tetrachlorodibenzofuran	Phthalates
2,3,4,7,8-pentachlorodibenzofuran	Benzylbutylphthalate
2,3,7,8-tetrabromodibenzofuran	Di-2-ethylhexylphthalate (DEHP)
2,3,7,8-tetrachlorodibenzofuran	Diisobutylphthalate
Hydroxy (hydro)-quinones	Di-n-hexylphthalate
Lead	Di-n-octylphthalate
Mercury	d-hydroxybenzoic acids (DHBA)
Methylcolanthrene (MCA)	Phenol
Polybrominated biphenyls (PBBs)	Polychlorinated diphenyl ether (PCDE)
Polychlorinated biphenyls (PCBs)	Radioactive iodine
2,2′,3,3′,4,4′-hexachlorobiphenyl (PCB 128)	Resorcinol
2,2′,3,3′,6,6′-hexachlorobiphenyl (PCB 136)	Styrenes
2,2′,4,4′,5,5′-hexachlorobiphenyl (PCB 153)	Tetrachloro-benzyltoluenes
2,3,3′,4,4′,5-hexachlorobiphenyl (PCB 156)	Thiocyanate
3,3′,4,4′,5,5′-hexachlorobiphenyl (PCB 169)	Vinyl acetate

dents or direct contamination from herbicide use, direct exposure to dioxins is not the major environmental concern. Instead, the transport on global air currents, eventual deposition onto soil or water, and the subsequent release into the food chain are the major concern. Indigenous populations such as the Inuit, who consume whale or seal blubber, have among the highest exposures in the world to these toxic chemicals. Dioxins also accumulate in breast milk lipids, where they pose a potential risk to the nursing infant. In developed countries, dioxin emissions have declined in recent years as a result of better industrial controls and of the introduction of alternatives to chlorine bleaching of paper. Worldwide, the total emissions of dioxins are continuing to rise.

In 1976, an explosion at a chemical factory in Seveso, Italy, exposed the nearby town to a cloud of dioxin and other contaminants. Four percent of the population, including many children, suffered chloracne, a disfiguring and persistent form of acne associated with exposure to dioxin. Persons residing in three zones of decreasing TCDD contamination and a reference population were followed up for cancer occurrence. Although the exposed population was not large, studies show elevated rates of hematologic neoplasms, sarcomas, non-Hodgkin lymphoma, and breast cancer in this cohort. In addition, the sex ratio of births to the most dioxin-exposed cohort was skewed significantly toward females, and women in this cohort tended to reach menopause at a slightly earlier age than unexposed women. Decreased IgG plasma levels evidenced immunologic effects. The mortality risk for diabetes, particularly for the women, and respiratory and cardiovascular mortality risks were increased 20 years after the accident.

Dioxin is a known endocrine disruptor. It acts primarily by binding to the aryl hydrocarbon (Ah) receptor, an orphan receptor that is found in most body tissues. Researchers believe that many of dioxin's complex effects stem from the activities of the Ah receptor, including suppression of immune function, promotion of tumor growth, and a cascade of effects on other hormone systems, such as an antiestrogenic effect and an antithyroid effect. Dioxin produces carcinogenic, immunotoxic, and teratogenic effects in laboratory animals at low doses. The lowest levels of dioxin in the pregnant rat necessary to cause adverse reproductive outcomes in the offspring (30–80 ng/kg) are within an order of magnitude of the current average background dose of dioxin in humans (5–10 ng/kg). The fact that dioxin produces adverse developmental and reproductive effects in fish, birds, and mammals suggests that it is likely to do so in humans.

The many Vietnamese exposed to dioxin from Agent Orange would be an excellent population for epidemiologic studies, but such studies have not been done. However, thousands of US service personnel also were exposed and are currently the subject of numerous studies. A National Academy of Sciences panel found that there is sufficient evidence of an association between Agent Orange exposure and three cancers: soft-tissue sarcoma, non-Hodgkin lymphoma, and Hodgkin disease. The panel was unable to verify a link to other cancers or problems such as birth defects and immune disorders.

Researchers are pointing out that, based on data from Seveso and several industrial cohorts, dioxin exposure levels close to those occurring in the general population may be carcinogenic. It appears that exposures during fetal development exert far more powerful effects than exposures during adulthood. This effect of timing could mean that adult workers and military personnel would be substantially less susceptible to dioxin toxicity than are infants in utero.

In Times Beach, Missouri, 10 years before the danger of dioxin was fully recognized, waste oils contaminated with dioxin were sprayed on roads to control dust. This created such outrage in the community— with extensive media coverage—that the EPA ordered the area closed, and the federal government paid for the evacuation and relocation of the residents. Breast-milk monitoring in southern Kazakhstan revealed some of the highest levels of 2,3,7,8-TCDD ever reported in the world. This cotton-growing region used Agent Orange as an herbicide. The resulting contamination of local fish from agricultural runoff into a lake resulted in a serious contamination problem. Follow-up studies have not been done to evaluate this population for health effects.

Dioxins are on the list of chemicals subject to international reduction efforts under the Stockholm Convention on Persistent Organic Pollutants, signed in May 2001.

Although dioxins cannot be banned because they are unintentional by-products, their release can be restricted or virtually stopped through the elimination of conditions that promote the formation of these chemicals.

REFERENCES

EPA: Exposure and human health reassessment of 2,3,7,8-tetra-chlorodibenzo-*p*-dioxin (TCDD) and related compounds, National Academy Sciences (NAS), www.epa.gov/ncea/pdfs/dioxin/nas-review/.

EPA: Questions and answers about dioxin, www.epa.gov/ncea/dioxinqa.htm#o0.

Eskenazi B: Serum dioxin concentrations and age at menopause. Environ Health Perspect 2005;113:858 [PMID: 16002373].

Steenland K: Dioxin revisited: developments since the 1997 IARC classification of dioxin as a human carcinogen. Environ Health Perspect 2004;112:1265 [PMID: 15345337].

Toft G et al: Epidemiological evidence on reproductive effects of persistent organochlorines in humans. Reprod Toxicol 2004;19:5 [PMID: 15336708].

Polychlorinated Biphenyls

PCBs are organochlorine chemicals with a variety of congeners depending on the number and location of chlorine atoms on the biphenyl rings. These chemicals are divided by toxicologists into two categories: those PCBs that assume a planar configuration because of the location of the chlorine substitutions and those in which the biphenyl rings assume a skewed configuration relative to one another. The coplanar PCBs are dioxin-like in their toxicology and generally are considered with the other dioxins. The noncoplanar PCBs have a distinct toxicologic profile and are discussed here. Commercial PCBs mixtures may contain chlorobenzenes, dioxins, and furans.

PCBs were manufactured in the United States between 1929 and 1977. Because of their stability, high boiling point, and low electrical conductivity, they were used primarily as coolants for electrical transformers, as dielectrics for electrical capacitors, and in stone-cutting oils, hydraulic fluids, and heat-transfer fluids. They also were used as plasticizers, in carbonless multicopy office forms, and as constituents of paints and objective immersion oils for microscopes. Although their manufacture is no longer permitted in the United States and many other countries, total PCBs currently in the environment exceed 500 million pounds, and 750 million pounds are still in use in capacitors and transformers. Obsolete stocks of transformer oils, capacitors, and transformers containing PCBs have been stored in developing countries, often in hazardous ways. PCBs are environmentally persistent, lipophilic, and accumulate by thousands of fold in the food chain. Almost everyone in the world now has detectable amounts of PCBs in their body. In many areas of the United States, there are advisories warning pregnant and breastfeeding women against eating local fish owing to PCB contamination.

Much of what is known about the acute toxicity of PCBs in humans resulted from an incident in Japan in 1968 and a similar incident in Taiwan in 1979, when an accidental leak in a rice-oil processing plant caused high levels of PCBs (and furans) in cooking oil. In a matter of weeks, consumers of the oil were ill and exhibited mild to severe chloracne; hyperpigmentation of the skin, nails, conjunctiva, and mucous membranes; liver disease, including necrosis; fatigue; headache; menstrual disorders; palpebral edema; and meibomian gland hypersecretion. In the Taiwan incident, there was a relatively high mortality rate from hepatomas, liver cirrhosis, or liver disease with hepatomegaly. Women had excess of stillbirths and deaths of offspring, and various birth defects also were observed, including growth abnormalities, hyperpigmentation, persistent conjunctival swelling, and abnormalities of nails, hair, teeth, and gums consistent with an acquired neuroectodermal dysplasia. Children born to affected women were shorter and lighter than controls. Delays of developmental milestones were observed, along with abnormalities on behavioral and developmental testing. Nursing infants who had not ingested the oil also showed symptoms, indicating that the mother's milk transmitted the toxicant.

Sport-fish consumption is estimated to deliver a dose of PCBs that is 4300 times greater than background exposure from inhalation or drinking water. Placental transport of PCBs and other organochlorine compounds has been demonstrated. PCBs and other organochlorine contaminants are associated with endocrine disruption, neurotoxicity, and developmental delay in humans and may be harmful to testicular function. Because PCBs can induce cytochrome P450, it has been suggested that the effect of PCBs on the reproductive system could be related to alterations in steroid hormones. Moreover, PCBs are mutagenic, with dose-related chromosome breakage in human white blood cell lines at low levels of exposure.

Among the environmental chemicals that may be able to disrupt the endocrine systems of animals and humans, PCBs are of considerable concern. PCBs appear to interfere with thyroid hormone. In human epidemiologic studies, higher levels of PCBs in breast milk correlate with elevated thyroid-stimulating hormone (TSH) in nursing infants. Decreased thyroid hormone in the first weeks of life is associated with increased risk of neurologic disorders, including the need for special education by age 9 years.

A Wisconsin cohort study of 212 children environmentally exposed to PCBs in utero because of maternal consumption of Great Lakes fish revealed delayed psychomotor development in those most highly exposed. At age 11 years, the most exposed children were more than three times as likely to perform poorly on IQ tests, were more distractible, and were more than twice as likely to be at least 2 years behind in reading comprehension. These results are consistent with the findings in two other cohorts of exposed infants, one in the Netherlands and one in New York State.

Researchers monitoring breast milk for PCB contamination identified polybrominated diphenyl ethers (PBDEs) at rapidly increasing concentrations in human milk samples. The PBDEs partially replaced PCBs as flame-retardant chemicals and have been used widely since the 1970s in polyurethane foam furniture, high-impact polystyrene electronics casings, and some fabrics. Preliminary testing indicates that the PBDEs are developmental neurotoxicants in rodents and behave similarly to PCBs in the environment and in the body. There already has been regulatory action in Europe and a voluntary agreement in the United States to eliminate some of the PBDEs from production.

REFERENCES

ATSDR: Toxicological profile on PCBs, www.atsdr.cdc.gov/toxprofiles/tp17.html.

Guo YL: Yucheng: Health effects of prenatal exposure to polychlorinated biphenyls and dibenzofurans. Int Arch Occup Environ Health 2004;77:153 [PMID: 14963712].

Hsu PC et al: Serum hormones in boys prenatally exposed to polychlorinated biphenyls and dibenzofurans. J Toxicol Environ Health A 2005;68:1447 [PMID: 16076757].

Yang CY et al: The endocrine and reproductive function of the female Yucheng adolescents prenatally exposed to PCBs/PCDFs. Chemosphere 2005;61:355 [PMID: 15885742].

Agricultural Contamination: Pesticides & Fertilizers

Since the introduction of dichlorodiphenyltrichloroethane (DDT) in 1939 and its successful use against mites, ticks, and mosquitoes during World War II, the production and number of synthetic pesticides have proliferated worldwide. In 1945, the world pesticide production was about 100 tons, mainly organochlorine compounds. In 2001, an estimated 2.6 million tons of active ingredients were produced, with some 1000 active ingredients marketed in the form of tens of thousands of commercial formulations. The United States and Europe are the largest producers, with six multinational corporations dominating 80% of the market. In 2004, global pesticide sales increased almost 5% to US$32,665 million, the increase in Latin America being 25%. Herbicides compose almost half the market value owing to increased use of herbicide-resistant genetically modified seeds, followed by insecticides

(28%), fungicides (22%), and other agrochemical compounds (5%). The International Fertilizer Industry Association reported that during the 2003–2004 growing season, 146 million kg of nitrogen, phosphate, potassium, and sulfur products were used globally, with highest demands from large-scale agriculture of corn, wheat, soybean, cotton, and rice.

The United States is one of the main pesticide users. The EPA reported that 900 million pounds of active ingredients of conventional pesticides were used in the United States during 2001, as well as 900 million pounds of wood preservatives and 1 million pounds of other biocides, such as disinfectants for water treatment. Still, this high amount of conventional pesticides, about 3 pounds on a per capita basis, is exceeded in some developing countries with intensive export agriculture, where use conditions are much worse. For example, in that same year, up to 4 kg per capita was used in some Central American countries.

Pesticides are employed mostly in agriculture but also in considerable amounts for domestic pest control, for vector control in public health programs, in food industries, and on recreational sites such as golf courses. Pesticides are also an important occupational health problem, especially in developing countries. The general population is exposed to a wide array of pesticides. The Third National Report on Human Exposure to Environmental Chemicals of the CDC stated in 2005 that more than 90% of U.S. residents have a mixture of pesticides in their bodies, with children having higher levels than adults. In 2005, a pilot analysis of the cord blood of 10 newborn babies in the United States detected 287 chemicals, on average 200 per baby, among them many pesticides.

The hundreds of commercially available pesticides have distinct toxicity, including acute and chronic poisonings, dermatitis, burns, eye injuries, neurotoxicity, cancer, neurodevelopmental effects, immune-system damage, birth defects, reproductive disorders, and endocrine disruption. A number of pesticides can be classified in chemical groups that share toxicologic properties. For example, all organochlorine compounds are neurotoxic and endocrine disruptors; they persist in the environment, accumulate in fatty tissues, enter the food chain, and continue to expose large populations many years after being banned. Organophosphate and carbamate pesticides generally are less persistent but, being inhibitors of the enzyme acetylcholinesterase, are acutely toxic, and cause many poisonings, especially in the occupational setting; also, long-term and delayed health effects such as nervous system illnesses, cancer, and reproductive disorders are becoming increasingly apparent. Pyrethroids, the next generation of insecticides, widely promoted as less toxic alternatives, have endocrine activity and produce allergies and possibly cancer.

Bipyridyl herbicides are a frequent cause of skin burns, may decrease respiratory capacity, and may be linked to Parkinson disease. Dithiocarbamate fungicides are allergenic, mutagenic, and carcinogenic and may produce reproductive effects; maneb has been associated experimentally with Parkinson disease. Major health-risk concerns with regard to fertilizers are their contamination of groundwater with nitrates and nitrites that are metabolized after ingestion to highly carcinogenic N-nitroso compounds, and greenhouse effects from emissions from nitrous oxide.

Although the recognition or corroboration of pesticide-related health effects is difficult, especially in developing countries, owing to methodologic limitations and scarce human and technical resources for epidemiologic studies, the body of evidence of serious health effects is ever-growing. Numerous studies of farm workers have found this population to be at increased risk of poisonings, cancer, neurologic illnesses, reproductive disorders, birth defects, and many long-term illnesses relative to the general population. Nonspecific symptoms are frequent manifestations of subclinical and chronic pesticide illness and usually are attributed to other causes. In Central America, almost 2% of the general population had an episode of poisoning symptoms after pesticide exposure in 2001. In Panama, 16% of banana workers were sensitized to one or more pesticides. Environmental exposure to endosulfan is suspected to have interfered with the synthesis of sexual hormones and delayed the sexual maturity in male Indian adolescents. In New York, babies' cord blood levels of organophosphate pesticides chlorpyrifos and diazinon were associated with reduced birth weight and length.

Many pesticide health effects have a long-lasting and profound impact on society. Dibromochloropropane, a nematocide used on banana and pineapple plantations during the 1970s, caused sterility of workers in Latin America, Southeast Asia, and Africa. In Central America, tens of thousands of these men, many abandoned by their wives and without children, are now too old and sick to be employed as banana workers and barely survive on day-to-day jobs. To solve pesticide-related environmental health problems, we need an ecosystem health approach, that is, assessing the environmental and health aspects together with the economic and social determinants and consequences.

Safe use of pesticides, a long-pursued goal of policy makers and industry, is difficult to achieve in industrialized countries and impossible in the poverty-stricken conditions of tropical developing countries. After 40 years of pesticide use, conditions have improved barely or not at all in the developing world, with continued use of highly toxic pesticides, faulty spraying equipment, inadequate or no use of protective equipment, and inadequate disposal of remnants and containers, resulting in severe contamination of workers, their families, and the environment.

Agricultural pesticides expose nearby populations through drift and runoff of recently sprayed fields, contaminating air and water sources. Workers take pesticides home on their clothing, shoes, and contaminated bodies, exposing family members. Mass poisonings, often involving children, have been documented after environmental exposures from spraying, fires in pesticide storehouses, and technical failures in pesticide industries. Infamous are the Seveso accident in Italy described earlier in this chapter and the Bhopal pesticide plant accident in India with thousands of deaths after inhalation of methyl isocyanate gas, a precursor in aldicarb production, and hundreds of thousands of people with severe long-term neurologic and respiratory sequelae.

Domestic pesticide use, principally insecticides and herbicides, may be very high. In the United States, homeowners use an estimated 10 times more chemical pesticides per acre than do farmers. Although pesticides marketed to consumers often are in a more dilute formulation, evaluation of risks to children have found that infants crawling on carpets or playing with family pets may be exposed to potentially unsafe levels of pesticides. In recent years, several organophosphate pesticides have been taken off the market for household use because of concerns about risks to children, especially neurodevelopmental effects. Domestic use of pesticides has been associated with various childhood cancers. The use of pesticides in public health to control diseases such as malaria and dengue fever exposes large populations, including the very young and old, the ill, and the immunologically depressed.

The impact of agricultural agents on human health through residues in drinking-water sources and food is a growing concern. Illness from pesticide residues in food is difficult to document. This is so because the clinical diagnosis is difficult to determine given that many of the health effects of pesticides are not acute and the symptoms are rarely pathognomonic of pesticide exposure. An example is the clinical diagnosis of low-dose exposures to organophosphate insecticides. Low doses may cause diarrhea, mood changes, and other neurologic symptoms. These nonspecific symptoms would not necessarily lead an individual to seek medical care and a clinician to order a test for one of the more than 300 pesticide compounds used on food. Human illnesses from consuming pesticides in food have been recognized in episodes where highly toxic compounds in foods led to acute manifestations. Two dramatic examples are the contamination of watermelons in the western United States by the the illegal use of the pesticide aldicarb and the probable food-tampering episode of

a frozen food with the organochlorine insecticide endrin. In both episodes, the public health problem was first identified by an alert clinician who notified public health officials.

The dramatic growth of the organic foods industry and the creation of new labels to promote foods grown using integrated pest management (IPM) techniques show that the general public has become concerned about some of the health and environmental problems associated with pesticides.

Pesticide food tolerances (legal pesticide residue limits) constitute the most important mechanism by which the EPA limits levels of pesticide residues in foods. A tolerance must be established for any pesticide used on any food crop. In the past, tolerances were based primarily on the results of field trials conducted by pesticide manufacturers and were designed to reflect the highest residue concentrations likely under normal conditions of agricultural use. Now pesticide tolerances are required to be set to offer a reasonable certainty of no harm to children. The determination of what might be a safe level of residue exposure is made by considering the results of toxicologic studies of the pesticide's effects on animals and, when data are available, on humans. Acute and chronic effects, including cancer, are considered separately. These data are used to establish human exposure guidelines (i.e., a reference dose) against which one can compare the expected exposure. Uncertainty factors generally are added to account for extrapolation from animal studies to humans and to account for population variability. A 1996 law, the Food Quality Protection Act (FQPA), which requires that pesticide tolerances be set at a level that protects children, also requires an additional uncertainty factor of up to 10-fold where there are data gaps relevant to the exposure or relative susceptibility of infants and children.

The implementation of FQPA has changed pesticide regulation dramatically in the United States. Not only does the law require for the first time that tolerances be set to protect children, but it also requires consideration of all aggregated exposures to the same pesticide (i.e., via food, water, household use, etc.). The law also requires consideration of the cumulative risk of all chemicals that act by a common biologic mechanism. This law has resulted in the cancelation of hundreds of pesticide tolerances and has limited the use of some of the most hazardous pesticides. Unfortunately, implementation of the law has been slow and inconsistent, and many pesticides still are regulated under the old standards. Registration procedures for pesticides in most developing countries continue to be highly deficient. Often the mere existence of a food tolerance in the country of origin is justification to allow any type of use in the developing country. Exposure conditions for developing countries are not considered, and true risk-assessment procedures are not carried out.

REFERENCES

Brent RL, Weitzman M: The current state of knowledge about the effects, risks, and science of children's environmental exposures. Pediatrics 2004;113:1158 [PMID: 15060213].

Calvert GM et al: Acute occupational pesticide-related illness in the US, 1998–1999: Surveillance findings from the SENSOR-pesticides program. Am J Indust Med 2004;45:14 [PMID: 14691965].

Colosio C et al: Low level exposure to chemicals and immune system. Toxicol Appl Pharmacol 2005;207:320 [PMID: 15992843].

EPA: Pesticide Web site, www.epa.gov/pesticides.

Fenske RA et al: Lessons learned for the assessment of children's pesticide exposure: Critical sampling and analytical issues for future studies. Environ Health Perspect 2005;113:1455 [PMID: 16203262].

Landrigan PJ et al: Children's health and the environment: public health issues and challenges for risk assessment. Environ Health Perspect 2004;112:257 [PMID: 14754581].

National Pesticide Information Center, http://npic.orst.edu/.

Pesticide Action Network: Pesticide database, www.pesticideinfo.org.

Ionizing Radiation

Ionizing radiation is electromagnetic radiation that has sufficient energy to separate electrons from their atomic or molecular orbits. Although natural radiation from both cosmic and terrestrial sources always has been part of the environment, technology has added other sources of exposure to ionizing radiation. The National Council on Radiation Protection estimates that 18% of the current average radiation exposure to people in the United States is due to human-created sources. Of this, 58% is ascribed to medical x-rays, 21% to nuclear medicine, 16% to consumer products, and the remaining 5% to occupational sources, fallout, and nuclear fuel. Obviously, there is considerable variability in exposures to specific individuals or populations.

At high doses, radiation can cause burns, hair loss, cancerous ulcers, sterility, immunologic dysfunction, bone marrow suppression, and death. At lower doses, the mutagenic effect of radiation can result in a wide array of cancers, genetic defects, and immune impairment.

A number of factors affect the severity of radiation damage, including age, physiologic variation, and differences between species. The usually long latency period of cancer development may mask other health effects when research objectives concentrate strictly on carcinogenic effects. For example, when immune repair mechanisms are damaged by radiation, many individuals may die earlier from infectious diseases, particularly pneumonia, so that only the most resistant individuals

would live long enough to be at potential risk for developing cancer.

Present knowledge of the health effects of radiation has been derived primarily from atomic bomb survivors in Japan and medical patients who have undergone radiation diagnostic studies or radiation therapy. Both these groups received high-level exposure. Consequently, the health risk level of low-dose exposure is not entirely clear and remains a major issue of controversy. Evaluations of cancer risk from ionizing radiation have undergone significant upward revisions compared with those published about a decade ago.

Both the A-bomb survivor cancer mortality and incidence data fail to suggest the existence of a threshold for cancer induction down to very low doses. Doses of 100 mSv—40-times the worldwide "background" exposure—have been associated with excess cases of leukemia among A-bomb survivors. Doses as low as 10 mSv have been associated with cancer after in utero exposure. Studies in survivors of Hiroshima and Nagasaki have failed to identify any threshold below which exposure was not associated with cancer.

Studies have found significant increases in specific types of cancer among exposed individuals, including lung, thyroid, bladder, and prostate cancers; multiple myeloma; lymphatic and hematopoietic neoplasms; and leukemia. In addition, there is some risk of increased cardiovascular morbidity and mortality with radiation exposure.

Levels of natural background radiation differ with geographic location. The type of soil in the area and the radionuclides present in soil affect the exposure. For example, while people living in Florida are exposed to about 2 mSv per year, those living in northeast Washington State are exposed to about 17 mSv per year. The difference is mostly due to radon levels. Overall, the dose-equivalent rate for the U.S. population is estimated to be approximately 3.0 mSv per year.

Uranium is a common constituent of rocks and soils throughout the United States. During the radioactive decay process, uranium decays to radium, which, in turn, decays to radon. Radon then diffuses out of the rocks and soils in which it is formed and undergoes further decay (with a half-life of 3.82 days) into a series of short-lived solid isotopes that commonly are called *radon daughters*. These radon-decay products, either free or attached to airborne particles, are inhaled and undergo further radioactive decay in lung tissue. During this radon-decay process in the lungs, high-energy alpha emissions penetrate the cells of the epithelium lining the bronchi and alveoli. Energy deposited in these cells during alpha radiation is believed to initiate the process of carcinogenesis. The EPA estimates that as many as 21,000 lung cancer deaths a year are attributable to radon, making it the second leading cause of lung cancer following tobacco smoking. Tobacco smoke has a synergistic effect with radon, increasing cancer risk by 10-fold over radon exposure alone.

The EPA estimates that as many as one 1 of every 15 homes throughout the United States has radon levels at or above the 4 pCi/L action level of radon. The EPA has recommended that homes below the third floor be tested for radon and that remediation be considered even at levels as low as 2 pCi/L.

The Bureau of Radiological Health has determined that x-rays used in patient diagnosis or treatment are the chief source of radiation exposure of the U.S. population. More than 300,000 x-ray units exist in the various health services, and an estimated 150 million people are exposed annually through medical and dental radiographs. Another important source of radiation exposure in health services is the use of radiopharmaceuticals, which more than 10,000 physicians in the United States are licensed to administer. Between 10 and 12 million doses of radionuclides are administered annually for diagnosis or treatment involving the brain, liver, bone, lung, thyroid, kidney, and heart. According to EPA estimates, this represents approximately 20% of the total radiation resulting from health services.

Prior to 1963, when most nuclear tests were performed in the atmosphere, large amounts of radioactive material were released, carried by the wind and brought to earth by rains. The first explosion at Bikini Atoll in 1954 exposed many in the area to radioactive fallout, including the inhabitants of surrounding islands. Among the Marshall Islanders, an unusual incidence of benign and malignant thyroid nodules, hypothyroidism, and growth retardation has been documented secondary to radioiodine exposure. These episodes indicate that significant harmful exposure occurs outside the prescribed "danger area" in part because of the unpredictability of atmospheric dispersion. Atmospheric tests conducted in Nevada during the 1950s and 1960s produced excessive levels of radioactivity in food and dairy products in many parts of the United States.

Several hundred nuclear reactors now exist in the United States for power production, scientific study, and other uses. Because of public indignation over the Three Mile Island and Chernobyl accidents, and because of the accelerating costs involved, the building of additional nuclear reactors remains in question. However, the existing reactors pose a risk to their workers as well as to populations in the area. Short of a full-scale "meltdown" with breach of the containment vessel, the major concern with possible reactor accidents relates to the emission of radioactive isotopes of iodine and their potential effect on the thyroid. Radioiodines, particularly ^{131}I, are the major public health risks fol-

lowing a reactor accident because they are readily volatilized and dispersed and rapidly taken up by the thyroid gland. The mining and milling of uranium to feed the reactors poses an ongoing risk to the inhabitants of several southwestern states in the United States, where 140 million tons of radon-emitting uranium mill tailings lie exposed to the atmosphere. Further risks are related to the disposal of radioactive wastes and to the flow of cooling water containing tritium, carbon-14, and krypton-85 into streams and rivers. These elements are nearly impossible to contain or remove and are capable of contaminating fish, drinking water, and the crops used for human consumption or animal feed that are irrigated with the water.

Because all possibilities cannot be included in any radiation research project, no reliable permissible dose equivalent has yet been established. Rather, the problem has been approached from risk-benefit considerations: How much radiation exposure are we willing to accept to achieve the benefits of nuclear energy? Most scientists would agree that no level of ionizing radiation is entirely safe or can ever be made so.

REFERENCES

Boice JD Jr: Radiation-induced thyroid cancer: What's new? J Natl Cancer Inst 2005;97:703 [PMID: 15900034].

Cardis E: Risk of thyroid cancer after exposure to I^{131} in childhood. J Natl Cancer Inst 2005;97:724 [PMID: 15900042].

Clapp RW: Nuclear power and public health. Environ Health Perspect 2005;113:720 [PMID: 16263488].

EPA Radon Information, www.epa.gov/radon/.

Mousseau TA et al: Don't underestimate the death rate from Chernobyl. Nature 2005;437:1089 [PMID: 16237420].

University of Michigan Health Physics Society: Radiation and health physics, www.umich.edu/~radinfo/.

Vastag B: Scientific, political debate continues on methods for estimating fallout exposure. J Natl Cancer Inst 2005;97:1240 [PMID: 16145038].

Wakeford R: The cancer epidemiology of radiation. Oncogene 2004;23:6404 [PMID: 15322514].

INTERNATIONAL ENVIRONMENTAL HEALTH

In a global trade economy, many occupational and environmental health problems have taken on an international dimension. This is reflected in the increasing concern about the migration of air and water pollutants across national boundaries and the effect that those pollutants can have on the public health and the environment of the affected country.

Concern about transboundary air and water pollution has led to several different international agreements to regulate such environmental degradation and its possible adverse health effects. These agreements have been spearheaded by the efforts of the United Nations, the World Health Organization (WHO), the International Labor Organization (ILO), the European Community, and the Organization for Economic Cooperation and Development (OECD) and by the trade provisions of the North American Free Trade Agreement (NAFTA) and the General Agreement on Tariffs and Trade (GATT).

The movement of hazardous waste across national boundaries has attracted special international attention. In 1989, the Basel Convention on the Control of Transboundary Movement of Hazardous Wastes and Their Disposal was adopted at a conference of more than 115 countries and went into effect in 1992. The Basel Convention permits movement and disposal of hazardous waste only if all involved countries—including any transit countries—give their written consent. More recent environmental treaties include the Rotterdam Convention on Prior Informed Consent. This treaty, adopted in 1998, requires exporters trading in a list of hazardous substances to obtain the prior informed consent of importers before proceeding with the trade. The convention establishes a first line of defense for developing countries by giving them the information they need to identify potential hazards and to exclude chemicals they cannot manage safely. If a country agrees to import chemicals, the convention promotes their safe use through labeling standards, technical assistance, and other forms of support. This treaty is designed to address the problem of companies in developed countries continuing to manufacture banned pesticides such as DDT for the export market.

PERSISTENT ORGANIC POLLUTANTS (POPS)

In 1997, following recommendations of the Intergovernmental Forum on Chemical Safety, the United Nations Environment Program (UNEP) Governing Council made the decision to reduce or eliminate through international action the emissions and discharges of an initial set of persistent organic pollutants (POPs) to protect human health and the environment. POPs are chemicals that remain in the environment without degradation for many years, are transported long distances and become widely distributed geographically, bioaccumulate through the food chain and are toxic for human health and wildlife. This resulted in the Stockholm Convention on Persistent Organic Pollutants in 2001, which establishes a commitment toward the global phase-out of 12 hazardous and persistent chemicals: aldrin, dieldrin, endrin, chlordane, DDT, toxaphene, mirex, heptachlor, hexachlorobenzene, PCBs, dioxins, and furans. This treaty also includes a mechanism for listing and phasing out additional persistent toxic substances that meet the criteria of persistence, bioaccumulation, and toxicity.

The Stockholm Convention came into effect in May 2004 when the fiftieth country ratified the treaty. Currently, over 100 countries have ratified the Stockholm Convention, not so the United States. Many of the POPs included in the Stockholm Convention are obsolete chemicals that are not actively in use anymore. However, the importance of addressing the reduction and elimination of persistent environmental levels on a global scale and in the context of international collaboration is unquestionable. For example, Inuit populations exceed tolerable intakes of persistent pollutants that have never been used in Arctic regions but entered the food chain. The continued use of DDT for malaria control is an issue of debate, where DDT is presented by public health officials as the only viable low-cost solution to prevent millions of deaths in the poorest countries, but sustainable pest control and underlying causes of the disease often are absent in the discussions. Delegates to the first Stockholm Convention meeting in Uruguay in 2005 agreed that current country-specific exemptions for the use of DDT for malaria control continue to be justified. But periodic reviews of the DDT exemptions are required, and countries using DDT must demonstrate that they are progressing with alternative pest control. The meeting also emphasized that the focus should be on integrated vector management and nonchemical controls and not on replacing DDT with other insecticides.

The tackling of the current 12 obsolete POPs is relatively easy, but future inclusion of new chemicals that are being produced in large amounts, such as certain flame retardants, will face industry resistance and needs more scientific assessment of deleterious health and environmental effects. In the meeting in Uruguay, four new chemicals were nominated for global elimination: the pesticides lindane and chlordecone and two brominated flame retardants, pentabromodiphenyl ether and hexabromobiphenyl. The Uruguay meeting established a new scientific body, the POPs Review Committee, with governmental and scientific representatives, to evaluate submissions of new chemicals. The process of adding a chemical to the treaty could take many years.

REFERENCES

Giles J: Treaty calls time on long-term pollutants. Nature 2004;427:768 [PMID: 14985725].

Tieyu W et al: Contamination of persistent organic pollutants (POPs) and relevant management in China. Environ Int 2005;31:813 [PMID: 15982740].

Van Oostdam J et al: Human health implications of environmental contaminants in Arctic Canada: A review. Sci Total Environ 2005;351:165 [PMID: 16297438].

Wong MH et al: A review on the usage of POP pesticides in China. Chemosphere 2005;60:740 PMID: 15949838].

www.pops.int.

SUSTAINABILITY

The last decade has witnessed a gradual shift in attitude toward sustainability. There has been a rise in corporate investments in sustainability programs, new types of environmental markets, and public demand for green products and investments. Once an afterthought, an annoyance, or a nonentity, sustainability is now sometimes an important objective for businesses. Some businesses are now viewing environmentally benign practices as a competitive advantage as they seek to win both stockholders and customers.

Efforts are underway to "internationalize" product quality standards through voluntary multinational agencies such as the International Standards Organization (ISO). ISO 9000 and 14000 standards are beginning to be used as benchmarks for the selling of products in the international marketplace. Structurally, the ISO 14000 series of environmental management standards (EMS) are a set of voluntary standards and guideline reference documents that include environmental management systems, environmental audits, ecolabeling, environmental performance evaluations, life-cycle assessments, and evaluations of environmental aspects in product standards. The EMS do not directly establish requirements for environmental compliance or specific levels of environmental performance. Rather, the emphasis is on management standards, much like the ISO 9000 quality management standards (QMS) series. However, the EMS specifications document addresses compliance indirectly through a commitment to both compliance with environmental laws and prevention of pollution.

Environmental certification is becoming the main tool for application of sustainable development principles. For decades, industry has been the main source of pollution in China. Determined to make changes, the mainland Chinese authorities have decided to promote mechanisms that incorporate environmental concerns into the internal management of enterprises. This is manifested in the rapid adoption of the ISO 14000 standards, including a significant increase in ISO 14001 registrations in China. The European Eco-Management and Audit Scheme and ISO 14001 both require for certification that companies adopt an environmental management system to prevent environmental impacts and to continuously improve environmental performance. For a good environmental performance evaluation (EPE), certification needs to use scientific methodologies and to interface with scientific research. Compared with the ready acceptance of the ISO 9000 quality standard, the ISO 14001 environmental management certification has been met with only moderate acceptance by industry. EMS certification does appear to signify a supplier who is managing the business well and exhibiting ethical responsibility. The European market is more environmentally conscious than those in other industrialized parts of the world. EMS offers a particularly valuable advantage for producers wishing to reach European markets. As policy makers seek to expand the voluntary adoption of EMS, a clear advantage for exporters should be noted by many industries.

There is now a general agreement that applying the "polluter pays" principle should solve environmental problems. As the cost of abatement increases, there is an incentive for firms to invest in either cleaner technology or more efficient abatement technology. There is also evidence that taxes and charges actually can affect trade. While it is true that stringent measures impose market access restrictions and cause limitations on competitiveness, this is much more widely felt by the developing countries because of lack of infrastructure and monitoring facilities, limited technology choices, inadequate access to environment-friendly raw materials, lack of complete information, presence of small-scale exporters, and emergence of environmental standards in sectors of export interest to developing countries. Small and medium-sized enterprises often divert sales either to the domestic market or to external markets where environmental requirements are less stringent in order to save on costs. In developing countries, 80% of the tanning industry is comprised of small and medium-sized enterprises processing raw to semifinished leather, usually less than 2 tons per day. In the developed countries, the small and medium-sized enterprises in the leather sector have vanished owing to strict environmental legislation, and this also likely will occur in developing countries. Environmental legislation has not always been practical either because the laws are too ambitious or unrealistic or because they have lacked effective institutional support and enforcement. Some environmental regulations have not succeeded because they do not match the technical requirements and economic reality of the country or region or because they do not take the institutional capabilities of the society that has to implement them into consideration. For the survival and sustenance of the small and medium-sized industry, it may be a viable alternative to carry out the tanning process in a decentralized fashion such that the raw to semifinished process is carried out in the large-scale sector, whereas the semifinished to finished process could be either reserved or open to competition as per the countries' requirements. But the issue of concern is whether it is fair that the raw to semifinished tanning process, containing 70% of the pollution discharge, should be undertaken by developing countries alone, especially if it is at the cost of their survival.

In the United States, it is clear that data collection on chemical risks and phase-outs of the most egregious chemicals alone will not achieve the goals of sustainable chemistry. These alone also will not internalize the cultural and institutional changes needed to ensure that design and implementation of safer chemicals, processes, and products are the focus of the future. A more holistic approach that involves not just chemical producers but also those who use and purchase chemicals is necessary. Some important lessons of the U.S. experience in chemicals management include (1) the need for good information on chemicals flows, toxic risks, and safer substances, (2) the need for comprehensive planning processes for chemical substitution and reduction to avoid risk tradeoffs and ensure product quality, (3) the need for technical and research support to firms for innovation in safer chemistry, and (4) the need for rapid screening processes and tools for comparison of alternative chemicals, materials, and products.

Efforts are also underway to harmonize the multitude of different occupational and environmental health and safety regulations that exist among the world's economies. However, harmonization may prove elusive. The GATT views stringent health and safety regulations as nontariff barriers, whereas others—concerned about exploited workers—view lax regulations as a subsidy to production. Another hurdle is that enforcement of environmental regulations is nonexistent in some countries and differs markedly even among industrialized countries.

The growing importance of technical regulation affecting the use and sale of chemical products is a topic of interest not only for the chemical industry but also for governments, nongovernmental organizations, consumers, and interested communities. The results of such regulation on behalf of the environment, health and safety of individuals, and its economic effects on industrial activity are well understood in the United States and in the European Union. In less developed countries, however, the general level of public understanding of these issues is still minimal. It is common knowledge that the so-called regulatory asymmetry between countries at different levels of development contributes to the establishment of technical barriers to trade. Such asymmetries, however, also have other impacts: the displacement of polluting industrial sectors to countries that have less demanding regulations, the concentration of unsafe and harmful environmental conditions in certain parts of the globe, and the competitive disadvantage for industries located in countries where control is more rigid.

Regulatory initiatives are emerging that require the electronics industry to incorporate environmental, health, and safety considerations into design and manufacturing decisions. Moreover, regulations governing the use, storage, transportation, and disposal of hazardous materials are beginning to influence the manufacturing process. It is hoped that by addressing environmental management issues, electronics manufacturers can reduce both hazardous materials and the generation of hazardous waste.

The electronics industry is preparing to comply with a number of restricted materials laws. In 2003, the European Union enacted the Restriction on Hazardous Substances (RoHS) Directive that bans the use of lead, mercury, cadmium, hexavalent chromium, and certain brominated flame retardants (BFRs) in most electronics products sold in the EU market beginning July 1, 2006. This directive, by banning the use of critical materials in electronics products sold in key world markets, may result in a significant change in the way products are designed for global sale.

The European Parliament and the European Council are considering legislation, Regulation, Evaluation, and Authorization of Chemicals (REACH), that will require industry to prove that chemicals being sold and produced in the European Union are safe to use or handle. REACH policy will require registration of all substances that are produced or imported into the EU. The amount of information required for registration will be proportional to the chemical's health risks and production volumes. Companies also will need to seek authorization to sell and produce problematic chemicals, such as carcinogens, mutagens, and teratogens. Toxic chemicals that persist in the environment or that bioaccumulate also will need authorization. The policy is slated for enactment in 2006.

The electronics industry also is beginning to take responsibility for its products at the end of their useful life. This responsibility also forms the basis for "take-back legislation" that is being implemented in the EU under the Waste Electrical and Electronic Equipment (WEEE) Directive, beginning in August, 2005. This directive encourages the design and production of electronics equipment to take into account and facilitate dismantling and recovery, in particular the reuse and recycling of electronics equipment, components, and materials necessary to protect human health and the environment.

REFERENCES

Bellesi F et al: Comparative advantage: the impact of ISO 14001 environmental certification on exports. Environ Sci Technol. 2005;39:1943 [PMID: 1587122].

EPA: International network for environmental compliance and enforcement, www.inece.org/pop1.html.

LaDou J: World Trade Organization, ILO conventions, and workers' compensation. Int J Occup Environ Health 2005;11:210 [PMID: 15875900].

Lopez AD: The evolution of the global burden of disease framework for disease, injury and risk factor quantification: Developing the evidence base for national, regional and global public health action. Global Health. 2005;1:5 [PMID: 15847690].

Pio Borges Menezes R et al: Using the WTO/TBT enquiry point to monitor tendencies in the regulation of environment, health, and safety issues affecting the chemical industry. Environ Int 2005;31:407 [PMID: 15734193].

Rotterdam Convention on prior informed consent, www.pic.int/.

Tickner JA et al: The US experience in promoting sustainable chemistry. Environ Sci Pollut Res Int. 2005;12:115 [PMID: 1585911].

United Nations Environment Program, www.unep.org/.

United Nations Environment Program: Basel Convention on the control of transboundary movements of hazardous waste, www.unep.ch/basel/.

United Nations Environment Program: Persistent organic pollutants, http://irptc.unep.ch/pops/.

World Health Organization, www.who.int/en/.

Routine Industrial Emissions, Accidental & Intentional Releases, & Hazardous Waste

38

Rupali Das, MD, MPH, Melanie Marty, PhD, & Marilyn Underwood, PhD

Over 23 million chemical compounds are known today. Of these, 70,000 are used regularly, and approximately 500 are introduced into the market every month. The processing, use, transport, and disposal of these chemicals present hazards to human health. This was painfully illustrated in 1985 when an accidental release of methyl isocyanate in Bhopal, India, caused death and injury to many thousands of people, resulted in increased public awareness of the effects of chemicals released into the environment, and sparked a host of international regulations aimed at preventing the recurrence of a similar tragedy. Routine and accidental releases of hazardous chemicals into air and releases of hazardous waste on land continue to occur. The sarin releases on the Tokyo subway in 1995, the attacks on the World Trade Center in New York City and the Pentagon in Washington, D.C., in 2001, and the spread of anthrax spores through the U.S. mail system the same year revealed the critical need for emergency preparedness for intentional releases of hazardous chemical and biologic agents. The tsunami off the coast of Indonesia in 2004 and hurricanes that hit the Gulf Coast of North and Central America in 2005 caused massive devastation and highlighted the additional need to better plan for natural disasters. Public health and emergency planners now focus on "all-hazards planning," including chemical, biologic, radiologic, nuclear, and explosions (CBRNE).

The United States and the European Union have the most comprehensive and complex environmental laws for the regulation of pollution. Environmental laws traditionally have been grouped according to both environmental media and the nature of pollutants: air pollution, water pollution, noise pollution, hazardous waste, hazardous materials management, remediation of contaminated soil and groundwater, and registration of toxic substances and pesticides.

This chapter discusses health hazards resulting from routine, accidental, and intentional releases of hazardous chemicals and waste material into the environment and the laws that are intended to regulate polluting industries and prevent adverse health effects from occurring. It is divided into three sections: routine industrial emissions, accidental and intentional releases, and hazardous waste. Each section discusses relevant health-based environmental regulations and the evaluation of potential health effects.

ROUTINE INDUSTRIAL EMISSIONS

In our modern technologic society, industries produce an enormous variety of products using vast amounts of chemicals and numerous physical processes. All industrial processes are associated with emissions of chemicals into the air, water, or land. In the 1970s, the United States began to seek information on the impacts of these emissions on human and ecologic health. This section focuses on available information on the extent and public health impacts of emissions into air.

Industrial emissions include a vast array of familiar and unfamiliar chemicals, few of which are well characterized toxicologically. While some epidemiologic studies have been useful for characterizing toxicity and the public health impacts of several air pollutants, most information comes from animal toxicology studies. Animal studies generally involve exposures of a genetically homogeneous population of rodents to one chemical at a time. Thus little knowledge exists about the interactions of chemicals or the consequences of exposure to many chemicals simultaneously in genetically heterogeneous human populations. Sources of airborne emissions are varied and range from large facilities such as oil refineries to small sources such as gas stations, auto body shops, and dry-cleaning operations. Emissions are somewhat characteristic for specific processes and source types.

TYPES OF SOURCES AND EMISSIONS TO THE AIR

Air pollutants have been characterized for regulatory purposes into two basic categories: criteria air pollutants (CAPs) and toxic air contaminants (TACs) [or hazardous air pollutants (HAPs) in U.S. federal programs]. The distinction is somewhat arbitrary in that both categories of emissions are toxic.

Criteria Air Pollutants

Criteria air pollutants (CAPs) are typical components of smog and were first identified by environmental scientists as posing public health risks in the 1960s. CAPs include chemicals emitted in large quantities and from many sources such as carbon monoxide (CO), sulfur oxides (SO_x), and nitrogen oxides (NO_x). The descriptor *criteria* refers to those chemicals for which there are regulatory standards determined by the U.S. Environmental Protection Agency (EPA) or, in some states, by state regulatory bodies. The standards are air concentrations that are designed to protect public health and which are not to be exceeded if an area is to be in compliance with the Clean Air Act or state regulations. Table 38–1 summarizes the federal ambient air quality standards.

Toxic Air Contaminants

Toxic air contaminants (TACs) are essentially everything else emitted into the air that is not a CAP and for which there is some regulatory concern. There are legal definitions for TACs (or HAPs) in both state and federal statutes, and the federal government and the State of California have lists of chemicals that have been formally identified as HAPs or TACs, respectively. Under EPA authority, HAPs are subject to specific regulatory requirements. Similarly, California has listed TACs (Table 38–2) that are subject to stationary and mobile source emissions controls. Cancer potency factors generated by the EPA or the State of California for some of the carcinogens can be used in risk assessments to estimate the cancer risk posed to the public from TAC emissions. The EPA has reference concentrations (RfCs) and the State of California has reference exposure levels (RELs) for some compounds that are useful in estimating public health impacts for noncancer toxicologic endpoints. Both RfCs and RELs can be viewed

Table 38–1. Ambient air quality standards.

Pollutant	Averaging[1] Time	National Primary Standards[2,3]
Ozone	1 hour 8 hours	0.12 ppm (235 $\mu g/m^3$) 0.08 ppm (157 $\mu g/m^3$)
Carbon monoxide	1 hour 8 hours	35 ppm (40 mg/m^3) 9 ppm (10 mg/m^3)
Nitrogen dioxide	Annual average	0.053 ppm (100 $\mu g/m^3$)
Sulfur dioxide	Annual average 24 hours	0.03 ppm (80 $\mu g/m^3$) 0.14 ppm (365 $\mu g/m^3$)
Respirable particulate matter (PM_{10})	24 hours Annual arithmetic mean	150 $\mu g/m^3$ 50 $\mu g/m^3$
Fine particulate matter (PM_{25})	24 hours Annual arithmetic mean	65 $\mu g/m^3$ 15 $\mu g/m^3$
Lead	30 day average Calendar quarter	1.5 $\mu g/m^3$

[1]National standards, other than ozone and those based on annual averages or annual arithmetic means, are not to be exceeded more than once a year.
[2]Concentration expressed first in units in which it was promulgated. Equivalent units given in parentheses are based upon a reference temperature of 25°C (77°F) and a reference pressure of 760 mm of mercury. All measurements of air quality are to be corrected to a reference temperature of 25°C (77°F) and a reference pressure of 760 mmHg (1013.2 mbar); parts per million (ppm) in this table refers to ppm by volume, or micromoles of pollutant per mole of gas.
[3]National Primary Standards: The levels of air quality necessary with an adequate margin of safety to protect the public health.
Source: California Air Resources Board, www.arb.ca.gov/aqs/aaqs2.pdf.

Table 38–2. Toxic air contaminants identified in California.

Acetaldehyde
Arsenic
Asbestos
Benzene
Benzo(*a*)pyrene (and related PAH)
Butadiene
Cadmium
Carbon tetrachloride
Chloroform
Chromium (+6)
Ethylene dibromide
Ethylene dichloride
Ethylene oxide
Formaldehyde
Lead
Methylene chloride
Nickel
Particulate matter from diesel-fueled engines
2,3,7,8-Tetrachlorodibenzo-p-dioxin (and related 2,3,7,8-chlorinated congeners)
Tetrachloroethylene
Trichloroethylene
Vinyl chloride

as exposure levels at or below which adverse health impacts are not anticipated. Modeled or measured air concentrations are compared with the RfC or REL to determine the potential hazard. For the most part, however, there are not enforceable ambient air quality standards for TACs.

Types of Sources

There are a great number of sources of airborne chemicals, which, for regulatory purposes, are divided into mobile sources (primarily cars, trucks, and buses) and stationary sources. The remainder of this section addresses stationary sources of airborne industrial emissions. Stationary sources traditionally are referred to as major or minor sources. Major sources include large industrial complexes such as refineries and aerospace and chemical manufacturing facilities. Major sources usually have large energy requirements and fulfill these demands via combustion of fuels, resulting in significant CAP emissions. Major combustion products include carbon monoxide and oxides of nitrogen and sulfur. Particulate matter is also emitted from combustion sources, particularly those that are poorly controlled. Refineries are some of the largest emitters of CAPs, releasing hundreds of tons per day of sulfur oxides and nitrogen oxides. Oxides of nitrogen react with hydrocarbons emitted into the air to produce

ozone on hot, sunny days. Thus ozone, a major component of photochemical smog, is not emitted directly but represents one reaction product from atmospheric transformation.

Minor sources usually are associated with lower emissions of CAPs than major sources. Yet minor sources can be important emitters of TACs, which are process-dependent. Specific industrial processes tend to use the same chemicals and result in similar emissions. Small dry-cleaning sources emit tetrachloroethylene, an animal carcinogen and probable human carcinogen. Incinerators, which can be found at both large and small facilities, emit an array of products of incomplete combustion ranging from carbon monoxide to complex chlorinated compounds such as the carcinogenic 2,3,7,8-tetrachlorodibenzo-*p*-dioxin (dioxin) and related congeners, as well as metals and acid gases. Polycyclic aromatic hydrocarbons (PAHs), some of which are carcinogens, are also high-molecular-weight products of incomplete combustion emitted by incinerators and combustion processes. Metal-finishing operations usually are small sources but may be associated with potentially significant public health impacts. The known human carcinogens hexavalent chromium and nickel are used extensively in metal-finishing operations, which are frequently associated with relatively high estimated near-source cancer risks (e.g., 10–100 in 1 million). Typically, regulatory agencies consider an excess individual cancer risk of 1 in 1 million for lifetime exposure to be de minimis. Regulatory activities, such as cleanup of hazardous waste sites or required air pollution controls, generally occur above this estimated level of cancer risk.

EMISSIONS DATABASES

The EPA maintains the Toxics Release Inventory (TRI), a database of stationary source emissions to air, water, and land, for specified compounds. In addition, the State of California maintains databases of emissions of toxic chemicals to the air from stationary sources. These databases are described below.

National Toxics Release Inventory

In 1986, Congress enacted the Superfund Amendments and Reauthorization Act (SARA) and added Title III, known as the Emergency Planning and Community Right-to-Know Act (EPCRA). Section 313 of SARA Title III created the TRI and gave the EPA authority to collect information quantifying emissions of more than 650 chemicals and chemical classes emitted by industrial sources. SARA Title III's passage was stimulated by the tragedy in Bhopal. Part of the premise for the statute is that citizens have a right to know about toxic materials used, stored, and released into the environment in their communities. The statute also mandates emergency planning for chemical accidents (see following section).

Facilities that need to report emissions to the EPA are those that produce, import, or process 25,000 pounds or more of a listed substance or use in any manner 10,000 pounds or more of a listed substance in a given reporting year. There are different reporting requirements for persistent bioaccumulative toxic (PBT) chemicals of 0.1 g for dioxins and dioxin-like compounds or 10–100 pounds for other PBTs. The facility must have a Standard Industrial Code (SIC) 20–39, which are the SICs for facilities engaged in manufacturing or fall into one of the following industrial categories: metal mining, coal mining, electric utilities that combust coal and/or oil, chemical wholesale distributors, petroleum terminals and bulk storage facilities, hazardous waste treatment and disposal facilities, and all federal facilities. The facility must have 10 or more full-time employees.

Emissions to air, wastewater discharges, disposal into on-site landfills, injection of liquid wastes into underground wells, transfer of wastes to publicly owned wastewater treatment works, and transfers of chemicals to off-site facilities for treatment, storage, or disposal all must be reported. Both routine releases and accidental spills are covered in the emissions reports. The Pollution Prevention Act of 1990 added further reporting requirements to SARA Title III that result in an ability to compare years by percent change and require the facility to estimate emissions for future years. In addition, the amended act allows information to be gathered regarding on-site or off-site recycling of chemical wastes and source-reduction practices and opportunities.

The TRI database and EPA's Annual Report are available online at www.epa.gov/tri/ and through the National Library of Medicine's TOXNET computer system. EPA's annual report includes state and county-level data and is available on CD-ROM and microfiche records in public libraries. The EPA provides a search tool, the TRI Explorer, on its Web page that can query the database.

TRI data are used for a variety of purposes. The EPA and state and local agencies use the data to identify potential exposures and risks and emissions-reduction opportunities and to track progress toward pollution reduction. Public interest groups use the data to help educate the public about toxics in their communities, to pressure industry into reducing toxic emissions, and to lobby the government to change policies. Industries use the information to help in pollution-reduction efforts.

In 2003, 23,811 facilities reported environmental releases for all TRI industries totaling 4.44 billion pounds. The manufacturing industries, metal mining, and electric utilities accounted for 44%, 28%, and 23%, respectively, of the total. On-site air emissions totaled 1.59 billion pounds, about half originating from manufacturing industries, including 15% from the chemical industry, 11% from the paper industry, and 45% from electric utilities. Approximately 2.2 million pounds of PBTs were emitted into the air, 0.5% of the total PBT environmental releases. PBT chemicals released into air included 5.41 pounds of dioxin and dioxin-like compounds, 138,387 pounds of mercury and mercury compounds, 1.3 million pounds of lead and lead compounds, 741,000 pounds of PAHs, and 436 pounds of polychlorinated biphenyls (PCBs).

Emissions from facilities reporting to TRI appear to have decreased over time. The TRI program motivates facilities to decrease their emissions. Poor public relations associated with being an emitter and a desire for more efficient operations and more recovery and recycling of waste have resulted in a decrease in overall emissions to the environment from the manufacturing sector. In 2003, 25.8 billion pounds of TRI chemicals were treated, recycled, landfilled into class 1 landfills or injection wells or combusted for energy recovery.

Changes in reporting requirements over the years complicate year-to-year comparisons for some compounds and industries. However, when comparing emissions of chemicals from manufacturing industries originally required to report in 1988 with the same chemical emissions in 2003, reported total releases dropped by 1.87 billion pounds. From 1998 to 2003 across all sectors, on-site and off-site releases decreased by 42 percent (2.87 billion pounds). Between 2002 and 2003, total air emissions decreased 3% (48 million pounds). Table 38–3 presents the 15 most common chemicals released into the air in the United States in 2003. Those carcinogens with reported releases into the air totaling over 400,000 pounds are presented in Table 38–4. The most commonly emitted chemicals have toxicity criteria developed by either the EPA or state agencies. These criteria are useful for estimating public health hazards through a risk-assessment process. Of the carcinogens in Table 38–4, benzene, formaldehyde, hexavalent chromium, nickel, ethylene oxide, and vinyl chloride are known human carcinogens. In addition, a number of occupations involving high exposure to PAHs are associated with elevated lung cancer risk.

The TRI data provide useful information on industrial releases into the environment. However, limitations in reporting may result in overall underreporting of total environmental releases, particularly to air, for some chemicals. Small facilities can be major contributors when their emissions are summed. Moreover, many large facilities emit substances into the environment but do not fall into the TRI reporting categories. It should be noted that mobile sources contribute a great deal to air-

Table 38–3. Top 15 TRI chemicals by volume of reported air emissions, 2003.

Chemical	Reported Total Air Emissions (million lb/yr)
Hydrochloric acid	594.7
Methanol	156.2
Sulfuric acid	141.2
Ammonia	120.8
Hydrogen fluoride	69.8
Toluene	55.2
Styrene	48.3
n-Hexane	41.6
Xylenes	37.5
Methyl ethyl ketone	24.6
Glycol ethers	23.4
Ethylene	22.2
Carbon disulfide	19.3
Acetaldehyde	13.0
Propylene	12.1

borne toxic chemicals. For example, benzene and 1,3-butadiene emissions reported in TRI represent a small fraction of total emissions into the air of these two chemicals that are emitted primarily from mobile sources. Finally, the toxic chemicals released from use of consumer products are not considered in TRI.

REFERENCES

Dolinoy DC, Miranda ML: GIS modeling of air toxics releases from TRI-reporting and non-TRI-reporting facilities: Impacts for environmental justice. Environ Health Perspect 2004;112:1717 [PMID: 15579419].

EPA: TRI Public Data Release Report, May 2005, www.epa. gov/tri/.

Touma JS et al: Air quality modeling of hazardous pollutants: Current status and future directions. J Air Waste Manag Assoc 2006;56:547 [PMID: 16739790].

California's Air Toxics Hot Spots Inventory

The California legislature passed the Air Toxics Hot Spots Information and Assessment Act in 1987 (Health and Safety Code Sections 44300 et seq.), partially in response to the Bhopal tragedy. The act allows the California Air Resources Board (CARB) to generate a comprehensive inventory of emissions of over 400 chemicals, including TACs, from stationary sources in the state and has a community right-to-know provision. The intent of the act is to gather information for cost-effective statewide toxics risk reduction, to provide citizens with information on toxics emitted into the air in their communities, and to require emissions reductions from facilities posing significant public health risks.

Emissions inventories are generated by the facilities and submitted to the local air pollution control district and the CARB. The districts prioritize facilities into categories of high, medium, or low concern based on the amount of pollutant emitted, toxic potency of pollutants, and proximity to populations. Facilities in the high-priority category are required to conduct a quantitative risk assessment of their airborne toxic emissions, which includes air-dispersion modeling and exposure estimates, and a quantitative assessment of the associated individual and population-wide health risks. If the facility is deemed by the district to pose significant risk, the facility must notify the community and engage in risk-reduction activity. The California hot spots program differs from the TRI in that there is a large risk-assessment and public-notification component.

The reporting triggers in the California program are considerably lower than for TRI; none is above 100 pounds per year. In addition, all types of facilities report their emissions, not just those that fall into the TRI categories. In this respect, the Air Toxics Hot Spots Inventory is quite comprehensive for California. Data are available for emissions from small facilities (e.g., dry cleaners and auto body shops) as well as from large-complex facilities such as refineries. However, unlike the TRI, the California program focuses only on airborne emissions, and there is no comparable database for land or water emissions in California. In addition, the TRI facilities are required to report yearly, whereas the California program only requires reporting every 4 years.

Of over 370 chemicals actually reported as emitted to the air in California in 2003, 90 are emitted in amounts greater than 10,000 pounds per year. Table 38–5 summarizes the top 25 chemicals by volume of emissions; Table 38–6 summarizes the top 25 carcinogens emitted by volume. Among these carcinogens, crystalline silica, formaldehyde, vinyl chloride, nickel, benzene, diesel engine particulate matter, radionuclides, and ethylene oxide are known human carcinogens. It is interesting to note that the most troublesome chemicals may not be those with a large volume of emissions. For example, emissions in pounds per year for hexavalent chromium are relatively small (586 lb/yr). Yet, because of the high potency estimates for this known human carcinogen, the near-source cancer-risk estimates can be relatively high. Compared with the California database, tetrachloroethylene emissions to air appear to be grossly underreported

Table 38–4. TRI carcinogens emitted into air in quantities greater than 400,000 pounds in 2003.

CAS Number	Chemical	Total Reported Air Emissions (thousand lbs/yr)
100-42-5	Styrene	48,284
75-07-0	Acetaldehyde	12,970
50-00-0	Formaldehyde	10,549
75-09-2	Dichloromethane	8,571
79-01-6	Trichloroethylene	6,876
71-42-2	Benzene	6,262
100-41-4	Ethylbenzene	5,929
108-05-4	Vinyl acetate	2,599
91-20-3	Naphthalene	2,042
127-18-4	Tetrachloroethylene	2,009
106-99-0	1,3-Butadiene	1,982
7439-92-1	Lead and compounds	1,239
7440-02-0	Nickel and compounds	1,073
67-66-3	Chloroform	927
126-99-8	Chloroprene	821
—	Polycyclic aromatic hydrocarbons (PAHs)[1]	741
7440-47-3	Chromium and compounds[2]	697
107-13-1	Acrylonitrile	636
75-01-4	Vinyl chloride	588
75-21-8	Ethylene oxide	441

[1]Reported total emissions of anthracene, benzo(g,h,i)perylene, phenanthrene, and the category polycyclic aromatic compounds.

[2]Hexavalent chromium is considered a human carcinogen; TRI only reports total chromium emissions; hexavalent will only be a portion of the total.

in TRI. Tetrachloroethylene emissions from dry cleaners and other sources in California totaled almost 1.8 million pounds, whereas TRI reports only 2 million pounds for the entire country. This is undoubtedly because many smaller operations use tetrachloroethylene and emit more overall than do those facilities required to report in TRI.

More than 850 risk assessments conducted by facility operators have been reviewed by the California EPA's Office of Environmental Health Hazard Assessment. Cancer risks estimated for facilities ranged from 1 in 1 million to 1 in 1000 for lifetime exposures to modeled airborne concentrations. This program demonstrates that a large number of facilities have risks greater than 1 in 1 million, the traditional de minimis

level for regulatory agencies. Initially, about 40% of evaluated facilities posed an estimated cancer risk greater than 10 in 1 million. Key chemicals that drive the cancer risk estimates in facilities posing cancer risks greater than 10 in 1 million include benzene, hexavalent chromium, tetrachloroethylene, PAHs, methylene chloride, arsenic, and formaldehyde. Many facilities have taken steps to reduce their emissions and associated risks. Thus the program is a successful motivating force for facilities to reduce emissions partly because of the public-notification provisions.

Facilities with relatively small emissions may pose high risks to a small number of people if the dispersion characteristics are poor. For example, cancer-risk estimates for

Table 38–5. Top 25 chemicals or chemical mixtures by volume of emissions in California's 2003 stationary sources inventory.

CAS Number	Chemical	Total Reported Air Emissions (thousand lbs/yr)
7664-41-7	Ammonia	23,835
7783-06-4	Hydrogen sulfide	4,949
108-88-3	Toluene	2,074
14808-60-7	Crystalline silica, respirable	2,053
127-18-4	Tetrachloroethylene	1,757
67-64-1	Acetone	1,700
—	Gasoline vapors	1,521
110-54-3	*n*-Hexane	1,417
50-00-0	Formaldehyde	1,355
1330-20-7	Xylenes (mixed)	1,285
7647-01-0	Hydrochloric acid	1,265
100-42-5	Styrene	1,061
1634-04-4	Methyl *tert*-butyl ether	872
71-55-6	Methyl chloroform	846
76-56-1	Methanol	818
—	Mineral oils	679
111-76-2	Ethylene glycol butyl ether	665
71-43-2	Benzene	541
78-93-3	Methyl ethyl ketone	525
67-63-0	Isopropyl alcohol	502
630-08-0	Carbon monoxide	416
75-09-2	Dichloromethane	405
115-07-1	Propylene	379
—	Fluorocarbons (chlorinated and brominated)	365
—	Diesel engine PM	241

dry-cleaning facilities are, in some cases, relatively large for nearby residents because the dry cleaner is located in close proximity to housing and the tetrachloroethylene emissions are poorly dispersed. Measures taken in California to reduce risks from tetrachloroethylene emissions include requiring solvent-recycling equipment and better ventilation and dispersion systems. Legislation enacted in 2004 phases out the use of tetrachloroethylene in dry-cleaning operations.

Large facilities such as refineries may emit large quantities of material but in some cases have lower can-cer-risk estimates than many smaller facilities because residences are located further away, and the materials are emitted from tall stacks, resulting in better dispersion. However, the number of persons exposed to that estimated cancer risk may be considerable.

California's Criteria Air Pollutant Emissions Inventory

California maintains an inventory of emissions of the criteria air pollutants: CO, NO_x, SO_x, and particulate

Table 38–6. Top 25 emitted carcinogens by volume in California's 2003 stationary sources inventory.

CAS Number	Chemical	Total Reported Air Emissions (thousand lbs/yr)
14808-60-7	Crystalline silica, respirable	2,053
127-18-4	Tetrachloroethylene	1,757
50-00-0	Formaldehyde	1,355
100-42-5	Styrene	1,061
1634-04-4	Methyl *tert*-butyl ether	872
71-43-2	Benzene	541
75-09-2	Dichloromethane	405
—	Diesel engine exhaust particulate matter	241
75-07-0	Acetaldehyde	217
100-41-4	Ethyl benzene	165
—	Polycyclic aromatic hydrocarbons (including naphthalene)	154
7440-02-2	Nickel (and compounds)	80.4
91-20-3	Naphthalene	76.3
75-56-9	Propylene oxide	69.8
79-01-6	Trichloroethylene	57.2
67-66-3	Chloroform	33.9
106-99-0	1,3-Butadiene	32.5
7439-92-1	Lead (and compounds)	22.2
75-01-4	Vinyl chloride	20.9
106-46-7	*p*-Dichlorobenzene	16.1
123-91-1	1,4-Dioxane	15.0
—	Radionuclides	13.8
108-05-4	Vinyl acetate	12.7
75-21-8	Ethylene oxide	10.0
107-06-2	Ethylene dichloride	5.2

matter less than 10 μm (PM_{10}) and less than 2.5 μm ($PM_{2.5}$) in diameter, as well as emissions of total suspended particulate matter (TSP), reactive organic gases (ROGs), and total organic gases (TOGs). ROGs and NO_x combine to form ozone; tracking these two categories of emissions is useful in predicting ozone concentrations. Table 38–7 summarizes the inventory for 2004. The category "Stationary Sources" represents a variety of industrial sources. Industrial emissions account for a significant proportion of total emissions of these pollutants into the air in the state. Emissions listed under "Area-wide" sources are dominated by consumer products use, architectural coatings, use of pesticides and fertilizers, residential heating, farming operations, and waste burning and disposal. Mobile sources are a major source of all these pollutants because of the combustion of fuels. In addition to tracking emissions of criteria air pollutants, ROGs, and TOGs, CARB also maintains a monitoring network to measure ambient air concentrations of these substances. This helps regulators to evaluate air quality,

Table 38–7. Statewide emissions of major components of smog in California in 2004 (tons/day).

	Stationary Sources[1]	Areawide Sources[2]	Mobile Sources[3]	Total Statewide
TOG	2490	2253	1418	6162
ROG	507	709	1302	2518
CO	406	2138	11,268	13,811
NO_x	507	93	2591	3191
SO_x	134	5	116	255
PM	214	3376	127	3717
PM_{10}	130	1852	125	2107
$PM_{2.5}$	86	593	102	780

[1]Emissions from stationary sources include those resulting from industrial processes, fuel combustion, waste disposal, cleaning and surface coating, and petroleum production and marketing.
[2]Emissions from areawide sources include those resulting from solvent evaporation, architectural coatings, pesticides/fertilizers, asphalt paving, refrigerants, residential fuel combustion, farming operations, construction and demolition, road dust, fires, cooking, and miscellaneous others.
[3]Emissions from mobile sources include those resulting from on-road motor vehicles, aircraft, off-road equipment and recreational vehicles, recreational and commercial boats and ships, fuel storage and handling, trains, farm-equipment, and miscellaneous other.
Source: From California Emissions Inventory Data and Retrieval System (CEIDARS), www.arb.ca.gov/html/database.htm.

particularly in metropolitan areas of the state, and the effectiveness of pollution-control efforts. Data on air quality are published both quarterly and annually and are available online at www.arb/ca/gov and on CD-ROM from CARB in the publication entitled *California Air Quality Data, Air Resources Board, California Environmental Protection Agency.*

REFERENCE

Air Resources Board: 2004 Estimated Annual Average Emissions Statewide, www.arb.ca.gov/app/emsinv/.

IMPORTANCE TO HEALTH CARE PERSONNEL

Epidemiologic studies of adverse health effects of air pollution have focused primarily on the major components of smog, such as ozone, particulate matter, nitrogen oxides, and carbon monoxide. A detailed description of studies is presented in Chapter 39. Recent studies indicate that children growing up in high-pollution areas of the United States (e.g., the Los Angeles Basin) suffer from reduced lung function, increased respiratory infections, and induction and exacerbation of asthma. Studies implicate ozone, particulate matter, acid aerosols, and NO_x in such respiratory effects. Ozone is a critical component of Los Angeles–type smog and contributes to respiratory and eye irritation. Particulate matter is associated in numerous studies with increased morbidity and mortality from respiratory and cardiac conditions.

To date, there are only a handful of published epidemiologic studies of the association between adverse health effects and exposure to TACs. In large part, this is a result of the difficulty of such studies, including a lack of exposure data and confounding by other air pollutants. Most of the health impacts of TACs have been inferred from occupational epidemiologic studies and toxicologic studies in experimental animals. A number of TACs are respiratory irritants. Exposure to TACs may contribute to respiratory disease and injury as well as result in systemic toxicity. There is increasing evidence linking exposure to TACs (e.g., acrolein, formaldehyde, PAHs, and diesel exhaust particles) to biochemical changes that are characteristic of allergic airways disease, including asthma, such as increases in proinflammatory cytokines and inflammatory cells in bronchiolar epithelium, increased mucin secretion, and elevated antigen-specific immunoglobulin (Ig) E. Risk assessments have indicated that certain industrial emissions may contribute to nonneoplastic respiratory or systemic adverse health impacts.

Risk assessments conducted for stationary sources in California under the air toxics hot spots program indicate relatively high (in an environmental context) excess individual cancer risks for people living near some facilities. Some of the estimated cancer risks from stationary source emissions are as high as 1 in 1000. There are a large number of causative agents of cancer, and chemical carcinogens emitted into the environment represent one source of these causal agents.

REFERENCES

Ernst KP et al: Releases from improper chemical mixing, Hazardous Substances Emergency Events Surveillance system, 1996–2001. J Occup Environ Med 2005;47:287 [PMID: 15761325].

Horton DK et al: Surveillance of hazardous materials events in 17 states, 1993–2001: A report from the Hazardous Substances Emergency Events Surveillance (HSEES) system. Am J Indust Med 2004;45:539 [PMID: 15164398].

Kaye WE et al: Surveillance of hazardous substance emergency events: Identifying areas for public health prevention. Int J Hyg Environ Health 2005;208:37 [PMID: 15881977].

Mindell J, Barrowcliffe R: Linking environmental effects to health impacts: A computer modelling approach for air pollution. J Epidemiol Community Health 2005;59:1092 [PMID: 16286501].

REGULATION OF STATIONARY SOURCES

State Regulations—California

The Toxic Air Contaminants Identification and Control Act (1983) created California's program to reduce health risks from air toxics. This was the first comprehensive state air toxics program to evaluate chemicals in the air and control sources of air toxics. CARB lists about 200 chemicals as TACs. Emissions of TACs from many source types are identified via the air toxics hot spots emissions inventory database and by a program that tests motor vehicle emissions. There are also statewide ambient air monitors that collect data on more than 50 chemicals. After formally identifying a substance as a TAC, CARB investigates the need, feasibility, and cost of reducing emissions of that substance. This process has resulted in air toxics control measures (ATCMs) to reduce emissions from the following sources: gasoline service stations (e.g., benzene and other volatiles), chrome plating and anodizing shops (e.g., hexavalent chromium), cooling towers (e.g., hexavalent chromium), sterilizers and aerators (e.g., ethylene oxide), medical waste incinerators (e.g., polychlorinated dibenzo-dioxins and dibenzofurans), serpentine rock in surfacing applications (e.g., asbestos), dry cleaning (e.g., tetrachloro-ethylene), metal melting (e.g., cadmium, nickel, and arsenic), and low-emission vehicle/clean-fuels regulations (e.g., benzene and 1,3-butadiene). A large effort is underway to reduce emissions dramatically from diesel-fueled engines, both stationary and mobile, resulting in reformulated diesel fuel and a number of ATCMs to curb diesel engine emissions.

At the local level, new and modified sources of air pollution are required to obtain operating permits from local air pollution control agencies. The goal is to ensure that new and modified devices are able to meet all air quality standards and not exacerbate air pollution problems in an area. In addition, the air toxics hot spots program risk-reduction provisions for existing facilities are enforced by local air districts and result in enforceable emissions reductions.

REFERENCE

The Toxic Air Contaminants Program, www.arb.ca.gov/html/brochure/airtoxic.htm#identification.

Federal Regulations

The federal Clean Air Act of 1990 represents a comprehensive statutory framework designed to reduce overall exposure to TACs, protect the stratospheric ozone layer, and reduce deposition of acidic constituents of air pollution (e.g., acid rain and acid snow). The Clean Air Act provides for use of market-based principles and other innovative approaches to reducing air pollution. Under Title III of the Clean Air Act, the EPA established a list of 189 HAPs. These HAPs are frequently referred to as *air toxics*. Technology-based standards have been promulgated by the EPA to control emissions of HAPs from major sources and "area" sources (defined by the EPA in this instance as minor sources). Residual risk (cancer and noncancer risks remaining after control devices have been put in place) is being assessed following the implementation of the technology-based standards of air pollution control. Further control measures may be developed if residual risks are considered by the EPA to be unreasonable.

REFERENCE

The Clean Air Act, www.epa.gov/air/oaq_caa.html/.

Worldwide Perspective

The concept of the EPA's TRI has attracted the attention of other countries. The Canadian government established a National Pollutant Release Inventory with many similarities to the TRI. Similarly, Mexico is formulating a pollutant-release inventory. The European Commission established a registry for pollutant emissions from industries. In addition, the Organization for Economic Cooperation and Development established a Pollutant Release and Transfer Register. Such developments on the international level facilitate pollution-control efforts on a global scale.

■ ACCIDENTAL AND INTENTIONAL RELEASES

The attacks on the World Trade Center and the Pentagon and ensuing rescue and cleanup efforts illustrated that health care providers, first responders (e.g., firefighters, police, emergency medical technicians, etc.), and public health agencies may be called on in the event of any large-scale accident. Health care providers gather information that is critical for assessing the public health effects of the release during their evaluation of potentially exposed persons. It is thus essential for health care personnel to be familiar with the health consequences of releases, reporting requirements, relevant regulations, and the steps involved in the public health assessment of chemical releases.

ACCIDENTAL CHEMICAL RELEASES & THE ROLE OF HEALTH CARE PROVIDERS

Accidental chemical releases may cause a variety of health effects (Table 38–8). However, it may be difficult to relate exposure from a release to alleged injury because preexposure health status information and exposure data may be unavailable. Much of the available information about the public health effects of chemical spills is based on reviews of medical records from initial clinic visits or medical consultations. In addition to providing immediate and continuing medical care, the information gathered can help to improve knowledge about long-term effects of chemicals released into the environment. When a victim of a hazardous substance exposure is evaluated, the following information should be recorded in the medical record:

- Subjective complaints
- General medical history, including the presence of preexisting medical conditions such as asthma and a history of smoking
- Occupational history, including potential workplace exposures unrelated to the release that might contribute to health complaints
- Exposure history
- Geographic and physical location of the individual relative to the site of the release
- The estimated length of time spent at any given location relative to the release during the incident
- Activities that may affect the exposure dose of chemical, such as strenuous exercise in the area of the chemical release or consumption of contaminated water or food
- Timing of onset of symptoms relative to potential exposure to accidentally released chemicals
- Identity of the substance(s) released
- Whether fires or explosions occurred as a result of the accident, which could involve exposure to combustion or pyrolysis products
- Physical examination
- Results of specific laboratory tests, such as spirometry, if relevant

Health care providers may play multiple roles following accidental releases of hazardous substances. In order to respond adequately, health care providers should

- Be prepared with an "all-hazards approach," relying on general principles of emergency management that can be applied to any natural or human-created incident
- Be familiar with chemical, biologic, radiologic, nuclear, and explosive (CBRNE) agents that have greatest potential for harm
- Be aware of required reporting of syndromes or illnesses to health agencies
- Develop and drill disaster response plans

ACCIDENT STATISTICS

Prevalence & Causes of Accidental Releases

The storage and transportation patterns of hazardous chemicals contribute to the high potential for accidental releases. Both worldwide and in the United States, chemical production continues to rise. Billions of pounds of hazardous chemicals are stored at manufacturing plants around the United States. More than a billion tons of hazardous materials are transported annually in the United States by trucks or railroad tank cars. The mate-

Table 38–8. Types of health effects reported following accidental releases of hazardous substances.[1]

Type of Injury	No. of Injuries[2]	Percent of Victims
Respiratory system	4200	52
Eye irritation	1529	19
Headache	1558	19
Dizziness or other central nervous system symptoms or signs	1380	17
Gastrointestinal problem	1340	17
Trauma	712	9
Skin irritation	730	9

[1]Based on 28,767 events with 8126 victims reported from 1998–2001 by 15 states to the Hazardous Substances Emergency Events Surveillance system.
[2]Since a person may have more than one type of health effect, the number of injuries exceeds the number of victims.

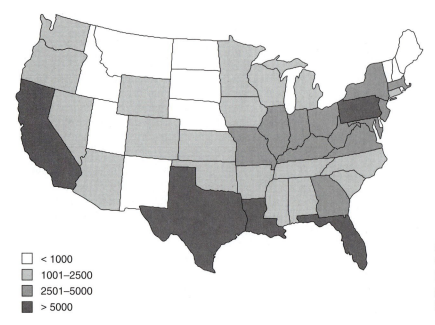

☐	< 1000
▨	1001–2500
▨	2501–5000
■	> 5000

Figure 38–1. Hazardous waste substances and oil releases reported to the Emergency Release Notification System, 1995–2000.

rials most often transported by rail are liquefied petroleum gas, chlorine, and anhydrous ammonia.

For the 10 years 1995–2004, more than 300,000 incidents involving hazardous substances, including intentional chemical releases, were reported to the National Response Center. In 2004 alone, more than 33,000 incidents were reported. Figure 38–1 provides a breakdown of accidents by state.

Accidental releases occur more commonly at fixed facilities (40%) than during transport (28%). Pipeline and storage-tank accidents also contribute to chemical releases. Overall, marine and offshore incidents are the most common causes of transportation accidents because petroleum products, which account for approximately 60% of accidental releases, are spilled most often in this setting. Transportation accidents involving nonpetroleum hazardous substances occur most commonly on highways. Transportation events are more likely to result in injury and death than are stationary source accidents; most deaths or injuries are a result of truck accidents. Hazardous substances releases at fixed facilities are most commonly a result of equipment failure (Table 38–9). Nonpetroleum hazardous substances account for approximately 20% of releases. Frequently released hazardous substances include ammonia, sulfur dioxide, and sulfuric acid (Table 38–10).

Public Health Consequences of Releases

The Agency for Toxic Substances and Disease Registry (ATSDR) maintains the Hazardous Substances Emergency Event Surveillance (HSEES) system to track public health outcomes of accidental releases. In 2004, 15 state health departments participated in this active surveillance system. During a 4-year period (1998–2001), 28,767 events were reported. The majority of the accidents reported to HSEES occurred at stationary facilities (75%), whereas 25% occurred during transportation.

From 1999–2001, injuries were reported in 9.1% of incidents. Most injuries (85.6%) occurred in stationary-facility incidents. Five hazardous substance categories accounted for more than 70% of injuries. In decreasing order, they were chlorine, ammonia, acids, pesticides, and bases. The most frequent cause of injury was chlorine, which was released in less than 2% of accidents but was responsible for 32.8% of injuries, indicating its high toxicity.

In addition to known hazardous substances, disasters may involve exposure to unknown substances and by-products of combustion, pyrolysis, and chemical reactions.

Table 38–9. Primary causes of accidental chemical releases at fixed facilities.[1]

Contributing Factors	N (%)
Equipment failure	9933 (46)
Human error	4483 (21)
Other factors (system/process upset, system startup/shutdown, etc.)	7182 (33)

[1]Based on 21,598 fixed-facility events reported by the Hazardous Substances Emergency Events Surveillance system, 1998–2001.

Table 38–10. Ten most frequently released hazardous substances.[1]

1. Ammonia
2. Sulfur dioxide
3. Sulfuric acid
4. Hydrochloric acid
5. Carbon monoxide
6. Sodium hydroxide
7. Nitric oxide
8. Mercury
9. Paint or coating, not otherwise specified
10. Ethylene glycol

[1]Based on 28,767 stationary-facility and transportation incidents reported by the Hazardous Substances Emergency Events Surveillance system, 1998–2001.

Effects of exposure to by-products are likely, especially if a release results in a fire or explosion. For example, pyrolysis products of methyl isocyanate unidentified to date may have contributed to the myriad and continuing health effects observed after the release of this gas in Bhopal.

Respiratory sequelae are the most common type of health effect reported following chemical releases (see Table 38–8). Trauma is more common in transportation-related incidents and generally is caused by mechanical events, not the hazardous substance released. Most victims of hazardous materials incidents are transported to a hospital and treated on an outpatient basis or treated at the scene of the incident. One in 10 individuals with illness or injury related to chemical releases is admitted to a hospital. Hazardous materials releases may result in fatalities among both employees and members of the public. Death occurs in 2% of injuries and often is the result of burns or trans-portation-related trauma.

Following accidental releases of hazardous materials, workers, including emergency-response personnel (such as firefighters and police), are injured most frequently, followed by the general public. In most cases, emergency responders are injured less frequently than other workers partly because they wear more protective equipment than other workers at the scene of a release. Most non-emergency-response employees (e.g., cleanup and construction workers) and 50% of emergency responders who are injured do not wear any personal protective equipment. Emergency responders are injured more often in transportation-related events than in fixed-facility releases, whereas non-emergency-response workers are injured more often in fixed-facility incidents.

REFERENCES

ATSDR: Hazardous Substances Emergency Events Surveillance (HSEES): Four-year cumulative report 1998–2001, www.atsdr.cdc.gov/HS/HSEES/Cum1998_2001.html.

Crabb C. Revisiting the Bhopal tragedy. Science 2004;306:1670 [PMID: 15576583].

Kaye WE et al: Surveillance of hazardous substance emergency events: Identifying areas of public health prevention. Int J Hygiene Environ Health 2005;208:37 [PMID: 15881977].

National Response Center. www.nrc.uscg.mil/nrsinfo.html.

Worker Health Consequences: The World Trade Center Attacks

Worker injuries and illnesses following the World Trade Center (WTC) attack on September 11, 2001, illustrate the general illness patterns outlined earlier (Table 38–11). During the first 24 hours following the collapse of the towers, 343 rescue workers died and an additional 240 sought emergency medical treatment. Traumatic injuries and systemic complaints of dehydration and exposure to debris accounted for the majority of medical diagnoses during the first 24 hours of response. Respiratory conditions comprised approximately one-fourth of illnesses diagnosed during this time period. Respiratory and mental health symptoms and lost work time have been reported by people work-

Table 38–11. Pattern of illness and injury among workers following the attack on the World Trade Center, New York City, September 11, 2001.[1]

	Rescue Workers[2]		Other Workers[5]
	First 24 Hours[3]	11-Month Follow-Up[4]	Postincident
Respiratory	25.7%	18.5%	65%
Trauma	38.1%		
Ophthalmic	10.4%		59%
Systemic	31.3%		
Psychological	3.3%	12.6%	34%

[1]CDC: September 11, 2002 (special issue): MMWR 2002;51:1.
[2]New York City Fire Department rescue workers who sought emergency medical care.
[3]N = 240; in the first 48 hours following the incident, 90% of 10,116 rescue workers complained of acute cough, often accompanied by nasal congestion, chest tightness, or chest burning.
[4]Follow-up was conducted at various times during the 11 months after the incident. Based on 10,116 rescue workers who sought medical care in the first 48 hours.
[5]Prevalence of symptoms among workers at one location in the vicinity of the WTC site (N = 224). The survey was conducted 4–6 months later, but referred to symptoms immediately following the incident.

ing near the WTC site but not involved in rescue, as well as by residents living near the site.

During the 11-month period following the incident, respiratory illnesses accounted for most of the illnesses among rescue workers who sought medical attention. Respiratory illnesses included eosinophilic pneumonia, pneumonia with lobar consolidation, and "WTC-related cough." Workers diagnosed with the latter condition had cough severe enough to require medical leave. It is estimated that 4% of the 11,336 rescue workers eventually may qualify for disability retirement because of persistent respiratory conditions. In addition to respiratory ailments, stress-related incidents accounted for a large number of reported medical conditions.

Industrial hygiene monitoring at the WTC site did not begin until 48 hours after the incident. During the first 48 hours, rescue workers most likely were exposed to high levels of respirable dust. Other chemicals detected 5–6 days after the incident included a complex mixture of building debris and pyrolysis and combustion by-products, including acid gases, asbestos, carbon monoxide, respirable silica, PAHs, and polychlorinated biphenyls. Induced sputum samples collected from highly exposed New York firefighters 10 months after the incident revealed inflammation and particles that were different from nonexposed controls and consistent with WTC dust exposure.

The observed pattern of respiratory illness among rescue workers may be partly attributed to inadequate use or availability of respirators. During the collapse of the towers, 52% of workers did not wear respirators; 38% did not wear respirators for the rest of the first day. Paper masks were the most commonly used respirators used during the first day. Although it is generally accepted that workers responding to accidental and intentional disasters should use adequate respiratory protection, the experience of the WTC response workers illustrates that barriers to use, such as heat stress, discomfort, communication, and training, must be addressed first.

REFERENCES

Banauch GI et al: Pulmonary disease in rescue workers at the World Trade Center site. Curr Opin Pulm Med 2005;11:160 [PMID: 15699790].

Landrigan PJ et al: Health and environmental consequences of the World Trade Center disaster. Environ Health Perspect 2004; 112:731 [PMID: 15121517].

Worker Education and Training Program: Learning from disasters: Weapons of mass destruction preparedness through worker training, www.wetp.org and www.wetp.org/index.cfm?fuseaction=wtc.

RESPONSE TO ACCIDENTAL RELEASES

Professionals essential in the response to accidental releases include health care providers, hospital staff, and emergency responders.

A. HEALTH CARE PROVIDER ROLE

In addition to providing medical information during a release and treating exposed victims, health care providers can act as reliable spokespersons on the potential health threat of toxic chemicals that are being used or stored at facilities in the community. Providing reliable toxicity information to first responders and the community in a timely manner should be one of the main goals of health professionals responding to a release.

When evaluating individuals for potential exposure to accidentally released chemicals, health care personnel first must identify the compound, consider decontaminating the individual, and decide on appropriate treatment measures. Online resources, material safety data sheets, and regional poison control centers should be consulted for substance identification and medical treatment options. If these sources do not have appropriate toxicity information, it may be necessary to contact the manufacturer directly. Manufacturers are allowed to withhold trade secrets about hazardous chemicals from the public, but they are required to provide this information to physicians or nurses who require it for the purpose of treating victims of exposure. Specific proprietary information can be obtained legally in order to render appropriate medical care, but the person receiving this information must agree to maintain this information confidential.

B. HOSPITAL ROLE

Following major chemical incidents, local hospitals may be overwhelmed by the volume of patients seeking acute care. To optimize response to these emergencies, hospitals should plan for response to accidental releases and establish policies specifying the scope and conduct of patient care to be provided at the facility. This includes determining methods to triage patients into mild, moderate, and severe injury categories; establishing treatment protocols; specifying decontamination methods to be used in treatment areas; and coordinating with other area hospitals and local and state agencies. Current toxicologic reference materials, including online databases and telephone numbers of the regional poison control center, should be readily available (Table 38–12). Information on referral and consultation services should be updated regularly.

Hospitals and other health care providers are part of a statewide emergency medical care system that coordinates patient distribution to hospitals and monitors medical resources during incidents (Table 38–13). The emergency medical care system also assists in planning and training, as well as certifying certain response personnel such as paramedics. Hospitals and emergency responders should coordinate drills and simulations to ensure optimal response during a large-scale emergency.

Table 38–12. Resources for planning for and response to accidental releases of hazardous materials.

SUBSTANCE IDENTIFICATION	
• National Fire Protection Agency labels	• Labeling system for describing chemical hazards
• US Department of Transportation (DOT) placards	• Warning placards for vehicles carrying hazardous materials
TOXICITY & RESPONSE INFORMATION **Databases**	
• Chemical Hazard Response Information System (CHRIS)	• Online information from the United States Coast Guard for emergency response for transportation accidents involving hazardous chemicals
• Integrated Risk Information System (IRIS), www.epa.gov/iris/	• Online health risk assessment information on chemicals from the EPA
• New Jersey Hazardous Substance Fact Sheets, www.state.nj.us/health/eoh/rtkweb/rtkhsfs.htm	• Online summarized information on hazards, safe storage, control, first aid, and emergency procedures for common chemicals
• Registry of Toxic Effects of Chemical Substances (RTECS), www.cdc.gov/niosh/rtecs.default.html	• Toxicity data from NIOSH for potentially toxic chemicals, including NTP test status
• Toxicology, Occupational Medicine, and Environment Series (TOMES) Plus System, www.micromedex.com/products/tomesplus/	• CD-ROM that brings together 14 different databases containing toxicity data, information for safe handling of chemicals, responding to hazardous chemical spills, and evaluation and treatment of persons acutely exposed
Manuals	
• Managing Hazardous Materials Incidents, Volumes I–III, ATSDR, www.atsdr.cdc.gov/mhmi.html	• Planning guides for emergency medical services, hospital emergency departments, and emergency department physicians
Telephone Resources	
• CHEMTREC (800) 424-9300	• 24-Hour hotline operated by Chemical Manufacturer's Association; provides information on identity and hazardous properties of chemicals; can put caller in touch with industry representatives and medical toxicologists
• Regional poison control center (800) 222-1222	• Provides information on immediate health effects, need for decontamination, protective gear, and specific treatment
REPORTING INFORMATION	
• National Response Center (800) 424-8802	• 24-Hour reporting system staffed by the United States Coast Guard which handles all significant hazardous materials spills under agreements with DOT and the EPA; relays calls to relevant response agencies

C. EMERGENCY-RESPONDER ROLE

Firefighters and emergency medical technicians usually are the first on the scene of an accident. By establishing protocols for decontamination, evacuating, or sheltering in place, emergency responders assist the injured, control the spread of chemicals, and minimize the impact on the surrounding community. Individual health care providers and hospitals should ensure that emergency responders are included in response plans as well as in drills.

REFERENCES

Braun BI et al: Hospital bioterrorism preparedness linkages with the community: Improvements over time. Am J Infect Control 2004;32:317 [PMID: 15454887].

Polatin PB et al: Bioterrorism, stress, and pain: The importance of an anticipatory community preparedness intervention. J Psychosom Res 2005;58:311 [PMID: 15992565].

Treatment

Following most cases of accidental exposure, symptomatic treatment will suffice. This entails choosing supportive or palliative treatment based on signs and symptoms and the route of exposure. Attempts should be made to distinguish symptoms caused by anxiety (worried well) from those caused by direct chemical effects. For some chemicals, clinical effects may not be obvious immediately, and delayed toxicity may need to be considered. For example, following phosgene inhalation exposures, patients should be monitored for 24 hours

Table 38–13. Guidance for emergency response.

Response Plan	Description	Web Site
Hospital Emergency Incident Command System (HEICS)	Incident command system-based crisis management plan for hospitals to use to coordinate their own response to emergencies or disasters	www.emsa.ca.gov/Dms2/heics3.htm
National Incident Management System (NIMS)	Federal system establishes standard protocols and procedures for incident managers and responders to work together to prepare for and respond to all incidents, including natural disasters and acts of terrorism	www.fema.gov/nims/
National Response Plan (NRP)	Establishes an all-hazards approach to manage domestic incidents; integrates best practices and procedures from disciplines, such as emergency medical services, law enforcement, first responder, public health and safety into a unified structure.	www.dhs.gov/dhspublic/interapp/ editorial/editorial_0566.xml
Standardized Emergency Management System (SEMS)	Incident command system-based plan for managing response to multiagency and multijurisdiction emergencies in California; consists of five organizational levels which are activated as necessary. Local governments must use SEMS to be eligible for funding of their personnel related costs under state disaster assistance programs.	www/oes.ca.gob/Operational/ OESHome.nsf/0/ B4943535210895448256C2A0071E0 38?OpenDocument

for onset of pulmonary edema. (See Chapters 19 and 20 for more detailed information on acute upper airway and pulmonary injury.) Only rarely are chemical-specific medications or antidotes available. For example, following inhalation or dermal exposure to hydrofluoric acid, treatment options may include nebulized or subcutaneous calcium gluconate in addition to corticosteroids; the oxime class of chemicals contains antidotes for organophosphate poisoning.

Decontamination

To minimize contamination of response personnel and treat exposed individuals most efficiently, the incident commander at a hazardous materials incident typically establishes a command post and creates hazard zones (Figure 38–2). The *hot zone*, also known as the *exclusion zone*, is closest to the spill, and only responders wearing personal protective equipment should be allowed to enter. Entry and exit are controlled through an entry point and a separate point of exit. Only rudimentary first aid is provided in this area. The *warm zone* provides a systematic way to lessen the exposure to the chemical hazard for those who have been in the hot zone and also serves to control the spread of contamination into the cold zone. Decontamination takes place in the warm zone and may extend into the cold zone. The *cold zone* is also termed the *support zone;* this area is theoretically safe from the chemical hazard and usually is set up a consid-

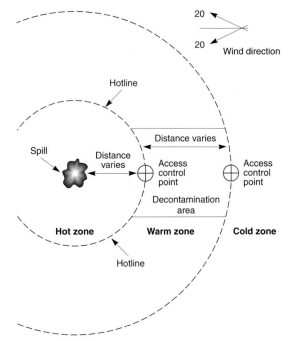

Figure 38–2. Schematic of hot, warm, and cold zones at a hazardous materials spill site. (Adapted from Olson KR, Mycroft FJ: Emergency medical response to hazardous materials incidents, in Olson KR (ed), *Poisoning and Drug Overdose*, 4th ed. New York: McGraw-Hill, 2004, Chap. 8.)

erable distance upwind of the spill. Command and control activities, first aid, and planning take place in the cold zone. Plume modeling may be used to map expected chemical concentrations to determine the different zones.

Many local jurisdictions have developed hazardous materials (HAZMAT) teams trained to identify and respond to hazardous materials incidents. Decontamination in the field is most likely to be performed by these teams. Guidelines exist for the decontamination of potentially exposed emergency responders. The Occupational Safety and Health Administration (OSHA) has issued requirements for emergency medical technicians and any other health care providers who may be required to respond to a hazardous materials spill. OSHA also requires that employers provide the necessary protective equipment and training to any employee who may encounter a situation involving hazardous materials. Guidelines for decontamination of the public also exist, but no uniform procedure is recommended by all agencies. Because the level of exposure often is unknown, it is considered good management to decontaminate at or near the site of the release.

Following exposure to a hazardous substance in liquid form, decontamination generally involves removing clothes and copiously rinsing the skin and eyes with water to remove chemical contaminants. Spills involving oily materials such as petroleum products may require the use of soap. Runoff water should be contained, if possible, to prevent the contamination of water sources. Decontamination with water may be harmful in some cases. For example, in the presence of water, metal phosphides such as aluminum, zinc, and magnesium phosphides hydrolyze to produce the toxic gas phosphine. If dermal exposure to a metal powder is suspected, the skin should be brushed off, and clothes should be aerated in a ventilated area. Clothes then should be laundered, and the contaminated bare skin should be washed thoroughly with soap and water.

An additional issue of occasional concern is that of secondary contamination of health care facilities and workers with toxic materials on the skin or clothes of accident victims or from toxic vomitus in the case of ingestion. An example of a substance that is of low risk for toxicity from secondary contamination is a gas such as chlorine. Substances of high risk for toxicity for secondary contamination require protection of both treatment facilities and medical personnel and include concentrated acids and bases and potent chemical carcinogens (Table 38–14).

Sheltering in Place versus Evacuation

In general, a decision to institute protective actions immediately following a spill is made by the emergency-response incident commander, such as a fire chief, police officer, or coast guard officer, in conjunc-

Table 38–14. Examples of substances that present low and high probability for secondary contamination of health care facilities and providers.

Probability of Secondary Contamination	Chemical or Substance Category
Low	Gases: chlorine, ethylene oxide Vapors: sulfuric acid mist (unless there has been significant exposure) Weak acids and bases: sodium hydroxide Most hydrocarbon products: gasoline
High	Strong acids and bases: hydrofluoric acid Volatile liquids: isocyanates, formaldehyde Potent pesticides Potent chemical carcinogens Radioactive materials Biologic agents

tion with local health personnel and elected officials. Few options are available for the protection of community residents after accidental releases. In the case of a release into water, residents may be cautioned to avoid contact with or consumption of the contaminated source. Following releases into air, the two alternatives for protective action are sheltering in place or evacuation. Little objective data exist to support one choice definitively over the other in a given release situation, although several theoretical guidelines are available. The decision to evacuate or shelter in place involves weighing many factors. For example, the characteristics of the chemical; the estimated concentration as a function of time; the source, size, and duration of the release; meteorologic conditions; and the intactness and infiltration rates of the structures used for protection all must be considered. Finally, the proximity of institutions that might require special attention during both evacuation and sheltering in place, such as schools, hospitals, and prisons, should be considered.

Theoretical research suggests that in-place protection is nearly always better than evacuation. It is of greatest benefit when the chemical's peak concentration, rather than its cumulative dose, presents the greater toxicity. Sheltering in place should be the initial response while any situation is being assessed. Buildings with ventilation systems turned off and with intact doors and windows closed may reduce exposure to half compared with unprotected outdoor exposures. Evacuation may be the preferred choice when there is the threat of a release, though none has yet occurred, or when the release may create an explosion or fire hazard. Evacuation usually is a time-consuming and confusing process and is the safest alternative only when it can be completed prior to the time when a toxic cloud reaches a populated area.

Both in-place protection and evacuation are most effective in protecting individuals from toxic exposure when the local population has received prior education about the proper procedures to follow in the event of an accidental release. Public education about toxic incidents should be coordinated with instruction on response planning for other natural and intentional disasters. Educational sessions should be held with the full participation of all agencies that might respond to an actual event. Chemical emergency planning is most effective when industry, government, the medical community, local community organizations, and public interest groups have established working relationships and coordinate their efforts to mitigate the effects of an accident.

REFERENCES

Edlich RF et al: Modern concepts of treatment and prevention of chemical injuries. J Long-Term Effects Med Implants 2005; 15:303 [PMID: 16022641].

Edkins A, Murray V: Management of chemically contaminated bodies. J R Soc Med 2005;98:141 [PMID: 15805553].

Jetter JJ, Whitfield C: Effectiveness of expedient sheltering in place in a residence. J Hazard Mater 2005;119:31 [PMID: 15752846].

OSHA: Safety and health topics: Emergency response, www.osha.gov/Publications/OSHA3114/osha3114.html.

Treat KN et al: Hospital preparedness for weapons of mass destruction incidents: An initial assessment. Ann Emerg Med 2001; 38:562 [PMID: 11679869].

PUBLIC HEALTH RISK ASSESSMENT AFTER ACCIDENTAL RELEASES

The Four Steps of Risk Assessment

During an actual release of a hazardous material, the health care provider must be prepared to assess the attendant risks and assist with the response. The National Academy of Sciences has defined the health risk assessment for toxicants as four steps: (1) hazard identification, (2) exposure assessment, (3) toxicologic and dose-response evaluation, and (4) risk characterization. Risk assessment is discussed in greater detail in Chapter 45. In theory, risk assessment is separated from risk management decisions made during an accidental release. In practice, however, because time constraints are imposed by the emergent nature of accidental releases, there is no clear separation of these four steps, and risk assessors may play a part in influencing man-

agement decisions based on the incomplete data available. Public health officials may act as either risk assessors or as risk managers, and multidisciplinary and interagency involvement is customary, even during small-scale chemical accidents. A large-scale accident may involve physicians, toxicologists, epidemiologists, emergency responders, and other staff from local, state, and federal agencies. The following sections examine the four steps of risk assessment as they apply to an accidental release.

A. HAZARD IDENTIFICATION

Hazard identification involves describing the released chemicals and determining their relative hazards in order to ascertain the immediate, delayed, and longer-term health risks posed by the release. The parent compound, as well as the breakdown products and other major ingredients in the formulation, must be identified, which can be done by using online government and chemical manufacturer databases. Identification of the spilled compound may not always be easy because rail tank car placards may be missing or inadequate toxicity testing may lead to failure to accurately categorize a chemical as hazardous. For new chemicals, health effects data may not be readily accessible. Information on breakdown products, chemical interactions, and nontoxicologic hazards, such as flammability, should be sought. In addition to causing thermal injury, explosions or fires may result in the release of a variety of toxic products of incomplete combustion, such as benzene, phosgene, or sulfur dioxide. When more than one substance has spilled, information regarding potential chemical interactions should be assessed to the extent possible.

B. EXPOSURE ASSESSMENT

Exposure assessment entails characterization of the source and location of the release, the potential pathways of human exposure, the population at risk, and the level of exposure. Exposures must be evaluated immediately following the release and levels predicted until the source is contained. In most cases, public health officials will need to rely on emergency responders for information on the exact location of the release, the time of the accident, whether the release has been contained, and the total amount spilled. The route of exposure to a hazardous substance often determines the types of health effects observed following its accidental release. Although routes of exposure often are obvious, such as when inhalation exposure follows a massive release into the air, this may not always be the case. For any particular spill, multiple routes of exposure may need to be considered.

Geographic information systems that take into account terrain, weather, and residential locations may be used to map spills and to predict the path of the chemical plume to better characterize potential exposures and identify the population at risk. Often, however, in the confusion that follows an accidental release, geographic information systems do not provide accurate, timely information to guide risk management decisions. Environmental monitoring of the released chemical and its breakdown products or other de novo toxicants is important to accurately determine the level of exposure; monitoring is essential in the case of a dynamic exposure source. The population at risk of exposure includes employees of the facility or transport mode responsible for the release; people at nearby facilities, residences, and businesses; and people in transit in their vehicles in the area of the release or in the path of the chemical plume. Although emergency responders are more likely to wear personal protective equipment than other workers or the general public, they usually are at greatest risk of exposure and adverse health effects.

C. DOSE-RESPONSE EVALUATION

Toxicologic and dose-response evaluation involves (1) identifying the toxicologic endpoints of concern from the published literature as well as unpublished documents, if available, and (2) characterizing the relationship between the exposure dose and the adverse health effects. Both animal and human data should be consulted because human testing often is inadequate. The results of acute, subchronic, and chronic carcinogenicity and reproductive toxicity testing should be obtained. When quantitative human data are unavailable, animal data are related to an equivalent human dose on a body-weight or surface-area basis.

D. RISK CHARACTERIZATION

Risk characterization involves (1) identification of health effects that may be expected from the release and of individuals or institutions at greatest risk of adverse health effects and (2) institution of emergency-response action levels to protect individuals from further exposure or to prevent injury.

1. Health effects—Health effects following accidental releases may be categorized into immediate, delayed, and carcinogenic. Table 38–8 lists the immediate health effects reported most commonly as a result of spills. While most health care providers evaluate and treat exposed persons for immediate effects, persistent or delayed conditions following exposure to accidentally released compounds may occur. For example, various reports exist in which reactive airways dysfunction syndrome has been described in police officers following a single exposure during transportation accidents. For the majority of hazardous substances releases, however, inadequate information is available on the long-term effects of acute exposures.

After a short-term exposure (up to 2 weeks), a quantitative evaluation can be made of certain potential long-term effects such as cancer based on the inherent toxicity of the compound, the exposure level, and the dose-response assessment. For most compounds, a short-term exposure would result in a negligible risk of cancer. If an accidental release results in chronic environmental or occupational exposures to relatively low levels of a contaminant, however, it is prudent to estimate risks of cancer or other long-term effects to guide surveillance, cleanup, and other response measures.

In addition to physical consequences of accidental chemical exposure, the psychological impact of accidental releases is an important factor to consider. Depression, anger, and anxiety are common in communities immediately following and as prolonged consequences of accidental releases. Health care providers and public health officials should recognize that exposed persons may need evaluation for and treatment of psychological problems. Additionally, anxiety about the possible effects of released chemicals may increase health care utilization by the "worried well," as well as by individuals considering litigation.

Persons who may be predisposed to adverse effects following exposure to accidentally released chemicals are termed *sensitive individuals,* some of whom are identified in Table 38–15. Institutions housing such individuals, such as schools, hospitals, or elderly care facilities, that are in the vicinity of an accidental release may warrant special mitigation measures. Public health officials may need to notify the public that certain sensitive subpopulations may be at an increased risk of specified health consequences.

2. Emergency-response standards—Emergency-response action levels are used to guide shelter-in-place or evacuation decisions; if evacuation has occurred, these levels may be used to determine when it is safe for community members to reenter the area. It is important to note that these levels are not used to predict health effects in a potentially exposed population. In general, a level defines the concentration and duration to which most individuals may be exposed without suffering from a designated health effect (e.g., mild, severe, or life-threatening). To derive an emergency-response level, the EPA recommends dividing the highest exposure dose that does not result in the health effect of interest (the no adverse or lowest adverse effect level) by uncertainty factors ranging from 1–10 to account for inadequacies in the database, incomplete scientific knowledge, and protection of sensitive subpopulations. The use of uncertainty factors offers a margin of safety for officials to consider when recommending responses to accidental releases. In the event of an accidental release, a variety of exposure reference levels may be used. These standards vary considerably in their use of accurate scientific methods and

Table 38–15. Examples of "sensitive individuals" with conditions predisposing toward adverse health effects following exposure to chemicals.

Sensitive Subpopulation	Proposed Reason for Increased Sensitivity	Chemical Examples
Infants and children	Age-related differences in anatomy and physiology, organ susceptibility, exposure	Pesticides; lead
Developing fetuses	Critically timed organogenesis extremely susceptible to disruption of normal events	Toluene
Asthmatics	Increased sensitivity to end-organ effects of substances	Ozone
Individuals with coronary artery disease	Increased sensitivity to end-organ effects of substances	Carbon monoxide

intent to protect public health. The EPA offers rough guidelines for "safe" 1-hour exposures for most members of a community (Table 38–16).

The preferred 1-hour levels on which to base emergency response actions are the Short-Term Public Emergency Guidance Levels and Acute Exposure Guidance Levels (AEGLs) developed by the National Academy of Sciences or the Emergency Response and Planning Guidelines-2 (ERPG-2) developed by the American Industrial Hygiene Association. Although relatively few substances have been addressed by these organizations when compared with the number of hazardous chemicals in use, guidance levels increasingly are available for some of the most commonly released substances.

If these levels are not available for a spilled chemical, the EPA recommends consultation with toxicologists (working in regulatory agencies) for advice based on a review of the toxicity of the material of concern. For example, even on an emergent basis, toxicologists may be able to derive exposure guidance levels based on literature review using uncertainty factors to account for data gaps such as interspecies and intraspecies differences. If this is not possible, the EPA recommends that other occupational standards be used to develop actions levels (see Table 38–16).

The EPA's focus is on events with the potential for outcomes similar in severity to the accident in Bhopal, as reflected in its emphasis on incidents that have high acute hazard potential. Incidents resulting in deaths, injuries, or

Table 38–16. The U.S. EPA's recommended hierarchy of emergency-response (1-hour) action standards for guiding actions during and after accidental releases.[1]

Name of Standard	Agency
Preexisting Levels (Preferred):	
1. Short-term Public Emergency Guidance Levels	National Academy of Sciences
2. Acute Exposure Guidance Levels-2	National Academy of Sciences
3. Emergency Response Planning Guidelines-2	American Industrial Hygiene Association
4. Levels based on comprehensive review of literature	State or local governmental agency
Levels Developed during Accident (If Above Are Not Available):	
5. Levels based on brief toxicity review	Government toxicologists
If Nothing Else Is Available:	
6. Threshold Limit Value—Short Term Exposure Limit	NIOSH
7. Threshold Limit Value—Time-Weighted Average multiplied by 3	NIOSH
8. Immediately Dangerous to Life and Health values divided by 10	NIOSH

[1]Based on the DOE: *Handbook of Chemical Hazards Analysis Procedures*, 2004, http://www.eh.doe.gov/techstds/standard/hdbk.

evacuations are given the highest priority, as is reflected in the accident definitions that guide emergency planning activities. The EPA defines *minor accidents* as those having low potential for serious human injuries and no potential for human fatalities. *Moderately severe accidents* are defined as having the potential to result in up to 10 fatalities, 100 injuries, and evacuation of up to 2000 people. The EPA does not claim that the recommended standards protect identifiable subpopulations that may be particularly susceptible to the adverse health effects of hazardous substances, such as asthmatics and persons with coronary artery disease (see Table 38–15).

REFERENCES

Jederberg WW: Issues with the integration of technical information in planning for and responding to nontraditional disasters. J Toxicol Environ Health 2005;68:877 [PMID: 16020182].

EPA: Acute exposure guideline levels (AEGLs), www.epa.gov/oppt/aegl/chemlist.htm

Woodall GM: Acute health reference values: Overview, perspective, and current forecast of needs. J Toxicol Environ Health 2005; 68:901 [PMID: 16020184].

Coordination of Multiagency Response

Several governmental agencies and professional specialties likely will be involved in the response to any major incident. Responses may be confusing, frustrating, and duplicative. To streamline response to major incidents, agencies should coordinate efforts to establish joint plans. Several levels of response may be activated as needed to deliver effective aid to multiagency and multijurisdiction emergencies. These levels are (1) field, (2) local government, (3) county, (4) region, (5) state, and (6) federal. Joint emergency management teams may operate under all kinds of emergencies, including intentional releases of hazardous substances and natural disasters. The National Response Plan is a federal document that establishes a comprehensive all-hazards approach to manage incidents. The plan integrates best practices and procedures from incident-management disciplines, such as emergency medical services, law enforcement, first responder, public health, and worker health and safety, into a unified structure. The National Incident Management System provides a framework for coordinating response to all major incidents (see Table 38–13).

REGULATIONS

General

Health care providers involved in the planning for or response to accidental releases should be aware of the complex regulations governing this area of environmental health and the sources of data for hazardous substance releases.

A. DEFINITION OF HAZARDOUS MATERIALS

Hazardous materials are defined as materials or substances in forms or quantities that, if released, might pose an unreasonable risk to health and safety or property. Chemicals listed under the Comprehensive Environmental Response, Compensation, and Liability Act of 1980 (CERCLA), also known as Superfund, are considered to be hazardous substances. Approximately 2400 materials are listed and are classified broadly into categories such as explosives, flammables, corrosives, combustibles, poisons, oxidizers, biologic agents, and radioactive materials. The transport of hazardous materials is regulated by the Department of Transportation (DOT) under the Hazardous Materials Transportation Act of 1975.

Stationary-Source Accidents

A. FEDERAL REGULATIONS

In general, stationary-source accidental release planning and response falls under the jurisdiction of EPA and transportation accidents under DOT. Mandatory emergency planning and reporting requirements for the manufacture, storage, and transportation of hazardous materials are determined by four major federal regulations: CERCLA and EPCRA, the Hazardous Material Transportation Act of 1974 (HMTA), the Clean Air Act Amendments of 1990 (CAAA), and the Clean Water Act (CWA).

CERCLA (42 CFR Chapter 103) requires that the EPA establish for each hazardous substance a reportable quantity (RQ) based on the substance's physical, chemical, and toxicologic properties, including aquatic and mammalian toxicity, ignitability, and reactivity, among other factors. Hazardous substance releases equal to or in excess of the RQ must be reported immediately to the National Response Center (NRC), as well as to state and local emergency-response officials. This notification is required for transportation incidents and releases from vessels, as well as stationary-source emergencies. Failure to report accidental releases can include civil and criminal penalties, including monetary fines, imprisonment, or both. There is no requirement to report non-CERCLA substances. The latter category includes chemicals for which there is inadequate toxicity information for characterization as hazardous materials. For example, there was little toxicity data on methyl isocyanate prior to its release in Bhopal.

EPCRA (40 CFR Part 355.40), or SARA Title III, requires that the release of an RQ or more of a hazardous substance that results in exposure of people outside a facility boundary be reported to state and local authorities. EPCRA also requires states to establish statewide and local emergency planning groups to develop chemical emergency-response plans for each community and requires facilities to provide material safety data sheets (MSDSs) or a list of hazardous materials on site to states, local planners, and fire departments and, through them, the public. In theory, EPCRA builds the foundation of the community emergency-response plan and public-industry dialog on accidental-release risk and risk reduction. EPCRA also requires facility operators to notify the state emergency-response commission (or its equivalent) of the type and quantity of hazardous materials stored in quantities equal to or in excess of the RQ. These regulations have resulted in increased notification of local, state, and federal governments about hazardous materials stored at facilities and improved knowledge of the patterns of accidental releases from both fixed and mobile sources. However, increased concerns for security as a consequence of actual and threatened terrorist events have resulted in reduced public availability of much of this information. In addition, local governments lack information about transportation of these substances through their jurisdictions.

HMTA (49 CFR Part 171.15) requires that the release of a hazardous material during transportation be reported to the NRC under certain circumstances, such as death, injury, significant property damage, evacuation, or highway closure.

Section 112r of the CAAA contains regulations aimed at preventing accidental releases of regulated materials and other extremely hazardous substances to the air and minimizing the consequences of releases by focusing preventive measures on chemicals that pose the greatest risk. It requires facilities to identify hazards resulting from releases, to design and maintain safe facilities, and to minimize the consequences of releases when they occur. In addition, the CAAA is unique among environmental regulations in that it requires the protection of not only the environment and the health of the public but also the health and safety of workers. To protect workers, OSHA has promulgated a chemical process safety standard to protect workers from chemical accidents at facilities using highly toxic, reactive, flammable, or explosive substances (57 CFR Part 6536). To protect the public, the EPA established a rule governing Risk Management Programs for Accidental Release Prevention (40 CFR Part 68). This rule requires facilities to prepare hazard assessments evaluating potential effects of an accidental release of any regulated substance. Based on these hazard assessments, facilities must develop programs aimed at prevention of and emergency response to accidental releases.

CWA (40 CFR Parts 110.10 and 300.300) requires that oil releases be reported to the NRC if the release (1) violates applicable water quality standards, (2) causes a film, sheen, or discoloration of the water or adjoining shoreline, or (3) causes a sludge or an emulsion to be deposited beneath the surface of the water or on the adjoining shorelines.

B. STATE REGULATIONS

A few states have regulations requiring facilities to prepare and implement plans for the prevention of chemical accidents and emergency response in the event of a release. The programs in two states are described briefly.

New Jersey's Toxic Catastrophe Prevention Act of 1987 is an excellent example of an effective accident-prevention program. Facilities that have "extraordinarily hazardous substances" equal to or in excess of a threshold quantity must prepare a risk-reduction program similar to that described earlier for the federal risk management program. One hundred and ten extraordinarily hazardous substances are defined and regulated based on their volatility and toxicity. In the 15 years since its inception, the Toxic Catastrophe Prevention Act has resulted in major reductions in registered inventories of extraordinarily hazardous substances through the substitution of less hazardous substances.

California's Risk Management and Prevention Program was enacted in 1986. This program's goal is to prevent accidental releases by anticipating their occurrence and requiring that preemptive actions be taken. This program requires the managers of a facility that handles a certain quantity of "acutely hazardous materials" to prepare documents reviewing its design and operations to determine potential sources of a chemical accident and the consequences such an accident could have on neighboring communities (an off-site consequence analysis). These documents are to be submitted for review to local "administering agencies" (e.g., fire departments and county health departments). The effectiveness of this program is limited by the technical expertise available in the local administering agencies, resulting in uneven review of such documents.

REFERENCES

Department of Energy (DOE): Hazardous Materials Transportation Act, www.eh.doe.gov/oepa/laws/hmta.html.

EPA: CERCLA overview, www.epa.gov/superfund/action/law/cercla.htm.

EPA: Consolidated list of chemicals subject to the Emergency Planning and Community Right-to-Know Act (EPCRA) and Section 112(r) of the Clean Air Act, 2006, EPA 550-B-01-003.

Kleindorfer PR et al: Drivers of accident preparedness and safety: Evidence from the RMP Rule. J Hazard Mater 2004;115:9 [PMID: 15518959].

SOURCES OF DATA

Various databases contain information about accidental releases, although no single source of information is comprehensive.

Hazardous Materials Information System

The Hazardous Materials Information System (HMIS) is a computerized information management system containing reports of transportation accidents involving hazardous materials. Transportation carriers are required to report by telephone whenever there is a significant hazardous materials incident during transportation or storage related to transportation, including those involving a death, an injury requiring hospitalization, property damage in excess of $50,000, an evacuation, the closure of a major transportation artery or facility, the alteration of the operational flight pattern or routine of an aircraft, the release of a radioactive material, or a situation that is judged by the carrier to merit notification even though it does not meet the specified criteria. Written reports must be filed by the carrier within 30 days of occurrence. The report identifies the mode of transportation involved, name of reporting carrier, shipment information, results of the incident, hazardous materials involved, nature of packaging, cause of failure, and narrative description of the incident. This information is available in the incident database approximately 3 months after receipt of the report.

Emergency Release Notification System

The Emergency Release Notification System (ERNS) is a computer database containing information on release notifications of oil and hazardous substances that have occurred throughout the United States and have been reported to the NRC and/or one of the 10 EPA regions. Data have been collected into ERNS since 1987. The EPA assigns each CERCLA hazardous substance an RQ that defines when a release must be reported to the NRC. ERNS contains various types of information on specific notifications of releases of oil and hazardous substances, including the following: discharger information, date of release, material released, cause of release, damage/injuries/deaths, amount released, source of release, incident location, response actions taken, authorities notified, and environmental medium into which the release occurred.

Limitations of this database include inadequate health data and the potential for duplicate reporting. In addition, because reports are made during the initial phases of an accident, are not verified, and are not subsequently modified after more thorough investigation, the information may not be entirely accurate or complete.

Hazardous Substances Emergency Event Surveillance System

Maintained by ATSDR since 1990, the Hazardous Substances Emergency Event Surveillance System (HSEES) actively collects information to describe the public health consequences associated with the release of hazardous substances. Information is verified using several different data sources. Because HSEES requires voluntary data gathering by state health departments, participation is limited. As of 2004, 15 states collect data for HSEES. Because few states participate, a single state with a large number of releases can skew the data.

State-Based Reporting Systems

In addition to the federal system, accurate information on accidental releases may be collected and used effectively by some states. For example, since 1988, any spill of a hazardous material in California must be reported to the Office of Emergency Services, and detailed information is compiled into the California Hazardous Material Incident Reporting System. This reporting system enables the examination of the factors most commonly associated with accidental chemical releases and facilitates planning for preventive measures to reduce their occurrence.

REFERENCES

ATSDR. Hazardous Substances Emergency Events Surveillance, www.atsdr.cdc.gov/HS/HSEES/.

California Office of Emergency Services: California hazardous material incident reporting system, www.oes.ca.gov/Operational/OESHome.nsf/1?OpenForm.

Department of Transportation, Office of Hazardous Materials Safety: Hazardous materials information system, hazmat.dot.gov/enforce/spills/abhmis.htm

EPA: Emergency release notification system (ERNS), www.nrc.uscg.mil/erns/epa.html.

New Jersey Department of Environmental Protection: Emergency response, www.state.nj.us/dep/srp/ber/.

CHEMICAL TERRORISM

Events over the past 10 years, such as the 1995 sarin gas release in the Tokyo subway, and continued concerns for national security have highlighted the need to prepare for chemical terrorism. Chemical terrorism may include the intentional release of chemicals, sabotage of chemical stationary facilities or transport, and covert contamination of the food or water supply. According to the World Health Organization (WHO), chemicals may be used deliberately in order to cause death or incapacitation; cut access to important areas; control movement of population groups; destroy crops, vegetation, or animals; induce terror and panic; and reduce or immobilize communications, health care, transport, and administrative and financial services. Chemicals also may be released into the environments as a result of natural disasters, such as earthquakes and floods. The all-hazards approach to emergency planning requires that preparation for response to chemical releases include both accidental and intentional releases, including chemicals released as a result of natural disasters. In the past, competing priorities and inadequate funding of the public

Table 38–17. Steps public health agencies should take in preparing for chemical terrorism.[1]

- Enhance epidemiologic capacity for detecting and responding to chemical attacks.
- Enhance awareness of chemical terrorism among emergency medical service personnel, police officers, firefighters, physicians, and nurses.
- Stockpile chemical antidotes.
- Develop and provide bioassays for detection and diagnosis of chemical injuries.
- Prepare educational materials to inform the public during and after a chemical attack

---

[1]CDC: Biological and chemical terrorism: strategic plan for preparedness and response. http:www.bt.gov/chemical/.

---

health infrastructure have resulted in incomplete preparation for response to accidental chemical releases. Recent initiatives have resulted in a general increase in funds available to the public health sector specifically for biologic and chemical terrorism and emergency-response activities.

Chemical terrorism preparedness should be part of a sound public health infrastructure (Table 38–17). Early detection and control of intentional chemical releases rely on a strong and flexible public health system at the local, state, and federal levels. As with any disaster, hospitals and clinics should participate in interagency chemical terrorism preparedness and coordination. In addition, health care providers should be trained to recognize and respond to chemical incidents because they probably will be the first to observe and report unusual illnesses or injuries. Training should include information on toxicity, clinical manifestations, treatment protocols, personal protective equipment, decontamination protocols for patients, staff, and equipment, and reporting requirements. Because chemical terrorism events cause both physical and psychological harm, disaster mental health assistance should be included in preparedness planning.

For medical purposes, the WHO classifies chemical weapons according to their effects as nerve agents, lung agents, systemic or blood agents, vesicants, sensory irritants (riot control), psychotropic, and antivegetation. They are also classified according to the degree of effect as harassing (causes discomfort), incapacitating (renders the person unable to function or move), or lethal. Using a modified classification system, the Centers for Disease Control and Prevention (CDC) has compiled a list of chemical agents (Table 38–18). This list contains a wide variety of substances, including common industrial chemicals, pesticides, and chemicals used only as weapons, and requires constant updating. The CDC also has developed case definitions to facilitate uniform reporting among local, state, and federal public health agencies of illness resulting from a chemical release.

Table 38–18. Substances that may be used as agents of chemical terrorism.[1]

Nerve agents
  Tabun (ethyl *N,N*-dimethylphosphoramidocyanidate)
  Sarin (isopropyl methylphosphanofluoridate)
  Soman (pinacolyl methyl phosphonofluoridate)
  GF (cyclohexylmethylphosphonofluoridate)
  VX (*o*-ethyl-[*S*]-[2-diisopropylaminoethyl]methylphosphonothiolate)

Blood agents
  Hydrogen cyanide
  Cyanogen chloride

Blister agents
  Lewisite (an aliphatic arsenic compound, 2-chlorovinyldichloroarsine)
  Nitrogen and sulfur mustards
  Phosgene oxime

Heavy metals
  Arsenic
  Lead
  Mercury

Volatile toxins
  Benzene
  Chloroform
  Trihalomethanes

Pulmonary agents
  Phosgene
  Chlorine
  Vinyl chloride

Incapacitating agents
  BZ (3-quinuclidinyl benzilate)

Pesticides, persistent and nonpersistent

Dioxins, furans, and polychlorinated biphenyls (PCBs)

Explosive nitro compounds and oxidizers
  Ammonium nitrate combined with fuel oil

Flammable industrial gases and liquids
  Gasoline
  Propane

Poison industrial gases, liquids, and solids
  Cyanides
  Nitriles

Corrosive industrial acids and bases
  Nitric acid
  Sulfuric acid

---

[1]CDC: Biological and chemical terrorism: Strategic plan for preparedness and response. Recommendations of the CDC Strategic Planning Workgroup. http://www.bt.cdc.gov/chemical/factsheets.asp

Although biologic agents are not considered in this chapter, some biologically derived agents may resemble chemical agents of terror. For example, ricin is a potent toxin derived from castor bean processing waste that may be used as a weapon. In early 2003, ricin and the equipment to make the poison allegedly were discovered by police in London. However, this was shown subsequently to be a false-positive finding.

REFERENCES

Belson MG et al: Case definitions for chemical poisoning. MMWR Recomm Rep 2005;54:1 [PMID:15660014]. www.cdc.gov/mmwr/preview/mmwrhtml/rr5401a1.htm.

CDC: Emergency preparedness and response: Chemical emergencies, www.bt.cdc.gov/chemical/.

CDC: Emergency preparedness and response: Protect yourself from chemicals released during a natural disaster, www.bt.cdc.gov/disasters/chemicals.asp.

Miyaki K et al: Effects of sarin on the nervous system of subway workers seven years after the Tokyo subway sarin attack. J Occup Health 2005;47:299 [PMID: 16096354].

Ohtani T et al: Post-traumatic stress disorder symptoms in victims of Tokyo subway attack: A 5-year follow-up study. Psychiatry Clin Neurosci 2004;58:624 [PMID: 15601387].

Oregon Department of Human Services: Guidelines for public safety, emergency medical service and health care personnel in chemical terrorism events, www.ohd.hr.state.or.us/acd/bioterr/chemterr.pdf.

WHO: Seven steps for preparedness in case of biological and chemical emergencies, w3.whosea.org/EN/Section23/Section1001/Section1470.htm.

WORLDWIDE PERSPECTIVE

Although it is clear that both major and minor chemical accidents are widespread, it is difficult to gain an accurate perspective of the magnitude of these incidents because reporting requirements and record keeping vary widely between countries. The following information aims to familiarize readers with situations in various countries, but it is not meant to be a comprehensive accounting of international programs.

Europe

In 1982, following accidents in Flixborough, United Kingdom, in 1974, and in Seveso, Italy, in 1976, the European Community (EC) initiated a directive (the Seveso Directive) on the major accident hazards involving dangerous substances. The Seveso Directive provides guidelines on risk management and emergency planning for the prevention of chemical accidents. The legislation's purpose is twofold. The first purpose is to incorporate control and safety measures into the design of a plant or process and to prepare emergency plans. The second purpose is to inform the general public about the following regarding their facilities: the substances on site that have the potential to cause a hazardous incident, possible harmful effects on humans and the environment, details regarding hazardous incident warning systems, and recommendations for actions to be taken in the event of a hazardous incident. In addition, it provides for notification of authorities if dangerous materials are stored, transported, used in operations, or released in an accident. The requirements regarding storage of hazardous materials, their potential risks, and on-site emergency plans for dealing with accidents apply to approximately 200 substances that are extremely toxic, carcinogenic, or explosive and whose amounts exceed specified thresholds.

A 1988 amendment to the Seveso Directive replaced the passive transfer of information on a need-to-know basis with a requirement for active provision of information to the public on a right-to-know basis. A 1997 revision of this directive (Seveso II) requires safety reports and accident-prevention and emergency-response plans.

There are several differences between the United States and Europe in planning for accidental releases. First, the terms of European directives are binding but leave member states free to choose forms and methods of implementation. Community directives become effective only when they become a part of national laws. Not all EC member states have incorporated the directives into their national legislation. Next, lists of hazardous substances that are subject to requirements contain different chemicals than those in the United States. Finally, the threshold amounts that trigger public notification and emergency planning are higher in Europe than in the United States.

A main difference between Europe and other nations is the physical planning required for plants near large housing districts. For example, in both the United Kingdom and the Netherlands, no new housing is allowed within a certain distance of plants that are considered hazardous. As attested to by the Bhopal release, this is a marked contrast from developing nations such as India.

Several separate systems exist for hazardous materials incidents reporting in Europe. The Major Accident Reporting System database, maintained in Ispra, Italy, contains reports of accidental releases from all EC states. Member nations are required to report incidents, but enforcement is variable, and the information is incomplete. The Hazardous Materials Accident Database maintained by the Netherlands since 1977 is the most complete. In the United Kingdom, the Major Hazard Incident Database Service records hazardous materials incidents worldwide, with most information coming from North America and Europe. Information on transportation accidents in the United Kingdom is also included in general accident statistics maintained by the Department of Transport. Canada's National Analysis of Trends in Emergencies System Database was established in 1974 for the voluntary reporting of pollution incidents involving hazardous substances, including oil spills.

REFERENCES

European Commission: Seveso II Directive, europa.eu.int/comm/environment/seveso/.

Major Accident Reporting System (MARS), mahbsrv.jrc.it/mars/Default.html.

Major Hazard Incident Data Service (MHIDAS), www.hse.gov.uk/infoserv/mhidas.htm

Asia

Exposures to hazardous materials as a result of both routine and accidental releases pose a large risk to public health and environmental integrity in some Asian countries. In countries such as China and Taiwan, economic reforms and rapid industrialization take precedence over the setting and enforcement of environmental and occupational standards. In contrast, industrially developed countries with greater resources, such as Japan and Singapore, pay more attention to controlling damage to the environment, including that caused by accidental releases.

A. CHINA

China's key agency for promulgating and implementing environmental policy is the State Environmental Protection Agency. Numerous regulations and orders have been promulgated to deal with air and water pollution and natural resources deterioration, among other environmental concerns. In reality, these regulations may be violated by government agencies as well as by joint ventures with foreign companies. Lack of enforcement also plagues the Republic of China's (Taiwan's) Environmental Protection Administration, which was created to ameliorate this country's highly polluted air and water. Novel approaches, such as incentives created by public disclosure, may reduce pollution in China significantly, even though environmental nongovernment organizations (NGOs) play little role, and there is no formal channel for public participation in environmental regulation.

B. INDIA

In the years following the Bhopal accident, the Indian government enacted a wide array of legislative and regulatory changes aimed at controlling pollution, protecting the environment, conserving natural resources, and improving safety-management practices in hazardous industrial facilities. For example, the Environment Protection Act requires firms to disclose detailed information on hazardous materials on site, air, and water pollution and investments in environmental protection and pollution control. The Public Liability Insurance Act requires plant owners to carry insurance to cover death, injury, or property damage resulting from an accident.

Other rules obligate plant managers to ensure the safety of all industrial activities, to prepare emergency-response plans, and to report "major accidents" to the "concerned authority." Managers are also required to report on-site storage of hazardous chemicals that are on a list of more than 400 substances defined on the basis of their acute toxicity, flammability, and explosiveness.

The effectiveness of this extensive legislation has been dampened historically by the lack of compliance by industry. For example, the National Safety Council of India reports that many factories with hazardous chemicals on site do not have emergency-response plans.

As with other developing nations, India does not maintain a nationwide database of accidental chemical releases. Instead, the high morbidity and mortality rate of such incidents can be gleaned from newspaper reports. The actual number of accidents and resulting morbidity and mortality rate are likely to be much higher.

International Programs

As a result of the incidents leading up to and shortly after the Bhopal accident, the United Nations Environment Program (UNEP) released the *Handbook on Awareness and Preparedness for Emergencies at Local Level* (APELL). The purpose of this handbook is to increase community awareness about local risks and hazards related to industrial operations, including accidental releases of hazardous substances, and to enable the development of emergency-response plans. This document is available in a number of languages. To complement the APELL program, the Organization for Economic Cooperation and Development (OECD) Environment Committee and the U.S. EPA prepared voluntary guidelines to provide a foundation to prevent, prepare for, and respond to chemical accidents throughout the world. The "Guiding Principles for Chemical Accident Prevention" was developed in cooperation with the International Labor Organization, UNEP, WHO, and the World Bank. The document describes the roles of industry, public authorities, employees, the public, and organizations in preventing and mitigating the effects of hazardous materials accidents. It is suggested that safety programs be aimed toward completely preventing harm to human health, environment, and property (zero risk) while recognizing that accidents still will occur. The "Guiding Principles" state that industries from OECD countries should operate with these same guidelines in their plants located in non-OECD (developing) nations. As of this writing, the "Guiding Principles" are being revised.

REFERENCES

Aldhous P. Energy: China's burning ambition. Nature 2005;435:1152 [PMID: 15988490].

Indian NGOs Environment Forum, www.indianngos.com/issue/environment/statistics/.

OECD: Guiding principles for chemical accident prevention, preparedness and response, www2.oecd.org/guidingprinciples/index.asp.

UNEP: Awareness and preparedness for emergencies at local level (APELL), www.uneptie.org./pc/apell/disasters.html.

Wang H et al: Environmental performance rating and disclosure: China's Green Watch program. J Environ Manag 2004;71: 123 [PMID: 15135947].

NUCLEAR ACCIDENTS

Although the detailed consideration of unintentional releases of radiologic material into the environment is beyond the scope of this chapter, the topic of accidental releases would not be complete without at least a brief mention of planning for and response to nuclear accidents. Nuclear accidents may occur anywhere radioactive materials are in use but may be more likely in countries with covert nuclear programs, where safety and early warning systems may be inadequately tested or nonexistent. While large-scale accidents are well publicized, numerous small accidental exposures, including military and hospital overexposures, may not be reported publicly for several years after their occurrence. Unlike the multiple reporting systems for accidental chemical releases, reporting systems for radiologic accidents in the United States are not standardized or easily accessible.

As mentioned earlier for chemical accidents, planning for response to nuclear accidents must include arrangement for medical services for contaminated victims. Hospitals should be prepared to assess, triage, and treat exposed individuals. Policies for triage of victims should be in place. Chapter 11 summarizes the medical consequences of exposure to ionizing radiation and treatment options.

Nuclear Regulation in the United States

A. AGENCIES INVOLVED IN ACCIDENT RESPONSE

Accidental exposure to radiologic material may be a result of situations as varied as nuclear reactor or nuclear power plant accidents, transport incidents involving radioactive material, spacecraft reentry, or fallout from atmospheric testing of nuclear devices. In the event of a radiologic accident, various federal agencies coordinate their efforts at the accident scene under the umbrella of the Federal Radiological Emergency Response Plan. The Federal Emergency Management Agency (FEMA) coordinates federal and state activities. The Nuclear Regulatory Commission (NRC) is the lead federal agency in an emergency at a licensed nuclear facility. The Department of Energy (DOE) is the lead agency in an emergency at one its nuclear facilities or in a transportation accident involving radiologic material in its custody. The EPA is the lead agency in an emergency involving radioactivity originating in a foreign country or in a domestic accident involving unregulated radioactive material. State and local governments are responsible for the health and welfare of the general public during an emergency.

The EPA has developed a system of protective action guides (PAGs) to help officials make critical decisions. These guidelines identify the radiation levels at which state and local officials should take actions to safeguard human health during an accident and direct the development of emergency response plans. The PAGs identify three phases of an emergency: early, intermediate, and late. In the early phase, which usually lasts from several hours to several days, evacuation and sheltering are the principal actions to insulate the public from exposure to direct radiation and inhalation of airborne radioactive material. In the intermediate phase, which can last from weeks to months, actions may include limiting food and water consumption to decrease ingestion of radioactive material and relocating people to minimize radiation exposure. Administration of stable iodine also may be considered in the early to intermediate phases. In the late phase, which can last from months to years, the PAGs address the decontamination of property. In an actual emergency, protective actions in addition to those addressed by the PAGs may be needed.

B. NUCLEAR REACTOR ACCIDENTS

There are currently more than 100 licensed reactors in the United States, and formal approval of emergency response plans is a condition for obtaining and maintaining operating licenses of these facilities. The NRC coordinates all off-site radiologic emergency preparedness efforts and evaluates state and local plans. Current regulations require that emergency planning be conducted at the facility with provisions for off-site emergency response, including arrangements for medical services for injured or radiologically contaminated individuals and training for those who may be called on to assist in an emergency.

The NRC has a nuclear plant emergency preparedness goal that sets health objectives in terms of probability of occurrence compared with other events. For example, the goal for severe accident prevention is a frequency of occurrence of less than 1 in 1 million per reactor per year; the risk to an average individual in the vicinity of a nuclear power plant of prompt fatalities that might result from reactor accidents should not exceed 0.1% of the sum of prompt fatality risks resulting from other accidents; and the risk to the population in the area near a nuclear power plant of cancer fatalities that might result from nuclear power plant operation should not exceed 0.1% of the sum of cancer fatality risks resulting from all other causes.

International Coordination

There are some efforts to institute international safety standards for nuclear reactors. OECD member countries account for approximately 85% of the world's installed nuclear capacity, and nuclear energy represents nearly a quarter of the electricity supply for these countries. Accident management activities exist in OECD countries, although there is significant variation among member countries as to what should be classified as severe accident management. The Nuclear Energy Agency, a panel of the OECD, has outlined existing programs in member countries and has encouraged further efforts at consistent emergency preparedness. However, among other issues, the lack of uniformity found in older reactors poses problems in the international safety regulatory arena.

There are separate regulations for emergency response planning for transport accidents involving radioactive material. It is estimated that more than 40 million shipments of packages containing radioactive material are made each year throughout the world, although there have been no reported transport accidents with serious radiologic consequences to date. The International Atomic Energy Agency has issued guidelines that have served for years as the basis for regulating the safe transport of radiologic materials worldwide. These universal recommendations are implemented by local authorities, taking into account the specific legislative structures and actual shipments.

REFERENCES

EPA Radiological emergency response: Protective action guides, www.epa.gov/radiation/rert/pags.htm.

Goans RE, Waselenko JK: Medical management of radiological casualties. Health Phys 2005;89:505 [PMID: 16217194].

Koenig KL et al: Medical treatment of radiological casualties: Current concepts. Ann Emerg Med 2005;45:643 [PMID: 15940101].

Nuclear Regulatory Commission: Federal Radiological Emergency Response Plan, www.fas.org/nuke/guide/usa/doctrine/national/frerp.htm.

OECD Nuclear Energy Agency, www.nea.fr/.

OSHA: Emergency preparedness and response, www.osha.gov/SLTC/emergencyresponse/index.html.

Waselenko JK et al: Medical management of the acute radiation syndrome: Recommendations of the Strategic National Stockpile. Radiation Working Group. Ann Intern Med 2004;140:1037 [PMID: 15197038] www.annals.org/cgi/content/full/140/12/1037.

■ HAZARDOUS WASTE

Concern about hazardous waste typically ranks at the top of the list when the public is polled about environmental concerns. The public is increasingly turning to physicians for advice and answers. A physician should have a working understanding of the health risks cre-

ated by hazardous waste and be able to take an exposure history. The ability to recognize when an exposure may be occurring is critical because environmental medicine, like occupational medicine, is prevention-oriented.

The following material on hazardous waste includes an overview of the nature and magnitude of the problem, the use of exposure assessment and health studies for studying the impact of hazardous waste facilities, and a synopsis of hazardous waste regulation and management. The focus is on chemical waste; however, radioactive waste and health care waste also are addressed. The last part provides a glimpse into hazardous waste issues at the international level.

DEFINING THE PROBLEM

The term *hazardous waste* is ambiguous. It more accurately should refer to hazardous chemicals because it is unclear when a hazardous chemical becomes a hazardous waste. For the most part, in U.S. regulation there is control over the storage, treatment, and disposal of hazardous waste, not hazardous chemicals. The single exception is the regulation of underground storage tanks. There are as many possible types of hazardous wastes as there are possible combinations of hazardous and toxic chemicals. These are the by-products of industry, home, agriculture, or the environment. Only a tiny fraction of chemicals in use have adequate toxicologic data. Data on interactions between different chemicals are even sparser.

Hazardous waste, as defined by U.S. legislation, is a subset of solid waste and can include solids, sludges, liquids, and containerized gases. These broad definitions have a myriad of exceptions, many being a result of the political influence of those who create the waste. Because the following materials are not considered solid waste, they are not listed as hazardous waste: domestic sewage, certain nuclear waste, in situ mining waste, and pulping liquors used in the production of paper in the kraft paper process. Household chemicals are also excluded from hazardous waste categorization, although there are many toxic chemicals in today's commercial products. Other hazardous waste exclusions include agricultural wastes used as fertilizers; mining overburden; discarded wood treated with arsenic; chromium wastes; petroleum-contaminated media from tank cleanup; specific ore-processing wastes; specific utility wastes; oil and gas exploration, development, and production waste; and cement kiln waste.

It is important to note that hazardous waste also excludes chemicals discharged directly into the air or water (i.e., releases allowed by permits under other federal pollution-control statutes such as the Clean Air Act and the CWA). Firms that generate small quantities of hazardous wastes can escape management requirements. Hazardous wastes mixed with fuel oils can be burned and released into the environment without adequate controls.

Americans are the largest producers of hazardous waste per capita; however, it should be noted that despite all the exceptions mentioned earlier, the definition of hazardous waste in the United States encompasses much more than that of any other country. In 2001, 19,024 large-quantity generators produced 41 million tons of hazardous waste, which is about 1 ton per 7 people. Chemical and petroleum/coal products manufacturing companies were responsible for most of the hazardous waste generation. Wastewater treatment and disposal accounted for the next most. The states generating the most hazardous waste were Texas, Louisiana, New York, Kentucky, Mississippi, and Ohio, which states accounted for over 50% of the national total quantity generated.

It is estimated that as many as 425,000 abandoned hazardous waste sites exist in the United States, although the EPA has inventoried only 46,000. As of October 2005, 1239 sites were on the EPA's National Priorities List (NPL). The EPA proposes sites for the NPL by applying a hazard-ranking system, which is an assessment of the relative public health, environmental, and ecologic threat posed by a given site. There are more than 158 sites owned by the federal government, primarily the DOE and the Department of Defense, on the NPL. These federal sites pose significant concern because of their large geographic areas and the complex mixture of waste that is contaminating them.

Health Care Waste

Health care waste is composed of waste that is generated or produced as a result of any of the following: diagnosis, treatment, or immunization of human beings or animals; research dealing with infectious agents; serums, vaccines, antigens, and antitoxins; waste that is biohazardous; or "sharps"—devices having acute rigid corners, edges, or protuberances capable of cutting or piercing, including hypodermic needles, syringes, blades, needles, and broken glass. Health care waste is generated by physician and dentist offices; by clinics, hospitals, skilled nursing facilities, research facilities, research laboratories, clinical laboratories, and other health care facilities; by illicit drug users; and by diabetics and others who depend on injections for health reasons.

Hospitals in the United States generate more than 2 million tons of waste each year. Only 20% of the waste is considered infectious, yet in the past, all waste was comingled. Similar practices were followed in other health care settings; however, hospitals, which comprise only 2% of the total number of generators, produce approximately 77% of the total infectious waste. As there has been increasing dependence in the medical community on disposable items, there has been an increase in the amount of health care waste being produced.

Radioactive Waste

The production of nuclear power and weapons creates hazardous waste from remnants left from uranium mining and routine radioactive waste at nuclear power facilities, weapons-production facilities, nuclear bomb testing locations, and cleanup at decommissioned nuclear power plants and military sites. Low-level radioactive waste (approximately 0.5 Ci/yd^3) results from radiologic uses at more than 20,000 facilities nationwide, such as hospitals, universities, biomedical research, pharmaceutical development, and other industrial sources. Civilian nuclear waste also arises from the 104 nuclear power plants in the United States. A large nuclear power plant produces 460 tons of low-level waste (approximately 1 Ci/yd^3) that includes contaminated trash, sludges and resins from the reactor, and irradiated reactor parts. Spent fuel from a power plant (approximately 27 tons per year) has a high level of radioactivity (689,999 Ci/yd^3 of waste). In addition, there are 12 nuclear reactors that are currently in shutdown mode and are being decommissioned. The decommissioning of these facilities produces spent fuel and low-level waste (approximately 76 Ci/yd^3).

The other major source of radioactive waste is from the production of nuclear weapons by the DOE for the Department of Defense. Defense waste is divided into low-level waste (1 Ci/yd^3), transuranic waste (4 Ci/yd^3), and high-level waste (approximately 780 Ci/yd^3).

In 1993, about 800,000 cubic yards of civilian low-level radioactive waste and 10,000,000 cubic yards of military low-level radioactive waste were produced. Approximately 3346 thousand cubic feet of low-level radioactive waste was disposed of in 2000. By 2005, there were approximately 52,000 tons of spent nuclear fuel stored at commercial power reactors. That same year, commercial nuclear reactors produced 28,000 metric tons of high-level waste (spent fuel) that accounted for 96% of the total radioactivity of all nuclear waste generated. The military produced 1,500,000 cubic feet of high-level and 1,110,000 cubic yards of transuranic waste. In addition to these wastes produced as a result of typical operating practices, the decommissioning of civilian reactors and military bases resulted in an additional amount of nuclear waste, primarily low-level waste.

REFERENCES

California Department of Health Services: Medical waste, www.dhs.ca.gov/ps/ddwem/environmental/Med_Waste/default.htm.

DOE: Office of Civilian Radioactive Waste Management, www.rw.doe.gov/.

EPA: National Priorities List, www.epa.gov/superfund/sites/npl/npl_hrs.htm.

EPA: Radioactive waste, www.epa.gov/.

EXPOSURE ASSESSMENT

Exposure assessment is the process of identifying all individuals or population subgroups that have been exposed to a chemical or chemicals. Based on demographic data available in the 1980s, the EPA estimated that approximately 41 million people live within a 4-mile radius of the 1134 NPL sites. Of course, residence near a hazardous waste site or a facility that handles hazardous waste does not necessarily translate to actual exposure to substances released from the site. For instance, completed exposure pathways were identified at only 45% of the NPL hazardous waste sites. A completed exposure pathway consists of the following five elements: a source of contamination, an environmental medium, a point of exposure, route(s) of exposure, and a receptor population. Table 38–19 lists some of the exposure pathways that should be considered.

At 91% of the NPL hazardous waste sites with completed exposure pathways, the exposure occurred through contaminated groundwater; at 46% of the sites, exposure occurred from contaminated soil; at 14% of the sites,

Table 38–19. Top 20 Hazardous substances at CERCLA sites.

Rank	Hazardous Substance
1.	Arsenic
2.	Lead
3.	Mercury
4.	Vinyl chloride
5.	Polychlorinated biphenyls
6.	Benzene
7.	Cadmium
8.	Polycyclic aromatic hydrocarbon
9.	Benzo(a)pyrene
10.	Benzo(b)fluoranthene
11.	Chloroform
12.	Dichlorodiphenyltrichloroethane (DDT)
13.	Arochlor 1254
14.	Arochlor 1260
15.	Dibenzo(a,h)anthracene
16.	Trichloroethylene
17.	Chromium, hexavalent
18.	Dieldrin
19.	Phoshorous, white
20.	Chlordane

exposure was via contaminated biota. However, these data need to be understood in the context of how they are collected by regulatory agencies. When hazardous waste sites are evaluated, the soil and groundwater almost always are sampled; however, air monitoring and sampling of biota are not usually conducted. Additionally, most environmental data are collected from the land immediately comprising the site and not from the surrounding neighborhood where potential exposed populations may be living. It is typical that community exposure is evaluated using models to estimate the fate and transport of chemicals from on-site to the neighborhood.

There are more than 600 unique substances found at waste sites in the United States; Table 38–19 lists the top 20 substances. The prioritization of the substances is based on three criteria: frequency of occurrence of a toxic substance at NPL sites, the substance's toxicity, and the potential for human exposure. Most hazardous waste sites are contaminated with a mixture of chemicals rather than a single chemical, and very little toxicologic information is known about mixtures.

People in communities are very suspicious of the modeled exposure and risk estimates used to assess the health impact. Communities that live around hazardous waste sites are increasingly asking for biologic monitoring investigations to ascertain their exposure.

Biologic monitoring measures exposure by monitoring body fluids (typically blood or urine) for the chemicals of interest. Biologic monitoring provides the best evidence of exposure and avoids many of the exposure assumptions and animal-to-human extrapolations that are used in traditional exposure/risk assessment. However, depending on the pharmacokinetics of the chemical, biologic monitoring may not provide the needed information about chronic exposure to chemicals from a hazardous waste site. For instance, volatile organic compounds such as vinyl chloride have very short half-lives (2–4 hours) in the blood, and thus a discrete blood sample analyzed for vinyl chloride may not reflect chronic, residential exposure. Unlike public health standards for allowable concentrations of a chemical in drinking water or soil, there are no accepted guidelines for the interpretation of biologic monitoring levels. Laboratories that conduct this type of testing define "normal," but these numbers have not been rigorously reviewed and typically are abstracted from one published study or from a straw poll of laboratory workers. Finally, if the chemical is detected above "normal," interpretation of the results to the community member or patient as a short- or long-term health impact is a huge unknown at this time.

Interpretation of biologic monitoring for individuals or communities surrounding a hazardous waste facility is greatly facilitated by the availability of large databases on the levels of chemicals in the "population," essentially "historical controls." The CDC publishes these data as a part of the National Health and Nutrition Examination Survey (NHANES), an ongoing survey of the general U.S. population. Levels of 27 chemicals from the blood and urine of 3812 people were collected as part of the most recent survey conducted in 1999. This national reference information was useful in finding that urine uranium concentrations from 85% of the individuals drinking private well water with high levels of uranium in South Carolina exceeded the 95th percentile of the national reference (NHANES). This elevated concentration still was seen 10 months after exposure had stopped, indicating that uranium in urine must have been mobilized from storage places in the body.

REFERENCES

Brown RV: Logic and motivation in risk research: A nuclear waste test case. Risk Anal 2005;25:125 [PMID: 15787762].

Burger J et al: The role of risk and future land use in cleanup decisions at the Department Of Energy. Risk Anal 2004;24:1539 [PMID: 15660610].

Metcalf S, Orloff KG: Biomarkers of exposure in community settings. J Toxicol Environ Health 2004;67:715 [PMID: 15192864].

National Center for Health Statistics: NHANES, www.cdc.gov/nchs/about/major/nhanes/.

Orloff KG et al: Human exposure to uranium in groundwater. Environ Res 2004;94:319 [PMID: 15016600].

HEALTH IMPACT OF HAZARDOUS WASTE

In general, little is known about long-term exposure to low levels of contamination in the environment. Various techniques have been used and are being used to study the health impact. However, the world of small-area epidemiology has all the usual problems of an uncontrolled or multivariable study, as well as several more. For instance, misclassification of exposure owing to inadequate exposure assessment can predetermine the findings of a null study. In addition, this aspect of hazardous waste has not been funded adequately. For example, approximately $4.2 billion is spent each year on hazardous waste sites in the United States, yet less than 1% has been devoted to the study of health risks at these sites.

Reviewing existing health outcome data often is the first step taken at a site. Data may be drawn from morbidity and mortality databases, birth statistics, medical records, tumor and disease registries, and surveillance databases. Reviewing such information for the small population around one site could not discriminate the risk from an environmental exposure unless the relative risk is high, for instance, similar to the relative risk for smoking causing lung cancer. However, reviewing available data sources over a larger area (called an *eco-*

logic study) has found significant effects from hazardous waste sources: increased hospitalization for coronary heart disease in areas near hazardous waste sites and increased risk of low birth weight and maternal residency near a polychlorinated biphenyl (PCB)–contaminated hazardous waste site in New York State.

Many disease- and symptom-prevalence studies have been conducted in response to community concerns about living next to hazardous waste sites. Many of these studies do not show statistically significant increases in adverse health effects. However, these studies often are plagued by inadequate study sample size, insufficient information about the level of exposure, and bias in self-reporting. Several investigations at specific sites have documented a variety of symptoms of ill-health in exposed persons, including low birth weight, cardiac anomalies, headache, fatigue, and respiratory and a constellation of neurobehavioral problems. It is more difficult to find an association with exposure and disease for health outcomes that are delayed in appearance, especially cancer.

Biomarkers of effect may be used to make comparisons of preclinical events rather than frank disease. This is an improvement over long-term, equivocal cancer-cluster or other endpoint studies. Biologic markers of effect are indicators of change or variation in cellular or biochemical components or processes, structures, or functions that are measurable in humans and, depending on the magnitude, are recognized as an established or potential health impairment or disease. A major limitation of the usefulness of biomarkers of effect to ascertain the health impact of hazardous waste sites exposures is that they are often not substance-specific; therefore, the adverse effect might be caused by factors other than the exposure of concern.

An assessment of 7307 individuals living in the Superfund site of Libby, Montana, found radiographic abnormalities greatest in former workers at the asbestos-containing vermiculite mines. Those individuals who lived with a former worker and may have gotten exposed to asbestos from take-home exposure also had increased association with pleural abnormalities. Playing in asbestos-containing piles of mine waste and longer duration of residency in Libby were associated with pleural abnormalities, even after controlling for occupational and take-home exposure.

Lack of good exposure information is common to most health studies of hazardous waste sites. This flaw reflects historical tendencies to collect data to conform to remediation efforts rather than health impact concerns. Site investigations historically have determined the extent of soil and groundwater contamination on the hazardous waste site only. Community exposure information then may be modeled, or surrogates for exposure may be used. In ecologic studies, exposure may equate to residency within a census tract or ZIP code. In symptom-prevalence studies, distance from the site or self-reported odor detection may be used. Exposure from groundwater contamination probably has been the most quantifiable, although this information is also based on several assumptions. The Massachusetts Department of Public Health constructed a water-distribution model to recreate exposure from trichloroethylene contamination in two of the eight municipal drinking water wells in Woburn and found a nonstatistical association with contaminated water exposure during maternal pregnancy and leukemia diagnosis for 21 children, whereas the child's exposure to contaminated drinking water from birth to age of diagnosis showed no association with leukemia risk.

Most hazardous waste site studies are restricted by the small size of the exposed community, which does not allow for an adequate study size. Use of meta-analyses to pool similar studies and the creation of exposure registries are two approaches that may help to deal with this problem.

Meta-analysis is a quantitative review and pooling of similar studies. The combination of studies of small populations into meta-analyses might generate sufficient power to reach conclusions, provided that the basic measures involved are comparable and that sound methods are used in all separate studies. The interpretation of meta-analyses is tempered by the awareness that reporting and publication biases can distort the sample of studies available for pooling. Meta-analyses have not yet been used for hazardous waste epidemiology as they have for clinical trials, but they may be useful in the future if there is consistency in environmental studies.

ATSDR was established, in part, to create registries of populations exposed to hazardous wastes and follow these populations over time to observe associated health effects. ATSDR has developed several specialized registries to study the long-term health effects of exposure to specific chemicals at hazardous waste sites, with the intention of combining data from several sites where similar exposures have occurred to achieve populations large enough that the associated health effects can be detected. Four hazardous substances have been selected for the chemical-specific registries: trichloroethylene (TCE), 2,3,7,8-tetrachlorodibenzo-*p*-dioxin (dioxin), benzene, and trichloroethane. ATSDR also has established two additional registries: individuals living in Libby, Montana (exposure from asbestos-containing vermiculite) and individuals most directly affected by the World Trade Center collapse.

An emerging condition reported from communities living next to hazardous waste sites is *sensitivity to chemicals*. This condition, frequently called *multiple chemical sensitivity* (MCS), is characterized by a wide variety of symptoms in response to extremely low levels of chemically unrelated, everyday substances. The most common symptoms appear to be fatigue, mood changes, and memory and concentration difficulties, followed by various muscular, airway, headache-related, and eye-irritation complaints. More than 120 substances, ranging from barbecue smoke and public restroom deodorizers to detergents, newspaper print, and marking pens, have been said to trigger these symptoms. There are no generally recognized physical signs or laboratory tests to describe this condition, thus MCS as a medical diagnosis is very controversial. MCS is, in essence, in the research phase, with many models and mechanistic hypotheses being put forward to explain it.

Psychological health effects are some of the most important effects observed in those living next to a hazardous waste site or a large facility that handles hazardous waste. While there has been some effort to scientifically study the physical health effects from living next to hazardous waste facilities, the psychological effects are unquantified and unsubstantiated except for anecdotal description. Research on the psychological impact of human-created disasters such as the effects of the *Exxon Valdez* disaster has shown that members of the high-exposure group were 3.6 times more likely to have generalized anxiety disorder and 2.9 times more likely to have posttraumatic stress disorder (PTSD). This acute environmental incident resembles a natural disaster more than the long-term stress impact from living next to a permanent potential or real health problem of an abandoned hazardous waste site.

Communities that experience chronic stress from living near a hazardous waste site suffer even more uncertainty than those involved in an acute disaster because there are so many more unknowns about how health will be affected in the future. There is also the feeling of a complete loss of control over the environment and their homes that once were a haven and subsequently are felt to be unsafe. In addition, unlike with a natural disaster, these communities are seen as hypersensitive because the outside world cannot see the devastation that natural or synthetic acute disasters incur. Documentation of the chronic psychosocial effects of living near a hazardous waste site is not yet available. Therefore, these communities are overlooked. Rather than joining as a community to react to an acute disaster, these communities tend to fragment, and individuals who are not directly affected view those who are suffering symptoms as overreacting. Built-in community support systems often break down in these situations.

Federal and most state laws do not provide a mechanism for compensating individuals who have developed illnesses from environmental exposures to hazardous waste sites. Instead, individuals must bring personal injury actions against firms shown to have caused disposal of the waste and must prove that a particular waste caused the illness. Despite the fact that these suits are difficult to win, thousands of plaintiffs are pressing such claims in the United States and in many other countries.

Health Care Waste

The primary health risks associated with infectious health care wastes are a result of occupational exposure for those who handle it, not for the general population. Treated health care wastes disposed of in a landfill pose some of the same potential impacts as solid waste if the landfill is not maintained properly. Contamination of the air can arise from incinerators burning health care waste. The EPA's 1995 dioxin emissions inventory estimated that health care waste incineration was the nation's third largest dioxin and furan source. The prevalence of chlorine-containing polyvinyl chloride (PVC) plastic products in health care waste is largely responsible.

The spread of hepatitis B virus (HBV) and the human immunodeficiency virus (HIV) through health care waste has become a public fear. Because of the extremely limited viability of HIV outside a living host, the potential for developing HIV infection from health care waste is remote. HBV has a more lengthy viability in the environment and therefore presents a slightly higher risk of infection from health care waste. Sharp objects pose the greatest concern because of their ability to puncture the skin and provide a portal of entry for disease transmission.

Radioactive Waste

For communities living next to nuclear waste facilities involved in nuclear power, disposal, or weapons production, the primary routes of exposure come as a result of using contaminated water for drinking, showering, or recreation; eating fish harvested as food habituating in the contaminated water; or consuming edible plants that were irrigated with the contaminated water and absorbed some of the radioactive substances. Additionally, there are low releases of radioactivity in the air emissions from most nuclear waste–generating facilities.

The main health effect associated with radiation exposure is cancer. In general, tissues with a high rate of turnover are more susceptible to the effects of ionizing radiation. Thus the thyroid, lung, breast, stomach, colon, and bone marrow have high sensitivity.

Another group of fast-growing cells susceptible to ionizing radiation is the germ cells. There is some evidence showing that parental exposure to ionizing radiation may result in increased cancer for offspring. In utero exposure to ionizing radiation also has been associated with spontaneous abortion, growth retardation, and congenital defects.

REFERENCES

Anderson BA et al: Exposure pathway evaluations for sites that processed asbestos-contaminated vermiculite. Int J Hyg Environ Health 2005;208:55 [PMID: 15881979].

deRosa CT et al: Implications of chemical mixtures in public health practice. J Toxicol Environ Health 2004;7:339 [PMID: 15371239].

Sergeev AV et al: Hospitalization rates for coronary heart disease in relation to residence near areas contaminated with persistent organic pollutants and other pollutants. Environ Health Perspect 2005;113:756 [PMID: 15929900].

Sivanesan SD et al: Genotoxicity of pesticide waste contaminated soil and its leachate. Biomed Environ Sci 2004;17:257 [PMID: 15602822].

Williamson DM et al: Including residents in epidemiologic studies of adverse health effects in communities with hazardous exposures. J Environ Health 2005;67:23 [PMID: 15690902].

HAZARDOUS WASTE REGULATION

The recognition of environmental problems in the United States historically has been a reactionary process. Reaction to the hospitalization of several people in 1972 in Minnesota resulting from drinking well water that had been contaminated with arsenic wastes resulted in the first legislation to address hazardous waste: the Resource Conservation and Recovery Act of 1976 (RCRA). RCRA requires that hazardous waste be identified and tracked as it is generated, ensures that it is contained and transported properly, and regulates the storage, disposal, and/or treatment of hazardous waste. This has been termed *cradle-to-grave hazardous waste tracking.*

In 1999, 1575 treatment, storage, or disposal facilities subject to RCRA permitting standards managed 26.3 million tons of hazardous waste. Land disposal accounted for 69% of the management total. Nationwide, 16 million tons of hazardous wastes were disposed of in underground injection wells, 1.4 million tons were disposed of in landfills, 705,000 tons were managed in surface impoundments, and 30,000 tons were managed by land treatment (land farming). Recovery (recycling) operations, including waste oil, solvent, and metals recovery, accounted for 8% of the national management total, and thermal treatment accounted for 11% of the national management total.

As a result of the discovery of the Love Canal dumpsite in 1975, the public became concerned about the past mismanagement of hazardous waste. Public pressure came to bear on the federal government to take regulatory action to protect public health. Health authorities and public health professionals were pressured to identify the actual and potential health problems that were associated with abandoned hazardous waste sites. CERCLA (Superfund) was created in 1980 to address inactive or abandoned waste sites. The Superfund derives its name from a large federal trust fund capitalized with a special tax on chemical and petroleum feedstocks, federal appropriations, penalties collected from firms found responsible for contamination, and interest earned on the fund balance.

While RCRA is a regulatory program that addresses current hazardous waste storage, treatment, and disposal, CERCLA deals with abandoned hazardous waste sites. The bulk of the CERCLA program requires private parties to remediate existing waste sites. CERCLA also causes hazardous waste producers to exercise great care in disposing of hazardous wastes to avoid the creation of a future Superfund site.

Many states have developed their own superfund programs, frequently by creating new environmental protection agencies. State hazardous waste site programs were largely modeled after the Superfund program.

Health Care Waste

In the late summer of 1987, a 30- to 40-mile stretch of beaches on Long Island and New Jersey was affected by trash washing ashore. The appearance of syringes and other health care wastes on the shore caused great alarm and resulted in the closure of some beaches. Even though the EPA, the National Institutes of Health (NIH), and CDC argued that health care waste constituted no more of a health hazard than any other form of municipally generated solid waste, the Medical Waste Tracking Act of 1988 was passed by Congress in less than 2 months. The legislation consisted of a demonstration tracking system for health care waste of limited duration and with voluntary state participation. The act was aimed at large generators of health care waste and as a result did not affect the home-care services or illegal drug activities that had been responsible for the "needles on the beach." The act expired in 1999, and health care waste disposal now is delegated to state authority.

Radioactive Waste

Following the Three Mile Island accident in 1979, the public became very concerned about radioactivity. Nuclear waste disposal became a liability for the few states that had been accepting waste from other states. In late 1979, two of the three low-level waste facilities in the United States announced their intention to close their doors to nuclear waste from other states. In response to the impending nuclear waste backlog, the Low-Level Radioactive Waste Act, a federal mandate that defined the states' responsibility for the low-level wastes produced within their borders, was passed by Congress in 1980. Because there was little progress toward the states acting independently, the Low-Level Radioactive Waste Amendment Act of 1985 placed the states in regional compacts for the purpose of sharing

the burden of disposal and set milestones for the construction of regional repositories. There are 10 compacts currently active, with the final compact waiting to be approved by Congress. Within each compact, there must be at least one site developed for disposal of low-level waste. At this time, there are only three active licensed low-level disposal sites: Barnwell, South Carolina, Hanford, Washington, and Clive, Utah, serving three compacts. Ward Valley, California, was licensed in 1993, conditioned on future ownership, but the opening of this site is still not settled. Three compact sites' licenses are currently being reviewed.

The Nuclear Waste Policy Act of 1982 specifies a detailed approach for high-level radioactive waste disposal, with the DOE having operational responsibility and the NRC having regulatory responsibility for the transportation, storage, and geologic disposal of the waste. This legislation requires that the health and environmental impact of a high-level disposal site be acceptable for thousands of years. The waste site must be in a solid form in a licensed deep, stable geologic structure. The Nuclear Waste Policy Amendments Act of 1987 designated a candidate site for a high-level waste repository at Yucca Mountain, Nevada. The DOE found the site viable and recommended to the president that the site be developed. In 2002, the Congress approved moving forward with Yucca Mountain.

HAZARDOUS WASTE PUBLIC HEALTH

Toxicologic animal studies that examine the mechanism, pharmacokinetics, and cell and organ impact of hazardous waste typically have been carried out within academic research institutions usually funded by the National Institute for Environmental Health Sciences (NIEHS) or the EPA. On the other hand, human-based studies of hazardous waste are carried out in the public health arena, historically by state health departments. The roles of the various public health levels of government in responding to the concern over the impact of hazardous waste on the health of the citizenry will be described in this section. Hazardous waste epidemiologic research also is now being conducted by environmental and occupational health clinics within academic institutions.

Local health departments are on the front line, along with physicians, in responding to environmental and public health concerns raised by citizens. The environmental and public health response at the local level is multifaceted, with hazardous waste issues being one aspect. Addressing the underground storage issues, tracking health care, and permitting and inspecting RCRA facilities are some of the responsibilities that generally are mandated for local health departments to regulate. Additionally, these same organizations often must be not only regulators but also public health officials. For questions and problems beyond its expertise or funding abilities, the local health department staff then refers issues to the state health department.

Many state health departments have specialized staff to deal with hazardous waste issues such as environmental toxicologists, epidemiologists, health educators, community coordinators, and physicians. State health departments play a supportive role for local health departments in addition to investigating alleged cancer and other disease clusters around hazardous waste sites.

Since 1987, the ATSDR has supported staff within the states to provide public health oversight at the hazardous waste sites, primarily the Superfund sites, in those states. This funding has greatly enhanced state efforts to address the health issues that confront them at Superfund sites.

At the federal government level, there are several groups that are concerned with the health effects of hazardous waste. These include the NIEHS, the National Center for Environmental Health (NCEH), and ATSDR. Superfund legislation (CERCLA) created ATSDR to address the health issues of hazardous waste to complement the regulatory mandate given to the EPA for overseeing cleanup. This pairing of a nonregulatory, scientific, fact-finding agency with a regulatory agency had been done previously with the pairing of National Institute of Occupational Health and Safety (NIOSH) and OSHA.

ATSDR's multipronged approach to dealing with hazardous waste sites includes reviewing and assessing the real health impact of each site, conducting or sponsoring epidemiologic and health studies of exposed communities, educating the community and health care providers about hazardous waste exposure and potential health impact, and reviewing the literature and identifying gaps in the toxicologic information about hazardous waste chemicals.

REFERENCES

ATSDR, www.atsdr.cdc.gov/.

Agramunt MC et al: Levels of dioxins and furans in plasma of nonoccupationally exposed subjects living near a hazardous waste incinerator. J Exp Anal Environ Epidemiol 2005;15:29 [PMID: 15635452].

Bakoglu M et al: An evaluation of the occupational health risks to workers in a hazardous waste incinerator. J Occup Health 2004;46:156 [PMID: 15090692].

CDC, www.cdc.gov/nceh/.

Silbergeld EK, Patrick TE: Environmental exposures, toxicologic mechanisms, and adverse pregnancy outcomes. Am J Obstet Gynecol 2005;192:S11 [PMID: 15891707].

Williamson DM et al: Including residents in epidemiologic studies of adverse health effects in communities with hazardous exposures. J Environ Health 2005;67:23 [PMID: 15690902].

DATA SOURCES

Information sources concerned with hazardous waste usually fall into two categories: those that deal with facilities or sites and those that deal with chemicals considered hazardous (see Table 38–19). To evaluate whether a site may be causing health effects in an individual living near a facility, it is necessary first to establish what chemicals may be stored, treated, or disposed of on the site and whether there is the possibility that these chemicals have migrated off-site. Site exposure information may be obtained from databases generated from government reporting systems that are available to the public. These databases include the Hazardous Substance Release Effects Database, TRI, the Biennial Reporting System, the Comprehensive Environmental Response, Compensation, and Liability Information System (CERCLIS) list, and the Nuclear Reactor List. Once exposure to chemicals of concern has been established, it may be necessary to research the toxicologic information about those chemicals. While basic toxicologic information may be found using Medline or by reading medical journals, there are several information sources that have compiled toxicologic and other chemical-specific information into a readily accessible and well-organized format. These toxicologic databases include the Hazardous Substance Release Effects Database and the Hazardous Substances Database (Table 38–20).

HAZARDOUS WASTE MANAGEMENT PRACTICES

Hazardous waste management is an attempt to achieve a balance between minimizing the environmental and health impact and costs of an industrial society and the economic and social costs involved in achieving these objectives. Management of hazardous waste involves recycling, treating the waste to reduce its volume or hazardous level, or disposal. All these activities are regulated, but there still may be some potential health risk posed. In addition, there is still the continued disposal mismanagement or accidental release by a few hazardous waste users.

Hazardous waste laws are based on the legal concept that generators of hazardous waste are liable for the long-term impact of their waste management practices, including their past practices. As a result, there has been an impetus for change in the waste management arena. One estimate puts the cost of cleaning up a hazardous waste site at 10–100 times greater than the cost of originally treating the wastes in the most efficient fashion. Now, most generators endeavor to minimize waste, and many manufacturers even factor waste management into the life cycle of their products (from research through manufacturing to use by the consumer and eventually ultimate disposition).

Reduction, reusing, and recycling of industrial waste are being actively pursued by many companies. This holistic approach to hazardous waste management is

Table 38–20. Hazardous waste databases.

Database Name/Location	General Description of Database	Specific Fields in Database
Hazardous Substance Release Effects Database (HazDat) www.atsdr.cdc.gov	A scientific and administrative database developed by ATSDR that provides information on the release of hazardous substances from Superfund sites or from emergency events and Substance-specific information for ATSDR's Priority List of Hazardous Substances (currently 250 hazardous substances + 11 chemical mixtures)	Site characteristics, activities and site events, contaminants found, contaminant media and maximum concentration levels, impact on population, community health concerns, ATSDR public health threat categorization, ATSDR recommendations, environmental fate of hazardous substances, exposure routes, physical hazards Health effects by route and duration of exposure, metabolites, interactions of substances, susceptible populations, and biomarkers of exposure and effects
Toxic Release Inventory (TRI) www.rtknet.org	Self-reported annual releases both accidental and permitted from industrial facilities to the air, water, land, or underground injection of more than 666 chemicals and chemical categories. TRI is built and maintained by the EPA and is authorized under the Emergency Planning and Community Right-to-Know Act of 1986 and expanded by the Pollution Prevention Act of 1990.	Facility name and address; latitude-longitude; parent company; description of chemical manufacturing, processing, or usage that occur at the facility; the quantity and type of chemical releases to the air, land, underground injection, surface water discharge, a publicly owned treatment facility (sewer system), or transfer offsite for disposal or treatment; description of on-site treatment method including air emission treatment and biological, chemical, physical, or thermal treatments
Hazardous Substances Database (HSDB) http://toxnet.nlm.nih.gov	Toxicity information for more than 450 chemicals. Database also contains other chemical-specific information. File is fully referenced and peer-reviewed. File is built and maintained by the National Library of Medicine and cosupported by ATSDR	Contains 150 data fields arranged in broad categories: substance identification; manufacturing/use information; chemical and physical properties; safety and handling; toxicity/biomedical effects; pharmacology; environmental fate/exposure potential/exposure standards and regulations; monitoring and analysis methods
Biennial Reporting System (BRS) www.rtknet.org	EPA's database of and information on 19,024 large-quantity generators of hazardous waste, 2499 facilities that are permitted to treat, store, or dispose and 18,860 shippers of hazardous waste (numbers are for 2001)	Facility name, waste type produced, tonnage of RCRA, managed waste, exempt managed waste, and state managed waste
Comprehensive Environmental Response, Compensation, and Liability Inventory System (CERCLIS) www.rtknet.org	EPA's database of hazardous waste sites that are recommended for further study and for eventual inclusion on the NPL. As of October 2005, there are 12,178 sites on CERCLIS	Site summary and location; EPA enforcement activities, events, and financial expenditures
Nuclear Reactor List www.nrc.gov	The Nuclear Regulatory Commission's database containing information on the 104 nuclear energy reactors and the 36 non-power reactors located in the United States	Facility statistics, emergency response information, plant description summary, simplified plant system diagrams, detailed plant system data

termed *industrial ecology*. Waste reduction requires changes such as product formulation, process modification, equipment redesign, recovery of waste materials for reuse, and waste separation for exchange or resale. Waste reduction may involve material substitution, process modification, equipment modification, or retraining personnel to get rid of wasteful habits and other housekeeping practices. Recycling consists of recovering and treating waste, and reuse means the recovery, without additional treatment, of hazardous waste that then can be used by the industry generating the waste or by another industry. Recycling of waste water, solvents, and used oil is commonplace now. As the costs of raw materials, waste treatment, and disposal rise, so has the popularity of industrial ecology. Waste exchanges, regional clearinghouses that facilitate the effective use of waste between various industries, began appearing in the late 1980s.

Treatment of Hazardous Waste

Treatment of hazardous waste that cannot be reused or recycled and remediation of contaminated hazardous waste sites involve a variety of methods: physical, chemical, biologic, and thermal treatment. Physical treatment does not reduce the toxicity of the waste but does transfer the waste into another medium or prevents the waste from migrating. Air stripping is one of the most common physical processes used for remediating groundwater contaminated with volatile organic compounds. Air stripping is a mass-transfer process that enhances the volatilization of compounds from water by passing air through water to improve the transfer between the air and water phases. The vapor may be released without treatment or may be passed through activated carbon before release. Similarly, contaminated soils may be cleaned using soil vapor extraction. Soil vapor extraction consists of passing an air stream through soil contaminated with volatile organic compounds, thereby transferring the contaminants from the soil matrix to the air stream.

Chemical treatment is used to alter the chemical structure of the waste constituents, thereby reducing the material's toxicity. The simplest example of this is the neutralization of an acidic or alkaline waste stream. Chemical oxidation using ozone, hydrogen peroxide, and chlorine is capable of destroying a wide range of organic molecules, including volatile organic compounds, mercaptans, phenols, and inorganics such as cyanide. Other chemical treatment methods include precipitation, ion exchange, and chemical dechlorination.

Stabilization, solidification, and fixation are physiochemical methods used to stabilize waste prior to disposal so that it is easier to handle and also as a remedy at abandoned hazardous waste sites that primarily keeps

the material from migrating and decreases the permeability, thereby reducing leaching.

Biologic treatment is the degradation of organic waste by the action of microorganisms with the aim of changing the molecular structure to create less toxic metabolites or completely breaking down the molecule to carbon dioxide, water, and inert inorganic residuals. Biologic treatment of almost any organic material can be accomplished because virtually all organic compounds can be degraded if the proper microbial communities are established, maintained, and controlled. Biologic treatment has been used for many years with municipal and industrial waste streams. In situ bioremediation means that biologic treatment is used to clean up contaminated groundwater and subsurface contaminants where they are found without excavating the overlying soil. *Natural attenuation* refers to using naturally occurring bacteria for the remediation, whereas *enhanced bioremediation* refers to the addition of nutrients or specifically chosen or genetically modified bacteria to the soil or water. Natural attenuation is often the choice for cleanup of low-level petroleum-contaminated groundwater. Thermal methods such as incineration and thermal desorption involve the use of heat to clean up contaminated soil. Incineration uses very high temperatures [760–982.2°C (1400–1800°F)] to alter the molecular structure to ideally reduce the toxicity. The soil typically becomes an ash. Incineration changes hydrocarbon molecules into carbon dioxide and water vapor. The combustion of wastes containing sulfur produces sulfur dioxide and sulfur trioxide. Halogen-containing wastes produce the corresponding acid halogen gas (e.g., hydrogen chloride or hydrogen bromide). Metals cannot be destroyed and are oxidized. The volatility of oxidized arsenic, antimony, cadmium, and mercury can create problems in the flue gas. Because of the tight regulations on incineration air emissions and concern from communities, on-site incinerators rarely are chosen as a remedy at hazardous waste sites.

Thermal desorption uses temperatures between 93.3 and 537.8°C (200 and 1000°F) to drive low-volatile compounds from contaminated soil. The compounds are then trapped, cooled, and recovered for proper disposal. Unlike incineration, the soil remains intact with thermal desorption.

DISPOSAL OF HAZARDOUS WASTE

Disposal means long-term storage in landfills, underground injection wells, or ocean dumping. Surface impoundments such as pits, ponds, and lagoons are storage facilities, not land disposal facilities.

In the past, it was cheap and simple to dig a hole in the ground, fill it with untreated waste, and cover the waste with clay to keep the rain out. However, chemicals in the waste leached from the fill, resulting in the contamination of groundwater and drinking water throughout the United States. Landfills still are the most popular method for disposal, but there are now strict guidelines for their construction. Federal regulation requires landfills to be double-lined, a leachate collection system to collect the inevitable migration of liquid through the liner and a groundwater monitoring system to check for failure of the leachate collection system. Additionally, waste may be disposed of in a landfill if it meets certain criteria related to corrosivity, reactivity, flammability, and toxicity. Thus waste often may be treated prior to its deposit in a landfill. The treatment method also may generate a by-product that must be disposed of as hazardous waste (e.g., incineration dust). As a result, even though landfilling of hazardous waste is discouraged, there always will be the need for some landfills.

Injection of waste into deep underground wells is also used for disposal of hazardous waste. Injection usually occurs below the deepest drinking-water aquifer, 1000–10,000 ft (304.8–3048 m) down. Modern deep wells use such safety features as double or triple casings and leak-detection systems. However, even if a leak is detected, remedying the problem may be impossible.

Ocean dumping has been a method of choice for disposal of dredge spoils, industrial waste, sludge from wastewater treatment plants, and radioactive waste but currently is being discouraged because of concern for ecologic damage and contamination of marine food chains.

Health Care Waste

Previously, every hospital had an incinerator in which it burned the infectious and noninfectious waste that was generated within the hospital. However, these incinerators had only rudimentary air pollution control devices, and heavy metals, acid gases, and dioxins release may have resulted. With the advent of stricter air pollution laws, many hospital incinerators were shut down. It is estimated that there were 6200 health care incinerators in 1988, and in 2003, there were around 100.

Many health care waste generators are using steam sterilization for certain health care waste. Steam sterilization does not create particulate emissions but does generate significant odors. Furthermore, it cannot be used to treat mixed waste, that is, infectious and radiologic and chemical. Since 1999, there has been a significant increase in the use of alternative technologies to treat health care waste: heat waste with microwaves and radiowaves; expose the waste to chemicals, bleach, or chlorine dioxide; subject the waste to heated chemicals; or expose the waste to irradiation sources.

Radioactive Waste

Radioactive wastes do not respond sufficiently to stabilization by chemical, physical, or biologic processes. Only time can render radioactive wastes inactive. At present, storage appears to be the only means of successfully solving the disposal problem.

Spent fuel from nuclear reactors can be reprocessed. This involves extracting the uranium and the plutonium, but this method results in concentrated fission process product wastes that also require disposal. In addition, because of the concern that plutonium, a by-product of reprocessing, could be diverted to produce nuclear weapons, reprocessing of nuclear fuel elements has been discontinued in the United States.

Radioactive wastes require confinement for shorter or longer periods of time depending on the characteristics of the radionuclides contained within them. The radioactivity of low-level waste will decline to safe levels in approximately 200–300 years, whereas intermediate-level waste will need safe containment for thousands of years. High-level waste, with half-lives of millions of years, requires special treatment.

Low-level waste disposal typically involves near-surface disposal facilities. Near-surface disposal facilities are required to be topped with an impermeable cover that will not allow air emissions and will keep rainwater from filtering through the waste. Still, the most likely mechanism for the release of radionuclides to the environment is transport in groundwater.

There are not yet any high-level or spent-fuel storage facility for the United States or worldwide. The quantities produced so far are being stored temporarily where they have been generated. A number of options have been proposed for storage of high-level waste; currently, the United States is pursuing disposal in a deep geologic formation, under the continental crust (Yucca Mountain, Nevada).

REFERENCES

Burger J et al: The role of risk and future land use in cleanup decisions at the Department of Energy. Risk Anal 2004;24:1539 [PMID: 15660610].

Liu L et al: An integrated subsurface modeling and risk assessment approach for managing the petroleum-contaminated sites. J Environ Sci Health A Tox Hazard Subst Environ Eng 2004; 39:3083 [PMID: 15533023].

Scott MJ et al: Modeling long-term risk to environmental and human systems at the Hanford Nuclear Reservation: Scope and findings from the initial model. Environ Manag 2005; 35:84 [PMID: 15984066].

INTERNATIONAL PERSPECTIVES

Other countries are also dealing with hazardous waste issues. The kind and size of each country's response to these concerns varies according to the social, political, and economic policies of the nation's government and people. Examining each country's approach to hazardous waste is beyond the scope of this chapter; however, the responses may be crudely reviewed according to developed, democratized countries, developing central and eastern European countries, and other developing countries.

The status quo of hazardous waste regulation and public health protection for these country groupings is likely to change tremendously in the coming years with globalization of the commercial enterprise and trade liberalization. There is concern that trade liberalization may encourage countries to set low levels of environmental protection, standards, and enforcement to reduce production costs and encourage foreign investment. In essence, lax regulations could be viewed as a production subsidy. Others see health and environmental protection as nontariff barriers.

Unlike any previous trade agreement, the North American Free Trade Agreement (NAFTA) does allude to environmental standards in its text, and a side agreement focuses on environmental issues. NAFTA, which was passed in 1993, encourages free trade between the signers: Mexico, the United States, and Canada. Because of the pollution problem along the border between Mexico and the United States, there was tremendous pressure by nongovernmental and governmental organizations in the United States to address environmental issues that go along with industrial development in NAFTA. NAFTA provides that obligations of international environmental agreements on hazardous wastes and other concerns take precedence over NAFTA obligations, subject to certain conditions. The conflict of environment and trade already has been seen. When the State of California banned the future use of methyl *tert*-butyl ether (MTBE) from gasoline because of its contamination of drinking water sources, a Canadian company involved in the production of MTBE sued the U.S. government saying that the ban violated the foreign-investment guarantees in NAFTA. The case is being heard in secret by a three-judge arbitration tribunal.

Developed Nations

Most industrialized nations have established a national regulatory program that is aimed at protecting human health and the environment from the mismanagement of hazardous waste. The major elements in a national control system for hazardous waste management are

- Developing an administrative definition for identifying and classifying hazardous waste to the particular level of detail necessary to support its legal procedures
- Defining the responsibilities placed on the waste generator
- Registering or licensing those involved in collection, transport, intermediate storage, treatment, and disposal of hazardous wastes

- Controlling transport, including importing and exporting, using a cradle-to-grave theory involving a manifest system
- Permitting of treatment or disposal facilities
- Developing a national strategy or plan for establishing facilities
- Addressing old or abandoned sites

In most developed countries, the responsibility for managing the national control system is shared among the national, regional, and local governments. While the details differ from country to country, the national government generally is responsible for establishing national standards, guidelines, or codes of practice. Regional and local governments often are responsible for enforcement and licensing activities.

Although most industrialized/developed nations have created hazardous waste management systems that include the elements just mentioned, there are differences in how these elements are implemented. Without examining each country's system in detail, the essence of the various differences can be represented by listing examples.

- From 1979 to 1984, European countries disposed of some 100,000 tons of waste at sea.
- Shallow-sea dumping is used in a number of countries; the United Kingdom dumped 260,000 tons at sea in 1985.
- Every national system differs in the detailed method for defining hazardous waste and in the breadth of waste included. For instance, *specifically controlled waste* is the term used for hazardous waste in Japan. Japan classifies fewer items as hazardous waste than any other developed country.
- Sewage sludge is specifically excluded in some countries' hazardous waste definition but not in others.
- It is extremely difficult to compare quantities of industrial or hazardous waste in different countries not only because of the various definitions but also because of inconsistent collection of statistics.
- Unlike many developed countries, the United States has not developed a national strategy for dealing with nonradioactive hazardous waste.
- In most developed countries, collection and transport of hazardous waste are carried out by private industry. In Sweden, collection and transportation of hazardous waste are handled through local utility companies run by the municipality.
- Hazardous waste in most developed countries generally is transported by road. The main exception is Denmark, where waste is transported primarily by rail.
- In most developed countries, hazardous waste may move freely across internal boundaries within the country. In Germany, a special permit is required be-

fore a shipment of hazardous waste is allowed to cross state boundaries.

- The United Kingdom is well known for its advocacy of codisposal of hazardous waste in municipal waste landfill sites.

- The Netherlands has an almost total absence of suitable sites for landfilling; thus landfilling of hazardous waste is prohibited unless specific exemption is granted.

- In Japan, vacant land is scare, so incinerating municipal and hazardous waste is a common means (78% of wastes) of disposal.

- In most developed countries, the primary means of encouraging waste avoidance or recycling is imposition of strict controls on hazardous waste disposal, accompanied by the charging of a stiff fee.

- Most countries have developed a national inventory and cleanup program of old or abandoned hazardous waste sites. One exception is Japan, where there is no general law governing the identification, assessment, and cleanup of contaminated soil, although many cases of such pollution have been identified.

Developing Countries

It is estimated that developing countries generate 20 million tons per year of hazardous waste. Of this amount, roughly 15 million tons are produced by the central and eastern European countries. Three primary sources of hazardous waste in developing countries are wastes generated by foreign-owned, state-owned, or joint-venture firms; wastes generated by small entrepreneurs, farmers, and householders; and wastes imported from other, usually more developed, countries. On the whole, major corporations have assumed responsibility for their own wastes. However, in cases where the industries are small or locally owned, adequate responsibility for treatment and disposal has not been assumed. Developing countries do not have resources to deal effectively with any of these sources.

Training, technical expertise, facility development, legislation, and the necessary governmental institutions, all in varying degrees, are inadequate in developing countries. Multinational companies may be expected to help, but they have a vested interest that would be expected to interfere with their dealing effectively with the full problem. Much assistance will need to be provided by developed countries.

To begin to fill the organizational void in these countries, information exchanges have been created by developed nations and international organizations. For instance, the UNEP has developed an International Register of Potentially Toxic Chemicals to identify all chemicals that have been banned or severely restricted

by five or more countries and is currently preparing guidelines to assist countries in developing environmental protection legislation.

Democratization and the end of one-party rule in most of eastern Europe are considered to have an important impact on hazardous waste issues in these developing countries. Most of the former socialized countries have well-developed occupational health services and rather poorly developed environmental health services and hazardous waste management programs. The ideology of the previous Communist governments may explain this pattern: Worker well-being was valued more than environmental quality, and most of the industry was owned and operated by the national governments. Toxicology, clinical occupational medicine, and some aspects of industrial hygiene have been relatively strong in many eastern European countries, whereas epidemiology, environmental engineering, risk assessment, and risk communication have not.

Unlike in the industrialized, developing countries of eastern Europe, hazardous waste concerns are a relatively new phenomena in the developing countries of Africa, Asia, and Central and South America. However, this is changing primarily as a result of exportation of hazardous waste and the transfer of hazardous industries from developed countries to the developing world. Environmental exposure to hazardous chemicals is increasing in developing countries. In many of the world's countries, there are no environmental regulations for hazardous waste, or if they do exist, there is little or no enforcement. The daily struggles for survival are the primary focus. Political agreements between developing and industrialized countries are critical to ensure that environmental and human health protection takes place in developing countries. Efforts at the international level have centered on controlling hazardous industries and hazardous wastes.

Thousands of tons of hazardous waste are shipped internationally each year. In 1989, 35 countries and the EC agreed to the Basel Convention, the first step toward regulating international transportation of hazardous waste. Currently, 163 countries have ratified the Basel Convention. The United States has signed but not ratified the Basel Convention. This treaty requires notification of intent of international hazardous waste transport and prior informed consent (PIC) by the receiving country. The original convention allowed hazardous waste transport to continue. A March 1994 addition to the Basel Convention immediately banned exporting hazardous wastes to developing countries for incineration or burial, and exporting of hazardous wastes for "recycling" was banned as of December 31, 1997.

The Lome IV Convention also banned hazardous waste export among more than 80 countries in Africa, the Caribbean, Europe, and the Pacific. Such international cooperation may be elusive. Various reports of countries redefining hazardous waste in order to avoid complying with the Basel Agreement are already surfacing. This is another reason that efforts such as those underway by the OECD to harmonize *hazardous waste* definitions into an international standard are so critical.

The transfer of hazardous waste technologies to developing countries is a consequence of stringent industrial and environmental regulations and increasing labor costs in the industrialized world. Alternatively, developing countries are attractive because of cheap labor and lack of (or poor implementation of) labor, environmental, and industrial regulations. Efforts to affect ethical behavior in the exporting of hazardous technologies to developing countries also have been attempted by international organizations: the OCED's *Guidelines for Multinational Enterprises,* the United Nations' *Code of Conduct on Transnational Corporations,* and the International Labor Organization's *Tripartite Declaration of Principles Concerning Multinational Enterprises and Social Policy.* Efforts to deal with transboundary hazardous waste and other pollution have been spearheaded by the United Nations, the WHO, the ILO, the European Economic Community, and the OECD.

Health Care Waste

Concern about air contamination coming from incineration of health care waste is a concern in other developed nations. In fact, it was research in Germany that showed that the levels of dioxins and furans in the fly ash collected from health care waste incinerators could be two orders of magnitude higher than the levels found in the fly ash of municipal waste incinerators. It was thought that health care waste may contain a greater percentage of plastic (~30%) than municipal waste (~7%) or that the municipal waste incinerators were equipped with better air pollution control and operated by better-trained professionals. In 2000, stricter emission limits for health care waste incinerators were introduced in the EU, resulting in the closing of many incinerators. Although alternative treatment technologies are increasing in number, incineration is still the prevailing method.

In developing countries, there are additional concerns, namely, exposure to untreated health care waste by landfill scavengers and waste pickers. The WHO indicates that there are many reports of needlestick injuries to waste workers and scavengers in dumpsites. Recently, children playing in garbage bins near a health center in Russia found discarded small pox vaccine ampules and became infected with the live-vaccine strain of the virus. Treatment of health care waste prior to disposal is needed to eliminate such risks.

Radioactive Waste

According to the International Atomic Energy Agency, about 10,000 m^3 of high-level radioactive waste accumulates each year in 25 countries with 437 nuclear reactors. This massive amount of radioactive material has no permanent home. Not a single country has implemented a long-term plan for its disposal; each relies on interim measures. Most countries are hoping to dispose of the high-level waste deep underground in geologically stable areas; eight countries are currently in the site-characterization phase of developing an underground storage facility. Other considerations for high-level radioactive waste disposal include permanent subterranean storage, entombment under the sea, and nuclear transmutation. Russia used ocean dumping extensively in the past and is responsible for most of the radioactive locations in the world's oceans. Although Russia is not officially dumping it now, it has imported and stockpiled large quantities of high-level waste that it is not capable of handling.

Historically, the primary mechanism of disposing of low-level radioactive waste by other countries had been sea dumping. However, the practice was discontinued in 1983 in part because of widespread public opposition and a nonbinding resolution passed by the signatories to the London Dumping Convention, which placed a de facto moratorium on sea dumping.

REFERENCES

Diaz LF et al: Alternatives for the treatment and disposal of health-care wastes in developing countries. Waste Manag 2005;25: 626 [PMID: 15993347].

International Network for Environmental Compliance and Enforcement: Network of government and non-government environmental compliance practitioners, www.inece.org.

Low-level radioactive waste, www.nirs.org/factsheets/llwfct.htm.

Misra V, Pandey SD: Hazardous waste: Impact on health and environment for development of better waste management strategies in future in India. Environ Int 2005;31:417 [PMID: 15734194].

Mitis F et al: Industrial activities in sites at high environmental risk and their impact on the health of the population. Int J Occup Environ Health 2005;11:88 [PMID: 15859197].

Palmer S et al: Risk of congenital anomalies after the opening of landfill sites. Environ Health Perspect 2005;113:1362 [PMID: 160203247].

International radioactive waste management information, www.radwaste.org.

Rotterdam Convention on Prior Informed Consent, www.pic.int/.

United Nations Environment Program, www.unep.org/.

United Nations Environment Program on Persistent Organic Pollutants and the Stockholm Convention, http://irptc.unep.ch/pops/.

World Health Organization: Health care waste, www.who.int/wate_sa.

Outdoor Air Pollution

39

John R. Balmes, MD

The dramatic air pollution episodes that occurred in the early part of the twentieth century in Belgium's Meuse Valley, Donora, Pennsylvania, and London, England, are not likely to occur in the world today. These episodes were caused by the large-scale burning of coal in the presence of "ideal" meteorologic conditions—atmospheric inversion leading to a stagnant air mass. A clearly evident excess mortality was observed during and after these episodes. Current air quality standards in North America preclude the development of episodes of this magnitude today. However, certain environmental air pollutants, such as ozone and respirable particles, do reach levels that may cause acute and chronic respiratory effects. Furthermore, in some eastern European and Asian countries where sulfur-containing fuels are burned without adequate air quality regulations, air pollution levels may be attained similar to those that were associated with excess mortality.

REGULATION OF OUTDOOR AIR POLLUTANTS

The Clean Air Act (CAA) was passed by the U.S. Congress in 1970 and last amended in 1990. It is the principal federal standard addressing outdoor air quality. It requires the Environmental Protection Agency (EPA) to list those pollutants for which there is sufficient scientific evidence documenting the risk to public health from unregulated exposure. To achieve this, the EPA periodically reviews a large body of scientific research dealing with the adverse health effects of pollutants. The subsequently produced documents are used in the development of a National Ambient Air Quality Standard (NAAQS) for each of the so-called criteria pollutants. Table 39–1 lists the six criteria air pollutants, their NAAQSs, and their principal adverse health effects.

The CAA mandates that the primary NAAQS be set to protect the health of all sensitive groups within the population. The EPA has identified children, people with a chronic respiratory disease such as asthma, and people with ischemic heart disease as constituting sensitive groups (i.e., that demonstrate a response to a pollutant at a lower level or to a greater degree than the average response of the general population).

TYPES & SOURCES OF EXPOSURE

Outdoor air contains an array of naturally occurring pollutants, including soil, dust, pollens, and fungi. In addition, human activity generates complex mixtures of pollutants. Much of the regulatory effort and scientific research have concentrated on the individual components of these complex mixtures. This chapter discusses the criteria pollutants (see Table 39–1) and acidic aerosols, a yet unregulated pollutant. It does not discuss highly toxic air pollutants, so-called air toxics, that are emitted from point sources and that are present in low concentrations in the environment (see Chapter 37).

The sources of outdoor air pollution usually are categorized as stationary or mobile. Stationary sources are primarily power or manufacturing plants and are responsible for most sulfur dioxide (SO_2) emissions, as well as considerable amounts of nitrogen oxides (NO_x) and particulate matter. In the eastern United States and Canada, atmospheric acidity is caused largely by the oxidation of SO_2 to sulfuric acid (H_2SO_4) and other acid sulfate species. The combustion of fossil fuel is the most important cause of stationary-source emissions, although release of volatile organic compounds (VOCs) by various industrial facilities can contribute to the generation of ozone (O_3) in the atmosphere.

In contrast with the pollution from stationary sources that characterizes eastern North America, southern California "smog" is derived primarily from automotive, or mobile-source, emissions. A large fraction of ambient O_3 is the product of complex photochemical reactions involving NO_x and VOCs emitted from automotive tailpipes. Nitric acid (HNO_3) is a more important contributor to atmospheric acidity than H_2SO_4 in southern California and is formed in the atmosphere from the reaction of NO_x with the hydroxyl radical (OH^-). Motor vehicle emissions are also responsible for much carbon monoxide and particulate pollution. A major success story in the control of the criteria pollutants involves the markedly decreased concentrations of lead in the ambient air of U.S. cities achieved as a result of removal of tetraethyl lead from gasoline.

PERSONAL EXPOSURE

Central stations monitor the ambient air for concentrations of the criteria pollutants. However, the regional

Table 39–1. Criteria air pollutants.

Air Pollutant	Standard	Principal Adverse Health Effect
Ozone	0.12 ppm as a 1-hour maximum concentration and 0.08 ppm as an 8-hour average concentration	Increased respiratory symptoms Decreased lung function Airway inflammation Increased airway responsiveness to nonspecific stimuli
Nitrogen dioxide	0.053 ppm as an annual arithmetic mean concentration	Increased respiratory symptoms and illnesses in children
Particulate matter (PM$_{10}$) (PM$_{2.5}$)	50 $\mu g/m^3$ as an annual arithmetic mean concentration and 150 $\mu g/m^3$ as a 24-hour average concentration 15 $\mu q/m^3$ as an annual arithmetic mean concentration and 65 $\mu g/m^3$ as a 24-hour average concentration	Increased respiratory symptoms Increased respiratory illnesses Increased respiratory morbidity in persons with asthma and COPD Increased cardiovascular morbidity in persons with ischemic heart disease Increased cardiopulmonary mortality in elderly persons
Sulfur dioxide	0.03 ppm as an annual arithmetic mean concentration and 0.14 ppm as a 24-hour average concentration	Increased respiratory symptoms Increased respiratory morbidity and mortality Decreased lung function in asthmatics
Lead	1.5 $\mu g/m^3$ as a concentration quarterly average	Cognitive deficits in children
Carbon monoxide	9 ppm as an 8-hour average concentration and 35 ppm as a 1-hour average concentration	Increased adverse reproductive outcomes Decreased exercise capacity in healthy adults Shorter duration to onset and increased duration of angina in people with CAD

COPD = chronic obstructive pulmonary disease; PM$_{10}$ = particulate matter <10 μm in diameter; PM$_{2.5}$ = particulate matter < 2.5 μm in diameter; ppm = parts per million.

average concentrations measured at such stations may not characterize personal exposures adequately. For example, local conditions will affect pollutant concentrations to the extent that areas downwind from major traffic congestion may have higher levels than those in the immediate vicinity of the congestion. How much time is spent outdoors is an important determinant of personal exposure. Most people spend most of their time indoors, where the concentrations of pollutants generally are lower than in the outdoor air. The concentration of NO$_2$, however, may be higher in indoor air largely as a result of natural gas–burning stoves. Individuals who spend a lot of time outdoors, especially if they are increasing their effective dose by means of increased minute ventilation from exercise, may sustain relatively high exposures to pollutants such as O$_3$ and particulate matter. Therefore, total personal exposure should be considered; this is estimated by the summation of the products of the concentrations of the pollutant

in various microenvironments with the duration spent in each.

Principles of Inhalational Injury

For any one individual, the total potential dose of a pollutant can vary depending on the preceding factors. Furthermore, pollutants in inhaled air are either gases or aerosols—droplets of liquid or particles suspended in gas—and their site of deposition after inhalation is determined largely by their water solubility. Gases that are extremely water-soluble, such as SO$_2$ and HNO$_3$ vapor, are deposited and removed primarily by the upper respiratory tract. Therefore, these water-soluble gases mainly induce toxic effects on the proximal airways and only damage the distal lung when inhaled in high concentrations. In contrast, gases that are of relatively low water solubility, such as NO$_x$ and O$_3$, may injure the distal lung predominantly. The less soluble the gas, the greater is the potential for damage at the level of the terminal respiratory unit.

The deposition of aerosols is determined by a number of factors, including the size and chemical characteristics of the aerosol, the anatomy of the respiratory tract, and the breathing pattern of the exposed person. The size of the droplet or particle usually is the primary factor affecting deposition, although the chemical nature of the inhaled pollutant can be important, especially if it is a water-soluble acid aerosol that can be neutralized by oral ammonia, such as a H_2SO_4 mist.

The majority of inhaled particles with a mass median aerodynamic diameter (MMAD) of more than 10 μm are deposited in the nasopharynx and will not penetrate below the larynx. Particles in the range of 2.5–6 μm deposit primarily in the conducting airways below the larynx, and particles in the range of 0.5–2.5 μm deposit primarily in the distal airways and alveoli. Many particles with a MMAD of less than 0.5 μm do not deposit in the alveoli and actually are exhaled. Particles less than 0.1 μm are called *ultrafine;* these particles are of considerable interest because there is evidence that they are especially toxic.

The site of particle deposition also is influenced by hygroscopic growth in the humidified environment of the airways, the shape and dimensions of the respiratory tree, the ventilatory pattern (respiratory rate and tidal volume), oral versus nasal breathing, and the amount and nature of respiratory tract secretions. Respiratory tract disease can affect particle deposition by altering airway dimension, airflow pattern, or respiratory secretions. Exercise increases oral breathing, bypassing the nasal scrubbing mechanism, and increases minute ventilation, thereby increasing particle velocity and inertial impaction. Both these changes result in greater particle deposition in the lower airways.

Clearance of inhaled pollutants occurs by several mechanisms. In general, highly water-soluble particles and gases are absorbed through the epithelial layer into the bloodstream near where they have been deposited. The clearance of insoluble particles depends on where they impact. Those deposited in the anterior nasal cavity are expelled by sneezing or rhinorrhea, whereas the remainder of particles deposited in the nose are cleared posteriorly to the pharynx. Particles deposited in the trachea, bronchi, or bronchioles, where there is ciliated epithelium and a layer of mucus, are transported up the mucociliary escalator to be expelled by coughing or swallowing. Particles deposited distal to the terminal bronchioles are cleared by alveolar macrophages and/or dissolution. Alveolar macrophages will ingest particles and migrate to the mucociliary escalator or into lymphatics. A small fraction of particles deposited in the alveoli will migrate through the alveolar epithelial layer directly into the lymphatic circulation.

REFERENCES

American Lung Association: Air quality, www.lungusa.org/air/.

Bernstein JA et al: Health effects of air pollution. J Allergy Clin Immunol 2004;114:1116 [PMID: 15536419].

Cohen AJ et al: The global burden of disease due to outdoor air pollution. J Toxicol Environ Health A 2005;68:1301 [PMID: 16024504].

EPA: National air quality status and trends, www.epa.gov/air/aqtrnd01/index.html.

SPECIFIC OUTDOOR AIR POLLUTANTS

In 1996, about 117 million people lived in counties in the United States with measured air quality above the primary NAAQSs. Therefore, from a clinical and public health perspective, such exposures continue to be of relevance. The health effects of outdoor air pollutants have been compiled by the interpretation of toxicologic studies (i.e., animal studies, in vitro studies, and controlled human exposure studies) and epidemiologic studies (i.e., ecologic, cross-sectional, and longitudinal designs). This section discusses each of the major air pollutants individually; however, it should be understood that exposures often occur to a mixture of pollutants, and separating out the individual contribution of each pollutant frequently is not possible.

Ozone

O_3 is a colorless, pungent, relatively water-insoluble gas that occurs with other photochemical oxidants and fine particles to form "smog." Tropospheric O_3, or ground-level O_3, is an environmental air pollutant and is distinct from the stratospheric O_3 that occurs at altitudes of greater than 10 km (6.2 mi) above the earth's surface. O_3 is generated by a series of sunlight-driven reactions involving NO_x and VOCs from predominantly mobile (i.e., motor vehicle) but sometimes stationary sources. The meteorologic conditions that tend to foster the generation of ozone typically are present from late spring to early fall. Peak concentrations of O_3 typically occur in midafternoon, after both the morning rush hour and several hours of bright sunlight. Indoor sources of O_3 include office equipment with electric motors or ultraviolet light, such as photocopy machines, and electrostatic devices, such as air purifiers and ion generators.

While O_3 has long been associated with southern California smog, many other areas of North America also experience high concentrations of this pollutant, especially Houston, Mexico City, and cities in the eastern United States and Canada during the summer months. In these areas, there are many days each year when the current NAAQS for O_3 is not attained.

Ozone is a potent oxidant and is capable of reacting with a variety of extracellular and intracellular molecules. When these molecules are unsaturated lipids, free radicals and toxic intermediate products are generated and can lead to cellular damage or cell death. Although direct cytotoxicity is clearly a necessary mechanism of O_3-induced tissue injury, secondary damage from the inflammatory response also may play a role.

Dosimetric studies indicate that much of the inhaled O_3 is deposited in the upper and proximal lower airways. However, because of its relative water insolubility, a considerable fraction does penetrate to the distal airways and alveoli, and the dose at the tissue level is highest at these sites. Increased inspiratory flow, such as with exercise, may overcome the upper airway "scrubbing mechanisms" and cause greater deposition of O_3 in the distal lung.

Most of the research on the health effects of O_3 has focused on short-term exposure. O_3 inhalation by healthy subjects causes mean decrements in forced expiratory volume in 1 second (FEV_1) and forced vital capacity (FVC) that correlate with concentration, exposure duration, and minute ventilation. These decrements in lung function are primarily a result of decreased inspiratory capacity rather than airways obstruction. The mechanism of the decreased inspiratory capacity appears to be neurally mediated involuntary inhibition of inspiratory effort involving stimulation of C-fibers in the lungs. Somewhat surprisingly, older subjects and those who are cigarette smokers demonstrate lower O_3-induced decrements in pulmonary function than healthy subjects. The acute decrements in pulmonary function induced by O_3 usually resolve within 24 hours.

Respiratory symptoms appear to be associated with these mean decrements in pulmonary function. There is a correlation between the decline in FEV_1 and the probability of developing lower respiratory tract symptoms (e.g., substernal chest discomfort, cough, wheeze, and dyspnea). Another adverse effect of short-term exposure to O_3 is enhanced airway responsiveness to nonspecific stimuli such as methacholine and histamine. This effect may persist longer than the acute decrements in lung function and may occur in individuals who do not experience a decline in their FEV_1.

Nasal inflammatory changes, type I alveolar and ciliated airway epithelial cell injury, infiltration of the airway mucosa by neutrophils, and increased bronchoalveolar lavage (BAL) fluid neutrophils and inflammatory mediators also have been observed after exposure. BAL evidence of inflammation has been demonstrated at effective doses allowable under the current NAAQS for O_3.

The effects of chronic O_3 exposure in humans have not been defined adequately. It has been hypothesized that chronic exposure would lead to emphysematous or fibrotic parenchymal changes; however, to date, animal toxicologic studies have failed to substantiate the induction of diffuse disease after long-term exposure to ambi-

ent concentrations. However, a recent study showed that ozone exposure of neonatal Rhesus monkeys led to abnormal development of conducting airways, especially with coexposure to house dust mite. In addition, there are several epidemiologic studies of young adults that do suggest that long-term residence of children in a high ambient O_3 environment can lead to remodeling of the small airways.

Because of their tendency to experience bronchoconstriction on inhalation of noxious stimuli, persons with asthma usually are more sensitive to inhaled irritants. Although studies of asthmatic and atopic subjects have failed to show enhanced spirometric responses to short-term O_3 inhalation, there are indications that asthmatics may experience a greater inflammatory response to exposure. Furthermore, there are several epidemiologic studies that show that high ambient O_3 concentrations are associated with an increased rate of asthma attacks and increased hospital admissions/emergency department visits for respiratory disease, including asthma. In addition to the exacerbation of preexisting asthma, there is also evidence that playing outdoor sports in a high ambient O_3 environment can lead to the onset of asthma. A newly documented effect of ambient ozone is an association with daily mortality that has been reported in both Europe and the United States.

Ozone toxicity may be enhanced by coexposure to other pollutants such as other oxidants, particulates, and atmospheric acidity commonly seen in urban smog. The mechanisms by which these cofactors may potentiate O_3 toxicity are poorly understood.

In summary, tens of millions of persons in the United States are exposed to levels of O_3 above the current NAAQS. This exposure is capable of inducing both acute decrements in lung function and respiratory symptoms. Although these effects are transient, acute respiratory tract inflammation also can be induced by short-term exposure to ambient concentrations of O_3 with exercise. The long-term consequences of this type of acute inflammatory response are not well understood, but there is epidemiologic evidence consistent with airway remodeling. Because O_3 inhalation can induce both airway inflammation and enhanced airway responsiveness, it is reasonable to expect persons with asthma to have greater susceptibility to this pollutant. Ozone is rarely the sole pollutant of concern in urban smog, and it is likely that environmental cofactors enhance its toxicity.

REFERENCES

Bell ML et al: Ozone and short-term mortality in 95 US urban communities, 1987–2000. JAMA 2004;292:2372 [PMID: 15547165].

Chan CC, Wu TH: Effects of ambient ozone exposure on mail carriers' peak expiratory flow rates. Environ Health Perspect 2005;113:735 [PMID: 15929897].

Tager IB et al: Chronic exposure to ambient ozone and lung function in young adults. Epidemiology 2005;16:751 [PMID: 16222164].

Nitrogen Dioxide

Most ambient nitrogen dioxide (NO_2) is generated by the burning of fossil-derived fuels, during which oxygen and nitrogen react to form nitrogen oxide (NO), which further reacts to form NO_2 and other NO_x. The principal source of NO_2 in outdoor air is motor vehicle emissions, but power plants and fossil fuel–burning industrial facilities also contribute. In most U.S. urban areas, ambient levels of NO_2 vary with traffic intensity. Annual average concentrations range from 0.015–0.035 ppm. Of all regions in the United States reporting NO_2 monitoring data in recent years, only the Los Angeles Basin exceeded the current NAAQS.

In contrast to other criteria pollutants, NO_2 is a common contaminant of indoor air, and indoor levels often exceed those found outdoors. Indoor sources of NO_2 include gas cooking stoves, gas furnaces, and kerosene space heaters. Because the majority of homes in the United States have gas cooking stoves and Americans spend a large proportion of time in their homes, the home environment is usually the most important contributor to total NO_2 exposure. High concentrations may be generated in a kitchen with a gas stove in use. Nitrous acid (HONO) and other NO_x are emitted by gas stoves, so health effects associated with the use of such appliances may not be a result of NO_2 alone.

Nitrogen dioxide, like O_3, is an oxidant, but it is less chemically reactant and therefore usually is considered less potent. Although both pollutants are relatively insoluble in water, the solubility of NO_2 is somewhat higher. When NO_2 is absorbed onto the moist surfaces of the respiratory tract, it can be hydrolyzed to evolve acidic species such as HONO and HNO_3. The potential for NO_2 to cause the local generation of hydrogen ions in the airways may be an important feature of its toxicity. Nitrogen dioxide and O_3 are frequent copollutants in southern California smog.

The annual averaging time of the NAAQS for NO_2 (as opposed to the 1-hour maximum for O_3) reflects an assessment that the health effects of this pollutant are determined more by chronic low-level exposure than by transient high-level exposures. Whether this assessment is correct or not has important consequences for individuals in the population with preexisting respiratory disease, such as those with asthma or chronic obstructive pulmonary disease (COPD) who are susceptible to the development of acute exacerbations. The lack of a short-term averaging time in the current NAAQS means that asthmatic persons are not felt to be at risk of developing acute exacerbations after brief exposures to NO_2.

The results of controlled human exposure studies have demonstrated no significant decrements in pulmonary function in normal, healthy subjects after exposure to NO_2 at low concentrations. Controlled exposure studies of subjects with asthma, however, have produced inconsistent results. Low-level NO_2 exposure was reported to have enhanced airway responsiveness after exposure. Unfortunately, subsequent studies produced conflicting results, so this issue has yet to be resolved. Perhaps the most intriguing finding from controlled studies of asthmatic subjects is that of enhanced bronchoconstrictor responses to inhaled allergen following NO_2 exposure. There are also animal studies that support an adjuvant effect of NO_2 exposure on allergic airway responses.

The toxic effects of NO_2 exposure have been studied extensively. There are abundant animal toxicologic data and reports of accidental human exposure that indicate that short-term inhalation of high concentrations of NO_2 can produce terminal bronchiolar and diffuse alveolar injury; exposure of humans to very high concentrations (i.e., >150 ppm NO_2) typically results in death. However, in contrast to what is seen with O_3, short-term exposure to NO_2 at concentrations in the ambient range does not induce airways inflammation.

Chronic exposure of animals to high concentrations of NO_2 has been shown to cause structural damage to alveoli with airspace enlargement, which is somewhat analogous to human emphysema. The terminal lung unit is the site of greatest NO_2-induced injury. Animal infectivity studies after NO_2 exposure have shown that high concentrations may impair respiratory tract defenses against some bacteria and viruses. The mechanisms of NO_2-induced enhanced microbial infectivity are not clearly understood but likely are caused by alveolar macrophage dysfunction. While some epidemiologic studies have shown a positive association between indoor NO_2 and respiratory illness, others have failed to demonstrate this finding. A meta-analysis using 11 cross-sectional and prospective studies of residential NO_2 concentrations in children estimated a 20% increase in risk of respiratory illness per 15-ppb increments in long-term NO_2 exposure. A more recent study of indoor NO_2 levels and respiratory symptoms failed to show an association between these factors. The inconsistency of this association in epidemiologic studies may be partly a result of methodologic factors such as different statistical power, confounding, and misclassification.

Somewhat surprisingly, given its lower potency than ozone as an oxidant gas, ambient NO_2 was significantly associated with a slower rate of growth of lung function in a large longitudinal study of school children living in 12 communities in southern California. As described previously for ozone, several epidemiologic studies have shown associations between ambient NO_2 and hospital admissions and emergency department visits for asthma.

In summary, NO_2 is a pollutant that is a ubiquitous component of urban smog. It is generated by combustion of fossil-derived fuels from both mobile and stationary sources. Indoor concentrations often exceed those outdoors primarily because of the use of gas stoves. Inhaled NO_2 penetrates to the deep lung because of the relatively low water solubility of the gas. Perhaps the most important effect seen in controlled human exposure studies of NO_2 is enhanced bronchoconstriction to inhaled allergen in specifically sensitized asthmatic subjects. Chronic exposure of experimental animals to high concentrations of NO_2 has caused emphysema-like changes and decreased resistance to bacterial infection. The applicability of these findings to ambient exposure of humans is not straightforward. Several epidemiologic studies show associations between asthma exacerbations or reduced growth of lung function and ambient NO_2 levels. Some investigators currently feel that these associations reflect the adverse health effects of traffic-related pollution and that NO_2 is merely a good marker of such pollution.

REFERENCES

Gauderman WJ et al: Childhood asthma and exposure to traffic and nitrogen dioxide. Epidemiology 2005;16:737 [PMID: 16222162].

Gauderman WJ et al: The effect of air pollution on lung development from 10 to 18 years of age. N Engl J Med 2004;351:1057 [PMID: 15356303].

Particles, Sulfur Dioxide, & Acid Aerosols

Particles, sulfur oxide(s), and acid aerosols are discussed as a group because they usually occur together as components of a complex pollutant mixture. Their production is primarily a result of sulfur-containing fossil fuel combustion. Particles and sulfur dioxide (SO_2) are the primary products of combustion, and acid aerosols are formed by subsequent atmospheric chemical reactions. This mixture of solid and liquid particles suspended in the air is termed *particulate matter* (PM); the constituent particles differ in size and composition. Particles with an aerodynamic diameter of more than 10 μm (PM_{10}) are the focus of regulatory interest because particles of this diameter may penetrate into and be deposited in the airways of the lower respiratory tract and the gas-exchanging portions of the lung. Acid aerosols usually are a complex and variable mixture and include dissolved gaseous pollutants.

Sulfur dioxide is a major air pollutant in many urban areas. The gas is emitted by coal- and oil-fired power plants and by industrial processes involving fossil fuel combustion. It leads to the secondary formation of acid aerosols. Because high-sulfur-content coal has

remained a relatively cheap fuel in regions where it is mined, SO_2 emissions generally have been more of a problem in the eastern United States than in southern California, where smog is primarily a result of photochemical reactions involving motor vehicle emissions. Unfortunately, the building of tall smokestacks to reduce the local concentrations of SO_2 around midwestern and eastern U.S. power plants has led to the long-distance transport of sulfur oxide pollutants and their progeny, acid sulfates, to New England and Canada (so-called acid rain).

Sulfur oxide emissions in the United States increased steadily during the twentieth century to a peak of 32 million tons in 1970. Exposure to high concentrations of SO_2 is highly localized to the vicinity [within 20 km (12.4 mi)] of major stationary sources. The initial clues that SO_2 might be an air pollutant capable of causing adverse respiratory effects came from the severe pollution episodes occurring earlier in this century. During these episodes, high ambient concentrations of SO_2, particles, and acid aerosols occurred and clearly were associated with increased mortality, primarily among persons with preexisting cardiopulmonary disease. During the 1952 air pollution episode in London, there were an estimated 4000 excess deaths. More recently, multiple epidemiologic studies have demonstrated an association between lower levels of particulate pollution and increased daily mortality from cardiopulmonary disease. The consistent finding of this association in studies conducted at various times and in diverse geographic locations makes it likely that there is a true causal relationship between respirable PM and daily mortality. However, the biologic mechanism underlying this association remains obscure, especially given the lack of toxicity of ambient levels of PM in animal studies.

Acute morbidity associated with lower-level particulate pollution has been examined using a variety of indicators, including measures of health care utilization by exposed populations, health status of exposed individuals, symptom questionnaires, and lung function tests. Use of these indicators has demonstrated that particle exposure has been associated with increased emergency room visits for respiratory illness, such as asthma and pneumonia; higher rates of hospital admissions for respiratory and cardiovascular illnesses; and increased daily mortality as a result of cardiovascular and respiratory diseases in elderly people.

Epidemiologic studies also show associations between exposure to particles and reports of respiratory symptoms severe enough to restrict activity. In smokers with COPD, declines in pulmonary function and daily emergency room visits for acute exacerbations have been positively associated with particulate air pollution. In children, studies have shown associations with particulate concentrations at levels commonly encountered today with respiratory illnesses, declines in pulmonary function, and aggravation of asthmatic attacks. In elderly people or patients with ischemic heart disease, decreased heart rate variability (a negative prognostic indicator), increased angina, and increased arrhythmias have been associated with ambient PM.

The chronic health effects of particulate air pollution are a more difficult endpoint to study. Despite this, a number of studies show an association between PM levels and the following: reports of chronic bronchitis, doctors' diagnoses of asthma, and in several prospective U.S. studies, an increase in city-specific cardiopulmonary mortality rates. The same study of southern California school children that found an effect of NO_2 on growth of lung function also showed similar effects of PM and nitric acid vapor. A recent report of a prospective U.S. study also showed an increased risk of lung cancer to be related to residence in metropolitan areas with higher particulate pollution.

From a toxicologic viewpoint, SO_2, particles, and acid aerosols have different mechanisms of action. Sulfur dioxide is highly soluble in water and is absorbed mostly in the upper airways. Although the nose effectively removes much of the inhaled gas, significant amounts may penetrate to the large airways. Here, the irritant molecules may act directly on smooth muscle or via sensory afferent nerve fibers to cause reflex bronchoconstriction. At high concentrations, SO_2 can cause epithelial sloughing in the trachea and proximal airways, leading to a bronchitis-like pathology. Despite the irritant potential of SO_2, studies fail to demonstrate effects on respiratory mechanics (at levels up to 1.0 ppm) in healthy people. However, in asthmatics, low-level exposure causes bronchoconstriction. This acute bronchoconstriction is observed within minutes of exposure and resolves within 1 hour after exposure ceases. While the mechanism of SO_2-induced bronchoconstriction is not fully understood, a reflex mechanism involving vagal afferent and cholinergic efferent nerves is postulated.

The toxicity of inhaled particles is determined by the physical and chemical nature of the particles, the physics of their deposition and distribution in the respiratory tract, and the biologic effect(s) of exposure. Particle toxicity often is complicated by the presence of other air pollutants that may cause interactive effects. Particle size is thought to be a critical determinant of toxicity. After exposure of animals to ultrafine particles (those with a diameter of 0.2 μm or less), acute lung inflammation has been noted. In vitro studies of the cytotoxicity of particles collected from polluted urban air also have demonstrated that such particles can be highly toxic to alveolar macrophages. The relative toxicity of the particles studied depended on both the metal and the combustion-derived organic content of the particles.

A particular type of ambient particles, diesel exhaust particles (DEPs), has been the focus of considerable research attention. Several studies involving animal models of allergic airways disease document an adjuvant effect of DEPs on both inhaled antigen-induced airway hyperresponsiveness and airway inflammation. Nasal instillation of DEPs in humans with allergic rhinitis confirms enhancement of antigen-induced inflammation. A recent study also showed that a common genetic variation of an antioxidant enzyme (GSTM1) resulting in absence of the protein is a major determinant of this effect of DEPs. What is not clear about DEPs is the importance of exposure to ambient concentrations regarding allergies and asthma among the general population.

In summary, particles, SO_2 and acid aerosols are a complex group of air pollutants that share a common origin. Epidemiologic studies consistently have shown that they exert adverse health effects on both respiratory and cardiovascular morbidity and mortality. In vitro and in vivo studies have attempted to study the mechanism(s) of these effects, but their interpretation is complicated by the difficulty in separating out the individual contributions and the potential synergistic interactions of the components.

REFERENCES

Enstrom JE: Fine particulate air pollution and total mortality among elderly Californians, 1973–2002. Inhal Toxicol 2005;17:803 [PMID: 16282158].

Gauderman WJ et al: The effect of air pollution on lung development from 10 to 18 years of age. N Engl J Med 2004;351:1057 [PMID: 15356303].

Gilliland FD et al: Effect of glutathione-S-transferase M1 and P1 genotypes on xenobiotic enhancement of allergic responses: Randomised, placebo-controlled crossover study. Lancet 2004; 363:119 [PMID: 14726165].

Jerrett M et al: Spatial analysis of air pollution and mortality in Los Angeles. Epidemiology 2005;16:727 [PMID: 16222161].

Lead

Lead continues to be recognized as a significant toxicant and is known to have adverse health effects on humans of all ages (see Chapters 27 and 37). However, the phaseout of the additive tetraethyl lead from gasoline in the United States as a result of the CAA has been associated with declines in ambient lead concentrations and blood lead levels in the population. Thus widespread airborne exposure to lead has ceased to be a major health problem in the United States. Airborne lead remains a serious problem in many developing countries.

Carbon Monoxide

Carbon monoxide (CO) is a colorless, odorless, nonirritating gas that is generated by the incomplete combustion of carbon-containing fuels such as oils, gasoline, coal, and wood. Because of these described properties, exposure to CO may be insidious; in fact, exposure to high levels of CO is the leading cause of poisoning deaths in the United States. Ambient environmental air pollution levels are unlikely to cause acute toxicity and death, although low-dose exposure may be associated with adverse health effects. The most common source of exposure in nonsmoking individuals is from vehicle emissions. Engine exhaust may cause local accumulation of CO, especially during periods of heavy traffic. In transit exposure assessments, commuting individuals have been shown to be exposed to high levels. In fact, in one study of commuters, levels as high as 50 ppm with mean values of 10–12 ppm were recorded. Emissions from nonvehicular sources such as lawn mowers, chain saws, space heaters, and charcoal briquettes also contribute to ambient CO exposure.

The toxicity of CO lies in its ability to bind strongly to hemoglobin and interfere with the transport of oxygen from the alveoli to tissues (see Chapter 30). The degree of exposure to CO may be determined by measuring the blood carboxyhemoglobin level. Normal levels in nonsmokers range from 0.3–0.7%. The NAAQS is 9 ppm as an 8-hour average, not to be exceeded more than once a year.

Because CO has no direct effect on the lungs, its principal adverse health effects are through its ability to cause or exacerbate diseases associated with impaired oxygen delivery. Effects on fetal development, cardiovascular disease, chronic respiratory diseases, and nervous system disease have been described.

Animal studies show that low-level CO exposure during pregnancy may have developmental effects on the fetus. Low birth weight, fewer successful pregnancies, and increased fetal and neonatal mortality have been observed. A series of epidemiologic studies conducted in the Los Angeles area demonstrated associations between ambient CO concentrations and adverse birth outcomes (e.g., low birth weight, preterm delivery, and cardiac malformations).

In healthy human subjects, controlled-exposure studies have shown that low-level CO exposure decreases exercise capacity. In individuals with ischemic heart disease, a shorter duration to onset and an increased duration of angina, as well as earlier ST-T changes (an objective measure of myocardial ischemia), have been observed with low-level CO exposure. Ambient levels of CO have not been shown consistently to cause ventricular arrhythmias. Several epidemiologic studies show an association between high ambient levels of CO and cardiorespiratory hospital admissions and cardiac deaths.

In summary, CO at ambient levels of exposure may exacerbate ischemic heart disease, increase cardiorespiratory morbidity and cardiac mortality, and lead to increased adverse reproductive outcomes.

REFERENCES

Brook RD et al: Air pollution and cardiovascular disease: A statement for healthcare professionals from the Expert Panel on Population and Prevention Science of the American Heart Association. Circulation 2004;109:2655 [PMID: 15173049].

Wilhelm M et al: Local variations in CO and particulate air pollution and adverse birth outcomes in Los Angeles County, California, USA. Environ Health Perspect 2005;113:1212 [PMID: 16140630].

Smoking & Occupational Health

40

Neal L. Benowitz, MD, & Fu Hua, MB, MPH, PhD

CIGARETTE SMOKING & DISEASE

The smoking of cigarettes and other tobacco products is the most significant preventable cause of sickness and death in the world today. It was ranked as fourth among 20 leading risk factors contributing to the global burden of disease and first in developed countries. Worldwide, 8.8% of deaths (4.9 million) and 4.1% of disability adjusted life years (59.1 million) are caused by tobacco. The fractions attributable to tobacco use were 66% for cancer of the respiratory tract, 38% for chronic respiratory disease, and 12% for vascular disease. In developed countries, over 90% of lung cancers in men and 70% in women are caused by tobacco smoking. Attributable fractions are 56–80% for chronic respiratory disease and 22% for cardiovascular disease. Smoking is also a major risk factor for infections, including tuberculosis. Table 40–1 lists major diseases related to cigarette smoking. For most smokers, smoking is a far greater risk to health than is the workplace.

Cigarette Smoking as a Form of Drug Dependency

Cigarette smoking is a form of drug dependency that appears to be motivated by the desire to partake of the pharmacologic actions of nicotine. Nicotine has multiple psychological effects, including euphoria, reduction of anxiety or tension, suppression of appetite, mood stimulation or relaxation, and improvement in performance and memory. The stimulant effects of tobacco use may be particularly useful for workers who perform repetitive tasks but need to remain vigilant. Smokers tend to regulate nicotine intake to maintain consistent levels from day to day. Smokers often find it extremely difficult to quit smoking, even when the motivation to do so, such as illness or social pressure, is high.

Components & Toxicology of Tobacco Smoke

Tobacco smoke is a complex mixture of chemical substances in the form of gases and particulates (Table 40–2). More than 3000 constituents have been isolated from tobacco and more than 4000 from the mainstream smoke of cigarettes. Toxic gases include carbon monoxide, which binds hemoglobin preferentially to oxygen and results in reduced oxygen delivery to tissues (see Chapter 30). Other gases, such as nitrogen oxides, are oxidizing agents or irritants and may contribute to chronic obstructive lung disease and atherosclerotic vascular disease. Hydrogen cyanide impairs ciliary function in the lung, which may predispose to pulmonary infection. Volatile nitrosamines and other gaseous substances, such as formaldehyde, may contribute to cancer formation.

The particulate phase of tobacco smoke includes the alkaloids—chiefly nicotine—and tar. Aside from its central nervous system actions, nicotine is a sympathetic nervous system stimulant that increases heart rate, blood pressure, and myocardial contractility and causes release of free fatty acids. Nicotine causes release of stress hormones such as cortisol and growth hormone as well as vasopressin and β-endorphin. As a consequence of the cardiovascular effects of nicotine, myocardial oxygen demand increases. Exposure to tobacco smoke results in reduced exercise tolerance in patients with angina pectoris and enhances the risk of acute myocardial infarction and sudden death in persons with coronary heart disease. Nicotine induces vasoconstriction and may contribute to coronary spasm as well.

Tar is a complex mixture of chemicals that includes most of the suspected carcinogens, cocarcinogens, and tumor promoters in tobacco smoke. These include benzo(*a*)pyrene and other polynuclear aromatic hydrocarbons, nicotine-derived nitrosamines, β-naphthylamine, polonium-210, and metals such as nickel, arsenic, and cadmium.

Sixty-nine carcinogens in tobacco smoke have been identified as of the year 2000, including 10 species of polynuclear aromatic hydrocarbons (PAHs), six heterocyclic hydrocarbons, four volatile hydrocarbons, three nitrohydrocarbons, four aromatic amines, eight *N*-heterocyclic amines, ten *N*-nitrosamines, two aldehydes, ten miscellaneous organic compounds, nine inorganic compounds, and three phenolic compounds. Eleven compounds classified as International Agency for Research on Cancer (IARC) group 1 human carcinogen have been found in mainstream smoke.

REFERENCES

Arcavi L, Benowitz NL: Cigarette smoking and infection. Arch Intern Med 2004;164:2206 [PMID: 15534156].

Table 40–1. Diseases associated with cigarette smoking.

Cancer, many types
Cardiovascular disease
   Sudden death
   Acute myocardial infarction
   Unstable angina
   Stroke
   Peripheral arterial occlusive disease
   Aortic aneurysm
Pulmonary disease
   Chronic bronchitis
   Emphysema
   Bronchiolitis
   Interstitial fibrosis
   Aggravation of asthma
   Increased susceptibility to pneumonia
   Increased morbidity from viral respiratory tract infections
   Increased susceptibility to pulmonary tuberculosis
Gastrointestinal disease
   Peptic ulcer
   Esophageal reflux
Reproductive disorders
   Reduced fertility
   Premature birth
   Low birth weight
   Spontaneous abortion
   Abruptio placenta
   Premature rupture of membranes
   Increased perinatal mortality
Other diseases
   Noninsulin-dependent diabetes mellitus
   Earlier menopause
   Osteoporosis
   Cataracts
   Macular degeneration
   Accidental injuries, including fire injuries
   Premature skin wrinkling
   Altered drug metabolism and effects

Oncken C et al: Knowledge and perceived risk of smoking-related conditions: A survey of cigarette smokers. Prev Med 2005; 40:779 [PMID: 15850879].

Weinstein ND et al: Smokers' unrealistic optimism about their risk. Tob Control 2005;14:55 [PMID: 15735301].

OCCUPATION & SMOKING BEHAVIOR

Worldwide, the total prevalence of tobacco use in 2000 was 28.9%—57.4% for men and 10.3% for women. Smoking rates vary considerably from country to country—in Africa 18.4%, eastern Mediterranean regions 21.0%, and in the western Pacific region 33.8%. A nearly twofold difference in men was found between the lowest levels in the eastern Mediterranean region (34.2%) and the highest in the western Pacific region (62.3%). The smoking rate for women in the western Pacific region (5.8%), however, is much lower than in the European region (23.4%). The distribution of smokers within various occupations is not homogeneous. In the United States, persons who are better educated and have white-collar jobs are less likely to smoke. Blue-collar workers, farm workers, and service workers are most likely to smoke and smoke, on average, more cigarettes per day than white-collar workers. The smoking rate among blue-collar workers is nearly double that among white-collar workers. Unfortunately, this group is also the one most likely to be exposed to occupational chemical carcinogens. Among blue-collar workers, workers in the restaurant, bar, and gaming industries are exposed to much higher levels of environmental tobacco smoke (ETS). According to a national survey in China in 1996, the standardized smoking rates in males by occupations from highest to lowest were for people who live on boats (69%), employees of private companies (68%), service people (65%), self-employed people (64%), farmers (64%), factory workers (63%), office workers (61%), medical workers (54%), researchers (53%), and teachers (44%). Among females, the highest smoking rates were for self-employed workers (5.6%) and people who live on boats (5.5%); the lowest rates were for teachers (0.8%) and researchers (0.9%).

The higher rate of smoking among blue-collar workers is a potential confounding factor in understanding the relationship between smoking, occupation, and disease. Smoking as a marker for lower socioeconomic class may be associated with dietary differences, greater consumption of alcohol, and greater air pollution in the home environment—because of both industrial pollution related to geographic location of housing and a higher probability of exposure to tobacco smoke in the home.

Table 40–2. Major toxic components of cigarette smoke.

Nicotine	Carbon monoxide[1]
Catechols	Acetaldehyde[1]
N'-Nitrosonornicotine	Nitrogen oxides[1]
Phenol[1]	Hydrogen cyanide[1]
Polynuclear aromatic hydrocarbons[1]	Acrolein[1]
Benzene[1]	Ammonia[1]
β-Naphthylamine[1]	Formaldehyde[1]
Nickel (carbonyl)[1]	Urethane[1]
Cadmium[1]	Hydrazine[1]
Arsenic[1]	Nitrosamines
Polonium-210[1]	

[1]Potential occupational and environmental exposures.

INTERACTIONS BETWEEN SMOKING & OCCUPATION

Cigarette smoking can interact with occupational exposures to cause disease in several ways:

1. *Contamination of tobacco products with toxic substances in the workplace.* For example, toxic exposures might occur when cigarettes become contaminated with pesticides, lead, or other chemicals.

2. *Pyrolysis of workplace chemicals into toxic chemicals, which then are inhaled by the smoker.* An example is polymer fume fever in workers who inhale fumes from heated Teflon in contaminated cigarettes. The syndrome can be quite severe, causing pulmonary edema and even death. Prevention of such diseases requires prohibiting smoking at work and encouraging hand washing before smoking.

3. *Additive exposures to toxic agents found both in the workplace and in tobacco smoke.* Most of the chemicals in tobacco smoke, with the exception of nicotine, may be found in work environments, particularly where there is combustion of organic material. Carbon monoxide is an example of a toxin for which there may be additive contributions of workplace and smoking. Habitual heavy smokers have blood carboxyhemoglobin concentrations of 5–10%. Similar increments may follow occupational carbon monoxide exposure owing to the presence of combustion engines or furnaces or to exposure to methylene chloride (which is metabolized in the body to carbon monoxide). A blood level of 5–10% occurring after either smoking or occupational exposure may be well tolerated, but a level of 10–20% resulting from combined exposure can cause headache, impair psychomotor function, and in high-risk patients, aggravate ischemic vascular disease.

4. *Additive or synergistic (multiplicative) effects of workplace and tobacco smoke toxins.* Effects of pulmonary irritants and carcinogenic compounds from cigarettes and the workplace may increase the risks of chronic obstructive lung disease or cancer. Synergistic interactions, such as the increased risk of lung cancer with exposure to cigarette smoke and asbestos, are particularly important. Control of smoking would prevent many such cancers.

5. *Accidental injury related to tobacco smoking.* This includes injuries from fires produced from cigarettes as well as vehicular, machinery, and other accidents occurring at a higher rate in smokers than in nonsmokers.

In addition to specific interactions, as discussed earlier, smokers are also more susceptible to and less well able to tolerate respiratory tract infections such as influenza. Smokers have more severe illnesses and prolonged disability after such infections. Smoking has adverse orthopedic consequences as well, including delayed healing of fractures, increased incidence of nonunion, and a greater risk of postoperative infection. From all causes, smokers have 50% more work-loss days than nonsmokers.

It is estimated—considering excess health insurance, fire loss, workers' compensation claims and workplace accidents, absenteeism, loss of productivity, and the health consequences of passive smoking—that employee smoking results in substantial costs to employers.

REFERENCES

Howard J: Smoking is an occupational hazard. Am J Indust Med 2004;46:161 [PMID:15273969].

Sorensen G et al: Reducing social disparities in tobacco use: A social-contextual model for reducing tobacco use among blue-collar workers. Am J Public Health 2004;94:230 [PMID:1479932].

SMOKING & OCCUPATIONAL CANCER

In 2004, the IARC concluded that tobacco smoking causes cancer of lung; oral cavity; naso-, oro- and hypopharynx; nasal cavity and paranasal sinuses; larynx; esophagus; stomach; pancreas; liver; kidney (body and pelvis); ureter; urinary bladder; uterine cervix; and bone marrow (myeloid leukemia). It is believed that tobacco smoking is responsible for approximately 25% of all cancer in men and 4% in women and in both genders approximately 16% of cancer in developed countries and 10% in less developed countries, although some estimates are as high as 30%. Lung cancer incidence data most clearly illustrate the smoking-cancer connection. The incidence of most types of cancer has been relatively constant in the United States since 1900, but the lung cancer rate has been rising steadily. The rise in lung cancer rate parallels the average per capita consumption of cigarettes, with a lag of 20–30 years. Smoking prevalence for men peaked in 1950–1960, but because of the lag, the lung cancer rate reached its peak in the late 1980s. Because women began smoking later than men, lung cancer rates in women began to rise sharply in the 1960s and continue to rise, having recently surpassed breast cancer as the greatest cause of cancer mortality in women.

How Does Cigarette Smoking Cause Cancer?

Cancer causation by tobacco smoke is most likely the result of the effects of the complex mixture of chemicals in smoke. According to a multistep model of carcinogenicity, the components of tobacco smoke directly cause the cellular changes that accumulate to drive the carcinogenesis process. Most chemical carcinogens in tobacco smoke require metabolic activation to exert a carcinogenic effect. The requisite enzymes are present in lung and other target organs. Individual risk may be affected by the activity and levels of enzymes such as glutathione-S-transderase, cytochrome P450 and N-acetyl transferase. In the course of metabolism, reactive forms of polycyclic aromatic hydrocarbons, nitrosamines, and aromatic amines are generated and become covalently bound to DNA in relevant tissues. Smoking produces some of the genetic and epigenetic changes affecting major pathways that must be disrupted for a normal cell to become a tumor cell. Epigenetic changes can trigger a complex cellular stress response. And genetic changes can endow some cells with a capacity to escape normal immunosuppression. Thus the changes in the cellular environment produced by tobacco smoke may select the emergence of cells that have acquired the capacity to undergo clonal expansion. This phenomenon can occur simultaneously at several sites within an exposed tissue field, resulting in multifocal lesions, some of which can progress to cancer.

Tobacco smoke carcinogens and occupational toxins may interact synergistically. Tobacco smoke also may be the vehicle for transmission of occupational carcinogens into the lung. Finally, cigarette smokers may be more tolerant of noxious substances in the air, allowing greater exposure to environmental carcinogens.

Asbestos, Smoking, & Lung Cancer

Lung cancer is a major type of cancer in asbestos workers. The interaction between smoking, asbestos exposure, and lung cancer is the best-studied example of the influence of smoking on occupational disease.

Studies of asbestos workers indicate a substantially increased risk of lung cancer, and lung cancers occur at greater than additive rates in persons exposed to both asbestos and cigarette smoke. The IARC Working Group concluded that the evidence supports synergism between asbestos exposure and smoking in causing lung cancer but noted that the degree of synergism remains uncertain.

Several mechanisms of interaction between asbestos and smoking are proposed: (1) Asbestos may act as a foreign body, resulting in chronic inflammation, with cell injury and repair, (2) tobacco smoke, acting as a tumor promoter, may impair the capacity of cells to repair injury, leading instead to cancer, (3) asbestos in the lung may attract pulmonary alveolar macrophages, which are capable of metabolizing polycyclic hydrocarbons to carcinogenic metabolites, and (4) asbestos fibers may adsorb, concentrate, and slowly release carcinogens from tobacco smoke.

The latency for lung cancer in asbestos workers is about 20 years. Although control of asbestos exposure has improved considerably in recent years, many workers have large body burdens of asbestos. The multiple-step carcinogenesis model strongly points toward smoking cessation as an intervention that could reduce the cancer risk prior to development of cancer. Thus, for workers already exposed to asbestos, the single most important way to decrease the risk of lung cancer is to stop smoking.

Smoking, Uranium Mining, & Cancer

Studies show a relationship between cumulative radiation exposure and the risk of bronchogenic cancer. Cigarette smoking substantially amplifies lung cancer rates, particularly at high radiation levels.

Uranium and other metal ores release radon gas, which decays to daughters, two of which are alpha-radiation emitters. The alpha-ray radiation, when present in close proximity to bronchial cells, causes local damage and ultimately neoplasm formation. Radioactive gases may adsorb onto particles, which then are inhaled and deposited in the lung. Cigarette smoke may be an important source of particles for delivery of radiation to the lung. Tobacco itself is also a source of polonium-210. Several studies indicated that smoking and radon could exert a synergistic but submultiplicative interaction. The carcinogenic effect of radiation is believed to be promoted by toxic materials in tobacco smoke, which would explain shorter onset and latency times to cancer development in uranium miners who are smokers.

Other Occupational Hazards

Studies of the combined effect of smoking and arsenic exposure in smelting or metal mining on lung cancer risk indicated that the risk was consistently greater than additive. In addition, occupational exposure to nickel also has a multiplicative effect on lung cancer risk in the presence of cigarette smoking. No consistent patterns of effect modification on lung cancer between silica exposure or silicosis and smoking are evident.

REFERENCES

Boffetta P: Epidemiology of environmental and occupational cancer. Oncogene 2004;23:6392 [PMID: 15322513].

Liang G et al: A functional polymorphism in the SULT1A1 gene (G638A) is associated with risk of lung cancer in relation to tobacco smoking. Carcinogenesis 2004;25:773 [PMID: 14688021].

Ruano-Ravina A et al: Occupation and smoking as risk factors for lung cancer: A population-based case-control study. Am J Indust Med 2003;43:149 [PMID: 12541269].

Schneider J et al: GSTM1, GSTT1, and GSTP1 polymorphism and lung cancer risk in relation to tobacco smoking. Cancer Lett 2004;208:65 [PMID: 15105047].

Wang LI et al: Asbestos exposure, manganese superoxide dismutase (MnSOD) genotype, and lung cancer risk. J Occup Environ Med 2004;46:556 [PMID: 15213518].

SMOKING & OCCUPATIONAL LUNG DISEASE

The major occupational chronic lung diseases are bronchitis, chronic obstructive pulmonary disease, pneumoconiosis (fibrotic disease of the lung parenchyma), and occupational asthma. Cigarette smoking is clearly the major cause of chronic bronchitis and chronic obstructive pulmonary disease and also may produce airway constriction in asthmatics. The net impairment of pulmonary function in workers is the sum of the influences of cigarette smoking, occupational exposures, and other factors such as genetic deficiency of α_1-antitrypsin.

Pathology & Pathophysiology of Smoking-Related Lung Disease

Chronic bronchitis—characterized by increased size of mucous glands, increased numbers of goblet cells, and mucus hypersecretion—is a nonspecific response to chronic irritant exposure. It may result either from cigarette smoking or from exposure to a variety of chemicals or dusts. The risks of chronic bronchitis from smoking and occupational exposure to dusts are additive in most studies, with the largest percentages of cases today attributable to cigarette smoking. Chronic bronchitis may be associated with reduced airflow at high lung volumes, consistent with large airway disease.

Chronic obstructive lung disease is the lung disease most specific for cigarette smoking. Small airways injury is common in smokers even without symptoms. Pulmonary function tests in smokers commonly reveal reduction of maximum midexpiratory flow rates, a manifestation of small airways disease.

Emphysema is a more advanced stage of smoking-related chronic lung disease in which destruction of alveolar walls results in airflow obstruction, increased lung compliance and total lung capacity, and decreased diffusing capacity for carbon monoxide. The pathophysiology of smoking-related emphysema is believed to involve exposure to oxidant gases with concomitant impairment of antioxidant protective mechanisms such as α_1-antitrypsin activity. Migration of neutrophils into the lung, which may be mediated in part by the effects of nicotine, may contribute to oxidant injury of membranes. Typically, the pattern of smoking-related emphysema is centrilobular.

Exposure to mineral dusts, such as coal or silica, also may produce small airways disease, with fibrosis of small airways and, later, focal emphysema. Typically, such disease is asymptomatic. Parenchymal lung disease with diffuse fibrosis may occur with asbestosis, silicosis, or coal miner's pneumoconiosis. Chest radiographs usually show parenchymal opacities ranging in size from less than 1 cm to massive fibrosis that involves large portions of the lung, and pulmonary function tests reveal severe restrictive disease, although there may be an element of obstructive disease as well. Findings of advanced pneumoconiosis generally are distinguishable from those associated with tobacco-related emphysema.

Cigarette smoking, including involuntary smoke exposure, may increase the degree of airway obstruction in asthmatics. Smoking increases the risk of sensitization to occupational allergies and would be expected to aggravate occupational asthma from any cause. Table 40–3 provides specific examples of interactions between occupational exposures and cigarette exposures in causing disease.

A good example of the interaction between smoking and occupation in causing acute respiratory disease is byssinosis in textile workers exposed to cotton dust. Some workers develop bronchitis or chest tightness after exposure to cotton dust, typically following a weekend or holiday when they have not been exposed. Pulmonary function tests indicate acute bronchoconstriction resembling asthma. The severity of symptoms is related both to the magnitude of cotton dust exposure and to whether or not the worker is a cigarette smoker. The symptoms and the magnitude of the pulmonary function test abnormalities are greatest in workers with higher dust exposure. Symptoms and manifestations are much more severe with the same level of cotton dust in smokers.

Although controversial, there are also reports of chronic airway disease in cotton textile workers, most severe in smokers but occurring also in nonsmokers. The interaction between smoking and cotton dust exposure has provoked debate concerning workers' compensation and regulatory issues; clearly, control of both risk factors should be goals of occupational health programs.

Asbestos exposure produces interstitial lung disease, which appears to be aggravated by cigarette smoking. For any given level of asbestos exposure, the asbestos-related abnormalities on chest radiograph are more severe in smokers. Smoking is a significant risk factor for interstitial lung disease in general, which may be contributed to by occupational exposures, such as to metal dusts.

REFERENCES

Samet JM: Adverse effects of smoke exposure on the upper airway. Tobac Control 2004;13:57 [PMID:14985618].

Vineis P et al: Environmental tobacco smoke and risk of respiratory cancer and chronic obstructive pulmonary disease in former smokers and never smokers in the EPIC prospective study. BMJ 2005;330:277 [PMID: 15681570].

Table 40–3. Interactions between occupation and cigarette smoking in causing disease.

Occupation	Exposure	Disease	Smoking-Occupation Interaction
Asbestos workers	Asbestos	Lung cancer	Multiplicative
		Chronic lung disease (restrictive, obstructive)	Additive
Aluminum smelter workers	Polynuclear hydrocarbons	Bladder cancer	Additive or multiplicative
Cement workers	Cement dust	Chronic bronchitis, obstructive lung disease	Additive
Chlorine manufacturing	Chlorine	Chronic obstructive lung disease	Additive
Coal miners	Coal dust	Chronic obstructive lung disease	Additive
Copper smelter workers	Sulfur dioxide	Chronic obstructive lung disease	Additive
	Arsenic	Lung cancer	Additive or multiplicative
Grain workers	Grain dust	Chronic bronchitis, obstructive lung disease	Additive
Rock cutters, foundry workers	Silica dust	Obstructive lung disease	Additive
Textile workers	Cotton, hemp, flax dust	Acute airway obstruction (byssinosis)	Possibly multiplicative
		Chronic bronchitis	Additive
Uranium miners	Alpha radiation	Lung cancer	Additive or multiplicative
Welders	Irritant gases, metal fumes, dusts	Chronic bronchitis, obstructive lung disease	Additive

INVOLUNTARY SMOKING

Involuntary (or passive) smoking is exposure to second-hand tobacco smoke (SHS), which is a mixture of exhaled mainstream smoke and sidestream smoke released from the smoldering cigarette or other smoking device and diluted with ambient air. Second-hand tobacco smoke consists of a gas phase and a particular phase. Secondhand tobacco smoke contains nicotine as well as oxidizing chemicals, carcinogens, and other toxins. Carcinogens include benzene, 1,3-butadiene, benzo(*a*)pyrene, 4-(methylnitrosamino)-1-(3-pyridyl)-1-butanone, and many others.

Evidence That Nonsmokers Inhale Cigarette Smoke

Many studies provide evidence of tobacco smoke components in the environment and in biologic fluids of nonsmokers. Biochemical measures include plasma, saliva, and urinary nicotine and cotinine (a metabolite of nicotine). Cotinine excretion in the urine of non-smokers exposed to other cigarette smokers in the home and in the urine of those exposed in the workplace are equivalent. Exposure in both places results in an additive increase in cotinine excretion. From urinary cotinine data, it is estimated that nonsmokers with exposure to secondhand tobacco smoke typically absorb a dose of nicotine equivalent to one-sixth to one-third of a cigarette; however, with heavy exposure to second-hand tobacco smoke, the amount of nicotine may be equivalent to as much as two cigarettes per day. There is overlap in the intake of heavily passively exposed nonsmokers and light primary smokers.

Health Hazards of Involuntary Smoking

A number of studies indicate that involuntary cigarette smoke exposure may present health hazards. Exposure of a nonsmoker to cigarette smoke is well known to be a source of annoyance primarily because of eye irritation, nose irritation, and malodor. That involuntary smoking may affect pulmonary function is supported by observations in children whose mothers smoke, that is, a higher incidence of respiratory infection during the first year of life, exacerbation of asthma, and evidence of reduced pulmonary function. In adults, involuntary smoke exposure may aggravate angina pectoris or asthma and may result in mild impairment of small airways pulmonary function, although the lifelong significance of the latter is unclear. Several epidemiologic studies have found an association between SHS exposure and an increased risk of myocardial infarction in nonsmokers with spouses who smoke. On average, SHS exposure is associated with a 30% increase in the risk of coronary heart disease, which has been estimated to cause as many as 37,000 premature deaths in the United States annually. Involuntary smoke exposure is associated with reduced birth weight in nonsmoking pregnant women.

Cancer & Involuntary Smoke Exposure

Many studies have reported an increased risk of lung cancer in nonsmokers who are involuntarily exposed to cigarette smoke. The first report was of a study of 142,800 women in Tokyo, of whom 91,500 were nonsmoking wives. In a 14-year follow-up prospective study, there were 346 cases of lung cancer, including 174 in nonsmoking wives. The relative risk for lung cancer in women who were smokers compared with women who neither smoked nor had a husband who smoked was 3.8. The relative risk of lung cancer in nonsmoking wives with husbands who smoke was 1.6 if husbands smoked fewer than 20 cigarettes a day and 2.1 if husbands smoked more than 20 cigarettes a day. Because most men in Japan at the time of the study smoked cigarettes and most women did not, involuntary smoke exposure appeared to be the most important cause of lung cancer in Japanese women.

Subsequently, more than 50 studies of involuntary smoking and lung cancer risk in never-smokers, especially spouses of smokers, have been published. Most studies found an increased risk of lung cancer in nonsmokers married to smokers when compared with those not married to smokers. Meta-analyses show that there is a statistically significant and consistent association between lung cancer risk in spouses of smokers and exposure to secondhand tobacco smoke from the spouse who smokes. The excess risk is on the order of 20% for women and 30% for men and remains after controlling for some potential sources of bias and confounding.

In 2004, the IARC Working Group noted that there is sufficient evidence that involuntary smoking causes lung cancer in human and that involuntary smoking is carcinogenic to humans (group 1).

REFERENCES

Brennan P et al: Secondhand smoke exposure in adulthood and risk of lung cancer among never smokers: A pooled analysis of two large studies. Int J Cancer 2004;109:125 [PMID: 14735478].

Vineis P et al. Environmental tobacco smoke and risk of respiratory cancer and chronic obstructive pulmonary disease in former smokers and never smokers in the EPIC prospective study. BMJ 2005;330:277 [15681570].

Involuntary Smoking & Workplace Illness

Workplace exposure to cigarette smoke can result in significant smoke intake, and involuntary smoke exposure may be related to impaired respiratory function and an increased risk of lung cancer in nonsmokers. For nonsmokers sharing a work environment with cigarette smokers, the workplace must be considered hazardous independent of any specific industrial toxic exposure. This risk is particularly important when a high percentage of the workers smoke or where smokers and nonsmokers work in poorly ventilated areas.

Another concern is that involuntary smoke exposure may act synergistically—as does primary smoking—with toxic industrial materials to amplify the dose-response curve for those substances. Although there is no empirical evidence to support this hypothesis at present, the possibility must be considered.

Asthma in adults has been reported to be aggravated by SHS, although research is conflicting. When exposed to SHS, nonsmokers often complain of eye irritation, nasal congestion, headaches, and coughing. Although these symptoms are prevalent in nonsmokers with exposure to SHS, they are more severe in people who have a history of allergies. The increased risk of respiratory tract infection, asthma, and middle ear effusion in infants and children exposed to SHS provides a basis for mandating that child-care facilities be smoke-free.

REFERENCES

Panagiotakos DB et al: Effect of exposure to secondhand smoke on markers of inflammation: The ATTICA study. Am J Med 2004;116:145 [PMID: 14749157].

Skeer M et al: Secondhand smoke exposure in the workplace. Am J Prevent Med 2005;28:331 [PMID:15831337].

Surgeon General's Report on the Effects of Secondhand Smoke, http://www.hhs.gov/news/press/2006pres/20060627.html

CONTROL OF SMOKING IN THE WORKPLACE

If the goal of an occupational health program is to prevent illness and disability, the most effective way to do so is by control of cigarette smoking. The importance of controlling exposure to potentially toxic industrial chemicals is obvious, but total elimination of exposure is often impossible. An optimal employee health program should include simultaneous control of toxic exposures and smoking. A smoking-control program should include both programs to encourage smoking cessation and environmental control measures to protect nonsmokers from tobacco smoke of their colleagues.

Workplace Tobacco-Control Strategies

The first strategy is restricting or prohibiting smoking in the workplace. Eighty percent or more of workplaces that employ 50 or more workers in the United States currently have formal workplace smoking policies. Most U.S. companies restrict smoking in common work areas. Many companies have complete workplace smoking bans. However, many small businesses do not have such restrictions. Of note, smoking restrictions in the workplace result in smokers smoking fewer cigarettes each day and increase the likelihood that smokers will quit.

The second strategy is the development of programs to encourage employees to quit smoking by physician counseling and educational activities and by either offering smoking-cessation programs on the job or by paid referral of workers to community smoking-cessation programs. Some businesses also offer various incentives for employees to quit smoking. Optimally, smoking-cessation programs should be sponsored jointly by management and labor. Another way in which employers can promote smoking cessation is by insisting that health care insurers cover smoking-cessation treatment as part of the worker's benefit package.

A third strategy is not to hire cigarette smokers. When the risks of smoking and occupational exposure are clearly synergistic, such as with asbestos exposure or uranium mining, not hiring smokers seems quite sensible.

Control of Involuntary Smoke Exposure

The concentration of tobacco smoke in a room depends on the size of the room, the number of smokers, the extent of ventilation, and other factors such as the nature of wall surfaces. Ventilation with outside air or the use of high-efficiency filtration systems substantially reduces smoke concentrations and is required at a minimum for workplace control of cigarette smoke. But even with good ventilation, such as with central air-conditioning systems, substantial concentrations of carbon monoxide and particulates are found in the workplace. Ventilation alone is inadequate.

Segregation of smokers and nonsmokers by space alone is partially effective but primarily for particulates. The greater the ratio of smoking to nonsmoking areas, the less effective the segregation. Placing physical barriers between smoking and nonsmoking areas may be more effective, but the effectiveness depends on the airflow between the segregated areas. If it is not possible to place smokers and nonsmokers in separate rooms, barriers are better than nothing.

Prohibition of smoking at the work site is the most effective way to reduce environmental smoke concentrations. Restricting workplace smoking so as to provide a smoke-free workplace for nonsmokers has been mandated legislatively in a number of communities. Compliance with such local ordinances has been good, and enforcement has not been a major problem.

Air quality standards and permissible occupational exposure levels relevant to tobacco-smoke components should be developed, monitored, and enforced. This may be an important area of activity for the Occupational Safety and Health Administration (OSHA).

Finally, where there is inadequate environmental control of cigarette smoke, nonsmoking workers should be advised of and given the opportunity to accept or reject the health risks of involuntary smoke exposure, as would be the case for workers in other hazardous environments.

REFERENCES

American Heart Association, Office on Smoking and Health, www.americanheart.org/presenter.jhtml?identifier=4673.

Bauer JE et al: A Longitudinal assessment of the impact of smoke-free worksite policies on tobacco use. Am J Public Health 2005; 95:1024 [PMID:15914828].

Moher M et al: Workplace interventions for smoking cessation. Cochrane Database Syst Rev 2005;2:CD003440 [PMID: 15846667].

Office of the Surgeon General: Reports on smoking and health, www.americanheart.org/presenter.jhtml?identifier=4673.

Building-Associated Illness

41

Michael L. Fischman, MD, MPH

The Clean Air Act, passed in the mid 1960s, focused national attention on cleaning up outdoor air but directed little interest toward improving the quality of indoor air—even though people spend only 10–20% of their time outdoors and the rest of their time indoors at home or at work. Studies conducted during the past three decades confirm that indoor air quality (IAQ) problems can cause or contribute to a variety of symptoms and sometimes illnesses in building occupants. Concentrations of some pollutants inside buildings may exceed standards established for outdoor concentrations.

The term *building-associated illness* is reserved for health problems that develop in nonindustrial settings customarily considered nonhazardous, such as homes, schools, and offices. Indoor air contamination is linked to a wide variety of building materials and consumer products.

TYPES OF BUILDING-ASSOCIATED ILLNESSES & HEALTH CONCERNS

It is possible to divide building-associated illnesses into two categories: (1) acute short-latency illnesses and (2) potentially chronic long-latency illnesses. The nature of the exposures that may give rise to each type differs substantially. Table 41–1 presents a classification scheme for building-associated illness. The principal focus of this chapter is on the acute short-latency illnesses.

The short-latency illnesses include sick-building syndrome, mass psychogenic illness, specific illnesses resulting from identifiable sources of noxious materials, certain infectious diseases, building-associated hypersensitivity pneumonitis, and dampness-associated asthma exacerbations. These conditions are characterized by a relatively acute onset, closely related in time to the individual's presence within the building and often relieved by removal from further exposure. Some of the building-related illnesses do not resolve promptly on leaving the building. In 1987, a committee on indoor air quality for the National Research Council defined *building-related illness* as those specific clinical syndromes resulting from exposure to indoor air contaminants, for example, hypersensitivity pneumonitis or Legionnaires' disease. In contrast, *sick-building syndrome* refers to the occurrence, in more than

20% of the work population, of a variety of nonspecific symptoms and minimal or no objective findings, wherein it is not possible to make a specific diagnosis.

In contrast, the long-latency illnesses include cancer and chronic pulmonary diseases perhaps resulting from long-term low-level exposure to contaminants in indoor air. Because of the long induction-latency periods for these conditions and their multifactorial origin, it is much more difficult to establish a causal link to the building exposure. Agents in indoor air that may be responsible for such illnesses include cigarette smoke, asbestos, radon gas, oxides of nitrogen, polycyclic aromatic hydrocarbons, and chlorinated hydrocarbon insecticides.

The relationship of these long-latency illnesses to indoor air pollution generally is speculative. Estimates of risk often are predicated on the basis of mathematical extrapolations from high-dose industrial or animal experimental exposures to substances encountered in much lower doses in building environments. There are more data suggesting a problem with cigarette smoke than with the other agents (see Chapter 40). Indoor asbestos exposure occurs at very low levels unless the insulation materials are disturbed or improperly removed. Exposure to low levels of radioactivity occurs in the form of radon gas from building materials and soil underlying basements or foundations. Polycyclic aromatic hydrocarbons are released into indoor air from wood-burning fireplaces and other sources. Based on the increased risk of lung cancer in much more heavily exposed asbestos workers, uranium miners, and coke oven workers, respectively, there is some concern about the impact of these agents on lung cancer incidence in the general population.

Certain products of combustion, such as oxides of nitrogen from unvented gas appliances, may pose long-term health risks. There is limited epidemiologic evidence suggesting increased respiratory infections, symptomatic worsening of asthma, and reduced performance on pulmonary function testing associated with exposure to gas stove emissions.

NATURE, SOURCES, & CONCENTRATIONS OF EXPOSURES

Potential sources of indoor air contaminants can be classified as follows: (1) contaminants released from the

Table 41–1. Types of building-associated illness.

Short-latency illnesses
  Sick-building syndrome
  Mass psychogenic illness
  Building-associated hypersensitivity pneumonitis
  Dampness-associated asthma exacerbations
  Building-associated infections
    Legionnaires' disease
    Pontiac fever
    Q fever
  Illnesses associated with specific contaminants
    Formaldehyde
    Carbon monoxide
Possible long-latency illnesses
  Lung cancer
  Chronic nonmalignant respiratory disease

building or its contents, including asbestos, formaldehyde, and radon, (2) contaminants generated by such diverse human activities as cooking, heating, cigarette smoking, and cleaning, and (3) infiltrated contaminants, that is, agents that enter the house or building along with the outside air but in lower concentration (typically by 25–75%).

The concentration of contaminants is influenced not only by the source of exposure but also by the exchange rate between indoor and outdoor air. The introduction of outdoor air into a home or building occurs either by implemented ventilation or by infiltration. Infiltration occurs through cracks or other leaks in the structure or through open doors and windows. The amount of infiltration depends on the type of building, the amount of insulation, and other weather-proofing and climatic conditions. Implemented ventilation, for example, forced-air heating or air-conditioning systems, may provide substantial amounts of outdoor air but also may be designed to recirculate preconditioned air with minimal fresh-air intake.

The amount of air exchange often is expressed in air changes per hour (ACH). ACH may vary from 0.2 in tightly sealed homes to 0.7 in an average home to 60 or more in some industrial settings with implemented ventilation. Alternatively, with implemented ventilation, the amount of outdoor air supplied may be expressed in cubic feet per minute (cfm) per occupant or liters per second per occupant.

The concentration of contaminants at any location within a building will be influenced by the location of the source and the degree of air mixing. In the case of reactive or particulate contaminants, the concentration will be affected by the rate of chemical reaction or the rate of deposition, respectively.

EVALUATION OF BUILDING-ASSOCIATED ILLNESS

Proper assessment of illnesses relating to indoor air quality involves both evaluation of the symptoms, usually by a physician, and assessment of the work environment, usually by an industrial hygienist. A symptom questionnaire may be helpful in establishing the nature, chronology, and frequency of complaints; the temporal relationship to presence in the building; the locations at which complaints arise; any incidents or activities that preceded the complaints; and the coexistence of any medical problems or risk factors that might account for some of the symptoms. Alternatively or in addition, personal interviews of affected employees may be useful; targeted physical examinations are less likely to be helpful. Analysis of the symptom data, with grouping of symptoms into categories and a search for factors associated with symptom occurrence across the population, is essential.

Industrial hygiene evaluation should begin with gathering of background information on the building, such as its age, type of construction, ventilation system design, and history of problems, renovations, and repairs. A walkthrough survey will permit an appreciation of the floor plan and the physical locations at which symptoms have occurred, as well as inspection of the ventilation system and any possible point sources of air contaminants, for example, blueprint machines, cleaning supplies, areas of microbial growth, and cafeteria equipment and exhaust (including cooking odors). A search for evidence of or a history of water intrusion that could lead to mold growth is also appropriate. A guideline jointly prepared by National Institute for Occupational Safety and Health (NIOSH) and Environmental Protection Agency (EPA) provides a thorough discussion of the approaches to prevention, investigation, and management of indoor air quality problems.

The American Society of Heating, Refrigerating, and Air Conditioning Engineers (ASHRAE) issued its most recent guideline for temperature and humidity control in 2004, designed to promote comfort for most (80%) occupants. The acceptable temperature range varies with the relative humidity. Thus, for office workers, at a relative humidity of 30%, the acceptable temperature lies between 20.5 and 25.5°C (69 and 78°F) during the heating season and between 24.5 and 28°C (76 and 82°F) in the cooling season. The desired relative humidity is between 30% and 60%. Relative humidity levels below 20% often result in drying of mucous membranes, with associated discomfort, whereas levels above 60% support mold growth. Depending on the ventilation system design, there may be localized areas within buildings that fall outside the comfortable range even though the rest of the building is controlled adequately.

ASHRAE also has issued guidelines for provision of adequate amounts of fresh outside air. In the current 2004 ventilation guideline, outside air should be provided in office areas at a rate of 17 cfm per occupant (slightly reduced from the prior guideline of 20 cfm per occupant), which amounts to about 8.5 L/s per occupant of outside air.

Limited environmental monitoring may be helpful in assessing the adequacy of ventilation—including the extent of fresh versus recirculated air—and temperature and humidity control. Minimal equipment is required for this monitoring—a room thermometer and relative humidity meter, smoke tubes to assess air movement, and direct-reading carbon dioxide colorimetric detector tubes.

Because carbon dioxide is a product of respiratory metabolism, its accumulation in office buildings reflects a balance between generation by building occupants and removal through ventilation and introduction of fresh outdoor air. Measurement of CO_2 levels aids in evaluating whether sufficient quantities of fresh air are being introduced into the building. The outdoor concentration of CO_2 varies typically from 250–350 ppm. The presence of CO_2 in concentrations above 1000 ppm inside the building suggests inadequate fresh-air ventilation. In prior building investigations, levels above 1000 ppm often were associated with perceptions of poor air quality and complaints of headache and mucous membrane irritation. Although the CO_2 itself is clearly not responsible for these symptoms, a high concentration suggests that other air contaminant levels are likely to be increased; in other words, the CO_2 level serves as a surrogate measure for the presence of other as yet unidentified contaminants likely to be the cause of these symptoms. A ventilation rate of 15 cfm per person generally will keep CO_2 levels below 1000 ppm. Indoor air quality complaints occur occasionally with concentrations of CO_2 as low as 700–800 ppm. Increasing the fresh-air ventilation rate to 25 cfm per person will reduce the CO_2 concentration below this level, often resulting in subsidence of symptoms. Table 41–2 lists some guidelines for factors having an impact on indoor air quality.

Further and more specific air sampling should be performed if significant sources of air contaminants are identified or suspected. In the absence of such point sources, however, it is quite unlikely that extensive untargeted industrial hygiene sampling will identify an unrecognized contaminant in concentrations sufficient to cause symptoms. Such sampling typically will be quite expensive. Moreover, in part because of the very high

Table 41–2. Relevant guidelines for indoor air quality.[1]

Factor	Guideline/Study Finding	Comment
Temperature	See text[2] 72°F	ASHRAE Standard 55, 2004 Reduced prevalence of sick-building syndrome symptoms
Relative humidity	30–60%	ASHRAE Standard 55, 2004
Fresh outside air	17 cfm per occupant	ASHRAE Standard 62.1, 2004
Carbon dioxide	≥ 1000 ppm ≤ 650 ppm	Perception of poor air quality and increased symptoms Improved occupant satisfaction
Carbon monoxide	9 ppm (8 hours)	Outdoor air standard from NAAQS/EPA[3]
Total volatile organic compounds (TVOCs)	No guideline	
Formaldehyde	0.1 ppm 0.05 ppm	Residential air quality guideline from Health Canada[1] Residential level to avoid irritation in allergic and asthmatic individuals from California Air Resources Board[1]
Particulates <2.5 μm <10 μm	 65 μg/m^3 over 24 hours 150 μg/m^3 over 24 hours	 Outdoor air standard from NAAQS/EPA[3]

[1]General reference source: ANSI/ASHRAE, Appendix B: Summary of Selected Air Quality Guidelines, Standard 62.1, 2004.
[2]See "Evaluation of Building-Associated Illness and Physical Factors" in text.
[3]National Ambient Air Quality Standards from U.S. EPA, www.epa.gov/air/criteria.html.

sensitivity of available analytic methodology, sampling invariably detects some contaminants, often in the low-ppb range. These results likely will raise concerns in building occupants but are not likely to explain symptoms or identify the cause of the building problem.

RESULTS OBTAINED FROM BUILDING INVESTIGATIONS

Analysis of accumulated experience from multiple IAQ investigations facilitates an understanding of the relative frequency of different causal factors, permitting prioritization of building investigation approaches. Investigators at the National Institute for Occupational Safety and Health (NIOSH) reported the results of over 400 evaluations conducted during the 1980s of buildings with indoor air quality problems. While dated, the analysis remains the largest published compilation of building investigations. Although they recognized that some of the problems may have had multiple causes, the NIOSH investigators were able to classify the results by the primary identified cause. In 32% of the evaluations, building ventilation was found to be inadequate, as evidenced by inadequate fresh-air intake, poor air distribution and mixing, draftiness, poor temperature and humidity control, pressure differences between office spaces, or air filtration problems. Inside contamination from various types of wet copiers, improper pesticide application, improper use of cleaning agents such as rug shampoo, tobacco smoke, combustion gases (e.g., from cafeterias), and the like accounted for 17% of the problems. Such contaminants were present at levels above the normal background but far below any permissible exposure limits. Outside contamination sources were the primary factor in 11% of the investigations, generally a result of entrainment of contaminated outside air as a result of improperly located exhaust and intake vents or contaminant generation near intake vents. A commonly identified source was the entrainment of vehicle exhaust fumes from parking garages into the air intake vent. Other contaminants included boiler gases, previously exhausted air, and asphalt from roofing operations. Microbiologic contamination accounted for 3% of the problems, resulting from standing water in ventilation system components or from water damage to carpets or other furnishings. A variety of disorders—including hypersensitivity pneumonitis, humidifier fever, allergic rhinitis, asthma, and allergic conjunctivitis—can arise from microbial contaminants. Building materials were the source of contaminants in 3% of the investigations, including such things as particle board, plywood, and some glues and adhesives. In 12% of the investigations, the factor or factors involved remained unknown. Recent data to establish the current frequency of causal factors do not exist, although more recent individual reports do not suggest a substantially different distribution of causes.

Although they did not list it as a primary cause, the NIOSH investigators indicated that tobacco smoke may have been a major contributor to indoor air quality problems largely because it contains numerous irritant compounds. Because of nonsmoking policies implemented in many workplaces and other locations in recent years, environmental tobacco smoke is now a less frequent contributor to indoor air quality problems in nonresidential buildings.

REFERENCES

Institute for Research in Construction: Indoor air quality and thermal comfort in open-plan offices, http://irc.nrc-cnrc.gc.ca/pubs/ctus/64_e.html.

NIOSH/EPA: Building air quality: A guide for building owners and facility managers, www.cdc.gov/niosh/baqtoc.html.

SHORT-LATENCY ILLNESSES

Sick-Building Syndrome

The term *sick-building syndrome* (SBS; previously referred to as *closed-building syndrome* or *tight-building syndrome* and sometimes referred to as *nonspecific building-associated illness*) denotes a characteristic set of symptoms, typically headache and mucous membrane irritation, recognized among occupants of nonindustrial buildings such as offices and schools. Despite the name, it is the occupants who are sick, with some factor about the building being the culprit.

In an effort to conserve energy, many sealed structures with centrally controlled ventilation were built in the 1970s and 1980s. Initially, SBS tended to occur in these buildings without operable windows. However, SBS problems continue to occur despite engineering changes in newer buildings to improve outside air ventilation.

A. OCCURRENCE & ETIOLOGY

The incidence of SBS is unknown, but the frequently reported outbreaks of illness consistent with this condition suggest that it is the most common building-associated illness. Symptoms that occupants relate to a building are common, even in buildings without recognized problems and with normal IAQ parameters. For example, in a questionnaire study of four nonproblem state buildings in Washington State, 55% of the 646 respondents reported recent upper respiratory symptoms temporally related to being at work, including dry eyes, nasal symptoms, and dry or sore throat. Forty-eight percent reported central nervous system symptoms, including commonly headache, unusual tiredness, tension, and mental fatigue. These symptoms were statistically associated with such factors as perception of the air as too dry, perception of too little air movement, and perception of the workspace as too noisy. Symptoms were not correlated with measured air contaminant levels.

Building outbreaks have occurred chiefly in government offices, business offices, and schools or colleges. There are a variety of known and suspected contributing factors to the development of SBS.

1. Physical factors—One common feature present in most afflicted buildings is a central ventilation system that depends on a significant proportion of recirculated air. Historically, these buildings often had low outdoor air ventilation rates, below 20 cfm per occupant (or about 10 L/s per occupant). However, SBS does occur in buildings that meet current ventilation and temperature control standards. A widely held theory is that suboptimal ventilation, in some cases below ventilation standards, permits the accumulation of low levels of many contaminants—volatile organic compounds, aldehydes, cigarette smoke, dust, microbial contaminants, and the like—that together induce the symptoms.

A recent consensus statement from EUROVEN concluded from a review of 22 properly conducted, peer-reviewed studies, including several experimental studies, that increasing fresh-air ventilation rates reduced the frequency and intensity of SBS symptoms and improved perceived air quality. Several studies also found improvements in productivity. These findings tend to support the hypothesis that at low outdoor-air ventilation rates, increases in the outdoor-air ventilation rates will reduce levels of contaminants and symptoms. The findings in these studies were largely but not universally consistent. The incomplete consistency probably reflects the substantial differences between buildings and the multitude of factors, in addition to outdoor-air ventilation rate, that may affect indoor air quality.

The EUROVEN consensus statement also reported that the presence of an air-conditioning system was associated in six of seven papers with increased reporting of SBS symptoms when compared with naturally or other mechanically ventilated buildings. The statement does, however, point out some potential confounding factors, such as building age, building materials, and operable windows that probably are associated with the presence (or absence) of air conditioning. The statement noted that one paper, a large study by NIOSH of 80 buildings, found an association between dirty heating, ventilation, and air-conditioning (HVAC) systems and SBS symptoms.

There is largely consistent evidence supporting an association of increased room temperature and SBS symptoms. A recent study by Reinikainen and Jaakkola demonstrated that temperatures in excess of 21–22°C (69.8–71.6°F) are associated with increased reporting of dryness and SBS symptoms. They reported that a similar association was observed in four of seven relevant studies, whereas no association was observed in three of seven studies. Elevated temperature, especially in conjunction with elevated relative humidity (RH; increased indoor air enthalpy), may reduce perceived air freshness and increase SBS symptoms. In a recent experimental study, Fang and associates found that perceived air freshness, acceptability, and SBS symptoms (e.g., fatigue, headache, and difficulty thinking) were favorably related to low temperature and relative humidity (20°C, 40% RH) compared with higher temperature and humidity (23°C, 50% or 60% RH). There is a strong inverse relation of temperature changes, even within the "comfort zone," on symptoms. Thus there is a need to consider the impact of temperature in all observational and experimental studies evaluating indoor air quality.

Dryness of the indoor air, both perceived dryness and actual dryness, may contribute to some of the symptoms of SBS. The sensation of dryness in many cases actually reflects the presence of higher air temperature and probably dust and air contaminants with a lesser impact of lower relative humidity.

Nevertheless, in some cases, increasing air humidity when the RH is low has reduced the sensation of dryness and symptoms related to dryness. For example, blinded experimental studies of office and hospital workers have demonstrated a reduction in symptoms of dryness of mucous membranes (eye and throat dryness or irritation) and skin (dryness, irritation, itching) with air humidification up to 35–45% as compared with control conditions of approximately 20–35%. There also was a reduction in perceived air dryness. In a subsequent randomized, blinded crossover trial of humidification (RH increased from baseline 22–29% to 28–37% depending on temperature), humidification reduced dryness symptoms (of skin and mucous membranes) and the sensation of dryness but did not reduce other SBS symptoms. The authors summarize the mixed results of earlier studies: In 5 of 11 studies, humidification reduced the prevalence of SBS symptoms or dryness, whereas in 3 of 11 studies, humidification increased such symptoms. Given that RH often falls in indoor environments during the heating season, low humidity may play a significant role in the induction of symptoms of SBS (particularly mucous membrane symptoms) in some situations.

On the other hand, high RH may lead to the apparent adverse impacts noted in some of the studies mentioned earlier and to increased fungal, other microbial, and dust-mite growth, which could contribute to SBS symptoms and other problems. Humidifiers provide a potential site for microbial growth. Thus moderate levels of RH, in the range of 35–45%, appear most desirable.

2. Chemical factors—It appears that low levels of chemical contaminants present in indoor air do contribute, in some cases, to SBS, but no specific chemical causes have been identified. Despite extensive measurements for a wide variety of possible contaminants, no substances have been found to be present consistently in concentrations judged sufficient to induce symptoms. There are a number of potential sources for air contaminants in the office environment. Formaldehyde is present in and will evaporate from resins in particleboard and plywood (used in furniture and construction materials) and furnishings (including carpets and draperies). Volatile organic compounds (VOCs) may evaporate from carpet glues and drying paints. Recently, Bako-Biro and associates reported from an experimental study that exposures to new computers increased air-quality complaints and SBS symptoms. The computers were shown to offgas a variety of VOCs at low levels. Releases from photocopiers and other office equipment also may contribute to the symptoms.

Chamber studies suggest that complex mixtures of VOCs at relatively low concentrations can lead to symptoms of mucous membrane irritation and perhaps other symptoms such as headaches. Some building studies have suggested a correlation between exposure to low-level VOC mixtures, particularly for those VOCs with stronger irritant properties, and irritant symptoms. There is evidence that VOCs react chemically with ozone and oxides of nitrogen in indoor air to form more irritating oxidized chemicals.

Moreover, odors from chemicals, including VOCs, and from other sources, including mold or other microbial growth, may contribute independently to SBS symptoms. Unpleasant odors are reported frequently by occupants of problem buildings. Odors are known to be capable of causing irritation, headaches, nausea, and other symptoms in the absence of a toxicologic effect.

The presence of increased dust in the indoor environment has been associated with increased reporting of SBS symptoms in some studies. For example, a large study of office workers in 14 buildings in Copenhagen (the Danish Town Hall Study) reported that symptoms of mucosal irritation and headache and fatigue were significantly correlated with some measures of dust contamination or accumulation. Cross-sectional studies have not documented a correlation between airborne particulate concentration, at least in the typical range, and SBS symptoms. There is some suggestion that symptoms may be associated with inadequate cleaning practices, as well as some evidence that thorough office cleaning may reduce SBS symptoms. However, some interventions to reduce dust, such as HEPA filtration of air, have not been shown to reduce symptoms of SBS.

3. Biologic factors—There is some evidence that exposure to damp buildings and to molds may be a contributor to symptoms of SBS. Some studies indicate an association between dampness and certain nonspecific symptoms, such as headache and fatigue. There has been some study of the potential role of exposure to mold and mold products—fungal glucans and microbial VOCs (responsible for some of the mold odor)—in the induction of SBS symptoms. These findings suggest a possible role for dampness and mold in the induction of SBS symptoms, at least in buildings with moisture problems. Several cross-sectional studies suggest an association between mold and some SBS symptoms, including cough, nasal and throat irritation, headache, difficulty concentrating, and nonspecific symptoms. One study found mucous membrane irritation symptoms, headache, and difficulty concentrating were associated with mold in floor dust in female (but not male) schoolteachers. Lung function tests and inflammatory mediators in nasal lavage fluid were not affected. Laumbach and Kipen, in a recent review, concluded that there is suggestive evidence for an association of bioaerosols with the development of SBS. However, they concluded that the role of mold exposures, including the role of mycotoxins and microbial VOCs, remains unclear, citing among other things significant limitations to existing studies and dose-response considerations.

4. Host factors—Individuals with atopy appear to develop more mucosal irritation symptoms, an observation supported by chamber studies demonstrating reactions to lower concentrations of irritants than for nonatopics. Contact lens wearers tend to be more prone to eye irritation. Women tend to report symptoms of SBS more frequently than men when both are present in a problem building.

5. Work organization and psychosocial factors—Studies, including the Danish Town Hall Study, have observed that a variety of work organization and psychosocial characteristics, including absence of varied work, dissatisfaction with the supervisor, little influence on the organization, high work speed, and reported general and work stress, were associated with the prevalence of symptoms, both mucosal irritation and general symptoms. However, in the Danish study, these factors could not fully account for the differences observed in the reporting of symptoms; indoor climate factors remained strongly associated with the symptoms. Other factors that have been identified as affecting the perception of the indoor environment include noise, overcrowding, the degree of management response to IAQ complaints, and the sense of empowerment to be heard or effect change.

Overall, these studies support the prevalent view that most episodes of SBS are multifactorial in etiology. They provide the rationale for a multidisciplinary approach to evaluation and management in the individual problem building. Some significant associations in these studies may not be causal because of the interrelationships between the many variables and the likelihood that some factors are merely surrogates for the actual underlying problem. Table 41–3 lists possible causative factors for the SBS.

B. CLINICAL FINDINGS

The most common symptoms are those associated with mucous membrane irritation and headaches. Eye irritation, difficulty in wearing contact lenses, nasal and sinus irritation and congestion, throat irritation, chest tightness or burning, nausea, headache, dizziness, and fatigue are common complaints. Some symptoms may be psychophysiologic in origin.

Symptoms typically occur shortly after entering the building and are relieved soon after leaving. Physical findings are nonexistent or minimal, consisting perhaps of mild injection of the oropharyngeal or conjunctival mucous membranes. Laboratory studies, including spirometry and chest radiographs, are normal. Atopic subjects, with a history or findings consistent with aller-

Table 41–3. Postulated causative or contributing factors to sick-building syndrome.

Category	Factor
Building factors	Contaminants
	Volatile organic compounds
	Formaldehyde
	Odors
	Organic dust
	Inorganic dust
	Microbial agents
	Other contaminants
	Inadequate fresh air ventilation
	Central ventilation system with no operable windows
	Elevated or reduced relative humidity
	High temperature
	Carpeting
	Noise
Host factors	Atopy (hayfever/asthma)
	Contact lens wear
	Female gender
	Psychological conditions
Work factors	Job stress
	Lack of control of work/environment
	Dissatisfaction with the supervisor
	Absence of varied work
	Job satisfaction diminished by quantity of work
	High work speed
	Little influence on the organization

gic rhinitis or asthma, in general seem to be more prone to develop symptoms in association with indoor air-quality problems.

C. TREATMENT & PREVENTION

For the individual patient, treatment consists of reassurance, with explanation of the apparent source and benign nature of symptoms, and temporary removal from the environment, if necessary. Fear about potential exposures, uncertainty about their health significance, and rumors about serious illnesses alleged to be related to the building in a population that is often medically and toxicologically unsophisticated may lead to considerable anxiety, which, in turn, may amplify or prolong the symptoms.

Findings from the studies cited earlier, which have been reasonably consistent, suggest a possible benefit from certain building interventions. Thus reduction in room temperature to the lower end of the comfort zone could be considered. If the outdoor-air ventilation rate is low (below 10 L/s, or about 20 cfm, per occupant), efforts to increase outdoor-air intake could be considered. Recommendations for the optimal outdoor-air ventilation rate vary. The EUROVEN consensus statement recommends outdoor-air ventilation rates at or above 25 L/s per occupant, although the investigators acknowledge that this measure would increase energy costs significantly. There is some support for conducting thorough cleaning of office areas, ideally during periods of low occupancy, and using cleaning materials with low volatility and odor. Limited information suggests a benefit from cleaning dirt and debris from dirty HVAC systems. There is some empirical support for "purging" the building, maximizing ventilation with the system set for maximum fresh-air intake, when the building is unoccupied. Depending on the nature of the problem identified, other changes may be necessary as well, such as relocation of air-intake vents or alteration in cleaning or pesticide application practices. Prevention would appear to require balancing energy-conservation concerns with the need to provide adequate fresh-air intake rates when designing ventilation systems. Open communications of findings and any remediation plans to the group and responsiveness to employee concerns should be considered important interventions for SBS.

REFERENCES

Ebbehoj NE et al: Molds in floor dust, building-related symptoms, and lung function among male and female school teachers. Indoor Air 2005;15:7 [PMID: 15926939].

Engvall K et al: Sick building syndrome and perceived indoor environment in relation to energy saving by reduced ventilation flow during heating season: A 1 year intervention study in dwellings. Indoor Air 2005;15:120 [PMID: 15737154].

Fang L et al: Impact of indoor air temperature and humidity in an office on perceived air quality, SBS symptoms and performance. Indoor Air 2004;14:74 [PMID: 15330775].

Laumbach RJ, Kipen HM: Bioaerosols and sick-building syndrome: Particles, inflammation, and allergy. Curr Opin Allergy Clin Immunol 2005;5:135 [PMID: 15764903].

Schiffman SS, Williams CM: Science of odor as a potential health issue. J Environ Qual 2005;34:129 [PMID: 15647542].

Shoemaker RC, House DE: A time-series study of sick building syndrome: Chronic, biotoxin-associated illness from exposure to water-damaged buildings. Neurotoxicol Teratol 2005; 27:29 [PMID: 15681119].

Mass Psychogenic Illness

Mass psychogenic (or sociogenic) illness is an illness of psychophysiologic origin occurring simultaneously in a group of individuals. Less-satisfactory terms include *mass hysteria* and *behavioral contagion*.

A. OCCURRENCE & ETIOLOGY

Episodes felt to represent building-associated mass psychogenic illness have occurred in office buildings, light industrial facilities, and electronics plants. The incidence of these illnesses is unknown. The precise cause, though unknown, would appear to involve the occurrence of an appropriate stimulus or trigger in a psychologically susceptible or anxious population. The trigger often is an unexplained odor. Concern that the odor represents a toxic gas or other threat may initiate psychophysiologic symptoms in some individuals. Individuals must perceive the threat to be credible in order to be affected. Because the trigger may be low levels of a respiratory irritant or an irritating odor, symptoms of SBS may occur concurrently. Thus SBS and mass psychogenic illness may occur simultaneously or sequentially in the same building incident. While SBS symptoms tend to occur in individuals who appear to be most exposed to the suspected environmental causal factors, building-associated mass psychogenic illness is transmitted within specific social networks in the workplace. In other words, friends of the initially affected individuals (index cases) are more likely to be affected.

Episodes of mass psychogenic illness have occurred in groups of workers in low-paying jobs they perceive as stressful, often with repetitive work and physical stress. Some evidence suggests that individuals who have lived and worked under high levels of stress and anxiety, often long prior to the illness outbreak, may be more prone to the development of mass psychogenic illness. These individuals then incorrectly attribute their symptoms of psychophysiologic origin to a possible toxic hazard from a problem building or a noxious odor. Since the attacks on the World Trade Center in September 2001, concerns about terrorist threats of a chemical or biologic nature have triggered episodes of mass psychogenic illness, even when no actual threat existed.

B. CLINICAL FINDINGS

Symptoms commonly reported in NIOSH investigations of outbreaks felt to represent mass psychogenic illness include headaches, dizziness, light-headedness, drowsiness, and nausea; dry mouth and throat; eye, nose, and throat irritation and chest tightness; and weakness, numbness, and tingling. It may be difficult to attribute particular symptoms in any given incident to mass psychogenic illness as opposed to SBS. Headache, dizziness, nausea, and numbness tend to predominate over symptoms of mucous membrane irritation in mass psychogenic illness when compared with symptom profiles in SBS. In mass psychogenic illness, symptoms are diverse in individuals in the group and occur or recur when the group is together both inside and outside the building. There are few or no physical or laboratory findings. Some subjects may be observed to hyperventilate. Of note, the illness in the index case or cases may be a result of actual exposure to an unpleasant odor or noxious substance or to a nonoccupational cause, for example, a viral syndrome.

In contrast to SBS, symptoms often do not resolve promptly when the individual leaves the building. One should use caution in applying the label of mass psychogenic illness to an outbreak of building-related symptoms, given the similarity of symptoms to those of SBS and the frequent occurrence of psychophysiologic symptoms in SBS.

Certain features strongly suggest the diagnosis of mass psychogenic illness. The symptoms are difficult to explain on an organic basis and are not consistent with the toxicologic properties of any suspected contaminants. There is a high level of anxiety in the group. The attack rate generally is higher among women than among men. There is a visual or auditory chain of transmission. In other words, subjects typically do not become ill unless they see or hear that others are becoming ill. Despite apparent severity and sudden onset of illness, the illnesses are consistently benign and without sequelae.

C. TREATMENT

Some investigation of the building is indicated to exclude the presence of significant contaminants. The scope of such an investigation will depend on the potential sources of exposure, which usually are limited in an office setting. An exhaustive search for every measurable chemical substance is a costly, low-yield effort. Because it typically takes time to conduct an investigation and obtain results, it may be necessary to consider closure of the building or area for a time if the symptoms and concerns warrant it. Removing employees from the area of concern also may reduce anxiety and transmission of symptoms to others.

Treatment involves primarily reassurance in a supportive environment. Early, open, and frequent communication with concerned individuals is important. Emphasis should be placed on the lack of physical findings and other abnormalities, the absence of evidence suggesting a significant toxic exposure, and the benign nature of the symptoms. Because many individuals potentially would be alienated by being told that their symptoms were psychologically mediated, it is important to be cautious about attributing symptoms to psychological factors or anxiety.

REFERENCES

Doyle CR et al: Mass sociogenic illness: Real and imaginary. Vet Hum Toxicol 2004;46:93 [PMID: 15080215].

Weir E: Mass sociogenic illness. CMAJ 2005;172:36 [PMID: 15632400].

Building-Associated Hypersensitivity Pneumonitis

Hypersensitivity pneumonitis is a form of interstitial lung disease characterized pathologically by lymphocytic and granulomatous infiltration of alveolar walls that results from inhalation of a variety of organic dusts. The prototype of this disease is farmer's lung, which results from inhalation of bacterial spores and antigens from stored moist hay. However, hypersensitivity pneumonitis has been described in a variety of occupational and avocational settings. Hypersensitivity pneumonitis has been reported in a number of individuals in homes or offices where mold or bacteria had been allowed to grow on humidifiers or air conditioners. Attack rates in such outbreaks have varied from 1–71% of the exposed population.

A. Occurrence & Etiology

Hypersensitivity pneumonitis is an immunologic disorder triggered by repeated inhalation exposures to a foreign antigen that probably results from a combination of immunopathogenic mechanisms. There is evidence to suggest a type III immunologic (immune complex–mediated) reaction with precipitating or complement-fixing antibodies to the offending antigen. Some antigens may be capable of direct complement activation. Type IV T-cell-mediated immune responses probably play a role in disease development, particularly in chronic hypersensitivity pneumonitis. In building-associated hypersensitivity pneumonitis, a number of agents and antigens are implicated, including bacteria (thermophilic actinomycetes such as *Thermoactinomyces vulgaris* and *Micropolyspora faeni*), fungi (*Aspergillus, Penicillium, Alternaria,* and others), and amebas (*Naegleria* and *Acanthamoeba*). The source of antigens usually is contaminated ventilation systems. Less commonly, persistently moist carpets, furnishings, and surfaces from water leaks in occupied areas are implicated.

B. Clinical Findings

There are both acute and chronic forms of hypersensitivity pneumonitis. The acute form presents typically with fever, chills, shortness of breath, nausea, myalgia, malaise, and cough without wheezing, usually developing 4–6 hours after exposure to the antigen. Symptoms may be attributed erroneously to an influenza-like illness. With the acute form, avoidance of exposure results in resolution of symptoms, and reexposure will result in recurrence of symptoms.

The chronic form of hypersensitivity pneumonitis typically is manifested by the insidious onset of fatigue, progressive dyspnea, nonproductive cough, and weight loss. A history of acute bouts of illness, as described earlier, may not be present. Physical findings may include fever, tachypnea, dyspnea, and bibasilar rales.

C. Diagnosis

Laboratory features may include leukocytosis with a leftward shift in acute bouts and chest radiograph and pulmonary function test abnormalities. Chest radiographs may be normal or may show increased interstitial markings or patchy, ill-defined densities. Pulmonary function tests may reveal a restrictive pattern, with reductions in vital capacity and total lung capacity. However, ventilatory abnormalities are not always present. The most consistent pulmonary function abnormality is reduction of diffusing capacity for carbon monoxide.

The presence of serum-precipitating antibodies to suspected antigens is of limited usefulness in that it documents intense and extensive exposure but does not indicate the presence of clinical pulmonary disease. Such antibodies may be seen in asymptomatic individuals, and some individuals with hypersensitivity pneumonitis may have negative precipitin tests. High-resolution computed tomographic (CT) scans, bronchoalveolar lavage (demonstrating a predominance of lymphocytes), inhalation provocation studies, and ultimately, lung biopsy may be useful in confirming a diagnosis.

In a study of hypersensitivity pneumonitis in office workers exposed to a contaminated air cooling system, shortness of breath and fever were present in all the affected individuals. If the onset of these two symptoms was in close temporal association with exposure to the workplace, this finding was even more suggestive of hypersensitivity pneumonitis. Because dyspnea and fever are uncommon in SBS, the presence of these symptoms in multiple individuals in a building should trigger concern about possible hypersensitivity pneumonitis.

D. TREATMENT

Avoidance of further exposure by removal from the environment usually results in resolution of symptoms and abnormalities. If symptoms fail to resolve following removal, a short course of corticosteroids—typically prednisone in high doses—is indicated. In some outbreaks, extensive cleanup efforts, including removal of contaminated items and alteration of ventilation systems, have allowed the return of affected workers without recurrence of symptoms.

REFERENCES

Greenberger PA: Mold-induced hypersensitivity pneumonitis. Allergy Asthma Proc 2004;25:219 [PMID: 15510579].

Jacobs RL et al: Hypersensitivity pneumonitis: Beyond classic occupational disease changing concepts of diagnosis and management. Ann Allergy Asthma Immunol 2005;95:115 [PMID: 16136760].

Mohr LC: Hypersensitivity pneumonitis. Curr Opin Pulm Med 2004;10:401 [PMID: 15316440].

Asthma and the Role of Building Dampness, Mites, & Molds

There is considerable evidence compiled in systematic literature reviews that dampness in homes or workplaces is associated with an increased risk of cough, wheeze, and asthma in both children and adults, with about 1.5- to 2-fold increased risks. Many of the studies also reported associations with allergy symptoms. One limitation to the conclusions is that either or both dampness indicators and health measures were self-reported in most of the studies in adults. The reviewers were unable to conclude what agent or factor associated with dampness led to the health effects, although available evidence tended to implicate mites, mite sensitization, and to a lesser extent, mold exposure. The appropriate measure of dampness to use to assess health risk is unclear, although high measured humidity in indoor air and evidence of moisture in construction materials both were regularly associated with symptoms and clinical findings. Indicators of the presence of mold, such as spores, sometimes were associated with wheeze, asthma, and related clinical findings.

Based on estimates of the prevalence of atopy and the prevalence of IgE antibodies to common molds in the population, approximately 5% of the general population would be expected to manifest allergic symptoms from mold exposure [American College of Occupational and Environmental Medicine (ACOEM)]. It is expected that most such symptoms would reflect outdoor exposure to mold.

A recent Institute of Medicine review concluded that there is sufficient evidence of an association between fungal exposure and exacerbations of asthma in sensitized asthmatics. Although there are a few studies that suggest that indoor fungal exposure can cause sensitization, the evidence is as yet inadequate to conclude that fungal exposure causes new onset of asthma.

Because of the potential for lower respiratory symptoms, allergy/asthma, and possibly other nonspecific symptoms, it is important to investigate dampness, water damage, and mold growth problems properly with a thorough search for indoor sources. Because of the lack of exposure limits for airborne fungi and the absence of known dose-response relationships for health effects, the value of air sampling for fungi is not clear. Air sampling may not be required, especially if the water damage and mold growth can be readily rectified. In the absence of exposure limits, the finding of higher concentrations [colony-forming units per cubic meter (CFU/m^3)] of fungi indoors compared with concurrent outdoor sampling suggests that there is a source of biomagnification/growth within the building that might require remediation. There is some agreement that levels below 500 CFU/m^3 probably pose no threat to healthy occupants.

A. CLINICAL FINDINGS & DIAGNOSIS

The clinical findings and diagnosis of asthma exacerbations related to dampness and exposure to mites and mold would be identical to those for other types of asthma, as discussed in Chapters 14 and 20. Diagnosis may be aided by performance of skin prick tests to detect IgE specific to fungal allergens or ELISA testing for IgE antibodies to fungal allergens, although such testing is limited by the availability of standardized fungal antigens, cross-reactivity among fungi, and the occurrence of false-positive and false-negative tests. These tests need to be interpreted carefully in conjunction with the history and physical findings. Documentation, through appropriate testing of the building, and of presumed exposure to the type of mold to which there appears to be IgE-mediated hypersensitivity may provide additional evidence of a connection between the asthma exacerbation and the building.

B. TREATMENT

Treatment for these exacerbations would involve the same therapeutic approaches employed in other cases of asthma. Removal from exposure also might be warranted, at least until remediation occurs. Remediation of any identified fungal growth by properly trained individuals using appropriate equipment and work practices also would be important, in addition to correcting structural problems leading to water intrusion.

Possible Health Effects of Mycotoxins

There has been considerable scientific inquiry and speculation, news media attention, and litigation regarding exposure to molds and fungal toxins (mycotoxins) in buildings and alleged illness. A number of common indoor fungi produce mycotoxins, including *Aspergillus, Cladosporium, Penicillium,* and *Stachybotrys* species. These mycotoxins are of high molecular weight and are not appreciably volatile; exposure requires aerosolization of spores or fungal fragments (ACOEM). *Stachybotrys chartarum* (or *atra*) has received considerable attention because of its possible role in an outbreak, reported by the CDC, of pulmonary hemorrhage in infants in Cleveland. However, after reevaluation, the CDC concluded that the evidence was insufficient to link exposure to *Stachybotrys* with the illnesses.

After thorough review of existing studies and building investigations, several recent reviewers have concluded that there is no scientific evidence linking inhalation exposure to mycotoxins (including *Stachybotrys* mycotoxins) in buildings with human disease. Those papers that have reported an association suffer from limitations in exposure assessment, dose-response assessment, documentation of health effects, and consideration of alternative explanations. Fung and Clark and the authors of the ACOEM statement suggest, based on mycotoxin content of fungal spores and dose-response considerations, that air concentrations substantially higher than those found in contaminated homes and offices would be required to induce health effects on a toxicologic basis. The ACOEM authors concluded that "current scientific evidence does not support the proposition that human health has been adversely affected by inhaled mycotoxins in home, school, or office environments." The recent comprehensive report from the Institute of Medicine, Damp Indoor Spaces and Health, provides further support for this position. Regarding mold in damp indoor environments, there are only five conditions or symptoms for which there is sufficient scientific evidence of an association: certain upper respiratory tract symptoms (nasal congestion, sneezing, runny or itchy nose, and throat irritation), wheezing, asthma symptoms in sensitized asthmatic individuals, cough, and hypersensitivity pneumonitis. While recommending further research, the authors were unable to conclude that mycotoxins are known to cause human illness from indoor inhalation exposures despite demonstrated illness from higher-dose ingestion exposures in other settings.

Trout and associates point out the limitations of immunoassays to detect fungal antibodies in assessing possible illness related to exposure to molds or mycotoxins. Because mold exposure is common, the presence of IgG antibodies only indicates apparent exposure at some time. These authors point out that many healthy individuals have such antibodies; for example, in one study, 65 of 132 blood donors not obviously exposed to fungi were found to have IgG antibodies to *S. chartarum*. Studies typically have not found correlations between exposure to fungi and levels of fungal antibodies or between fungal antibody levels and illness. Further issues with assays are immunologic cross-reactivity between different fungi, the absence of standardization of fungal extracts, technical problems with assay methodology, reproducibility, and quality control, and selection of an appropriate comparison population. The authors indicate that there is currently insufficient scientific evidence to warrant the use of these immunoassays for assessing fungal exposures or possibly related health effects.

REFERENCES

Bornehag CG et al: Dampness in buildings as a risk factor for health effects. Indoor Air 2004;14:243 [PMID: 15217478].

Edmondson DA et al: Allergy and "toxic mold syndrome." Ann Allergy Asthma Immunol 2005;94:234 [PMID: 15765738].

Fung F, Clark RF: Health effects of mycotoxins: A toxicological overview. J Toxicol Clin Toxicol. 2004;42:217 [PMID: 15214629].

Khalibi B et al: Inhalational mold toxicity: Fact or fiction? Ann Allergy Asthma Immunol 2005;95:239 [PMID: 16200814].

Other Building-Associated Hazards and Illnesses

Certain infectious diseases that are noncommunicable may be transmitted in indoor air. Legionnaires' disease—a multisystem disease dominated by pneumonia—is caused by the bacterial organism *Legionella pneumophila* and occasionally other *Legionella* species. Pontiac fever, also caused by *L. pneumophila*, is an influenza-like illness characterized by fever, chills, headache, myalgias, and sometimes cough and sore throat. Most reported cases are sporadic, with only about 11% of cases associated with an outbreak of illness.

Most commonly, building-associated outbreaks result from contaminated aerosols, usually disseminated in the ventilation system from cooling towers, evaporative condensers, humidifiers, and air-conditioning systems. Other sources of aerosols include decorative fountains, whirlpool hot tubs, and produce misters in grocery stores. *Legionella* species can be cultured in up to 40% of cooling towers, although infections stemming from exposure to the aerosols are reported uncommonly. *Legionella* bacteria thrive in water systems maintained at warm temperatures between approximately 26.7°C (80°F) and 48.9°C (120°F). Proper cleaning and maintenance of these potential sources is critical in preventing outbreaks of Legionnaires' disease.

The appropriate investigation and management of a building and its occupants, when one or more individuals is found to have *Legionella* infection, often will find the source of exposure to be in the community outside the workplace. Nevertheless, it is appropriate to begin a building investigation and to inquire about compatible illnesses in other building occupants, referring those with symptoms for medical care. Investigation of the building involves identification of relevant elements in the water and ventilation systems, particularly those from which aerosolization could occur, and testing the water by culture for *Legionella*. Any likely source then should be cleaned properly and decontaminated with chlorine or other biocides. If such decontamination can occur promptly, the facility typically can remain open and operational while the investigation proceeds. Characterization of isolated organisms from water systems and from the case patient by species and serogroup may provide evidence for or against a link with the building.

Q fever, caused by the rickettsial organism *Coxiella burnetii*, has been responsible for several building-associated outbreaks. The animal reservoirs for this infection typically are sheep, goats, and cattle and less commonly cats, dogs, and rabbits. Airborne transmission of organisms from animal excreta and products of parturition to humans has occurred via ventilation systems in animal-handling and medical research facilities.

Certain hazardous materials whose presence is not suspected routinely in nonindustrial buildings have been linked to building-associated symptoms or illnesses. Elevated levels of formaldehyde have been found in mobile homes and other buildings, in which large quantities of urea-formaldehyde insulation or pressed-wood products (i.e., plywood, particleboard, and fiberboard) made with formaldehyde-containing resins have been used. When present in concentrations at or above 0.1 ppm, it may cause symptoms of eye, nose, and throat irritation and nausea.

Carbon monoxide in buildings may be the cause of mild symptoms, such as headache and nausea, or more severe, potentially life-threatening intoxication. Incomplete combustion in defective gas furnaces or unvented gas stoves and other appliances, typically in residences, occasionally may be the source of significant indoor emissions of carbon monoxide. In addition to the potential for acute intoxication, long-term low-level exposure can cause recurrent subacute symptoms. Attentiveness to these symptoms, when temporally related to presence in a building, may help to identify and correct previously unrecognized CO exposures. Less commonly, carbon monoxide may be entrained from the outside via air intakes in the vicinity of vehicle loading docks.

There is some evidence for an increased risk of the common cold associated with shared office space and mechanical ventilation. Some authors, including Hodgson, have reported about 1.5-fold increased rates of upper respiratory infections in such offices after controlling for other factors that were associated with the risk for colds. While not conclusive, these findings provide some validation for the frequent complaint of employees in problem buildings that they catch colds more frequently.

REFERENCES

Arts JH et al: Inhaled formaldehyde: Evaluation of sensory irritation in relation to carcinogenicity. Regul Toxicol Pharmacol 2006;44:144 [PMID: 16413643].

Chan GM: Carbon monoxide poisoning, myocardial injury, and mortality. JAMA 2006;295:2601 [PMID: 16772620].

Pedro-Botet ML, Sabria M: Legionellosis. Semin Respir Crit Care Med 2005;26:625 [PMID: 16388431].

EPA: Sources of indoor air pollution—Formaldehyde, www.epa.gov/iaq/formalde.html.

Vorobeychikov E et al: Evaluation of low concentration aerosol for infecting humans with the Q fever pathogen. Ann N Y Acad Sci 2005;1063:466 [PMID: 16481561].

Water Pollution

Daniel T. Teitelbaum, MD, & Tushar Kant Joshi, MBBS, MS, MSc

42

Demand for water to sustain the world's people is projected to double by 2025. By that date, nearly half the estimated world's population of more than 6 billion will be living in countries where either the quantity or the quality of water supplies will have sunk to levels ranging from inadequate to economically crippling.

BIOCONTAMINATION OF WATER SUPPLIES

Biocontamination of water supplies used or intended for human drinking water represents the most immediate waterborne threat to human health. A growing understanding of the epidemiologic characteristics and patterns of disease associated with human pathogens distributed in drinking water has led to the development of infrastructure for potable and waste water collection, storage, treatment, disinfection, and distribution in the urban areas of most developed countries. As the microbiologic integrity of the supply of potable water has improved, a significant reduction in human disease caused by waterborne pathogens has occurred. Nonetheless, recent experience has demonstrated that the potable water supply throughout the world is always at risk. Serious waterborne disease epidemics with recognized and new pathogens continue to occur in both developed and developing areas of the world.

The most common effect of waterborne biocontamination is acute diarrheal disease. This disease is characterized by loose or watery stools, and it is often accompanied by vomiting and fever. Many of these diarrheal episodes are the result of waterborne infection with bacteria, viruses, or parasites or the ingestion of their enterotoxins. Cholera, shigellosis, salmonellosis, coliforms, yersiniosis, giardiasis, campylobacteriosis, cryptosporidiosis, and viral gastroenteropathies produce diarrheal signs and symptoms. Careful evaluation of the patient and the water supply using newer laboratory tests permits the correct etiologic diagnosis of diarrhea in more than 70% of cases in developing countries. Unfortunately, the resources and equipment for such evaluations often are not available. The vast majority of the waterborne outbreaks are caused by contaminated groundwater supplies.

Effective methods of microbiologic and chemical treatment and surveillance of water supplies are in place in most public water supplies in developed countries. However, the water disinfection process is not without its risks. Although it is vital to the provision of pathogen-free potable water, it produces by-products that carry long-term risks of chronic illness. Chlorination processes to disinfect water are associated with increased risks of bladder cancer and may be associated with other cancers. When used alone or in combination with chlorine disinfection, ozonation contributes to a reduction of toxic trihalomethanes in the treated water and may have an independent beneficial risk by reducing the mutagenicity of the treated water. There is a relationship between disinfection by-products and adult leukemia and chronic myeloid leukemia. In less-developed and developing countries and in rural areas of developed countries where raw or untreated water from surface or groundwater sources is used as potable water, effective control of microbiologic water contamination is not always ensured. Despite the technological sophistication of civil engineering of water and waste water supplies, outbreaks of waterborne disease occur frequently in both developed and developing countries. Epidemics of waterborne disease in developed countries often are the result of technical flaws or unusual and unforeseen climatologic events that disrupt the normal potable water supplies. In the Indian subcontinent, the substitution of tube-well technology for surface waters as the source of drinking water to reduce the risk of waterborne pathogen disease has resulted in a major disaster through the use of arsenic-contaminated but biologically acceptable sources for potable water.

Municipal drinking water supplies can be contaminated by viruses both from surface waters and from unidentified sources. These viruses include hepatitis A, enteroviruses, echoviruses, and coxsackie viruses.

In less-developed countries, the proximity of human residence, agriculture, animal husbandry, and unprotected potable water sources typically are the cause of epidemic waterborne disease. In some areas, the use of waste water containing human excreta as agricultural irrigation water greatly increases the risk of contamination of local drinking water supplies and the transmission of enteric and other diseases through the consumption of food crops contaminated with pathogens.

The use of waste water for irrigation purposes was and is recommended in certain areas of the world where water resources are very limited. Originally developed in Europe and North America in the nineteenth century, sewage farming was conceived as an efficient and economical way to dispose of urban waste water. Rainwater was allowed to enter the rivers from which drinking water traditionally was drawn, and waste water was applied to the fields, where natural biologic processes were expected to purify the water before it reached the rivers and reentered the potable water resources. As long as there was enough agricultural land in close proximity to large urban centers, this system was useful. However, as the proximity of agriculture and urban life diminished, the usefulness of the sewage farming techniques also decreased. However, in arid lands, the economic advantages of waste water farming remain. Properly employed, waste water farming can be both safe and economically attractive. The Engelberg Guidelines for the microbiologic quality of treated waste water used for crop irrigation were developed by the World Health Organization (WHO) for use in developing areas where the scarcity of water dictates the reuse of waste water for agricultural purposes. They are based on extensively studied use of waste water in agriculture. The Engelberg Guidelines suggest that a geometric mean of 1000 coliforms per 100 mL of irrigation water for unrestricted crop use is safe, based on epidemiologic outcome studies. The guidelines also create, for the first time, appropriate controls on the presence of helminth eggs in irrigation water. Varying country requirements may alter the suitability of treated or partially treated waste water for irrigation purposes, but altering the seasonal procedures of the treatment plant my offer an opportunity to provide safe and nutrient-rich irrigation for agricultural purposes.

Worldwide, explosive population growth, expanding poverty, urban migration, and increased international travel affect the risk of exposure to waterborne infectious disease. These emerging diseases include waterborne cryptosporidial diarrheal disease and cholera, *Escherichia coli* 0157:H7 diarrheal disorders, *Mycobacterium avium* complex, *Legionella* species, *Helicobacter pylori*, and *Cyanobacteria* species. *Cyclospora* species, *Cryptosporidia,* and *Giardia* continue to be parasitic threats to potable water supplies. Coccidia and other protozoans are common food and waterborne pathogens throughout the world. Toxoplasmosis has been identified as a result of waterborne *Toxoplasma gondii.* Hemorrhagic fevers, tuberculosis, and hantavirus infections may have waterborne sources. Norwalk virus, rotavirus, caliciviruses, adenoviruses, and hepatitis A virus are well-identified viruses transmitted through consumption and use of contaminated water supplies. Major climatologic changes, such as drought and flooding, also contribute to disruption of the normal supply of water in all countries. Abnormal events such as earthquakes, hurricanes, tornadoes, snowstorms, and similar phenomena cause disruption of normal potable water supplies and may result in epidemic disease in humans. In all such events, increased surveillance of water supplies and rapid response with appropriate public health measures are indicated. Such responses include "boil water" advisories, temporary shift of water supplies to uncontaminated resources, and microbiologic assessment of the supply for viral, bacteriologic, parasitologic, and helminthic contamination. In addition, facilities and supplies for the immediate assessment and treatment of victims of waterborne epidemics, which may include typhoid, cholera, hepatitis, and other diseases, should be prepared and put in place.

REFERENCES

Environmental Protection Agency (EPA): Drinking water and ground-water statistics, www.epa.gov/safewater/data/00factoids.pdf.

WHO: DDC: Implementation of epidemic control actions, www.afro.who.int/emc/implementation.html.

WHO: IPCS: *New Drinking Water Guidelines,* www.who.int/pcs/newsletter/ipcs-04.pdf.

CONTROL OF MICROBIOLOGIC WATER CONTAMINATION

BOD, COD, TOC, & TSS

Conventional management of potable water and waste water supplies involves separation of the flow of the two fluid streams and protection of the potable water supply from contamination with the contents of the waste water stream. Conventional waste water treatment systems are developed to remove organic matter from waste water on the basis of their biochemical oxygen demand (BOD) or chemical oxygen demand (COD). The BOD is a measure of the load placed on the oxygen resources of the receiving waters, usually as a result of microbiologic growth. Treatment efficiency is evaluated on the basis of BOD removal by the treatment facility. Unless otherwise stated, BOD signifies the biochemical oxygen demand for 5 days at 20°C (68°F).

The BOD is useful to determine the extent to which oxygen can be used by a supply of microbial life. The test is most important in the management of waste water and in food manufacturing and drinking-water preparation facilities. High concentrations of dissolved oxygen predict that oxygen uptake by microorganisms is low and that the breakdown of nutrient resources in the water by microorganisms is also low. Low concentrations of dissolved oxygen signify high microorganism demands and imply contamination of the water.

COD is also employed in the assessment of water quality. This test determines the quantity of oxidizable material in the water. It varies with the composition of the water, temperature, concentration of the reagent, period of contact, and other factors. Generally speaking, the COD, BOD, and the total organic carbon (TOC), a quick method of estimating organic contamination of water, are correlated. Treatment facilities are also designed to remove total suspended solids (TSSs) to a level that is both microbiologically and aesthetically acceptable. Recently, tertiary treatments facilities have been designed that improve pathogen removal to produce finished water with very low pathogen counts.

Water & Waste Water Treatment

Conventional waste water treatment systems that employ sedimentation, activated sludge, biofiltration, aeration, and oxidation, combined with chemical disinfection, produce water with coliform counts that are very low. In the absence of a disinfection step, low coliform counts may not be achieved. Without slow-sand filtration of water and waste water, protozoa, viruses, and other pathogens also may remain in the finished water. The use of slow-sand filtration should control the waterborne spread of the various hepatitis viruses, including hepatitis E, which is currently a major problem in many parts of the world.

The intensity of water treatment for a particular supply and distribution area must depend on the nature and quality of the source. The degree of contamination will determine the required treatment. Multiple treatment barriers are recommended by the WHO for contaminated water sources to prevent the spread of pathogens.

Typical treatment processes for urban water drawn from lowland sources include impoundment and reservoir storage. If needed, predisinfection is applied during impoundment. Impoundment and storage in reservoirs may result in a 99% reduction in fecal indicator bacteria, *Salmonella,* and enteroviruses. During storage and impoundment, the microbiologic environment changes as a result of natural sedimentation, the lethal effect of ultraviolet light on the surface layers of the water, the deprivation of nutrients required by the organisms, and predation. Following impoundment and storage, coagulation, flocculation, and further sedimentation or flotation to remove solids are employed. Filtration and disinfection complete the cycle of typical urban water treatment. Aeration to improve the aesthetic quality of the final product also may be used. This typical system meets the multiple barrier requirements of WHO's *Water Quality Guidelines.*

In rural and remote areas, multiple barrier concepts also may be used. Typical protocols dictate impoundment and protection of the water, sedimentation and screening, gravel prefiltration and slow-sand filtration, and a final disinfection step.

The efficacy of these treatment protocols may be expected to be high, and the quality of the finished water is likely to be excellent. Monitoring of the results of urban water treatment is required under the Safe Drinking

Water Act in the United States and under various state and local regulations. In other countries, specific guidelines for monitoring treated water have been adopted. WHO recommends that public water supplies be sampled monthly. The number of recommended samples varies with the size of the water system.

Pharmaceutical products for humans or animals, as well as their related metabolites, contaminate the aquatic environment. Low concentrations of pharmaceuticals are detectable in municipal waste water, surface water, groundwater, and drinking water. Little is known about the health effects of long-term exposure to low concentrations of pharmaceuticals for humans or aquatic organisms. The precautionary principle—or possibly new scientific evidence—may give rise to more stringent demands on waste water treatment in the future. A combination of biologic treatment with high sludge residence times and ozonation of the effluent seems to be the most promising technology to control pharmaceutical product contamination.

REFERENCES

Alonso E et al: Microorganism regrowth in waste water disinfected by UV radiation and ozone. Environ Technol 2004;25:433 [PMID: 15214448].

Bomo AM et al: Bacterial removal and protozoan grazing in biological sand filters. J Environ Qual 2004;33:1041 [PMID: 15224942].

Derksen JG et al: Diffuse pollution of surface water by pharmaceutical products. Water Sci Technol 2004;49:213 [PMID: 15053118].

Hong SW et al: Pilot testing an alternative on-site waste water treatment system for small communities and its automatic control. Water Sci Technol 2005;51:101 [PMID: 16104411].

Jones OA et al: Potential ecological and human health risks associated with the presence of pharmaceutically active compounds in the aquatic environment. Crit Rev Toxicol 2004;34:335 [PMID: 15328767].

Taghipour F: Ultraviolet and ionizing radiation for microorganism inactivation. Water Res 2004;38:3940 [PMID: 15380984].

PATHOGEN-CAUSED WATERBORNE DISEASES

Waterborne bacterial disease includes the most classic infections of large populations: enterocolitis caused by coliforms, cholera, typhoid and paratyphoid fevers, shigellosis, and salmonellosis. *Campylobacter* infections also have become significant in recent years. Many new pathogens have emerged as widespread causes of waterborne disease outbreak.

The most common identified organism continued to be *Cryptosporidium parvum* in treated water and *E. coli* 0157:H7 in freshwater venues. Other reported illnesses were caused by *Naegleria fowleri,* amebic meningitis, leptospirosis, and Pontiac fever.

Campylobacter Diarrhea

Campylobacter species are believed to cause 5–14% of cases of diarrhea worldwide. In developed countries, children and young adults have the highest frequency of disease. Several *Campylobacter* species are associated with infection in homosexual men. In developing countries, the illness occurs primarily in children younger than 2 years of age. The use of unchlorinated drinking water is highly associated with *Campylobacter* infection.

Cholera

Cholera remains a threat throughout the world. Recent outbreaks of cholera in Ecuador with characteristic acute massive diarrhea were highly associated with the drinking of unboiled water, the drinking of beverages supplied by street vendors, and the eating of raw seafood. Always drinking boiled water at home was protective against the illness, as was the use of soap in the home. The cholera strain identified in this outbreak also demonstrated multiple-antibiotic resistance. A recent large outbreak of cholera in Colombia was directly associated with contamination of the municipal water supply. This outbreak was highly associated with the consumption of unchlorinated and unboiled water from the piped municipal water system.

Management of cholera cases requires strict oral-fecal precautions and other measures designed to confine the spread and mitigate the illness. Oral rehydration is effective in most cases, as in rehydration with polyelectrolyte solution that contains glucose. The effect of zinc supplementation started during diarrhea rehydration was dramatic. The administration of zinc for 7 days during each episode of diarrhea shortened the duration and reduced the occurrence of complicating respiratory disease. The addition of zinc to the rehydration regimen proved to be an inexpensive and effective addition to the control of diarrheal disease because morbidity and mortality in the zinc-treated group were decreased significantly.

In the oral rehydration regimen, volume-for-volume replacement should be undertaken after existing losses at presentation have been corrected. Antibiotic treatment or mass prophylaxis generally is not useful. However, some experienced physicians recommend the use of tetracycline or cotrimoxazole prophylaxis in family outbreaks. Immunization of contacts is not indicated in epidemic situations. Nor do the available vaccines seem to be useful in areas where the disease is endemic because the best of those available seems to offer protection for no more than 2 years with a single dose or for 5 years with a booster. On the other hand, for travelers to areas where the disease is endemic, for those who must work in areas of potential exposure, and for health care workers who may be sent to assist in acute outbreaks, the vaccine may offer worthwhile protection. Some countries where cholera is endemic continue to require vaccination for travelers. The protective value of the procedure is uncertain. Prophylaxis must rest on the avoidance of ambient unpurified water, food (in particular "street foods and drink"), and hand-to-mouth contact, as in any oral-fecal-transmitted disease.

Typhoid Fever & Paratyphoid Infections

Disease caused by waterborne *Salmonella typhi* is quite rare in developed countries, and when it occurs, it is usually associated with a particular food-borne event. Outbreaks of typhoid fever in the United States are accompanied by significant morbidity. Most outbreaks are small, they are often food-borne, and they require thorough investigation.

In endemic areas where sanitation is poor, many cases of typhoid fever occur annually. The disease has a case fatality rate of 10%, although appropriate treatment with antibiotics results in a case fatality rate of less than 1%. Ten percent of patients discharge the bacterium for up to 3 months after infection. A chronic carrier state may be established among 2% of patients, who become infected in middle age. Women with a history of gall bladder disease seem most likely to develop the carrier state. Available laboratory tests permit identification of the responsible organism and permit distinction between typhoid and paratyphoid disease.

Vaccination against typhoid generally is not employed in developed countries. Currently, it is recommended that travelers to endemic areas who have significant potential for exposure as a consequence of their occupation be vaccinated. The primary series of inoculations requires two injections several weeks apart. Booster doses every 3 years are also recommended. An oral vaccine is available that causes considerably less reaction than the traditional injectable vaccine. The Ty21a oral vaccine is available in two forms: an enteric-coated capsule and a liquid formulation reconstituted from a lyophilized organism with buffered water. The oral formulations should be used as a control measure in areas where the incidence of typhoid fever is high and the *S. typhi* varieties are antibiotic-resistant.

Treatment of most cases of typhoid fever is accomplished readily at home with bed rest, fluid replacement, and several antibiotic regimens. In uncomplicated cases, and when fully susceptible strains of *S. typhi* are present, treatment with fluoroquinolone drugs as the drug of choice if it is available or with chloramphenicol, amoxicillin, or trimethoprim-sulfamethoxazole is indicated. When multidrug resistance is noted, fluoroquinolone as the first-line drug, and azithromycin or a third-generation cephalosporin is indicated. When quinolone resistance is found, azithromycin or a third-generation cephalosporin is the regimen of choice.

Other drugs, including amoxicillin, cotrimoxazole, or tetracyclines, are also effective.

The emergence of some resistant strains of *S. typhi* is a continuing challenge. Usual and customary management may not be effective in cases of typhoid fever caused by resistant organisms. In that instance, and for the carrier state, if the fluoroquinolones are ineffective, chloramphenicol may be indicated. The use of chloramphenicol carries a significant risk of irreversible aplastic anemia, and the drug should be employed only when no other antibiotic is suitable.

Systemic paratyphoid fever occurs frequently but may not be reported. The case fatality rate is much lower than in typhoid fever. Epidemiologic parameters are similar to those of typhoid fever. The infection may be caused by several different organisms and many phage types. When the infection is confined to the gastrointestinal tract, the illness is more properly called *salmonellosis*. Chronic carrier states do not occur. No vaccination is available for paratyphoid fever.

Nontyphoidal Salmonellosis

Disease caused by nontyphoidal *Salmonella* strains occurs frequently but is rarely reported unless very large numbers of people are involved. Industrial cattle and chicken breeding and food production facilitate the waterborne spread of nontyphoidal *Salmonella*. In immunocompromised patients, these disorders can be life-threatening, although most patients recover fully without treatment.

SHIGELLA & OTHER PATHOGENIC BACTERIA

Shigella sonnei and other related *Shigella* strains often are responsible for diarrheal diseases that occur under adverse conditions. On the Navajo Reservation in the southwestern United States, families who live outside of organized settlements and use well water or surface water sources for potable water have frequent episodes of *Shigella*-induced diarrhea. These episodes are rarely reported. In a recent program of surveillance of *S. sonnei* isolates in southwestern Korea, the organisms responsible for the outbreak were found to vary in microbial susceptibility from year to year. These variations seemed to have been the result of antibiotic selective pressure, which caused the emergence of resistant integrins. In Israel, *Shigella* isolates from 1998–2000, when compared with isolates from 1991–1992, were dramatically less susceptible to tetracycline, trimethoprim-sulfamethoxazole, and ampicillin. Moreover, emerging resistance to quinolones also was seen. Local monitoring of antibiotic resistance should be continuous in order to determine appropriate therapy in *Shigella* outbreaks.

In 2001, approximately 10,000 cases of *S. sonnei* diarrhea occurred in the United States. These infections usu-

ally occurred among young children and were associated with poor hygiene or unsanitary conditions. Although shigellosis is usually a waterborne disease, outbreaks of *S. flexneri* disease have been increasing among men who have sex with men. An outbreak of *S. flexneri* disease in 2000 demonstrated the need for increased surveillance and renewed efforts at prevention of this sexually transmitted disease. The Centers for Disease Control and Prevention (CDC) also reports an increasing number of cases of shigellosis, hepatitis A, and cryptosporidiosis among child-care workers in recent years. Elsewhere in the world, *S. dysenteriae* type 1 causes large numbers of cases of diarrhea in children who live in crowded and unsanitary conditions and who drink water from ad hoc and untreated water supplies. The case fatality rate in *S. dysenteriae* infection is particularly high in children.

Escherichia coli Diarrhea

E. coli are frequently responsible for diarrheal episodes. *Traveler's diarrhea* is often the result of *E. coli* infection. Most episodes are not etiologically identified, although abnormal coliform counts in a water supply during such episodes are the rule rather than the exception. *E. coli* can cause a variety of syndromes. Water and food are common vehicles of transmission of *E. coli*. The gastrointestinal and systemic disease may present in one of five forms:

1. Enterotoxigenic (ETEC).
2. Enteroinvasive (EIEC).
3. Enteropathogenic (EPEC).
4. Enterohemorrhagic (EHEC).
5. Enteroaggregative (EAggEC).

The largest outbreak of waterborne *E. coli* 0157:H7 disease in the United States occurred in upstate New York following a county fair. The coliform organism was isolated from 128 specimens obtained from 775 persons. Not surprisingly, *C. jejuni* also was isolated from this outbreak. In one case, both organisms were isolated from a single patient. The sources of the infection appeared to be water drawn from an unchlorinated well that was contaminated by a nearby septic tank.

Recent reports have identified the enterotoxigenic strain of *E. coli* 0157:H7 that was responsible for a disastrous food-borne epidemic from undercooked hamburger in the northwestern United States as the cause of an outbreak of waterborne diarrheal disease. In 2002, a major outbreak of *E. coli* 0157:H7 infection developed in Colorado and surrounding states from contaminated ground beef. Among the 28 cases reported by the CDC in this outbreak, there were 7 cases severe enough to require hospitalization, and 5 cases of hemolytic-uremic syndrome. Another outbreak of *E. coli* 0157:H7 disease was reported among 51 visitors to a dairy farm from contact with calves and the barn environment. Most patients were 4 years of age or younger, and 8 developed hemolytic-uremic syndrome; 13% of the cattle on the farm were infected with the coliforms.

The management of severe illness caused by *E. coli* 0157:H7 is complex. Unlike traveler's diarrhea, this life-threatening disease often requires hospitalization and treatment with appropriate antibiotics and hydration and may require dialysis and other critical-care management if the hemolytic-uremic syndrome develops. Because of emerging antibiotic resistance, the usual management of coliform-induced disease with trimethoprim-sulfamethoxazole may not be effective. Quinolone antibiotics may be needed, and even these new-generation drugs may be ineffective in particular cases because of emerging resistance.

Prophylaxis of traveler's diarrhea can be accomplished with bismuth subsalicylate taken orally for several days prior to travel, through the period of travel, and then for 2–3 days after travel is completed. The only complication of this regimen is black stool from the bismuth. Adequate fluid intake must be maintained during the use of this medication because of the salicylate load. Prophylaxis with norfloxacin, 400 mg daily, is also effective. Most often, hydration alone is indicated for treatment of the infection and diarrhea that results. In severe cases, particularly in children, early treatment of infection with cotrimoxazole, trimethoprim-sulfamethoxazole, or other antibiotics also may be indicated. No vaccines are available.

Waterborne *Legionella* Illness

Legionella species have been identified repeatedly as the cause of outbreaks of the respiratory disease known as *Legionnaires' disease.* Water droplets contaminated with the *Legionella* organism transmit the disease. Hot tubs, cooling-tower aerosols, air-conditioning systems, and other water-facilitated machinery have been the source of the aerosol that carries the pathogen.

Recent reports of major outbreaks of Legionnaires' disease among cruise ship passengers who favored the use of the whirlpool spa, either by immersing themselves in the spa or by sitting beside it, suggest a need to alter the management of water resources aboard cruise ships. In this outbreak, a clear dose-response curve was demonstrated that associated hours at the spa with risk of Legionnaires' disease.

Of great concern is the newly recognized role of waterborne nosocomial infections in immunocompromised hospitalized patients. In addition to *Legionella*-induced waterborne nosocomial diseases, 1400 deaths a year occur in hospitalized patients as a result of waterborne nosocomial *Pseudomonas aeruginosa* pneumonia. The epidemic of waterborne nosocomial infections is blamed on failures to enforce water-quality standards by the relevant public health agencies.

Cyanobacteria and Related Microcystins (Blue-Green Algae–Like) Enteritis

Among the emerging waterborne pathogens are the blue-green algae of the *Cyanobacterium* genus. A major problem with the delineation of the pattern of disease associated with this *Cyanobacterium* relative is the delay commonly noted to occur between ingestion of the putative carrier food and onset of the disease. As much as a week may pass before the severe repetitive and troublesome diarrhea develops. To date, fatalities have not been reported. However, in animal studies and in a few human cases, severe gastroenteritis, hemorrhagic liver failure, and allergic and irritant reactions have been reported. Severe infections with microcystins may be treated with rifampin, which appears to be effective in both prophylaxis and treatment in animal experiments.

Cyclospora and Related Protozoa

Recent reports associate *Cyclospora* species with outbreaks of food-borne enteritis. The food that carries this emerging bacterial pathogen has variously been identified as strawberries and raspberries.

Patients who have traveled to tropical destinations in developing countries who present with persistent mild diarrhea that is unresponsive to the usual antibiotic therapies should be studied for the presence of these protozoa. Control of the organism is readily accomplished with current therapy. If control of the diarrhea is not accomplished with fluoroquinolones or cotrimoxazole, the use of metronidazole may be tried. Although there has been concern that land farming of dried sewage wastes might contribute to the transmission of disease caused by this group of organisms, recent studies indicate that *Cyclospora* and *Microsporidium* are unlikely to survive the processes of anaerobic digestion used in the preparation of biosolids for land-farming purposes.

REFERENCES

Garg AX et al: A gradient of acute gastroenteritis was characterized, to assess risk of long-term health sequelae after drinking bacterial-contaminated water. J Clin Epidemiol 2006;59:421 [PMID: 16549265].

Gascon J: Epidemiology, etiology and pathophysiology of traveler's diarrhea. Digestion 2006;73:102 [PMID: 16498258].

Hrudey S: Drinking-water risk management principles for a total quality management framework. J Toxicol Environ Health A 2004;67:1555 [PMID: 15371201].

Krewski D et al: Managing the microbiological risks of drinking water. J Toxicol Environ Health A 2004;67:1591 [PMID: 15371204].

Riddle MS et al: Incidence, etiology, and impact of diarrhea among long-term travelers. Am J Trop Med Hyg 2006;74:891 [PMID: 16687698].

Robben PM, Sibley LD: Food- and waterborne pathogens: You are (infected by) what you eat! Microbes Infect 2004;6:406 [PMID: 15101398].

Yates J: Traveler's diarrhea. Am Fam Phys 2005;71:2095 [PMID: 15952437].

OTHER PROTOZOA-CAUSED WATERBORNE DISEASES

Among the traditional and emerging waterborne diseases, protozoan-induced illness has become the major threat to human health. While amebiasis, which was once a major cause of diarrheal and systemic disease, is now rare in developed countries, other organisms, such as *C. parvum* and *G. lamblia*, now exact a heavy toll.

Amebiasis

Amebic dysentery and systemic amebiasis are ubiquitous. Outbreaks are reported regularly on every continent and in both developed and developing countries. The most common source of infection is the ingestion of oocysts from contaminated water sources. Fortunately, it is now rarely detected in settled populations in developed countries because of the use of slow-sand filtration in the preparation of potable water. However, in immunocompromised patients and in newly arrived immigrants in the developed countries, acute and chronic infection with amebae occurs. In human immunodeficiency virus (HIV)–infected patients in the United States, the incidence was found recently to be low, 13.5 cases per 100,000. The source of amebic infection in these patients was most often sexual transmission. In newly arrived immigrants, 22% of refugees had intestinal parasites detected. The most commonly reported parasites were *Giardia* and *Trichuris*, although amebiasis, hookworm, schistosomiasis, and ascariasis also were detected.

Most infections with ameba are asymptomatic, although severe enterocolitis and systemic disease may occur. *Entamoeba histolytica* is the usual cause of the disease, although other pathogenic amebae are recognized. *Acanthamoeba* and *Leptomyxid amoebae* cause progressive granulomatous encephalitis in immunosuppressed hosts. Five cases of disseminated cutaneous amebiasis without central nervous system (CNS) findings were noted recently in acquired immunodeficiency syndrome (AIDS) patients. Amebic keratitis has been reported in immunocompromised and nonimmunosuppressed individuals who wore disposable contact lenses. The pathogens in these cases were not the usual *Acanthamoeba* species but rather *Vahlkampfia* and *Hartmannella* species, two other free-living amebae.

Other nonpathogenic amebae may be found in the intestine and should not be confused with the pathogenic species. The disease is always waterborne. Acutely ill individuals are only of limited danger to others because they do not excrete the infectious cysts, and the live trophozoite does not survive for a long period in stools, water, or food. Chronic carriers of amebic cysts may pass the cysts for years and are infectious throughout this period.

Treatment of intestinal and tissue stages of *E. histolytica* generally is accomplished with metronidazole or other 5-nitroimidazoles. However, for ocular infection with *Acanthamoeba* or *Naegleria*, which may involve the eyes or the brain, no drug of choice is favored.

Cryptosporidium parvum Diarrhea

Many outbreaks of cryptosporidiosis have been reported in developed countries. The most dramatic epidemic occurred in Milwaukee, Wisconsin, affecting almost half a million people. Both primary and secondary cases of the disease occurred. The source of this epidemic was fecal contamination of the drinking water, which is river-drawn from areas in which cow manure entered the river. Inadequate sand filtration probably allowed the protozoan pathogen to enter the drinking water supply. Unfamiliarity with the disease and its transmission probably contributed to the delay in recognition of the epidemic and prolonged its persistence.

A study of the presence of cryptosporidial organisms in the tap water of AIDS patients who developed cryptosporidial disease demonstrated a significant association with the highest doses of tap water consumed within the home. A lower association was demonstrated with tap water consumed outside the home. Immunocompromised patients may need to consider avoiding tap water. *C. parvum* is highly resistant to chlorination and must be filtered out of the water.

Cryptosporidial outbreaks have been reported in many regions. In each case, the likely source of the original pathogen appears to have been cattle feces from which infective oocysts reached the potable water supply because of a breakdown in filtration procedures or because of their absence in the multiple barriers system.

Giardiasis

Giardiasis is a major waterborne protozoal disease. Often reported in cold countries, outbreaks have occurred in Vail, Colorado, and Zermatt, Switzerland. Both these towns are high-altitude winter resorts where water is drawn from cold surface mountain sources believed to be pure. Prior to these outbreaks of disease, the survival of the protozoan in cold mountain streams was not recognized. In the United States, 75% of the waterborne gastrointestinal disease outbreaks are caused by either *Giardia* or *Cryptosporidium*.

Recent outbreaks of giardiasis in Canada were shown to be waterborne. Contaminated community drinking water was identified as the source in a community in British Columbia, where two successive outbreaks were traced to the same strain of *Giardia* by enzyme-linked immunosorbent assay (ELISA) techniques.

Recent studies of internationally adopted children show that 19% of the children studied had evidence of *G. lamblia* infection. A study conducted along the United States–Mexico border in households lacking municipal sewer and water demonstrated hyperendemic *Cryptosporidium* and *Giardia* infection. Most of the families were chronically infected but asymptomatic. At particular risk were children younger than 5 years of age. When households purified their drinking water, there was a significant reduction in the rate of infection with *Cryptosporidium*, but no effect on *Giardia* infection was noted.

Campers and backpackers who use surface-water sources for potable water during their travels should be particularly careful to use filters and treatment systems that are now available commercially to remove *Giardia* organisms from drinking water. Treatment of giardiasis is accomplished with metronidazole, although the diagnosis is sometimes difficult to confirm by stool examination. Severe diarrhea in a camper or backpacker who has been using surface water for drinking should alert the physician to the possibility of giardiasis. Empirical treatment with metronidazole then may be appropriate.

Toxoplasmosis

Toxoplasmosis is transmitted occasionally through a waterborne route. British Columbia identified the source of an outbreak of toxoplasmosis as a municipal drinking water supply. Studies completed recently demonstrated *Toxoplasma gondii* infection both in domestic and wild cats in the watershed area and in cougars in the watershed. The cougars and deer mice in the watershed were found to shed *T. gondii* oocysts near the water's edge. These animals were believed to be the source of the Victoria, British Columbia, outbreak. Future outbreaks may be anticipated because of the endemic nature of the sylvatic and domestic infection.

A major outbreak of highly endemic waterborne toxoplasmosis also has been described in north Rio de Janeiro State, Brazil, where 84% of the population in the lower social classes was seropositive for *T. gondii*, whereas 62% of the middle class and 23% of the upper class were seropositive. Drinking unfiltered water in this community in Brazil was highly associated with *T. gondii* seropositivity.

REFERENCES

Dubey JP: Toxoplasmosis: A waterborne zoonosis. Vet Parasitol 2004;126:57 [PMID: 15567579].

Savioli L et al: Giardia and Cryptosporidium join the 'Neglected Diseases Initiative'. Trends Parasitol 2006;22:203 [PMID: 16545611].

Sopwith W et al: The changing epidemiology of cryptosporidiosis in North West England. Epidemiol Infect 2005;133:785 [PMID: 16181496].

Yakoob J et al: Giardiasis in patients with dyspeptic symptoms. World J Gastroenterol 2005;11:6667 [PMID: 16425362].

WATERBORNE VIRAL DISEASES

Enterovirus (Picornavirus) Hepatitis A

Waterborne hepatitis epidemics are common throughout the world. In developed countries, hepatitis A frequently is spread from a single case through food-borne means; however, waterborne transmission is reported. Most often, waterborne transmission of hepatitis A in developed countries occurs as a result of sewage contamination of potable water supplies. In less developed countries and in the rural areas of developed countries, waterborne transmission of the hepatitis A virus is common. In countries where environmental sanitation is poor, infants and children frequently contract hepatitis A, and the survivors become immune. In more developed areas, where environmental sanitation is better, a reservoir of nonimmune adults is found, and epidemic disease in adults may be seen. In the United States, epidemic hepatitis A occurred in waves during the 1980s. Large epidemics are now infrequent but may occur from time to time. Outbreaks in nurseries and day-care centers and as a result of food and water contamination occur sporadically.

Identification of the disease is helpful in order to distinguish it from hepatitis E, which has a similar course and indistinguishable epidemiologic pattern. Serologic diagnosis is available, which uses either ELISA or radioimmunoassay (RIA) techniques. Positivity may linger for months. Most young persons recover with little or no sequelae. However, a case fatality rate of 0.6% is noted. Most fatalities occur in adults who have fulminant disease. No specific treatment is available for hepatitis A. Hyperimmune globulin usually has been given as prophylaxis if exposure to hepatitis A becomes known and the disease is not yet symptomatic. The current availability of a well-tested and effective antihepatitis A vaccine throughout the world should help to reduce the remaining pool of susceptible persons and limit the epidemic nature of the disease. Travelers and workers who plan to work in areas with high rates of endemic hepatitis A should be vaccinated in accordance with CDC recommendations long enough in advance of the trip to allow buildup of adequate antibody before departure to the endemic area.

Hepatitis E

Like hepatitis A, hepatitis E is an enterically transmitted viral infection of the liver. The causative organism has not been fully characterized, although recent studies identify it as a single-strand polyadenylated RNA virus. Hepatitis E disease is often called *enterically transmitted non-A, non-B hepatitis* to distinguish it from hepatitis A and from the blood-borne hepatitis B. It also has been called *fecal-oral non-A, non-B hepatitis*.

Hepatitis E is an acute infection that causes mild to severe disease with varying case fatality rates. It occurs commonly in the 15–40-year-old age group in developing countries, where it is an important cause of morbidity and mortality. In the general population, case fatality rates of 0.5–3.0% are noted. Pregnant women appear to be particularly sensitive to the effects of hepatitis E infection. In several reported studies, case fatality rates as high as 20% have been reported among pregnant women, although overall mortality in the same epidemic is very much lower. Transmission of hepatitis E is almost invariably through contaminated water, although person-to-person transmission also may occur.

A serologic test to determine the presence of hepatitis E is available. Recent studies indicate that 2–3% of blood donors in the United States and in northern Europe are positive for hepatitis E antibodies, 6.8% of blood donors in Spain carry anti–hepatitis E antibodies, and 70% of blood donors in Thailand carry the antibody. In India, during identified outbreaks of hepatitis E, 85% of the affected individuals lacked evidence of antibodies either to hepatitis A or B, and 84% were positive for antibodies to hepatitis E virus.

No specific treatment is available for hepatitis E, and no vaccine is yet available. Immune globulin is not currently indicated for prophylaxis of the disease. Chlorination of water cannot be relied on to reduce the risk of waterborne hepatitis virus. Slow-sand filtration is required to remove the causal organisms.

Other Waterborne Viral Infections

Other viruses are associated with waterborne epidemics from time to time. Poliovirus, the cause of poliomyelitis, has long been suspected of being transmissible through water routes, but there is little credible evidence to support this view. In the developed world, where wild-type poliomyelitis is now virtually eradicated, spontaneous cases of polio usually are associated with vaccines.

Norwalk virus has been identified as a cause of epidemic enteritis in New South Wales, Australia. From time to time, many other waterborne epidemics of viral disease occur. The sporadic episodes usually are due to breakdown of the multiple barriers system in developed countries and the use of fecally contaminated water in less developed areas for the potable water supply.

REFERENCES

Ehlers MM et al: Detection of enteroviruses in untreated and treated drinking water supplies in South Africa. Water Res 2005;39:2253 [PMID: 15919105].

Fong TT, Lipp EK: Enteric viruses of humans and animals in aquatic environments: Health risks, detection, and potential water quality assessment tools. Microbiol Mol Biol Rev 2005; 69:357 [PMID: 15944460].

Lodder WJ, de Roda Husman AM: Presence of noroviruses and other enteric viruses in sewage and surface waters in The Netherlands. Appl Environ Microbiol 2005;71:1453 [PMID: 15746348].

Maunula L, Von Bonsdorff CH: Norovirus genotypes causing gastroenteritis outbreaks in Finland. J Clin Virol 2005;34:186 [PMID: 15914082].

WATERBORNE TREMATODE & HELMINTH INFECTIONS

Schistosomiasis (Bilharziasis)

Schistosomiasis caused by *Schistosoma hematobium* is a major problem throughout Africa. *S. mansoni* causes the disease in the Arabian Peninsula, South America, some of the Caribbean Islands, and in areas of the Middle East. *S. japonicum* is endemic in Asia. A number of other schistosomes are found regionally and locally. A blood fluke (trematode), the schistosome lives in blood vessels of the host for long periods of time.

Three forms of schistosomiasis are recognized: swimmer's itch or cercarial dermatitis, acute schistosomiasis, and chronic schistosomiasis. Chronic schistosomiasis causes severe illness in the host. Bladder, kidney, and other infections have been reported. Fibrosis, granulomas, obstructive uropathy, and bladder cancer may result from schistosomiasis. Bilharziasis, an older name for the same disease, is favored as the disease designation in South America and in other parts of the world.

The schistosomal infection is acquired from water containing the free-swimming larval form, the cercariae. The life cycle is complex, but in most mammals, the eggs leave the hosts in the urine, hatch in the water, and then are carried in snail hosts. From the snail host, the cercariae are released into water, from which they penetrate the skin of human waders or swimmers, and the cycle progresses.

Schistosomiasis is not transmissible from person to person, but infected persons are able to transmit the disease through excretion of infective eggs in urine for a lifetime. Prophylaxis depends on avoiding exposure to contaminated water.

Soldiers who serve under difficult conditions in endemic areas are at particular risk for schistosomiasis. In addition to the known endemic areas in Africa, schistosomiasis has been endemic in China and the Philippines. A large project in China sponsored by the World Bank has managed schistosomiasis successfully in humans but has not controlled the snail host of the intermediate forms successfully.

Praziquantel is the drug of choice for treatment of all species of schistosome infection. Other drugs are also available and sometimes are effective in treating the disease.

Ascariasis

Roundworm, or *Ascaris lumbricoides*, generally causes an asymptomatic infection of the intestinal tract. The organism is ubiquitous. In tropical countries, infection rates of up to 50% have been noted. Some patients develop pulmonary ascariasis and are symptomatic. Fever, cough, wheezing, and other pulmonary symptoms may occur. Ascariasis may contribute to nutritional deficiency.

Although soil contaminated with the eggs of the worm is the usual mode of transmission, waterborne transmission also has been reported. Effective treatment is available with mebendazole, although reinfection occurs commonly. Mebendazole is contraindicated during pregnancy. Pyrantel also has been reported to be effective in single doses against ascariasis. A number of other drugs are also reported to be safe and effective in treatment of the infestation.

REFERENCES

Cardosco FC et al: Human antibody responses of patients living in endemic areas for schistosomiasis. Clin Exp Immunol 2006; 144:382 [PMID: 16734606].

Hagan P et al: Schistosomiasis control. Trends Parasitol 2004; 20:92 [PMID: 14747023].

Utzinger J, Keiser J: Schistosomiasis and soil-transmitted helminthiasis: Common drugs for treatment and control. Expert Opin Pharmacother 2004;5:263 [PMID: 14996624].

CHEMICAL WATER CONTAMINATION

Chemical contamination of water is a worldwide problem. The prospect for remediation of existing chemical water pollution problems is not hopeful in the near term. For example, studies of trout and perch in Scandinavia show that decreases in mercury tissue concentration since the 1970 ban on the use of phenyl mercury in pulp and paper production have been very slow. Even though a river habitat is involved in their studies, 15 years is required for mercury levels in trout in the mercury-polluted waters downstream from a pulp and paper plant to fall to a level equal to that in the trout upstream of the plant. Similar long delays in the remediation of water quality have been noted for arsenic, chromium, and other metals and persistent organics.

The opportunity for primary prevention of further deterioration in the universal water supply by intervention in agricultural and industrial activities that contribute to the load of biologically unacceptable materials in water is significant.

HUMAN DRINKING WATER REQUIREMENTS

Human drinking water requirements are well defined. Studies in temperate conditions demonstrate that acclimatized adults consume approximately 2 L of water per day. Under more extreme conditions, such as desert environments, or under heavy work, human water consumption and water loss may rise precipitously. The average acclimatized 70-kg (154.3-lb) human living in a temperate climate and at rest consumes 800–1000 mL of water per day as water in food and generates 300–400 mL of water from oxidation of food. Also, 1–2 L/day is consumed as liquid, some of which reasonably may be expected to be tap water. To balance this intake, 800–1000 mL of water is insensibly lost in exhaled air, and approximately 200 mL is evaporated as sweat. A total of 100–200 mL of water is lost in the feces, and 1–2 L of urine is produced per day. Thus a balance at 2100–3400 mL of water intake and output is normal.

In addition to the dosage of water that is ingested daily, humans are exposed to water vapor, aerosols, and mists of water on a continuous basis. While this exposure to atmospheric water vapor and aerosols may contribute little to the water balance of the exposed humans, soluble organics and inorganics in this inhaled water may increase the dose of toxic material that is absorbed through the respiratory system substantially. In addition, water that is on the skin may contain dissolved material that can penetrate the epidermis and dermis and thus be absorbed. Dermally absorbed organics also may contribute significantly to the total dose of toxic substances delivered to humans from contaminated water sources. The Agency for Toxic Substances and Disease Registry (ATSDR) estimates that in circumstances where humans use water contaminated with partially soluble organic materials such as halogenated hydrocarbons for all ordinary domestic purposes, consumption, cooking, and hygiene, one-third of the absorbed dose of toxic materials comes from the water they drink, one-third from inhaled water vapor and aerosol, and one-third from dermal contact. The dose of hydrocarbons absorbed by inhalation of contaminated water used for showering and bathing may exceed the dose consumed by the same individuals by an order of magnitude.

THE WATER CYCLE & SOURCES OF HUMAN DRINKING WATER

The earth's water is constantly in a cycle of evaporation and precipitation. Once deposited on the earth's surface, water may run off, be impounded, or percolate through various layers of soil, sand, and rock to become free-flowing water or confined water. Deep aquifers often are confined. They do not participate in the evaporation and precipitation cycle unless the confining zone above them has been penetrated and fluids extracted from them. Evaporation from saline water sources, the oceans, and large salt marshes also contributes to the total air-borne water vapor that eventually may precipitate to the earth's surface. The process of evaporation and precipitation has the potential to cleanse water of organic and inorganic contaminants, as does percolation of water through sand and soil and the action of humic bacteria and other mechanisms. Unfortunately, soluble organics that may escape the soil/sand adsorption process or that may be resistant to bacterial degradation may be evaporated with water, separately and at different rates, only to redissolve in the water-air mass. While much of this organic load is the result of industrial and agricultural activity, a very significant portion may be volatile halomethanes of several different structures produced in finished drinking water that has been chemically disinfected with chlorine- or bromine-based disinfection systems. The most prominent of these halomethanes is chloroform, a proved animal and probable human carcinogen. Other closely related halo-organic species also occur in finished water and in the air as a result of water disinfection processes. Bromomethanes, chloramines, and other closely related chemicals have been identified in finished disinfected water.

Airborne particulate matter, which is produced by the combustion of fossil fuels, may carry high loads of oxides of sulfur. These sulfur compounds are either adsorbed to the particulate's core or are dissolved in the aerosols that oxidative combustion produces. Acid particulates contribute an acid load to atmospheric water, which may become acid precipitation. Because these acidic materials are quite stable in water, they progressively acidify the surface and groundwater into which they are mixed. Smokes, aerosols, mists, and vapors all may contribute organic materials and inorganic substances of varying toxicologic significance to the air. In the vicinity of some coal-fired power plants and some other solid or beneficiated fuel-fired facilities, alkaline fly ash is deposited, which produces paradoxical alkalinization of the soil and adjacent surface water and groundwater. Much of the particulate-bound load is partially water-soluble. It will reprecipitate to the earth's surface as atmospheric conditions change and rain falls. Oxynitrogenated organics, partially soluble polynuclear organics, and metallo-organics may participate in the evaporation-precipitation cycle to contaminate surface and subsurface waters.

REFERENCES

Kasim K et al: Chlorination disinfection by-products in drinking water and the risk of adult leukemia in Canada. Am J Epidemiol 2006;163:116 [PMID: 16319293].

Koudinonou BK, Lebel GL: Halogenated acetaldehydes: Analysis, stability and fate in drinking water. Chemosphere 2006; 64:795. [PMID: 16376407].

Nikolaou AD et al: DBP levels in chlorinated drinking water: Effect of humic substances. Environ Monit Assess 2004;93:301 [PMID: 15074622].

Song W et al: Polybrominated diphenyl ethers in the sediments of the Great Lakes. Environ Sci Technol 2005;39:3474 [PMID: 15954222].

Villanueva CM et al: Total and specific fluid consumption as determinants of bladder cancer risk. Int J Cancer 2006;118:2040. [PMID: 16284957].

SIGNIFICANT POLLUTANT SOURCES & INPUT TO SURFACE & GROUNDWATER SOURCES

Surface waters and groundwater are particularly vulnerable to pollution by the direct influence of anthropogenic wastes. Figure 42–1 demonstrates many of the inputs and outputs of the water cycle. Agricultural chemicals, industrial chemicals, mining wastes, septic tank and landfill leakage, and direct sewage discharge to surface or groundwater may contaminate drinking water resources. Small-scale inputs of agricultural chemicals from domestic lawn and garden care with herbicides such as 2,4-dichlorophenoxyacetic acid (2,4-D) can pollute large quantities of drinking water. In the early 1970s, 2,4,5-trichlorophenoxyacetic acid (2,4,5-T), a phenoxy herbicide closely related to 2,4-D, which was a component of Agent Orange, the defoliant used in Vietnam by American military forces, was deregistered for domestic lawn care purposes because of its potential to contaminate water in or around homes with materials that were believed teratogenic or embryotoxic to humans.

Halogenated solvents, paints and varnishes, carburetor cleaners, and gasoline may become troublesome if released to the groundwater or surface waters in quantities below those that are regulated and reportable. These chemicals are a significant source of local and regional surface and groundwater pollution. Large-scale contaminant discharges often are sudden and clearly are recognized by those responsible for the release. Large releases must be reported to state and federal environmental agencies when the discharge is recognized. However, smaller-scale backyard and garage contamination sources may be equally dangerous. Although unrecognized and unreported, these releases will appear quite soon afterwards in the water supply of the local districts.

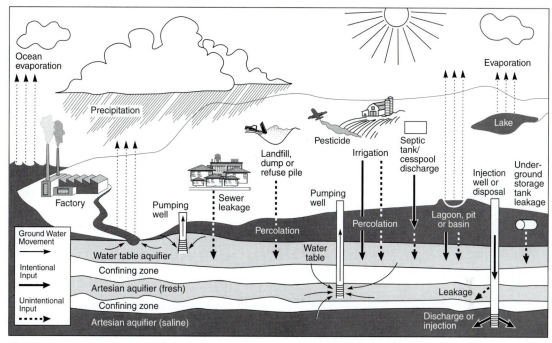

Figure 42–1. How waste-disposal practices can contaminate the groundwater system.

Extensive contamination of water resources with persistent organic chemicals is a worldwide problem. The North American Great Lakes and many local rivers and streams have been heavily polluted with polychlorinated compounds. These compounds include the polychlorinated and polybrominated biphenyls used extensively in twentieth century industrial processes. Huge expenditures to remove and remediate these waters have been made, and more are underway. The ultimate removal of these materials from the environment will take many years. The problem is not confined to North America or western Europe.

Surface water and groundwater contamination from industrial disposal practices was common in the United States until the passage of the Clean Water Act. Prior to that time, there was rampant disposal of many persistent organic compounds into surface and groundwater supplies. In recent years, dumping of agricultural and industrial chemicals has been greatly reduced. In the future, new major pollution problems may not occur as a result of deliberate disposal practices in the United States because of enforcement of the Clean Water Act.

The right to discharge materials into the environment is granted under a permitting process that is administered by state, local, and federal authorities. The permits that are granted specify the quantities of pollutants that may be discharged, the conditions under which they may be discharged, and the time of discharge. They also establish the monitoring and other activities that must be carried out to ensure compliance with the permit. These National Pollutant Discharge Elimination System (NPDES) permits are designed to keep information flowing about environmental contamination. They help to ensure that a responsible standard is applied uniformly to all who discharge hazardous materials and who contaminate water resources, soil, or air.

REFERENCES

Chemyak SM et al: Time trends (1983–1999) for organochlorines and polybrominated diphenyl ethers in rainbow smelt. Environ Toxicol Chem 2005;24:1632 [PMID: 16050579].

Hickey JP et al: Trends of chlorinated organic contaminants in Great Lakes trout and walleye from 1970 to 1998. Arch Environ Contam Toxicol 2006;50:97 [PMID: 16328618].

Rajendran RB et al: Distribution of PCBs, HCHs and DDTs, and their ecotoxicological implications in Bay of Bengal, India. Environ Int 2005;31:503 [PMID: 15788191].

Ripa MN et al: Agricultural land use and best management practices to control nonpoint water pollution. Environ Manage 2006;38:253 [PMID: 16779698].

Xing Y et al: A spatial temporal assessment of pollution from PCBs in China. Chemosphere 2005;60:731 [PMID: 15964056].

SPECIFIC SOURCES OF WATER POLLUTANTS

Pulp & Paper Industry

Some permitted specific industrial sources of water pollutants are still worrisome. Among these are the river and stream discharges of the pulp and paper manufacturing industry. This industry discharges large quantities of toxic persistent and complex organics directly into surface waters, albeit with fully permitted facilities that generally operate close to or within their permitted limits. In addition to abietic acids, lignins, and other organic extracts, chlorine-based pulp bleaching plants discharge 2,3,7,8-tetrachlorodibenzo-*p*-dioxin (2,3,7,8-TCDD) and its congeners to streams and rivers throughout the United States. These highly persistent organics are transferred to silt, sediment, and biota. From the silt, toxics are transferred to fish in the stream ecosystem. The pollutants may be concentrated many-fold within the fish before humans or animals consume the chemicals. When sportsmen or subsistence fishermen consume contaminated fish, they may further concentrate the toxins. The fishermen and their families subsequently may develop illnesses caused by the chemical of interest.

Bioconcentration of lipophilic organics, metals, and other substances has been well studied. In recent times, newer processes have reduced the number and concentration of persistent organics and dioxins produced in the pulp and paper industry. The increasing use of chelating agents, including ethylenediaminetetraacetic acid (EDTA), has altered the amount of free and available metal in environmental media. The increased solubility of various metals, which results from the use of EDTA, appears to have the potential to increase eutrophication of the downstream environments. The continuing use of oxidation ponds to manage paper mill wastes has not been adequate to control the contamination with metals at concentrations well above the European Union's acceptable levels.

Petrochemical Exploration, Refining, & Distribution

Large-scale chemical disposal problems with prominent water pollution components arise in the petrochemical industries. Both surface contamination and groundwater pollution occur as a result of losses and spills in petrochemical extraction, refining, distribution, and utilization. Control of production and distribution wastes has improved in the petrochemical industry. However, wetlands in the south-central and southwestern United States in Texas, Louisiana, California, and elsewhere have both brackish and sweet-water resources

contaminated with oil production and refining wastes. At the oil field level, abandoned drilling mud, a complex semifluid material that may contain barium, chromium, asbestos, and many other substances, may be found. Many of these substances, including the hexavalent chromium used in the ferrochrome component of the drilling fluid, are water-soluble. They may enter the human drinking water supply. Waste crude oil and wellhead condensate often were dumped on-site at drilling locations. Such materials have penetrated to drinking water in some areas of the "oil patch."

During petrochemical refining and transport, spills of intermediates and final product occur. The *Exxon Valdez* crude oil spill, the fifty-fifth largest oil spill on record, in Alaskan coastal waters is a dramatic example of the problem. More common are the small spills from barges, trains, trucks, and other transport vehicles reported in the media around the world on an almost-daily basis.

Leakage of gasoline products from underground storage facilities continuously inputs significant quantities of toxic and carcinogenic hydrocarbons such as benzene, toluene, and xylene, as well as the newer and relatively poorly understood MTBE (methyl *tert*-butyl ether), into groundwater and surface waters that become the human drinking water supply. These volatile hydrocarbons are also released into the air of the homes of persons who live above contaminated groundwater plumes. Contaminant plumes may be the cause of human illnesses such as immunologic impairment, neurologic and cognitive deficits, birth defects, and cancers characteristic of exposure to these substances.

Current regulations prohibit the disposal of oily wastes to groundwater or surface water sources or the placement of these materials in landfill or municipal-controlled solid waste sites. Impoundment and cleanup/purification and treatment of oily and sour-water wastes are required before these materials may be released to sewage systems. However, past practices and current breaches of operating rules in the petrochemicals industry continue to contribute significant levels of hydrocarbons to the drinking water supplies of residents who use well water that is collected in the vicinity of these operating units.

Land Farming & Sludge Applications

The practice of land farming or sludge disposal from industrial and municipal waste plants is common in western Europe, the United States, and Canada. It is used increasingly in Japan and other developed and developing countries. The application of sewage sludge, "biosolids," and processed industrial wastes to uncontaminated land and to agricultural soils presents a complex balance of risks and benefits. Of particular concern is ecologic damage from the elevated concentrations of metals in the sludge materials. While the impact on humans is of equal concern, only a minimal database on the human impact of biosolid use is available.

Municipal treatment plant sludge, which is high in both organic and inorganic materials, as well as in semidry biologic products and bacterial contaminants, is applied to soil. Sludge frequently contains dioxins and related products, metals, and other persistent toxins. Land-farming practices are permitted by the EPA and by state and local environmental authorities because of their potential for soil beneficiation. Most companies and municipalities try to operate within the limits of their permits for sludge application. However, the safety of land farming as a waste-disposal method for sludge that contains persistently toxic, partially soluble organics, metals, and bacterial contaminants of significant long-term toxicity, even at quite low concentrations, is unclear.

In contrast to the apparently favorable indications of studies on the ecologic effects of sewage sludges, the impact on humans is less favorable. The EPA found that direct adverse effects were noted in persons living within 1 km (0.6 miles) of a biosolids application area. Rashes; burning of the eyes, throat, and lungs; and an increased incidence of *Staphylococcus aureus* infection from the colonic bacteria in the solids dust were reported. Two fatalities occurred. The EPA concluded that the application of sewage sludge contaminated with low levels of irritant and toxic chemicals and with low levels of pathogens and endotoxins may have an adverse impact on nearby residents. There is significant resistance among farmers and consumers in France to the use of sewage sludges on agricultural soils. Of particular concern to European scientists is the possibility of spread of enteric diseases such as *Taenia solium* and *T. saginata* infections and of cysticercosis.

Deep-Well Injection of Toxic Materials

Direct injection of waste chemical materials into deep saline aquifers continues to be a permitted method of disposal of hazardous chemicals in some areas of the United States and elsewhere in the world. This process of injection of materials into the deepest saline water resources was acceptable for many years. Unfortunately, penetrations into the deep artesian sources for petroleum exploration purposes have made this practice unwise because the waste materials do not remain inaccessible. They may be pumped for various purposes. Thus saline water may be moved to freshwater aquifers that provide drinking water supplies.

Mining & Minerals Production and Natural Mineral Deposit Impact

On a global basis, mining and minerals production and the processing and fabrication of the final metallic products constitute one of the largest sources of water pollutants. Exploitation of mineral resources results in the transfer of large volumes of metals from relatively protected deep mineral deposits to surface areas. Natural migration and solvation of metals from mineral deposits to drinking water can result in human poisoning. This process is responsible for areas of endemic blackfoot disease caused by arsenic in well water in Taiwan. In these areas, liver, kidney, lung, and bladder cancer appear to be elevated. Extrapolation of the Taiwanese data to the concentrations of arsenic present in drinking water supplies in the United States suggests that the risk of cancer caused by arsenic may be comparable with that caused by environmental tobacco smoke and radon.

Acute arsenic poisoning from environmental sources in the United States also has occurred. However, most metal pollution of water resources is the result of working mineral deposits. Extraction of the minerals of interest and preparation of the economic product introduce large volumes of metals and the chemicals used to extract them to the surface and groundwater resources.

The most dramatic occurrence of arsenic poisoning from naturally tainted water source consumption has occurred on the Indian subcontinent. In West Bengal, India, and in Bangladesh, many thousands of cases of arsenical poisoning of a chronic nature, with skin disease, skin cancer, and visceral cancers, have occurred as a result of the natural contamination of the "safe drinking water" wells constructed in the area. These tube wells, which were built to United Nations' specification, were to replace surface water supplies that were heavily contaminated with pathogens. The tube wells proved to be contaminated with natural arsenicals at highly toxic levels.

Fifty percent of Bangladesh's population (57 million) is at risk of arsenic poisoning from naturally occurring arsenic in well water. The WHO predicts that 1 in 10 adults residing in southern Bangladesh could die of arsenic-related cancer within a few years, and it is believed that about 6.5 million people are drinking contaminated water with arsenic levels above 50 μg/L in the affected districts of West Bengal, with an additional 32 million people in Bangladesh.

The direct extraction of metals produces water pollutants. Acid mine drainage also contributes significantly to water pollution in the downstream areas. Acid mine drainage has affected stream ecosystems significantly, contaminated fish populations, and increased stream mineral loads. Aluminum at toxic levels also has been detected in surface waters draining acid-sensitive watersheds. The source of this aluminum may be mine wastes, or it may occur naturally. The acid load is derived both from mine drainage and from acid rain precipitation from fossil-fuel burning.

Lead, zinc, copper, nickel, vanadium, manganese, and iron compounds at toxic concentrations have been demonstrated in surface water and groundwater adjacent to and downstream from mines and minerals extraction facilities. Drinking water wells in mining areas or highly mineralized areas should be tested for metal content as well as for extraction chemicals such as phosphates, nitrates, and cyanides because these materials readily enter the water table from leaky extraction facilities. Tailing ponds, tailing piles, slag heaps, and other abandoned mineral-rich waste collections often weather under the influence of rain and other water flows, and relatively insoluble mineral forms such as galena (lead sulfide) are converted to lead carbonate, which then migrates into drinking water wells. Other mining-associated materials that have been identified in surface and groundwater sources for drinking water include polychlorinated biphenyls and sulfuric acid.

Studies of the biologic impact of marine environmental contamination with mercury have been conducted on populations of the Seychelles Islands, the Faeroe Islands, and elsewhere. While the data support an adverse effect on the intelligence quotient of children born to mothers who consumed mercury-contaminated seafood of many sorts, there is considerable controversy on the degree of impairment, its origin, and its prognosis. That mercury-containing mine waste is highly toxic to humans has been demonstrated repeatedly. Studies in Brazil and Spain strongly support the adverse consequences of soil and water pollution with mercury-containing mine wastes. In Almaden, Spain, the location of the world's largest mercury mine, sediment concentrations of mercury ranged between 5 and 1000 μg/g. These concentrations of mercury are one to four orders of magnitude greater than regional background concentration. Water concentrations have been as high as 20 μg/L. In marine bivalves, mercury concentrations between 1 and 4 μg/g dry weight were found; 30% of the mercury in the bivalves was present as highly toxic methyl mercury.

Other mining wastes, including zinc, tungsten, and rare earths, have been found in elevated concentrations in water and soils in copper, lead, and zinc-mining areas.

Asbestos and other mineral fibers contaminated the Great Lakes from taconite (iron ore) mining operations. Studies of the effect of asbestos contamination of the Great Lakes found associations between asbestos fibers in drinking water and cancer incidence or mortality at many body sites, including the esophagus, stomach, small intestine, colon, and other organs.

In the Balkan states, Balkan nephropathy has been identified and associated with mineral nitrogen, which probably arises in the course of minerals extraction. Studies of nitrite water contamination in the former Yugoslavia and its associated interstitial nephritis have raised concerns about the effect of these compounds on renal health. Cadmium-induced nephropathies, and itai-itai ("ouch-ouch"), a cadmium-induced systemic disease, occurred in Japan as a result of the contamination of estuarine waters that provided most of the dietary fish to a large population.

Radionuclides

Radioactive minerals extraction used during cold war military activities and for the purposes of fueling nuclear power plants has led to surface and groundwater contamination with radionuclides. These radioactive materials include radium, uranium, and their decay products. The water may release radon gas. In a number of areas, water has been significantly contaminated with tritium and alpha emitters as a result of these activities. In some localities, these elevated concentrations of waterborne radionuclides are believed to be responsible for elevated childhood leukemia rates.

Natural radioactivity also leads to contamination of groundwater and drinking water sources. Drinking water contaminated by naturally radioactive derivatives of the uranium and thorium decay series accounts only for a very small portion of the total annual dose of radiation for most humans. In some situations, the risk of leukemia and other cancers is elevated for those who live above or drink from groundwater sources that contain higher than normal radionuclide decay products including radon. Extensive study of the quantitative cancer risk associated with radon in groundwater and drinking water has been undertaken. In some studies, the risk is considered to be formidable. Regulations to limit radon concentrations in drinking water have been proposed in the United States, but formal adoption of these rules has not yet been completed.

High-Technology Industries

High-technology industries such as semiconductor manufacturing plants, which are now proliferating in both the developed and developing areas of the world, use large quantities of water. They may then return large quantities of potentially contaminated water to the sewage systems. The materials used in these facilities include large quantities of halogenated organics such as trichloroethylene, trichloroethane, perchloroethylene, and carbon tetrachloride. Many complex organics are used as photoactive agents in photoresists. Metals and metalloids such as arsenic, selenium, beryllium, cadmium, and lead are also in use in these plants. Semiconductor facilities have plating sections where cyanides and metallic plating solutions containing hexavalent chromium and other carcinogenic metals are in use. Many of the materials are in water-soluble formulations. They may enter the waste water discharge systems of the facilities either by design or in error. Although on-site treatment is required in the United States and other Western countries, it is not enforced so effectively as to prevent the accidental contamination of groundwater. In less developed countries, a far more serious problem exists. The costs of treatment on site must be borne by the manufacturers. In the absence of rigorous enforcement, it is probable that releases of semiconductor manufacturing chemicals to the environment will occur.

Groundwater and drinking water contamination from high-technology industries has occurred in areas where groundwater sources are important contributors to drinking water supplies. Groundwater contamination problems occurred in the Silicon Valley of California as a result of semiconductor industry chemical use. These instances represent only a portion of the contaminated groundwater problems that exist in the United States, Japan, and other countries.

Simple loss of hazardous materials from the waste water systems of industrial facilities through leaky pipes and other problems continues to occur. Recently built treatment facilities and remediation of existing contaminated sites under and adjacent to these and many other high-technology plants eventually may provide a source of clean water to the contaminated communities. At the present time, however, many people are drinking water contaminated with halocarbons and other materials that probably originated in these plants.

The current situation is worrisome because the majority of the chemicals that have been leaked by these plants are of the same general type as the halohydrocarbons produced in the disinfection of drinking water. Thus the concern about long-term carcinogenic and other effects from disinfectant chemical residues, which at this time are inevitably present in community water supplies, is accentuated by the consumption of this high-technology chemical cocktail.

The greatest concern must be directed toward bladder and colon cancer, which are increased in communities where there is long-term consumption of water with elevated concentrations of halohydrocarbons. Recent studies add to the rising concern that lifetime or long-term consumption of water contaminated with halohydrocarbons significantly increases cancer rates. Because it appears that water-disinfection technology is not sufficiently developed to permit abandonment of the chlorination procedures currently in use, the added burden of halohydrocarbons in the drinking water supply from industrial sources is a serious public health problem.

Power Plants & Cooling Towers

Thirty-eight percent of all water used in the United States is employed to cool machinery used in the pro-

duction of electrical power. Much of this water is used as cooling water for coal- and other fossil-fuel-fired plants. Some water is used for cooling water for nuclear power facilities. Many of these electrical power facilities are private plants developed by large industrial facilities such as refineries, chemical plants, heavy manufacturing facilities, and municipalities. In countries other than the United States, such local power facilities are the rule rather than the exception. In eastern and central Europe, every large and many smaller industrial facilities have their own on-site power-generation facilities.

Each of these facilities must treat its water to prevent corrosion of the cooling towers and to arrest growth of bacteria, such as the *Legionella* genus, and fungi in the cooling water. For many years, the principal materials used to prevent cooling-tower corrosion were hexavalent chromium compounds. Organic mercurials were the rule for cooling-tower biocides. These materials are no longer used in the United States for these purposes in cooling system. Elsewhere in the world, hexavalent chromium corrosion inhibitors continue to be used, as do mercurial biocides. These highly toxic materials may be disposed of directly to the water systems. At best, they are impounded and evaporated. From impoundment ponds they may reach the groundwater after subsequent leaching caused by rain and runoff. In California, at least one community groundwater supply was severely contaminated by the practice of disposal of cooling-tower wastes from a natural gas compression plant containing hexavalent chromium into waste water ponds. Hexavalent chromium, which is a class 1 human carcinogen, later leached into the domestic wells of the surrounding residences. Concentrations of chromium hundreds of times above California's standards were measured in some of the wells. It is hoped that in these situations the hexavalent chromium eventually will be transformed to trivalent chromium by natural reductive processes. However, local conditions are so variable that there is substantial risk that carcinogenic chromium will be distributed in the drinking water, along with organic mercurial biocides and other substances from cooling-system chemicals.

Agricultural Chemicals

Agriculture is the largest user of water resources around the world. It is also the industry with the most direct access to surface and groundwater resources. Because agriculture is universally chemically intensive and the chemicals generally are applied in solution, suspension, or as wettable concentrates and powders, agricultural chemicals have the greatest potential to produce serious water pollution problems. No area of the world is free of agricultural chemical contamination of surface and groundwater resources.

In the past 50 years, the development of chemically intensive agriculture in every country has led to the contamination of water supplies with many evanescent and persistent chemicals of considerable acute and chronic toxicity. Contamination of individual and community water supplies with every agricultural chemical that has been introduced has occurred.

In the 1960s, water pollution from organomercurial seed-coating fungicides used on the Indian subcontinent led to the contamination of deep-sea tuna with levels of mercury that were unacceptable to Western countries. The source of this organic mercury was the fungicidal substances that were applied to rice seed. Because the use of organomercurials produced an 1800% increase in rice yield per acre, it was inevitable that those countries in the Indian subcontinent that depend on rice to prevent starvation would continue to use the mercurials. Only recently have runoffs from the rivers of Asia had reduced levels of mercury.

Organic mercury contamination from seed-coating fungicides, paper-pulp fungicides, and cooling-tower biocides has been a major cause of water pollution in Japan, the Indian Ocean, and Scandinavia.

Perhaps of even greater significance is the current widespread contamination of drinking and groundwater supplies of wells and rivers throughout Europe, Asia, and North America with herbicide chemicals of every structure. The most widely used chemicals lead the contaminant list. Atrazine, a triazine herbicide used for weed control, appears in virtually every well in every area of the United States where it has been used. Other materials have similar widespread distribution. Chlorophenols, fluorinated compounds, chlorothalonil, dinoseb, metribuzin, linuron, monuron, glyphosate, and others all have been identified in public and private drinking water supplies.

The widespread contamination of agricultural water resources with herbicides such as 2,4-D and atrazine, among many others, may be causally associated with the worldwide epidemic of non-Hodgkin lymphoma that has been underway for several years. Abnormalities of human lymphocytes occur at concentrations of atrazine and linuron similar to those found in drinking water supplies. In California, groundwater contamination with aldicarb, a powerful carbamate insecticide, has resulted in statistically significant lymphocyte CD2:CD8 ratio changes in women who consumed the groundwater.

In many parts of the world, dibromochloropropane (DBCP) contamination of groundwater has occurred as a result of the direct injection of this carcinogenic compound into the soil for the control of nematodes in bananas, pineapples, and sugar beets. Dibromochloropropane causes male sterility in agricultural and manufacturing workers who make or apply it. The widespread contamination of groundwater with this reproductive toxin in Costa Rica, Honduras, the Philippines, Ivory Coast, and California is very serious. Contamination of surface and groundwater with nitrates used as fertilizers has led to serious and even fatal acute illness in children who consumed this water in infant formula. Studies in eastern and central Europe and the United States confirm that agricultural nitrate runoff has reached levels that are capable of causing methemoglobinemia in children. In addition, these nitrates are the substrate for further biologic alteration to nitrosamines, which are carcinogenic.

The finding of other persistent and transient elevations of water pollutants in groundwater and drinking water makes imperative the development of newer techniques to control waterborne exposure to chemicals in agriculture. Peroxide and ultraviolet treatment of waste water significantly degrades pesticide residues.

REFERENCES

Ball P: Arsenic-free water still a pipedream. Nature 2005;436:313 [PMID: 16034383].

Barringer JL et al: Mercury in groundwater, septage, leach-field effluent, and soils. Sci Total Environ. 2006;361:144. [PMID: 15996719].

Brugge D et al: Exposure pathways and health effects associated with chemical and radiological toxicity of natural uranium: A review. Rev Environ Health 2005;20:177 [PMID: 16342416].

Cornel P, Weber B: Water reuse for irrigation from waste water treatment plants with seasonal varied operation modes. Water Sci Technol 2004;50:47 [PMID: 15344772].

Hanf RW, Kelly LM: An assessment of drinking-water supplies on the Hanford site: An evaluation conducted at a federal nuclear facility in southeastern Washington state. J Environ Health 2005;67:44 [PMID: 15794463].

Horn RC et al: Determination of sediment mutagenicity and cytotoxicity in an area subjected to petrochemical contamination. Mutagenesis 2004;19:445 [PMID: 15548755].

Kowalska E et al: H_2O_2/UV-enhanced degradation of pesticides in wastewater. Water Sci Technol 2004;49:261 [PMID: 15077981].

Murshed R et al: Clinicians' roles in management of arsenicosis in Bangladesh: Interview study. BMJ 2004;328:493 [PMID: 14988183].

Shanley JB et al: Physical controls on total and methylmercury concentrations in streams and lakes of the northeastern USA. Ecotoxicology 2005;14:125 [PMID: 15931963].

CHEMICAL AND BIOLOGIC TERRORISM DIRECTED AT WATER INFRASTRUCTURE AND SUPPLIES

National and international unrest, war, and terrorist activities have brought the unthinkable possibility of deliberate widespread chemical and biologic contamination of water infrastructure and potable water supplies to the fore. The possibility of an attack on water supplies is significant. In many jurisdictions, the water resources are largely insecure, and a determined terrorist could readily attack reservoirs, collection and distribution centers, and water-treatment facilities. Although considerations of dilution, half-life in water, target populations, and other issues make an attack on general water supplies more impractical than not, an attack on a small water system that supplies a critical facility such as a hospital, a government building, or a military installation seems feasible. Many states and the EPA have developed protocols for the evaluation of the security of public water supplies.

All public water systems must complete a security assessment in order to meet EPA water-supply guidelines. There are also requirements for small water systems. Much of this work has been developed in response to the Homeland Security Act. Steps are now underway to harden the perimeters of many water infrastructure facilities and to increase the vigilance of the security services over these institutions.

REFERENCES

EPA, Office of Water: *Water Vulnerability Assessment Factsheet,* www.epa.gov/ogwdw/security/index.html.

Magnuson ML et al: Responding to water contamination threats. Environ Sci Technol 2005;39:153 [PMID: 15871218].

Meinhardt PL: Water and bioterrorism: preparing for the potential threat to U.S. water supplies and public health. Annu Rev Public Health 2005;26:213 [PMID: 15760287].

DRINKING WATER REGULATORY CONSIDERATIONS

It is estimated that close to 350 billion gallons of water are used in the United States each day. This total of approximately 1400 gallons of water per capita is the highest in the world. Only 10% of the total water usage in the United States each day is for drinking-water purposes: Eleven percent is for industrial purposes, 38% is used to cool electric power generating plants, and 41% is used for agricultural purposes. Each of the major water-consuming segments contributes significant waste water to the U.S. water supply; many contribute substantial contaminant loads to it as well.

Public drinking water systems supply much of the drinking water in the United States and elsewhere around the world. The sources for these drinking water systems vary widely. Surface waters, such as rivers, streams, lakes, and reservoirs, and shallow and deep groundwater aquifers may be used. These water systems generally are regulated by local or national regulatory bodies, which set specific standards for water quality. Standards include treatment requirements and the concentration of contaminants and pathogens that are allowed in the finished drinking water. In the United States, local governments most often are responsible for the provision of finished drinking water.

The Safe Drinking Water Act limits total halomethanes in finished, disinfected drinking water to 100 ppb. This is a performance-based standard that does not take into account the health effects of the halomethanes. Rather, it considers the technologic and economic infeasibility of water engineering systems and practices to achieve a lower level of disinfectant by-products at the present time. Other water contaminants are limited in finished drinking water by the Safe Drinking Water Act. Metals such as arsenic, lead, and barium; pesticides such as aldicarb, 2,4-D, and chlorinated organics and nonhalogenated substances such as benzene and other aromatic and aliphatic compounds are regulated. The Safe Drinking Water Act regulates the amount of radioactivity in water supplies and the concentration of certain inorganic ions such as cyanide and nitrate, as well as pathogenic organism counts.

The EPA enforces the Safe Drinking Water Act. The EPA sets two standards for each regulated pollutant. The first standard, called a *maximum contaminant level goal* (MCLG), is set at a concentration that is not expected to cause adverse health effects over a lifetime of consumption of water at that concentration. A substantial safety margin for this MCLG is included in each unenforceable standard. There is no penalty assessed for violation of the MCLG concentration by a public water supply system. In addition to the MCLG, the EPA has promulgated enforceable standards called *maximum contaminant levels* (MCLs) for each regulated contaminant. Regulated suppliers of drinking water must comply with the MCLs. By law, the EPA must attempt to set the MCL as close to the MCLG as is technologically and economically feasible. In almost all cases, the enforceable MCL is higher than the MCLG. Safe Drinking Water Act amendments also banned the use of lead pipe or soldered connections in any public drinking water system in order to reduce lead contamination of water that may affect the intellectual development of infants and children. Suppliers of public drinking water must comply with these regulations as well.

MCLs apply only to public drinking water supplies in the United States. MCLs for noncarcinogenic compounds are believed to be protective of the most sensitive human populations that may be exposed to them. Details of the protective factors and diseases or effects protected against may be found for each substance in the EPA Integrated Risk Information System (IRIS) database, which is accessible through the National Library of Medicine's online TOXNET system. Only two current MCLs, those for bacteria and nitrate, would cause acute illness if they were exceeded. All others consider chronic or long-term adverse effects.

MCLs for carcinogens are considered by EPA to be protective to a level where the allowed concentration of the regulated contaminant in water would not cause a human population risk of cancer greater than 1 in 100,000. Details of the carcinogenesis decision-making bases for each MCLG and MCL are also found in the IRIS online database. The decisions for short- and long-term water standards are based on calculations of NOAEL (no adverse effect levels) and LOAEL (low adverse effect levels). The Office of Drinking Water of the EPA calculates acceptable daily intakes (ADIs) from these data. The process has a high level of uncertainty, which is adjusted for to some degree in the calculations. The regulations often are based on indirect evidence of questionable relevance. From the available data, the EPA also calculates 1-day health advisories for noncarcinogenic effects for children, 10-day health advisories for children, and 1-day, 10-day, and lifetime health advisory (HA) levels for 70-kg (154.3-lb) adults. These calculations are used as informal guidelines to municipalities and other institutions in the event of emergency chemical spills and in other contamination situations. Recent attempts by the EPA to revise its approaches to the calculation of waterborne chemical risks and their implications for regulatory policy are well illustrated in the work that has been done on trichloroethylene.

MCLs do not apply to private drinking water wells, which are estimated to supply 15% of the U.S. population, or 40 million people, with their daily drinking water supplies. Neither MCLGs nor MCLs apply to bottled water, which is often used as a substitute for contaminated public drinking water supplies. If the bottled water is drawn from private wells or springs, as is often the case, only the supplier's goodwill protects the ultimate consumer of the water from consumption of contaminants that would not be permitted in a public water supply. No contaminant concentration limits exist for the use of groundwater, recreational water, springs, streams, lakes, or ponds as drinking water supplies.

Additional regulatory proposals have been made for materials for which no enforceable MCLG or MCL exists. These proposals are not legally enforceable. They are often health- rather than performance-based guidelines. Because of the limited toxicologic database on which these suggested guidelines are based, or for other economic and regulatory considerations, MCLs have not been officially adopted as binding for many known toxic water contaminants. These documents provide detailed assessments of the contaminants and their toxic profiles. Unfortunately, the information that is available on many water contaminants is incomplete and inconclusive. Uncertainty limits the ability to regulate the chemicals in water, even though the evidence is suggestive that chronic consumption of these materials produces disease in animals and humans.

REFERENCES

EPA: Ground Water and Drinking Water Contaminants and MCLs, www.epa.gov/safewater/mcl.html.

Reimann C, Banks D: Setting action levels for drinking water. Sci Total Environ 2004;332:13 [PMID: 15336887].

Renzetti S, Dupont D: The performance of municipal water utilities: Evidence on the role of ownership. J Toxicol Environ Health A 2004;67:1861 [PMID: 15371221].

US Code Collection: National Drinking Water Regulations, www4.law.cornell.edu/uscode/42/300g-1.html.

Ward MH et al: Drinking-water nitrate and health. Environ Health Perspect 2005;113:1607 [PMID: 16263519].

Williams PR et al: The risk of MTBE relative to other VOCs in public drinking water in California. Risk Anal 2004;24:621 [PMID: 15209934].

Multiple-Chemical Sensitivity

43

Robert J. Harrison, MD, MPH

Clinicians have been challenged by the individual with multiple complaints relating to low-level occupational or environmental exposures. Patients report respiratory, central nervous system, musculoskeletal, gastrointestinal, and systemic symptoms after exposure to common environmental irritants such as perfumes, cigarette smoke, home or office furnishings, household cleaners, and a host of other petrochemical products. Upper respiratory (e.g., nasal congestion, dryness, or burning), central nervous system (e.g., concentration problems, memory difficulties, insomnia, drowsiness, irritability, and depression), and vegetative (e.g., fatigue, headache, arthralgias, and myalgias) symptoms predominate. Symptoms occur with exposures well below thresholds permitted by federal or state regulatory agencies as causing acute adverse effects in humans, resulting in significant impairment, lost work time, complete job loss, or major alterations in social and family functions. Individuals may report symptom onset following acute or chronic low-level occupational or environmental exposures, with persistent symptoms that are triggered by subsequent environmental contaminants. Often patients seek help from multiple health care providers who suggest psychiatric etiologies or treatment, obtain toxicologic or immunologic test batteries, or initiate a variety of empirical treatments. Workers' compensation or disability claims often are disputed, and employers often have difficulty accepting or accommodating clinician or patient requests for alternative work environments. As a result, frustration, anger, hostility, and suspicion may confront the clinician when significant impairment continues despite lengthy and expensive consultations.

Some controversy continues to surround the etiology, case definition, diagnosis, and treatment of individuals with *multiple-chemical sensitivity* (MCS). The specialty of clinical ecology that emerged in the 1960s adopted theories of causation that differ from those of traditional allergy, immunology, and toxicology, thereby laying the basis for medical and legal disputes regarding legitimate or acceptable forms of treatment, medical or workers' compensation insurance reimbursement, and disability benefits. As a result, some clinicians believe that etiologic theories, diagnosis, and the clinical management of MCS are inconsistent with sound medical

science. In more recent years, however, important progress has been made in elucidating and defining the nature of this condition. The combined efforts of several disciplines, including toxicology, psychology, and physiology, have suggested a multifactorial explanatory model for this condition. To guide the clinical evaluation of individuals with this disorder or to respond to requests for epidemiologic investigation, the health care practitioner should be aware of current controversies, including knowledge gaps and the need for further research.

EPIDEMIOLOGY & CASE DEFINITIONS

The term *multiple-chemical sensitivity* was defined in 1987 as an acquired disorder characterized by recurrent symptoms, referable to multiple organ systems, occurring in response to demonstrable exposure to many chemically unrelated compounds at doses far below those established in the general population to cause harmful effects. These seven criteria should be met:

1. The disorder is acquired in relation to some documentable environmental exposure(s), insult(s) or illness(es).
2. Symptoms involve more than one organ system.
3. Symptoms recur and abate in response to predictable stimuli.
4. Symptoms are elicited by exposures to chemicals of diverse structural classes and toxicologic modes of action.
5. Symptoms are elicited by exposures that are demonstrable (albeit at low level).
6. Exposures that elicit symptoms must be very low, by which is meant standard deviations below "average" exposures known to cause adverse human responses.
7. No single, widely available test of organ function can explain the symptoms.

Previous terms for this disorder included *environmental hypersensitivity* and *environmental illness*. Environmental hypersensitivity was defined as a chronic (i.e., continuing for more than 3 months) multisystem disorder usually involving symptoms of the central nervous system and at least one other system. Affected persons are frequently intolerant to some foods and react adversely to some chemicals and to environmental agents, singly or in combination, at levels generally tolerated by the majority. Affected persons have varying degrees of morbidity, from mild discomfort to total disability. On physical examination, the patient usually is free from any abnormal objective findings. Improvement is associated with avoidance of suspected agents, and symptoms recur with reexposure. The term *environmental illness* (EI) has been described as an acquired disease characterized by a series of symptoms caused and/or exacerbated by exposure to environmental agents. Symptoms involve multiple organs in the neurologic, endocrine, genitourinary, and immunologic systems.

A panel of the World Health Organization (WHO) recommended that the terms MCS and EI be replaced by *idiopathic environmental intolerance* (IEI), arguing that use of the word *sensitivity* may be construed as connoting an allergic cause and that the link between symptoms and exposure is unproven. Other names for this disorder have been used in the published literature, including *chemical intolerance* and *toxicant-induced loss of tolerance*. However, none of these terms has been adopted universally.

Patients with MCS should be distinguished from those with acute occupational diseases such as acute solvent intoxication, occupational asthma, and allergic rhinitis/sinusitis. In these conditions, there usually are objective findings, and the relationship between the condition and exposure is more readily apparent. Several medical organizations, including the American Academy of Allergy and Immunology, the American College of Physicians, the American College of Occupational and Environmental Medicine, and the Council of Scientific Affairs of the American Medical Association, have issued position statements about the causal etiology of MCS. These organizations have not found evidence to link MCS with toxic chemical exposures and have suggested that MCS is primarily a psychological or behavioral disorder.

The epidemiologic and clinical case definitions for MCS have been refined by researchers over the past few years, and certain subsets of questions can provide high specificity for the diagnosis. In one study, combinations of four symptoms (having a stronger sense of smell than others, feeling dull/groggy, feeling "spacey," and having difficulty concentrating) successfully discriminated MCS patients from controls. In another study, self-reported reactions to copy machine emissions, marking pens, aftershave, window cleaner, nylon fabric, pine-scented products, and Rayon material were significant in a discriminant matched-pair analysis of MCS cases and controls. Other studies report overlap between these symptoms and those reported by patients with other conditions of unexplained etiology, such as chronic fatigue syndrome, fibromyalgia, irritable bowel syndrome, and temporomandibular disorder.

A population-based survey in California found that 6.3% reported physician-diagnosed "environmental illness" or "multiple chemical sensitivity," and 15.9% reported being "allergic or unusually sensitive to everyday chemicals." Hispanic ethnicity was associated with physician-diagnosed MCS, and female gender was associated with self-reported sensitivity. Significant functional impairment in terms of physical, occupational, and social functioning was reported among individuals with MCS. Another population-based survey in Georgia found that 12.6% reported increased sensitivity. Among these individuals reporting hypersensitivity to common chemical products, the most common triggers of symptoms were cleaning products, tobacco smoke, perfume, pesticides, and car exhaust. Lifestyle modifications were reported frequently, including change in household cleaning/personal hygiene products, home water- and/or air-filtration systems, and location of residence. Self-reported chemical sensitivity was found among 9% of respondents in a population-based survey in Germany.

No single chemical exposure or workplace process is more prevalent in association with the onset of MCS. Records-based reports from an allergy practice, academic occupational medicine clinic, and environmental health center suggest that individuals with MCS are predominantly women (70–80%) in the 30–40-year-old age range, with a disproportionate number from service industries. MCS patients in these reports tend to be of higher socioeconomic status, more highly educated, and had a diversity of both occupational and environmental exposures. In a Canadian survey, symptoms such as difficulty concentrating, fatigue, forgetfulness, and irritability were reported at the start of illness. Symptoms related to respiratory irritation such as sneezing, itchy or burning eyes, and hoarseness or loss of voice were reported commonly after subsequent exposure to environmental irritants. Several populations have been identified that may develop symptoms of MCS, including industrial workers, occupants of "tight buildings" such as office workers and school children, residents of communities whose air or water is contaminated by chemicals, and individuals with unique, personal exposures to various chemicals in domestic indoor air, pesticides, drugs, or consumer products. Workplace exposures to poor indoor air quality, pesticide exposure, and remodeling have been associated with the onset of MCS. Other diagnostic subsets have been reported among individuals with solvent-associated psycho-organic syndrome, chemical headaches, and intolerance to solvents.

Symptoms of MCS also resemble those of sick-building syndrome, a constellation of excessive work-related symptoms related to an indoor office environment (e.g., headache; eye, nose and throat irritation; fatigue; and dizziness) without an identifiable etiology. MCS has been reported to follow pesticide exposure among employees in a casino and among several office workers following a large-scale outbreak of sick building syndrome. Several symptoms included in the Centers for Disease Control and Prevention (CDC) case definition of chronic fatigue syndrome (i.e., fatigue, confusion, memory loss, sleep difficulties, myalgias, and headaches) also are common among individuals with MCS, and affected individuals may be concerned about occupational or environmental etiologies for chronic fatigue syndrome. Aside from symptom overlap, there is currently no evidence linking chronic fatigue syndrome to occupational or environmental chemical exposures.

A number of epidemiologic surveys have been performed among symptomatic veterans of the Gulf War and Cambodia peacekeeping operations. In most studies, veterans report poorer general health, more cognition difficulties, and a higher prevalence of chronic fatigue syndrome, posttraumatic stress disorder, irritable bowel syndrome, and MCS. One study reported a prevalence of symptoms consistent with MCS in 13.1% of Gulf War veterans. Another study of Gulf War veterans found a higher prevalence of MCS than among non–Gulf War military personnel (5.4% versus 2.6%), with greater sensitivity to organic chemicals, vehicle exhaust, cosmetics, and smog. The prevalence of MCS among British Gulf War veterans was significantly associated with exposure to pesticides. Among Cambodian peacekeeping operations veterans, significantly more MCS subjects reported having used insect repellants that contained N,N-diethyl-metatoluamide (DEET). However, the proportion of Cambodia peacekeeping veterans with symptoms of MCS was relatively low.

ETIOLOGY

The major theories of pathogenesis of MCS can be divided into those that center on a physiologic or toxicologic mechanism and those that ascribe MCS to psychological or behavioral determinants.

Toxicologic Mechanisms

Studies of symptoms in MCS patients are focused on responses below those seen with classic higher-dose exposures because workplace or environmental exposures in this population are considerably lower than those expected to cause end-organ toxicity based on known dose-response relationships. In some studies, no specific reactions to the type or level of chemical exposures have been found in controlled environments, suggesting that autonomic arousal mechanisms in response to odors may play an important role in mediating symptoms. In these studies, MCS subjects do not demonstrate lower olfactory threshold sensitivity or enhanced ability to identify odors accurately. This suggests that nonsensory factors (e.g., attention, bias, and personality) can alter the self-reported impact of exposure to volatile chemicals. In a recent study of Gulf War veterans with chemical sensitivity compared with healthy veterans, MCS subjects exposed to low levels of chemicals (i.e., diesel vapor with acetaldehyde) reported significantly increased symptoms such as disorientation, respiratory discomfort, and malaise.

Psychiatric Mechanisms

Several studies suggest that anxiety and depression are significant contributors to the physical and cognitive symptoms of MCS subjects. Data from some clinical and epidemiologic studies show an association between lifetime psychiatric disorder, particularly mood, anxiety, somatoform, and personality disorders. Many patients with MCS are reported to have psychiatric conditions (e.g., psychoses, affective or anxiety disorders, or somatoform disorders–somatization, conversion, and hypochondriases) with symptoms well before their diagnosis of environmentally related illness. Some patients with persistent or recurrent medically unexplained symptoms may have an atypical posttraumatic stress disorder, where specific and recurrent somatic symptoms follow acute or chronic chemical exposures, with subsequent experience of symptoms repeatedly triggered by low-level environmental irritants.

Patients with MCS display high anxiety sensitivity and in response to laboratory carbon dioxide inhalation tend to experience heightened anxiety and panic attacks. Patients with self-identified chemical sensitivity exhibited a positive symptomatic response to sodium lactate compared with placebo infusion, suggesting that MCS may have a neurobiologic basis similar to that of panic disorder. MCS subjects in one study scored significantly higher than controls on standardized psychological questionnaires for agoraphobic conditions and agoraphobia. One study has shown a significantly higher prevalence of the panic disorder–associated CCK-B allele 7 in subjects with MCS.

Prolonged physical symptoms and sensitivity to common environmental irritants have been described as a behavioral conditioned response or an "odor-triggered panic attack." Several authors suggest that the development of MCS in some individuals may be a result of, at least in part, pavlovian conditioning processes in which the expression of overt symptoms to certain substances reflects classically conditioned responses to previously neutral olfactory and contextual stimuli. Specific cognitive and behavioral interventions such as systematic desensitization, relaxation techniques, self-hypnosis, and biofeedback have been suggested as treatment strategies for these patients. Some MCS patients have been described as primarily ideational (obsessive-compulsive) or phobic in character, requiring a different psychotherapeutic approach focusing on the effect of physical symptoms on psychological function, stress associated with physical and interpersonal isolation, or the frustration of multiple physician consultations.

Neuropsychological measures [e.g., electroencephalography (EEG), scalp electromyography, and skin resistance] during relaxation in individuals who attribute medical and psychological symptoms to chemical exposures have been compared with subjects with primary psychological disorders and with a control group. MCS patients did not differ from psychological subjects, and both were significantly different from controls, suggesting that individuals with MCS may have primary emotional, anxiety, attentional, or personality disorders. The MCS group had a higher somatization score on a standard self-report symptom inventory, and a subset of these patients had a history of early childhood sexual abuse. Patients recruited from the practice of a community allergist with a reported diagnosis of chemical sensitivity were compared with control patients from a university-based occupational musculoskeletal and back-injury clinic. Patients with MCS reported a higher prevalence of current psychological distress (i.e., depression, anxiety, and somatization) and somatization symptoms preceding the onset of sensitivity symptoms. Neuropsychological performance did not differ when adjusted for the level of psychological distress.

In one case series of patients referred for outpatient evaluation for MCS, three-quarters met DSM-IV criteria for at least one psychiatric disorder, and over one-third had somatoform disorders. Subjects with a diagnosis of environmental illness had a higher prevalence of affective disorders (particularly major depression), anxiety, and somatoform disorders compared with controls, and more environmental illness subjects met lifetime criteria for a major mental disorder. Both asthmatics and MCS subjects performed significantly higher than controls on scales of chemical odor intolerance and anxiety sensitivity, and anxiety and depression were significant contributors to the physical and cognitive symptoms of MCS subjects. Individuals with environmental illness filing workers' compensation claims had a greater prevalence of prior psychiatric morbidity (i.e., anxiety, depression, and somatization trait) and higher self-reported measures of somatization and hypochondriasis.

Although many studies find that MCS is a psychological disorder with a belief system characterized by the toxic attribution of symptoms and disability, some stud-

ies suggest that psychiatric and psychological disorders may be a consequence, rather than a cause, of MCS. Among subjects referred to an occupational medicine clinic who met the case definition for MCS, psychiatric evaluation did not suggest any premorbid psychiatric diagnosis or a premorbid tendency toward somatization. Clinically significant psychiatric symptoms of depression and anxiety were present among most subjects, with a subset performing poorly on tests of verbal performance. Despite a preponderance of psychiatric symptoms among MCS patients, psychiatric diagnoses were uncommon, and most did not suffer from a diagnosable psychiatric disease. In a population-based survey of Georgia residents, among individuals reporting hypersensitivity to common chemicals, only 1.4% had a history of prior emotional problems, whereas 37.7% developed these problems after physical symptoms began.

Immunologic Mechanisms

Environmental and occupational chemical exposures may affect the immune system, with a variety of cellular and cell-mediated immunologic effects established in both animals and humans. Xenobiotics may produce immunosuppression and alter host resistance in experimental animals following acute or subchronic exposure, and immunologic effects in humans have been reported in association with dusts (e.g., silica and asbestos), polyhalogenated aromatic hydrocarbons (e.g., dioxins, furans, and polychlorinated biphenyls), pesticides, metals (e.g., lead, cadmium, arsenic, and methyl mercury), and solvents. However, neither experimental immune dysfunction nor epidemiologic evidence of altered immunity has been correlated with clinical disease.

MCS has been postulated to be an immunologic disorder, with generalized immune dysregulation as a result of free-radical generation and alkylation, structural alteration of antigens, or hapten/carrier reactions. Chemicals are hypothesized to alter immune responses, triggering lymphokines and leading to clinical symptoms of cell-mediated immune response. Chemically sensitive patients are reported to have altered T- and B-lymphocyte counts, abnormal helper-suppresser ratios, and antibodies to a variety of chemicals. Patients with building-related illness have been reported to have an abnormal antibody response and altered cellular immunity to formaldehyde, although these findings have not been confirmed using controls, and clinical correlation is absent. MCS also has been hypothesized to be the result of an interaction between the immune and nervous systems.

Studies of patients with MCS have found no consistent abnormalities in immunoglobulins, complement, lymphocytes, or B- or T-cell subsets. A study of patients with MCS found no evidence of increased autoantibodies, lymphocyte count, helper or suppresser cells, B or T cells, or

TAI- or interleukin-2-positive cells compared with control subjects. Absence of objective evidence for immunologic abnormality distinguishes patients with MCS from those with other allergic disorders, autoimmune diseases, and congenital or acquired immunodeficiencies.

Respiratory Mechanisms

Many individuals with MCS report a heightened sense of smell or develop symptoms at low levels of environmental irritant exposure. MCS has been hypothesized to represent an amplification of the nonspecific immune response to low-level irritants. Altered function of C-fibers, respiratory epithelium, or neuroepithelial interaction is postulated to result in increased symptom reporting correlated with physiologic abnormality. Neurogenic inflammation mediated by cell-surface enzymes could play a role in upper respiratory symptoms reported by MCS patients. Subjects with MCS were reported to have a significant decrease in flow values with anterior rhinomanometry, independent of substance or doses, compared with controls. Subjects with MCS showed greater respiratory symptom scores with controlled exposures to test irritants. Capsaicin inhalation provoked more respiratory symptoms in subjects with MCS than controls, suggesting that neurogenic factors may be of importance. Patients with MCS were found with rhinolaryngoscopy to have marked cobblestoning of the posterior pharynx, base of the tongue, or both.

Olfactory-Limbic Mechanisms

MCS has been postulated to be the result of environmental chemical exposure, with the triggering or perpetuation of affective and cognitive disorders as well as somatic dysfunction in vulnerable individuals via sensitization of the central nervous system. The neural sensitization model may incorporate both physical and psychological stressors that are elicited following chemical exposure. This theory proposes that MCS may result from neural sensitization, with excessive or altered neurotransmitter activity and/or alterations of the blood-brain barrier. There are anatomic links between the olfactory nerve, limbic system, and hypothalamus that could explain how odor or irritation of the respiratory tract indirectly results in multiorgan symptoms. Animal models have been developed recently to study the effects of repeated formaldehyde exposure on the hypothalamus-pituitary-adrenal axis and behavioral sensitization. Interactions between environmental chemicals and the vomeronasal organ also have been postulated to play a role in altered chemosensory function.

Kindling is a type of time-dependent sensitization of olfactory-limbic neurons by drug or nondrug stimuli, with activation of neural structures such as the amygdala

and hypothalamus. Limbic structures are among the most susceptible to kindling-induced seizures, and persistent cognitive and emotional sequelae have been associated with temporal lobe epilepsy in humans and kindling in animals. The vanilloid receptor also has been proposed a possible CNS target in MCS. In this model of MCS, sensitization to food or chemicals parallels the phenomenon of time-dependent sensitization from drugs or nondrug stressors, with heightened sensitivity to stimuli, gradual improvement following withdrawal, and reactivation of symptoms following reexposure. Time-dependent sensitization has been studied as a possible model for cacosmia (subjective sense of feeling ill from odors) among nonpatient populations, which may have relevance to similar symptoms reported by MCS patients. It also has been hypothesized that shy individuals may have hyperreactive limbic systems and may self-report greater symptoms of illness owing to chemical exposures. Laboratory studies have demonstrated sensitization in individuals with MCS for variables such as electroencephalographic activity and increased heart rate and blood pressure. In this model, low-level chemical exposure among susceptible individuals could result in affective spectrum disorders with various cognitive and somatic symptoms. This theory attempts to unify physiologic and psychological theories, suggesting that altered neurotransmitter activity may be the underlying mechanism for both affective and somatic symptoms seen among MCS patients.

CLINICAL MANAGEMENT
History & Physical Examination

A careful, thoughtful, and compassionate exposure and psychosocial history is critical. Although the etiology of MCS is controversial, the patient may be suffering from disabling symptoms and frustrated by the lack of definitive answers from clinicians and sometimes is desperately seeking advice and counsel regarding treatment. Approaching the history with the suspicion that the patient with MCS is suffering from a psychiatric disorder, is malingering, or is seeking monetary benefits is not helpful in establishing a therapeutic relationship. Acknowledgment of symptoms and the establishment of a trusting relationship should not necessarily be avoided because the etiology is uncertain or patient motivation is suspect. Where the diagnosis is suspect or contested, an adversarial relationship sometimes may emerge in the provider-patient context that may erode trust, challenge the provider's capacity to treat the patient, and interfere with the therapeutic goals.

A history should be obtained of symptom onset in relationship to acute or chronic exposures. One standardized questionnaire called the Quick Environment

Exposure Sensitivity Inventory (QEESI) has been developed that can assist clinicians in evaluating patients and populations for chemical sensitivity. Attention should be paid to respiratory, dermal, neurologic, and systemic symptoms. Most patients with MCS report general systemic symptoms such as difficulty concentrating, fatigue, lethargy, forgetfulness, and irritability. Myalgias, gastrointestinal complaints, headache, burning eyes, and hoarseness or loss of voice also are reported commonly. These various symptoms are provoked by exposure to low-level airborne contaminants such as perfumes, colognes, cleaning solutions, smoke, gasoline, exhaust fumes, and printing inks. Duration and severity of symptoms should be recorded, particularly in relationship to repeated exposures in the workplace or environment (e.g., improvement away from work or on weekends/vacations with worsening symptoms at work). An occupational history should be obtained, including past employment and exposure to chemicals, dusts, or fumes. Recent and past chemical exposures should be identified by product names or material safety data sheets, and any environmental monitoring data should be reviewed if available.

Symptoms of headache, fatigue, lethargy, myalgias, and trouble concentrating may persist for hours to days or even weeks, with typical "reactions" reported after exposures to airborne chemicals. Often the individual with MCS will have already identified a variety of chemicals that result in symptoms and will have initiated an avoidance regimen. Varying degrees of restrictions in social and work activities may be reported, including problems driving an automobile, grocery shopping, wearing certain types of clothing, or staying away from office buildings or other workplaces.

The physical examination often is normal in patients with MCS, but particular attention should be paid to examination of the respiratory tract, skin, and nervous system.

Diagnostic Tests

Although routine laboratory evaluations usually do not reveal any consistent diagnostic abnormalities, it is essential to rule out other nonoccupational diseases through a comprehensive history, review of previous records, and appropriate diagnostic studies. The presence of asthma and/or allergic disorders should be considered carefully and an appropriate workup undertaken. A few patients may have increased airway responsiveness and develop symptoms of chest tightness or shortness of breath on exposure to low-level environmental contaminants. Pulmonary function testing with nonspecific airway challenge testing may be indicated depending on history and symptoms. As suggested by the clinical history, confirmatory serologic and/or skin testing for common aeroallergens may be useful. If contact dermatitis is suspected, diagnostic level IV patch testing should be performed.

If a focal neurologic defect is suggested by history or physical examination, additional neurodiagnostic testing may be indicated. One patient with symptoms of altered odor sensitivity was found to have papilledema and a visual-field defect and was determined to have a treatable occipital lobe meningioma. Single-photon-emission computed tomographic or positron-emission tomographic studies of brain perfusion, computerized electroencephalographic analysis, or visual-evoked response and brain stem auditory-evoked response have not revealed consistent neurotoxic or neuroimmunologic brain changes in patients with MCS and should be used primarily to confirm clinical findings.

Additional psychological evaluation should be considered if the history suggests the presence of significant psychiatric disorder. Psychiatric consultation and/or treatment may be advised regardless of the etiology of MCS because many patients may have significant psychiatric morbidity with this disorder. Caution is advised in the interpretation of neuropsychological test results because these techniques are very sensitive but not specific. Abnormal test results could be a result of a neurologic, medical, or neuropsychiatric disorder. Neuropsychological studies have not shown significant differences between MCS patients and controls on tests of verbal learning, memory functioning, and psychomotor performance.

The capsaicin inhalation test has been used to assess sensory hyperreactivity in patients with MCS, but this test is not widely available for routine use, and its correlation with symptoms and response to treatment has not been confirmed. There is no convincing evidence that MCS is caused by a disturbance of heme synthesis, and tests for porphyrin metabolism in blood, urine, or stool specimens have not been correlated with clinical symptoms.

Several controversial techniques have been employed for the diagnosis of MCS, including provocation-neutralization testing, chemical and food challenges, inhalant challenges, serologic testing for Epstein-Barr virus antibodies and various autoantibodies, blood testing for organic hydrocarbon and pesticides, and hair testing for heavy metals. Many of these tests have no diagnostic utility. There is no evidence linking MCS to past infection with the Epstein-Barr virus. There is no association between MCS and levels of organic hydrocarbons or pesticides in blood or fatty tissue, and knowledge of minute residues of these chemicals may serve only to mislead and alarm the patient. The use of biomarkers (e.g., detailed profiles in serum of lipid-soluble toxins and their metabolites or heavy metals in the hair matrix) have no role in the diagnosis of patients with MCS. These tests have not been correlated with any pathologic consequences in MCS or control groups.

Blinded provocation testing has been employed in research studies but has not been evaluated rigorously as a useful diagnostic technique for individual patients. Immunologic testing has not been shown to be diagnostic for specific chemical exposure or associated illness.

In the absence of other concurrent medical conditions suggested by history, physical examination, or routine laboratory testing, the diagnosis of MCS relies on the patient's history of multiple symptoms triggered by low-level chemical exposures.

Treatment

Patients with MCS should be advised that, as with a chronic illness, treatment is not directed at a "cure" but rather at accommodation. Care should emphasize relief of symptoms and a return to active work and home life. These treatment strategies entail a treatment alliance between patient and clinician without judgment regarding the etiology of MCS. Ethnographic studies have shown that many MCS patients manage their symptoms through a combination of prevention/avoidance, detoxification, and emotional self-care. In addition to symptoms and the ongoing difficulty in living with this condition, social relationships and daily life may be affected greatly. For some individuals, education regarding general principles of toxicology (e.g., routes of exposure of toxic chemicals and routes of elimination) may be reassuring if they are concerned about long-term storage of chemicals in the body and the fear of ongoing damage. Elimination of exposures at home, workplace, or school through a variety of strategies (including room air filters) often is implemented by patients. In one case series of MCS patients from an occupational health practice, improvement in symptoms was associated with self-reported avoidance of specific substances or materials. Two of the three most highly rated treatments as reported by a large series of MCS patients were creating a chemical-free living space and chemical avoidance. While many patients report empirical improvement of symptoms, avoidance of low-level irritants has not been tested in controlled scientific studies. In some patients, avoidance may reinforce the notion of disability and lead to further isolation, powerlessness, and discouragement.

Although it is not clear whether psychological symptoms are the cause of MCS or simply accompany the diagnosis, specific cognitive and behavioral interventions may be most useful in the treatment of MCS. A biopsychosocial model of illness conceptualizes a close correlation between physical and psychological diseases. MCS may be a heterogeneous disorder with more than one causal mechanism. Significant psychophysiologic symptoms may occur after exposure to low-level volatile compounds in persons with and without coexisting or preexisting psychiatric illness. Similar to techniques used in other functional syndromes, behavioral strategies such as response prevention,

systemic desensitization, graduated exercise regimens, and progressive relaxation may help patients to regain normal activities, minimize role impairment, and curtail sick behaviors.

Improving the patient's understanding of the role of stress on illness and enhancing coping mechanisms for the impact on daily life may be helpful. Biofeedback-assisted relaxation training and cognitive restructuring have been reported with some success in MCS patients. Treatments with demonstrated efficacy in panic disorder also may be of benefit in MCS, and conversely, treatments that reinforce anticipatory anxiety and avoidance behavior may be detrimental.

Pharmacologic treatment for specific symptoms suggestive of depression or anxiety, in conjunction with other behavioral techniques, may offer some relief as part of an overall treatment program. In addition, antidepressants sometimes alleviate somatic symptoms (particularly pain and insomnia) and may improve the functional status of some MCS patients. One case report demonstrated dramatic improvement in a patient with MCS who received a selective serotonin reuptake inhibitor.

Patients in whom panic responses may be at least a contributing factor to symptoms might be responsive to intervention with psychotherapy to enable their desensitization or deconditioning of responses to odors or other triggers. These patients also may be helped by anxiolytic medications, relaxation training, and counseling for stress management.

A number of controversial methods have been used for the treatment of MCS, including elimination or rotary diversified diets, vitamins or nutritional supplements, oxygen, antifungal and antiviral agents, thyroid hormone supplement, supplemental estrogen or testosterone, transfer factor, chemical detoxification through exercise and sauna treatment, intravenous gamma-globulin, and intracutaneous or subcutaneous neutralization. A specially designed chemical-free environmental control unit has been used as a method to decrease blood pesticide levels and improve symptoms as well as intellectual and cognitive function. Controversial treatment methods offer hope of improvement to many individuals with MCS, and some patients do report symptom improvement over time. Many of these treatment methods are expensive and rarely are covered by health insurance. These treatment methods have not been validated through carefully designed, controlled trials, may have unwanted side effects, and may serve to reinforce counterproductive behaviors. Patients should be advised that such treatments are controversial, have not been subject to controlled clinical trials, and are not recommended by most medical professional organizations.

Follow-up studies indicate that up to half of MCS patients may improve over a period of years, but the majority continue to remain symptomatic with a major impact on career, marriage or family and other common daily activities.

REFERENCES

American College of Occupational and Environmental Medicine: Evidence-based statements: *Multiple Chemical Sensitivities: Idopathic Environmental Intolerance,* www.acoem.org/guidelines/article.asp?ID=46.

Caress SM, Steinemann AC: Prevalence of multiple chemical sensitivities: A population-based study in the southeastern United States. Am J Public Health 2004;94;746 [PMID: 15117694].

Hausteiner C et al: Self-reported chemical sensitivity in Germany: A population-based survey. Int J Hyg Environ Health 2005; 208:271 [PMID: 16078641].

Richardson RD, Engel CC Jr: Evaluation and management of medically unexplained physical symptoms. Neurologist 2004;10;18 [PMID: 1472031].

National Institute for Environmental Health Sciences: Health topics: *Multiple Chemical Sensitivities Syndrome,* http://www.niehs.nih.gov/external/faq/mcss.htm.

Occupational Safety and Health Administration: Safety and health topics, www.osha.gov/SLTC/multiplechemicalsensitivities/index.html.

Disease Surveillance Systems

Ana María Osorio, MD, MPH, & Peggy Reynolds, PhD, MPH

This chapter presents an overview of surveillance systems dealing with diseases related to occupational or environmental exposures. The use of population-based disease surveillance systems is an increasingly cost-effective means for investigating initial concerns about human health effects from workplace or environmental hazardous agents or for initial identification of unusual patterns of morbidity or mortality. The various kinds of surveillance systems currently available offer a wide variety of opportunities to both better understand the patterns of disease occurrence and plan for primary and secondary disease-control measures. Surveillance, medical monitoring, and the components of a surveillance system are discussed. Information is presented about how to classify a diagnosis of environmental or occupational intoxication, formulate a case definition, and investigate potential disease outbreaks. Examples illustrate current surveillance for environmental and occupational disease. This information should assist individuals seeking to develop a surveillance system, to evaluate an existing system, or to gain a better understanding of data derived from these types of systems.

DEFINITIONS

The National Centers for Disease Control and Prevention (CDC) provides the following definition:

> Public health surveillance is the ongoing systematic collection, analysis, interpretation and dissemination of data about a health-related event for use in public health action to reduce morbidity and mortality and to improve health.

Different attributes need to be considered in line with the overall goals of the system: monitoring of health outcomes versus hazardous exposures, collecting information for a general population versus medical monitoring of a workforce, systems that focus on just environmental or occupational health conditions, and case ascertainment which may include active collection of health data and/or passive receipt of case reports.

In recent years, the threat of terrorism and emerging diseases (such as SARS) have created expectations for public health surveillance to provide timely detection of outbreaks. *Syndromic surveillance* refers to the systematic gathering and analysis of prediagnostic health data to rapidly detect clusters of symptoms and health complaints suggestive of an infectious disease outbreak or other public health threat.

For the purposes of this review, *surveillance* refers to the ongoing standardized system of data collection, analysis, interpretation, dissemination, and where appropriate, follow-up intervention for a given health outcome (in this case, environmental or occupational disease). Public health surveillance systems are used for planning, implementing, and evaluating public health intervention and control programs, as well as hypothesis-generating studies that may lead to more in-depth epidemiologic research. In some situations, *registry* may be used instead of the term *surveillance system* (e.g., cancer registry). On a smaller scale, certain components of a surveillance system may be applied to a specific workplace or community population (which is in the form of a medical monitoring program). In addition, all surveillance systems should be reviewed periodically to ensure their optimal performance and usefulness. Examples of both environmental and occupational disease surveillance will be discussed.

REFERENCES

CDC: Updated guidelines for evaluating public health surveillance systems, www.cdc.gov/mmwr/preview/mmwr/rr5013a1.htm.

CDC: Framework for evaluating public health surveillance systems for early detection of outbreaks, www.cdc.gov/mmwr/preview/mmwr/rr5305a1.htm.

COMPONENTS OF A SURVEILLANCE SYSTEM

Surveillance systems are developed for a target health event of public health importance. Characteristics of such target illnesses or injuries may include incidence rate (for acute illness), severity of health effect, preventability, effective interventions, associated disparities or inequities associated with affected population, societal cost of an untreated health event, and public interest. The following items constitute the key components of a public health disease surveillance system.

- *Objectives of system.* These objectives may include detection of disease outbreaks, monitoring of trends, generation of hypotheses about disease etiology, development of research studies, and evaluation of intervention efforts.
- *Case definition.* The definition usually will include details on person, time, and place characteristics that will designate an individual as a confirmed surveillance case. These factors may include pesticide exposure history, geographic coverage, time period, clinical symptoms, physical findings, laboratory results, and environmental sampling. It should be noted that a surveillance case definition may not require the same degree of diagnostic information as that of a clinical diagnosis of a patient.
- *Organized flow of information.* Figure 44–1 provides an example of a surveillance system flow diagram.
- *Population under surveillance.* This may include the geographic area or defined workforce covered by the reporting system.
- *Time period for data collection.* Surveillance may be an ongoing system or set up for a finite period.
- *Data collection.* Type of case information being collected.
- *Data sources.* Identified case-reporting sources.
- *Data management.* This includes confidentiality, records management, data storage, and system security procedures.
- *Analytic methods.* Procedures for analyzing surveillance data.
- *Reporting of findings.* Periodic publication of surveillance data, such as an annual report.
- *Dissemination plan.* Procedures for getting the surveillance information to the key stakeholder groups.
- *Evaluation plan.* This includes assessment of simplicity and ease of operations, flexibility in responding to changing conditions or informational needs, acceptability by participating groups (e.g., medical community), sensitivity and predictive value positive (Table 44–1), representativeness of data in comparison with what is known of the target population and health event under study, timeliness of individual components and overall system, and stability of the system over time.

REFERENCE

CDC: Updated guidelines for evaluating public health surveillance systems, www.cdc.gov/mmwr/preview/mmwr/rr5013a1.htm.

INFORMATIONAL SOURCES FOR CASE ASCERTAINMENT

Understanding the utility as well as limitations of the various sources used for identification of cases is critical in disease surveillance. Table 44–2 illustrates the relative degree of diagnostic confirmation and population-based information associated with typical case-report sources.

Vital Records

The most prevalent source of health outcome information is vital records. Registration of basic birth and death information is available for local, national, and international populations. Information on causes of death is categorized by a general coding system, the International Classification of Diseases (ICD). Basic demographic information is collected on newborns and their parents and on decedents. These data have the advantage of being population-based and standardized within certain minimum parameters. In summary form, the data can provide valuable initial impressions on regional variations and secular trends in patterns of population change and mortality. They can be useful for looking at broad measures of adverse reproductive outcomes or cause-specific mortality. Although they have the advantage of broad coverage, vital records data typically have the disadvantage of a lack of detailed information on diseases of interest and provide rather indirect evidence for the actual incidence of most disease endpoints. While some vital records systems contain information on multiple causes of death, most are restricted to underlying cause-of-death information. As such, they provide a good indirect tool for measuring incidence trends in diseases with high case fatality rates (such as lung cancer) but do not provide good descriptive information on incidence for diseases associated with good survival.

Hospital Records

Institutional sources of targeted morbidity information are commonly available for special purposes. Hospitals typically maintain a diagnostic index or discharge summary that reflects the census of inpatients by presenting conditions for a particular period of time. In some cases, this information is aggregated for a broad geographic area to reflect the pattern of hospitalizations across institutions. Information from such sources serves as a valuable planning tool for within-institution resource allocation or for characterizing some between-institution differences. This information also may serve as an indicator or early-warning sign for health outcomes of special concern. It does not, however, provide a broad view of morbidity for the population of interest. Hospital discharge data may provide valuable insights into the profile of clientele and service needs. For many conditions, however, discharge data tend to represent the extremes or episodes of illness severe enough to require hospital admission. This information also may include multi-

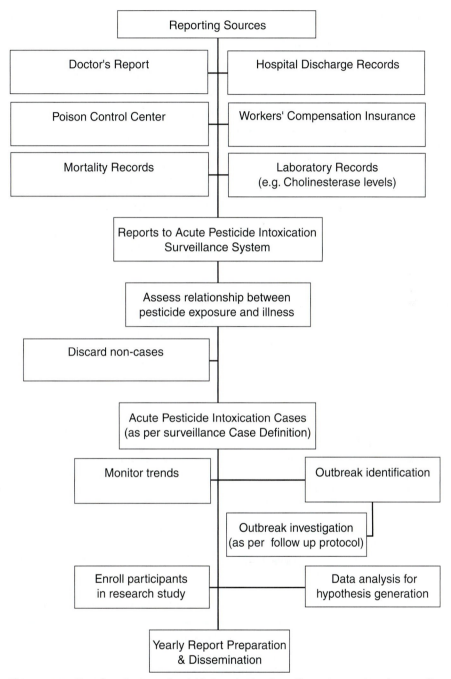

Figure 44–1. Flowchart for Acute Pesticide Intoxication Surveillance System. Need to specify target population, geographic area, and time period. Overall system should be reevaluated every 2 years.

Table 44–1. Analysis of sensitivity[1] and predictive value positive (PVP)[2] for a disease surveillance system. The sensitivity measures how well the surveillance case reflects the number of true cases in the target population. On the other hand, the PVP identifies the degree to which a surveillance case represents a true case.

	True API Case	True Noncase	Total
Surveillance API case	A	B	A + B
Surveillance noncase	C	D	C + D
Total	A + C	B + D	A + B + C + D

Abbreviation: API = acute pesticide intoxication.
[1]Sensitivity of case reporting = A/(A + C).
[2]Predictive value positive (PVP) = A/(A + B).

ple case reports of the same individual with recurrent episodes of illness rather than a unique hospital discharge for a patient. Unique personal identifiers for each case may not be available owing to confidentiality issues. These data may better reflect the urgent care needs of a small subgroup rather than the incidence or prevalence of diseases of interest.

Workplace Records

Some employers maintain medical monitoring information on their employees. This information reflects anything from voluntary use of in-house medical services for minor ailments to mandatory injury and disease reporting for certain events of interest to the company. Also, some employers offer medical screening programs for various conditions that may be more prevalent because of certain occupational hazards or simply as part of a larger workplace wellness program. Some of the workplace medical screening results are used for regional surveillance systems. For example, mandatory reporting of blood lead testing by physicians and laboratories occurs in various state-run lead intoxication surveillance programs.

Other Sources

In addition to hospital discharge data or a hospital's diagnostic index, there are a number of other sources of administrative data that can facilitate health studies. These include pharmacy databases, health care maintenance organization records, and other large-scale medical care programs that serve targeted populations such as the U.S. Centers for Medicare and Medicaid Services (CMS, formerly Federal Health Care Financing for the Aged) or various state-based Medicare programs. Although these programs are designed for medical delivery rather than research, they also can serve as valuable resources for health care research and other types of epidemiologic investigation. To a limited extent and for specific subgroups, such sources of information may serve as the source for integrated socialized health care information for some European countries. Although the health outcome information may be limited, these programs are virtually population-based for identified groups and can form the basis for preliminary indicators of health patterns or for selection into more in-depth studies. For example, in case-control studies of cancer, the HCFA files (which include individuals older than age 64 years) are used commonly to identify potential population-based controls in older age groups much more cost-efficiently than other procedures such as random-digit dialing. These databases also can be used to examine purely ecologic associations. Information on trends for sales of the conjugated estrogen Premarin in the 1970s was temporally associated with an epidemic of endometrial cancer in postmenopausal women in California. Increased use of screening mam-

Table 44–2. Different types of information used in disease surveillance systems.

Diagnostic Confirmation	Population-Based Data	
	No	Yes
Low	• Workplace medical monitoring • Lead screening programs	• Vital records • Health administrative data bases • Pesticide illness reporting
High	• Hospital discharge records	• Communicable disease reporting • Cancer registries • AIDS registries • Birth defects surveillance registries

mography during the late 1980s was associated with an increased incidence of early-stage breast cancer. Both these ecologic associations were demonstrated later to be consistent with the evidence from more in-depth case-control and cohort studies.

REFERENCE

CDC: Health topic: Surveillance resources, www.cdc.gov/health/surv_resources.htm.

EXAMPLES OF DISEASE SURVEILLANCE SYSTEMS

Acute Pesticide Intoxication Surveillance

California has required physician reporting of pesticide illnesses since 1971. *Pesticide* is defined as any substance that controls pests such as insects, fungi, weeds, rodents, nematodes, algae, viruses, bacteria, or adjuvants (substances added to enhance the efficacy of pesticides). Physicians are required to report any suspected case of pesticide-related illness or injury by telephone to the local health officer within 24 hours of examining the patient. Data sources for the Pesticide Illness Surveillance Program include (1) the Pesticide Illness Report filled out by the health officer receiving the doctor's case report, (2) the Doctors' First Report of Occupational Illness and Injury, which is required for workers' compensation claims, and (3) the California Poison Control System, whereby poison-control staff fill out a case report for physicians calling for assistance with a pesticide case.

The county agricultural commissioner is responsible for the investigation of all pesticide exposure incidents in the commissioner's geographic area. Specialized state-based laboratories provide analytic assistance for the pesticide exposure investigations. Criteria are used to indicate a high-priority incident needing immediate attention: human health effects (e.g., death, hospitalized cases, or episode with five or more medically diagnosed illness), special incidents (e.g., involvement of neighboring states or Mexico), environmental effects (e.g., special air, water, animal, and land contamination scenarios), and property loss or damage (e.g., depending on extent of financial loss). Yearly summary reports are produced that highlight important investigative findings.

Table 44-3 illustrates results from 4 years of acute pesticide intoxications (API) surveillance, 2000–2003. There were 3627 cases evaluated as being pesticide-related, with 99 (2.7%) hospitalizations and 13 (0.3%) deaths. Most of the cases presented with systemic symptoms (64.3%) and involved occupational exposures (72.8%). The two most frequent activities at the time of exposure were pesticide application (18.5%) and field work (14.9%).

For the period 1982–1998, the most common pesticides involved in occupational episodes were sodium hypochlorite, chlorine, and chlorpyrifos (for systemic effects) and sodium hypochlorite, quaternary ammonia, and propargite (for eye and dermal effects) (Table 44-4). The nonoccupational cases had metam-sodium as the most common pesticide exposure, partly as a consequence of a large environmental outbreak.

Because of the broad scope and long duration of this surveillance system, the API database has been used extensively in health policy development, rule making, research, risk assessment, intervention programs, and evaluation efforts. Several problems exist that potentially may cause underreporting of certain API cases: lack of physician recognition of APIs, subtle and early manifestations of API may not cause an individual to seek medical care, some residents or workers lack medical insurance and do not seek medical care until severe symptoms develop, some residents or workers lack residency documents and do not feel empowered to complain about health problems or seek medical care, some individuals are binational and receive medical attention in their native country (e.g., Mexico), and the migratory nature of some individuals does not allow follow-up or continuity of medical care, which would aid in the medical diagnosis of more subtle or chronic disease. With respect to the surveillance system, some question the strictness of the case definition that may discard some cases that may be true APIs, language and cultural barriers at the employer, medical community and surveillance staff level that may pose a problem in light of the diverse population in California (especially among high-risk groups), and the fact that some of the nonpriority investigations take a long time to be initiated, which may compromise the data collection.

In addition to California, 11 other states have API monitoring activity: Arizona, Florida, Iowa, Louisiana, Massachusetts, Michigan, New Mexico, New York, Oregon, Texas, and Washington. The National Institute for Occupational Safety and Health (NIOSH), in collaboration with the Environmental Protection Agency (EPA), provides funds to 8 of these states and coordinates standardization of data collection and reporting among all 12 states.

REFERENCES

California Department of Pesticide Regulation, Worker Health and Safety Branch, www.cdpr.ca.gov/docs/whs/whs_hoempage.htm

CDC, NIOSH: Pesticide Illness and Injury Surveillance, www.cdc.gov/niosh/topics/pesticides/.

Kass DE et al: Devloping a comprehensive pesticide helath effects tracking system for an urban setting. Environ Health Perspect 2004;112:1419 [PMID: 15471736].

Table 44–3. Selected data from the California Pesticide Illness Surveillance Program for the period 2000–2003.

Year	2000	2001	2002	2003	1997–1999 Period (% of Total Cases)
Total reports received	1104	979	1859	1232	5214
Pesticide-related cases[1]	893	616	1316	802	3627
Number of men	494	375	665	450	1984 (54.7)
Category of cases[1]					
Definite/probable	637	430	1025	614	2706 (74.6)
Possible	256	186	291	188	921 (25.4)
Hospitalizations	36	29	25	9	99 (2.7)
Fatalities					
Suicides	5	0	0	4	9 (0.2)
Unintentional	0	0	3	1	4 (0.1)
Health effects of cases					
Systemic	503	284	592	302	1681 (46.3)
Respiratory	103	103	221	141	568 (15.7)
Dermal/ocular	288	229	503	359	1379 (38.0)
Circumstances of exposure[2]					
Agricultural exposure	417	192	702	405	1716 (47.3)
Occupational setting	656	408	1025	553	2642 (72.8)
Selected activities among occupationally exposed					
Pesticide application	175	132	168	196	671 (18.5)
Field work	161	57	240	81	539 (14.9)
Mixing/loading pesticides	54	52	69	65	240 (6.6)
Packaging/processing	42	11	137	18	208 (5.7)
Transport/storage/disposal	28	23	19	14	84 (2.3)
Emergency response	10	10	5	12	37 (1.0)
Manufacturing/formulation	2	3	5	3	13 (0.3)

[1]Pesticide-related indicates that the relationship between pesticide exposure and resulting symptoms was one of the following:

Definite—High degree of correlation with both medical evidence (e.g., cholinesterase inhibition, positive allergy test, signs observed by clinician) and physical evidence of exposure (e.g., environmental or biological samples and exposure history).

Probable—Relatively high degree of correlation with either medical or physical evidence being inconclusive or unavailable.

Possible—Some degree of correlation with both medical and physical evidence inconclusive or unavailable.

[2]Categories not mutually exclusive.

Osorio AM: Surveillance systems for pesticide intoxications. Int J Occup Environ Health 2002;8:1 [PMID: 11843434].

Cancer Registries

Early concerns about basic public health disease control gave rise to legally mandated population-based reporting requirements for targeted infectious diseases. For noninfectious diseases, the best-established model for such systems has come from population-based cancer registries. These were primarily voluntary reporting systems, but in recent years, many local governments have enacted mandatory cancer-reporting requirements similar to those for infectious diseases. In the United States, population-based cancer registration dates back to 1935 when the Connecticut Tumor Registry initiated a surveillance system for all newly diagnosed malignancies among residents of the state. The Con-

Table 44–4. List of pesticides associated with at least 100 acute pesticide intoxication cases identified by the California Pesticide Illness Surveillance Program, 1982–1998. These cases were determined to be definitely, probably, or possibly related to pesticide exposure.[1]

| | Occupational Setting | | | | |
| | Systemic | | Eye/Skin | | |
Pesticide	Definitive/Probable	Possible	Definite/Probable	Possible	Total
Sodium hypochlorite	847	243	1711	215	3016
Sulfur	118	114	326	492	1050
Quaternary ammonia	46	30	717	64	857
Chlorine	531	99	98	75	803
Chlorpyrifos	341	289	113	44	787
Propargite	19	20	490	150	679
Glyphosate	32	76	354	152	614
Diazinon	188	167	65	29	449
Malathion	187	104	40	18	349
Glutaraldehyde	87	22	205	17	331
Propetamphos	156	82	8	4	250
Cyanuric acid	68	13	142	23	246
Methyl bromide	66	55	86	10	217
Metam-sodium	103	20	71	18	212
Methomyl	94	69	20	22	205
Phenolic disinfectants	15	10	153	16	194
Aluminum phosphide	100	47	6	28	181
Calcium hypochlorite	71	19	69	10	169
Parathion	75	69	9	5	158
Mevinphos	74	68	10	5	157
Cyfluthrin	89	28	11	16	144
Dimethoate	78	35	17	10	140
Propoxur	55	46	28	8	137
Creosote	8	2	82	27	119
Paraquat	15	25	59	13	112
	Nonoccupational Setting				
	Systemic		Eye/Skin		
Pesticide	Definitive/Probable	Possible	Definite/Probable	Possible	Total
Metam-sodium	341	83	54	2	480
Diazinon	73	39	4	10	126
Chlorpyrifos	57	60	3	1	121
Malathion	87	22	9	1	119
Chlorine	94	12	8	0	114

[1]Strength of relationship between pesticide exposure and resulting symptoms:

Definite—High degree of correlation with both medical evidence (e.g., cholinesterase inhibition, positive allergy test, signs observed by clinician) and physical evidence of exposure (e.g., environmental or biologic samples and exposure history).

Probable—Relatively high degree of correlation with either medical or physical evidence being inconclusive or unavailable.

Possible—Some degree of correlation with both medical and physical evidence inconclusive or unavailable.

Table 44–5. Age-adjusted Surveillance Epidemiology and End Results (SEER) incidence and death rates for United States (years 1995–1999 by primary cancer site and gender). SEER data include reports from 13 participating areas: Alaska, Atlanta, Connecticut, Detroit, Hawaii, Iowa, Los Angeles, New Mexico, rural Georgia, San Francisco/Oakland, San Jose/Monterey, Seattle/Puget Sound, and Utah. Rates are per 100,000 residents and are age-adjusted to year 2000 U.S. standard population.

Cancer Site	Mortality		Incidence	
	Female	Male	Female	Male
Bones/joints	0.4	0.5	0.7	1.0
Breast	26.4	0.3	134.4	1.2
Digestive	37.0	60.3	75.2	111.2
Endocrine	0.8	0.8	11.7	4.8
Eye/orbit	0.1	0.1	0.6	0.9
Genital	16.7	30.8	50.7	180.2
Leukemia	5.8	10.2	9.4	15.9
Lymphoma	7.0	10.8	18.2	26.3
Mesothelioma	—	—	0.4	1.9
Myeloma	3.2	4.7	4.5	6.9
Nervous system + brain	3.7	5.6	5.3	7.6
Oral/pharynx	1.6	4.2	6.4	15.5
Respiratory	41.7	79.4	51.0	85.4
Skin[1]	2.2	5.3	15.4	24.2
Soft tissue[2]	1.2	1.5	2.4	3.5
Urinary	5.2	14.0	17.6	53.4

[1]Excludes basal and squamous cell skin cancers.
[2]Includes heart.

necticut Tumor Registry has been operating continuously since then and is one of the most valuable, and one of the only, sources of information for long-term cancer incidence trends.

Until the 1970s, the National Cancer Institute (NCI) conducted a series of national cancer surveys in targeted areas of the United States to assess patterns of incidence. During the same time, the NCI collected patient treatment and follow-up information from a series of hospitals throughout the country. These hospitals volunteered to contribute to the End Results Program, which formed the basis for information on differences in expected survival for various types of cancer. Following the Third National Cancer Survey (for the years 1969–1971), the NCI initiated an ongoing surveillance system that integrated elements of both the national surveys and the End Results Program. This program, called the Surveillance, Epidemiology and End Results (SEER) Program, collects and maintains an integrated system of information on newly diagnosed cancers, as well as on basic treatment and follow-up survival. Operating in several designated areas of the United States, the SEER system was not designed to be representative of the total population but rather to reflect the population diversity of the United States. SEER data come from 14 population-based cancer registries and three supplemental registries in the following states: Alaska, Arizona, California, Connecticut, Georgia, Hawaii, Iowa, Kentucky, Louisiana, Michigan, New Jersey, New Mexico, Utah, Washington, and the Commonwealth of Puerto Rico. Currently, the SEER Program covers approximately 26% of the U.S. population and is the primary basis for national statistics on cancer incidence and survival. By the end of 2002, the database contained more than 3.2 million in situ and invasive cancer cases, with some diagnoses dating from 1973. Annually, approximately 170,000 new cases are added from the areas covered by the registries.

Table 44–5 provides an overview of cancer rates by organ system for the most recent time period from the SEER Program. During the period 1998–2002 in the United States, the primary cancer site with the highest incidence rate for males was prostate (173.8 per 100,000) and for females was breast (134.4 per 100,000). In contrast, lung cancer was the primary cancer site with the highest mortality rate for both genders (males: 76.3 per 100,000; females: 40.9 per 100,000). Using a cancer thought to be largely caused by environmental/occupational exposures as an example, Figure 44–2 shows the incidence trend for invasive mesothelioma among men. This cancer is known to have a

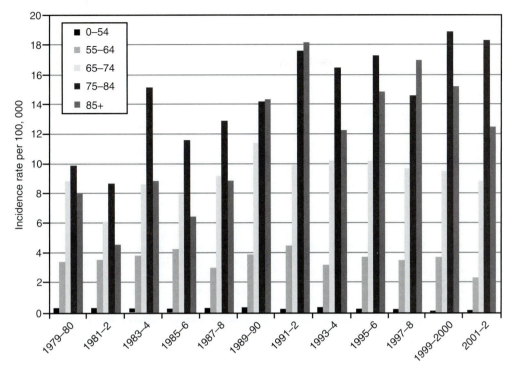

Figure 44–2. Age-adjusted Surveillance Epidemiology and End Results (SEER) incidence for invasive mesothelioma among men (years 1979–2002). Incidence rates are per 100,000 male residents and are age-adjusted to year 2000 U.S. standard population.

lengthy latency period of 20+ years between onset of exposure to asbestos and development of clinically detectable disease. There is a much lower incidence rate with relatively small variation for females for this same time period. For males, there is a striking increase in the incidence rate in the older age ranges, especially for those aged 55 years or older. In addition, there is an upward trend in the incidence over time. As men reached their fifth decade of life, sufficient time has elapsed from the original asbestos exposure in the workplace to allow the clinical manifestations of mesothelioma to become apparent. Subsequent cohorts of workers had increased exposure to asbestos, and this also may contribute to the increasing incidence rates across this time period.

The United States is not unique in supporting population-based cancer registration systems. Many countries throughout the world have done likewise, although many of those cancer reporting systems are not as old and not as detailed. The International Agency for Research on Cancer (IARC; formed in 1965 by the World Health Organization) has published a series of monographs of international incidence data called *Cancer Incidence in Five Continents*, which began in 1966

and was published by a predecessor organization, the International Union against Cancer. The latest monograph contains cancer information from 50 areas of the world. These monographs are designed to be representative, rather than comprehensive, of the world's populations and include data from registries that meet the IARC's standards of data quality. Over the last several decades, these monographs have been the single most valuable source of information on international variations in cancer incidence.

In the 1980s, there was a great deal of local interest in developing legislation to mandate statewide cancer registries throughout the United States and Canada. During this time, there was a rapid proliferation of population-based cancer reporting. By the late 1980s, the American Association of Central Cancer Registries, an organization of state and local cancer registries in the United States, was formed. This organization, now called the North American Association of Central Cancer Registries, plays an active role in setting data standards and establishing a minimal data set across registries and also has begun to generate summary data for its 72 U.S. and 12 Canadian registry members.

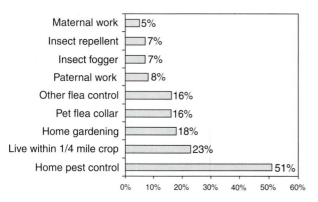

Figure 44–3. Percentage of women with pesticide exposure during pregnancy for case or comparison child in pesticide birth defects study. California Birth Defects Monitoring Program (*N* = 1299 cases and 734 comparison babies).

REFERENCES

CDC: National program of cancer registries, www.cdc.gov/cancer/npcr/.

IARC/WHO and International Association of Cancer Registries: *Cancer Incidence in Five Continents,* www.iacr.com.fr/statist.htm.

National Cancer Institute, SEER Cancer Statistics Review, http://seer.cancer.gov/csr/1975_2003/.

North American Association of Central Cancer Registries, www.naaccr.org/.

Birth Defects Surveillance

Approximately 1 in 33 babies born in the United States has a birth defect, but an individual type of defect is a rare event. Thus pooling of case-report information between registries is needed to study a given birth defect of interest. In 1996, Congress authorized CDC funding to establish "centers of excellence for birth defects prevention research." In addition to the Metropolitan Atlanta Congenital Defects Program at the CDC, there are research centers in Arkansas, California, Iowa, Massachusetts, New York, North Carolina, Texas, and Utah. The issues addressed by these centers include the expansion and improvement of existing birth defects surveillance systems, as well as participation in the National Birth Defects Prevention Study. This national multicenter collaboration is a case-control study of infants born with major congenital anomalies and includes assessment of both environmental and occupational exposures. Also, CDC funds other states or territories to improve the timeliness of the data collection and conduct intervention activities for major birth defects: Arizona, Colorado, Florida, Illinois, Michigan, Minnesota, New Hampshire, New Jersey, Ohio, Oklahoma, Puerto Rico, Rhode Island, Vermont, and Virginia.

One of the largest of these registries is in California. Using birth registration data (which provides the denominator for rates of birth defects), this registry has provided important descriptive and analytic information on the occurrence of a wide spectrum of birth defects. One example is a study dealing with pesticide-associated risk factors for birth defects in California. Researchers interviewed 1299 women with babies born with oral clefts, neural tube defects, conotruncal heart defects, or limb defects and 734 women with comparison babies lacking birth defects. Contact with pesticides during pregnancy was reported in 78% of the women interviewed, with residential pest-control activity being the most common type of exposure (Figure 44–3). Elevated risks were observed for oral clefts, neural tube defects, heart defects, and limb defects among women exposed to household gardening and neural tube defects among women living within a quarter mile of agricultural crops.

REFERENCES

California Birth Defects Monitoring Program, www.cbdmp.org.
CDC: Birth defects registry, www.cdc.gov/ncbddd/bd/bdsurv.htm.

ASSESSMENT OF RELATIONSHIP BETWEEN DISEASE AND EXPOSURE

Surveillance systems depend mostly on clinician reporting of cases, so it is critical for health care providers to diagnosis environmental and occupational illnesses accurately, especially the more readily detected acute intoxications. Because environmental and occupational exposures may be associated with nonspecific medical complaints (especially in the early stages of intoxication), it is very useful to link the traditional medical review of organ systems with an exposure history (see Chapter 2).

In evaluating the association between a given toxicant exposure or physical hazard in the occupational or environmental setting and an acute clinical condition, key questions to consider include

- Are the symptoms and physical signs appropriate for the exposure agent being considered?
- Are there coworkers or others in the surrounding environment who are ill (e.g., workplace, residence, school, neighborhood, and recreational areas)?

- Do the timing of the exposure episode and the onset of health problems make sense?
- Is there confirmation of physical exposure to the pesticide (e.g., history of activity with direct contact or exposure with agent, dermal residue sampling, proven agent contamination of work clothes or other personal protective equipment)?
- Is there any record of environmental monitoring data (e.g., bulk sampling, air, soil or water tests)?
- Is there any record of biologic monitoring results?
- What is the biologic plausibility of the resulting health effect given the exposure scenario?
- Can one rule out other nonagent exposures or preexisting health problems?

A concurrent nonagent exposure either can have no effect, can exacerbate, or can be the sole cause of the health condition under study. It is inappropriate to automatically eliminate occupational or environmental exposure as a possible contributory factor when underlying or concurrent nonpesticide exposures exist. Consultation with an occupational and environmental health specialist may be needed for patients with complicated mixed-exposure scenarios or multiple concurrent disease situations.

INVESTIGATION OF DISEASE CLUSTERS

An important activity associated with surveillance systems is the rapid identification and investigation of disease outbreaks or clusters. These investigations can be time-consuming and often require a team approach with various types of health and safety professionals. Thus a protocol usually is developed with action criteria for when a follow-up investigation should occur. The following outline covers the major steps involved in investigating a disease outbreak:

Medical Diagnosis

- Formulate a tentative medical diagnosis.
- Confirm diagnosis of identified cases.
- Review medical records (clinic, hospital, company).
- Review any biologic tests (e.g., blood, urine, or exhaled air testing or parent compound or metabolite).
- Review decontamination procedure for the patient, facility, and transport system.
- Consult with treating health care providers.

All these initial cases represent the group of "index cases."

Identify Unrecognized Cases

- Interview cases and other exposed individuals.
- If feasible, interview nonexposed individuals as possible comparison group.

- Interview health care providers at clinics and hospitals in area of outbreak to detect any other cases.
- If this is an occupational setting, then conduct interviews with coworkers, company management, and union representative (if unionized workforce). Also interview company medical care provider and determine whether any medical monitoring exists for the pesticide-exposed workers.

Case Definition

- Develop a working case definition that includes the following aspects: (a) exposure setting, that is, one or more suspected agents or high-risk activity, population group, location, and time period, (b) expected physical signs and symptoms, and (c) pertinent biologic or environmental tests. Table 44–6 contains an example of a case definition used for a recent pesticide intoxication outbreak in Central America.

Exposure Information

- Evaluate the following outbreak information: formulation and physical form of agent(s) involved, timing

Table 44–6. Example of a case definition used in a recent pesticide intoxication outbreak.

A case is defined as a farm worker who was present during a recent half-day application of a carbamate pesticide (Temik) at a banana plantation and who has one or more symptoms consistent with cholinesterase inhibition (see table below). For those workers receiving medical attention, reversibility of symptoms after atropine treatment provides confirmation for cholinesterase inhibition.

Category of Health Effect	Physical Signs and Symptoms
Early onset	Headache, nausea, dizziness, hypersecretion
More severe, later onset	Muscular twitch/fasciculations, weakness, tremor, incoordination, vomiting, abdominal cramps, diarrhea
Ocular	Miosis
Neuropsychiatric	Anxiety, restlessness, depression, memory loss, confusion, toxic psychosis
Respiratory	Bronchorrhea, bronchospasm, pulmonary edema, respiratory depression and arrest
Cardiovascular	Bradycardia and sinus arrest, tachycardia and hypertension, myocardiopathy
Advanced neurologic	Loss of consciousness, incontinence, convulsions

Table 44–7. Example of a line listing of subjects for an outbreak investigation among banana workers involved in pesticide applications. All exposed workers were male and of Hispanic origin. Backpack application of Temik (a carbamate nematocide) occurred for approximately 5 hours partly during heavy rains.

Name	Age	Job Title	Onset of Symptoms	Symptoms (Sx)	Treatment	Activity at Time of Exposure	PPE Use[1]
Worker 1	27	Backpack applicator	End of application	Dizzy, weak, diarrhea, vomiting	Atropine response, hospital × 1 day	Applying Temik	Yes
Worker 2	21	Backpack applicator	30 minutes after application ended	Severe headache	None	Applying Temik	Yes
Worker 3	31	Backpack applicator	Within 1 hour of end of application	Dizzy, weak, diarrhea, nausea, vomiting	Atropine response, hospital × 1 day	Applying Temik	Unknown
Worker 4	24	Backpack applicator	Within 1 hour of end of application	Dizzy, anorexia, abdominal pain, diarrhea	Atropine response, hospital × 1 day	Applying Temik	Unknown
Worker 5	Unknown	Backpack applicator	Within 1 hour of end of application	Nausea	Observed in emergency room for approximately 5 hours	Applying Temik	Unknown
Worker 6	Unknown	Backpack applicator	Within 1 hour of end of application	Nausea	Observed in emergency room for approximately 5 hours	Applying Temik	Unknown
Workers 7–15	Approximately 20–40	Backpack applicator	No symptoms reported	No symptoms reported	None reported	Applying Temik	Unknown

[1]Personal protective equipment (PPE) used by worker included boots, overalls, cartridge mask, and gloves.

and duration of exposure, delivery system, personal protective equipment used, weather conditions, and general circumstances of the exposure event.

- Determine how many individuals were involved (include those directly and indirectly exposed).
- Inspect any machine/apparatus used, original containers and labels or material data safety sheets, and personal protective equipment, if available.
- Review any past exposure or biologic monitoring records and environmental sampling results.

Characterize Cases

- Create a listing of index cases, additional cases, and exposed individuals. Table 44–7 illustrates the line listing created for the banana worker outbreak example.

Epidemic Curve

- Plot out the incidence on a graph comparing number of cases versus time of symptom onset (Figure 44–4).

Dose-Response Relationship

- Determine severity of cases and compare with intensity of exposure. In this way, one can determine whether a dose-response relationship exists (cases with higher levels of exposure also have a more severe clinical presentation).

Incidence Rate

- Derive an incidence rate for the outbreak: (Number of cases/number of individuals exposed) × 100. In the case of the banana worker episode, the incidence rate is 40% [(6/15) × 100]. Even if one only accepts cases that were reported by clinicians, the incidence rate is still quite high at 33.3% [(5/15) × 100].
- Finally, one can compare the outbreak incidence with the general population incidence and conduct a test for statistical significance to assess whether this elevated rate is likely to be real or a chance result.

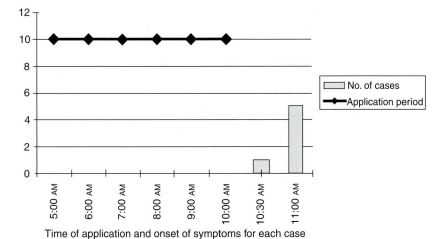

Figure 44–4. Epidemic curve for banana worker outbreak (6 cases per 15 exposed workers).

Report with Recommendations for Intervention

Summarize all the information gathered during the investigation in a report and present to all key stakeholders (e.g., workers, community residents, company representatives, medical community, and governmental agencies). This report should state clearly the extent of the disease, the etiologic factors, and how to prevent or control the present exposure situation, as well as make recommendations for ways to prevent such episodes in the future. While all individuals evaluated should receive their personal test results, one needs to ensure that all public reports and communications with stakeholders maintain the confidentiality of the participants.

Cluster investigations for chronic disease (e.g., cancer) may follow a slightly different evaluation process. Many state and local health departments respond to inquiries regarding potential disease clusters. Only approximately 5–15% of the reported clusters result in a statistically elevated cancer rate. Even in these situations, it is usually not possible to ascertain the causative exposure owing to the latency problem and the long time that prior exposure would have occurred. Some examples where the difficulty in evaluating cancer clusters was overcome include scrotal cancer in chimney sweeps exposed to coal dust, osteosarcoma in watch radium painters, mesothelioma and lung cancer in asbestos workers, and hepatic angiosarcoma among chemical workers exposed to vinyl chloride.

EXPOSURE MONITORING

Although the focus has been on disease surveillance systems, there are population-based exposure monitoring programs that complement disease-based efforts. One example is the ongoing biomonitoring survey conducted by the National Center for Environmental Health within CDC. This program conducts exposure assessment by analyzing selected toxicants in biologic samples from the general population. The *Third National Report on Human Exposure to Environmental Chemicals* provides the latest findings of the ongoing assessment of 148 chemicals. One group of chemicals of great interest are the organophosphate insecticides and their urinary metabolites. The survey obtained urine samples from the National Health Nutrition and Examination Survey (NHANES) for the years 2001–2002. This survey is a continuous national sample of the U.S. population. NHANES conducts a standardized health interview, physical examination, and testing of biologic fluids. For organophosphates, the assessment included various urinary metabolites. Of interest is the metabolite indicative of chlorpyrifos and chlorpyrifos-methyl: 3,5,6-trichloro-2-pyridinol (TCP). While use is restricted in the home environment, chlorpyrifos and chlorpyrifos are still used extensively in agriculture (especially chlorpyrifos). In looking at the values in Table 44–8, there does not appear to be much difference in concentration by gender, but there is a threefold increase in child urinary levels as compared with adults. This finding was observed in both surveys and merits further study. This type of pesticide exposure trend at relatively modest levels in the population would only have been identified using the more precise biologic exposure assessments seen in the National Exposure Survey. This exposure tool promises to be a more precise assessment of population body burden than the usual measurement of pesticide sales or agricultural pesticide applications available in some states.

Table 44–8. Distribution of 3,5,6-trichloro-2-pyridinol urine concentrations (μg/g creatinine) for 1999–2000 and 2001–2002 National Health and Nutrition Examination Surveys of U.S. population aged 6–59 years. This analyte is the primary metabolite of chlorpyrifos and chlorpyrifos-methyl. Geometric means (GM) and 95% confidence intervals (CI) are provided.

	1999–2000 Survey			2001–2002 Survey		
Population	**GM (CI)**	**95th Percentile**	**Number of Samples**	**GM (CI)**	**95th Percentile**	**Number of Samples**
Total group	1.58 (1.35–1.85)	8.42	1994	1.73 (1.49–2.01)	9.22	2508
Age range						
6–11	3.11 (2.31–4.19)	14.0	481	3.48 (2.80–4.32)	16.9	573
12–19	1.60 (1.34–1.91)	6.16	681	2.09 (1.72–2.55)	10.3	822
20–59	1.41 (1.23–1.62)	6.42	832	1.49 (1.30–1.71)	7.44	1113
Gender						
Female	1.48 (1.27–1.72)	7.63	972	1.71 (1.47–2.00)	10.3	1183
Male	1.69 (1.42–2.01)	8.44	1022	1.75 (1.49–2.07)	8.98	1325

REFERENCES

CDC: *Third National Report on Human Exposure to Environmental Chemicals,* www.cdc.gov/exposurereport/3rd/.

Thun MJ et al: Understanding cancer clusters. CA Cancer J Clin 2004;54:273 [PMID: 15371285].

LINKAGE OF DISEASE DATA SETS

By themselves, disease surveillance systems serve an important function in providing descriptive information on the geographic/demographic scope and temporal changes in the occurrence of diseases. In combination with other sources of information on population groups defined geographically, occupationally, or with respect to some other common characteristics, surveillance also offers a powerful tool for better understanding the causes or natural history of disease.

Geographic Linkage

Disease registry information has been an important resource for better understanding of disease spatial patterns and as an important planning tool for secondary prevention programs. Population-based registries typically collect address information that can be geocoded to various levels of detail with geographic coverage ranging from state, county, Zip code, Census tract, or block group to actual real-world coordinates (provide information on the exact location of an event within a city block). The increasing availability of geographic-based reference information based on Census characteristics of the population, environmental exposure measures, physical geography, and increasingly sophisticated geographic information system (GIS) technology pro-

vides opportunities to evaluate patterns of disease in the context of a wide range of factors.

These tools provide the basis for ecologic studies of disease. These include studies that correlate differences in disease rates with such population characteristics as socioeconomic status or environmental characteristics such as land use. Well-known examples include general studies of the association of skin cancer rates with sunny climates or specific studies of various cancer types by the proportion of petrochemical industries by U.S. county. More recently, improvements in GIS methodology have allowed more detailed evaluation of differences in incidence rates for certain malignancies by geographic characteristics. For example, childhood cancer rates that vary between neighborhoods with different levels of exposure to various environmental hazards such as motor vehicle emissions or agricultural pesticide use. Such studies do not in themselves make a case for disease causation, but such observations can provide valuable evidence for developing hypotheses that can be tested in other, more complex study designs. Likewise, these tools have proved to be a valuable adjunct to studies of disease clusters or in evaluating the potential health impact of identified environmental hazards on the health of a community.

Ecologic studies are not new. They date back at least as far as John Snow's classic observations about the eight- to ninefold higher rate of cholera deaths among London residents served by the Southwark and Vauxhall water company in the mid-1800s. Inferences drawn from that observation led to swift public health intervention, removal of the Broad Street Pump handle, and the introduction of legislation requiring London water companies to filter their water. Notably, this occurred nearly 20 years *before* Koch's identification of the cholera vibrio.

Some of the simplest geographic studies are those that merely examine rate differences associated with other area differences and have served to stimulate active areas of epidemiologic enquiry. Studies that have reported the correlation of higher heart disease and breast cancer mortality rates in countries with higher levels of dietary fat consumption have provoked more sophisticated assessments of these associations. Studies that have noted striking international differences in stomach and colon cancer rates between Japan and the United States, with intermediate rates evident for migrant populations, have served as the basis for studies of the influence of diet and other cultural differences as possible risk factors for these gastrointestinal malignancies.

Occupational or Environmental Linkage

Occupational cohorts or other defined cohorts also can be linked to disease outcome registries. Such linked data sets have proved to be a valuable source of hypothesis generation for a variety of suspected exposure-disease relationships. A widely reported example is the Swedish Cancer Environment Registry, which has linked individual information on occupation and residence from the national 1960 census to 20 years of follow-up information from the population-based cancer registry and has provided extensive information on environmental, socioeconomic, and occupational risk factors for a variety of cancers. Sweden also maintains a linked registry between the national census data and its medical birth registry, which has formed the basis for studies of adverse reproductive outcomes among certain employment groups. A recent report from this linked registry suggested that infants born to mothers working in chemical industries experienced higher rates of several adverse outcomes, including low birth weight, short gestational age, and infant mortality.

Similarly linked national registers have been reported from Denmark and Great Britain. The Danish registry additionally has linked its census-cancer registry to more detailed work-history information from a variety of Danish industries, providing valuable background information for such major international efforts as the IARC's monograph series entitled the *Evaluation of Carcinogenic Risk to Humans.*

Linkage efforts such as these, which represent the full universe of a population at risk linked to a system of completely ascertained disease reporting, represent an ideal resource for preliminary evaluations of suspected risk associations. As a result, they are a first step in the search for causality. Provocative risk associations can be followed up in nested case-control studies with study subjects selected from a well-defined and well-characterized universe.

Although not all places offer such universal opportunities for evaluation, similar approaches have proved useful in the evaluation of cancer risks in cohorts of individuals selected in other ways, particularly in a wide spectrum of occupational cohorts in the United States. Such an approach was taken in the late 1970s when clinicians in the small California community of Livermore noted an apparently high frequency of malignant melanoma of the skin occurring in patients who were employees of the Lawrence Livermore National Laboratory (LLNL), a U.S. Department of Energy high-energy physics research facility in Livermore and a primary local employer. The LLNL medical staff was aware of some of the melanoma cases but was not sure how many additional cases there might have been nor how many might have been expected in the laboratory workforce, which consisted primarily of white men. Because the San Francisco Bay Area, including Livermore, was covered by population-based cancer registration, it was possible to use computerized linkage methods to match the historical LLNL employee roster with the cancer files to fully ascertain the number of melanomas occurring among members of the LLNL workforce. The number of observed cases was roughly four times that which would have been expected when compared with the same age, race, sex, and areas of residence of the laboratory employees. Furthermore, an analysis of adult melanoma rates in Livermore suggested that they were slightly higher than might be expected based on prevailing rates for the county but that when LLNL employees were removed from the numerator and denominator of the community rates, they were indistinguishable from rates elsewhere in the county. This initial evaluation was conducted fairly quickly because of the availability of the population-based cancer registry. Subsequent studies have been undertaken to evaluate the degree to which workplace or other factors may explain this apparent disease excess.

The most widely reported health outcomes in these studies have been cancers of various types. This is so because population-based cancer registries are more common than registries for other chronic disease outcomes, and incidence data are considered somewhat more reliable and relevant than mortality data. Nonetheless, similar approaches also have been reported for various adverse birth outcomes and, in some Scandinavian countries, even for registration of cardiovascular events.

REFERENCE

Boscoe FP et al: Current practices in spatial analysis of cancer data: Data characteristics and data sources for geographic studies of cancer. Int J Health Geograph 2004;3:28 [PMID: 15574197].

ADVANTAGES OF SURVEILLANCE SYSTEMS

Completeness of Ascertainment

A primary advantage of surveillance systems is that unlike the perceptions that may be developed based on patients from a given clinical practice, they provide an opportunity to evaluate the full spectrum of specific disease outcomes. Particularly in the case of population-based surveillance, great emphasis is placed on the ability to collect and maintain health outcome information for all members of a temporally and geographically defined population at risk.

Definition of Disease

Another advantage of disease surveillance systems is that they use explicit decision rules for disease classification. Cause-of-death information typically is coded centrally by a nosologist trained to use standard decision criteria for underlying and contributing causes of death noted on the death certificate. Cancer registries use specially trained tumor registrars to abstract and code diagnostic detail on newly identified cases, using standard criteria for malignancy, subsite distribution, and multiple primaries. While there may be many gray areas of definition within the medical community, most disease surveillance systems use documented consensus criteria that allow for comparisons across treatment facilities, states, or countries.

Secular Trends

Because disease surveillance systems use standard procedures for identifying and classifying a disease in a defined population, it is possible to examine changes in incidence, mortality, prevalence, or survival over time. Changes in the observed occurrence of various disease outcomes in hospital settings, for example, easily could be a function of changes in the institutional catchment area, referral patterns, or reimbursement criteria rather than changes in the underlying disease experience of the population. While changes in diagnostic conventions can affect both kinds of reporting systems, temporal correction factors can be applied to surveillance data.

Comparison Groups

Another particularly valuable contribution of population-based disease surveillance systems is the ability to compare health outcomes in subgroups of interest. Disease registries are a valuable tool in secondary prevention (disease control) and can provide an important early-warning signal when subgroups defined by age, race, sex, geography, or time demonstrate a disproportionate disease burden compared with normal levels in the general population. A study that first linked records from local acquired immunodeficiency syndrome (AIDS) and cancer surveillance systems in San Francisco provided valuable information on concerns about the trends in Kaposi sarcoma incidence

among the city's residents. This study also identified Hodgkin disease as another sentinel cancer for AIDS in young men.

LIMITATIONS OF SURVEILLANCE SYSTEMS

Behavioral Risk Factors

An important limitation of studies based on record linkage between a cohort and disease surveillance systems is the lack of individual risk factors that may mediate the apparent association between a suspected occupational or environmental risk factor and a specific disease outcome. For example, numerous studies suggest that a variety of blue-collar occupations are associated with a higher risk for lung cancer. But unless such studies are designed to adjust for the effect of active smoking, the apparent occupational associations are less convincing. Typically, personal risk factors are either unavailable or not available in sufficient detail in either cohort or surveillance files to be able to assess the role of such factors in record linkage studies.

The influence of some of these factors can be assessed indirectly by using external information sources. One approach is to use group attributes available at the Census tract or block group level to indirectly adjust for such effects. This approach is used commonly in geographic studies. A similar approach can be used by applying group summary information to other identifiable groups, such as an occupational cohort. This latter approach was used in a study of occupational mortality in California in which standardized mortality ratios were estimated for broad occupational categories, indirectly adjusting for smoking, alcohol consumption, and socioeconomic status. In addition, a linked exposure-outcome file can be used as the basis for selecting cases and controls from which to collect additional risk-factor information for follow-up studies.

In some areas, cancer registry programs have initiated a complementary risk-factor surveillance program to enhance the ability to evaluate potential risk associations for various cancers. The general approach is one of a random-digit dialing population survey for targeted risk factors of interest that can serve as a comparison group for specially collected information on cases in the registry. One well-known model for this type of program is from the Detroit Cancer Registry, which instituted a system of collecting occupational information from a community survey that then could be compared to occupational data from the registry. This occupational risk-factor surveillance system, in combination with occupational data collected by the cancer registration process, has provided some provocative evidence for higher risks for certain cancers in several occupational groups (e.g., cancer elevations among certain types of workers in Detroit's automotive industry). This is a cost-effective way to generate hypotheses that can be pursued in more in-depth studies of occupational risks for cancer.

Temporal/Geographic Associations

While the availability of computerized cohort and disease surveillance systems offers a marvelous opportunity for hypothesis generation about disease causation and identification of high-risk subgroups, inferences from such studies need to be interpreted cautiously with respect to the temporal association between exposure and disease. Because of the relative newness of most computerized population-based disease surveillance systems, particularly for long-latency diseases such as cancer, it has not been possible to evaluate apparent occupational or environmental associations with disease over as long a time period as may be desirable.

Similarly, because address information in surveillance systems typically represents location at the time of diagnosis, admission, or death, geographic information from such sources is limited and does not necessarily represent an individual's long-term residence. Importantly, address at the time of a health event, particularly in increasingly mobile populations, may be unlikely to represent locations associated with location at the time of significant exposure.

An important exception to these constraints is offered by the model of cancer-environment surveillance systems in some of the Scandinavian countries. In the case of the Swedish cancer-environment registry, in which 1960 census information on individuals was linked to persons diagnosed with cancer during a follow-up period (1961–1979), it was possible to evaluate differences in disease rates by occupational affiliation. This has been the source of a number of studies of occupational associations and cancer. Interestingly, it also has provided the basis for evaluating the degree to which childhood socioeconomic status (as defined by father's occupation) is a predictor of cancer risk in later life.

Confidentiality Concerns

While the use of disease surveillance systems provides the opportunity to better understand disease association risks, it raises special concerns about the confidentiality of the identity of individuals in each record system, especially those that involve linkage between a cohort and outcome file. These are important concerns, with the enabling legislation for most population-based disease surveillance systems including provisions for maintaining confidentiality. Because of the possible breach of confidentiality, many Scandinavian countries recently enacted strict restrictions on the uses of surveillance data that virtually preclude access to many potential investigators. With the increasing sophistication of geographic information system technology, the potential to identify individuals from characteristics associated with rare events at smaller levels of geographic detail also has caused concern. There are confidentiality concerns about mapped data presentation even when individual identities are unknown. Thus restrictions have been placed on precise geographic information for rare events in many public-use data sets derived from surveillance systems.

In 1996, the Health Insurance Portability and Accountability Act (HIPAA) was enacted. This regulation provides protection for personal health information (individually identifiable health data). Public health surveillance uses this type of information extensively. Detailed discussion of the applicability of HIPAA for public health practice is contained in a guidance document issued by the CDC, and information on this topic is found on the Department of Health and Human Services Web site (maintained by the Office of Civil Rights).

REFERENCES

CDC: HIPAA privacy rule and public health, www.cdc.gov/mmwr/preview/mmwr/m2e411a1.htm.

Department of Health and Human Services, Office of Civil Rights, www.hhs.gov/ocr/hipaa/.

Diagnostic/Treatment Detail

Typically, disease registries are designed to provide information that can guide primary treatment decisions and profile the incidence of disease occurrence. To do this, data must be collected with sufficient detail and accuracy to fully characterize the heterogeneity of broad classes of disease. Cancer registries, for example, collect detailed information on the anatomic subsite, cell type, laterality, and staging for most tumors. Quality-control procedures generally require a high percentage of histologic confirmation for diagnosis. Studies that have compared death certificate information on cancer type with that from registry data for decedents suggest that death certificates provide less reliable information on the type of cancer that may have been the underlying cause of death. For some cancers in particular, death certificate information may systematically misrepresent the distribution of underlying disease. Unfortunately, with the need for large-scale standardization, registries sometimes fall behind in the ability to characterize what may be considered state-of-the-art disease-specific markers. For cancer, these include important site-specific information such as microstaging for malignant melanoma or estrogen receptor status for breast malignancies.

CONCLUSION

Disease surveillance is not a new concept. Some idea of a defined population at risk and the incidence of disease in that population dates back to the earliest efforts to control the spread of infectious diseases. In more recent years, similar tools have been applied to understanding the scope of noninfectious diseases, particularly cancer. Vital records provide the most basic model for population-based disease surveillance. While hospital-based or occupation-based disease monitoring provide similarly useful information, population-based disease surveillance systems used in conjunction with geographic, occupational, or environmental information on defined cohorts of interest provide a less biased view of their underlying disease experience. Disease surveillance systems are somewhat limited by the breadth and depth of information on diagnostic detail and relevant risk factors. By virtue of their standards for completeness and consistency, however, they offer a valuable means for assessing important population variations in disease that can be used as the basis for designing more in-depth epidemiologic studies of disease etiology or intervention efforts for disease control.

Health Risk Assessment

Michael J. DiBartolomeis, PhD, DABT

Most people generally are aware that voluntary or involuntary exposure to chemicals and other hazardous substances can cause harm to their health or to the health of their children and the unborn fetus. Taken at the proper dosages, however, some chemicals, such as medicines, are also beneficial to human health. Manufacturing with chemicals has resulted in some new products and technologies that have, arguably, benefited society as a whole by creating new jobs, developing less costly and more durable consumer products and building materials, and improving communication and transportation. However, the true cost of the production, use, and disposal of these synthesized chemicals to the environment and human health is unknown. Furthermore, we know that hazards in the workplace associated with chemical exposure often are greater than the hazards from exposure to environmental pollutants. Many other factors also play a role, including poverty and employment status, which affect nutrition and access to health care, violence, smoking, and drug use. Scientists still do not know the exact degree to which human health problems can be attributed to environmental pollution and how much should be attributed to other environmental factors or lifestyle choices.

In the early 1970s, the level of concern for the safety of the food supply, air, drinking water, and working environment intensified, and new laws were passed and regulations promulgated to help control and restrict the level of pollutants released into the environment (U.S. Environmental Protection Agency, www.epa.gov/epahome/laws.htm). Many of these regulations were based on observed or predicted human health effects of exposure to hazardous materials either in the environment, in the food or water supplies, or in the workplace. Despite these efforts, some contend that not enough is being done to clean up and maintain a healthy environment, whereas others believe that these concerns are exaggerated or unwarranted.

Given the scientific uncertainties involved in evaluating the impact of environmental stressors on human health, it is prudent public health practice to reduce or eliminate preventable exposures to hazardous substances when an activity raises the risk of harm to human health or the environment, even if cause-and-effect relationships have not been fully established. This is the guiding principle behind the precautionary approach to risk management, a familiar component of international and European environmental law. Furthermore, environmental protection programs should effect empowerment within individuals and communities and raise the consciousness about their health, their environment, and multicultural issues. In the United States, these are particularly important given the rapidly changing demographic face of the nation, the ongoing problems associated with environmental pollution, and the increased production and use of chemicals.

RISK AS A DECISION-MAKING FACTOR

Environmental decision making is a multidimensional process. Policies and laws that are written to address concerns about environmental pollution, occupational hazards, and the protection of human health usually rely on information taken from a myriad of sources, some of which are process-based and others of which are value-based or based on a systematic analysis. Table 45–1 provides examples of some factors that might be considered in formulating a decision on an environmental problem.

Although it is only one tool that might be used in the overall decision-making process, government agencies more often than not consider risk first when making decisions on mitigation, control, enforcement, or regulation of chemicals released into the environment. By definition, *risk* is the probability or chance that a desired or unwanted action, circumstance, or event will result in loss or harm. It can apply to almost any activity or event, such as the likelihood for injury when playing a sport or driving a car, the chance for developing a disease from exposure to pathogens or chemicals, or the possibility for property damage from a natural catastrophe. This chapter focuses on human health risks and how to evaluate risk. Risk assessment methodology also has been developed and applied to evaluate the impact of pollution on the environment and ecosystems and, to a lesser degree, on quality-of-life issues. However, a discussion of these applications of risk assessment is beyond the scope of this chapter. In the context of human health, risk is the probability that adverse health effects, ranging from death to subtle biochemical

Table 45–1. Examples of decision-making factors that might be considered in formulating environmental policy.

Process	Value-Based	Analysis
Negotiation (consensus and compromise)	Popular opinion (e.g., from media accounts and polls and surveys)	Availability of or lack of relevant scientific data
Voting (i.e., number of votes, majority versus minority)	Cultural diversity (e.g., traditions, religious beliefs)	Demographics of impacted area
Application of existing laws, statutory mandates or legal precedence	Ethical considerations (e.g., who benefits and who is harmed?)	Geographic location of impacted area
Political pressure (e.g., lobbying, campaign contributions)	Public perception	Quantified exposures (measurement of environmental levels, biomonitoring)
Precaution (take all necessary action to protect from known or potential harm)	Education (presentation of factual materials that raise the level of knowledge about a particular issue)	Risk (absolute, excess, or relative)
Sustainability (conserving resources for future generations)	Quality of life (e.g., aesthetics, peace of mind, health status)	Economics (cost and benefit analysis)
Urgency (e.g., response to an emergency)	Voluntary versus involuntary (in terms of use of exposure)	Technical feasibility (e.g., laboratory capability, existence of efficient mitigation technology)
Unification (e.g., labor and community activism)	Justice (application of laws and practices regardless of socioeconomic status, race, gender, etc.)	Prevention (e.g., reduce or eliminate exposures)
History or convention (continue practices that have been used in the past)	Right to know (knowledge is powerful)	Development and use of alternative (safer) technologies

changes, may occur because of exposure to a hazardous substance. Risk also might be thought of as voluntary or involuntary. Smoking, for example, is both a voluntary and an involuntary risk. It is voluntary because the smoker might choose to begin smoking. It is involuntary because second-hand smoke can cause harm to nonsmokers and also because nicotine is addictive, and it is difficult to stop smoking even if the user wants to.

Risk assessment is a means or methodology to quantify risk, but it is important to recognize that it is a process and not a science. The process of risk assessment uses scientific data, statistical and mathematical methodology, and expert judgment to characterize the probability for an adverse outcome. In its most basic form, risk assessment is the process through which toxicology data collected from animal studies and human exposure studies are combined with information about the degree of exposure to predict the likelihood that a particular adverse response will be seen in an individual or a population.

Historically, the results of risk assessments have been used to regulate chemical production, use, and release into the environment or food supply. For example, risk assessment methodologies have been used to set stan-

dards for pesticide residues in food, chemical contaminants in drinking water, indoor and ambient air standards, and exposure limits for contaminants found in consumer products and other media. However, risks might be assessed differently among agencies, and there are actually only a few "environmental agencies" that assess environmental or occupational health risks. These agencies attempt to make decisions based on data supported with scientific judgment. Some agencies also are mandated to consider future or multiple risks. With the exception of the application of pesticides in agriculture, risk assessment has not been used widely as a basis for setting workplace exposure standards.

GENERAL RISK ASSESSMENT PROCESS

Elements of the Model

The risk-based model for environmental priority setting generally follows a two-tiered approach. The first tier is to evaluate the size and scope of the potentially hazardous situation and quantify the level of risk posed by the hazard (risk assessment). The National Research Council defines *risk assessment* as a four-step process devel-

Table 45–2. Standard steps to conducting a health risk assessment.

Risk Assessment Step	Examples of Questions Asked by the Risk Assessor
Hazard identification	What substances harm humans, and what kind of harm is it? Of all the substances involved in a problem area (e.g., air pollution) which substances will we look at in this analysis?
Dose-response assessment	What could happen to humans if they are exposed to different levels of these compounds? What are the cancer-causing effects and non-cancer-causing effects?
Exposure assessment	What are the sources and duration of exposures to this substance? How many people are exposed to the hazardous substance? What range of doses do they receive?
Risk characterization	Given all we have learned so far, what are the human health impacts of current exposures? What is the risk to an individual? What is the risk to an entire population? Are any subpopulations more impacted than others? How confident are we in the overall analysis?

oped to aid in the evaluation of the safety of synthetic chemical use or the exposure to humans from chemicals in the environment. The four steps of risk assessment are hazard identification, dose-response assessment, exposure assessment, and risk characterization. In conducting health risk assessments, a number of representative questions about each environmental problem are asked (Table 45–2).

The results of a risk assessment then are used to help determine which risks need to be addressed or managed. This second process is called *risk management,* and it uses a value-based approach to determine what level of risk to human health will be considered significant and to formulate options for identifying, selecting, and implementing actions to prevent, reduce, or maintain risks below that level. Risk management considers risk along with other technical, economic, legal, and social factors.

A third element of the risk assessment model, *risk communication,* was added later with the intent of linking risk assessors with the public by presenting information in the most effective way. In communicating risk to the public, some questions that might be asked include: Is the information clearly relevant to and understandable by the affected public? Does the information respond to the public's concerns? What are the limitations of the risk assessment? Despite the best efforts of the risk assessors to communicate the results of a risk assessment to the public, it is clear that risk communication is an afterthought in the process. More recently, as the emphasis for addressing environmental pollution issues has been placed on the affected communities (i.e., disproportionate risk and environmental justice), the importance of involving the public earlier in the process has been realized.

Scope of Risk Assessment

Health risk assessments can be conducted for any hazard for which there are adequate toxicologic (from ani-

mal or human exposures) or epidemiologic data and either measured or estimated exposure in an individual or population. The spectrum of health effects described in toxicologic and epidemiologic studies is quite broad and might include acute, subchronic, and/or chronic effects following exposure to a chemical or chemical mixture. Acute adverse health effects usually are observed a few hours after a single high-level exposure (or dose) or after several high-level exposures over a short period of time. Although some health effects, such as delayed neuropathy or developmental toxicity, might be observed days or even months after a single high-level exposure to a chemical, chronic health effects usually are observed following repeated low-level exposures over many years (up to a lifetime in animals), and subchronic health effects usually are observed from repeated doses over 30 to 90 days in animals and for up to about 1 year in humans.

Table 45–3 presents some typical toxicologic endpoints used for risk assessment. It should be mentioned that for some toxic effects, the length and level of exposure might not be limited to any one category, and in fact, there is some overlap. As a general rule, a risk assessment does not exclude any toxicologic effect that is clearly caused by the chemical exposure. In cases when there is ambiguity in the data or the data are incomplete, it is generally a responsible approach to assume that the health effect is related to the chemical exposure until more data become available that clearly show an alternative cause of the adverse health effect.

RISK ASSESSMENT STEPS

Hazard Identification

To begin a risk assessment, hazard identification is the step in which it is determined whether exposure to an agent could (at any dose) cause an increase in the incidence of adverse health effects (e.g., cancer, birth

Table 45–3. Common toxicologic endpoints reported in animal and human exposure studies that are used for quantitative health risk assessment.

Toxicologic Endpoint	Exposure Duration		
	Acute	**Subchronic**	**Chronic**
Clinical signs and overall abnormal appearance of test animal (general malaise)	++	++	++
Clinical signs and symptoms (reported in human exposures)	++	++	+
Abnormal results of gross pathologic and histopathologic examinations	+	++	++

Neurologic effects:
  (a) Cholinergic signs, cholinesterase inhibition, tremor, incoordination
  (b) Delayed neuropathy[1]
  (c) Behavioral effects (e.g., attention deficit, lethargy)
	++	++	++

Changes in absolute body weight, or body weight gain	+	++	+
Respiratory airway dysfunction and/or irritation	++	±	±
Dermal or ocular abrasion or irritation	++	+	–
Sensitization (dermal or upper airway)	+	+	±
Change in absolute or relative organ weight	–	++	++
Developmental (e.g., birth defect, frank toxicity, lower body weights, spontaneous abortion)	–[2]	++	±
Reproductive effects (e.g., decreased fertility, testicular atrophy or degeneration)	–	++	++
Changes in normal physiology and function (e.g., changes in hormone production, transient or irreversible effects on the immune system)	–	++	++

Altered clinical lab values:
  (a) Biochemical (e.g., changes in hepatic enzyme levels)
  (b) Blood (e.g., increased white blood cell count)
  (c) Urine (e.g., proteinuria or hematuria)
	–	++	++

Evidence for cellular degeneration, changes in cellular metabolic activity	–	+	++
Genotoxicity[3]	+	±	±
Increased incidence of tumors	–[4]	–[5]	++

Decreased survival:
  (a) Lethality studies
  (b) Increased morbidity, premature death (decreased survival)
	++	+	+

Legend: + = Common part of examination and frequently observed result for this type of study; ++ = common part of examination and frequently observed result for this type of study and endpoint is often the most sensitive for risk assessment; ± = might be part of examination and result might be reported for this type of study but not frequently; – = not usually part of examination and not usually reported for this type of study.
[1]By definition, the effect is delayed but it is usually the result of an acute high-level exposure.
[2]Not usually reported/observed after an acute exposure, however, a single in utero exposure at a specific time during pregnancy can result in a birth defect.
[3]Genetic toxicity endpoints are often used in risk assessment as supplemental data but not as a quantitative end point. Nevertheless, there are numerous in vitro and in vivo assays to assess the genotoxic potential of a chemical that usually fall into three categories: (1) mutations in genes usually in mammalian cells, bacteria, fruit flies, or yeast; (2) chromosomal effects usually in mammalian cells; and (3) DNA damage (usually assayed by measuring rate of unscheduled DNA repair).
[4]Single-dose irradiation can be oncogenic (e.g., leukemia in atom bomb victims in Hiroshima).
[5]Unusual occurrence, but might be early onset caused by, for example, in utero exposure to diethylstilbestrol (DES).

defects, or neurotoxicity) in humans. Many factors are considered in this determination, and depending on the toxicologic endpoint of concern, there might be specific additional factors to consider. If human exposures and toxicity are well documented, identification of a hazard is relatively easy; it can be more complicated when only experimental data in animals are available. In general, the criteria used in a risk assessment to identify a threat to human health from animal data include the number of animal species affected, the dose at which the animals are affected, the existence of a dose-response relationship, the severity of the effect, and for some agents, whether the toxicity observed in the animal is relevant to humans.

For individual chemicals and chemical mixtures, multiple health effects frequently are observed following dosing in animals or exposure to humans. For example, as required under the Federal Insecticide, Fungicide and Rodenticide Act (FIFRA), registrants must submit data from a standard battery of experimental toxicity tests that include acute, subchronic, and chronic studies for all pesticide active ingredients. Each pesticide usually exhibits some consistent toxicologic effects in different species that are related or unrelated to the pesticidal action of the chemical. In addition, there also might be either nonspecific toxicity or species-specific effects that occur at comparable doses or at higher or lower doses than the consistent toxicologic effects. The spectrum of toxicity exhibited by a chemical in a battery of tests can be considered a "hazard profile" that might or might not be consistent with other structurally related chemicals or chemicals that exhibit comparable mechanisms of action.

For some toxicologic endpoints, additional consideration needs to be given to fully characterize or profile the hazard. For carcinogens, it is also important to consider the number and types of tumors occurring in the animals, the target organs affected, the background incidence (usually regarded as historical controls), the time-to-tumor response, the formation of preneoplastic lesions, and the genotoxicity (including mutagenicity) of the chemical. For carcinogens, there might not be consistency among species for tumor type, and there might be positive data in one species and negative data in another. Depending on the final use of a risk assessment, it is often prudent to accept the results from positive studies even if there are negative studies in order to take a precautionary approach to protecting public health.

To address the concern of equivocal data, a "weight of evidence" approach might be taken. A weight-of-evidence approach considers the complete data set (including all negative and positive results) as a whole in order to gain an appreciation of the scientific certainty of the identification process. This process includes all available data, regardless of the source, and evaluates the results of the studies in a qualitative manner to develop a sense of consistency or inconsistency in the data set. A meta-analysis approach, on the other hand, involves compiling data from comparable experiments (i.e., similar experimental design, statistical power, reporting details, and overall quality) and evaluating the data set in a quantitative, statistical context. Epidemiologic data from several comparable studies sometimes are examined using meta-analysis, as are data from multiple carcinogen bioassays in animals.

In the hazard identification phase of a health risk assessment, there is often a need to separate statistical significance from biologic significance. Statistical significance might exclude effects of biologic significance, and in the case where several studies demonstrate comparable biologic effects with varying statistical significance, the effect still might be considered for risk assessment. In the dose-response assessment step, other criteria would be applicable to help discern the mechanism of toxic action and the use of the data for quantitative purposes. Furthermore, there are toxicologic endpoints for which biologic relevance is not known or difficult to define (e.g., increased immunologic activity without obvious clinical signs of toxicity). Therefore, the risk assessor might attempt to define the term *adverse effect* or at least segregate an effect that is clearly adverse from one for which the data are equivocal. The validity of this exercise is open to scientific debate, and there are many examples where the difference between adverse and nonadverse is not at all clear for a toxicity endpoint.

Dose-Response Assessment

Dose-response evaluations define the relationship between the dose of an agent and the observance or expected occurrence of a specific toxicologic effect. A dose-response evaluation usually requires extrapolation from doses administered to experimental animals to the exposures expected from human contact with the agent in the environment or in the workplace. When evaluating toxicologic effects in animals, it is generally assumed that at a given dose the animal response to a chemical will be nearly identical to the human response. This approach is reasonably accurate for chemicals that exhibit a threshold dose-response curve and which are eliminated from the body fairly rapidly (i.e., short biologic half-life). If available, human exposure/dosing data from occupational or environmental exposures might be useful to better characterize the dose-response relationship of a chemical and its toxic effect. Data from human volunteer studies for exposure to hazardous substances are less desirable because of the generally poor study design, inherent bias of the subjects or the investigators, lower statistical power, and questionable ethical context.

Chemicals are thought to exhibit two types of dose-response relationships, those exhibiting a threshold for toxicity and those that do not. For chemicals that exhibit a threshold, the basic principle is that a specific dose level can be identified below which no toxic effect would be observed. The conventional approach to selecting dose levels for risk assessment of chemicals that exhibit a threshold for toxicity is to first identify the most sensitive endpoint from all studies and then to identify the highest no-observed-adverse-effect level (NOAEL) for that endpoint from the data collected from comparable studies. If no NOAEL can be identified (because of a dose selection that did not find a dose level at which no effect was observed), then the lowest observed adverse effect level (LOAEL) is substituted. In the case where a LOAEL and not a NOAEL is used for risk assessment, additional uncertainty is inherent in the calculation of risk that should be accounted for in the risk characterization step (see "Risk Characterization" below).

Alternatively, for chemicals that exhibit a toxicity threshold, a benchmark dose (BMD) methodology might be better suited with certain data sets in which a NOAEL cannot be clearly established. In this method, a toxicologic effect is first identified, such as a percentage of animals exhibiting a response or a percentage of decrease or increase in an enzymatic activity. Second, a benchmark response level is selected (e.g., a response rate of 5% or 10%), and a mathematical model is applied to the data. The fitted curve then is used to designate the corresponding BMD. A lower limit on the BMD confidence level often is chosen as the NOAEL equivalent. This BMD confidence level then is used for risk assessment calculations by applying the appropriate safety/uncertainty factors.

The methods for dose-response extrapolation employed for carcinogens are different. It is widely assumed that for chemicals that induce tumors, no threshold for toxicity exists. However, we do not fully understand the mechanism(s) of action for all chemical carcinogens. Chemical initiators and promoters have been identified in experimental studies, and for these, a postulated genotoxic mechanism of action appears to be reasonable. For other chemicals that induce tumorigenesis in laboratory animals, the evidence supporting a genotoxic mechanism of action is equivocal or negative, and other mechanisms, such as cytotoxicity or disruptions in physiologic processes that affect hormone levels or immunologic response, have been postulated.

To describe the dose-response curve for carcinogens at the low doses expected for human occupational or environmental exposures, it is often necessary to extrapolate from the relatively high doses used in cancer bioassays (typically in rodents).

Most low-dose extrapolation models are derived from assumptions of the statistical distribution of the data (e.g., log-probit, Mantel-Bryan, logit, and Weibull), the postulated mechanism of carcinogenicity (e.g., linear

one-hit, gamma multihit, and Armitage-Doll multistage), or some other parameter (e.g., time to tumor, pharmacokinetic, and biologically based). The carcinogenic process typically is described mathematically by a set of elementary biologic events, most often as part of a multistage process, and the effect of carcinogens on these processes is assumed to be the simplest possible (e.g., described by a chemical reaction rate). Therefore, the dose-response relationship described by these mathematical models usually will be as arbitrary as the assumptions made for the biologic processes.

There are several mathematical models that usually will fit the animal cancer bioassay data. Because these models use different formulas and assumptions for predicting the chemical's carcinogenic potency, they might yield different results at the doses to which humans are exposed depending on the characteristics of the dose-response curve and the assumed mechanism of carcinogenicity (Figure 45–1). For most carcinogens, the one-hit and linearized multistage models are applied to the animal cancer bioassay data in order to estimate cancer potency in humans. These models were developed based on our understanding that ionizing radiation and genotoxic chemicals exhibit a linear, or nearly linear, response in the low-dose region. When presenting the results of the dose-response assessment for carcinogens, the upper-bound risk from the cancer models are provided as well as the upper and lower bounds of the risk. The objective of the bounding techniques is to attempt to account for the statistical uncertainty in the results of the animal tests.

There are chemicals for which there are positive cancer bioassay data but negative or equivocal genotoxicity data. There is an ongoing debate in the scientific community as to the mechanism of tumorigenesis for these agents. For example, the chloro-s-triazine herbicides (e.g., atrazine, simazine, and cyanazine) induce mammary tumorigenesis, but the data for genetic toxicity are equivocal. There is some evidence that these chemicals disrupt endocrine function at the level of the hypothalamus-pituitary-ovarian axis, although they do not bind estrogen receptors. Therefore, a threshold dose-response for the triazine herbicides has been proposed, but no clear mechanism of action has been demonstrated. Other examples of chemical carcinogens for which there is ongoing debate as to the mechanism of action include chlorinated solvents such as chloroform and chlorinated polycyclic aromatic compounds such as 2,3,7,8-tetrachlorodibenzo-p-dioxin.

Physiologically based pharmacokinetic (PBPK) models are used by some risk assessors to predict the human response from rodent data. These models attempt to quantitatively account for the various differences between the test species and humans by considering body weight, metabolic capacity and products, respiration rate, blood flow, fat content, and a number of other parameters (Figure 45–2).

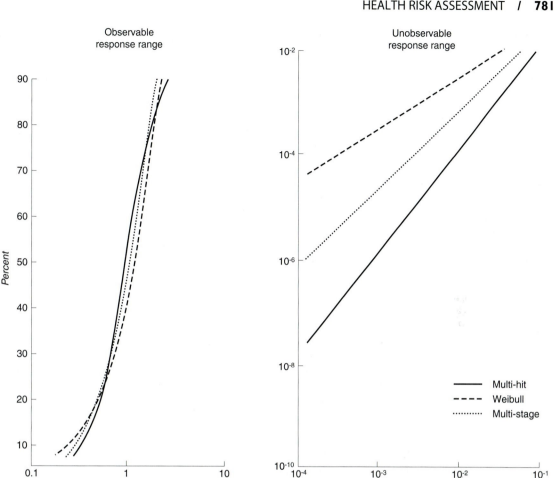

Figure 45–1. The fit of most dose-response models to data in the observable range is generally similar (*left plot*). However, because of the differences in assumptions on which the equations are based, the risk estimates at low doses can vary dramatically between the different models (*right plot*).

Confidence in the results of physiologically based pharmacokinetic models often relies on some untestable assumptions, such as the delivered dose of an unstable metabolite to a target organ. While PBPK models have been developed for a variety of industrial chemicals (e.g., chlorinated solvents) and pesticides (e.g., malathion), application of the results of these analyses for risk assessment is still not clearly defined. Biologically based approaches to estimating cancer risk are also being developed that allow for the incorporation of biologic factors such as the number of mutations required for malignancy and the role of target-cell birth and death processes in the accumulation of these mutations. A key element is a quantitative description of how the carcinogen affects the cellular birth, death, and mutation rates. At this time, however, most of the information needed to perform these analyses is not yet available.

The results of human exposure (e.g., epidemiology) studies also might provide useful data to supplement the animal cancer bioassay data or offer an independent assessment of the dose-response of a chemical and its effect in humans. The design of human exposure studies, however, often limits use of the results of such studies for risk assessment purposes because the degree of uncertainty in estimating exposures is greater and the statistical power of the studies is usually lower than for experimental animal studies.

REFERENCE

EPA: *Guidelines for Carcinogen Risk Assessment*, 2005, http://cfpub.epa.gov/ncea/cfm/recordisplay.cfm?deid=116283.

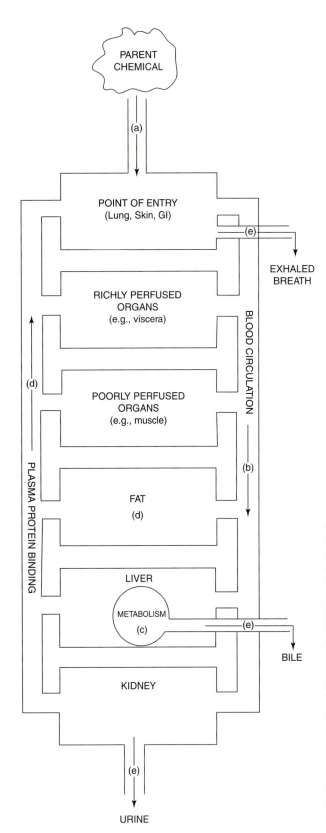

PARENT
CHEMICAL

(a)

POINT OF ENTRY
(Lung, Skin, GI)

(e)

EXHALED
BREATH

RICHLY PERFUSED
ORGANS
(e.g., viscera)

BLOOD CIRCULATION

POORLY PERFUSED
ORGANS
(e.g., muscle)

(d)

(b)

FAT
(d)

PLASMA PROTEIN BINDING

LIVER

METABOLISM
(c)

(e)

BILE

KIDNEY

(e)

URINE

Figure 45–2. Simplified diagram of a general compartmental physiologically based pharmacokinetic model. The (*a*) absorption, (*b*) distribution, (*c*) metabolism, (*d*) storage, and (*e*) elimination of an internalized xenobiotic are described by a series of mathematical interrelationships. Physiologically based pharmacokinetic models yield information such as the predicted change in the amount of a chemical in a given organ over time depending on the data input (e.g., rate constants for transport, distribution, respiration, metabolism, and excretion, as well as the chemical and physical properties of the chemical). The compartments are intended to represent, as best as possible, actual anatomic structures, defined with respect to their volumes, blood flows (perfusion rate), chemical binding (partitioning) characteristics, and ability to metabolize and excrete the chemical of interest. For risk assessment purposes, these models are used primarily to predict and compare target tissue doses for different exposure situations in different animal species.

Exposure Assessment

For there to be a health risk, there must be both inherent toxicity and exposure to a chemical. In other words, the prevention or elimination of the exposure to a toxic substance would result in zero risk. Because the total elimination of chemical exposure often is not feasible or practical, the exposure assessment step in a risk assessment is used to estimate the magnitude and probability of uptake from the environment by any combination of oral, inhalation, and dermal routes of exposure. The results of the exposure assessment are quantitative doses presented in the amount of the chemical per unit of body weight per unit of time (e.g., mg/kg per day).

Early in the exposure assessment, the population at risk needs to be identified by determining who would be exposed to the chemicals of concern. The size of the exposed population depends on the proximity of the population to the source. For example, there is a high potential for exposing large numbers of people if the chemical is in drinking water or air. On the other hand, if the contamination is confined to an enclosed area (e.g., indoor workplace), the population affected is likely to be smaller. In characterizing an exposed population, it is important to consider age, gender, health status, and race and cultural diversity within that population because individuals differ in sensitivity and susceptibility to a chemical hazard.

The primary routes of exposure to chemicals in the environment are inhalation of particulates, dusts, and vapors; dermal contact with contaminated surfaces (e.g., soils or contaminated vegetation); use of consumer products (e.g., paints and plastic containers); and ingestion of contaminated food, water, and contaminated surfaces (i.e., hand-to-mouth transfer). Workplace exposures also result from inhaling, ingesting, and making contact not only with contaminated media but also with concentrated solutions or mixtures of industrial chemicals. Despite recent advances in protective clothing and gear, labeling instructions, and properly engineered ventilation systems, the potential for workplace exposures is still significantly higher than most environmental exposures.

Estimates of human exposure might be based on analytic measurements of samples taken from environmental or workplace monitoring, direct measurements of human exposure, or mathematical (predictive) models. Although direct measurements of human exposure are the most precise methods for detecting exposure in an individual or population, these methods are costly, require specialized instruments, and are time-consuming. More frequently, exposure estimates are based on mathematical models. Numerous methodologies for estimating the human uptake of contaminants have been proposed and refined in recent years. Models have been developed and used to predict the movement of chemicals in the environment (e.g., in air, groundwater, or surface water), transfer from contaminated surfaces (e.g., carpet or clothing, hand-to-mouth), and deposition onto edible fruits and vegetables. Physiologically based pharmacokinetic models also are used to predict the rate of absorption, metabolism, and distribution of a chemical in the body. Some retrospective studies of human exposure rely on surveys and the recall of the exposed persons. This latter method, while often necessary, is the least reliable and one reason that data from some epidemiologic studies cannot always be used for quantitative risk assessment.

In quantifying exposure doses, the number of exposed persons at each of the anticipated dose levels is described, as well as the upper and mean estimates of exposure. The best approach is to develop exposure scenarios that examine a range of potential or actual exposures for individuals, populations, and subpopulations. Depending on the use of the risk assessment, it might be adequate to estimate only doses from a single chemical exposures from a single source of the chemical. More often, multiple chemical exposures from multiple sources should be evaluated and aggregated, despite the relative complexity of doing this.

Formulas for estimating exposures from environmental and workplace chemicals can be applied in order to quantify dose levels for risk assessment. These formulas require entering values for physiologic and activity parameters such as breathing rate (resting and/or under exertion), daily water ingestion, food intake, body weight or size, and other factors that depend on the age, gender, physical well-being, and habits of the individual. Factors such as drug interactions, physical debilitation, stage in development (e.g., fetus, perinatal, or infancy), and smoking status, for example, might increase susceptibility and sensitivity to a chemical exposure and should be documented and considered in the exposure assessment if possible. Values for body weight, breathing rate, and body size are obtained from tables that normalize the data and present mean and statistical bounds on the data. Often, values for parameters such as water ingestion and food intake are obtained from regional or even national surveys and therefore are not specific to a particular community, ethnicity, or lifestyle. For a more precise or defining exposure assessment for a specific population or individual, it is necessary to gather more specific data for entering into the exposure formulas.

Application of statistical analyses to the exposure data set might be necessary to determine the distribution of data because environmental and occupational data might be log-normally distributed rather than conform to a Gaussian distribution.

Depending on the exposed population and the problem, exposure estimates might need to be made for different subpopulations (e.g., children and infants, pregnant women, and the infirm) because these individuals are differentially susceptible, exhibit different activities patterns, or are particularly sensitive for a number of reasons. For a purely statistical description of a population, stochastic or "likelihood of risks" approaches were developed to characterize exposures using models that replicate randomness in exposure. The probabilistic techniques can characterize a range of potential exposures and their likelihood of occurrence.

Some chemicals persist for many years in the environment, whereas others degrade rapidly. The environmental fate of chemicals depends on several factors, for example, the chemical and physical properties of the substance, the potential for movement through various environmental media (e.g., groundwater and porous soils) or storage (e.g., binding of chemicals to sediments), the rate of degradation in the environment (e.g., by sunlight, soil and water microbes, and evaporation), and the potential for bioaccumulation and biomagnification. Some chemicals such as the polychlorinated aromatic hydrocarbons [e.g., polychlorinated biphenyls and dichlorodiphenyltrichloroethane (DDT)] can persist in the environment for 50 or more years, whereas other chemicals (e.g., some organophosphorus pesticides) degrade relatively rapidly and will persist for weeks or a few months. Lipophilic chemicals (e.g., methyl mercury) in the environment are stored in the tissues of animals, most notably fish and, through a process called *biomagnification*, increase (sometimes to concentrations hundreds of times greater than the original environmental levels) as the stored chemicals move up the food chain. Therefore, although direct human exposures to chemical contaminants might be reduced when chemicals are degraded rapidly, there is certainly significant exposure potential for even those chemicals that exist for only a few days in the environment (e.g., agricultural workers) or that start out at low concentrations but bioaccumulate in the food chain (e.g., contaminated fish).

New technologies and advances in analytic instrumentation and methodologies now allow for the detection of very small quantities of exogenous (xenobiotic) chemicals in blood, urine, hair, feces, exhaled breath, and fat and other tissues (i.e., biomonitoring). Measurement of chemical residues at parts per trillion (ppt) levels and even lower is now possible in biologic tissues (as well as in environmental media). For many chemicals, biomonitoring results represent a direct indicator of either acute or chronic exposure to a chemical. These direct measurements offer a better alternative to assessing exposure than using any mathematical models. Furthermore, environmental monitoring also has benefited from these advances in technology, although the presence of mixtures of chemicals and the matrices in which these chemicals reside tend to complicate and interfere with environmental measurements at low

levels. As field measurement techniques are further refined, less reliance will need to be placed on mathematical models for predicting the distribution of chemicals in the environment.

Risk Characterization

In the risk characterization, the risk assessor summarizes and interprets the information collected from the previous three steps, presents a quantitative estimate of the human health risk(s), and identifies (and quantifies when possible) the uncertainties in these risk estimates. This process allows the risk assessor to identify the greatest individual and population health risks and promulgate health-based action levels to protect individuals and populations from further exposure or to prevent immediate- or long-term injury. Estimated risks depend on the measured or estimated exposure duration and can be calculated either retrospectively (i.e., the release of the chemical or the exposure has already occurred) or prospectively (i.e., as a means to prevent a release or the exposure from happening). It is appropriate and often necessary in a risk characterization to estimate both noncancer and cancer risks for a chemical exposure and to evaluate multiple exposure scenarios to aid in the determination of the necessary mitigation steps.

For chemical toxicity endpoints that clearly exhibit a threshold dose-response curve, reference exposure levels (RELs), defined as threshold exposure levels below which no adverse health effects are anticipated, can be calculated. These reference levels are comparable with the EPA's reference doses (RfDs) or reference concentrations (RfCs).

RELs are derived by identifying and dividing the NOAEL (or BMD) by uncertainty factors to account for inadequacies in the database, incomplete scientific knowledge, and protection of more sensitive individuals (Table 45–4). The application of uncertainty factors offers a margin of safety to consider when developing mitigation options or regulatory standards. Some uncertainty factors can be considered default values when adequate physiologic or toxicologic information does not exist to provide a more precise estimate of uncertainty.

For carcinogens, unless a threshold for toxicity is clearly demonstrated, it is assumed that the dose-response is linear with no "no risk" level. For these chemical agents, a cancer potency is calculated, and the probability for excess individual cancer risk is estimated based on exposure estimates. The determination as to what is an "acceptable" (or *de minimis*) cancer risk is a value-based decision, and often a range of risk is presented for comparative purposes.

Documented differences in physiology and toxicology between species may be used to modify RELs and,

Table 45–4. Uncertainty factors that may be applied in calculating risk-based exposure levels.

Data Gap or Methodologic Consideration	Uncertainty Factor (Range)
Data extrapolation from acute to chronic	100
Data extrapolation from subchronic to chronic	10
Human (intraspecies) variability	10
Animal to human (interspecies) variability	10
Increased sensitivity or susceptibility (e.g., children)	(1–10)
Conversion of LOAEL to NOAEL	(3–10)
Evidence for genotoxicity (no cancer data)	(1–10)
Reported NOAEL may be a LOAEL	(1–10)
Extrapolation from subchronic to acute	1
Structure activity relationship	Varies with potency
Inadequate experimental design	(1–10)
Pharmacokinetic corrections	Varies with parameter measured or modeled

to a lesser degree, cancer risk estimates to better reflect the human exposure and predicted response to the chemical. The concept of ensuring a margin of safety between exposure and toxicity still should apply, however, even when a more precise estimate of uncertainty can be made. In particular, some subpopulations (e.g., the developing fetus, infants, and children) may be more sensitive or differentially susceptible to a chemical exposure. It is difficult to predict with accuracy the effects of a chemical exposure to such an individual compared with the average, healthy adult in the population. Frequently, gender, race, or other genetic traits also may affect an individual's sensitivity. The risk characterization step should take into account the differences in individuals and subpopulations and uncertainties in the data and methodology.

In general, a thorough characterization of risk also should discuss background concentrations of the chemical in the environment and in human tissue, pharmacokinetic differences between the animal test species and humans (the results of a PBPK or another biologically based model are useful here), the effect of selecting specific exposure parameters, the level of uncertainty in the methods (i.e., calculations and statistical analyses), and other factors that can influence the magnitude of the estimated risks. Furthermore, areas for which additional research is needed also should be identified (e.g., data gaps).

EXAMPLE OF THE APPLICATION OF RISK ASSESSMENT METHODOLOGY

The general approach to calculating risk for noncancer and cancer endpoints is illustrated below for the pesticide and environmental contaminant dibromochloropropane (DBCP). California promulgates maximum contaminant levels (MCLs) for drinking water contaminants that are based in part on public health goals. In deriving an MCL, which is a regulatory standard, costs, benefits, and technical feasibility (e.g., of detection or mitigation) must be considered. A public health goal is developed based on a risk calculation, consideration of the uncertainty in the methods and the data, and taking into account the most sensitive or susceptible individuals (e.g., infants and children). The public health goal is developed in order to protect public health, but it is not a regulatory standard like an MCL and therefore is not enforceable.

DBCP was used extensively as a soil fumigant and nematocide in the United States until 1977, when its registration as a pesticide was suspended. Although it is no longer manufactured commercially or used in this country, groundwater contamination still exists in the San Joaquin Valley and other agricultural regions in California. Exposure to DBCP occurs from the use of tap water as a source of drinking water, as well as in preparing foods and beverages. It is also used for bathing or showering and for washing, flushing toilets, and other household uses resulting in potential dermal and inhalation exposures.

Noncancer Health Effects

DBCP induces testicular damage and infertility, as evidenced by numerous studies of occupational exposures, described as reduced (oligospermia) or no sperm counts (azoospermia), altered sperm motility, damage to the seminiferous tubules, and hormonal disruption. Testicular toxicity is reported most frequently and appears to occur at lower exposures than that of other noncancer endpoints (i.e., it is the most sensitive noncancer toxicity endpoint). In experimental animal studies, the highest NOAEL of 0.025 mg/kg per day is identified for adverse testicular effects in the male rabbit. Using this information, the calculation of an REL (or public health goal), in this case defined as C mg/L for a non-carcinogenic effect of DBCP, follows the equation

$$C = \frac{NOAEL \times BW \times RSC}{UF \times W}$$
$$= \frac{0.025 \, mg/kg - day \times 70 \, kg \times 0.8}{1000 \times 6 \, Leq}$$
$$= 2.3 \times 10^{-4} \, mg/L = 0.2 \, ppb \, (rounded)$$

where NOAEL is no observed adverse effect level, BW is body weight [a default value of 70 kg (154.3 lb) for an adult male is used], RSC is relative source contribution (the sole anticipated source of exposure is groundwater, and therefore, 80% is used as input for DBCP), UF is the uncertainty factor (10 to account for interspecies extrapolation, 10 for use of subchronic NOAEL, and 10 for potentially sensitive human subpopulations), and W is daily water consumption rate [a daily water consumption rate of 6 liter equivalents (Leq) is used because direct ingestion accounts for approximately one-third of the total exposure from household use of DBCP contaminated water, and the remaining two-third is from dermal and inhalation exposure].

The risk of noncancer health effects from drinking DBCP-contaminated water can be determined by calculating the hazard index, which is the ratio of human exposure to the REL. If the hazard index is less than 1, an adequate margin of safety exists. If the hazard index is equal to or greater than 1, the estimated exposure is equal to or greater than the REL, and further examination of the public health implications is required. Applying this method for DBCP, a hazard index of greater than 1 would be achieved when drinking water levels exceed 0.2 ppb.

Carcinogenic Effects

DBCP also causes cancer in experimental animals, and there is some suggestive evidence from human exposure studies. For risk assessment purposes, the development of squamous cell carcinomas of the stomach in female mice is used to calculate a carcinogenic potency of 7 (mg/kg-day)$^{-1}$. To calculate the cancer potency, the multistage model was fit to the animal carcinogenicity dose-response data, and the 95% upper confidence limit on the linear term (q1*) was used. This estimate in animals is adjusted to a lifetime potency, assuming that potency tends to increase with the third power of the observation time in a bioassay. The estimate of lifetime animal carcinogenic potency is converted to an estimate of potency

in humans by the factor (70 kg/animal body weight)$^{1/3}$. This conversion follows from the assumption that a dose rate calculated as daily intake of DBCP divided by (body weight)$^{2/3}$ has the same potency in rodents and humans. Using this cancer potency, the calculation of an REL (C) for DBCP in drinking water using the cancer endpoint follows the equation

$$C = \frac{R \times BW}{CSF \times W}$$
$$= \frac{10^{-6} \times 70 \, kg}{7 \, (mg/kg\text{-}day)^{-1} \times 6 \, Leq/day}$$
$$= 1.7 \times 10^{-6} \, mg/L = 1.7 \, ppt$$

where BW is adult body weight [the default of 70 kg (154.3 lb) for an adult man], R is *de minimis* level for lifetime excess individual cancer risk (a default of 10^{-6}), CSF is cancer potency (q1*) of 7 (mg/kg-day)$^{-1}$ for the development of squamous cell carcinomas of the stomach in female mice, and W is daily volume of water consumed in liter equivalents (Leq) per day.

Therefore, for DBCP, an individual excess cancer risk of 1×10^{-6} (1 in 1 million) would be exceeded when drinking water levels are above 1.7 ppt. It is clear from the results of this risk assessment that the drinking water level considered more health protective is the one based on the cancer endpoint.

DISCUSSION

Quantitative risk assessment has been the foundation for environmental decision making in the United States for more than 30 years. If risk assessment and risk management are to remain the key factors in environmental decision making, "value" choices in the risk evaluation process should be made explicit, and policymakers must recognize the limitations of quantitative risk assessment. Furthermore, the design and results of the risk assessment must be described clearly in the context of the environmental problem. In other words, the context within which the "science" of risk assessment is performed should shape how scientific information is used and interpreted.

Limitations of Using Risk Assessment for Environmental Decision Making

There is an ongoing debate concerning the limitations of using risk assessment results in environmental decision making. The primary complaints include

1. Risk assessment is not solely "science based" but incorporates judgments and values that are limited by a high degree of uncertainty.

2. Conventional risk assessment methods do not account for the disproportionate risk burdens borne by certain communities, nor do they account for the impacts of cumulative and multiple exposures in toxic hot spots or to groups of people (e.g., farm workers and their families).

3. Risk assessment as a two-tiered approach separates risk assessment from management as a means to insulate the "objectivity" of risk assessment from value-laden management decisions. This approach is criticized by scientists and philosophers of science for being unrealistic in that no practice of science is purely objective. Some social scientists argue that risk assessors cannot be completely immune to the political factors of the institutions within which they operate.

4. Risk assessment leads to regulatory delays; that is, "paralysis by analysis."

5. Focusing on the quantitative aspects of risk does not provide enough information on the qualitative aspects, such as anxiety about the future, involuntariness of exposure, and equity concerns.

6. Risk assessment is used primarily to justify certain amounts of pollution, whereas the goal should be pollution elimination, prevention, or environmental sustainability (i.e., leaving sufficient resources and a clean environment for future generations).

7. The process is disempowering (undemocratic) and often neglects the public participation and social values needed to make good decisions about environmental priorities. Inclusion of "risk communication" in the latter stages of the risk assessment process not only is a poor use of an important information resource (i.e., the affected community itself), but it also clouds the process, making it difficult to understand and reproduce.

8. Environmental decisions based on risk comparisons with regulatory benchmarks often are viewed with skepticism by those who are affected the most.

Individual versus Population Risks

Some risk assessments or decisions based on risk assessments rely on measures of population risks; that is, measures of the additional incidence of some adverse impact in the affected population. In this situation, assessing and comparing risks for a potentially hazardous situation using population risks alone might not identify it as an environmental priority. For example, if arsenic were to leach from an abandoned toxic waste site into a nearby waterway, it could present alarmingly high individual risks. The total population risk associated with this situation, however, might be very small if only a small number of people depended on that water supply. A circular construct emerges: Waste sites and industrial facilities that often are located in poor communities and communities of color are not subject to stringent intervention or remedial action because the population risks (as opposed to individual risks of those exposed) are seen as minimal. By using population risk as the benchmark, policymakers might justify not taking action on the basis of the lesser benefits of mitigation to the overall population. Using average population risk for ranking without also looking at maximum individual risk is an economic or policy choice, not a "scientific" decision.

The use of aggregate statistics and population risk measures does not routinely account for "hot spots," that is, geographic areas where residents experience greater environmental risks or locations where multiple exposures to hazardous substances and associated risks occur over time. In addition, risk assessments do not routinely account for differences in individual susceptibilities to toxic substances and chemical-chemical interactions in mixtures. Some attempts have been made by the EPA to develop guidance to incorporate these and other considerations in the risk assessment process. Nevertheless, inclusion of these issues is not yet widely practiced.

Public Involvement

Collaboration among the business community and industrial sector, the general population, and government agencies is required for effective involvement of the public. Although public participation is now generally accepted in diverse policy fields, it is still not addressed adequately in science-based environmental decision making such as risk assessment and risk management.

Environmental agencies should develop and implement plans to involve the public in the decision-making process and recognize that public participation can be seen as a solution to some environmental problems in and of itself, but only when the public is involved as a full and equal partner, not as an adversary. This includes maximizing meaningful participation in the review of agencies' activities and progress in accomplishing the objectives of promoting long-term planning for sustaining a healthy environment and workplace. To accomplish this, public participation needs to be initiated early in the hazard evaluation process and incorporated into the decision-making process. Furthermore, education is a key component to effective public involvement, and therefore, technical information should be easily accessible to the public and translated, if necessary, into the residents' and workers' primary language(s).

Research Needs

More research needs to be done to better understand the risks that environmental and workplace pollution poses, including

1. Completing the toxicity database for many substances released in large quantities into the air, water, land, and workplace or as contaminants in food and other consumer products.
2. Making available data describing actual human exposures to most pollutants.
3. Developing risk assessment methods further. For example, methods to assess cumulative risk from multiple chemical exposures and the effects of chemicals on the endocrine, nervous, and immune systems are necessary to understand better the full spectrum of hazards posed by environmental pollutants and occupational hazards.
4. Considering subpopulations that bear disproportionate risks (that is, "hot spots"), which must be incorporated into any new and/or existing site-specific risk assessments.
5. Developing methods to assess the societal distribution of environmental and occupational health risks in the context of achieving environmental justice.
6. Devoting resources to measuring population exposures to toxicants, including from microenvironments, from accidental releases, and among highly exposed groups.
7. Increasing the capacity to identify and prevent future impacts on public health and the environment from emerging risks.

Other Models for Environmental Decision Making

Applying scientific knowledge and judgment to address environmental issues requires universal strategies as well as some fundamental changes in the status quo of environmental decision making. In other words, more consideration should be given to alternative science or value-based processes proposed or used to address environmental and occupational hazards.

One alternative model used to support environmental decision making, predominantly in European countries, is the precautionary principle. This approach does not exclude making estimates of risk, but the burden of proof is levied on the polluter rather than the affected public. In fact, it has been argued that the precautionary principle should be viewed as a complement to science to be invoked when a lack of scientific evidence means that the outcomes are uncertain. In applying the precautionary principle, ethical and value-based aspects should be weighed equally with the science. The key element to the precautionary principle is that action should be taken in the face of uncertainty rather than delaying action until more "evidence" is generated.

Other options include technology-based approaches that require retooling or reformulating industrial processes to use fewer or lesser amounts of hazardous materials or by substituting them with safer alternatives. The EPA is already mandated to incorporate pollution prevention into its implementation plans under the Toxic Substances Control Act and the Clean Air Act, whereas the reduction or elimination of hazardous pesticide use has lagged behind. These approaches apply the principles of hazard identification without necessarily relying on a risk-based assessment because the ultimate goal is to achieve elimination of hazardous materials and prevention of environmental and workplace exposures. In banning the chemicals DDT, polychlorinated biphenyl (PCB), and lead in gasoline, pollution prevention is achieved without allowing for some level of "negligible risk."

Public pressure, public right-to-know laws, and civil suits also have achieved a certain degree of success in influencing environmental decision making. For example, California's Proposition 65, approved by a wide margin in 1986 as an initiative to address growing concerns about exposures to toxic chemicals, is an example of a public right-to-know law that also empowers citizens to "blow the whistle" on polluters. Currently, more than 700 chemicals are listed as reproductive or developmental toxicants or carcinogens. Proposition 65 is an effective mechanism for reducing certain exposures that may not have been controlled adequately under existing federal or state laws. It also provides a market-based incentive for manufacturers to remove listed chemicals from their products. Furthermore, because of Proposition 65, information regarding the dangers of exposure to certain chemicals in more susceptible subpopulations is widely disseminated.

REFERENCES

OEHHA: Proposition 65, www.oehha.ca.gov/prop65.html.

OEHHA: Public health goal for 1,2 dibromo-3-chloropropane in drinking water, www.oehha.ca.gov/water/phg/allphgs.html).

United Nations Educational, Scientific and Cultural Organization: The precautionary principle, 2005, http://unesdoc.unesco.org/images/0013/001395/139578e.pdf.

Biostatistics & Epidemiology

Marc B. Schenker, MD, MPH

It is apparent to anyone who reads the medical literature today that some knowledge of biostatistics and epidemiology is a necessity. This is particularly true in occupational and environmental health, in which many of the findings are based on epidemiologic studies of subjects exposed to low levels of an agent. Research has become more rigorous in the area of study design and analysis, and reports of clinical and epidemiologic research contain increasing amounts of statistical methodology. This Appendix provides a brief introduction to some of the basic principles of biostatistics and epidemiology.

▌ I. BIOSTATISTICS

DESCRIPTIVE STATISTICS

Types of Data

Data collected in medical research can be divided into three types: nominal (categorical), ordinal, and continuous.

Nominal (categorical) data are those that can be divided into two or more unordered categories, such as gender, race, or religion. In occupational medicine, for example, many outcome measures, such as cancer rates, are considered separately for different gender and race categories.

Ordinal data are different from nominal data in that there is a predetermined order underlying the categories. Examples of ordinal data include clinical severity, socioeconomic status (SES), or ILO (International Labor Office) profusion category for pneumoconiosis on chest radiographs.

Both nominal and ordinal data are examples of discrete data. They take on only integer values.

Continuous data are data measured on an arithmetic scale. Examples include height, weight, blood lead levels, or forced expiratory volume. The accuracy of the number recorded depends on the measuring instrument, and the variable can take on an infinite number of values within a defined range. For example, a person's height might be recorded as 72 inches or 72.001 inches or 72.00098 inches depending on the accuracy of the measuring instrument.

Summarizing Data

Once research data are collected, the first step is to summarize them. The two most common ways of summarizing data are measures of location, or central tendency, and measures of spread, or variation.

A. MEASURES OF CENTRAL TENDENCY:

1. Mean—The mean ($\bar{x}$) is the average value of a set of interval data observations. It is computed using the following equation:

$$\bar{x} = \frac{\sum_{i=1}^{n} x_i}{n}$$

where *n* is sample size and x_i is a random variable, such as height, with $i = 1, \ldots, n$.

The mean can be strongly affected by extreme values in the data. If a variable has a fairly symmetric, or bell-shaped, distribution, the mean is used as the appropriate measure of central tendency.

2. Median—The median is the "middle" observation, or 50th percentile; that is, half the observations lie above the median and half below. It can be applied to interval or ordinal data. When there is an odd number of observations, the median is merely the middle observation. For example, for the following series of observations of subjects' weights (in pounds): 124, 138, 139, 152, and 173, the median is 139. When there is an even number of observations, the median is the mean of the two middle numbers. Using a similar example of subject weights, for the following series of weights: 124, 138, 139, 152, 173, and 179, the median is (139 + 152)/2 = 145.5. The median does not have the mathematical niceties of the mean, but it is not as susceptible as the mean to extreme values. If the variable being measured has a distribution that is asymmetric or skewed—that is, if there are a few extreme values at one

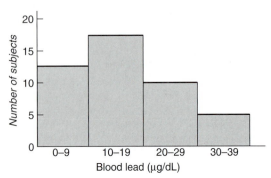

Figure A-1. Frequency distribution of subjects by blood lead category.

end of the distribution—the median is a better descriptor than the mean of the "center" of the distribution.

3. Mode—The mode is the most frequently occurring observation. It is used rarely, except when there are a limited number of possible outcomes.

4. Frequency distribution—In discussing measures of location or spread, we often refer to the frequency distribution of the data. A frequency distribution consists of a series of predetermined intervals (along the horizontal axis) together with the number (or percentage) of observations whose values fall in that interval (along the vertical axis). An example of a frequency distribution is presented in Figure A–1.

B. MEASURES OF VARIATION:

1. Range—The range is the simplest measurement of variation and is defined as the difference between the highest and lowest values. Disadvantages of the range are that it is sensitive to a single extreme value, and it tends to increase in value as the number of observations increases. Furthermore, the range does not provide information about the distribution of values within the set of data. The interquartile range (25–75th percentiles) is sometimes used because it is less influenced by extreme values.

2. Variance—The sample variance (s^2) is a measure of the dispersion about the mean arrived at by calculating the sum of the squared deviations from the mean and dividing by the sample size minus 1. The equation for deriving sample variance is as follows:

$$s^2 = \frac{\sum_{i=1}^{n}(x_i - \bar{x})^2}{n-1}$$

Variance can be thought of as the average of squared deviations from the mean, or more simply, variance

tells you how spread out the distribution of the observations is.

3. Standard deviation—The sample standard deviation (s) is equal to the square root of the sample variance. Basically, it tells you how tightly clustered all the observations are around the mean of a set of data.

$$s = \sqrt{\frac{\sum_{i=1}^{n}(x_i - \bar{x})^2}{n-1}}$$

See Table A–1 for examples of the calculation of mean, median, mode, variance, and standard deviation.

Variability in data may be a result of the natural distribution of values or of random factors produced by errors in measurement. The variance or standard deviation does not distinguish between different sources of variability.

Table A-1. Calculation of mean, median, mode, variance, and standard deviation ($n = 10$ workers).

x_i = Number of Years of Exposure to Asbestos.			
Worker	x_i	$(x_i - x)$	$(x_i - x)^2$
1.	$x_1 = 4.0$	−2.2	4.84
2.	$x_2 = 4.5$	−1.7	2.89
3.	$x_3 = 5.0$	−1.2	1.44
4.	$x_4 = 5.0$	−1.2	1.44
5.	$x_5 = 6.0$	−0.2	0.04
6.	$x_6 = 6.5$	+0.3	0.09
7.	$x_7 = 7.0$	+0.8	0.64
8.	$x_8 = 7.5$	+1.3	1.69
9.	$x_9 = 8.0$	+1.8	3.24
10.	$x_{10} = 8.5$	+2.3	5.29
Total:	$\Sigma x_i = 62.0$		$\Sigma(x_i - x)^2 = 21.6$

Mean: $\bar{x} = \dfrac{62.0}{10} = 6.2$

Variance $= \Sigma(x_i - x)^2/(n - 1) = 21.6/9 = 2.4$
Standard deviation $= \sqrt{2.4} = 1.55$

Median:
1. Order the observations from lowest to highest.
2. Median $= \frac{1}{2}\left(\left[\dfrac{n}{2}\right]\text{observation} + \left(\left[\dfrac{n}{2}\right] + 1\right)\right.$

   $\left.\text{observation}\right) = 1/2$ (5th observation + 6th observation)
3. Therefore, median $= \frac{1}{2}(6.0 + 6.5) = 6.25$

Mode:
Most commonly occurring observation is 5.0, because it occurs twice and all other observations occur once.

Sample versus Population Descriptive Statistics

The descriptive statistics discussed thus far are sample estimates of true population values or parameters. Because we usually do not have the resources to measure the variables of interest on entire populations, we instead select a sample from the population of interest and then estimate the population mean from the sample mean or the population variance from the sample variance. The population mean usually is represented by the Greek letter μ and the population variance by the Greek letter σ^2. One almost never knows the true population values for these parameters and is almost always conducting sample surveys to estimate them.

The Normal Distribution

The most important continuous probability distribution is the normal, or Gaussian, distribution, also known as the *bell-shaped curve*. Many quantitative variables follow a normal distribution, and it plays a central role in statistical tests of hypotheses. Even when one is sampling from a population whose shape departs from the normal distribution, under certain general conditions, it still forms the basis for statistical testing of hypotheses.

We often transform data to make them more normal in distribution. The normal distribution has several nice properties that make it amenable to statistical analysis, and variables that follow a normal distribution are for that reason preferred. For example, in occupational exposure studies, the log dose often is used rather than the actual dose because the log dose more closely approximates a normal distribution. A particular normal distribution is defined by its mean and variance (or standard deviation). Two normal distributions with different means but the same variance will differ in location but not in shape (Figure A–2). Two normal distributions with the same mean but different variances will have the same location but different shapes or "spreads" about the mean value (Figure A–3). Note that the normal distribution is unimodal

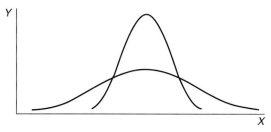

Figure A–3. Two normal distributions with identical means but different standard deviations.

(has one value occurring most frequently), bell-shaped, and symmetric about the mean.

The population encompassed by one standard deviation (σ) on either side of the mean in a normally distributed population will include approximately 67% of the observations in that population (Figure A–4); the population between 2σ on either side of the mean will include approximately 95% of the observations; and that between 3σ on either side of the mean encompasses more than 99% of the observations in the population (see Figure A–4). This property of the normal distribution is particularly useful when a researcher or clinician is trying to identify patients with high or low values in response to a certain test. If one knows the mean for that particular test and has a good estimate of what the standard deviation is, the range within which one would expect (let us say) 95% of patients to fall can be determined, and a patient with values outside this range might need to be examined further.

To use this property of the normal distribution, the sample should be large enough to provide reasonably certain estimates of the mean and standard deviation.

Example I: *If the mean hematocrit value in a clinical population is 42% with a standard deviation of 3%—and assuming hematocrit values follow a normal distribution—one would expect 95% of the clinic population to have hematocrit values between 42% ± (2 × 3%) or (36, 48)%. A patient falling outside this range could be identified for further testing.*

Another principle relevant to the normal distribution is the central limit theorem, which holds that no

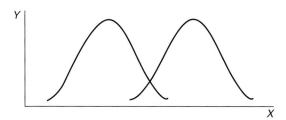

Figure A–2. Two normal distributions with different means but identical standard deviations.

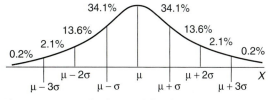

Figure A–4. Standard normal distribution.

matter what the underlying distribution of x, the particular variable of interest, the sample mean ($\bar{x}$) will have a normal distribution if the sample size (n) is large enough. Thus, if $\bar{x}$ itself comes from a population with a mean value μ and population standard deviation s, then $\bar{x}$ (calculated from a sufficiently large sample of size n) will have a normal distribution with the same population mean μ and a smaller population standard deviation equal to $\sigma/\sqrt{n}$. One then can test hypotheses concerning the sample mean $\bar{x}$ because it is known to have a normal distribution, and its mean and standard deviation are also known. The standard deviation of $\bar{x}$ is called the *standard error of the mean* (SEM).

Because one is usually concerned with estimating the true population mean μ from the sample mean $\bar{x}$, it is important to know how good an estimate the sample mean is of the true mean. Every time a sample of size n is selected from the population and $\bar{x}$ is calculated, a different value for $\bar{x}$ will be obtained and thus a different estimate of μ. If this were done over and over again and many $\bar{x}$ values were generated, the $\bar{x}$ values themselves would have a normal distribution centered on with standard deviation equal to $\sigma/\sqrt{n}$. In practice, one does not calculate several $\bar{x}$ values to estimate μ; only one is calculated. The SEM quantifies the certainty with which this one sample mean estimates the population mean. The certainty with which one estimates the population mean increases with sample size, and it can be seen that the standard error decreases as n increases. It also can be seen that the standard error increases as σ increases. This means that the more variability in the underlying population, the more variable will be the estimate of μ. The "true" SEM is $\sigma/\sqrt{n}$, and the sample estimate of the standard error of the mean is $s/\sqrt{n}$, where s is the sample standard deviation. An investigator wanting a more precise estimate of the mean (smaller SEM) could either increase the sample size n or try to decrease σ.

Many investigators summarize the variability in their data with the standard error because it is smaller in value than the standard deviation. However, the standard error does not quantify variability in the population; it quantifies the uncertainty in the estimate of $\bar{x}$, the population mean. An investigator describing the population sampled should use the standard deviation to describe that population. The SEM is used in testing hypotheses about the population mean.

Example II: Suppose that blood lead is measured in 20 patients. Assume that the sample mean ($\bar{x}$) equals 20 µg/dL and that the sample standard deviation (s) equals 5 µg/dL with a sample size (n) of 20. If blood lead has a normal distribution in this sample, one would expect 95% of the population to lie within 2s of the mean. Thus, if the investigator's sample was a representative one, 95% of the population will have blood leads between 20 ± (2 × 5) (i.e., between 10 and 30 µg/dL). These numbers quickly summarize the distribution and give the reader a range against which to compare the reader's own patients. However, investigators often summarize their data with the mean and the standard error of the mean and report, "Blood lead in this sample population was 20 ± [2 × (5/√20)]." This would lead a reader to believe that 95% of blood lead values are expected to fall between 17.8 and 22.2 µg/dL if one did not know the difference between the standard deviation and the standard error of the mean. In reality, 17.8 and 22.2 µg/dL describe a quantity known as the 95% confidence interval for the true mean blood lead ; it does not describe a range of expected values. The reader of the report usually wishes to compare a patient's blood lead with an expected range of values for blood lead, that is, the mean ± 2s.

INFERENTIAL STATISTICS

In general, there are two steps to be followed in data analysis. The first is to describe the data by using descriptive statistics such as the mean, median, variance, and standard deviation. The second step is to test specific hypotheses that were formulated before conducting the research project. This is done by formulating a null hypothesis and an alternative hypothesis, where the null hypothesis is "no difference exists" and the alternative hypothesis is "difference exists."

An example of a null hypothesis might be, "There is no difference in pulmonary function between groups of underground miners and surface miners." The alternative hypothesis would be, "There is a difference between the two groups."

Once the hypotheses are formulated, the appropriate statistical test can be performed. Some of the most commonly used methods are discussed below.

The Case of Two Groups: The *t*-Test

In many instances an investigator is interested in comparing two groups to determine whether they differ on average for some continuous variable. For example, an investigator might be interested in determining whether exposure to organic solvents has an effect on psychomotor performance such as reaction time. To do this, one would select a sample of a group of industrial painters who are exposed to such solvents and compare their test performances with those of a group of workers not exposed to such solvents. Obviously, even if there are truly no differences between two employee groups in how they perform on such a test, the sample mean test scores probably will be unequal simply because of random fluctuation.

The main question is, "Are the differences larger than one would expect by chance if there truly is no difference in the reaction times?"—that is, do the samples come from one underlying population, not two? The null hypothesis in this situation is that the true mean reaction time in the painter group equals the true mean reaction time in the nonpainter group.

The alternative hypothesis is that the underlying true means are unequal. This is usually called a *two-sided* alternative hypothesis because we are not specifying the direction of the inequality. In the example, average reaction time in the painter group might be faster or slower than average reaction time in the nonpainter group. Differences in either direction are examined by testing the null hypothesis.

The appropriate statistical test in this situation is the two-sample *t*-test. Two independent samples have been drawn; that is, the individuals in one sample are independent of the individuals in the other. The *t*-test has the following form:

$$t = \frac{\bar{x}_1 - \bar{x}_2}{SE(\bar{x}_1 - \bar{x}_2)}$$

where $\bar{x}_1$ is the sample mean in group 1 and $\bar{x}_2$ is the sample mean in group 2.

Note that the numerator is the difference of sample means, and the denominator is the standard error of this quantity. Dividing by the standard error standardizes the difference in sample means by the variability present in the data. If the difference in the means was very large but the data from which it was calculated were highly variable, the *t*-statistic would reflect this and would be adjusted accordingly.

Use of the *t*-statistic assumes that the two samples have the same underlying population variance s_p^2. Thus a pooled estimate of the variance is calculated and substituted into the *t*-statistic. This pooled estimate s_p^2 has the following form:

$$s_p^2 = \frac{(n_1 - 1)s_1^2 + (n_2 - 1)s_2^2}{(n_1 + n_2 - 2)}$$

Therefore, the two-sample *t*-statistic is as follows:

$$t = \frac{\bar{x}_1 - \bar{x}_2}{\sqrt{\left(\frac{s_p^2}{n_1}\right) + \left(\frac{s_p^2}{n_2}\right)}}$$

Note that the pooled estimate of the variance is simply a weighted average of the variances from sample 1 and sample 2. Thus, if one sample is much larger than the other, more weight is given to its estimate of σ^2 because it is assumed to be more reliable given that it is

based on a larger sample size. Note further that if the two samples are of equal size, the pooled variance is simply the sum of the two sample variances divided by 2. From the format of the *t*-test, one can see that if the two sample means are similar in value, the numerator of *t* will be close to zero—and consequently, the value of *t* would be small—leading to the conclusion that the null hypothesis is true and that there is probably only one underlying distribution from which the two samples come. If one obtains a large value for the *t*-statistic, it is likely that the two samples come from two different underlying distributions, and one therefore would want to reject the null hypothesis.

How large does *t* have to be to reject the null hypothesis? Tables of the t-statistic indicate what value of *t* would cause the null hypothesis to be rejected. Even when the null hypothesis is true and there really is no difference between the groups being compared, there is the possibility that a large value of *t* might occur owing to random chance alone. One would like the probability of this occurrence to be small, that is, less than 5%.

To find the proper cutoff value of *t* (to reject the null hypothesis) for a particular study, it is necessary to know the number of degrees of freedom. The degrees of freedom are equal to $(n_1 + n_2 - 2)$. This may be thought of as the number of observations that are free to vary once the mean is known. Once the degrees of freedom are known, the value of *t* may be obtained from the *t*-table and compared with the *t*-statistic calculated in the study. If the study *t*-statistic is larger than the tabled cutoff value, one can conclude that this is unlikely to have happened under the null hypothesis, which is therefore rejected.

Bear in mind that the alternative hypothesis was the two-sided alternative, meaning that the two group means were simply different but not specifying the direction of the difference. Consequently, in the *t*-table, two cutoff points actually are obtained because both very large negative and very large positive values of *t* are of interest. The *t*-distribution is symmetric, so the two cutoff points are simply ±*t*. If the study *t*-value is larger than +*t* or smaller than −*t*, the null hypothesis is rejected.

Example III gives the flavor of the *t*-test and how it is used.

Example III: *Two-sample t-tests. The following tabulation presents the mean change in plasma cholinesterase concentration from baseline levels for 15 pesticide applicators and 14 unexposed controls.*

	N	Mean Decline (%)	Standard Deviation
Applicators	15	25	11
Controls	14	10	8

Do the data present sufficient evidence from which to conclude that the mean decline in cholinesterase is different for the two groups?

The null hypothesis is that there is no difference in cholinesterase change between the two groups. The alternative hypothesis is that there is a difference in cholinesterase change between the two groups.

First calculate s_p^2:

$$s_p^2 = \frac{(n_1-1)s_1^2 + (n_2-1)s_2^2}{(n_1+n_2-2)}$$

$$= \frac{(15-1)\,11^2 + (14-1)\,8^2}{(15+14-2)}$$

$$= 90.21$$

Substitute into the formula for t:

$$t = \frac{\bar{x}_1 - \bar{x}_2}{\sqrt{\left(\frac{s_p^2}{n_1}\right) + \left(\frac{s_p^2}{n_2}\right)}}$$

$$= \frac{25-10}{\sqrt{\left(\frac{90.21}{15}\right) + \left(\frac{90.21}{14}\right)}}$$

$$= \frac{15}{\sqrt{12.458}}$$

$$= 4.25$$

Therefore, $t = 4.25$ and $df = n_1 + n_2 - 2 = 27$.

The study t-value of 4.25 with 27 degrees of freedom is compared with the tabled t value of ± 2.05, which has a 5% chance of occurring when the null hypothesis is true. Because $+4.51$ is larger than $+2.05$, the null hypothesis is rejected; that is, there is a statistically significant difference in the mean change in plasma cholinesterase from baseline between the two study groups. In other words, this difference is unlikely to have occurred by chance.

This result also can be expressed as the confidence interval or maximum range of the true change in cholinesterase. In this case, the 95% confidence interval is 16.5–33.5. Stated another way, the probability is approximately 0.95 that the true mean decline in plasma cholinesterase concentration in the applicators is within the range 16.5–33.5.

Paired t-Test

The preceding discussion concerns the two-sample t-test and is appropriate for the situation in which two independent groups are being compared. Another common situation occurs when there are paired samples; that is, the two observations are not independent of one another.

For example, suppose that a researcher is measuring change in pulmonary function [e.g., forced expiratory volume in 1 second (FEV_1)] over a work shift and there are 20 subjects in the study (see the example below). The researcher would measure FEV_1 among the subjects before and after the work shift. Clearly, the before and after measurements are not independent, and one would like to take advantage of the fact that all individual (nonexposure) characteristics have been controlled. To do this, the difference in FEV_1 (before − after) is calculated for each subject. Because the difference is the only observation made per subject, the data set now has gone from 40 observations (2 per subject) to 20 observations (1 per subject). If there is no effect of work shift on FEV_1, one would expect the difference in FEV_1 for each subject to be small in value or close to zero. If the null hypothesis is not true and work shift exposure does change FEV_1, the differences will not be close to zero. The t-statistic calculated in this situation is known as the *paired* t-statistic and has the following form:

$$t = \frac{\bar{D}}{(s_D / \sqrt{n})}$$

where $\bar{D} = \dfrac{\Sigma D_i}{n}$ = **average difference and**

s_D = **standard deviation of differences.**

$$= \sqrt{\frac{\sum_{i=1}^{n}(D_i - \bar{D})^2}{n-1}}$$

The appropriate null hypothesis is that the true mean of the differences is zero, and the appropriate alternative hypothesis is that the true mean of the differences is not zero. Again, it is a two-sided alternative, and one is looking for large positive or large negative differences. Small absolute values of the t-statistic would indicate that the null hypothesis is probably true, and large absolute values of t would lead to rejection of the null hypothesis. One goes to the t-table or computer program to determine how large a value of t is needed to reject the null hypothesis. To obtain the correct value, one needs to know the appropriate degrees of freedom. In the paired t situation, there are $n - 1$ degrees of freedom, or the number of pairs minus one.

Common Errors in Use of the t-Test

EXAMPLE: Paired t-test

A study of painters involved measuring pulmonary function (FEV, liters) at the beginning (A) and end (B) of a work shift. The results were as follows:

Case #	A_1	B_1	$D_1=(A_1-B_1)$	$(D_1-\overline{D})$	$(D_1-\overline{D})^2$
1	3.14	3.01	0.13	0.10	0.010
2	2.85	2.80	0.05	0.02	0.000
3	2.50	2.30	0.20	0.17	0.029
4	3.01	3.15	−0.14	−0.17	0.029
5	1.55	1.55	0.00	−0.03	0.001
6	2.21	2.15	0.06	0.03	0.001
7	2.81	2.68	0.13	0.10	0.010
8	3.25	3.34	−0.09	−0.12	0.014
9	2.66	2.56	0.10	−0.07	0.029
10	1.95	1.90	0.05	−0.02	0.000
11	3.50	3.46	0.04	0.01	0.000
12	3.95	4.06	−0.11	−0.14	0.020
13	4.10	3.90	0.20	0.17	0.029
14	3.60	3.56	0.04	0.01	0.000
15	2.80	2.90	−0.10	−0.13	0.017
16	2.50	2.50	0.00	−0.03	0.001
17	2.10	2.16	−0.06	−0.09	0.008
18	3.70	3.61	0.09	0.06	0.004
19	2.92	2.86	0.06	0.03	0.001
20	3.31	3.42	−0.11	−0.14	0.020
			0.54		0.198

$$\overline{D} = \frac{\Sigma D_i}{n} = \frac{0.54}{20} = 0.027$$

$$s_D = \sqrt{\frac{\sum_{i=1}^{n}(D_i-\overline{D})^2}{n-1}}$$

$$= \sqrt{\frac{0.198}{19}} = 0.102$$

$$t = \frac{\overline{D}}{(s_D/\sqrt{n})} = \frac{0.027}{0.102/\sqrt{20}} = 1.18$$

Compare the calculated t of 1.18 to the tabled t of 2.093. Since the calculated t is less than the t in the table, the null hypothesis (of no change in function over work shift) is not rejected.

A common mistake made with the *t*-test is known as the *multiple-comparison problem*. The problem arises when an investigator has several groups to compare and proceeds to compare them in groups of two, using the *t*-test each time. In other words, group 1 is compared against group 2 using the *t*-test, then group 2 against group 3, then group 1 against group 3, and so on. The problem with proceeding in this fashion is that overall there is *more* than a 5% chance of erroneously rejecting the null hypothesis even though there is only a 5% chance of making this mistake with each individual comparison. This increased probability of making a mistake occurs because multiple tests increase the likelihood that an error will occur. Thus the chance of erroneously rejecting a null hypothesis is greater than the 5% risk of mistakenly rejecting each comparison taken by itself, even if all the hypotheses are true. There are many ways of adjusting for this situation, known as *multiple-comparison procedures.* What is important to remember is that if one does enough of such two-group comparisons, the probability of rejecting the null hypothesis incorrectly at least once increases with the number of such comparisons made and can be quite a bit greater than 5% unless the investigator uses an appropriate adjustment for multiple comparisons.

Analysis of Variance (ANOVA)

When the variables under study are continuous in nature and there are more than two groups being studied, the investigator usually is concerned with whether the means in the groups are different from one another. An appropriate statistical method to answer this question is to use *analysis of variance* (ANOVA).

Suppose that one were studying three groups of workers occupationally exposed to three different gases. One might want to test whether the particular gases affect mean FEV_1 levels differently in the three groups. In this example, individual FEV_1 values would be adjusted for nonexposure determinants (i.e., age, gender, height, or race). The null hypothesis is that the group means for FEV_1 are equal, that is, that a particular exposure has no effect on FEV_1 values. Obviously, there will be differences between the sample means in each group owing to random fluctuations in FEV_1 among individuals.

Are the differences observed in the sample means merely a result of random fluctuations, or are they a consequence of true differences in FEV_1 caused by the gas exposures? To answer this question, one examines whether the data are consistent with the assumption that the gas exposure has no effect and that the three groups are really random samples from the same underlying population. The null hypothesis assumes that any observed differences in the sample means and standard deviations are due simply to random sampling. ANOVA tests this null hypothesis by estimating the true population variance in two different ways and comparing these two estimates of the variance. If the three samples do indeed come from the same underlying population, these two estimates of the variance will be very close in value. If the three samples do not all come from the same underlying population, these two estimates will be further apart in value, and this variation is what one hopes to detect.

Certain statistical assumptions are made when an ANOVA test is performed on a set of data: (1) It is assumed that groups have been randomly assigned to receive the treatment or exposure and that the groups are independent; (2) the underlying variance (σ^2) in each group is assumed to be identical (even though the true group means may be different and the sample variances may differ slightly); and (3) the random variable under study—for example, FEV_1—has a normal distribution.

Conceptually, the method of ANOVA proceeds as follows: Once the null hypothesis is formulated, the sample variance (s^2) is computed within each exposure group, and each of these s^2 estimates is unaffected by differences among the group means. These s^2 estimates are averaged to obtain one "within group" variance estimate. The values of the individual exposure group means then are used to arrive at a second "between group" variance estimate of σ^2. In this "between group" estimate of σ^2, differences (or variability) among the group means will affect the overall estimate of σ^2. For example, if a particular gas exposure has no effect on FEV_1, both estimates of σ^2 should be similar. To test the null hypothesis, a statistic known as the F statistic is calculated. The value of F is simply the ratio of the "between group" variance estimate to the "within group" variance estimate. Because both numbers estimate the same parameter (σ^2), if the null hypothesis is true, the value of F should be close to 1. If F is significantly larger than 1, you should reject the null hypothesis and conclude that the exposure groups are different with regard to FEV_1.

How does one determine how large F must be in order to reject the null hypothesis? Because of random fluctuations in the data, it is possible that a large F statistic might result even when the null hypothesis is true. However, one would like the chance of this happening to be very small. Tables of the F statistic are available to assist the investigator in selecting a value of F against which the F statistic calculated from the data can be compared. The tabled value of F is one that would occur less than approximately 5% of the time if the null hypothesis were true. If the F statistic calculated from the researcher's data is larger than the one found in the table, the results are less than 5% likely to have occurred by random chance, even if the null hypothesis (no difference in sample groups) is true. Because the observed results therefore are very unlikely to have happened by chance under the null hypothesis, the researcher is justified in rejecting the null hypothesis and saying that there is a difference among the groups. The 5% cutoff point is an arbitrary one, and depending on the individual situation, one could set the cutoff at one or 10%; however, the conventional cutoff point is 5%.

When one is studying more than two groups and the data involved are continuous (e.g., FEV_1 or blood lead concentration) and the question of interest is whether the groups all come from the same underlying population— that is, have the same mean for the variable of interest— ANOVA is the most appropriate method to use for initial testing of the null hypothesis. If one fails to reject the null hypothesis with the F statistic, no further tests of the null hypothesis are necessary. There are no differences among groups. On the other hand, if one performs ANOVA on the data and rejects the null hypothesis, then differences in the outcome (FEV_1 or blood lead level) among the study groups associated with the particular exposure may exist. One then can use multiple-comparison tests to identify exactly which group or groups are significantly different.

This is a simplified discussion of ANOVA meant only to introduce the concept of this important statistical method. We have not provided enough details for the reader to be able to perform this test accurately. The purpose is to identify situations in which ANOVA is appropriate as an initial analytic procedure (see References).

Analyzing Rates & Proportions: The Chi-Square Test

In preceding sections we described methods of analysis for continuous types of data. This section begins a discussion of the analysis of categorical data. The following table of cigarette smoking history and lung cancer cases and controls (persons without cancer) presents an example of categorical data.

	Lung Cancer	Controls
Cigarette smokers	450	225
Nonsmokers	20	225
Total	470	450

It is immediately apparent, without doing any statistical tests, that there is an association of cigarette smoking and lung cancer. The row variable, cigarette smoking, is associated with the column variable, lung cancer. A simple calculation of the proportions of lung cancer cases and control cases who smoked confirms this association. Of the lung cancer cases, 450/470 = 95.7% smoked cigarettes, whereas 225/450 = 50% of the controls smoked cigarettes.

However, suppose that the table was of mesothelioma (a very rare type of lung cancer) and cigarette smoking, and the following results were obtained:

	Mesothelioma	Controls
Cigarette smokers	80	200
Nonsmokers	40	104
Total	120	304

In this example, the ratio of cigarette smokers to nonsmokers among the mesothelioma cases (80/120 = 66.6%) and the controls (200/304 = 65.8%) is nearly the same, with approximately twice as many smokers as nonsmokers for both the case and control groups. In this case, one would say that there is no association between the column variable (mesothelioma) and the row variable (cigarette smoking). The null hypothesis in this example would be that there is no association between mesothelioma and cigarette smoking, and one could not reject the null hypothesis owing to the similarity of the proportions of smokers in the mesothelioma and the control groups.

Most situations with categorical data are not as clear-cut as these two examples. In most cases, one cannot simply "eyeball" the data to determine whether the two variables are independent or not. The statistical test one uses to determine whether or not there is an association in such data is known as the *chi-square test*. Example IV is a situation in which the chi-square test is applied.

Example IV: *Three groups of farm workers are studied for the occurrence of new skin rashes during the growing season. The three groups are involved in growing and harvesting (1) grapes, (2) citrus crops, and (3) tomatoes. The workers are followed for the growing season, and the occurrence of new rashes in the three groups is compared to determine if there is an association between exposure (crop) and outcome (rash).*

Crop 1, N = 100
Crop 2, N = 200
Crop 3, N = 200

Response	Exposure (Crop)			
	1	2	3	Total
Rash	30	40	32	102
No rash	70	160	168	398
Total	100	200	200	500

The null hypothesis in this situation is again the hypothesis of "no difference," only it is phrased as no association between the row variable (rash) and the column variable (crop).

One can quickly compute from the table that the percentage working on crop 1 with a rash is 30/100 = 30%; on crop 2, it is 40/20 = 20%; and on crop 3, it is 32/200 = 16%. By just quickly observing the data, one might think that crop 1 is different from crops 2 and 3. However, the null hypothesis is that there is no association between crop worked and rash development. Thus the question is whether the observed differences in response are simply a result of random variation in the data or are

larger than one would expect by chance alone if the null hypothesis were true. To test this, a chi-square statistic is calculated. As with the *t*-test and *F*-test, one determines whether this chi-square value is unlikely to have occurred by chance alone under the null hypothesis. The calculation of the chi-square involves first determining an "expected" value for each cell in the table. The expected value is the value one would "expect" to see in the cell if there were no association between row (rash) and column (crop exposure) variables, that is, that value one would "expect" to see if the null hypothesis were true. The expected value is obtained as follows.

According to the null hypothesis, we would expect the same proportion to develop a rash in each group. If this is true, the best estimate of the expected proportion with rashes in each exposure group comes from the overall information given by the total number of workers with rashes divided by the total number of workers in the study; that would be 102/500 = 0.204. Then, for crop 1, one expects that 0.204 of the 100 people in crop exposure group 1 will develop rashes, that is, 20.4 people; for crop 2, one expects that 0.204 of the 200 people working with crop 2 will develop rashes, that is, 40.8 people; and for crop 3, one expects that 0.204 of the 200 people will develop rashes, that is, 40.8 people. In other words, because under the null hypothesis there is no association between exposure and percentage developing a rash, one expects the same percentage to respond favorably (or unfavorably) in each group. The expected proportion of workers not developing rashes is obtained in the same manner. The best estimate of the proportion not developing a rash in each group is the total number not developing a rash divided by the total number of workers, which equals 398/500 = 0.796. This gives an expected frequency of 100 × 0.796 = 79.6 working with crop 1 not developing rashes, 159.2 working with crop 2 not developing rashes, and 159.2 working with crop 3 not developing rashes. Putting the expected values in parentheses alongside the observed values, the table now looks like this:

Response	Exposure (Crop)			
	1	2	3	Total
Rash	30 (20.4)	40 (40.8)	32 (40.8)	102
No rash	70 (79.6)	160 (159.2)	168 (159.2)	398
Total	100	200	200	500

To test the null hypothesis, one looks at the observed and expected numbers in each cell to see how close together the two values are. If the values are close together, one may decide that the null hypothesis is true. If they are very different, one may decide that the null hypothesis is not true. To decide whether the observed and expected values are close together, the chi-square statistic is calculated. It has the following form:

$$\chi^2 = \sum_{i=1}^{n}\left[\frac{(O_i - E_i)^2}{E_i}\right]$$

where E_i is the expected value in cell i, O_i is the observed value in cell i, $i = 1, \ldots , n$, and n is the number of cells in the table.

Large chi-square values indicate a lack of agreement between observed and expected values; small chi-square values indicate close agreement.

How does one determine what constitutes a large chi-square value? As in the preceding discussions about t- and F-tests for continuous data, one consults a table of chi-square values. The table identifies the chi-square value that would occur less than 5% of the time if the null hypothesis (no association) were true, and this is compared with the study chi-square value. If the study-chi square is larger than the table cutoff value, the null hypothesis is rejected because this is known to occur less than 5% of the time when the null hypothesis is true. If the study chi-square value is smaller than the table cut-off value, the null hypothesis is not rejected. Alternatively, one could calculate the exact probability, or P value, of the study chi-square statistic. To use the chi-square tables, the degrees of freedom are needed to select the proper value from the table. The degrees of freedom in the chi-square situation are equal to (number of rows – 1) × (number of columns – 1). When there are two rows and three columns in a table, the degree of freedom is (2 – 1) × (3 – 1), which equals 2 degrees of freedom. One thing to remember is that the chi-square statistic works only when the sample is sufficiently large. A rule of thumb is that the chi-square test yields good results when the expected values in each cell are greater than or equal to 5.

Calculating the chi-square statistic for the preceding example, the following results are obtained:

$$\chi^2 = \frac{(70 - 79.6)^2}{79.6} + \frac{(160 - 159.2)^2}{159.2}$$
$$+\frac{(168 - 159.2)^2}{159.2} + \frac{(30 - 20.4)^2}{20.4}$$
$$+\frac{(40 - 40.8)^2}{40.8} + \frac{(32 - 40.8)^2}{40.8}$$
$$= 8.08$$

The tabled value of chi-square to which the calculated value is compared is 5.99. Because 8.08 is larger than 5.99, the null hypothesis is rejected.

Calculating the chi-square statistic is only one method for analyzing categorical data. It is, however, one of the most common statistical tests found in the medical literature.

The *P*-Value & Statistical Significance

An important quantity in all statistical hypothesis tests is the P-value. The P-value is the probability of observing a particular study result (e.g., t-statistic calculated from study data) by chance alone when the null hypothesis is really true. In the examples thus far, the P-value of the test statistic actually has been used without calculating its exact value. The procedure has been to calculate, for example, a t-statistic from the study data. A computer program then would compare the t-statistic observed with the t-statistic known to have a P-value of 5%.

If the value of the t-statistic computed for the sample is smaller than the 5% value, the null hypothesis is not rejected. When the computed sample t-statistic has a value larger than the 5% P-value, the null hypothesis is rejected. The exact P-value of the sample t-statistic also can be obtained from tabulated values so that one can report P-values less than other cutoff values, for example, 1% ($P < 0.01$). When the P-value is less than 5%, the result is commonly referred to as being *statistically significant.* However, statistical significance may not be the same as clinical or public health significance because the former is affected by the size of the study population and may reflect differences that have no biologic importance.

Another way to express the statistical significance of an observed result is the confidence interval (CI). The CI provides a range and the probability that this range includes the true population mean. For example, a 95% CI is calculated as the sample mean plus or minus two standard errors of the mean. The CI is interpreted as giving a 95% probability of including the true population mean. A 99% CI is the sample mean plus or minus three standard errors of the mean.

It should be noted that the width of the CI will decrease as the sample size increases; that is, we are more confident of knowing the true population mean when it is estimated from a larger sample. The degree of certainty is also inversely related to the width of the confidence interval. For example, we can be more precise (narrower CI) in estimating the 95% CI than the 99% CI for the same sample size.

The CI is generally preferred to the P-value because it gives the range of values observed with a select level of statistical confidence (e.g., 95%) and not just a single determination of whether the observed result is above or below the P-value.

The researcher in a typical study is interested in comparing an exposed group to a control group and using the observed difference in proportions or mean values to estimate the effect of the exposure. For example, let's say one is interested in determining delta (δ), where δ equals the true mean value of sperm concentration among workers exposed to heavy metals minus the true mean value of sperm concentration in unexposed workers. One then wishes to test whether $\delta = 0$; that is, one may wish to determine whether the (true) proportion with disease from one exposure is equal to the (true) proportion with disease under a second exposure or control. One can then calculate δ as the difference between these two proportions, again testing to see whether $\delta = 0$.

Even if the treatment and control groups in the study are truly being sampled from one underlying population (i.e., if there is no real difference between treatment and control), some differences between the two groups will occur by chance alone. If the observed difference in sample means or proportions has a small probability of occurring by chance alone (assuming no true underlying difference), then the null hypothesis that $\delta = 0$ is rejected. The "rule" for deciding how small that probability has to be before rejecting the null hypothesis is known as the *level of significance* of the statistical test and is designated as alpha (α).

Thus the procedure in a typical study is to formulate a null hypothesis (H_0), and usually,

H_0: $\mu_1 = \mu_2$
also written as H_0: $\delta = \mu_1 - \mu_2 = 0$

for example, H_0: mean sperm concentration with exposure 1 (heavy metals) = mean sperm concentration with exposure 2 (no exposure), or

H_0: $p_1 - p_2 = 0$
also written as H_0: $\delta = p_1 - p_2 = 0$

in other words H_0: proportion with disease in exposure (P_1) = proportion with disease in exposure (P_2).

The (two-sided) alternative hypothesis is

H_A: $\mu_1 \neq \mu_2$
also written as H_A: $\delta = \mu_1 - \mu_2 \neq 0$

that is, H_A: the mean sperm concentrations are not equal under treatments 1 and 2, or

H_A: $p_1 \neq p_2$
also written as H_A: $\delta = p_1 - p_2 \neq 0$

that is, H_A: the proportions with disease are not equal under treatments 1 and 2 ($P_1 = P_2$).

After completion of the study, sample estimates of μ (or p) are calculated for the two exposure groups. The probability is calculated that a difference as large as the one observed in the study would occur if the null hypothesis were true. This probability is the *P*-value of the test. If the *P*-value is less than α (the significance level), the null hypothesis is rejected. If the *P*-value is not less than α, the null hypothesis is not rejected. A CI also can be calculated for proportions as it can be for means, and one can determine the probability that the true proportion is within the calculated CI.

THE TYPES OF MISTAKES ONE CAN MAKE IN DOING A RESEARCH STUDY

There are two main categories of errors one can make in deriving inferences from a typical research study. They are known as *type I* and *type II errors.*

Type I Error

A type I error occurs if one decides to reject the null hypothesis and declare the two groups different when in fact they really are from the same underlying population. Type I error is equal to the significance level α, and the significance level must be established before the study is conducted. Thus α equals the probability that one will reject the null hypothesis when the null hypothesis is true, that is, when the investigator decides what chance of making this kind of mistake is acceptable and sets the α level accordingly. For example, an investigator may decide that it is extremely important not to declare that a disease (e.g., cancer) is associated with an exposure unless there is overwhelming evidence of an association from the study. In this case, the α level might be set at 1% instead of 5%, where 5% is the value for α used in most studies.

Type II Error

A type II error occurs if a researcher decides not to reject the null hypothesis when, in fact, there is a difference between the two groups; that is, a true difference between the two groups has been missed. Type II error is usually designated by β.

In a research study, the type II error is not a single value. If the null hypothesis is false, this means that outcomes seen in the exposure group are not equivalent to those seen in the control group; that is, δ is not equal to 0. There are an infinite number of values that this difference could take on. For each value of the difference δ between the exposed and control groups, there is a different value for the type II error. If one is interested in determining the probability that one would miss a true difference between exposure and control groups, the exact value of the difference being examined must be specified. Once this is done, the probability that one would fail to reject the null hypothesis given the true nonzero difference between the two groups can be calculated.

The Power of a Study

One of the most important quantities calculated for a research study is the power of a particular study. The power is the probability that one will correctly reject the null hypothesis when the null hypothesis is truly false. In other words, the power is the probability of correctly recognizing a true difference between the two groups. The power of a study is actually the complement of the type II error β, that is, power = $1 - \beta$. Thus the power of a study is different for every different value of β that occurs. To calculate the power, one must specify a particular alternative. Power is particularly important when one is evaluating a negative study—a study that finds no difference between the groups.

Suppose that the power of a specific study is 40%. This means that the researcher has only a 40% chance of discerning that a true difference exists between the exposure groups. Therefore, if no difference between exposure groups is found and the power of the study is reported as 40%, a reader might wonder whether that particular study had any real chance of finding a difference between exposures even if the exposures were truly associated with the different outcomes. In practice, it is much more common to use 80% or 90% for the power of a study so that you have a reasonably good probability of detecting a difference between exposures if one truly exists.

The power of a statistical test is determined or affected by three quantities: (1) the magnitude of the type I error α, (2) the size of the exposure effect δ the researcher is interested in detecting, and (3) the sample size of the study. Quantities (1) and (2) can be used to estimate the sample size needed in a study for a specified study power.

As the size of the type I error becomes smaller, the power of the study likewise becomes smaller. Remember, the type I error is the probability of incorrectly declaring a difference when none actually exists. As it becomes less likely to make this mistake (i.e., α is smaller), it becomes less likely the null hypothesis will be rejected in general, and power involves correctly rejecting the null hypothesis.

When a study is set up to look for a very large exposure effect δ, it is relatively easy to detect this large effect, and the chances are great that the null hypothesis will be correctly rejected. The opposite occurs when one is looking for a very small δ. Thus power increases as δ increases.

As sample size increases, the variability of the measure of exposure effect decreases. Consequently, the test statistic increases in value, making it easier to exceed the cutoff point for rejecting the null hypothesis. This increases the chances of correctly rejecting the null hypothesis, and so power increases as sample size increases.

A handy table for remembering the quantities discussed in this section is shown below:

	H_0 true (no difference)	H_0 true (difference exists)
H_0 study (declare no difference)	Correct decision	Type II error β
H_0 reject (declare a difference)	Type I error α	Power $1-\beta$

REFERENCES

Centers for Disease Control and Prevention: www.cdc.gov/publications.htm (free software download: epi info, epi map).

Minitab: www.minitab.com (a general statistical program, used for teaching and research; good graphics; PC and Mac).

Stata (Stata Corporation): www.stata.com (general purpose statistical software; PC and Mac).

Statistics.com: www.statistics.com (free software, commercial products, and Web-based resources).

University of Glasgow Department of Statistics: www.stats.gla.ac.uk/cti/links_stats/software.html.

■ II. EPIDEMIOLOGY

Epidemiology is the study of the distribution and determinants of health- and disease-related conditions in populations. It is concerned with both epidemic (excess of normal expectancy) and endemic (always present) conditions.

The basic premise of epidemiology is that disease is not randomly distributed across populations. Not only is it important to know what sort of disease a particular person has, but it is also necessary to know what sort of person has a particular disease. While the practice of much of occupational medicine is concerned with the pathogenesis (development) of disease and the treatment of individuals with diseases, the focus of occupational epidemiology is on groups of individuals—with or without diseases—in an attempt to infer the causes that precede specific disease conditions and to determine what occupational or other lifestyle factors can be manipulated to eliminate specific diseases or reduce the prevalence of the disease.

There are three major types of epidemiologic studies: descriptive, analytic, and experimental.

Descriptive epidemiologic studies characterize person, place, and time: (1) Person: What are the characteristics of people who get a particular disease (e.g., age, race, gender, occupation, socioeconomic status, immune status)? (2) Place: Where do they live, work, or travel (e.g., international, national, and local comparisons; urban

Table A–2. Measures of mortality.

$$\text{Crude death rate} = \frac{\text{Number of deaths in year (all causes)}}{\text{Total population}} \times 1000$$

e.g., US 1977 = 8.8 ÷ 1000 population or 878.1 ÷ 100,000 population

$$\text{Cause - specific death rate} = \frac{\text{Number of deaths from specific cause in year}}{\text{Total population}} \times 100,000$$

e.g., cancer in US 1977 = 178.7 ÷ 100,000 population

$$\text{Age - specific death rate} = \frac{\text{Number of deaths among persons of specified age group in year}}{\text{Population in specified age group}} \times 100,000$$

e.g., cancer in age group 1–14 years = 4.9 ÷ 100,000

$$\text{Infant mortality rate} = \frac{\text{Number of deaths among children younger than 1 year of age in year}}{\text{Number of births in year}} \times 1000$$

e.g., US 1977 = 14.1 ÷ 100,000 live births (12.3 for whites; 21.7 for blacks and others)

versus rural populations; climate; altitude)? (3) Time: When does the illness occur (e.g., temporal variation, seasonal fluctuations)? Descriptive studies are not used to test hypotheses but nevertheless are powerful tools for characterizing disease distributions and associations.

Analytic studies attempt to determine the etiologic factors associated with a disease by calculating estimates of risk: (1) What exposures do people with the disease have in common (e.g., smoking, exogenous hormone use, diet, exposure to radiation or asbestos)? (2) How much is disease risk increased by such exposures (using relative risk as the measure of excess risk? (3) How many cases could be avoided if the exposure were eliminated (using attributable risk as the appropriate measure)? Analytic studies involve testing specific hypotheses.

Experimental studies involve a search for strategies for altering the natural history of disease. Examples of experimental studies are intervention trials to reduce risk factors, screening studies aimed at identifying the early stages of disease, and clinical trials of different treatment modalities to improve prognosis.

MORTALITY & MORBIDITY

The two basic measures of disease in a population are mortality (death) rates and morbidity (disease) rates.

Table A–2 provides examples of different types of mortality rates and how each is calculated. Morbidity is measured by calculating either prevalence or incidence rates. *Prevalence* is the number of existing cases of a disease at a given time divided by the population at risk for that disease at that time. This result is commonly multiplied by 100,000 to derive the prevalence rate per 100,000 population.

For purposes of etiology, the *incidence rate* is a more important measure of morbidity and is equal to the number of new cases of a disease occurring over a defined interval divided by the midinterval population at risk for that disease (multiplied by 100,000).

While worldwide mortality data are available—at various degrees of precision depending on the quality of death registration systems—incidence rates can be calculated only for those diseases for which there are population-based registries or for which special studies have been conducted. The National Cancer Institute has a program of cancer registries around the United States that provides information on cancer incidence covering approximately 10% of the U.S. population. Accurate enumeration of the population at risk—available from Census data—is vital for deriving valid estimates of both mortality and morbidity rates. Rates can be specific to any subgroup of interest, defined by age, gender, race, or other characteristics. For example, the age-adjusted incidence rate for cervical cancer among white women in the United States was 8.7 per 100,000, compared with 11.1 per 100,000 among black women and 15.8 per 100,000 among Hispanic women. One must remember that in calculating a rate, the events in the numerator must be drawn from the population specified in the denominator; that is, those in the denominator must be at risk for the disease. Thus, for cervical cancer, men would not be included in the denominator.

Some problems to keep in mind about current disease data sources include the following:

1. The only complete cause-specific disease registry is for deaths, and the cause-of-death assignment on the death certificate is often inaccurate. In addition, for a disease whose case-fatality ratio is low (i.e., a disease unlikely to result in death when it occurs), the death rate is a gross underestimate of the incidence of the condition in the community. An example of this is nonmelanoma skin cancer, which has a high incidence but low mortality rate.

2. Morbidity reports, even when legally mandated, as is the case for certain infectious diseases (e.g., tuberculosis and sexually transmitted diseases), often are incomplete because of severe underreporting.

3. Complete and accurate population-based morbidity registries are limited in geographic coverage.

ADJUSTMENT OF RATES

In attempting to compare disease rates across population groups or assessing changes in rates over time, the effect of differential age distributions in two populations whose rates are being compared should be taken into account. Disease risk almost always is a function of age; differences in crude rates (i.e., rates not adjusted for age) across populations may reflect age differences rather than differences in occupational or environmental factors of interest.

Age-specific rates are not subject to this drawback, provided the range in each age group, or age stratum, is relatively narrow. It is cumbersome, however, to compare rates among populations across many age strata. Age adjustment or standardization provides a summary measure of disease risk for an entire population that is not influenced by variations in age distribution.

There are two methods for age adjustment: a direct method, which applies observed age-specific rates of death or disease to a standard population, and an indirect method, which applies age-specific rates of death or disease from a standard population to the age distribution of an observed population. In discussing the methods for adjusting rates, cancer will be used as the disease of interest.

The direct method of age adjustment is appropriate when each of the populations being compared is large enough to yield stable age-specific rates. For example, the direct method is used for comparison of cancer rates over time in the United States. Crude mortality rates showing a dramatic increase in cancer over the past few decades would seem to provide strong evidence of a cancer epidemic. It needs to be ascertained, however, to what extent the aging of the country's population has contributed to the apparent epidemic or to what extent other factors, such as an increase in cancer-causing agents in the environment, might be responsible.

The first three columns of Table A–3 show the actual age distributions of the U.S. population in 1940 and 1970, the percentage of the population in each group in the two periods, the corresponding number of actual cancer deaths, and the age-specific death rates. Crude death rates per 100,000 population were 120.2 for 1940 and 163.2 for 1970, an increase of more than 30%. Comparison of the age-specific rates, however, shows only minor increases between the two time periods. It should be noted that the percentage of the population in all age groups over 40 was higher in 1970 than in 1940.

To remove the variable effect of age using the direct method of adjustment, a "standard" population is chosen. The number of people in each age group of the standard population then is multiplied by the appropriate age-specific rate in each of the study populations. This generates the number of deaths or cases of disease one would expect in each age group if the populations had similar age distributions. The expected number of deaths or disease cases then is summed over all age groups, the sum is divided by the total standard population, and the result is multiplied by 100,000. The choice of a standard population is arbitrary; it might be the combined population of the two groups whose rates are being compared, only one of those populations, or any other population.

In our example, the standard was the combined population of the United States in 1940 and 1970, shown in column 5 of Table A–3. The age-specific rates for each period (column 4) were applied for each age group to the standard population, yielding the expected number of deaths shown in column 6. Age-adjusted rates then are calculated by dividing the sum of expected deaths for each period by the total standard population. The resulting adjusted rates are 139.8 per 100,000 for 1940 and 149.9 per 100,000 for 1970. Thus the magnitude of the increase in the crude rates has been reduced from about 30% to 7%. It can be concluded that age is an important factor in the increased cancer rates in the United States, although age alone does not entirely explain changes over time.

Table A–3. Age adjustment by direct method, using cancer mortality data for the United States, 1940 and 1970.

Age Group	Actual Population (1)	(2)	Number of Cancer Deaths (3)	Age-Specific Death Rates Per 100,000 (4)	Standard Population (5)	Expected Number of Cancer Deaths (6)
1940						
< 40	87,737,829	66.7	10,283	11.72	217,093,330	25,443
40–49	17,053,068	13.0	18,071	105.97	41,149,961	43,607
50–59	13,100,511	10.0	33,279	254.03	34,177,557	86,821
60–69	8,534,997	6.5	43,686	511.85	24,143,606	123,579
70–79	4,073,514	3.1	38,160	936.78	13,352,179	125,080
80+	1,139,143	0.9	14,721	1,292.29	4,934,355	63,766
Totals	131,639,062	100.0	158,200[2]		334,850,988	468,296[2]
1970						
< 40	129,355,501	63.7	16,096	12.44	217,093,330	27,006
40–49	24,096,893	11.9	26,075	108.21	41,149,961	44,528
50–59	21,077,046	10.4	61,143	290.09	34,177,557	99,146
60–69	15,608,609	7.7	90,099	577.24	24,143,606	139,367
70–79	9,278,665	4.6	88,826	957.31	13,352,179	127,821
80+	3,795,212	1.9	49,333	1,299.87	4,934,355	64,140
Totals	203,211,926	100.0	331,572[1]		334,850,988	502,008[1]

[1]Crude death rate = [sum of column 3 + sum of column 1] × 10^5 = 163.2 per 100,000 population. Age-adjusted death rate = [sum of column 6 + sum of column 5] × 10^5 = 149.9 per 100,000 population.
[2]Crude death rate = [sum of column 3 + sum of column 1] × 10^5 = 120.2 per 100,000 population. Age-adjusted death rate = [sum of column 6 + sum of column 5] × 10^5 = 139.8 per 100,000 population.

When the group of interest is relatively small and thus likely to have unstable age-specific rates, it is more appropriate to use the indirect than the direct method of age adjustment. This is commonly the situation with investigation of cause-specific mortality in an occupational cohort. The indirect method is employed frequently to compare the cancer incidence or follow-up experience of a study group with that expected based on the experience of a larger population or patient series. With the indirect method, the age-specific rates from a standard population are multiplied by the number of person-years at risk in each group in the study series. The number of observed deaths then is compared with the number expected by means of a ratio.

The standardized mortality ratio (SMR) is an example of indirect standardization. In calculating an SMR, the age-specific rates from a standard population (e.g., county, state, or country) are multiplied by the person-years at risk in the study population (e.g., industry employees) to give the expected number of deaths. The observed number of deaths divided by the expected number (times 100) is the SMR (see the example in Table A–4). An SMR also may control for time-specific mortality rates by indirect standardization.

Thus the equation for an SMR is as follows:

$$SMR = \left[\frac{\Sigma\, a_i}{\Sigma\, E(a_i)} \right] \times 100$$

$$= \left[\frac{Observed}{Expected} \right] \times 100$$

where a_i is the number of people with a specific cause of death in the ith stratum of age, and $E(a_i)$ is the expected number of deaths based on the age-specific rates in the reference population.

The result is multiplied by 100, so when observed deaths equal expected deaths, the SMR is 100, and the differences from 100 represent the percentage difference in mortality in the study population compared with that of the reference population.

Indirect standardization also may be used to adjust incidence rates for age or other factors. Thus incident cases of a disease within a workplace could be expressed as the standardized incidence ratio (SIR), as follows:

$$SIR = \left[\frac{Observed\ number\ of\ new\ cases}{Expected\ number\ of\ new\ cases} \right] \times 100$$

Table A–4. Age adjustment by indirect method in computation of standardized mortality ratio (SMR).

Age (Years)	Observed Deaths (1)	Person Years (2)	US Population Rates (per 10⁵) (3)	Expected Deaths = (2) × (3)
20–29	1	5,000	20.6	0.1
30–39	0	15,000	22.7	0.3
40–49	4	60,000	45.3	2.7
50–59	2	40,000	94.3	3.8
60–69	12	70,000	224.4	15.7
Σ Obs = 19				Σ Exp = 22.6

SMR = [Σ Obs/Σ Exp] × 100 = [19/22.6]100 = 84

Although it is most common to adjust rates for age and time, the direct and indirect methods of adjustment can be used to adjust for population differences in other factors as well, such as gender, race, socioeconomic status (SES), and stage of disease.

Design Strategies for Analytic & Experimental Studies

Descriptive epidemiology provides disease rates for different groups. It identifies segments of the population—by age, gender, occupation, marital status, geographic area of residence, or other parameters—whose unique experience suggests etiologic hypotheses worthy of pursuit through rigorous analytic studies. Descriptive epidemiology tells who gets the disease where and when and is the basis of analytic epidemiology, which, in turn, focuses on specific questions, such as the following:

- What exposure do people with the disease have in common as compared with people without the disease?
- Why does exposure induce or promote disease?
- How much is disease risk increased by such exposure?
- How many cases might be avoided were the exposure eliminated?

The last question addresses the ultimate objective of epidemiologic research: to identify risk factors so that intervention might either prevent the occurrence of the disease (primary prevention) or lead to early detection (secondary prevention).

The three basic strategies for analytic epidemiology are (1) the cohort study, (2) the case-control study, and (3) the experimental study (clinical trial).

Cohort and case-control studies are observational: The investigator does not control exposure or modify behavior of the study subjects. In the experimental study, the investigator intervenes by introducing treatment or other exposures to study their impact on the disease experience.

TYPES OF EPIDEMIOLOGIC STUDIES

1. The Cohort Study

In the design of a cohort study, a disease-free group of individuals (a cohort) characterized by a common experience or exposure of interest is identified and followed forward over time, or prospectively, to determine whether disease occurs at a rate different from that in a cohort without the exposure. The relative risk (RR) of disease associated with the exposure then can be calculated:

$$RR = \frac{\textit{Incidence rate in the exposed group}}{\textit{Incidence rate in the nonexposed group}}$$

A frequently cited example of the prospective cohort design is the follow-up study of British physicians whose smoking habits were ascertained by means of a mailed questionnaire. The doctors were grouped according to smoking habits, and their deaths were subsequently monitored. Lung cancer rates for those exposed to various levels of smoking then were compared with the rates for nonsmokers by means of the relative risk. Other examples of cohort studies include investigations of long-term cancer incidence among atomic bomb survivors exposed to varying degrees of radiation and deaths among British coal miners.

Theoretically, the prospective cohort study is ideal because the hypothesized cause or exposure precedes the effect or disease. It is also valuable because disease rates and relative risks can be calculated directly, provided that a suitable comparison group is built into the study or is otherwise available for calculation of rates in the nonexposed population. In addition, the exposure of interest can be recorded accurately at the time of exposure; it is not based on recall of past events. This approach has been popular in occupational studies in which the disease experience of workers exposed to putatively hazardous substances has been compared with that of other workers without the exposure or compared with that of the general population.

In practice, however, because of the expense, the time involved, and the number of subjects required, the model prospective cohort study is relatively rare. To avoid some of these constraints, a historical cohort study might be done, whereby a group of persons who in the past experienced an exposure of interest is identified, and their disease record up to the present is investigated. An example is the follow-up of mortality among insulation workers exposed to asbestos. The population of union insulation workers in the 1940s was identified, and their cause-specific mortality rates through the 1970s were determined. Mortality rates for lung cancer and other causes in this

Table A–5. Presentation of data from a cohort study.

		Disease		
		Present	Absent	
Exposure $\{$	Yes	a	b	$a+b$
	No	c	d	$c+d$

population were tabulated and compared with those expected on the basis of mortality rates for all U.S. men. Because the historical cohort study is really a retrospective approach, the terms *cohort study* and *prospective study* should not be used synonymously.

Measures of Association in a Cohort Study

Measures of association illustrate the statistical relationship between two or more variables, and three important measures of association will be discussed using the symbols and numbers provided in Tables A–5 and A–6. Let us assume that one is doing a study of smokers and nonsmokers and following them to see who develops lung cancer over a defined period of time.

A. RELATIVE RISK

Relative risk (RR) is the risk of disease among people exposed to a factor relative to the risk among people not exposed and is a measure of the strength of association between an exposure and a disease.

$$RR = \frac{\textit{Disease rate in the exposed population}}{\textit{Disease rate in the nonexposed population}}$$

$$= \frac{\dfrac{a}{a+b}}{\dfrac{c}{c+d}} = \frac{\dfrac{63}{10^5}}{\dfrac{7}{10^5}} = 9$$

An RR greater than 1 implies a positive association of the disease with the exposure of interest; an RR less than 1 implies a negative association (or protective effect) between the disease and the exposure.

Table A–6. Example of data collected in a cohort study of lung cancer and smoking.

	Develop Lung Cancer	Do Not Develop Lung Cancer	
Smokers	63	99,937	100,000
Nonsmokers	7	99,993	100,000

The results in the preceding example suggest that the risk of lung cancer among smokers is nine times greater than the risk for nonsmokers. RR is important for testing etiologic hypotheses.

B. ATTRIBUTABLE RISK

Attributable risk (AR) is the rate in the exposed population minus the rate in the nonexposed population.

$$AR = \frac{a}{a+b} - \frac{c}{c+d}$$

$$= \frac{63}{10^5} - \frac{7}{10^5} = \frac{56}{10^5}$$

It indicates the rate of occurrence of death or disease that is caused by a specific exposure factor.

Of the 63 lung cancer deaths that occur annually among 100,000 smokers, 56 (89%) are attributable to smoking. Because a disease may have multiple risk factors that interact with each other, the sum of attributable risks may be greater than 100%.

AR can be an important tool for counseling individuals with specific risk factors because it helps give an idea about the amount of disease that could be avoided by reducing risk factors in individuals.

C. POPULATION ATTRIBUTABLE RISK PERCENTAGE

Population attributable risk (PAR) *percentage* is the proportion of a disease in a population related to (or "attributable to") a given exposure.

$$PAR = \frac{P_e(RR-1)}{P_e(RR-1)+1}$$

where P_e is the proportion of the population exposed to the risk factor, and RR is relative risk.

Assuming that 40% of the population smokes (P_e) and that the relative risk (RR) of lung cancer associated with smoking is 9, then

$$= \frac{0.4(9-1)}{0.4(9-1)+1} = \frac{3.2}{4.2} = 76.2\%$$

That is to say, 76% of cases of lung cancer in the general population are attributable to smoking. PAR is important for public health policy and planning, that is, in estimating what percent of cases in a population could be eliminated by removing an exposure.

2. Case-Control Study

The case-control study is a frequently used design in analytic epidemiology. It determines the risk factors associated with a particular disease by comparing a group of subjects who have the disease (cases) with one or more groups composed of subjects who do not have the disease (controls). Risk factors studied may be permanent, such as gender or race; they may be current, such as present drug use; or they may be historical, such as previous employment. The difference in the frequency distribution of the risk factors between the case and control groups is examined, and the magnitude of the association of these factors with the disease under study is estimated.

Case-control studies are a commonly used design in occupational epidemiology to evaluate multiple exposures associated with a single outcome. For example, an investigator may be interested in the many occupational and nonoccupational causes of lung cancer. Conversely, a study of many health outcomes associated with a single exposure or workplace would best be investigated using a cohort design.

The case-control study is always retrospective. The investigator starts by identifying diseased and nondiseased individuals (i.e., the effect) and looks backward for the presence or absence of exposures (i.e., the causes) in these individuals.

For example, to study the relationship between asbestos exposure and mesothelioma, a case-control study would compare the history of asbestos exposure in a group of mesothelioma patients with the history of asbestos exposure in a group of subjects who do not have mesothelioma. The cohort study, in contrast, first identifies a group of disease-free individuals classified for absence or presence of the risk factor or exposure of interest and then follows these individuals over time to compare the incidence of disease in the exposed and unexposed groups. A cohort study of the relationship between asbestos exposure and mesothelioma first would classify a group of nondiseased persons according to their asbestos exposure and follow them to determine whether the asbestos-exposed subjects had a higher incidence of mesothelioma over time than the nonexposed subjects.

Case-control studies generally can be done more rapidly and less expensively than cohort studies. The time required to complete the study is the time needed to assemble the necessary data; the investigator does not need to wait for cases of the disease to appear. This usually results in lower costs because fewer study personnel and subjects are necessary to test a hypothesis.

For example, suppose that half the general population is exposed to a risk factor (e.g., cigarette smoking) and half is not. If a disease (e.g., lung cancer) has an annual incidence rate of 100 per 100,000 in the exposed population and 10 per 100,000 in the nonexposed population, a study of 100 cases and 100 controls probably would reveal the increased risk of disease associated with exposure to the factor. Uncovering 100

cases of disease in a cohort study would mean following 10,000 exposed people for 10 years. The more rare the disease, the greater the relative advantage of the case-control study.

Source & Selection of Cases

In defining a case, the diagnostic criteria should be clear and permit selection of a homogeneous group of cases. For example, in cancer studies, microscopic confirmation of the presence of disease and clearly defined criteria for classification by a pathologist of the type of cancer greatly enhance the validity and generalizability of the study findings. The case group usually is composed of (1) all persons with the disease seen at a particular medical facility or group of facilities in a specified period or (2) all persons with the disease found in a community or in the general population in a specified period. Whatever the source of the cases, they should be newly diagnosed (or incident) cases of the disease. Inclusion of prevalent (diagnosed in the past) cases will increase the sample size but can complicate analysis and interpretation of results. Prevalent cases are "survivors" and therefore may not be representative of all people who develop a given disease. Inclusion of prevalent cases inadvertently may identify factors that result from the disease rather than factors that are causally related to its development.

Source & Selection of Controls

The four most common sources of the control group are (1) the general population, (2) hospital patients, (3) relatives of cases, and (4) associates or friends of cases.

The general population control group is appropriate if all or most cases occur in a specific geographic area—for example, a county—because in this situation the controls represent the same target population as the cases. Using general population controls, however, presents certain problems: potentially lower response rates than from other types of control groups and from the case group, differing quality of information if the interview setting differs for the cases and the controls, and higher costs for obtaining information.

The hospital patient control group is selected from patients at the same hospital or clinic that the cases attended. This control group may share the selective factors that influenced the cases to come to a particular hospital or clinic, such as residence, ethnicity, or income. These patients (the controls) are readily available, often have the time to accommodate study interviewers, and can be more cooperative. The disadvantage of the hospital control group is that it is composed of people with an illness who may differ from the general population with regard to factors often associated with disease, such as smoking habits and/or drug use. In addition, the factors that cause patients to attend a particular hospital may not be the same for all diseases. For example, a hospital with a national reputation for treating Hodgkin disease may have patients with this disease from all over the country, whereas its population of coronary disease patients may come only from the region surrounding the hospital; thus the two patient groups may differ greatly. Similarly, healthy people attending a hospital screening clinic may differ markedly in ethnic, socioeconomic, or other factors from the inpatient population of that hospital. One consideration in selecting controls is whether to draw them from the hospital's entire patient population or to exclude patients who have diseases related to exposure factors under study. For example, in a case-control study of the relationship between lung cancer and smoking, it would seem logical to exclude from the control group persons who have emphysema because emphysema is related to smoking, the exposure factor under study. There also may be the problem of a lack of knowledge of whether factors being studied are related to diseases present in hospital controls. Selecting controls with differing types of diseases would minimize this problem.

Spouses and siblings are the relatives used most commonly as controls because of similarity in ethnicity and environment with the case group. Moreover, sibling controls genetically are similar to the cases. Spousal controls are appropriate if there is an approximately equal number of male and female cases, and the age range of cases is such that a high proportion of spouses are likely to be alive. When siblings are the controls, one sibling should be selected per case; using all available siblings would result in the control group having many characteristics related to family size, which may confound any observed associations between the exposure factor and the disease. In contrast, cases with no siblings would have to be excluded from the study (for lack of an equivalent control), which may result in biased study results.

A control group of associates of cases such as neighbors, coworkers, friends, or schoolmates has the advantage of being composed of generally healthy individuals who are similar to the case group with regard to lifestyle characteristics; for example, neighborhood controls are usually of the same SES as the cases. However, such associates might be more similar to cases than members of the general population with respect to risk factors under investigation, thus impairing the ability of the study to detect true differences in exposure between people with and without disease. Other disadvantages of associates as controls are the effort necessary to identify them, a response rate different from that of cases,

and probable variations in the quality of information obtained from cases and controls.

Sampling

Once the source of the control group has been determined, one must decide on the method of selecting the controls. Either all eligible individuals are selected from a specific group—although this is usually not required—or a sample is selected. Whenever sampling is employed, its protocol should be defined and adhered to throughout the sampling period. Examples of common sampling strategies are (1) random sampling, (2) systematic sampling, and (3) paired sampling.

In random sampling, each member of the source group has an equal chance of being represented in the control group. For example, all individuals might be assigned a number, and the sample would be selected using a table of random numbers.

In systematic sampling, the source group for controls is assumed to have an ordered sequence, and every nth individual is selected. As long as the sequence of the source group is not related to an important study variable (e.g., age), the resulting characteristics of a systematic sample are similar to those of a random sample.

In addition to random or systematic sampling, a popular method of selecting controls is paired sampling. In paired sampling, one or several controls are selected for each case based on a predefined relationship to the case. For example, if hospital controls are used, the person who was admitted immediately before or after the case might be chosen for the control group. The investigator may choose to select for each case one or more controls who are individually matched with the case on characteristics such as gender, age, or SES—which, if not controlled, might lead to spurious associations in the final results. For example, as a neighborhood control, the resident of the nearest dwelling to the right of the case's house who is of the same gender and age (±5 years) as the case might be selected. Such matching at the outset of the study is one way of taking into account any variables known to be associated with both the disease and the exposure of interest.

Sources of Bias

Bias must be acknowledged as a potential issue for nearly every type of epidemiologic study design. It is defined as a systematic error in the design, execution, or analysis of a study that results in an erroneous estimate of the effect of an exposure of interest to the risk of an outcome or disease.

While bias is more common in case-control studies, it also may occur in cohort studies; for example, information about outcome measures may be obtained differently in exposed and unexposed subjects. However, the underlying principle is the same: Any difference in the way information is obtained from the study groups may bias the results of the study.

There are two main categories of bias to be aware of: selection bias and information bias (or measurement error).

A. SELECTION BIAS

The appropriate control group should be chosen judiciously because when a systematic error is made in the selection of one or more study groups, selection bias may result. Under the null hypothesis, cases and controls have been equally "exposed" to the study factor. Therefore, selection of the cases and controls must use similar eligibility criteria to ensure that both groups are comparable and therefore more likely to be representative of the same underlying population so that if we reject the null hypothesis and determine that cases differ from controls on the study factor, it is not because we selected them to be different by using a biased procedure. Because the case group usually is chosen first, selection bias is avoided by a careful choice of the appropriate control group.

As an example of how selection bias can occur, suppose that the study is about the relationship between Alzheimer disease and previous exposure to lead. The case group is chosen from the inpatient population of a private hospital and the control group from the outpatient clinic of the same hospital. Once the cases and controls are selected, it is discovered that they differ dramatically with respect to SES—the inpatient population being predominantly upper middle class and the clinic population predominantly lower class. Thus, if the study finds that the cases and controls differ in terms of prior lead exposure, it would not be known whether this is a true difference or whether the difference is a consequence of other factors related to SES.

Selection bias also can occur if the control group is composed of people who volunteer for the study, because volunteers differ in significant ways from nonvolunteers; for example, they may be more educated, more active in community affairs, or less likely to be smokers.

B. INFORMATION BIAS

In interviewing study subjects about past exposures or events, the interviewer who knows the disease status of the individual (case or control) may pose questions unconsciously or probe for answers in a different manner, commonly referred to as *interviewer bias*. For example, in a case-control study of factors related to lung cancer, an interviewer might pursue in greater depth questions concerning asbestos exposure when obtaining work or environmental histories from cases than from controls.

To avoid this bias, the procedure used to collect information should be identical for cases and controls. Ideally, the data collector is unaware of the hypotheses being tested and whether the subject is a case or control; however, in collecting information of a medical or personal nature, it is often difficult to avoid learning of the person's disease status. Every effort therefore must be made to keep interviews as comparable as possible (e.g., place, length, and format of questionnaire; attempts to gain cooperation and accurate information; and other aspects of the interview), and each interviewer should see an equal number of cases and controls.

Another source of information bias can occur when a study subject is asked to recall past exposures or events because recall might depend on the person's current disease status. For example, a person with lymphoma is more likely to recall remote exposure to pesticides than a control subject without cancer. To minimize recall bias in this instance, one might try to obtain independent verification of previous exposure. It is also advantageous to use information recorded before the time of diagnosis wherever possible. In using data from interviews in which the case has a serious illness and the control has not, the items on which cases and controls can be compared with the greatest confidence are those least subject to recall bias. For example, prior surgery is a more objectively reported event than prior drug use.

Misclassification of study subjects also can bias study results owing to inaccuracies in the methods by which data are gathered from study subjects or methods by which information is abstracted from various sources. Misclassification bias comes in two forms—differential and nondifferential. Differential misclassification that is related to disease or exposure status can lead to the appearance of a relationship between exposure and disease where one does not truly exist, or perhaps more unsettling, it can mask a true association. Nondifferential misclassification is not related to exposure or disease status and tends to attenuate any association between exposure and disease.

Confounding

The phenomenon of *confounding* is another explanation for an apparent association between an exposure and a disease and also may cause no association to be observed when a true association exists. As with bias, confounding may occur in any type of analytic epidemiologic study. By definition, a factor that is associated with the exposure of interest and is also an independent cause of the disease being studied is a confounder. When confounding occurs, an observed association between an exposure and a disease is in fact due wholly or in part to the association of the exposure with the confounding factor, which, in turn, is itself a cause of the disease. If the suspected confounder is not differentially associated with the exposed subjects or is not a cause of the disease, it cannot be considered a confounding factor.

An example of a confounding factor is cigarette smoking in a study of an occupational exposure and lung cancer. Cigarette smoking is a known cause of lung cancer. If the cigarette smoking prevalence were greater (or less) in the population exposed to the occupational exposure agent, failure to control for smoking in the study design or analysis would lead to an apparently greater (or lesser) association between the occupational exposure and lung cancer.

Analysis of Case-Control Studies

Data from the case-control study are conventionally arrayed so that cases and controls can be compared on exposure to a hypothesized etiologic factor:

		Disease Status	
		Cases	Controls
Exposure }	Yes	a	b
	No	c	d
		a + c	b + d

The incidence of disease among the exposed and nonexposed cannot be calculated by using case-control data because the cases and controls in the study rarely reflect the true proportions of diseased and nondiseased persons in the population. [The investigator usually selects roughly equal numbers of cases ($a + c$) and controls ($b + d$) in the study, whereas there are likely to be many more nondiseased than diseased people in the general population.] Therefore, the relative risk (RR) of disease associated with exposure cannot be calculated directly in a case-control study, as it was for the cohort study. However, an estimate of the RR, known as the *odds ratio* (OR), can be calculated if the proportion of diseased people in the general population is small compared with the proportion of nondiseased (almost always true). Recall that the true RR using data from a cohort or incidence study is as follows:

$$RR = \frac{\frac{a}{a+b}}{\frac{c}{c+d}}$$

where a is the number of cases among the exposed group in a cohort study, b is the number of noncases among the exposed group, c is the number of cases among the nonexposed group, and d is the number of noncases among the nonexposed group.

In a cohort study, as in the general population, a is very small relative to b. Similarly, c is very small relative

to d. Thus, in the general population (and the usual cohort study), $a/(a + b) \approx a/b$ and $c/(c + d) \approx c/d$. Consequently, the formula for relative risk reduces to

$$\frac{\frac{a}{b}}{\frac{c}{d}} = \frac{ad}{bc} = \text{odds ratio (estimated relative risk)}$$

Example: *One hundred men with lung cancer and 100 controls are interviewed regarding smoking history:*

	Cases	Controls
Smokers	80	30
Nonsmokers	20	70
	100	100

$$\text{Odds ratio} = \frac{ad}{bc} = \frac{80 \times 70}{30 \times 20} = \frac{5600}{600} = 9.3$$

Because the OR is an estimate of RR, one can conclude that these data show a ninefold increased risk of lung cancer in smokers compared to nonsmokers.

PAR (i.e., the proportion of all instances of the disease in the population that can be attributed to the exposure of interest) can be estimated from case-control studies by using the following equation:

$$PAR = \frac{p\,(OR - 1)}{p\,(OR - 1) + 1}$$

where p is the proportion of the population with exposure of interest [estimated from controls as $b \div (b + d)$], and OR is the estimated RR (OR) associated with the characteristic.

Matched Case-Control Studies

Controls frequently are selected in a case-control study so as to be individually matched to the cases as to characteristics such as age, gender, race, or SES that are known to be related to the disease. Matching helps to make the two groups similar with respect to factors other than the exposure of interest in the study and thus serves to reduce the likelihood of spurious associations. The investigator must be careful not to overmatch, that is, to match cases and controls on factors related to the exposure of interest; overmatching can artificially reduce—and may even eliminate—true exposure differences between diseased and nondiseased individuals in the study. It should be obvious that cases and controls cannot be compared in the analysis with respect to any characteristics on which they have been matched.

The data in a matched-pairs analysis are organized as shown below:

		Controls	
		Exposed	**Not exposed**
Cases	**Exposed**	r	s
	Not exposed	t	u

where r is the number of pairs in which both case and control are exposed to the factor (concordant), s is the number of pairs in which the case but not the control is exposed to the factor (discordant), t is the number of pairs in which the control but not the case is exposed to the factor (discordant), and u is the number of pairs in which both case and control are not exposed to the factor (concordant).

To compute the OR (estimated RR) for a matched-pairs study, only the discordant pairs enter into the calculation:

$$\text{Odds ratio} = \frac{s}{t}$$

$$\text{where } t \neq 0$$

Example: One hundred seventy-five children age 5–15 years admitted to hospital in 1968 with acute asthma were matched on age, gender, race, and date of admission to 175 controls. All children in the study or their parents were interviewed regarding personal habits and home characteristics during the month preceding admission. The results regarding environmental tobacco smoke (ETS) exposure were as follows:

		Controls		
		Yes ETS	**No ETS**	**Totals**
Cases	**Yes ETS**	10	57	67
	No ETS	25	95	108
		35	152	187

$$\text{Odds ratio} = \frac{s}{t} = \frac{57}{25} = 2.3$$

These data show that children who have asthma have a 2.3 times greater odds of environmental tobacco smoke exposure than do children without an acute asthma admission. Show the calculation for how you arrived at the answer by way of example.

3. The Experimental Study

The experimental study is the type of design most familiar to clinical investigators, but it is rarely encountered in occupational epidemiology. Unlike the cohort and case-control studies, which are observational in nature—that is, the investigator observes exposed individuals for the development of disease or diseased individuals for past exposures—in an experimental study, the investigator manipulates exposures and studies the impact on disease. The intervention can occur at different points in the natural course of the disease. Subjects are normally randomly assigned to the different interventions in an experimental study. Ideally, study outcomes also should be determined by individuals blind to the exposure status of the subjects.

Experimental clinical trials often are undertaken among individuals with the same disease who are assigned to different treatment groups. An example is the Carotene and Retinol Efficacy Trial (CARET) study, in which men with asbestos exposure, who are at increased risk of lung cancer, were randomly assigned to receive beta-carotene or a placebo. The study was undertaken to determine whether beta-carotene decreases the risk of developing lung cancer.

Alternatively, intervention might occur in the form of a screening program offered to one group of people at risk of disease and not to another similar group. An example of this type of intervention study is the National Cancer Institute's Cooperative Screening for Early Lung Cancer Program. Men aged 45 years and older with a history of heavy cigarette smoking were assigned to a dual-screened group receiving chest radiographs and sputum cytologic testing or to a group receiving only chest radiographs. The objective was to determine whether the addition of sputum cytologic testing to regular chest radiography resulted in earlier detection and improved lung cancer survival.

CAUSAL ASSOCIATION

An epidemiologic study may demonstrate an association that is not valid because of chance, bias, or confounding, as discussed previously. If the association is believed to be valid—that is, the disease occurrence is in fact not equal among the exposed and unexposed subjects—and the observed association cannot be explained by chance, bias, or confounding, the investigator must consider whether the data support a cause-and-effect association.

This process involves consideration of the study itself and all existing data on the subject. Factors that should be considered in evaluating whether an association is causal include (1) the strength of the association, (2) whether dose-response relationships are present, (3) consonance with existing knowledge (i.e., other studies demonstrating the same finding), (4) biologic plausibility (i.e., whether there is a proposed biologic mechanism), and (5) the temporal sequence of events (i.e., cause precedes effect).

While uncertainties always will exist following an epidemiologic study, action on the findings of a study will depend in part on how strongly the data support a causal association and on the need for action versus the consequences of obtaining more data.

REFERENCES

Epidemiology Software

Epi Info 6, Epi Map 2, www.cdc.gov/epiinfo/Epi6/EI6.htm (Epi Info is designed for public health professionals. It is easy to use and comes free from CDC. The package includes word processing, data management, and epidemiologic analysis programs. Epi Map is a program for displaying counts or rates on geographic maps. For PC only.).

EpiCalc 2000,:www.brixtonhealth.com/ (An easy-to-use statistical calculator; can be customized for languages other than English. For PC. Available for free with other epidemiologic and statistical programs.).

Vitalnet, www.ehdp.com/vitalnet/index.htm/ (A data-analysis program for analysis of mortality and population data. It provides the data analysis/data dissemination infrastructure for a national, state, or city. Runs locally or over the Internet.).

The R Project for Statistical Computing, R 2.2.1, www.r-project.org/ (R is a free software environment for statistical computing and graphics. It compiles and runs on a wide variety of UNIX platforms, Windows, and Mac OS.)

Index

Note: Page numbers followed by *f* or *t* indicate figures and tables, respectively.